ALEXANDER'S CARE OF THE PATIENT IN SURGERY

# Alexander's Care of the Patient in Surgery

**WALTER F. BALLINGER, M.D.**

Bixby Professor of Surgery and Head of the Department, Washington University School of Medicine, St. Louis, Missouri

**JACQUELYN C. TREYBAL, R.N.**

Assistant Director, Barnes Operating Rooms, Barnes Hospital, St. Louis, Missouri

**ANN B. VOSE, R.N., B.S.N., M.S.**

Director, Department of Nursing Service, University of Michigan Medical Center, Ann Arbor, Michigan; formerly Director, Department of Nursing, Barnes Hospital, St. Louis, Missouri

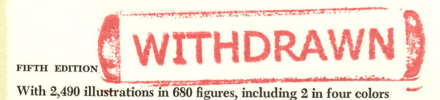

**FIFTH EDITION**

With 2,490 illustrations in 680 figures, including 2 in four colors

## The C. V. Mosby Company

Saint Louis   1972

# COLOR ILLUSTRATIONS

ALEXANDER'S CARE OF THE PATIENT IN SURGERY

Within an effective organization, the member groups fit together with collective tolerance.

Thus an effective organization consists of three components: (1) the arrangement of the parts, (2) the specifications of the individual parts, and (3) the ability to act as one body.

To organize nursing services effectively, the nursing staff should be concerned essentially with the group members, with patients, and with their relationships to each other in a given situation. The effectiveness of the nurses is dependent on understanding, accepting, and teaching all employees an awareness of their duties and relationships to each other and the organization.

## Centralization or decentralization

In fitting the parts of an organization together, evidence seems to indicate the need for both centralization and decentralization. The balance between them becomes a managerial decision. Trends influencing centralization are (1) size of the units, (2) capital costs of consolidation of expensive equipment in one area, (3) operational costs—locating specialized services in one unit rather than in several functional areas, and (4) use of mechanized administrative tools such as installation of computers. Decentralization provides for flexibility and better communication within the group involved. Some authorities apply Newton's third law of motion to other spheres. The mechanical analogy is the design of a wheel. If the diameter and the circumference of a wheel are increased, the hub and the spokes must also be strengthened. The movement toward centralization should be accompanied by approximately an equal and opposite trend toward decentralization.

Specialization in medicine, nursing, and administration also affects the organizational structure. Gardner[13] states, "Specialization is a universal feature of biological functioning, observable in the cell structure of any complex organization—in insect societies and in human social organization."*
Because of expanding specialization in surgery, the professional nursing staff must select certain independent functions and delegate other functions to the allied health group members. For both management and professional roles, specialization involves learning one thing in depth. The cardiovascular or plastic surgeon achieves excellence of performance through intensive training in a narrow segment of his potentialities. In the same vein the professional nurse achieves excellence of performance through intensive training in depth in his or her particular specialty. Bryson[11] said, "The purpose of a democratic society is to make great persons. . . . a democratic way of doing anything is a way that best keeps and develops the intrinsic powers of men."†
Thus the dynamic content of an organization is provided by people who have the capacity to function as generalists, by people who are specialists, by other combinations of internal groups, and by the external environmental forces.

## A dynamic structure

A dynamic organization is the outcome of a continuous evaluation process that changes with the existing circumstances and personalities operating within the organizational structure. A rigidly maintained structure or an aging one usually has an oppressive effect on creative ideas, hampering new and productive developments. In such situations, the new employee may hear the statement, "You just have to understand how we do it here." A dynamic organization encourages individual development and expression of ideas.

A dynamic nursing service organization provides for the following: (1) safe, continuous, and effective therapeutic patient

---

*From Gardner, J. W.: Self-renewal—the individual and the innovative society, New York, 1964, Harper & Row, Publishers, p. 23.

†From Bryson, L.: The next America, New York, 1952, Harper & Row, Publishers, p. 8.

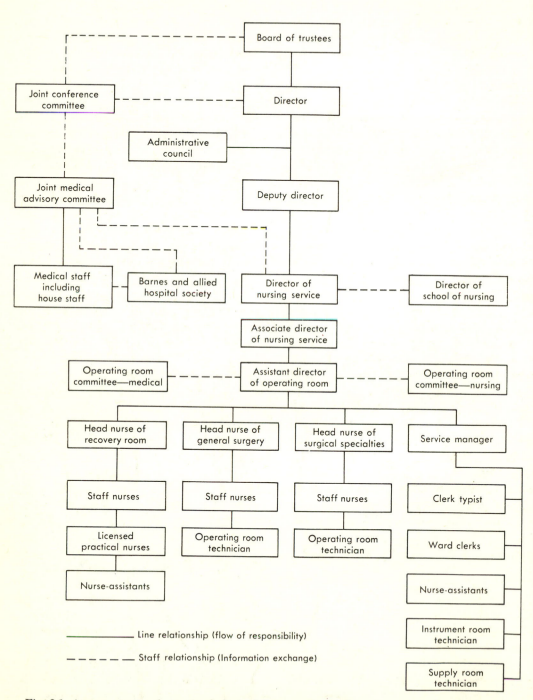

**Fig. 2-1.** An organizational structural chart of the operating and recovery rooms demonstrating the line and staff responsibility and relations and information exchange among nursing service groups, nursing service staff, and other group members of the institution.

# CONTRIBUTORS

**RONALD M. BURDE, M.D.**

Assistant Professor of Ophthalmology, Washington University School of Medicine, St. Louis, Missouri

**RICHARD E. CLARK, B.S.E.(Chemistry), M.S., M.D.**

Assistant Professor of Surgery and Biomedical Engineering, Division of Cardiothoracic Surgery, Washington University Schools of Medicine, Engineering, and Applied Science, St. Louis, Missouri

**ELIZABETH COLTER, R.N.**

Head Nurse, Barnes Operating Rooms, St. Louis, Missouri

**BARBARA ROSENBERG GRANA, R.N.**

Head Nurse, Operating Rooms, Ellis Fischel Missouri State Cancer Hospital, Columbia, Missouri; formerly Staff Nurse, Barnes Operating Rooms, St. Louis, Missouri

**DORINDA HARMON, R.N.**

Head Nurse, Labor and Delivery Rooms, St. Louis Maternity Hospital, St. Louis, Missouri

**VIRGINIA HIGGINS, R.N.**

Nursing Team Leader, Barnes Operating Rooms, St. Louis, Missouri

**DORRIS JACKO, R.N., A.A.**

Staff Nurse, Barnes Operating Rooms, St. Louis, Missouri

**JUDITH YVONNE JACOBS, R.N.**

Instructor, Operating Room Nursing, Barnes Hospital School of Nursing, St. Louis, Missouri

**JUDITH A. JONES, R.N.**

Staff Nurse, Barnes Operating Rooms, St. Louis, Missouri

**PEGGY E. LILES, R.N., B.S.**

Instructor, Operating Room Nursing, Barnes Hospital School of Nursing, St. Louis, Missouri

**MAXINE LOUCKS, R.N.**

Assistant Director, Nursing Service, McMillan Operating Rooms, St. Louis, Missouri

**EILEEN MOEHRLE, R.N.**

Instructor, Operating Room Nursing, Department of Staff Development, Department of Nursing, Barnes Hospital, St. Louis, Missouri

**JUNE MUSTERMAN, R.N.**

Staff Nurse, Barnes Operating Rooms, St. Louis, Missouri

**LINDSAY L. PRATT, M.D.**

Assistant Professor of Otolaryngology, Washington University School of Medicine, St. Louis, Missouri

**BETTY J. DAVIES TAGUE, R.N.**

Staff Nurse, Barnes Operating Rooms, St. Louis, Missouri

**PATRICIA TIPPETT, R.N.**

Staff Nurse, Barnes Operating Rooms, St. Louis, Missouri

**PAUL M. WEEKS, M.D.**

Professor of Surgery (Plastic and Reconstructive), Washington University School of Medicine; Plastic Surgeon-in-Chief, Barnes Hospital, St. Louis, Missouri

# PREFACE

The fifth edition of *Care of the Patient in Surgery* has been completely revised by the operating room nurses of Barnes Hospital in order to update the content of the text and to prepare a basic reference for the technological care of the patient undergoing surgery. The fundamental principles and scientific concepts for administering safe patient care in the operating room, as seen in Barnes Hospital, are encompassed in the text. Specific operative techniques are presented in detail, thus providing the nursing team with basic knowledge for planning individualized patient care.

This book is designed for all operating room personnel. The professional staff will appreciate its use as resource material for those nurses desiring to specialize in or to teach the care of the patient in surgery. Nonprofessional personnel will appreciate its sequential explanation of each procedure, thus enabling them to participate as more competent team members.

Chapters 1 through 5 and Chapter 7 present fundamental operating room principles that ensure a safe environment for all patients. The beginning chapters focus on the principles to be considered in planning for (1) safe, efficient facilities for patients and personnel, (2) the bacteriological factors that influence the selection and methods for providing a clean, safe environment, and (3) the principles underlying an effective system of organization and management. Chapters 4, 5, and 7 describe the general principles applied in the preparation of the patient for surgery and the selection of equipment and supplies in relation to the position and kind of body structure and tissues involved in operative procedures.

Chapters 8 through 25 are concerned with various surgical procedures organized according to anatomical and physiological specialties. In addition to revising and updating the original text, we have included material on new procedures or techniques in all chapters; for example, microsurgical techniques in cardiothoracic surgery and neurosurgery, total hip replacement, and cesarean section. New chapters are devoted to plastic and reconstructive surgery and pediatric surgery. Individually these chapters present the purpose and methods specific to procedures. The contents serve as a guide in orientation and clinical training for operating room personnel or may be utilized as a reference in the development of nursing care plans.

We are most grateful for permission given by other authors and publishers to reproduce their illustrations and express our sincere appreciation to the many surgeons of the Washington University Center and to the nursing staff of Barnes Hospital Operating Rooms who have given of their time and knowledge concerning the preparation of this edition.

We wish to express our appreciation to the many surgical instrument equipment and supply houses for supplying illustrations and giving their permission for us to reproduce other illustrations.

We also appreciate the valuable photographic reproductions and photographs

vii

produced by Mr. K. Cramer Lewis, Director of the Department of Illustrations, Washington University School of Medicine, and the pen-and-ink illustrations drawn by Miss Annette Porter, Medical Illustrator for the Department of Surgery, Washington University School of Medicine. We also thank Mrs. Karol Johnson, who patiently assisted all by typing the manuscript, and Mrs. Eileen Moehrle, who followed through on many of the details of its preparation.

Most of all, however, we wish to express a special appreciation to the inspired, enthusiastic, and dedicated contribution of Mrs. Marie Rhodes, Associate Director of Nursing Service, Barnes Hospital, without whom this text would undoubtedly never have achieved publication. Her continued support, pressure, and guidance made it into a text *about* nursing *by* nurses. This, perhaps, is the most important aspect of this text.

**Walter F. Ballinger**
**Jacquelyn C. Treybal**
**Ann B. Vose**

# CONTENTS

# CHAPTER 1

# Design of the surgical suite

RICHARD E. CLARK

The renovation of old hospitals and the building of new ones are accelerating at the present time and are likely to continue for the next decade in response to an increased need, rapid population growth, population shifts, and federal governmental funding. Surgeons and operating room personnel are frequently requested to provide advice on a new surgical suite. The purpose of this chapter is to outline an approach to a thoughtful analysis of surgical suite design by the operating suite nursing division. It includes consideration of systems analysis, suite and operating room configuration, environmental control, and safety. The end result, however, will be a compromise of the ideal because costs, prejudices, and outdated building codes alter the best of plans.

## APPROACH TO THE ANALYSIS

The request for an analysis by the operating room nurses is usually initiated by the architect through the hospital and nursing administrators. However, the nursing division may be consulted only after the fact, for example, after plans have been drawn by the architect and approved by the hospital administration or renovation and building committees. This is unwise. Initiative, assertion of the right to advise, and well-defined proposals promptly submitted are necessary if a functional, technologically efficient, and cost-effective new surgical suite is to meet patient and nursing needs.

To begin the analysis, determine the requirements necessary to perform the type and number of surgical operations anticipated. Consider the total number of planned or present acute care beds and the types of surgical services available in the community. Ask whether additional surgical specialties or new procedures are likely to be added. About 2.5% of the total number of acute care beds is a reasonable estimate of the number of operating rooms required if the minor surgical rooms are excluded.

The second consideration is the materials-handling systems in use. If a renovation of existing facilities is planned and the central supply section will be unchanged, the flow and work patterns of personnel may be dictated, in part, by the way materials enter and leave the suite. Include an analysis of instrument cleaning, sterilization systems, storage of disposable and recycled goods, decontamination methods, and delivery systems.

The third consideration is the needs of the persons involved: patients, nurses, surgeons, anesthesiologists, and orderlies. Lack of in-depth analysis of the characteristics of surgical personnel, actual human activity patterns, and time-efficiency data has resulted in dissatisfaction with new or renovated facilities. Analysis depends, in part, on the organization of the surgical suite nursing personnel. If the unit system is used, in which each operating room group is independent, constantly together,

1

and has its own hierarchy and in which duties and responsibilities are fairly constant and well defined, suggestions should come up the line through each head nurse to the room group supervisor and then to the director of the surgical suite. Studies should be made of the activity patterns of each operating room crew. Inefficient movement results in slower case turnover and increased costs. Where large anesthesia and nursing staffs exist, anesthesia induction rooms should be considered and the two-surgical-team approach used. This increases efficiency, and fewer new operating rooms are required.

## OPERATING ROOM SYSTEMS

Once the general requirements for the performance of surgery in the community and hospital have been considered, the analysis may be carried into more detail and specificity by reducing the surgical suite activities into four major systems[1]: (1) traffic and commerce (activities), (2) surgical support systems (the environment), (3) communication and information (record), and (4) administration (management).

### Traffic and commerce

Specific traffic patterns must be determined. These are dependent on the entrances and exits for both personnel and materials. Renovation planning of existing facilities should consider renovation of central supply and storage areas to bring these as close to the point of utilization as possible. Where entirely new wings, buildings, or entire hospital complexes are being considered, there is opportunity to design traffic, materials-handling, and storage systems around the requirements of the surgical suite. Traffic control design is aided by designating the four zone concept.[1, 7, 18] The four zones are the protective area, the clean area, the sterile area, and the dirty area. The protective area includes the patient reception area, the locker rooms, lounges, and offices. The clean areas include induction rooms, clean storage areas,

scrub areas, and recovery rooms. The sterile areas are the operating rooms and the sterile supply storage areas. The dirty area is the disposal area, where all utilized materials and linen are gathered, packaged, and sent to appropriate areas. Newer surgical suites have utilized two control desks to handle communications and traffic. The external desk directs patient and personnel flow and screens incoming calls; the internal desk controls and directs the activities within the operating room suite.

Materials-handling systems are difficult to integrate into the desired traffic pattern. Three options are available: a horizontal system in which all materials handling is on the same floor, a stacked or vertical system in which materials travel by elevator or dumbwaiter, or a combination of the two. The decision as to which system to use may be determined by vertical versus horizontal construction costs, the degree of automation of the material delivery systems that will be employed, and the cost of storage of disposable as opposed to recycled items. Some modifications of complete unitized surgical packs have been developed,[15] although these systems have not been employed widely as yet. Conveyor systems have proved time saving and cost effective.

Careful consideration must be given to disposal systems. Both individual room and grouped room systems have been proposed for clean and contaminated linen and disposable materials. If possible, a separate exit method should be arranged to avoid contamination of incoming supplies. This is not necessary if all items are carefully packaged and handled.

### Surgical suite design

Suite design is dictated in part by the number of operating rooms required. In hospitals with 100 beds or less, many functions (sterilization, storage, delivery) can be carried on within the same area of the surgical suite. The single-corridor or L-shaped designs are applicable for two to three operating rooms and support-areas

In hospitals with 500- to 600-bed capacities, twelve to fifteen operating rooms will be required, and the double-corridor U-shape or T-shape suites are more suitable. In larger hospitals, all these have been used, as well as the cluster, circular, or rectangular patterns with either central core and radial distribution or the peripheral corridor plan. However, the peripheral corridor scheme tends to be more expensive because of excessive corridor space. The large passageway becomes a storage area for movable equipment. A recent study of newly constructed surgical suites revealed three basic faults: insufficient and poorly organized storage space, poorly designed traffic patterns, and inefficient materials handling.[10] None of the suites examined were failures. In fact, they handled considerable surgical loads with fair efficiency in the performance of successful surgery. Laufman[9] has noted, "It is this wide margin of permissible error in operating rooms design which permits equally good surgery to be performed in so many different designs."

## Operating room design

Operating rooms have been built in a myriad of shapes, but the rectangle or square remains the most practical, flexible, and least expensive.[8] Ovoid and multifaceted rooms have not offered significant advantages over simpler designs that lend themselves to modular and prefabricated constructional techniques.

There is controversy about the ideal size of an operating room. A 400-square foot area is satisfactory except when procedures require extensive peripheral equipment such as a heart-lung machine. Open heart procedures require an area of 600 to 800 square feet.[2] Similarly, endoscopy, cystoscopy, and outpatient minor surgical rooms require half the floor space. Thus a modular unit system can be devised that will accommodate each need by halving or doubling the basic unit for special applications.

The interior of the operating room has special requirements for environmental control. The ceilings should be smooth, washable, and preferably sound absorbent. They should be a minimum of 9 feet in height and preferably 10 feet to accommodate ceiling-mounted surgical lighting fixtures. Room lighting should be flush mounted in the ceiling and should have prismatic lenses and fixtures solidly grounded for elimination of transient radio frequency interference.

Walls no longer have to be tiled. The plaster between the tiles is porous and can harbor bacteria. New paneling materials and flexible wall coverings, together with new adhesives, permit completely sealed wall, ceiling, and floor joints so that these surfaces may be washed with all types of bactericidal chemical solutions. Some coverings such as Tedlar permit steam cleaning.

All cabinets, view boxes, and receptacles should be recessed. No windows should be installed.

Floor coverings must have the same requirements as the wall surfaces but, in addition, must be highly wear resistant. At the present time, building codes require conductive flooring.[11-14] New national meetings and conferences are in progress that may yield decisions that will obviate conductive flooring for special application rooms where a high degree of monitoring is required. In this situation the patient would become a ground center to which all ground lines are referenced.

Doors should be of the sliding type, if possible, but of the type that slides against a wall so that all surfaces may be washed.[9] All door frames should be a minimum of 5 feet in width.[1] Swing doors produce a high degree of air turbulence. Studies show a markedly increased count of both total particles and bacteria when swing doors are opened or closed.[4, 5]

Color requirements of the ceiling, walls, doors, and floors are few. Obviously, the hue decided on must be generally acceptable. Most new European surgical suites have used warmer tones, whereas the

United States has used the cool pastels of the spectrum. Similar or the same color hues throughout give a sense of increased space.

The surgical specialties will require consideration of special needs. For example, flush-mounted snap-lock water connections for the heart-lung machine, x-ray facilities, space for neurocryosurgery, and special outlets for air-powered equipment may be required. Some specialties will use fiber-optics, a laser apparatus, or special built-in television or film-loaded cameras. Each service should be consulted for any anticipated special needs that will require preparation, operation, or maintenance by the nursing service.

## ENVIRONMENTAL DESIGN

Environmental design aids in the control of surgical infections. The average new operating room is now required to have eighteen to twenty-five room changes of air per hour, five changes of which must be fresh air. The average new system has inlet vents in the ceiling and return air ducts in the hall. Each room can be made to have ¼ inch water pressure greater than the hall. Dispersion of the inlet air should be in the central portion of the ceiling and not near the walls.[17] Some have noted that when the number of room air changes exceeds thirty per hour, the turbulence created tends to sweep the floor and cause settled particles and bacteria to rise and swirl about the operative team.[17] Temperature should be controlled between 68° and 72° F. and humidity at 50% to aid in the control of bacterial growth and the suppression of static electricity.[6, 17] In the past few years, laminar flow systems have come into vogue as a result of the use of such systems by NASA for the assembly of highly intricate electronic parts. A volume of 500 to 600 room air changes per hour is utilized through an entire ceiling covered with HEPA (high efficiency particulate absorbent) filters.[6] Special lint-free clothes and entrance and exit high-flow air locks are used. Such an installation is costly to build and maintain; however, the results in the space program have merited the expense. Fewer than 100 particles (viable and nonviable) per cubic foot of air can be obtained. It has been found that the count of viable particles (bacteria and macroviruses) parallels the total particle count in the range of one bacterium per 100 to 100,000 particles.[4-6] The average surgical suite corridor, anesthesia induction room, scrub sink areas, and adjacent rooms contain 200,000 to 500,000 particles per cubic foot of air.[4] To date, there has been no proof that reduction in total particles bears any relationship to the wound infection rate. At present, few hospitals have permanent laminar flow systems and there has been too little time for sufficient data to accumulate. However, one study has shown that a marked reduction in airborne bacteria can be accomplished with a temporary laminar flow system in an old hospital. Volume room air changes of 100 to 130 per hour with laminar flow have reduced bacterial counts to one bacterium or less per cubic foot of air.[5] The general approach is excellent in theory, but laminar flow systems have not been made cost effective as yet. An example of a renovated 40-year-old operating room is shown in Fig. 1-1. Because of the recurring replacement cost of ceiling-mounted HEPA filters, a ducted system using a false ceiling plenum was utilized in this renovation and a series of filters incorporated into the air-handling system. The final filter removes 99.97% of all particles 0.3 micron or greater. The maximum volume rate is 100 room air changes per hour through 96 square feet of perforated screen. Return air is handled by four corner-mounted ducts. In summary, laminar flow systems will provide a cleaner operating room environment, but the necessity for this has not been shown for all types of operations. This system will virtually remove airborne infections but is recommended only for high-risk operating rooms where prosthetic materials are employed, that is, cardiac, neurosurgery, orthopedic, and plastic surgery areas.

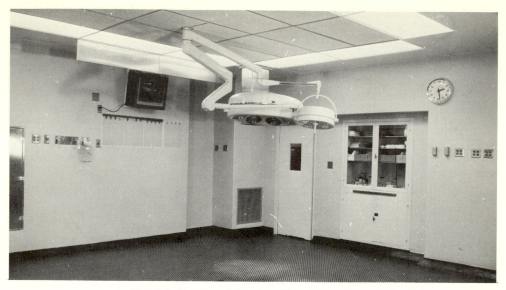

**Fig. 1-1.** Renovated 40-year-old operating room.

A laminar flow system will have little effect on the rate of wound infections even in these areas but should significantly lower the infection rate from prosthetic appliances. Of far greater importance in the control of wound infections is the strict maintenance of sterile technique, preoperative elimination of clinical and subclinical infection in the patient, control of the shedding phenomena from facial hair and skin, and the removal of bacterial carriers from the operating room team.

Lighting is an important aspect of the operating room environment. Only recently have any standards been adopted.[3] Illumination at the field from the ceiling lights alone should be 200 to 300 footcandles. The surgical light should be a single post, ceiling-mounted unit. Satellite spotlights may be added. Lights traveling on tracks should not be employed for two reasons. First, ceiling tracks are inaccessible for cleaning and will harbor bacteria. Second, the track lights have a handle that is initially sterile when applied by a member of the surgical team but likely to become contaminated. Recent bacteriological studies on such light handles at the completion of operations have shown that over 50% are contaminated.[3] The concentration of the surgical

light in the surgical wound should not be so intense as to provide a sharp contrast between a small intense light field and a surrounding large dark zone because this results in visual fatigue and depth perception abnormalities.[9] Peripheral lighting should uniformly and adequately illuminate all necessary work areas.

## SAFETY DESIGN

Safety design incorporates features that prevent or control the foreseeable hazards of infection, flame, explosion, and electricity. The control methods for infection have already been detailed. Well-devised traffic patterns, materials-handling systems, disposal systems, strict adherence to sterile technique, clothing control of shedding, control of carriers, positive-pressure and well-dispersed clean ventilation, and high-flow laminar flow systems for special applications all contribute to a safe surgical environment. Flame and explosion hazards have been decreasing in recent years. This can be traced directly to the use of noninflammable anesthetics. Greater use of new gaseous and especially intravenous agents can be expected to reduce the hazards of flame and explosion from anesthetic causes to almost nonexistent levels. The single

greatest hazard to the life of the surgical patient at the present time is the electrical one.[16] This increasing hazard has evolved because greater loads have been put on antiquated wiring systems and because of the use of two-pin plugs rather than three-pin grounded system plugs. The present problems revolve about the grounding systems and the increasing use of extensive monitoring. If a voltage exists between any two electrical conductors touching the patient, an electric current will flow. This can lead to ventricular fibrillation and sudden death. It is imperative that each operating room have an isolated electrical system and that each ground is referenced to a common ground. The maximum point-to-point resistance of the systems should be less than 50 milliohms. An insulated stranded AWG 4 ground conductor is the minimum required. The static electricity hazard has been greatly reduced with control of the humidity at 50%, nonexplosive anesthetics, and use of disposable non-woven and polymer products that resist generation of static electricity.

The extensive use of electronic monitoring for cardiac patients has led to wider application of its use in all surgical specialties. Only the electrocardiogram is electively monitored in most routine operations. However, electronic measurement of vascular pressures requires the use of voltage in most pressure transducers. Damaged transducers can cause current flow in the patient and result in disaster. Thus special attention must be directed to those rooms that will require special engineering to yield a safe environment for the surgical patient.[16] In such rooms a dynamic ground detector system and expanded irradiated insulation on conductors should be installed. The older static detector systems will not activate at 20-microampere current leakage, which can be fatal.

The last important design safety feature is in the communications system. An analysis of the number of telephone lines required both to the central desk and to the surgical suite administrative offices is necessary. A reliable intercommunications system is required from each operating room to the central desk and from there to the blood bank, operating room director, recovery room, intensive care unit, surgical pathology department, x-ray department, central supply service, housekeeping department, maintenance department, and computer center. Pneumatic tube systems have been of value as an accessory supply and communications network in some suites, although there is potential hazard of environmental contamination.

## SUMMARY

An approach to analysis of the requirements of a surgical suite in terms of systems, materials, and human needs has been outlined. Specificity of design can be determined with consideration of the four major surgical suite systems: traffic and commerce, surgical support systems, communication and information, and administration. Specific suite design depends on the number of operating rooms involved. Single-corridor and L-shaped configurations are most applicable to smaller suites, whereas the double-corridor T and U shapes are more appropriate for larger units. The circular or rectangular designs are under development but have not yielded the high efficiency and safety first envisaged. The principal faults of recent designs have been poor traffic patterns, insufficient storage areas, and inefficient materials-handling patterns. The rectangular- or square-shaped operating room has been found most useful; an average unit size of 400 square feet is required. Specialty rooms may require half to twice the unit size. Uniform size and shape aid in cost control in construction. All interior surfaces must be washable. Conventional tile walls are not recommended. Doors should be of the sliding type, and the requirement that the floors be conductive may not be necessary in the future. The special needs of neurosurgical and cardiac operating rooms are emphasized. Environmental design includes consideration of highly filtered center ceil-

ing distribution with eighteen to twenty-five room air changes per hour. Relative humidity should be closely controlled at 50% with the temperature between 68° and 72° F. Laminar flow ventilation systems remain experimental and appear justified only for protection of prosthetic materials from airborne contamination. Single post, ceiling-mounted surgical lights are suggested, as is adequate room illumination to avoid sharp contrast of lighting zones. Finally, safety design has emphasized the electrical hazards to the patient and the necessity of assuring that all electrical units carry a ground wire and that all conductive surfaces touching the patient are referenced to a common ground.

## REFERENCES

1. Alexander, E. L., Burley, W., Ellison, D., and Valleri, R.: Care of the patient in surgery, including techniques, St. Louis, 1967, The C. V. Mosby Co.
2. Beall, A. C., Jr.: The ideal operating room environment for open heart surgery, Bull. Am. Coll. Surg. 55:42, July-Aug., 1970.
3. Beck, W. C.: Operating room illumination, Bull. Am. Coll. Surg. 54:277, Sept.-Oct., 1969.
4. Clark, R. E.: Laminar flow ventilation for a cardiac operating room, A.O.R.N. Journal 15: 61, May, 1972.
5. Coriell, L. C., Blakemore, W. S., and McCarrity, E. J.: Medical applications of dust-free room. II. Elimination of airborne bacteria from an operating theater, J.A.M.A. 203:134, 1968.
6. Goodrich, E. O., Jr., and Whitfield, W. W.: Air environment in the operating room, Bull. Am. Coll. Surg. 55:7, June, 1970.
7. Jacobs, R. H., Jr.: Surgical suite locker room design and procedure, J. Am. Inst. Architects 38:83, Sept., 1962.
8. Laufman, H.: Planning tomorrow's surgical care facilities, J. Assoc. Adv. Med. Instru. 2:1, 1967.
9. Laufman, H.: Developments in operating room design and instrumentation, Chicago, 1971, Year Book Medical Publishers, Inc.
10. Laufman, H.: Critical survey of surgical suites (in press).
11. National Electrical Code, 1971, a U.S.A. Standard.
12. NFPA Code No. 56A: Code for flammable anesthetics, Boston, 1971, National Fire Protection Association.
13. NFPA Code No. 70: Recommended safe practice for hospital operating rooms, Boston, 1968, National Fire Protection Association.
14. National Institutes of Health, Public Health Service: Electronics for hospital patient care, pub. no. 1807, Washington, D. C., 1967, U. S. Government Printing Office.
15. Swenson, O., and Grana, L.: A new and improved sterilization and set-up technique for the operating room, Bull. Am. Coll. Surg. 55:17, March, 1970.
16. Walter, C. W.: Safe electric environment in the hospital, Bull. Am. Coll. Surg. 54: 4, July-Aug., 1969.
17. Walter, C. W., Kundsin, R. B., and Brubaker, M. M.: The incidence of airborne wound infection during surgery, J.A.M.A. 196:908, 1963.
18. Wheeler, E. T.: Infection control through design of operating room (an architect's view on asepsis), Hosp. Top. 42:89, Nov., 1964.

# CHAPTER 2

# Administration of operating room nursing services

ANN B. VOSE

The complexity and continuity of health programs for patients and families require a hospital team approach. It is the operating room nurses' responsibility to work with the medical staff in the surgical treatment of patients and to maintain team relationships with other hospital departments that render related institutional services.

## THE TEAM APPROACH FOR QUALITY NURSING CARE

The hospital team approach should radiate from the controlling body of the hospital downward and laterally. A team approach involves various groups who are delegated specific functions in the care of patients.

The professional nursing staff should continually develop knowledge and skills to accept responsibilities associated with new surgical concepts in the treatment of patients. The professional nursing staff should work with other groups who are skilled in managerial and general hospital services. With the ever-increasing benefits derived from medical, nursing, and technological research, the increase in health insurance enrollment, the growing concept of the "people's right to adequate health care," and the increase in capital and operational hospital costs, operating room graduate nurses are obligated to consider and implement new approaches to provide nursing services to patients.

## STANDARDS FOR ORGANIZED NURSING SERVICES

The quality of nursing care and related institutional nursing services is dependent on the establishment and observance of accepted standards. A standard may be considered a pattern for guidance in providing quality, quantity, and correctness of *nursing care*. A standard provides a basis for appraisal. To give patients the best possible nursing services, standards of organized nursing services should be dynamic. They should be reviewed periodically and revised in light of new medical and nursing knowledge and techniques and methods of organization and management.

The Committee on Nursing Service of the American Nurses' Association formulated *Standards for Organized Nursing Services*,[6] which can serve as guidelines for the nursing department of any type of health care facility. This committee also identified the purposes of the standards, developed assumptions on which to base them, and designated criteria for each statement. These statements should be reviewed as an invaluable guide for formulating operating room nursing service standards.

The Committee on Quality of Organized Nursing Service, appointed by the De-

partment of Hospital Nursing Steering Committee, developed the statement *Criteria for Evaluating a Hospital Department of Nursing Service.*[18] These criteria are also helpful guides in evaluating the department.

Lesnik's and Anderson's *Nursing Practice and the Law*[16] is a helpful tool in defining the dependent functions of nursing. The seven nursing functions that focus on the patient and his care are as follows:

1. Application and execution of the physician's order
2. Observation of symptoms and reactions
3. Supervision of the patient
4. Supervision of those participating in care
5. Reporting and recording facts
6. Application and execution of nursing procedures and techniques
7. Promotion of physical and emotional health by direction and teaching

Operating room nursing care encompasses all of the preceding functions.

Standards for the practice of nursing are intended to provide safe individualized patient care, detect inadequacy of care, prevent legal complications resulting from alleged nursing malpractice or negligence, and improve the integrated health program offered to each patient. The professional operating room nursing staff should develop a specific method of auditing operating room nursing care.[20] The National League for Nursing statements entitled *In Pursuit of Quality Hospital Nursing Services*[18] should be reviewed in developing nursing service operating room standards.

## PHILOSOPHY, PURPOSE, AND DEVELOPMENT OF OBJECTIVES OF OPERATING ROOM NURSING
### Philosophy

The philosophy of operating room nursing should blend with that of the hospital's controlling body, the general and specialty surgical programs, and the training and research programs of medical and nursing services.

One philosophy of operating room nursing service and the constituent parts of operating room nursing may be summarized as follows.

1. Operating room nursing is a dynamic, behavioral, and highly technical process directed toward participation in the surgical team for the accomplishment of treatment for each patient.

2. Operating room nursing service provides for nursing care of patients before surgery, during surgery, and immediately after surgery, with continuous awareness of the human dignity of man and his physical, emotional, and spiritual needs.

3. Operating room nursing service promotes knowledge and skills of its members as a means of meeting technical and scientific progress in the health and hospital fields.

4. Operating room nursing service continually adjusts its organization and functions in accordance with current acceptable health and educational programs.

The philosophy defined by the professional operating room nursing staff should be approved by the department of nursing service and hospital administration. The philosophy of an operating room department in any type of hospital should encourage all employees to accept responsibilities and perform them effectively.

### Purpose

Operating room nursing is designed to provide assistance to the medical staff in meeting the emergency, preventive, and restorative health needs of patients, regardless of race, color, creed, national origin, social status, and economic status and is planned and administered in combination with related services to render a safe, comfortable, and therapeutic environment for patients.

### Development of objectives

The objectives of an operating room department should be practical, specific, and attainable for the persons performing nursing functions. They should be detailed

statements supporting the defined philosophy. Effective objectives are developed and changed through the cooperative efforts of the director, supervisors, and other members of the staff. If the controlling body of the institution approves the establishment of an extensive program in the treatment of cancer or cardiac patients, the objectives of the operating room nursing department would include new predetermined quality and quantity nursing service specifications. Frequently, difficulties arise in the delegation, coordination, and establishment of standards in the absence of unified objectives of the various groups.

In developing objectives, the professional nursing service group should consider the following factors:

1. The overall objectives of the department of nursing services should be the core around which the operating room nursing staff work.

2. Objectives should be written in positive "doing" terms to help all staff members achieve them. For example, the operating room department may initiate a surgical technician program or an open heart surgical program. The objectives should clearly state the overall functions of the groups concerned, the limits of authority, and the managerial and training functions of the various group members.

3. Objectives should provide for assignment of duties to permit personnel to perform at their highest potential and provide a means for the staff to broaden their knowledge and skills.

4. Objectives should be reasonable and attainable in the light of existing and foreseen conditions such as availability of trained personnel, facilities, operating scheduled time, and operational costs.

5. Overlapping of objectives within the institution should promote cooperation between group members and coordination between the departments. From the institutional aspects of operating room nursing, the housekeeping department has similar objectives concerning the prevention and control of infection and of electrical explosive hazards.

6. Objectives should be written for, freely available to, and understood by all personnel. A positive attitude on the part of the administrator, supervisors, head nurses, and employees is essential to the fulfillment of the objectives. The nursing service staff should be encouraged through daily conferences and training programs to help set realistic goals to meet the objectives.

7. Objectives should be reviewed periodically and revised to bring about necessary changes in the standards of operating room nursing service.

## Sample objectives of operating room nursing

1. Provide sufficient experienced nursing staff to assist with patient care.

2. Provide a safe therapeutic environment for patients and staff.

3. Provide suitable equipment and supplies in good, safe condition for all elective and emergency procedures.

4. Evaluate and revise nursing standards in accordance with medical and nursing concepts.

5. Instruct and teach others to perform at a high level of proficiency.

6. Enhance the nursing service department by contributing ideas.

7. Coordinate responsibilities of other departments with those of the operating room.

## PURPOSE OF ORGANIZATION

An organization may be defined as a framework within which *human beings* in various groups perform certain jobs with the assistance of *things* to accomplish the desired goals of the institution.

The words *to organize* mean to arrange the parts so that the whole shall act as one body. It is easy to assemble the parts of a piece of equipment so that it operates smoothly and effectively, but it is more difficult to arrange the activities of people and have them coordinate their activities effectively for the ultimate good of patients.

are; (2) an effective communication system to facilitate flow of instructions and information through the vertical and horizontal lines of the organizational structure; (3) a system for collecting and recording up-to-date facts concerning the quality and the quantity of the services rendered; (4) a smooth, economical, effective procedure of operation; and (5) a demarcation of responsibilities and authority that states in detail the *line* and *staff* responsibilities of groups for obtaining instructions, reporting facts, appraising situations, and taking decision-making actions.

## Organizational chart

The organizational chart is a valuable tool for formative discussion during construction and revision of an organization and for simple presentation of the jobs and lines of authority. An organizational chart is a static diagnostic statement of formal relationships between groups who act to achieve the established objectives in a specific situation. The chart should show the pattern of administrative control in an orderly fashion, linking together the different levels of responsibility and authority (Fig. 2-1).

The levels of authority are shown vertically. Each employee has an immediate superior who is delegated to give orders and guidance.

The term *line responsibility* stems from the chain of command that is transferred from the top administrator down the line of assistants, supervisors, head nurses, and general duty graduate nurses to other individual employees. Line functions consist of action-producing duties on the job.

The term *staff responsibility* within the diagonal structure may be advisory in nature, or it may be a direct responsibility delegated by the controlling body to a committee, to an administrative professional group, or to an individual within the organization. The medical, administrative, and nursing groups have both line and staff functions within an organization. For example, the director of surgery has professional supervisory relations and direct responsibility relations for the care of patients. Through staff responsibilities, the professionals work as a team to meet the needs of patients and raise the standards of patient care. In appraisal of care, they may make recommendations for improvement of patient care services to the infection control committee, to the director of a service, to administration, or to the faculty curriculum committee of an educational program (Fig. 2-1).

Horizontal (diagonal) coordination of activities results between departments and other professional groups within the hospital hierarchy.

The *committee* or *conference* structure of the hospital and department should not perform functions that can be performed by established departments for which individuals can be held accountable.

There are advantages and disadvantages of committee action. Advantages of committees are that they (1) disseminate information and ideas, (2) provide for integration of ideas, (3) deter quick decision-making actions, (4) provide for coordinated action by individuals having line and staff responsibilities, and (5) broaden viewpoint of individuals pertaining to a specific problem or plan. The disadvantages of committee action are (1) difficulty in achieving control of action, (2) time of people needed to achieve general agreement of the group, (3) difficulty in getting members to attend, especially when emergency decision-making action is needed, and (4) difficulty in appraising results because of diffusion of responsibilities within the group.[17]

Within a department in the hospital, committees—administrative, advisory, judicial, executive, and others—combine a number of functions and characteristics. Organizationally, a committee may have line or staff responsibility. A line or staff committee may be delegated decision-making or enforcement responsibilities established by the controlling body. For ex-

ample, the administrative supervisor of the operating room department, as a member of the steering (executive) nursing service committee, has a staff responsibility for decision-making in accordance with the established functions of the committee. The administrative supervisor of the operating room, because of her line responsibility, may become a staff advisor as a member of the operating room committee.[2]

A formal or standing committee has a permanent place in the organizational structure of the hospital and department. The informal, temporary, or special *ad hoc* committee does not have a permanent place in the organizational chart. In developing or revising the committee structure, the following factors should be considered: (1) the purposes of each committee should be stated in writing; (2) the functions of each committee should be established; (3) the rules and regulations pertaining to selection of members, their responsibilities to provide effective functioning, and the responsibilities of the committee chairman should be determined; and (4) the committee structure should be approved by the controlling body.

### Meetings

The three major types of meetings are informational, advisory, and problem-solving. Before a meeting is scheduled, several decisions must be made: (1) the purpose of the meeting, (2) selection of people who should attend, always considering their responsibility and authority, (3) who shall conduct the meeting, and (4) how it shall be conducted.[9]

## BASIC ELEMENTS OF PROFESSIONAL MANAGEMENT

The highest efficiency in organized nursing services is obtained by providing the necessary quantity of nursing staff, of the required quality, at the required time, and by the best and most economical way.

Regardless of the graduate nurse's position in the organization or in the hierarchy

of responsibilities for patient care, the nurse performs five basic functions: planning, organizing, staffing, directing, and controlling.

*Planning* consists of determining in advance an outline of what should be done. Planning is an intellectual process. It consists of selecting a framework of action using the objectives, policies, programs, procedures, or other means to achieve the objectives. Knowledge, facts, judgment, insights, intuition, and resources are used.

*Organizing* means the establishment of a structure of authority through which work is subdivided for determining and enumerating the necessary activities and things that are required to achieve the objectives. This includes grouping activities, assigning activities to group members, delegating necessary authority, dividing the work, defining relationships, procuring equipment and materials the employees will need, and guiding them through planned meetings and conferences.

*Staffing* involves selecting and training of personnel, formulating methods of operational procedure, appraising operational efficiency, and determining the number, quality, and type of persons needed to staff the department.

*Directing* involves decision-making, guiding, teaching, coaching, and supervision of others through written and verbal instructions and orders to get the best results from their efforts.

Successful direction depends on the actions and attitude of both the individual who is being directed and the individual who is directing. The inexperienced "director" may remark, "I prefer to do it myself; it is easier and faster to do the job than to train another to do it." Successful leaders observe intelligently, analyze their own jobs, and explore the reasons for specific reactions and results. Each may ask: Should I have been more explicit? How could I have gained better cooperation? Was I too critical of the performance? Is there a better way to do the job?

*Controlling* is seeing that the work pro-

:eeds and is coordinated to meet the ituation.

Cooperation, coordination, construction, und occasionally controversy are necessary elements to ensure that policy decisions are :arried out and that objectives and stand-urds are attained in an economical and effective manner.

Coordination is the orderly synchroniza-ion of efforts of all the workers to provide he proper amount of service at the re-quired time and the quality of performance o that their unified efforts lead to the tated objective—namely, adequate, safe vatient care. Tead[23] describes coordination s the effort that assures that the end purpose of an organization will be realized vith minimum friction and maximum ef-ectiveness of the varied component parts.

The controlling body should make cru-ial decisions pertaining to major policies nd developments. The executive level in he professional nursing hierarchy de-ermines the time and resources to be pent in different functions. The many sser decisions should be made at the epartmental and supervisory levels be-ause these groups know the details of a ituation and, together, have more collec-ve brain power, perspective, and experi-nce to determine an effective decision.

## EVELOPING JOB DESCRIPTIONS OR OPERATING ROOM URSING POSITIONS
erminology

In the preparation for job analysis and 1e resultant job description, the staff 1ould use common definitions and under-and the terminology.

A *task* is a unit of work or human effort :erted to achieve a specific purpose. Ex-mples are checking identification bands of atients, checking patient charts to ensure fety of each patient, and assembling sur-cal instruments in a metal sterilizer tray. hese are called tasks, or duties. When a fficient number of similar tasks have de-loped, a position is created for one orker.

A *function* is a group of tasks (duties) with closely related similarities and char-acteristics that logically fall into a uni-fied unit of work for the accomplishment of a responsibility delegated to a worker or a department. An example is to pre-plan, organize, and control the staffing pattern to ensure effective utilization of personnel in meeting the required nursing care of a group of patients. This function comprises several tasks performed by the clinical nursing supervisor or head nurse.

A *position* is a collection of tasks and responsibilities rendered by one worker who is delegated to perform specific func-tions.

A *job* refers to a group of positions that involve the same duties, skills, knowledge, and responsibilities.

A *job description* is a statement describ-ing the title of the position, the department where the position is located, and the char-acteristics, functions, and duties of a specif-ic job.

In defining organizational responsibili-ties, the functions should be described in clear divisional terms. They should state who does what, with whom, where, and how often and provide a plan of contacts occurring on a daily, weekly, or monthly basis. The actual plan of work is described in terms of people who have to carry out duties.

The *job specifications* refer to a written statement of the minimum qualifications or standards that must be met by the applicant for a specific position. These requirements include experience, educa-tion, training, physical and mental activi-ties, and so forth.

*Job relationships* refer to other workers within and outside the department who have similar duties or joint responsibili-ties to achieve specific objectives.

*Job analysis* is a technique of getting in-formation about the work performed in a job. Four basic ways to get information are questionnaire, observation, interview, and experience.

A job analysis helps determine how the

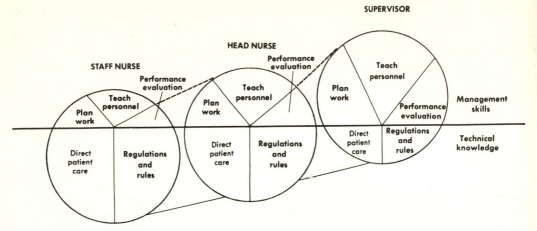

**Fig. 2-2.** Allocation of functions and responsibilities of staff nurse, head nurse, and supervisor in relation to planning of work, teaching, direct patient care, and rules and regulations.

job will be developed. The industrial analysis formula to get facts is what the worker does, how it is done, why it is done, and the skills involved.

An effective job analysis program is dependent on several important factors, as follows:

1. The individual who does the job analysis should have the ability to get along with people and be able to express ideas effectively in an analytical manner.

2. The program must be planned in detail as far as possible.

3. The program must be approved and supported by the administration.

4. The workers concerned must understand the purpose and mechanics of the program.

5. The supervisory staff must review the collected data.

6. The analyst must observe and interview the workers, write the first draft, and review it with the supervisory staff—then revise the draft until it is accepted by the department head.

## JOB DESCRIPTIONS IN OPERATING ROOM NURSING

The professional graduate nurse, regardless of her position in the nursing service hierarchy, performs clinical, managerial, and operational nursing service duties. In the upward progression of the hierarchy, the clinical leadership duties increase and operational (doing) duties decrease. The functions of the administrative supervisor involve almost entirely clinical leadership duties. In many hospitals the service manager system has been implemented to assume clerical and management functions now being performed by the professional nurse. At the lower level the job of a paramedical worker involves "doing" duties (Fig. 2-2).

The number and type of jobs required to meet the nursing care of patients in the operating room and recovery room suite depend on the size and complexity of the surgical services offered to patients, the jobs of other departments in performing related duties, and the type of organizational structure of the institution.

**Job title:**    Director, Assistant, operating room
**Department:**   Nursing service
**Job code no.:**    **Job grade:**

**Job summary**

Under the general direction of an associate director of nursing service, is responsible for the direction and guidance of the operating room suites. Adapts the philosophy and objective

of the department of nursing to the operating room. Implements standards that ensure safe and therapeutically effective nursing care of patients. Maintains good interdepartmental and intradepartmental relationships. Keeps the associate director informed of all activities in her area and seeks guidance from administrative or staff personnel as needed. Evaluates nursing care and plans the kind and amount of nursing care in relation to objectives of the department and the institution. Works closely with staff development in orientation and educational programs for personnel (both professional and nonprofessional). Continues individual education for growth and development. Promotes good public relations within her department, participates in hospital activities related to the community, and is active in professional organizations.

**Operational guidelines**

1. Responsible to an associate director of nursing service for the proper functioning of the operating rooms, including personnel and supplies.
2. Interviews applicants, guides staff members, and prepares performance evaluations as well as wage change recommendations for her employees.
3. Interprets and upholds policies and procedures as determined by the administrative body.
4. Communicates problems and recommended solutions to an associate director by weekly meetings.
5. Meets collectively with all head nurses in her area on a scheduled basis and individually as necessary.
6. Evaluates effectiveness of the assignment plans on a daily and weekly basis to determine reasons for operational delays and then takes necessary action to solve problems.
7. Plans and establishes a master staffing pattern within the geography of the area in accordance with established budgetary allowance and personnel policies to ensure effective coverage to meet nursing care requirements. Is responsible for adequate staffing.
8. Delegates and coordinates the clinical, managerial, and operational duties to the head nurse to ensure a consistently high level of nursing practice.
9. Utilizes daily rounds in the operating room suites to observe quality of nursing care in relation to medical and aseptic techniques, safety of patients, management of operating rooms, and use of equipment and supplies.

10. Coordinates and evaluates orientation and staff development programs.
11. Participates with the head nurses and service manager in the preparation of a budget that will allow for adequate personnel, supplies, and equipment, as well as physical facilities.
12. Reviews, with head nurses and service manager, monthly reports on operational costs and compares figures with estimated budget. Is responsible for operating within budgetary limitations.
13. Participates in the planning and renovation of operating room suites.
14. Constantly evaluates the quality and quantity of nursing care being given by utilizing appropriate administrative tools and recommends changes and programs to accomplish patient care objectives.
15. Prepares and submits an annual report for the director of nursing from the nursing area, which includes past performance and future goals.

**Qualifications**

1. Graduation from an accredited school of professional nursing. Bachelor of Science in Nursing preferred.
2. Experiences in which progressive leadership, administrative, educational, and clinical competencies have been demonstrated, preferably with 2 years' experience in the operating rooms.
3. Current licensure by the state board of nursing.

**Job title:** Nurse, Head, operating room
**Department:** Nursing service
**Job code no.:** **Job grade:**

**Job summary**

Under the general guidance and direction of the assistant director in charge of the operating rooms, directs, supervises, plans, staffs, coordinates, and controls the functions of assigned areas of responsibility. Plans and directs the activities of the operating room suites in accordance with established nursing and hospital policies. Adapts philosophy and objectives of the department of nursing to the operating room. Implements standards that ensure safe and therapeutically effective nursing care of patients. Keeps assistant director informed of all activities in her areas and seeks guidance from administrative nursing personnel as needed. Analyzes and evaluates performance of personnel and makes recommendations for promotions. Participates in the preparation of a budget that will allow for adequate personnel, supplies, and equipment, as well as physical facilities. Maintains good interdepartmental and intra-

departmental relationships. Active in the professional organizations, as well as keeping informed on current developments related to operating room nursing care.

## Operational guidelines

1. Interprets and upholds policies and procedures as determined by the administrative body.
2. Promotes and maintains good relationships within the nursing department and with other hospital departments, as well as correlating nursing service in the operating room area with the working activity of other departments.
3. Plans and directs the staffing assignments in accordance with objectives and established staffing pattern and policies to ensure required coverage and effective utilization of workers for 24 hours per day, 7 days a week.
4. Coordinates and organizes activities within the operating room with surgical staff and anesthesia department to provide an efficient free-flowing schedule.
5. Coordinates with the appropriate hospital departments the flow, availability, and operational efficiency of equipment and supplies within the operating room needed in the treatment of patients.
6. Observes how equipment and supplies are utilized and handled; observes techniques followed by workers in preparation, cleaning, and storing equipment, and takes action to improve techniques and methods.
7. Interviews and selects personnel, prepares and reviews performance evaluations, and recommends promotions, transfers, or termination of employees of the department.
8. Communicates problems and recommended solutions to the assistant director.
9. Identifies and studies patient care problems and assists in their solutions.
10. Consults with and assists department heads (for example, central supply, laundry, housekeeping, maintenance, purchasing) who perform specific services for the operating room.
11. Maintains a bacteria-free, safe physical environment for patients and workers in accordance with sanitation, housekeeping, electrical, and fire codes and established hospital standards.
12. Works with staff development in planning orientation of new personnel and in-service development programs.
13. Utilizes resource persons who are available within the department of nursing.

## Qualifications

1. Graduate of an accredited school of professional nursing.
2. Bachelor of Science in Nursing preferred.
3. Experiences in which progressive leadership, administrative and clinical competencies have been demonstrated, preferably with 2 years' experience in the operating rooms.
4. Current licensure by the state board of nursing.

**Job title:**      Nursing team leader
**Department:**   Nursing service (operating room)
**Job code no.:**        **Job grade:**

## Job summary

Under the guidance and direction of the head nurse, is responsible for the nursing care of patients and the management of assigned personnel in a specific area of responsibility. Plans, organizes, directs, and controls the quality and quantity of nursing care given within a specialty area according to hospital policies and established nursing and management practices. Assists in the implementation of standards that ensure safe and therapeutically effective nursing care of patients. Keeps head nurse informed of all activities of area and seeks guidance from administrative nursing personnel as needed. Maintains good interdepartmental and intradepartmental relations. Assumes responsibilities of the head nurse when authorized to do so. Maintains a knowledge of patients' conditions at all times to ensure maximum care and determines need for additional or modified service. Participates in the development and implementation of nursing policies and procedures as related to patient care and personnel. Active in the professional organizations, as well as keeping informed on current developments related to operating room nursing care. Continues individual education for growth and development.

## Operational guidelines

1. Interprets and upholds policies and procedures as determined by the administrative body.
2. Ensures availability of supplies and equipment. Informs appropriate personnel when supplies are needed.
3. Counsels and evaluates personnel according to hospital personnel policies.
4. Assists in orientation of professional and nonprofessional personnel and nursing students to the basic procedures and techniques of the specialty.
5. Observes medical and surgical aseptic techniques, rules, and regulations of the operating room and takes appropriate action.
6. Responsible for planning daily work as

signments within a specialty area according to the qualifications of personnel and standards of the hospital.

7. Assists the head nurse and staff development in planning orientation of new personnel and in-service development programs.
8. Responsible for supervising all personnel, instruments, techniques, equipment, supplies, and cleaning in area to ensure and maintain quality care for patients.
9. Promotes and maintains good relationships both interdepartmentally and intradepartmentally and correlates nursing service in area with the working activity of others.
10. Identifies and studies nursing care problems and assists in their solution.
11. Responsible for accurate reporting and recording of patients' identification, reactions, and progress.
12. Observes and maintains knowledge of patients' conditions at all times and determines need for additional or modified service.
13. Responsible for seeing that incident reports are initiated as indicated.
14. Attends in-service, grand rounds, or any other educational programs pertinent to the operating room nurse.

## Qualifications

1. Graduate of an accredited school of professional nursing.
2. One year minimum experience as a staff nurse in the operating room in which leadership and administrative and supervisory abilities have been demonstrated.
3. Current licensure by the state board of nursing.

**Job title:** Staff nurse, operating room
**Department:** Nursing service
**Job code no.:** **Job grade:**

## Job summary

Under the guidance and direction of the team leader, is responsible for the direct and indirect nursing care of patients within an assigned area. Plans and participates in patient care as a circulating nurse, scrub nurse, or a teacher to ensure safe and therapeutically effective nursing care. Keeps team leader informed of all activities and seeks guidance and assistance as needed. Maintains good intradepartmental relations. Assumes duties of team leader when authorized to do so. Maintains a knowledge and awareness of the patient's condition at all times to effect maximum care. Maintains nursing policies and procedures as related to patient care and personnel. Active in the professional organizations, as well as keeping informed on current developments related to operating room nursing care. Continues individual education for growth and development.

## Operational guidelines

1. Demonstrates knowledge of general nursing theory and principles and practices of operating room nursing.
2. Interprets and upholds policies and procedures as determined by the administrative body.
3. Ensures availability of supplies and equipment. Informs appropriate personnel when supplies are needed.
4. Assists in orientation of professional and nonprofessional personnel and nursing students to the basic procedures and techniques of the assigned area.
5. Utilizes knowledge of medical and surgical aseptic techniques, rules, and regulations while acting as a circulating nurse, scrub nurse, or teacher.
6. Ensures quality nursing care through the maintenance of instruments, techniques, equipment, supplies, and cleaning in the assigned area.
7. Maintains good intradepartmental relationships while working with others.
8. Identifies and studies nursing care problems and assists in their solution.
9. Responsible for accurately maintaining operative records.
10. Exhibits knowledge and awareness of the patient's condition and modifies nursing care accordingly.
11. Initiates incident reports as indicated.
12. Performs a wide variety of repetitive tasks rapidly and accurately.

## Qualifications

1. Graduate of an accredited school of professional nursing.
2. Current licensure by the state board of nursing.
3. Experience optional.

**Job title:** Technician, operating room
**Department:** Nursing service
**Job code no.:** **Job grade:**

## Job summary

Performs scrub, circulating, and supply duties under the supervision of the staff nurse in the area. Keeps the staff nurse informed of any problems that may arise. Demonstrates good knowledge of principles and practice of aseptic technique. Demonstrates knowledge of equipment, instruments, procedures, and supplies used in the operating room. Is alert to proper identification and the immediate condition of the patient. Func-

tions well with other team members and shows initiative and judgment in anticipating needs of team members. Helps to sustain the quiet, orderly environment of the department. Accepts responsibility for activities performed, works under pressure, and works in situations where maintaining good interpersonal relationships may demand much patience and tact. Reliable in attendance and duties performed. Adheres to the dress policies and deportment established by the department. Continues individual education for growth and development.

**Operational guidelines**
1. Functions as a circulating or scrub nurse.
2. Cleans, replenishes, and sterilizes instruments and supplies as needed.
3. Demonstrates an understanding of aseptic technique.
4. Renders effective nursing care to meet the patient's physical, psychological, and spiritual needs.
5. Identifies, prepares, and sends specimens and cultures to the respective departments.
6. Prepares and maintains adequate operative records.
7. Moves and positions patient before, during, and after surgery using any special equipment as needed.
8. Attends conferences, in-service programs, and meetings as scheduled.
9. Upholds and functions according to hospital policies.
10. Performs other duties as directed.

**Qualifications**
1. High school graduate. Graduate of an approved operating room technician program with a certificate preferred.
2. Good physical and mental health. Should have the ability to tolerate long hours of standing, walking, or any other physical exertion required in the operating room. Good coordination and dexterity are pertinent. Should have the ability to work in stressful situations.

**Job title:**    Manager, Service
**Department:**    Nursing service
**Job code no.:**      **Job grade:**

**Job summary**

Under the general direction of the special services coordinator, directs and is responsible for the nonnursing managerial functions of the operating room on a 24-hour basis. Maintains suitable environment for patient care by coordinating all defined activities with other departments in the medical center affecting the patient unit and works in cooperation with nursing service personnel. Institutes and observes policies and procedures as defined by nursing service and hospital administration. Interviews and employs new personnel for the service area. Orients, tours, and trains personnel under administrative jurisdiction with the assistance of staff development. Evaluates, counsels (developmental and disciplinary), transfers, and terminates service personnel. Directs all clerical functions, daily housekeeping functions in auxiliary service areas, and daily dietary food service to patients as it is related to the patient unit. Arranges hours for nursing personnel coverage by using head nurse's planned pattern. Arranges nursing personnel vacation schedule as directed by head nurse of the unit. Maintains needed supplies and equipment for patient care and operation of a defined unit. Keeps historical data so that more realistic standards of stock drugs, general supplies, medical and surgical supplies as well as linen may be studied and maintained. Establishes a budget for unit in cooperation with head nurse and acts as consultant for supplies. Checks monthly budget and gives explanation for differences. Holds regular meetings for communication purposes with service personnel and meets regularly with head nurse for the purpose of coordinating nursing and nonnursing functions. Participates in research activities. Also may participate in the development of staff on request.

**Operational guidelines**
1. Manages the nonnursing functions of a patient unit on a 24-hour basis.
2. Plans, develops, coordinates, and evaluates all aspects of the service area.
3. Maintains a suitable environment in a defined area so that a high standard of clinical medicine and nursing may be practiced.
4. Provides and maintains a qualified service staff to perform the necessary service functions in the area.
5. Cooperates with nursing service in formulating budget for the area and operating within its limits. Acts as consultant to the head nurse when necessary in this regard.
6. Develops and maintains rapport and good interdepartmental and intradepartmental relationships.
7. Plans and attends meetings involving the unit.
8. Plans the time schedule for nursing personnel in the operating room unit.

**Qualifications**
1. High school graduate required. One or more years of college preferred.

2. Experience in the supervision of six or more people with the ability to coordinate productively the activities of others.
3. Must be able to work for 8 hours with physical endurance in performance of required duties.
4. Must possess maturity, interest, and ability to get along with people.
5. Must be creative, demonstrate considerable initiative, willingness to work variable hours, and the desire to be permanent on the job.
6. Must possess some knowledge in budgets and accounting.

**Job title:** Volunteer, operating room
**Department:** Volunteer service
**Job code no.:** **Job grade:**

#### Job summary

Under the direction of the volunteer service chairman and director of volunteers, is responsible to the assistant director of the operating rooms. In a quiet and willing manner, assists the operating room secretary and other operating room personnel with patient transportation and relaying messages, small supplies, and surgical supplies and equipment between the operating room and related services.

#### Operational guidelines

1. Posts messages on operating room doors.
2. Escorts female patient with orderly to and from operating rooms.
3. Delivers cultures to the bacteriology laboratory on request.
4. Delivers specimens from operating room area to pathology substation.
5. Obtains emergency items from pharmacy, central service, and blood bank.
6. Assists operating room personnel in the instrument room in washing and wrapping instruments for sterilization.
7. Assists in meeting the needs of children and other patients awaiting surgery in the suite.
8. Prepackages and makes small supplies to be sterilized.
9. Makes up stretchers.
10. Delivers sterile supplies and instruments to the operating rooms from the general supply area.

#### Qualifications

1. Familiarity with the hospital complex.
2. Able and willing to perform varied assignments in an atmosphere of controlled stress.
3. Courteous and reliable.
4. Able to undertake work that entails much walking and light physical activity.

### HOSPITAL, MEDICAL, AND NURSING POLICIES, RULES, AND REGULATIONS

The controlling body of the institution delegates to the medical board the administration of the medical treatment of patients and to the hospital personnel, through the executive administrative staff, clearly defined functions and lines of authority concerned with meeting the needs of patients.

The personnel who care for patients in the operating rooms and recovery room require written information in the form of directives, rules, and regulations. This information should be available in separate manuals covering administrative policies, medical policies, nursing service standards, and procedures. Each institution should establish a general format, using simple, concise language, grouping related materials together, and providing an effective index suitable to the needs of the staff.

Manuals aim to provide for consistent interpretation and administration of policies for uniform quality of practices, for direction and controls for use by the nursing staff of the department. The directives, rules, and regulations should be reviewed periodically and revised to meet new medical, nursing, and managerial concepts.

The policies affecting operating room and recovery room patient care should be formulated by representatives of the groups concerned through appropriate committees within the organizational structure of the surgical service and hospital professionals. The number of committees, the line and staff responsibility relationships, and the functions of each committee depend on the type and needs of the institution (Fig. 2-1).

The *operating room committee* (surgical committee) may be delegated to recommend policies concerned with operating room services to patient, standard procedures and techniques in the therapeutic aspects of patient care, and managerial policies such as allocation of space and time to members of the surgical staff.

The membership of this committee should include representatives of the surgical staff, anesthesia staff, and hospital and nursing service administrative staff. The nursing service administrator has an opportunity and an obligation to seek guidance and to keep interested groups informed of acceptable nursing care practices and standards.

The graduate nurses of the operating room department should have permanent representation on the nursing service committees such as the steering committee, the staff development committee, and the procedure (nursing practice) committee. Suggested methods of communication are shown in Fig. 2-1. Within the operating room department itself, the personnel should participate as members of committees or conference groups to improve operating nursing practices and their own knowledge and skills.

### Administrative hospital policies

The objectives of hospital policies are to protect patients and personnel from injury and to meet medical and sanitation codes, local, state, and federal government laws, and the *Standards for Hospital Accreditation of the Joint Commission on Accreditation of Hospitals*. The laws concerning negligence, legal obligations, and grounds for liability may vary from state to state. The directives should interpret the existing laws and those policies that affect the hospital, the patient, and the workers.

The operating room policy manual should include directives, procedures, rules, and regulations concerning the following.

1. *Safety of patients and workers.*
   a. Fire regulations: Procedure for operating room staff, rules concerning the types of inflammable materials permitted and their use, methods for handling and storing them, and smoking regulations.
   b. Explosion hazard regulations: Procedure for handling, use, and storage of explosive agents, procedures for use of electrical surgical equipment such as operating room battery head lamps, electric outlets, and cauteries and for grounding of the patient, and procedures for cleaning and testing of the conduction of flooring and metal furniture in the operating rooms, induction areas, and recovery room units.
   c. Cleanliness and sterility of air circulation and of equipment and supplies: Directives should include the responsibilities delegated to various departments that provide services to the operating room department on daily, weekly, and monthly schedules, the methods for testing the effectiveness of the air conditioning and ventilation system, and the method for testing and reporting at stated intervals sterility of surgical equipment and supplies and the operational efficiency of sterilizers.
   d. Method for reporting accidents involving injuries to patients, visitors, physicians, and hospital personnel.
   e. Disaster procedure in event of a local or general disaster: The directive should state functions, lines of authority, communications, and possible types of patients to be cared for in the surgeries and recovery room.
   f. Handling of radioactive materials: The directives should include how to obtain and handle the various types of materials and safety prevention methods required for patients and workers. Generally, these policies are formulated by the radioactive isotope committee or in consultation with the head of the x-ray department.
2. *Admission of patients.* The rules and regulations concerning patients for surgery include the following.
   a. Types of laboratory tests and other procedures required for hospital admission and for a specific kind of surgery.
   b. Consent for operation: Policies should state the responsibility of the patient, the surgeon, the admitting officer, and the nursing personnel and the types of consent necessary for adults and minors having routine or special surgical services such as a dismembering operation or emergency care. The directives should give key points involving legal implications.
   c. Screening of patients for the recovery room: The policies should state the types of patients to be admitted and those who may not be admitted. For example, the directive may state that patients with a contagious disease, patients with an infected wound, and patients requiring iso-

lation techniques shall not be admitted to the recovery room.

Other patients shall be admitted to the recovery room, regardless of age, sex, race, and operative procedure if they have received a general, spinal, or regional anesthetic, or if they have had a local anesthetic and the medical staff considers recovery room care necessary.

3. *Visitors and visiting hours.* The policies should provide for necessary limitations and restrictions affecting specific selected group members such as physicians, clergymen, nurses, and students; who will grant permission; and circumstances that may warrant admission such as consulting surgeon or clergyman and member of immediate family if patient is critically ill in the recovery room.

4. *Public relations.* The policy should include rules for releasing information to the press, police, and visitors concerning a patient's condition or an incident involving patients or staff members and for communicating incidents and information to the hospital administration, head nurse in the unit, and hospital public relations staff.

5. *Records.* The directive should include information on kinds of records required, including the following.

   a. The operative record: The directive should include information to be completed such as patient's name, hospital number, date of operation, names of surgeon and assistants, anesthesiologist, nursing team members, preoperative and postoperative diagnoses, operative procedure performed, time operation started and ended, types of drains or medium inserted in the patient, and the surgeon's description.

   b. The anesthesia and recovery room form.

   c. Other records: Included are the narcotic record, physician's record and orders, nursing notes, tissue reports—all are part of the patient's chart.

6. *Disposition of tissues or dismembered part or parts of the body.* The directive should include information concerning the types of forms used, persons who must complete forms, and procedure for handling and disposing of specimens in accordance with established policies of the hospital pathology department and state laws.

The operating room staff needs to know specific rules for the identification, preservation, handling, transfer, and recording of routine specimens, of other specific types of tissue, of cultures, of smears, of frozen sections, of dismembered specimens, and of stillbirths.

7. *Notification of death and care of body.* The hospital directive should give procedure for handling the patient who expires in the operating room or recovery room, including the persons to be notified by nursing personnel, by hospital administration staff, and by surgical staff, the kind of forms to be completed, by whom, and the routing of the forms, and the care and disposition of the body. Death of a patient in the operating room department automatically becomes a case for the medical examiner.

8. *Surgical staff membership and privileges.* The listing of surgical staff members and their standing responsibilities and privileges should be kept up-to-date. (Directives for house staff concerning who may assist, who may operate, and what procedures they may perform are formulated by the surgical staff and are approved by the directors. Generally this information appears under surgical procedural policies.)

9. *Scheduling policies, rules, and regulations.* The directives for booking of patients for elective or emergency procedures are formulated by representatives of the surgical staff, administrative staff, anesthesiology staff, nursing staff, and the admitting office. The directives should include the following: available operating hours and days for use of various rooms during each 24 hours Monday through Friday and on weekends and holidays, the method for booking elective surgery on private and ward patients, responsibilities and authority of appropriate group members such as the surgeon, operating room supervisor, booking secretary, and admitting officer, rules for unused time and for cancellation of clinic services' time for elective surgery, rules for scheduling emergency procedures, rules for requesting x-ray and other diagnostic tests and examinations and for securing blood from blood banks, and rules for application of plaster casts.

Clearly defined scheduling policies, rules, and responsibilities promote effective, economical services to patients and provide all surgeons an equitable opportunity to use the facilities. Davis and Reed[11] report on a study to determine variability controls to provide maximum operating room utilization. The researchers and consultants appear to agree on several factors affecting scheduling controls:

1. Scheduling of operations must be under the control of one scheduler.

2. Specific facts are needed, that is, age, male or female, slight or heavy, and special limitations: (a) personnel staff available, (b) written classification of urgency for various types of operations to be booked, (c) estimated operating time required for specific kinds of procedures, (d) average set up and cleanup time for operations, and (e) existing restrictions of hours when surgeons are not available to operate and of the medical specialists and anesthetists.

A system of measurements and controls should be initiated to enhance the daily effectiveness of the scheduling policies. Data should be collected at periodic intervals concerning the following: (1) the variations of actual numbers of operations per week from predicted scheduling policies, (2) the total hours of actual operating room time used, showing the range between maximum and minimum hours used each week, (3) the average set up time and the average terminal cleanup time, and (4) the unused operating room time, resulting from variations in the schedule or improper observance of rules.

Collection and analysis of data assist the group members and the controlling body to determine methods to decrease excessive expenditures for staffing and equipment that result from the practice of staffing based on maximum for existing case load rather than on the expected demand for services.

## Surgical staff policies, rules, and regulations

Policies pertaining to dependent functions of the medical staff are formulated by a representative committee and are recommended to the administrative staff for approval by the controlling body. There are many policies and rules that relate to the interdependent functions of medicine and nursing. The surgical staff and administrative nursing staff have joint responsibilities in formulating overall policies related to therapeutic aspects of patient care. In the nursing procedure manuals, the directives, rules, and regulations are described fully in a concise, clear, step-by-step descriptive manner.

1. *The responsibilities and respective privileges of attending, associate, and consultant physicians.* These are defined and approved by the executive medical board and the board of trustees of the institution. The operating room supervisor should have a listing of the surgical staff and their privileges. For example, the directives may state the following facts.
   a. The surgeon shall be responsible for the total medical care of his patient and retains all the obligations and authority pertaining to the care of his patient in the operating room and in the recovery room.
   b. The anesthesiologist shall be responsible for those aspects of the patient's care pertaining to administration of anesthetics and their effects.
   c. The nurse anesthetist shall be responsible to the anesthesiologist and shall assist him in the anesthesia related to the care of patients.
   d. The house staff shall assist the surgeons in the care of patients in accordance with the scheduling policies for cases and the scheduled assignment plan. This plan shall be posted in the operating room, recovery room, and patient units.
2. *Reporting postoperative infections.* The directives should include the procedure for professional personnel to follow pertaining to reporting and recording all apparent postoperative infections and breaks in technique.
   A hospital control committee under the direction of the medical staff should be composed of professional group members concerned with all phases and problems of medical and surgical asepsis.
3. *Controlling entrance of individuals with acute infections.* The surgical staff assists the medical health director in determining health policies for personnel. For example, the rules may state that individuals with acute nasal or throat conditions or an abscess shall have cultures taken and if these show the presence of coagulase-positive *Staphylococcus aureus* or *Streptococcus* beta-hemolytic organisms, the individual shall not be permitted in the operating room or recovery room units. (See Chapter 3.)
4. *Surgeons' owned equipment.* The directives should describe the method of use in the care and maintenance of the equipment. The policy should clarify the responsibility

of the hospital for general repair or replacement of parts of the equipment.

5. *Consents for operation.* The surgical staff assists the hospital administration in formulating policies pertaining to the types of consents for specific procedures, as described previously under hospital policies.

6. *Surgical techniques.* The directives should provide general rules for positioning patients, emergency treatments such as for cardiac arrest, and preventive measures to prevent the spread of pathogenic organisms during surgery, such as in open heart procedures.

7. *Medical and surgical aseptic standards.* Many of the procedures, rules, and regulations are described in detail in the nursing procedure manual. Physicians, nurses, and other professionals concerned formulate the overall policies and directives. Some of the policies requiring joint approval include the following.

   a. The type of operating room apparel required for entrance of an individual in a specific operating room area or in the recovery room. The donning and removal of operating room apparel such as caps, masks, surgical gowns and gloves, shoe protectors, surgical suits and dresses, and visitors' gowns.

   b. Definition and handling of patients in the operating room who have infectious or communicable diseases.

   c. Skin cleaning procedures: The directives should include the extent of body area to be prepared for the different kinds of operations and diagnostic procedures, the kinds of disinfectants and germicides to be used, and the general scrubbing rules (Chapter 4).

8. *Standardization and selection of equipment.* The selection of new equipment for specific use and care and handling procedures should be defined by the surgical committee. The surgical staff collaborates with the nursing staff in the establishment of standard setups for all procedures.

9. *Sponge count.* The directive should include the types of materials to be used, operations for which counts are required, procedure for detecting a missing sponge, and reporting and recording a sponge count error or deficiency. This procedure usually appears in the nursing procedure manual. (See Chapter 5.)

## Nursing procedural manual

The procedure manuals for the operating room and for the recovery room should include the purpose, tools required, major principles and techniques, and step-by-step descriptions of those procedures adopted for use by nursing personnel in patient care.

Many nursing functions are interdependent; others are independent functions of nursing. Procedure manuals provide for uniform, consistent practices and instruction on how to reduce errors and provide up-to-date, accurate information to workers.

Some of the information in the general procedure manual includes the following:

1. *Procedures for scrub-up and attire* (Chapter 4).

2. *Procedures for preoperative preparation of skin* (Chapter 4).

3. *Procedures for draping and positioning the patient for different types of operations* (Chapters 5 and 7).

4. *Surgical nomenclature and setups for different types of operations, including instruments, textiles, sponges, sutures, drains, and so forth* (Chapter 5).

5. *Surgeons' card file.* The directives should state what information is to be recorded in file and how and when file is to be used and revised.

6. *Sterilization and disinfection procedures.* The directives should include the items prepared for use by moist heat, chemical disinfection, or gas sterilization (Chapter 3). Rules should describe in detail how equipment is to be operated, how and when it should be tested, and the routing of the results of tests.

7. *Terminal procedure for handling soiled and unusual equipment and textiles.* The procedure should be described in detail: the various personnel duties, the care and handling of big and delicate items, the operation of the washer-sterilizer or ultrasonic cleaner, and the assembling and storing of clean equipment.

8. *Procedures for care and handling of all types of specimens.* The policies should classify the types of specimens that may be collected, the forms or records to be completed, and the labeling and transporting procedure in routine cases and in emergency care.

9. *Sponge count.* The directive should include the types of sponges available for different kinds of procedures (Chapter 5).

10. *Admission of a patient.* The procedure should include identification of the patient and his chart, safety measures to be taken, and so forth.

11. *Administering of narcotics.* The nursing service policies for handling narcotics should be

carried out, including cocaine and other agents used for local anesthesia.

12. *Recording nursing information.* The nursing notes of the chart should be used.

## Nursing service administrative manuals

The administrative manual should include the philosophy and objectives of operating room nursing, the qualitative nursing standards to meet the nursing care of the patients, procedures for the control of equipment and supplies, quantity standards, the types of records and reports, budgetary information (costs and expenditures) organizational chart, committee structure of the department and related departments, and personnel policies. This material will vary if a service unit management system is in effect.

The personnel policies, including job descriptions, master staffing, work plan assignments, on-call system, appraisal of performance, and the like, may be in a separate manual entitled *Personnel Policies.*

The staff development manual should include the purpose, content, methods of instruction, hours, length of the program for orientation of various categories of workers, on-the-job training, and leadership staff development.

## REFERENCES

1. Alexander, E. L.: Nursing administration in the hospital health care system, St. Louis, 1972, The C. V. Mosby Co.
2. American Hospital Association: Automatic data processing in hospitals, Hospitals **38**:77, Jan., 1964.
3. American Management Association: Supervisory management (monthly issues), New York, 1965, The Association.
4. American Nurses' Association: Standards for organized nursing services, New York, 1965, The Association.
5. Association of Operating Room Nurses' Statement Committee: Definition and objectives for clinical practice of professional operating room nursing, A.O.R.N. Journal **10**:43, Nov., 1969.
6. Bender, W. B.: Industrial engineers seek better methods (definitions of industrial engineering terms included), Mod. Hosp. **102**:91, April, 1964.
7. Blocker, T. G., Elrod, J. T., Lewis, S. R., Grant, D. A., and Lynch, J. B.: Motion and time analysis of operating room procedures, Plast. Reconstr. Surg. **32**:82, July, 1963.
8. Bryson, L.: The next America, New York, 1952, Harper & Row, Publishers.
9. Coughlan, R. J.: Meetings—three major types and key factors, prepared for and presented at Institutes on Nursing Service Administration, 1965, sponsored jointly by the American Hospital Association and the National League for Nursing.
10. Creighton, H.: Law every nurse should know, ed. 2, Philadelphia, 1970, W. B. Saunders Co.
11. Davis, J. G., and Reed, R.: Variability control is the key to maximum operating room utilization, Mod. Hosp. **102**:113, April, 1964.
12. Fox, M. L.: Role of a committee member, Chicago, 1964, American Hospital Association (presented at regional conferences).
13. Gardner, J. W.: Self-renewal—the individual and the innovative society, New York, 1964, Harper & Row, Publishers.
14. Hayt, E.: Current status of medical liability problems in the United States, Hosp. Manage. **105**:18, April, 1968; **105**:18, May, 1968.
15. Lambertsen, E. C.: Nursing definition and philosophy precede nursing goal development, Mod. Hosp. **103**:136, Sept., 1964.
16. Lesnik, M. J., and Anderson, B. E.: Nursing practice and the law, Philadelphia, 1955, J. B. Lippincott Co.
17. National League for Nursing: A method for rating the proficiency of the hospital general staff nurse, New York, 1964, The League.
18. National League for Nursing: Criteria for evaluating a hospital department of nursing service, New York, 1965, Department of Hospital Nursing, The League.
19. National League for Nursing: Is there a new design for the functions of nursing services? New York, 1970, The League, #20-1387.
20. Phaneuf, M. C.: A nursing audit method, Nurs. Outlook **12**:42, May, 1964.
21. Rosenthal, G. D.: The demand for general hospital facilities, Chicago, 1964, hospital monograph series no. 14, American Hospital Association.
22. Swansburg, R. C.: Team nursing, New York, 1970, G. P. Putnam's Sons.
23. Tead, O.: Administration: its purpose and performance, Hamden, Conn., 1968, The Shoe String Press, Inc.
24. Wessel, L.: Does your operating room have a philosophy? A.O.R.N. Journal **10**:61, July, 1969.

# CHAPTER 3

# Cause and prevention of infections; sterilization and disinfection methods

PEGGY E. LILES

How can the surgical patient be assured of a bacteria-free operating room? How can surgical asepsis be maintained? How can the patient be protected against hospital-acquired infection? The answers to these questions are based on extensive scientific information and principles of microbiology and bacteriology.

Regardless of the architectural design to control infection, effective hospital and operating room control programs must be carried out by all persons who help care for patients. Control programs involve methods of housekeeping and maintenance of the facilities; cleanliness of the air in the suite and of the skin and apparel of patients, surgeons, and personnel; sterility of surgical equipment; strict aseptic technique; and careful observance by all the staff of well-defined written procedures, rules, and regulations.[1, 2]

A control program is based on a knowledge of the nature and characteristics of microorganisms that are capable of producing infection in the surgical patient and an understanding of their transmission in the environment and wound. An ongoing and up-to-date control program requires study and critical analysis of the latest accepted information to provide effective methods that will destroy or in-

hibit specific microorganisms in particular situations.

## DEFINITION OF TERMS RELATED TO BACTERIOLOGY

Definition of terms should be agreed on and clarified. It is important that each worker have some understanding of the nature and characteristics of pathogenic and nonpathogenic organisms.[5]

### Terms related to infection and infecting agents

*Pathogens* are organisms that are capable of producing disease. In man, a satisfactory balance may be reached between the invading pathogens and the host, resulting in no noticeable ill effects. The aggressiveness and virulence of pathogens, the size and composition of the microbial population, the physical environment, and the susceptibility of the host determine the occurrence of an infection.

Most pathogenic bacteria are capable of leading a parasitic or saprophytic existence. Some pathogens reside naturally on or within man without producing disease until the opportunity arises. For example, the enteric organisms are a large group of gram-negative, nonspore-forming bacilli whose natural habitat is within the lumen

of the intestine of man and animals. *Escherichia coli,* one of the enteric bacilli, is capable of producing infection on entrance into the peritoneal cavity.

*Parasites* are organisms that reside on or within the bodies of living organisms called *hosts* in order to find the environment and food they require for life and reproduction. Some organisms are obligatory parasites, meaning that they are dependent on their hosts for survival and reproduction. Other organisms are facultative parasites, meaning that they normally reside on dead matter but may receive nourishment from living matter. All disease-producing organisms are parasites; however, not all parasites are disease producing.

*Saprophytes* are organisms that reside on dead or decaying organic matter. They are found in water, soil, and debris—wherever the process of decay occurs. They reduce decaying matter to simple soluble compounds, which in turn become available to bacteria. For example, *Clostridium tetani,* which causes tetanus (lockjaw), cannot survive in healthy tissue but requires dead (necrotic) material. Some organisms are facultative saprophytes, meaning that they usually obtain their nourishment from living matter but may obtain it from dead organic matter.

Certain bacteria, members of the genera *Bacillus, Clostridium,* and *Sporozoa,* form and develop specialized structures called *spores* (endospore) within the cell under specific conditions. One cell generally produces one spore. The specific environment that starts sporulation is still unknown. When conditions are again favorable for growth, the spore germinates to produce one vegetative cell. The spore appears to possess a large number of active enzymes and is especially resistant to heat, chemicals, and drying.

So-called *transient microorganisms* are those having a very short span of life, such as the normal flora present on the skin surface of man.

*Resident microorganisms* are those that habitually live in the epidermis, deep in the crevices and folds of the skin.

Most bacteria produce one or more poisonous materials known as *toxins.* The term *exotoxin* refers to specific injurious toxins that are formed by certain microorganisms and diffuse freely from the organisms into the environment. *Clostridium tetani, Clostridium botulinum,* the sporulating anaerobes isolated from gas gangrene such as *Clostridium perfringens, Streptococcus pyogenes,* and *Staphylococcus aureus* are some of the organisms with this property.

*Endotoxins* are toxins that are part of the cell wall of some organisms. Endotoxic substances are not secreted to a significant degree into the environment but are released after death and dissolution of the organisms. Their poisonous effect depends on the species. *Salmonella typhosa* and *Neisseria meningitidis* are endotoxic pathogens.

Bacteria differ from one another in their relationship to molecular oxygen. The strictly *aerobic* (obligatory type) bacteria are unable to live and produce without access to free atmospheric oxygen. *Mycobacterium tuberculosis, Vibrio comma* (agent of Asiatic cholera), *Bacillus subtilis,* and *Corynebacterium diphtheriae* are aerobic bacteria. The strictly *anaerobic* bacteria can live only in the absence of air; atmospheric oxygen is poisonous to them. The facultative pathogenic bacteria, such as *Clostridium tetani, Clostridium botulinum,* and *Clostridium perfringens,* are anaerobic bacteria. However, many bacteria have enzyme systems that permit them to live and produce with, without, or with a very small amount of free oxygen.

The term *infectious agent* refers to a microorganism (bacterium, spirochete, fungus, virus, or any other type of organism) that is capable of producing infection. Infection is the process by which living pathogenic microorganisms enter the body of the host under conditions favorable for their growth and by the production of toxins may act injuriously on the tissues of the host.

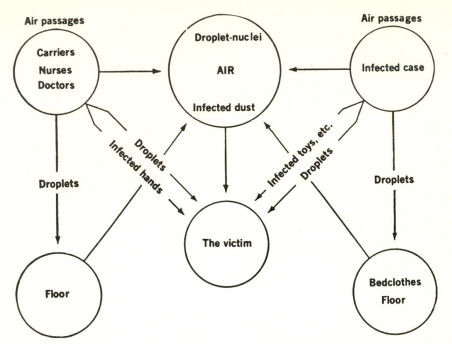

**Fig. 3-1.** Diagram showing how infections may be accidentally spread in hospitals. (From Medical Research Council War Memorandum no. 11. Reproduced by permission of the Comptroller of His Britannic Majesty's Stationery Office.)

The term *source* refers to the object, substance, or individual from which an infectious agent passes to a host. In some cases, transfer is direct from the reservoir, or source, to the host. The source may be at any one point in the chain of transmission. For example, the nose of an individual may be the reservoir, or source; his hands, his clothing, or mask may become the intermediate mechanism for the transfer of the agent to the host.

*Hospital-acquired infection,* as defined by Williams,[23] is as follows: "Any infection that is acquired in a hospital, whether from ordinary risk or from one peculiar to hospitals, whether the results appear in the hospital or after the patient has gone home, thus including infections from one person to another (cross infection), and infection from one tissue to another in the same person (self-infection)."* (See Fig. 3-1.)

*From Williams, R. E., Blowers, R., Garrod, L. P., and Shooter, R. A.: Hospital infection—causes and prevention, Chicago, 1966, Year Book Medical Publishers, Inc.

A *carrier* is a person who harbors one or more specific pathogens in the absence of discernible clinical disease. Carriers may be classified into three groups: convalescent carriers who continue to harbor or shed organisms for variable periods after recovery from the disease, chronic or permanent carriers who harbor organisms usually for the duration of life, and transitory or temporary carriers who, without a recognized attack of the disease, harbor organisms for short periods.[7, 9]

The term *contamination* refers to the presence of pathogenic organisms on or in an animate or inanimate vector. It generally is used in reference to a specific object, substance, or tissue that contains microorganisms, especially disease-producing organisms. For example, a person's skin or an instrument may be contaminated (by contact) with pathogenic organisms, but it is not infected.

*Inflammation* is a defense reaction by the body to an injury or abnormal stimulation caused by a physical, chemical, or biological agent. Frequently the tissue of the

host cells, assisted by phagocytes, localize and destroy the pathogenic invader. This reaction is observed as a local inflammation. Nature provides many barriers for protection against disease-producing organisms, such as intact skin and mucous membranes.

A *local* infection is one in which the causative agent is limited to one locality of the body and becomes circumscribed in a boil or abscess. *Primary* infection is the first infection that develops after microbial invasion. In *secondary* infection the organisms invade tissues where there is an existing primary infection. When the infectious agents spread throughout the body tissues, the condition is termed a *systemic* infection. "The dissemination of microorganisms by a distributing focus results in either a bacteremia or a septicemia. In a bacteremia the primary focus distributes bacteria once or intermittently, resulting in their transient appearance in the blood. When it distributes organisms more or less constantly, their continual presence in the bloodstream is known as septicemia. The old concept suggested that the actual growth or reproduction of bacteria within the circulating bloodstream was a septicemia in contrast with a bacteremia in which microorganisms found it impossible to reproduce in the circulating blood. The newer concept indicates that the difference is in the rate of dissemination from the distributing focus, it being more or less constant in a septicemia and intermittent or single in a bacteremia."*

*Sepsis* is a generalized reaction to pathogenic organisms, their poisons, or both. The septic condition may be evident clinically by the signs of inflammation and the systemic manifestations of the patient.

Normally the leukocytes (white blood cells) remove debris, including bacteria,

from the blood by devouring these foreign particles. This process is called *phagocytosis,* and the devouring cells are called *phagocytes.* In some cases the white cells are killed in the process and accumulate at the site of the infection. This accumulation of decayed cells and serum is called *pus.* The inflammatory battle is an overall reaction of the body to injury. The action of the phagocytes, the bactericidal substances in the blood, and the desire of the tissues to localize the infection result in production of the cardinal inflammatory signs of redness, heat, swelling, and pain.

An *antigen* is a foreign substance in the body that encourages specific immunity by production of specific substances called *antibodies.* General antibodies, which are protein, appear to be produced mainly in the spleen, lymph glands, and bone marrow.

## Terms related to destruction of microorganisms

To prevent infection in man, specific microorganisms must be destroyed, removed, or inhibited by one of several methods, depending on the circumstances.

*Sterile* means that the object or substance is completely free of all living microorganisms and is incapable of producing any form of life. *Sterilization* refers to the process of destroying all organisms and spores that are present. The term is sometimes used in reference to the destruction of all forms of life, including fungi, viruses, spores, and other types of organisms.

### Surgical asepsis

In 1867 Lister realized that a patient's wound could become infected by organisms floating in the dust through the air and by organisms settling on instruments that later came into direct contact with the wound. Lister's objective was to make the air aseptically clean and free of disease-producing organisms by spraying the air and the skin with phenol solution.

---

*From Altemeier, W. A., and Culbertson, W. R.: Applied surgical bacteriology. In Moyer, C. A., Rhoads, J. E., Allen, J. G., and Harkins, H. N., editors: Surgery principles and practice, ed. 3, Philadelphia, 1965, J. B. Lippincott Co., p. 46.

This marked the beginning of the antiseptic era. The term *asepsis* means the absence of any infectious agents. Asepsis is directed at cleanliness and the elimination of all infectious agents. It produces sterility in a specific area by elimination of all living microorganisms. Aseptic techniques exclude microorganisms present in the environment and prevent those living harmlessly within or on the body from reaching the open wound so that healing may take place by first intention. Modern surgery is aseptic in the use of sterile instruments, sutures, dressings, gloves, linens, and so forth.

### Germicide, bactericide, and disinfectant

Germicides, bactericides, and disinfectants are agents, usually chemical substances, that destroy or inhibit pathogens and nonpathogens but do not kill spores. In practice the term *bactericide* and *germicide* are generally used synonymously, most often in reference to agents applied to inanimate objects.

The term *disinfectant* usually refers to an agent having the properties that kill infectious organisms. The agent may be capable of destroying some pathogens and other harmful organisms but not the spores. *Disinfection* refers to any chemical or physical process that results in the destruction or removal of infectious agents outside the body. The term is not synonymous with *sterilization.*

*Concurrent disinfection* refers to the immediate disinfection process following discharge of infectious materials from the body of an infected person or after contamination of articles by an infectious agent. *Terminal disinfection* is the process of rendering all articles and materials and their immediate physical environment incapable of conveying infectious agents to other persons after the patient has left the room.[14, 19]

### Antiseptic

An antiseptic is an agent that arrests the growth of microorganisms either by inhibiting their activity or by destroying them. For example, a germicide may be an antiseptic, depending on the strength of the solution, the period of action, and the nature of the organism. An agent that destroys organisms in a given period of time may only inhibit their growth if the exposure time is shortened. Thus an agent may be a germicide in one situation and an antiseptic in another. Some organisms are less resistant to toxic agents than are others. For this reason, a substance may be a germicide against one organism and an antiseptic against another.

### Chemotherapeutic agent

A chemotherapeutic agent is one that in vivo effectively limits bacterial growth or is bactericidal at concentrations that are nontoxic for the parasitized host.

## ORGANISMS THAT CAUSE INFECTION
### Staphylococci

There are two recognized species of staphylococci: *Staphylococcus aureus* and *Staphylococcus epidermidis.*

Numerous disease processes are associated with *Staphylococcus aureus.* There are several portals of entry: the skin, the respiratory tract, and the genitourinary tract. Staphylococci survive for long periods of time in the air, in dust, in debris, in bedding, and in clothing. Pathogenic staphylococci grow in the sweat, urine, tissue, and skin of man. They are resistant to heat and chemicals, including high concentrations of sodium chloride. They are more difficult to destroy than many other nonspore-forming organisms.

Staphylococci are called *coagulase-positive* (pathogenic) when they are capable of clotting plasma and, conversely, are called *coagulase-negative* (usually nonpathogenic) when there is clumping by the plasma. *Staphylococcus aureus* is hemolytic, parasitic, pathogenic, and coagulase-positive. *Staphylococcus epidermidis* is parasitic, less pathogenic, and coagulase-negative.

In studying the response of staphylococci to various bacteriophages, it was found that certain strains have epidemic potentials and that some are particularly virulent and drug resistant. Two strains classified in this manner that are known to be highly virulent are 80/81 type and 77 type. In the past there were only one or two epidemic strains, whereas today there are several. Staphylococci vary in their resistance to antibiotics. For example, resistance of staphylococci to penicillin differs from their resistance to other antibiotics. Many strains formerly nonpathogenic are now disease-producing organisms.

Pathogenic staphylococci are capable of causing rapid suppuration. In many cases the staphylococci have a tendency to remain localized as an abscess and then break through to the outside. Eventually healing occurs. Wound sepsis is not the only manifestation of staphylococcal infection. Patients may suffer staphylococcal pneumonia, enterocolitis, urinary tract infection, or skin infection. Patients who undergo operations on the heart and great vessels seem to be particularly susceptible to coagulase-negative staphylococci.

Staphylococcal pneumonia may develop in patients who contract influenza in the hospital, especially those surgical patients with advanced chronic bronchitis, uremia, or some other type of debilitating disease. If the pneumonia has been classified as caused by an epidemic strain of staphylococci, the patient may become a potent source of infection for other persons. A patient with enterocolitis may suffer an acute onset of tachycardia, fever, and profuse diarrhea after surgery. For this reason terminal disinfection and zoning environmental principles, including adequate air changes, are important factors in an infection control program.

The skin surface is the most common site of staphylococci. Studies indicate that 5% to 10% of persons carry staphylococci on their skin, which may lead to contamination of clothing and dispersal of the organisms.

Persons who are skin carriers of staphy-lococci differ in their ability to shed the organisms, for no known reason. There appears to be no obvious difference between light and heavy shedders in hygiene and skin condition, and no other contributing factor is apparent. Heavy shedders appear to be in normal good health.

The nasal and throat cavities are the most important reservoirs that continually replenish the external environment. Studies indicate that 40% of adults and 60% of persons under 20 years of age are carriers. Colonization of staphylococci occurs within eight days after birth in 80% of infants. Among hospital staffs (particularly among nurses), 50% of the staff are temporary carriers, 35% are persistent carriers, and 15% never become carriers. Carriers usually harbor either coagulase-positive (pathogenic) or coagulase-negative (nonpathogenic) staphylococci, seldom both types, and rarely more than one strain.[6] Since an individual may be a carrier of staphylococci one day and a noncarrier the next day, frequent swab testing of the nose as a check to the spread of the organisms is impractical.[23] Cleanliness of the environment, proper handling and sterilization of linens and equipment, and adherence to adequate washing techniques are important controls to prevent transmission of infection.

The severity of a staphylococcal infection in human beings is determined by many factors: the type and size of the invading population, route of transmission, properties of the toxic products, and previous exposure and susceptibility of the host. Other contributing factors are the amount of physical trauma and the general health and nutritional state of the patient, as well as the possibility of allergic states or the presence of uncontrollable diabetes or toxemia.

### Streptococci

Most streptococci are generally gram-positive, nonmotile, nonspore-forming organisms. Streptococci are classified according to their action on red blood cells (alpha, beta, or gamma hemolysis), their

resistance to physical and chemical factors (for example, growth at 45° C., growth in 6.5% NaCl), and biochemical tests (for example, group-specific C carbohydrates). Alpha-hemolytic streptococci produce a number of toxic substances resulting in partial hemolysis of red blood cells. When alpha-hemolytic streptococci are present, a greenish discoloration surrounds the colony. Beta-hemolytic streptococci produce toxins that completely hemolyze red cells and when they are cultured on blood agar plates (preferably containing sheep blood), there is a complete clear zone around the colony. Gamma-hemolytic streptococci do not hemolyze blood.

According to immunological differentiation proposed by Lancefield, group A hemolytic streptococci are primarily pathogens of man, whereas group C hemolytic organisms are occasionally pathogens of man. Other species are entirely saprophytic for man. Virulent streptococci are more serious invaders than are staphylococci because the former tend to involve wide areas of tissue and to cause necrosis without localization. However, this is partially counterbalanced by the fact that these virulent streptococci are usually sensitive to penicillin, whereas this may not be the case with staphylococci. Streptococci also occur in mixed infections with other pathogens.

In wounds, a streptococcal infection is introduced via the skin and spreads through the lymph vessels and nodes, resulting in inflammation, cellulitis, and sometimes suppuration. Alpha-hemolytic, or viridans type, streptococci, which normally reside in the respiratory tract or throat of man, may produce a localized infection such as an abscess in the gums or teeth or subacute bacterial endocarditis. Alpha-hemolytic streptococci may also produce meningitis, although they are not very virulent in contrast to pyogenic beta-hemolytic streptococci. Nonhemolytic streptococci or enterococci may occasionally produce atypical pneumonia, endocarditis, or urinary tract infection.

Transmission of streptococci from the infected person to the susceptible host is accomplished in part by direct contact and in part by contamination of the environment. Direct contact may be by inhalation of infectious droplets expelled from the nose and mouth or by hand-to-hand contact. Indirect contact is by means of infected air and dust in the environment. Most upper respiratory tract infections appear to be airborne. The nasal carrier is by far the most dangerous because he is a contributor of large numbers of streptococci to his environment (Fig. 3-1).

Prevention of streptococcal infections, via persons and via wounds, can be accomplished by adherence to aseptic techniques, including proper handling of contaminated clothing and masks, adequate ventilation with frequent air changes, exclusion of personnel with acute sinusitis from the patients, and effective sterilization of supplies and instruments.

*Streptococcus (Diplococcus) pneumoniae* is a nonmotile, generally gram-positive, nonspore-forming diplococcus that produces no toxins of real significance. Pneumococci are the normal inhabitants of the upper respiratory tract of man. Between 40% to 60% of persons are at some time carriers of pneumococci. The carrier state is not permanent, but sporadic and intermittent. A majority of carriers tend to carry the less virulent types of organisms (type IV). An individual may carry two or more types simultaneously. A healthy carrier is more important in dissemination of infection than is an infected patient.

Pneumococci are the chief cause of lobar pneumonia in man. In this disease, pneumococci do not remain in the lung but migrate from the source of infection through the nasal passages or are distributed by means of the vascular system to other parts of the body, appearing as a localized infection. Sinusitis, parotitis, conjunctivitis, peritonitis, and pyogenic infection such as arthritis are frequently caused by pneumococci.

Pneumococci are transmitted chiefly by direct contact with the infected person or carrier and by inhalation of droplets ex-

pelled from the throat into the air.[5] Prevention of pneumococcal infection is accomplished through environmental sanitation, exclusion of carriers from the operating room, effective care of patients, strict adherence to surgical and medical asepsis, and use of chemotherapy.

### Neisseria

*Neisseria* species are gram-negative, nonmotile, nonspore-forming diplococci. *Neisseria catarrhalis* is found frequently in the nasopharynx of healthy persons and in persons with colds and other respiratory infections. *Neisseria sicca* is present on the mucous membrane of the respiratory tract and may be a causative agent of kidney infection.

*Neisseria gonorrhoeae* usually gains entrance to the tissues after being deposited on and by burrowing through the mucous membranes, from which it is spread by the lymphatic or blood vessels. It may invade the bloodstream by means of local lesions. Gonorrheal vulvovaginitis is transmitted by bedding, clothing, and other inanimate vectors, whereas gonorrhea is spread by direct contact. Prophylaxis and control are accomplished by environmental sanitation and chemotherapy.

*Neisseria meningitidis*, the meningococcus, is a pathogenic organism capable of producing acute meningitis in man. Meningococci may gain access to the central nervous system via the nasopharynx. The method whereby the meningococci leave the nasopharynx, invade the bloodstream, and reach the central nervous system is not known. Meningococcal meningitis is disseminated by direct contact and by droplet infection from secretions of the mouth, nose, and throat. Some persons are temporary carriers, whereas others are chronic meningococcal carriers.

### Clostridium

Members of the genus *Clostridium* are anaerobic, spore-forming bacilli, many of which are pathogenic for man. The species include *Clostridium tetani, Clostrid-* *ium perfringens, Clostridium novyi, Clostridium histolyticum, Clostridium septicum,* and *Clostridium botulinum. Clostridium sporogenes* is one of the nonpathogenic species.

*Clostridium tetani* produces tetanus (lockjaw) in man. The bacilli normally reside in the soil and in the intestinal contents of some animals and man. Tetanus toxin is a potent poisonous substance to man. Tetanus is characterized by spasms of the voluntary muscles, particularly those of the jaw and neck—thus the name lockjaw. The bacilli gain entrance to the tissues by way of a deep, dirty wound and set up a localized infection. The toxin is disseminated throughout the body, and when it reaches the nervous system, lockjaw occurs. Surgical tetanus may occur postoperatively and is usually due to faulty sterilization of equipment or dressings. Tetanus that follows a puncture wound facilitates multiplication of anaerobic bacilli. Tetanus of the newborn (tetanus neonatorum) may follow infection of the umbilicus. Treatment includes the use of antitoxin and an active immunization program.

Gaseous gangrene is produced by spores of *Clostridium* species present in contaminated wounds, especially those involving fracture or extensive tissue necrosis. Accidental injuries, puerperal sepsis, and ruptured appendix may be accompanied by gas gangrene. It is usually formed by anaerobic, toxin-producing, spore-forming bacilli. The gangrenous process results from the activity of the sporulating obligate anaerobes and the exotoxins they produce. There are several species of *Clostridium* that may infect wounds and produce gas gangrene. The most frequent are *Clostridium perfringens, Clostridium novyi, Clostridium septicum,* and *Clostridium histolyticum. Clostridium sporogenes,* although considered nonpathogenic, is found in many cases.

*Clostridium perfringens* is an anaerobic pathogen capable of producing gaseous gangrene alone or with other anaerobic

organisms in a closed abscess in uterine, gastrointestinal, genitourinary, or biliary infections. This organism is a normal inhabitant of the intestinal tract of man. Entrance of *Clostridium perfringens* into a wound does not always produce gas gangrene. The pathogenicity of a *Clostridium* species depends on the amount of powerful exotoxins it produces either within the body or in circumscribed tissues. In gas gangrene, the gas in the tissues causes them to expand. This creates pressure, thereby decreasing the flow of blood to the tissues, and necrosis results. The powerful exotoxins also weaken the general condition of the patient.

## Pseudomonas aeruginosa

The best-known pathogenic aerobic species of *Pseudomonas* for man is *Pseudomonas aeruginosa*. It is frequently found in soil, water, sewage, debris, and air and occasionally in the normal flora of the skin and intestines. Its incidence increases in the intestine when the coliform organisms are suppressed. Until recently, it was considered a harmless saprophyte or possibly a microorganism of slight pathogenic power. It is now known that this bacillus may be associated with a great many suppurative infections in man. *Pseudomonas aeruginosa* appears to be a pathogen only when it is introduced into areas devoid of normal defenses, when it is superimposed on staphylococcal infection, or when it is present in a mixed infection. It may attack a debilitated patient with extensive burns or traumatic injuries.

*Pseudomonas aeruginosa* is resistant to most antimicrobial agents. Environmental sanitation and strict adherence to aseptic techniques are important preventive measures.

## Salmonella

*Salmonella* species are members of a large general classification of organisms that are often called *enteric* (or coliform) bacilli because they inhabit the intestinal tract of man. These organisms are gram-negative, nonspore-forming aerobic bacteria. Other well-known members are *Shigella* species (the dysentery bacilli), *Escherichia* species, and *Proteus* species (the paracolon bacilli).

*Salmonella* species are all pathogenic to a greater or lesser degree and are non-spore-forming, gram-negative, motile bacteria. They do not form exotoxins, but all possess endotoxins. *Salmonella* infection in man is acquired by ingestion of the organism, usually by means of contaminated food or water. These bacteria may produce either clinical or subclinical infection. The three major diseases for which they are causative organisms are enteric fever, gastroenteritis, and septicemia.

*Salmonella typhosa* is the causative agent of typhoid fever. About 3% of patients with typhoid fever become carriers for some time. The bacteria remain in the gallbladder and intestine and occasionally in the urinary tract.

## Escherichia

*Escherichia coli* is one of the most common causes of septicemia, inflammation of the liver, and gallbladder and urinary tract infection, especially when the host's defenses are inadequate, as in infants or elderly patients with terminal disease. These organisms may also cause infection following radiation treatment and may escape through the wall of the bowel, causing secondary peritonitis. However, most strains of *Escherichia coli* are non-pathogenic in the normal, healthy host.

## Proteus

*Proteus vulgaris* is often associated with *Pseudomonas aeruginosa*. *Proteus* organisms are gram-negative, motile, aerobic bacilli, usually found free living in water, soil, dust, and sewage.

*Proteus vulgaris* is frequently found in the normal fecal flora of the intestinal tract. These bacilli also produce infection in man only when they leave the intestinal tract. This species may become the causative agent of cystitis and is most resistant

to heat and antimicrobial agents. Specific antibiotics are active agents against *Proteus*.

## Mycobacterium

*Mycobacterium tuberculosis* is a non-spore-forming aerobic bacillus. Disease is produced by establishment and proliferation of virulent organisms and interactions with the host. Tubercle bacilli spread in the host by direct extension through the lymphatic channels and bloodstream and by way of the bronchi and gastrointestinal tract. These bacilli can infect almost any tissue, including skin, bones, lymph nodes, intestinal tract, and fallopian tubes.

Tubercle bacilli are transmitted directly by means of discharge from the respiratory tract, less frequently through the digestive tract, by inhalation of droplets expelled during coughing, or by kissing and indirectly by means of contaminated articles and dust floating through the air. Prevention and control programs include rigid environmental hygiene, disinfection and sterilization of contaminated equipment, and isolation of individuals with active infection.

## STERILIZATION AND CLEANING METHODS FOR PREVENTION OF INFECTION

Modern surgery demands increasingly intricate and delicate instruments and more efficient dry goods, utensils, and fluids. Methods of sterilization of surgical items must result in complete destruction of all microbial life and absence of toxic residue on the objects, as well as little or no deterioration or damage to heat- and moisture-sensitive instruments and other items.

### Steam sterilization

Pressure steam is recognized as the safest, most practical means of sterilizing surgical dry goods, fluids, the majority of instruments, and other inanimate objects. Steam under pressure permits permeation of moist heat to porous substances by condensation and results in destruction of all microbial life.[15]

As stated by Perkins,[16] "Steam is water vapor and as such, it presents a physical state of water as truly as ice does, but as a gas it may be near or far away from its condensing temperature."* Saturated steam exerts the maximum pressure for water vapor at a given temperature and pressure.

### *Theory of microbial destruction*

It is believed that microorganisms are destroyed by moist heat through a process of denaturation and coagulation of the enzyme-protein system within the bacterial cell. Microorganisms are killed at a lower temperature when moist heat is used than when dry heat is used. This fact is based on the theory that all chemical reactions, including coagulation of proteins, are catalyzed by the presence of water.

Compressed steam results in effective sterilization because moisture and heat are always present. When steam comes in contact with a cold object, condensation takes place immediately. As the steam condenses, it gives off latent heat and results in heating and wetting of the object; in other words, both moisture and heat are provided.

### *Principles and mechanism*

Pure steam at sea level atmospheric pressure has a temperature of 212° F. (100° C.). When water is boiled in a vessel from which the steam cannot escape, a higher temperature is reached. To attain steam under pressure, a vessel that can be closed tightly must be used. A home pressure cooker generates steam from the water inside the tightly closed vessel when it is placed over a gas flame or electric plate. In the hospital autoclave, the steam coming from the boilers is compressed, thus giving off latent heat.

---

*From Perkins, J.: Sterilization by heat, 1957, Becton, Dickinson & Co. Lecture.

The higher the steam pressure, the higher the temperature becomes. The steam is the sterilizing agent, not the compressed hot air. If steam is mixed with air at the same pressure, the temperature will be lower than pure steam at atmospheric pressure. For example, if the mixture is two-thirds steam and one-third air, the temperature at 15 pounds pressure per square inch (psi) will be 240° F. (115° C.) instead of 250° F. (121° C.). The air acts as a barrier to steam penetration.

The *autoclave,* generally speaking, consists of two metal cylinders (the shell and the chamber), one within the other. Between the cylinders is an enclosed space (jacket) in which steam and heat can be maintained at a considerably high pressure. The autoclave is fitted with various gauges, pipes, valves, clocks, wheels, thermometers, and the like.

In the conventional steam sterilizer the sterilization process may be divided into five distinct phases:

1. Loading phase, in which the objects are packaged and loaded in the sterilizer.
2. Heating phase, in which the steam is brought to the proper temperature and allowed to penetrate around and on the objects in the chamber.
3. Destroying phase, or the time-temperature cycle, in which all microbial life is exposed to the killing effects of the steam.
4. Cooling and drying phase, in which the objects are cooled and dried, clean air is introduced into the chamber, the door is opened, and the objects are removed and stored.
5. Testing phase, in which the efficiency of the sterilizing process is checked.

PHASE 1. Packaging and wrapping of surgical supplies and loading them in the sterilizer are important factors that govern the effectiveness of steam sterilization. Textiles must be freshly laundered to assure sufficient moisture content of the fibers to prevent superheating and absorption of the sterilizing agent.

The size and density of the dry goods pack must be restricted to ensure uniform steam penetration. The largest bundle should not exceed 12 × 12 × 20 inches and should have an average weight of 12 pounds. Today, paper sheets and towels have advantages in regard to density of the pack. All wrappers must protect the materials or objects from contamination in handling and must serve as effective dust filters; therefore wrappers must be checked for torn areas and holes before they are used. A double-thickness muslin wrapper, thread count 140, has good filtering qualities and permits the passage of steam to the inner contents of the bundle during sterilization. To hold wrappers in place on bundles and packages, pressure-sensitive (indicating) tape can be used. This tape will seal the wrapper and also indicate that the package has been subjected to a certain degree of temperature in the chamber.

Owen and others[14] have found that cotton, when surrounded by an atmosphere containing vapor of water, will take up or give off vapor until a condition of equilibrium is reached. Moisture has a profound effect on cotton fibers. The rate of evaporation depends on both the amount of water in the fibers and the temperature. Laundering of dry goods between sterilizing exposures reduces the deterioration rate of cotton materials.

Tubes, needles, and drains must have moisture in the lumen that can turn to steam and prevent trapping of air, which creates a barrier against effective sterilization. The container must be covered with a material that permits penetration of steam to all inside surfaces of the container.

In assembling the items in the bundle, the lighter materials should be placed near the center of the bundle. The alternate layers of dry goods should be crossed to promote free circulation of steam and removal of air.

Dating the package serves to assure that storage is not prolonged. Long shelf life exposes goods to the hazards of dust, ex-

cessive handling, and accidental contamination.

When the chamber of the sterilizer is loaded, the bundles and packages should be arranged so that there is little resistance to the passage of steam through the load from the top of the chamber toward the bottom of the sterilizer. All packages should be placed in the sterilizer on edge in a vertical position.

A second or upper layer may be placed crosswise on the first or lower layer. Packs should be in loose contact with each other to promote free circulation of moist steam and heat through each entire pack.

All jars, tubes, canisters and other nonporous objects should be arranged on their sides with their covers or lids removed to provide a horizontal path for the escape of air and free flow of steam and heat.

Instruments are placed in trays that have mesh or perforated bottoms. They may be autoclaved while unwrapped and used immediately, or they may be wrapped in double-thickness muslin wrappers and sterilized for later use.

To guard against superheating, the surgical packs should not be subjected to preheating in the sterilizer with steam in the jacket only prior to sterilization.

PHASE 2. When the steam enters the autoclave, it will at first be at the same pressure as that of the atmosphere. With closure of the valves and doors communicating with the outside, the pressure of the steam inside rises, resulting in an increase in the temperature of the steam.

Gauges on traditional autoclaves register the pressure in both the jacket and the chamber. Most vacuums are designated in terms of inches of mercury. A perfect vacuum is represented by a column of mercury 29.92 inches high. Standard gauges indicate vacuum starting with zero (at room or normal atmospheric pressure). As the air is removed, the gauge registers down to 30 inches.

Evacuation of air from the conventional sterilizer is necessary to permit proper permeation of steam. The most common method for removal of air is the downward or gravity displacement method. This method is based on the principle that air is heavier than steam. The steam that is piped into the sterilizer through a pressure-reducing valve is introduced into the chamber. The steam forces the heavier air ahead of it, down and forward, until all the air is discharged from a line at the front of the sterilizer. If a sterilizer is improperly loaded, mixing of air with steam acts as a barrier to steam penetration and prevents the attainment of sterilization temperature.

PHASE 3. The destruction period is based on the known time-temperature cycle necessary to accomplish sterilization in saturated steam. Authorities have shown that the order of death in a given bacterial population subjected to a sterilizing process is determined by definite laws. If the temperature is increased, the time may be decreased. The minimum time-temperature relationships in terms of sterilizing efficiency are as follows:

> 2 minutes at 270° F. (132° C.)
> 8 minutes at 257° F. (125° C.)
> 18 minutes at 245° F. (118° C.)

To provide a safety margin, the minimum estimated exposure period is extended to cover the lag between the attainment of chamber and load temperatures.

The recording thermometer, not the pressure gauge, is the important guide to the sterilizing phase. The recording clock on the sterilizer gives information about the run of the load and to what temperature the goods were exposed. The temperature inside the chamber must be maintained throughout the determined time of exposure.

PHASE 4. At completion of the sterilization cycle, the steam inside the chamber is removed immediately so that it will not condense and wet the packs. To assist in the drying process, the jacket pressure may be left on to keep the walls of the chamber hot as the steam from the chamber is exhausted to zero gauge pressure.

When chamber pressure has been exhausted, the door may be opened slightly to permit vapor to escape. Another method is to introduce clean filtered air by means of a vacuum dryer (ejector) device in conjunction with the operating valve on the sterilizer. The minimum drying time for all methods is approximately 15 to 20 minutes.

The freshly sterilized packages should not be placed on cold surfaces such as metal tabletops. The sweating that occurs on the cool table will form pools of water that may pick up contamination. This contaminated water may be reabsorbed by the dry goods. Bacteria are capable of passing through layers of wet cotton. Freshly sterilized packs should be left in the loading carriage for 15 to 20 minutes or should be placed on edge in wire mesh containers that are lined with several layers of muslin to absorb the sweating moisture.

Sterilized packs should never be stacked in close contact with each other. Their arrangement on the shelves should provide for air circulation on all sides of each package. The freshly dated sterile packages are placed behind those already on the shelving.

The length of time a pack is considered to remain sterile depends on the filtering qualities of the cover, the kind and extent of contaminating influences present in the storage area, the changes in atmospheric conditions surrounding the packs, the handling of the packs, and the presence or absence of outer protective plastic coverings. Sterile packages wrapped in muslin should remain sterile for 3 to 4 weeks. Because of many hazards, standards should be established providing for the use of all items within 3 weeks.

PHASE 5. Checks on the mechanical function of equipment such as autoclaves must be made regularly, and reports must be issued by the person responsible. There are several methods of keeping a constant check on the proper functioning of a sterilizer and ensuring the efficiency of the sterilizing process.

Mechanical controls such as thermometers and automatic controls assist in identifying and preventing malfunction of the sterilizing equipment and operational errors made by the personnel.

Indicating thermometers, located on the discharge line of the sterilizer, indicate the temperature throughout the sterilizing cycle on a dial on the front of the sterilizer. This device indicates a drop in temperature when and if it occurs and can act as a warning of sterilizer failure. Because the lowering of the temperature may be intermittent and is not recorded permanently, it must be seen by those responsible for operating the sterilizer. This device cannot detect air pockets within the load or pack. Air is a poor conductor of heat; therefore it is one of the greatest causes, other than human error, of sterilization failure.

Recording thermometers indicate and record the same temperature as the indicating thermometers. They record the time the sterilizer reaches the desired degree of temperature and the duration of each exposure. The recording thermometer can be helpful if there are several individuals using the sterilizer or if the operator should forget to time the load. Its recordings will act as a daily proof that exposure time of loads have been correct, as well as showing that proper temperature limits have been maintained. The daily record should show the number of the sterilizer, the time, and the date and provide evidence that can be used to correct discrepancies should errors occur. Like the indicating thermometer, the recording thermometer does not detect cool air pockets; therefore additional controls are necessary for complete safety.

Automatic controls are devices that, by a predetermined plan, will control all phases of the sterilizing process. The controls allow the steam to enter, time the sterilizing cycle, exhaust the steam, and allow drying. Some will lock the door so that it cannot be opened until the cycle is complete.

A thermocouple may be placed within the pack or load and will indicate whether

the required degree of temperature has been reached and maintained within the contents throughout the sterilizing cycle. Although this device records the temperature and the length of time it has been maintained, it does not assure sterility of the item if, like petrolatum, it cannot be penetrated by steam.

Thermal controls, sometimes referred to as sterilizer controls or sterilizer indicators, such as sealed glass tubes, pressure-sensitive (indicating) tape, and color-change cards and strips can be used to detect cool air pockets inside the sterilizer chamber. They can be useful in checking packaging and loading techniques on a package-by-package or load-by-load basis, as well as the mechanical functioning of the sterilizer. However, they do not "prove" sterilization because some of them will react even when the temperature is inadequate for sterilization. A method of checking thermal controls is to expose them to steam in a sterilizer set at 115° C. (240° F.) for 30 minutes. This temperature is inadequate for sterilization, therefore the controls should not react.

One thermal control is a sealed glass tube with a heavy thread securely fastened to one end to facilitate handling that contains a pellet that melts on reaching the sterilization temperature. These tubes are placed in the center of each linen pack or package. Another tube may be placed among the packs, with the thread visible, after the sterilizer is loaded. A melted pellet will indicate that the temperature has been reached in the place where the indicator was placed and that the items have been exposed to sterilizing conditions.

Pressure-sensitive (indicating) tape, used most often to secure wrappers on packages, has light lines, squares, or wording that turns dark when exposed to the sterilizing agent (steam or gas) for a time and at a temperature that will effect the color change. It is valuable in differentiating packages that have been exposed to sterilization from those that have not; however, it is not a check on the sterility of the contents of the package because it cannot indicate conditions in the center of the package. These tapes should be removed from the muslin wrappers when packages are opened because they create laundry problems such as stopping up screens and filters. In some cases the tapes leave a dye on the wrappers that may cause deterioration of the material.

Color-change cards and strips are made of a heavy paper imprinted with a special ink that will change color when exposed to moist heat. Disadvantages are that some of these will change color under conditions less than adequate for sterilization and others emit acid fumes. Because these fumes can damage sterilized materials, these indicators must be placed in metal holders designed for this use.

A biological control is the most accurate method of checking sterilization efficiency. Commercially prepared spore strips and ampules that have been approved by the Biological Division of the National Institutes of Health are available. They contain a known population of *Bacillus stearothermophilus,* a highly heat-resistant, spore-forming microorganism that does not produce toxins and is nonpathogenic. The spore strips or ampules should be placed in test packs of linen of the largest density and in the areas of the sterilizer least accessible to the steam. When spore strips or ampules are removed, they are sent to the bacteriology laboratory, a commercial laboratory, or the manufacturer for results. Tests should be conducted at least once a month but more often if there is a rapid turnover of personnel operating the sterilizer or if sterilizers are old and known to function improperly at times. When possible, the tests should be unannounced and unknown to the personnel operating the sterilizer. The incubation period for the test is usually 7 days, although "positive readings" are sometimes available sooner. Negative reports indicate that wrapping techniques, loading procedures, and sterilizing conditions are correct and that the sterilizer is functioning properly.

Spore control ampules are used for steam sterilization only and cannot be used in

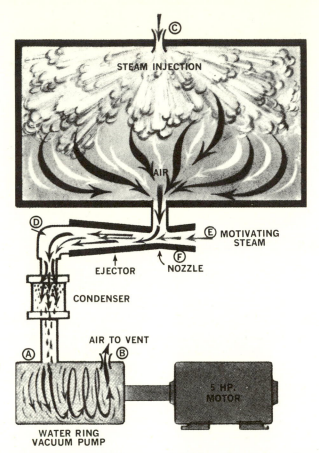

**Fig. 3-2.** Vacamatic vacuum system. This type of sterilizer features simultaneous vacuum and steam injection. Air evacuation from chamber and load prior to sterilization is accomplished by means of high vacuum, coupled with simultaneous steam injection. This conditioning of load eliminates possibility of temperature lag when exposure period starts. Saturated steam enters chamber and penetrates densest packs in load, heating them rapidly to from 272° to 276° F. Water-ring vaccum pump, together with steam ejector, forms direct, balanced, quiet element. Air to be evacuated from chamber is drawn into pump through an opening, **A,** and is exhausted through opening **B.** As air is being evacuated, "conditioning steam" is injected into chamber through **C,** thus diffusing air in space surrounding fabrics. Conditioning steam assisted by partial vacuum diffuses rapidly through fibers, thereby completely releasing absorbed air by displacement. Water-ring pump creates vacuum of about 50 mm. Hg absolute at base of steam ejector, **D.** Steam from sterilizer jacket enters ejector through **E.** Incoming steam expanding through nozzle, **F,** creates tremendous velocity, which draws with it air from sterilizer chamber out to condenser and through pump. (Courtesy American Sterilizer Co., Erie, Pa.)

hot air (dry heat) sterilizers, since 121° C. (250° F.) would also sterilize them, without sterilizing the load itself. In general, hot-air sterilization is not as good as either steam or ethylene oxide and should be avoided whenever possible. Spore strips containing *Bacillus subtilis* should not be used to check steam sterilizers because they are not heat resistant enough. However,

they may be used with ethylene oxide (gas) sterilization, since they are very resistant to gas sterilization.

### Prevacuum, high-temperature method

In recent years the automatic, prevacuum, high-temperature sterilizer has been developed by researchers in both Great Britain and the United States.[8, 14]

The downward displacement method has been replaced in many instances by an automatic, prevacuum, high-temperature method. This method is usually accomplished by means of an air-blasted, oil-sealed rotary pump, protected by a condenser and coupled with an automatic control mechanism (Fig. 3-2).

Air removal is accomplished by means of a powerful vacuum pump that draws a near-absolute vacuum in the chamber in the first 5 minutes of the cycle, before the steam is introduced. This new system aims to reduce the time necessary to accomplish all phases of the sterilizing process.[14] Reports indicate that the effect of saturated steam temperatures (250° F. versus 270° F.) on the tensile strength of cotton fabrics produces no marked difference in deterioration. Gloves subjected to 270° F. showed less tensile loss than those exposed to 250° F. steam temperature.

The prevacuum, high-temperature steam sterilizer provides a system that is automatically controlled and reduces the total cycle time to 14 minutes. The usual cycle of a prevacuum high-temperature sterilizer is (1) prevacuum (98% air removal) for 5 minutes, (2) heating for 2 minutes, (3) timing for 3 minutes at 135° C. (275° F.), (4) postvacuum for 3 minutes, and (5) return to atmospheric pressure for 1 minute. The cycle will vary with the size of the sterilizer, the adequacy of the steam, and the supply of water. Faulty packaging and overloading or incorrect placement of objects in the chamber is not likely to interfere with air removal, and full heating of the load will take place more rapidly than with the downward displacement method. The prevacuum, high-temperature sterilizer will permit more supplies to be sterilized within a given time.

### Moist heat, high-temperature method

The high-speed pressure (usually automatic) instrument sterilizer is adjusted to operate at 270° F. (130° C.) and 27 pounds pressure per square inch (Fig. 3-3).

The operational process consists of the following steps:

1. Maintain steam in the jacket of the sterilizer just prior to and during the daily operating schedule.

2. Clean soiled instruments with warm tap water containing a detergent and then rinse them thoroughly in a fat-solvent solution.

3. Place the opened instruments in a perforated metal tray, position the tray in the sterilizer, and close and lock the door of the sterilizer.

4. Open steam of the chamber valve or of automatic set timer for a 3-minute exposure period and turn the selector switch to fast exhaust setting.

5. Turn the operating valve to sterile setting. Time exposure period begins when the thermometer records 270° F.

6. On completion of the exposure period, close steam to the chamber valve and open the exhaust valve.

7. Open the door when the exhaust valve registers zero.

8. Remove the instruments and deliver them to the operating room table.

### Boiling water (nonpressure)

Boiling does not sterilize instruments or other inanimate objects. The boiling point of water varies at different altitudes. For example, at sea level the boiling point of water is 100° C. (212° F.); at 589 feet above sea level the boiling point is 99° C (210° F.); and at 10,000 feet above sea level the boiling point is 94° C. (201° F.). Heat-resistant microorganisms, bacterial spores, and certain viruses can withstand boiling water at 100° C. (212° F.) for many hours.

### Ultrasonic cleaner

An instrument that is to be sterilized must first be thoroughly clean. The cleaning method must provide protection from damage to the instrument, cross contamination, and injury to the worker and must be economical.

The ultrasonic cleaning process is based on electronic engineering principles. An electric current, usually 230 volts and 60 cycles, is fed into an electronic generator.

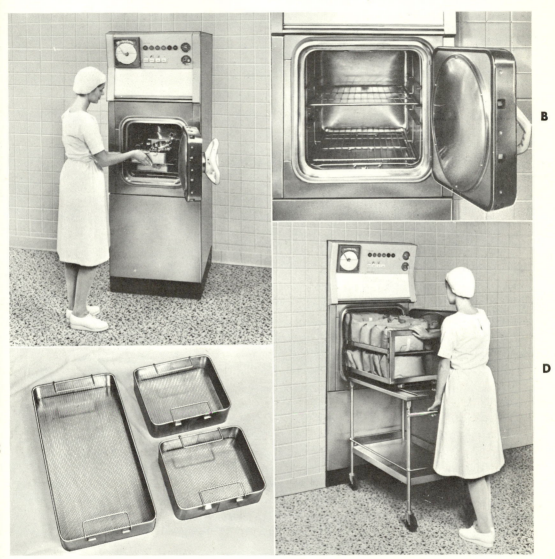

**Fig. 3-3. A,** General purpose high-speed sterilizer is designed for sterilization at 250° to 270° F. It sterilizes instruments, wrapped and unwrapped packs, utensils, and flasked solutions. The productivity of this high-speed cycle falls approximately halfway between standard gravity units and mechanical air removal (vacuum) high-temperature sterilizers. **B,** Adjustable loading rack with four shelf positions. Shelves are removable and designed to permit maximum loading efficiency for variety of mixed or single-item loads. **C,** Instrument trays that feature perforated bottom, foldover, and hinged handles and are available in full-tray or half-tray lengths. **D,** It is ideal for central service use with added feature of a high-speed, automatic, programmed cycle for fabrics. All human-engineered aspects of control panel have been zoned and color-coded for simplified selection of time, temperature, and cycle. Mechanism protects cycle from being changed while in progress. Mechanical timer permits timing from 0 to 60 minutes. Dual purpose transfer carriage is used as portable cart when loading is inside 20 × 20 × 38 inch sterilizer chamber. Locking mechanism with release button holds car securely to transfer carriage. (Courtesy American Sterilizer Co., Erie, Pa.)

where the frequency is raised to a rate of 18,000 to 20,000 cycles per second. This electrical energy then flows into a magnetic device known as a transducer, which converts the electrical energy into mechanical energy. The ultrasonic waves pass through the fluid in the bath. When passing through the fluid of the bath, the ultrasonic waves form very small bubbles that collapse quickly, thus creating a negative pressure action on all surfaces of the instruments in the bath. By means of this pulling action, called the *cavitation process,* debris and material are removed from all surfaces of the instruments without damage to the instruments.

The ultrasonic process has been used effectively to clean delicate and routine general surgical instruments, but this process is not a means of sterilization.

### Manual washing of instruments

Soiled instruments should be cleaned as soon as possible to prevent blood and other substances from drying on the surfaces or in the crevices. If soiled instruments cannot be washed immediately, they should be submerged immediately in a warm detergent solution. Abrasive compounds should never be used.

To wash soiled instruments manually, the following steps should be observed:

1. Release all catches or joints of instruments and open hinged instruments.

2. Place instruments in a deep basin or tray and cover them with water at 125° F. that contains a noncorrosive detergent that will loosen fats, minerals, dried blood, and other substances. The type of detergent to be selected is influenced by the hardness of the water supply.

3. Soak instruments 10 to 45 minutes, depending on the kind and amount of soilage and the composition of the instruments.

4. Using gloves, scrub the instruments with a fairly stiff hand brush.

5. Drain off the detergent solution, rinse instruments, and then immerse them for a few minutes in boiling water. Dry instruments at once—preferably sterilize them in a high-speed autoclave. Inspect and return them to trays or storage.

### Mechanical washing of instruments

The horizontal type of pressure instrument washer-sterilizer (Figs. 3-4 and 3-5) (cabinet design) can be used to wash soiled instruments and to sterilize them after a clean or septic case.

When this sterilizer is used, the instruments are cleaned with the aid of a mechanically agitated water bath containing a detergent. The water is removed from the sterilizer, and the instruments are sterilized for 3 minutes at 270° F. Sterilizers of this type help control the spread of

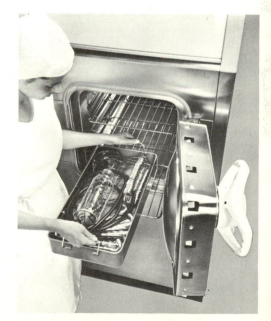

Fig. 3-4. Automatic washer-sterilizer. This type of sterilizer is used to clean and decontaminate instruments and utensils immediately after any surgical procedure, as routine protection to personnel and further safeguard against contamination. It is designed specifically for this function; however, it may be used in supplementary capacity for automatically programmed 3-minute and 10-minute sterilization of surgical instruments and utensils. Pullout shelves permit modern aseptic technique for handling instrument trays. Operator grasps the two hinged handles on new instrument tray and transfers it to table. (Courtesy American Sterilizer Co., Erie, Pa.)

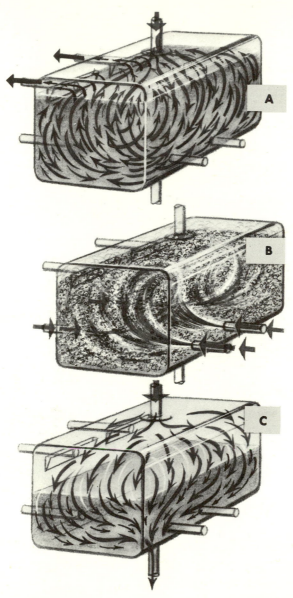

**Fig. 3-5.** Automatic washer-sterilizer. Washing action attained in washer-sterilizer is created by unique combination of high-velocity jet streams of steam and air, which develops violent underwater turbulence. **A,** Cold water filling chamber, covering load to overflow. This cold water, with aid of a detergent, begins to loosen and dissolve gross soil such as blood, tissue, and foreign matter. **B,** Four powerful jet streams of steam and air located near bottom of chamber drive water into violent turbulence to continue cleaning process. **C,** Water temperature rises to 145° to 155° F. This expanding water causes upward flow, which carries loosened debris to water line. Steam is activated into top of chamber, thereby forcing wash water out through bottom drain. Steam under pressure floods chamber, and temperature holds at 270° F. for not less than 3 minutes. Then steam is exhausted through automatic condenser exhaust, and audible signal indicates unit is ready for unloading. (Courtesy American Sterilizer Co., Erie, Pa.)

bacteria, reduce labor costs, and conserve time.

The efficiency of the process depends on the kind of foreign material present and the number of instruments in the load. Complete removal of all soil from the serrations and crevices of instruments depends on the construction of the instrument, the time of exposure, and the pH and efficiency of the detergent solution. Soiled grooved instruments such as the von Petz anastomosis clamp, blood vessel clamps, and scissors should be soaked immediately in a detergent-germicide solution to prevent foreign material from drying into the grooves. They should be processed as soon as possible in the pressure instrument washer-sterilizer. The worker should always follow the operational instructions prepared by the manufacturer. If proper precautions are taken in using the equipment, questions about sterility will not arise.

### Hot air (dry heat) sterilization

When the physical characteristics of certain materials such as powders, grease, and anhydrous oils do not permit permeation of steam, dry heat sterilization may be used. As the proteins become dry during exposure to dry heat, their resistance to denaturation increases. For this reason, at a given temperature, dry heat sterilization is much less effective than is moist heat.

Dry heat sterilization is accomplished by means of a mechanical convection hot oven at a temperature of 320° F., for an exposure period of an hour or longer. The hot oven should be equipped with a blower for forced air circulation. Today, gas sterilization is replacing dry heat sterilization.

An autoclave can be used on a temporary basis as a hot air sterilizer. It is important to remember that the maximum temperature that can be maintained in the chamber is 250° F. and the minimum exposure time is 6 hours, preferably longer. It is also difficult to determine the true temperature of the chamber because the thermometer on the autoclave does not record temperature when moist heat is not present in the chamber.[16]

Incineration, or actual burning of materials, is the most drastic application of dry heat. It is used for the disposal of contaminated gloves, dry goods, and other inorganic and organic wastes and materials.

Direct flaming or dipping in alcohol allows bacteria to be burned off. This is an uncontrollable, unsafe practice and has no place in the operating room!

### Gaseous sterilization

Gaseous sterilization refers to a chemical technique of destroying bacteria, viruses, and other microorganisms. In this form of sterilization the chemicals are gases instead of liquids or solids in solution.[17] Gaseous sterilization is sometimes called *chemical sterilization* and is frequently referred to as *cold sterilization*. This latter term refers to the temperature of 38° C. (100° F.) to 54° C. (130° F.) of the gas sterilization as compared to the 121° C. (250° F.) to 132° C. (270° F.) temperatures of steam sterilization.

In recent years, gaseous sterilization has had considerable application in sterilization of intricate, delicate surgical instruments, large pieces of equipment used in the hospital, plastic and porous materials, and electrical instruments, which are difficult to sterilize without deterioration and damage.[17, 21]

*Ethylene oxide* is the most commonly used gas. It is colorless at ordinary temperatures, has an odor similar to ether, and has an inhalation toxicity similar to that of ammonia gas. Another toxic effect of ethylene oxide is that the vapors can cause large blisters if they are in contact with the skin over a period of time. Pure liquid evaporates too fast to cause harm to the skin unless it is confined by clothing or other means. It is easily kept as a liquid that will boil at 10.73° C. (51.3° F.) and freeze at −113.3° C. (−168.3° F.).

Ethylene oxide is highly explosive and very flammable in the presence of air. These hazards have been greatly reduced

by diluting the ethylene oxide with inert gases such as carbon dioxide or fluorinated hydrocarbons (Freon). Neither of these two inert gases appears to affect the bactericidal activity of the ethylene oxide but serves only as an inert diluent that prevents the flammability hazard.[17]

Kereluk and Lloyd[11] and other investigators have proposed several theories on how ethylene oxide kills bacteria. It is generally believed that the killing rate of bacteria is relative to the rate of diffusion of the gas through their cell walls and the availability or accessibility of one of the chemical groups to react with the ethylene oxide. The killing rate is also dependent on whether the bacterial cell is in a vegetative or spore-forming state. Destruction takes place by alkylation through chemical interference and probably inactivation of the reproductive process of the cell.

As a sterilizing agent, ethylene oxide has the advantages that it is easily available; is effective against all types of microorganisms; penetrates through masses of dry material easily; does not require high temperatures, humidity, or pressure; and is noncorrosive and nondamaging to items.

Gas sterilization with ethylene oxide also has the disadvantages[17] that long exposure time makes it a lengthy process; it is expensive when compared with steam sterilization; an aeration period of 6 hours for nonporous materials to 7 days for tubings used in heart surgery and items sealed in plastic is required; skin irritation, burns of body tissue, and hemolysis of blood result when materials are not aired sufficiently after sterilization; diluents used with ethylene oxide cause damage to some plastics; and human error and mechanical breakdown are more likely to occur.

Factors affecting sterilization with ethylene oxide are time of exposure, gas concentration, temperature, humidity, and penetration. The time exposure that is required depends on temperature, humidity, gas concentration, the ease of penetrating the articles to be sterilized, and the type of microorganisms to be destroyed. Manu-

facturers of gas sterilizers have developed recommended exposure periods for various ethylene oxide concentrations in relation to the material to be sterilized. In general, an exposure period of 3 to 7 hours is necessary for complete sterilization. Exposure time is set for absolute destruction of the most resistant microorganisms, which is a very slow process.

Gas concentration is affected by the temperature and humidity inside the sterilizing chamber, which also affects the exposure period. Concentration is considered effective within the margin of 400 mg. to 1500 mg. per liter of chamber space. If the concentration of gas is doubled, the exposure time may be shortened.[9] The concentration and pressure of the ethylene oxide gas varies with types of sterilizers used; therefore manufacturer's instructions should be followed.

Temperature has a marked influence on the destruction of microorganisms. It is important in gaseous sterilization with ethylene oxide gas because it affects the penetration of the ethylene oxide through bacterial cell walls, as well as through wrappings and packaging material. The temperature for sterilizing is 21° C. (70° F) to 60° C. (140° F.), and automatically controlled ethylene oxide sterilizers are usually preheated to 54° C. (130° F.). Small canister-type ethylene oxide sterilizers can be operated at the temperature and relative humidity of the room for a standardized time cycle. A higher gas concentration is used to compensate for the lower temperature.

Humidity of 40% to 60% is recommended with ethylene oxide to ensure enough moisture to kill microorganisms. Dry spores are most difficult to kill, but, when moistened, their resistance to gas penetration is lowered. Dehydration makes some microorganisms nearly immune to ethylene oxide sterilization, whereas too much moisture can slow the action of the gas below the lethal point. Ethylene oxide sterilizers with automatic controls most often provide for moisture injection to

raise the relative humidity within the chamber, but less automated sterilizers require vials of water or soaked sponges to provide the necessary moisture.

Penetration throughout the load is essential. Items to be sterilized must be thoroughly cleaned of soil before being placed in any type of sterilizer. Lumens of tubing, needles, etc. should be dry. The packaging material must be permeable to moisture as well as to the gas to make it more effective. Sufficient space for gas sterilization is necessary if materials are to be penetrated properly. Care should be taken not to overload the sterilizer. Compression of packages will prevent penetration of the gas, and if packages are plastic wrapped, compression will hinder evacuation of air and cause packages to open during the decrease in chamber pressure when a vacuum is drawn.

Sterilizers range in size from small tubular devices (canisters) that operate under manual control at room temperature to large chambers equipped with completely automatic controls (Fig. 3-6). The automatic control cycle of the sterilizing process consists of air evacuation, humidification, sterilization, gas evacuation, and vent to atmosphere.

Beta-propiolactone is an excellent sterilizing agent, but it is unstable, expensive, and vesicant. In a gaseous form it can be used much the same as formaldehyde. It is well suited to treating large enclosed areas that need not be hermetically sealed, such as laboratories. It is unsuited as a replacement for ethylene oxide because it lacks a high degree of penetration and effectiveness at low relative humidity.

## CHEMICAL DISINFECTION

In recent years, physicians and hospital staffs have been faced with a continuous array of new germicides and disinfectants, many of which it is claimed are ideal for diverse purposes. Research data, however, do not support these claims.

The terms *disinfectant* and *antiseptic* are applied to antimicrobial activity. By

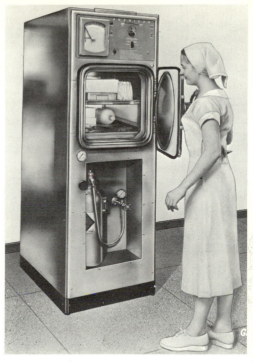

Fig. 3-6. Cryotherm gas sterilizer designed for cold sterilization of delicate steel and plastic eye, neurosurgical, and cardiovascular instruments, electric cords, and catheters. This sterilizer uses cylinders of Pennoxide Oxyfume-7 or 12 or Benvecide or Cry-oxcide, which are highly efficient sterilizing agents. They are nonflammable and nonexplosive. Operator loads sterilizer, sets control for desired exposure period, and presses start button. The control system draws vacuum into chamber, admits gas, and governs proper temperature-pressure-humidity balance. At conclusion of selected exposure period, gas is exhausted, and vacuum is drawn to remove residual gas. Sterile air is then admitted through bacteria-retentive filter, and buzzer and light signal that machine is ready to unload. (Courtesy American Sterilizer Co., Erie, Pa.)

usage, they have come to mean different things. As previously discussed, a disinfectant is a potent chemical that is applied to inanimate objects, whereas an antiseptic refers to a chemical that is nontoxic when applied superficially to living tissue. To be meaningful, the terms must be defined in relation to the microorganisms against which a specific chemical substance is expected to be used.

## Disinfection process

Disinfection is brought about by one of a limited number of types of reactions or by combinations of these. These include denaturation of proteins in the cell, halogenation, poisoning of vital enzymes, hydrolysis, oxidation, and combination with proteins to form salts. The microbial destruction depends on the concentration of the chemical and the effects on the specific bacteria.

## Selection of disinfectant

Selection of a disinfectant depends on the nature and population of microorganisms to be killed. For disinfection purposes, microorganisms may be grouped into three classes: nonsporulating, vegetative bacteria, which possess the least resistance; tubercle bacilli, which have more resistance than the vegetative organisms; and spores, which are extremely resistant to any disinfectant.

Most disinfectants are capable of destroying vegetative bacteria and tubercle bacilli but not spores. The vegetative forms of molds and yeast, as well as animal parasites, are susceptible to disinfectants. Some fungi and antibiotic-resistant staphylococci have been shown to be as resistant as bacterial spores. Data indicate that viruses vary in their resistance to disinfectants.[20] At present there is no disinfectant that will destroy with certainty the hepatitis virus.

A strong concentration kills more rapidly than a weak one. According to Burrows,[7] a disinfectant is primarily bacteriostatic when the range of concentration over which inhibition of growth occurs is a relatively wide one and is primarily bactericidal when the range is narrow. When the microorganisms are killed within a short period of time, the antimicrobial activity is termed lethal. When the rate of microbial death is slow, some microorganisms survive for a considerable time without multiplication. For those surviving, the antimicrobial activity is termed growth-inhibiting or bacteriostatic.

A disinfectant should be used at the lowest effective bactericidal concentration. A rapidly lethal concentration for the microorganisms may cause corrosion and dullness of the blades of delicate instruments. On the other hand, in a weak concentration, its disinfecting power is ineffective.

The larger the number of microorganisms present, the longer the disinfection time required to kill the resistant cells present. According to genetic principles, when the population is large, the proportion of highly resistant bacteria is correspondingly greater than it is when the population is small. However, when the size of the population is *extremely* large, there may be fewer highly resistant cells.

## Temperature and surface tension of disinfectants

Increased temperature accelerates the rate of disinfection. The only practical value of this fact is in disinfection of inanimate objects. With some disinfectants, antimicrobial activity is increased when the chemical agent is added to warm or boiling water. The surface tension (wetness) of a disinfectant or antiseptic promotes contact between the agent and the microorganisms. A tension-reducing disinfectant, when combined with other chemicals, enhances the disinfecting power of that solution, thus decreasing time-exposure rate. Friction applied to the skin when an antiseptic is used enhances its effectiveness.

## Construction and condition of objects

An object must be thoroughly clean to provide for effective disinfection. Construction and composition of the object influence the disinfection time. A hard, flat, smooth-surfaced object requires less disinfection time than an uneven-surfaced object or material of porous composition. The disinfectant coagulates the proteins in blood and other organic debris present on the object. Thus organic material creates a barrier on the object against the disinfecting solution. At present there is no ideal all-purpose disinfectant.

## Bactericidal effectiveness of some disinfectants

The various disinfectants on the market may be divided into five major groups: halogens and halogen compounds, heavy metals, phenols and their derivatives, synthetic compounds, and alcohols.[11, 19]

### Halogens and halogen compounds

Of the halogen compounds, the hypochlorites and iodines are widely used in hospitals. The hypochlorites are available as powders containing calcium hypochlorite and sodium hypochlorite, in combination with hydrated trisodium phosphate, and as liquids containing sodium hypochlorite. Preparations containing calcium hypochlorite (chlorinated lime) have been replaced by other detergents for cleaning purposes because of the former's unstable characteristics.

*Chlorine* acts primarily by oxidation, and its odor may therefore be objectionable. The many organic chlorine compounds that liberate their chlorine more slowly (chloride of lime) are effective as mild disinfecting agents. Inorganic chlorine is valuable in the disinfection of water.

*Iodine* acts directly by iodination and oxidation reactions. It can change spontaneously into a vapor state without first passing through a liquid phase.[19] Iodine, the most active antimicrobial of the halogens, combines readily with organic material. Because of its insolubility in water, it is prepared in various ways; the tinctures (or alcoholic solutions) are the most common forms. The standard solution of 7% iodine and 83% alcohol has proved to be too caustic and coagulative. The modern iodine tincture (U.S.P. XVIII) contains 2% iodine, 2.4% sodium iodide, and 44% to 50% alcohol by volume. Price[18] recommends 1% to 2% iodine dissolved in 70% ethyl alcohol by weight as a skin antiseptic. Iodine is a good bactericide but stains fabric and tissue. In combination with alcohol, iodine is tuberculocidal and appears to increase the efficiency of the alcohol as a skin antiseptic.

Aqueous iodine solution (N.F. XIII) contains 2% iodine and 2.4% sodium iodide in water. This solution is preferred by many surgeons. Aqueous iodine spreads on the skin evenly, dries slowly, and evaporates without leaving a ring of concentrated iodine to irritate or burn the skin. Iodine, tincture or aqueous, may be irritating to some tissue; it may also be allergenic. It corrodes metals and stains skin and clothing.

Several syntheses of many organic iodine compounds in which iodine is held in dissociant complexes are available. The iodophors are iodine-detergent combinations capable of killing vegetative bacteria and tubercle bacilli if used in sufficient concentration (450 ppm of available iodine). Iodophors are not good sporicides. The iodophors do not stain clothing, are nonirritating, and are virtually odorless. The iodophor releases the iodine slowly and lowers the surface tension of the solution. Of the many commerical iodophors, Betadine as a skin antiseptic and Wescodyne as a disinfectant for floors and walls have gained popularity.[13]

### Heavy metals

All metallic ions inhibit microorganisms if applied in sufficiently high concentrations. Mercury, silver, and copper (to a lesser degree) have inhibiting power in low concentrations.

The ions of the heavy metals have such a strong affinity for proteins that the bacterial cells absorb them out of the solution. However, the property that makes these ions appear lethal limits their usefulness because their activity is reduced in the presence of organic matter. The ions are also irritating to tissues and poisonous.

Attempts have been made to decrease the toxic corrosive and irritating qualities of mercuric disinfectants by incorporating mercury in complex organic molecules in preparations known as Mercurochrome, Merthiolate, and Metaphen. Data indicate that aqueous solutions of both inorganic

and organic mercurials are ineffective in reducing cutaneous flora. Mercurials are poor disinfectants and have no place in modern surgical disinfection.

## Phenols and their derivatives

Phenol in pure state (carbolic acid) is not used as a disinfectant because there are many derivatives that are more effective. Like phenol, its derivatives act mainly by coagulation and partly by lytic and toxic effects that are not clearly understood. Since phenols appear to have a greater affinity for nonaqueous media than for aqueous media, it is believed that their action is dependent on their selective concentration at cell surfaces, resulting in the denaturation of proteins and an increase in permeability.

The aliphatic homologs of phenol have greater antimicrobial power than does phenol itself. Of this group, the methyl phenols—orthocresol, metacresol, and paracresol—and the halogenated phenols have phenol coefficients of three or more, but they are poorly soluble in water. The bisphenols have become the most useful of the phenolic antiseptics. The most important of these compounds are ortho-hydroxydiphenyl and chlorinated methylene and sulfur compounds. Of the chlorophenes, hexachlorophene is commonly used in soap. It is capable of retaining, to a large degree, its antibacterial activity when incorporated in soap. The bisphenols are relatively insoluble in water but are soluble in dilute alkali and in many organic solvents.

Hexachlorophene is popular as a skin antiseptic. It is virtually insoluble in water, but it is soluble in alkali, acid, and acetone and retains its antibacterial potency when kept in solution of soap. Hexachlorophene does not act as quickly as alcohol does.

If the skin surface is washed frequently each day with hexachlorophene, a relatively low flora population may gradually be achieved and maintained.[18] Studies indicate that the use of a mixture of hexa-

chlorophene and pHisoderm as a scrubbing solution for hands of the operator prevents rapid growth of remaining bacteria under rubber gloves. It is an effective preoperative skin agent when it is applied several times a day for 4 or 5 days prior to surgery. In preparation for operations on the face, feet, perineum, and other areas of the body that are difficult to disinfect, cleansing with hexachlorophene is effective if it is done as previously described.

## Synthetic detergent disinfectants

The quaternary ammonium compounds (often called *quats*) are among many surface-active detergents. These compounds are amines that contain pentavalent nitrogen and may be considered derivatives of ammonium chloride in which certain radicals are substituted for the hydrogen.[5] There are three types of quaternary ammonium compounds: those in which the organic radical is a cation, those in which the organic group is the anion, and those that do not ionize (nonionic).

These compounds possess bacteriostatic power in high dilutions and are not highly irritating or toxic. They are effective surface-tension reductants. Their antimicrobial activity is affected by the kind of water (acid, alkaline, hard, or soft) to be used and the material or substance involved. In the presence of hard, acid, or iron-rich waters the antimicrobial activity is lowered, especially for the cationic compounds.

Benzalkonium chloride (Zephiran), a cationic detergent, gained acceptance in 1948 as a skin antiseptic. It has marked incompatibility with anionic-type soaps and cationic-type detergents because in mixture the antibacterial activity disappears. The nonionic detergents do not react in this way. For example, quaternary ammonium compounds may be mixed with nonionic detergents that have good solubilizing activity to provide an effective cleansing detergent.

Benzalkonium chloride in a concentration of 1:1000 is nonirritating and possesses anti-

septic action. It is bacteriostatic to vegetative bacteria but has no effect on tubercle bacilli or spores. Much of the antibacterial action of the tincture of benzalkonium chloride is due to the solvent (alcohol or acetone).

### Alcohols

Ethyl (grain) alcohol and isopropyl (rubbing) alcohol are much more useful as antiseptics than as disinfectants. Alcohol is a rapid bactericide and a most active germicide against tubercle bacilli in concentrations of 70% to 90%, but it is not sporicidal.

Frequently, alcoholic solutions are prepared by volume instead of by weight. The latter is the more accurate method of preparation. Alcohol is lighter than water and expands in the presence of heat. Evaporation is by two fractions—the alcohol fraction (about 95%), which vaporizes fairly rapidly, and the water fraction, which evaporates more slowly. The effectiveness of isopropyl alcohol as a skin disinfectant increases when its concentration is increased, in contrast to ethyl alcohol, whose effectiveness is not influenced by an increase in strength.

Ethyl alcohol is nontoxic, colorless, tasteless, and nearly odorless and acts by denaturation of proteins. It may precipitate a protein covering around bacterial cells present in blood, pus, and mucus. Ethyl alcohol is less effective as a fat solvent than is isopropyl alcohol.

A 70% solution of ethyl alcohol by weight is a satisfactory disinfectant for ordinary vegetative bacteria. It spreads easily, dries slowly, is not too expensive, is readily available, and is easy to prepare and store. Because it is a poor fat solvent, adequate contact between it and the bacteria, sufficient time for antimicrobial activity, and friction with gauze should be provided to produce effective results.

### Formaldehyde

An aqueous solution known as *Formalin* is highly germicidal and sporicidal in a strong concentration. When a combination of 8% formaldehyde and 70% isopropyl alcohol is used, the action is even greater. Tubercle bacilli and viruses (except the hepatitis virus, whose destruction with certainty is not known) are promptly killed and sterility can be expected in 3 hours.

Irritating fumes limit formaldehyde's usefulness. It is also toxic to tissues; therefore materials treated with formaldehyde must be thoroughly rinsed before use.

*Glutaraldehyde* is a relative of formaldehyde but is more active. An aqueous solution of 2% is equivalent to an 8% solution of formaldehyde and alcohol. It is a high-level disinfectant, destroying tubercle bacilli in a few minutes and spores in 3 hours. It is useful in disinfecting lensed instruments.[20]

### REFERENCES

1. Adams, R.: Prevention of infections in hospitals, Am. J. Nurs. **58**:344, 1958.
2. Altemeier, W. A., and Culbertson, W. R. Applied surgical bacteriology. In Moyer, C A., Rhoads, J. E., Allen, J. G., and Harkins, H. N., editors: Surgery: principles and practice, ed. 3, Philadelphia, 1965, J. B Lippincott Co.
3. American Hospital Association: Control of infections, Chicago, 1962, The Association.
4. Aseptic Thermo-Indicator Company: Principles and practice of ethylene oxide sterilization, North Hollywood, Calif., 1971, The Company.
5. Becton, Dickinson, & Co. Lectures: Sterilization, 1957-1959.
6. Burnett, G. W., and Scherp, H.: Oral microbiology and infectious disease, Baltimore 1962, The Williams & Wilkins Co.
7. Burrows, W.: Textbook of microbiology, ed 18, Philadelphia, 1963, W. B. Saunders Co
8. Farringer, J. L.: Control of hospital infections, J. Tenn. Med. Assoc. **53**:507, Dec. 1960.
9. Ginsberg, H.: High-vacuum sterilizers help meet increased demands for efficiency, Mod Hosp. **102**:130, April, 1964.
10. Hare, R.: Bacteriology and immunity for nurses, London, 1961, Longmans, Green & Co., Ltd.
11. Kereluk, K., and Lloyd, R.: Ethylene oxide sterilization, a current review of principle and practices, J. Hosp. Res. **7**: Feb., 1969
12. La Salle, A. J.: Fundamental principles o

bacteriology, New York, 1961, McGraw-Hill Book Co.

3. Lawrence, C. A., Carpenter, C. M., and Naylor-Foote, A. W. C.: Iodophors as disinfectants, J. Am. Pharm. Assoc. Chemical Abstracts **46**:500-505, Aug., 1957.

4. Owen, T. B., Perkins, J. J., Irons, A. S., Reichert, A. W., and Mannarino, S. J.: Prevacuum high-temperature steam sterilization, Erie, Pa., 1963, American Sterilizer Co.

5. Perkins, J.: Principles and methods of sterilization, Springfield, Ill., 1956, Charles C Thomas, Publisher.

6. Perkins, J.: Sterilization by heat, 1957, Becton, Dickinson & Co. Lecture.

7. Phillips, C. R.: Gaseous sterilization, 1958, Becton, Dickinson, & Co. Lecture.

8. Price, P.: Surgical scrubs and skin disinfection, J. Hosp. Res. **5**: Dec., 1967.

19. Reddish, G. F., et al.: Antiseptics, disinfectants, fungicides, and chemical and physical sterilization, Philadelphia, 1957, Lea & Febiger.

20. Spaulding, E.: Chemical disinfection in the hospital, J. Hosp. Res. **3**: Jan., 1965.

21. Synder, C. C., Wardlaw, E., and Kelly, N.: Gas sterilization of cartilage and bone implants, Plast. Reconstr. Surg. **28**:568, Nov., 1961.

22. Watson, D. C., and Kabat, H. F.: Sterilizing techniques with ethylene oxide, Hospitals **37**: 81, Sept., 1963.

23. Williams, R. E., Blowers, R., Garrod, L. P., and Shooter, R. A.: Hospital infection—causes and prevention, Chicago, 1960, Year Book Medical Publishers, Inc.

# CHAPTER 4

# Skin cleansing and disinfection; gowning and gloving procedures

PEGGY E. LILES

To prevent bacteria on the skin surfaces from entering the surgical wound, it is necessary to cleanse and disinfect the skin area of and around the proposed incision, as well as the hands and forearms of the members of the operating team. Proper skin cleansing and disinfection depend on knowledge of the physiology and bacteriology of the skin and on knowledge of the action of soaps, detergents, and antiseptic agents.

## OBJECTIVES AND INFLUENCING FACTORS

Methods of skin preparation may vary; however, all are based on the same principles and share the same objectives— namely, to control the normal epidermal flora, to remove as many microorganisms as possible, and to recondition the skin.

The same general principles of skin cleansing apply, whether the situation is preparation of the patient's skin at the operative site or preparation of the hands and arms of the members of the operating team. In either case, factors to be considered in skin disinfection are (1) the condition of the involved area, (2) the number and kinds of contaminants, (3) the characteristics of the skin to be disinfected, and (4) the general physical condition of the individual.

## STRUCTURE AND PHYSIOLOGY OF THE SKIN

The skin consists of two distinct layers: (1) the epidermis, a stratified squamous epithelium, and (2) the true skin, or dermis. The outer layer, or epidermis, is the tissue to be treated by cleansing and disinfecting procedures (Fig. 4-1).

The *epidermis* constantly sheds the cells that form its horny outer layer, which are replaced by the multiplication and upward movement of cells from the lower levels. There are no blood vessels in the epidermis, although the hair shafts, the glandular ducts, and fine nerves reach through it. The *dermis* is a connective tissue containing blood and lymph vessels, sweat and sebaceous glands, nerves, and hair follicles.

Bacteria are found in all levels of the skin. Those that inhabit the deep structures of the dermis, the glands, and the hair follicles are considered the resident flora. They tend to move out and are shed with the old cells and skin secretions. The epidermal layers contain this debris from the dermis as well as soil and bacteria picked up by contact with various objects.

The resident flora of the skin are forced to the surface with perspiration and other secretions. This action is one way in which

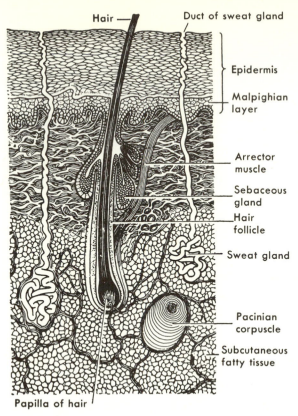

Fig. 4-1. Vertical section of skin (schematic). (After Cunningham; from Zoethout, W. D., and Tuttle, W. W.: Textbook of physiology, ed. 15, St. Louis, 1965, The C. V. Mosby Co.)

the skin disinfects and reconditions itself. The bacteria accompanying these secretions from the deep layers may, however, become a source of infection. The activity of sweat glands is increased by external heat, emotional stress, and certain diaphoretic drugs.

Generally, the acidity of perspiration acts as a protective barrier against the growth of certain organisms. But the perspiration in axillary and pubic regions has a higher pH and may permit more bacterial growth. Bacteria are also protected by the folds, ridges, and crevices of the skin whence detritus is not so readily shed as from smoother surfaces.

## AGENTS FOR SKIN CLEANSING AND DISINFECTION

There are many soaps and detergents available for skin cleansing. Although most of them produce similar results in the immediate removal of soil and microorganisms, certain factors need further consideration in selecting a product for surgical use.

### Action of soaps and detergents

Most soaps and detergents emulsify and peptize other waste products and oils that are absorbed in surface soil and permit the detritus to be rinsed off the skin with running water. The product selected should hydrolyze in the presence of water and yield a pH that corresponds to that of the average, normal skin. An odorless agent that produces a good lather for easy, comfortable use is usually preferred. It should not irritate the skin or in any way interfere with normal functioning. Careful rinsing and drying will help minimize skin irritation resulting from frequent scrubbing.

Hexachlorophene added to agents used for cleansing and lubricating the skin has been found to suppress bacterial growth on the skin. Hexachlorophene is a chlorinated phenol compound that is insoluble in water but soluble in alcohol. Hexachlorophene retains its antibacterial power in the presence of soap and is combined with it in liquid or solid form in products available for the surgical scrub.

Hexachlorophene forms a long-lasting, imperceptible bacteriostatic film on the skin and develops a cumulative suppressive action with routine use. For this reason, an agent with hexachlorophene added, and no other soap, should be used daily by persons who scrub for surgery in order to obtain the best effect and to reduce the bacterial population of the skin significantly.

In the preoperative preparation of a patient's skin, it is similarly useful to begin the regular use of a hexachlorophene compound for washing in the days immediately prior to surgery in order to take advantage of its suppressive bacteriostatic effects. This is usually possible in elective cases and is highly desirable in preparation for orthopedic surgery, since infections of the bones and joints may be particularly serious in terms of prolonged or permanent dysfunction.

It is impossible to sterilize the skin because chemicals that have the power to destroy bacteria are also injurious to the living tissues of the skin. Thus new bacterial populations are constantly being brought to the surface of normal skin.

### Antiseptic agents

Many antiseptic agents are useful, however, in reducing large numbers of pathogenic organisms on the skin surface or in inhibiting their reproduction. Among these are the quaternary ammonium germicides such as 1:750 solution of aqueous benzalkonium (Zephiran) chloride, alcohol, and iodine.

Benzalkonium is effective against staphylococci and streptococci, the common contaminants of normal skin, but in aqueous preparations it is ineffective against *Mycobacterium tuberculosis*. Some tinctures of these chemicals have been found to be effective against tubercle bacilli (Chapter 3).

Alcohol is a good antiseptic. Studies indicate that 50% to 95% solutions of isopropyl alcohol have more germicidal action, more fat solvent action, and lower surface tension and cost less than ethyl alcohol of the same concentrations. Since alcohol is a protein precipitant, it is not used in an open wound nor applied to mucous membrane (Chapter 3).

U.S.P. tincture of 1% or 2% iodine dissolved in 70% alcohol provides a "wetting" agent for the iodine, and the combination is an effective skin antiseptic. Iodine is highly irritating. The solution should be lightly applied and allowed to dry. The excess should be removed to leave a uniform stain on the skin. (See Chapter 3.)

Iodine and other halogens such as fluorine and bromine are combined with organic compounds or detergents for use as antiseptics. One of these new compounds is povidone-iodine, a complex of polyvinylpyrrolidone and iodine. Povidone-iodine is a topical antiseptic agent that possesses the potent germicidal effect of iodine without many of its irritating properties. The activity of this agent is prolonged because it is released from the binding polymer gradually as the brownish iodine color fades from the skin. It is effective in the presence of pus, whereas the activity of the iodine complex is of somewhat shorter duration in the presence of blood or serum. Wounds with necrotic tissue will usually require repeated applications. It is nonstaining and can be safely used on mucous membrane. It should not be allowed to pool on the skin or in the body cavities.

## PREOPERATIVE SKIN PREPARATION
### Nursing considerations

The preoperative skin preparation is a treatment ordered by the physician, and

it requires consideration in the preparation of each patient.

If the preoperative skin preparation is done when the patient is awake, the nurse has the opportunity to explain to him the purpose and method of the procedure. Every effort should be made to allay any fears he may express and to answer his questions in a reassuring manner. During the procedure, the nurse observes the patient's general condition, particularly the condition of the skin under treatment. If there is any contraindication to the procedure because of an abnormal skin condition, lesion, allergy, irritation, or adverse reaction by, or injury to, the patient, the nurse should report to the physician for further directions.

In carrying out the procedure the nurse provides for the comfort, safety, and privacy of the patient. She also maintains the body in good alignment and uses special supports for positioning, as indicated.

Since the procedure may be alarming, embarrassing, or uncomfortable for the patient, every effort should be made to minimize these features by proceeding in a considerate, methodical, and professional manner.

## Initial preparation of the operative area

In the immediate preoperative period, the skin of the involved part of the body is prepared by special cleansing. This preparation consists of careful washing and shaving of the proposed site of incision and the surrounding area. Shaving is not necessary for all operative sites, such as the abdomen of small children, but it is necessary where coarse long hairs are present. The removal of hair ensures cleanliness and prevents bits of hair from being carried into the wound as foreign bodies or carriers of bacteria. When shaving the site, great care should be taken to avoid scratching, nicking, or cutting the skin because cutaneous bacteria will proliferate in these areas and increase the chances of infection.

The skin preparation may be carried out in the operating room or in the patient's unit. The decision of where, when, and by whom the procedure is performed depends on the time it is to be done, the facilities and personnel available, the patient's reactions, and the philosophy and policies that have been determined and established by the surgical committee.

There are advantages and disadvantages of preparing the skin for surgical procedures in the operating room suite. Theoretically, it is advantageous to do the shave as close to the scheduled time of surgery as possible to minimize the regrowth of hair and bacteria. Also, special equipment needed for positioning the patient, as well as better lighting facilities, is available and should be an aid in minimizing abrasions of the skin. Nicks and cuts made at this time can be regarded as clean wounds. (Decontamination concepts are described in Chapters 1 and 5.)

Patients with traumatic injuries that may be excessively painful, such as fractures, burns, and soft tissue lacerations, may require anesthesia for skin preparation. If possible, the preparation should be done in an anesthetizing area or preparation room rather than the operating room per se.

Skin preparation in the operating room has the disadvantages that the patient's anesthesia time is prolonged, optimum use of the operating room is infringed on, loose hair remaining on the surrounding linen may get into the wound, and water used to wash the skin can result in sterile drapes becoming wet. Hence many hospitals arrange to do the initial skin preparation for elective surgery in the patient's unit on the day before surgery.

### Procedure for preoperative shave

Individual sanitary supplies are used for each patient. Commercially prepared kits that contain the basic essentials for shaving the site of incision are available. The use of disposable sets and razors can help ensure a safe, personal technique. The use of rubber or plastic disposable gloves is

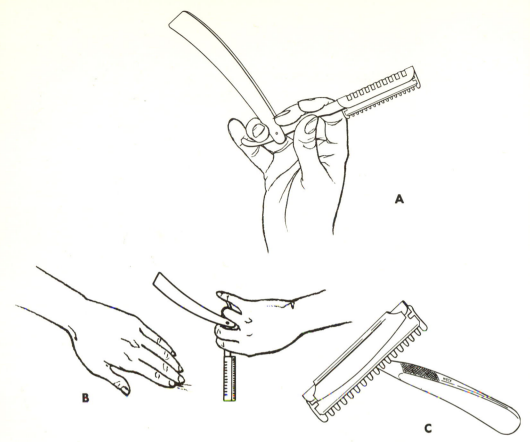

Fig. 4-2. Skin-cleansing equipment. With traction on skin and proper type of razor in correct position, hair will be shaved clean, and skin will not be injured. **A,** Straightedge for barber-style razor with replaceable blade is preferred to remove horny layer of skin and long hair. **B** illustrates correct finger hold for straight razor. Razor with short blade and tooth guard is preferred for general use in difficult areas around eyes and perineum. **C,** Safety or hoe-type razor is used to remove hair on smooth surfaces. (From Pate, M. O.: The preparation manual, Long Island City, N. Y., 1963, Edward Weck & Co., Inc.)

an additional safeguard for the patient and for the worker and is often esthetically desirable.

SETUP. In the nursing unit or decontamination area, blankets and supports for the patient's position, as well as the necessary lighting and handwashing facilities, are provided.

**Basic equipment**

Gloves
Basins with water and soap
Razor, as selected (straightedge, safety, or disposable) (Figs. 4-2 and 4-3)
Sponges for washing
Draping, as needed (towels and waterproof pads)

**Accessory equipment**

Brushes
Files or orangewood sticks for cleaning nails
Scissors and clippers for trimming long hair and nails
Applicators
Solvents for removal of adhesives and nail polish

*Note:* The use of volatile liquids such as alcohol, ether, benzine, and acetone should be strictly regulated in anesthetizing areas or where cautery or other electrosurgical equipment is in use because of the danger of fire, burns, and explosions.

METHOD. Apply soap or detergent to

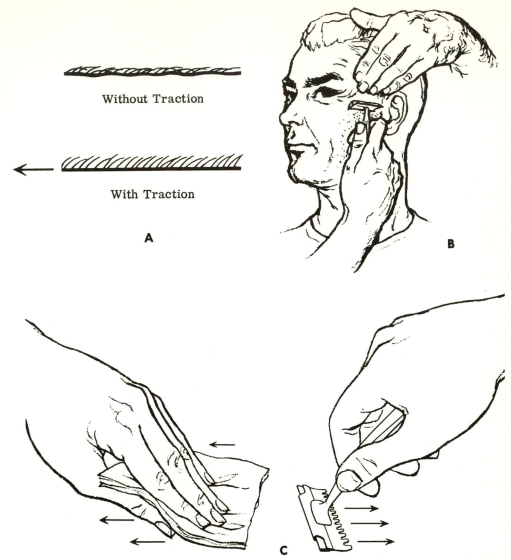

Without Traction

With Traction

**A**

**B**

**C**

Fig. 4-3. Skin cleansing. To shave skin area, worker must do the following. **A,** Provide skin traction with free hand in direction opposite to slant of hairs in order to tighten and smooth skin and raise hairs in more upright position. **B,** Shave off hair and horny layer of skin. **C,** Apply traction with sponge and hold hoe-type razor head against skin, as shown in **A.** (From Pate, M. O.: The preparation manual, Long Island City, N. Y., 1963, Edward Weck & Co., Inc.)

the skin area using sponges moistened with water. Using a circular motion and light friction, work up a lather. Begin with the proposed site of incision and work toward the periphery of the area. The principle is to avoid contaminating cleansed areas with uncleansed areas. As sponges become soiled, discard them and continue with fresh sponges.

Difficult areas in folds of skin, the umbilicus, and axillary and pubic hair may benefit from longer soaking as well as being held taut while washing. Cotton-tipped applicators are needed to clean the umbilicus thoroughly, and a brush may be required for nails and calloused skin of the hands and feet.

Sensitive or denuded areas should be

gently soaked with detergent and then rinsed or irrigated with sterile water.

A new or sterilized razor with a sharp new blade is used to shave off the lathered hair. Holding soft areas and loose skin taut with the free hand will raise the hair and permit easier accessibility to the area. A clean shave can be obtained without injury to the skin by gently stroking in the direction of the hair growth (Figs. 4-2 and 4-3). Nicks or cuts resulting from the shave should be reported as incidents and the surgeon notified.

After the shave, scrub the prepared area a second time for a full 3 or 4 minutes. Rinse carefully and blot the skin dry to prevent chapping and irritation.

At the conclusion of the preparation, the patient is made comfortable, the unit is left in order, and the equipment is cared for and cleaned.

Reusable items are washed and sterilized. Expendable materials are disposed of according to the prevailing regulations. The worker follows the principles of good aseptic technique for the removal of gloves and for terminal handwashing before proceeding to the care of other patients.

## Final skin disinfection of the operative area

### Considerations

After the patient has been positioned on the operating table, final skin cleansing and disinfection are performed. This procedure is essentially the same as the initial cleansing. A wash with a cleansing agent containing an antibacterial such as hexachlorophene is the preliminary step. While this is being carried out, the shave can be inspected and touched up or extended as needed. Skin cleansing is followed by disinfection with the selected germicide.

When there is a preparation area adjacent to the operating room, the preliminary skin wash can be done there, using the basic equipment already described. It may be necessary, or even preferable, as in the preparation of traumatic wounds or for head, eye, or ear surgery, to perform the wash in the operating room itself. The operator who is to carry out the procedure scrubs and dons sterile gloves.

### Method

The supplies required for the final skin preparation may be arranged on a separate sterile preparation table. The items include stainless metal cups for water or saline solution, the cleansing agents, the selected germicide, gauze sponges, and sponge-holding forceps if desired.

The wash begins at the line of the proposed incision and proceeds to the periphery of the area. The sponges used in washing are discarded as they become soiled, and fresh ones are taken. Thus a soiled sponge is never brought back over a washed surface. The lather is wiped off, using dry sterile sponges. The area is rinsed, using sponges saturated with sterile water or normal saline solution, and the area is blotted dry.

The germicide is applied, using sponges held in sponge forceps or in the gloved hand. The operator who has prepared the skin then removes the gloves he wore during preparation and dons sterile gown and gloves to join the surgical team.

### Extent of skin preparation for various procedures

Although specific orders for the skin preparation are written by the surgeon on the chart of the individual coming for an operation, a manual with diagrams and instructions concerning the preoperative skin shave is useful for the guidance and information of the personnel to whom the task is delegated (Figs. 4-4 to 4-13).

### Influencing factors

The extent of the area to be shaved is determined by the site of incision and the nature of the operation. A generous area surrounding the area of incision is prepared. This provides a wide margin of safety and ensures that the skin adjacent

*Text continued on p. 74.*

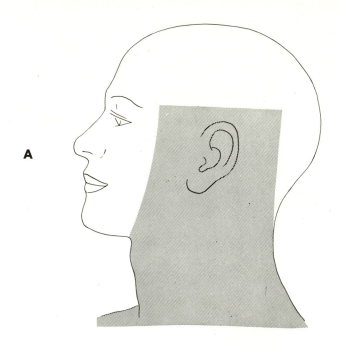

A

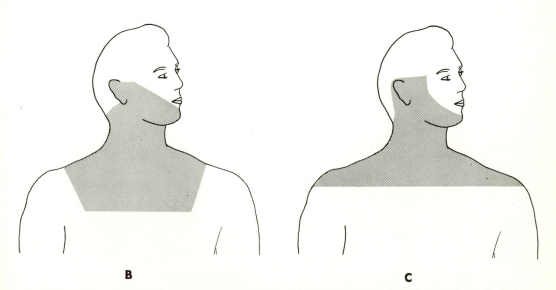

B                                                                    C

**Fig. 4-4.** Preparation for neck and ear surgery. **A,** For major otological operations. **B,** For submaxillary operations. **C,** For removal of lesions of neck and glands. (From Pate, M. O.: The preparation manual, Long Island City, N. Y., 1963, Edward Weck & Co., Inc.)

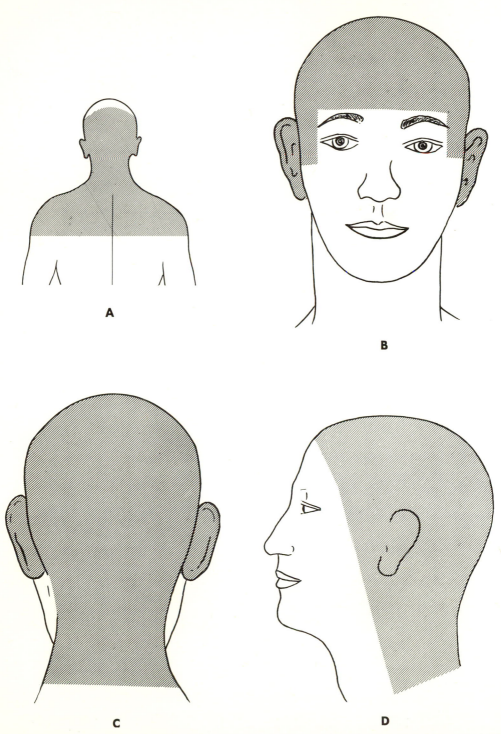

**Fig. 4-5.** Preparation for head and major neck surgery. **A,** For posterior craniotomy. **B** and **C,** For craniotomy, frontal tumor excision. **D,** For major scalp surgery. (From Pate, M. O.: The preparation manual, Long Island City, N. Y., 1963, Edward Weck & Co., Inc.)

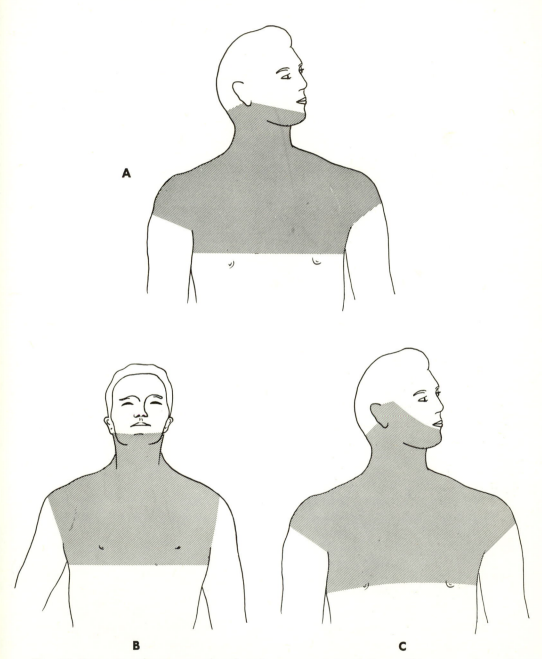

**Fig. 4-6.** Preparation for surgery of neck and uppermost part of thorax. Skin area is cleansed and disinfected from earline to nipple line anteriorly and midline posteriorly. **A,** For esophageal diverticulectomy, esophagotomy, scalenectomy, cervicothoracic anterior approach, and thyroidectomy. **B,** For laryngectomy. **C,** For radical neck dissection. (From Pate, M. O.: The preparation manual, Long Island City, N. Y., 1963, Edward Weck & Co., Inc.)

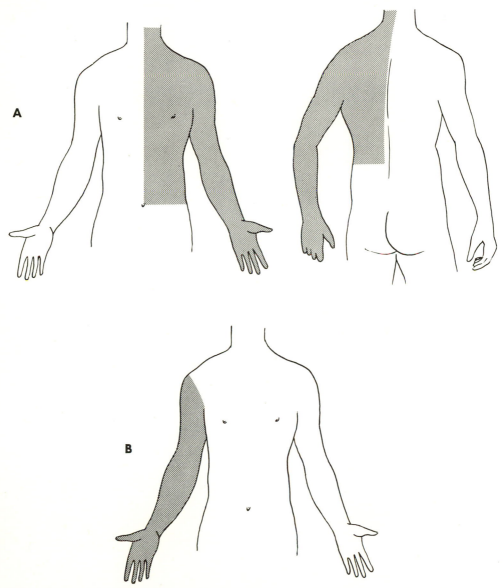

**Fig. 4-7.** Preparation for major surgery on shoulder, arm, or hand. **A,** For unilateral shoulder operations, skin area is prepared from affected neckline to umbilicus, as well as axilla, arm, and hand, front and back 3 inches beyond midline. **B,** For operations on elbow, preparation is done anteriorly and posteriorly. **C,** For chest and unilateral operations, for radical mastectomy, affected chest, shoulder, and forearm are prepared. **D,** For combined thoracoabdominal operations, for cardiac surgery, chest and shoulder are prepared bilaterally and both anteriorly and posteriorly. (From Pate, M. O.: The preparation manual, Long Island City, N. Y., 1963, Edward Weck & Co., Inc.)

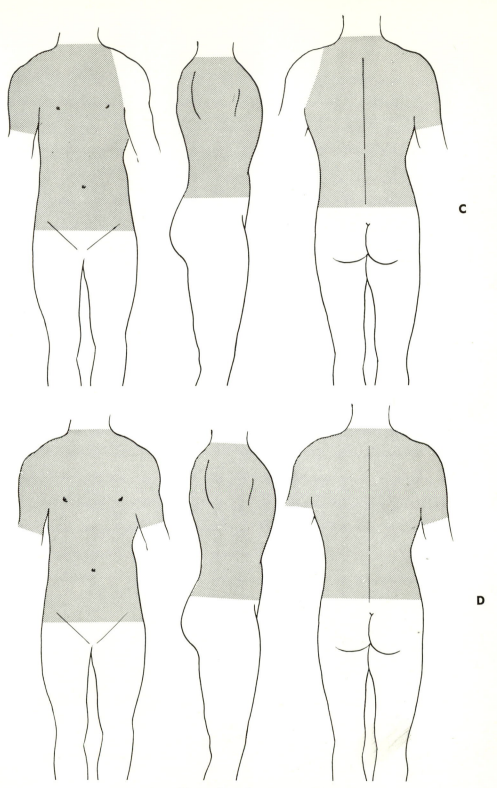

Fig. 4-7, cont'd. For legend see opposite page.

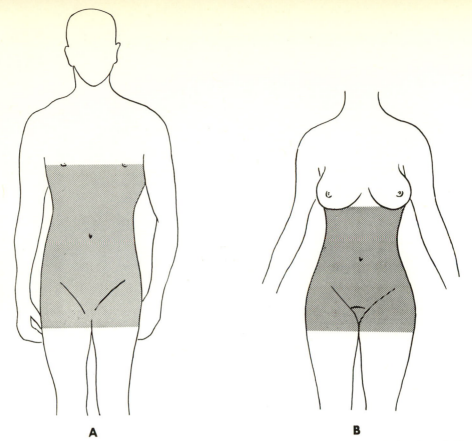

**A**                                    **B**

Fig. 4-8. **A,** Preparation for abdominal surgery. Skin area is cleansed and disinfected from nipple line to 3 inches below pubes, including external genitals to bedline. This preparation is done for operations such as gastrointestinal, biliary, liver, splenectomy, and to reach great vessels of trunk. **B,** Preparation for appendectomy, hernia, and some pelvic surgery. (From Pate, M. O.: The preparation manual, Long Island City, N. Y., 1963, Edward Weck & Co., Inc.)

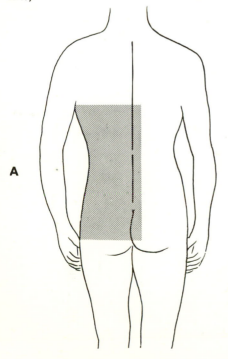

**A**

Fig. 4-9. Lateral preparation. **A,** Unilateral operations for posterior lumbar region. **B,** For lumbar sympathectomy. **C,** For operation on kidney and upper ureter. (From Pate, M. O.: The preparation manual, Long Island City, N. Y., 1963, Edward Weck & Co., Inc.)

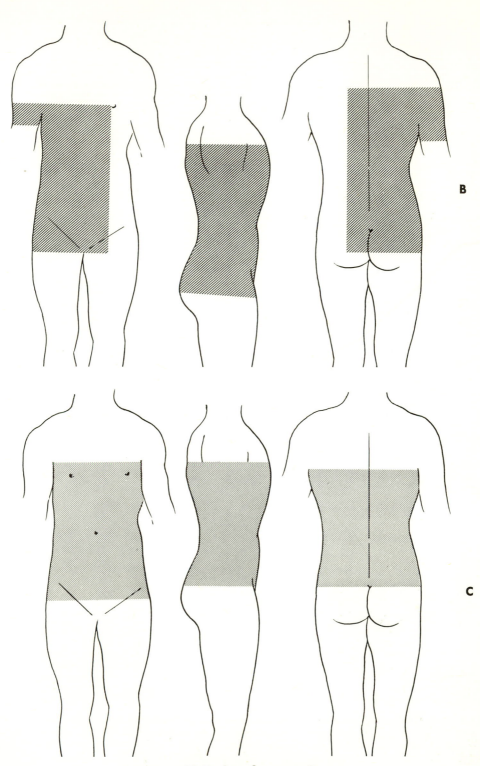

**Fig. 4-9, cont'd.** For legend see opposite page.

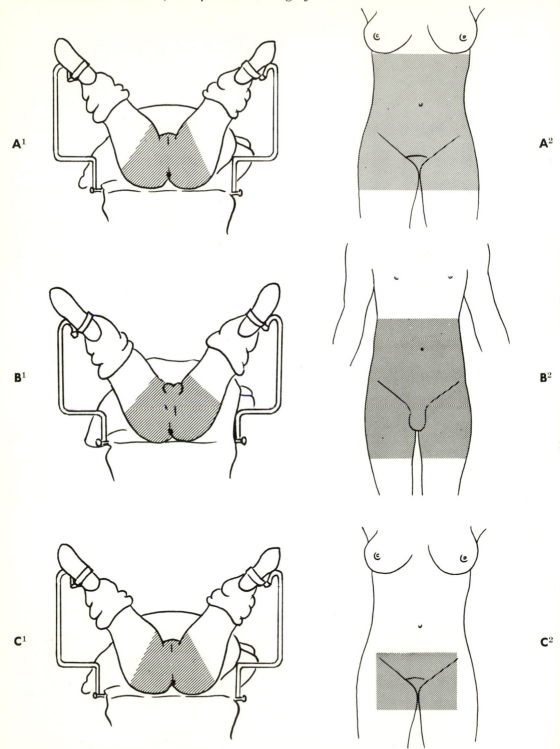

**Fig. 4-10.** Pelvic and perineal preparation for gynecological and genitourinary operations. **A**[1] and **A**[2], Preparation for combined vaginal and abdominal operations. **B**[1] and **B**[2], Preparation for suprapubic prostatectomy and bladder operations. **C**[1] and **C**[2], Preparation for minor vaginal and rectal operations. (From Pate, M. O.: The preparation manual, Long Island City, N. Y., 1963, Edward Weck & Co., Inc.)

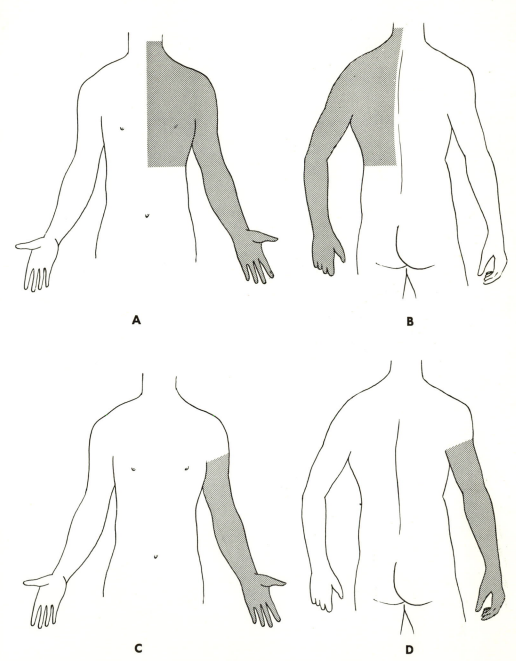

**Fig. 4-11.** Preparation for surgery of upper extremity. **A** and **B,** For major operations on shoulder and uppermost part of extremity, skin area is prepared from neckline to elbow line and axilla to midline anteriorly and posteriorly. **C** and **D,** For operations on forearm, preparation includes fingertips and axilla. (From Pate, M. O.: The preparation manual, Long Island City, N. Y., 1963, Edward Weck & Co., Inc.)

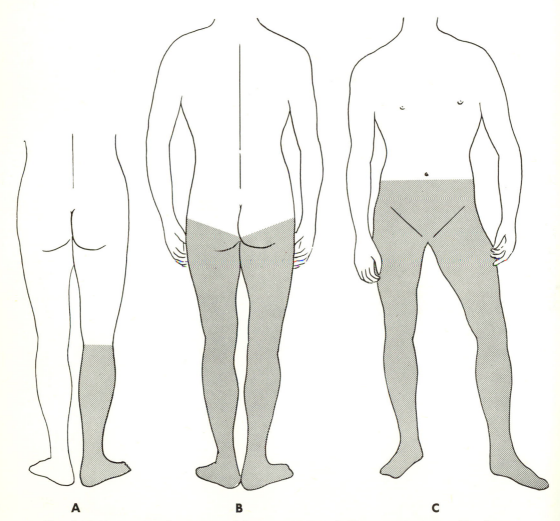

**A**                    **B**                    **C**

**Fig. 4-12.** Preparation for surgery of lower extremity. **A,** For operations on ankle, foot, or toes, area is prepared anteriorly and posteriorly. **B** and **C,** For bilateral leg operations, that is, varicose vein ligation and skin and bone grafts. **D,** Operations on foot and lower leg. **E,** Unilateral hip operations. **F,** Unilateral leg operations, anteriorly and posteriorly. **G,** Unilateral operations involving hip and thigh. (From Pate, M. O.: The preparation manual, Long Island City, N. Y., 1963, Edward Weck & Co., Inc.)

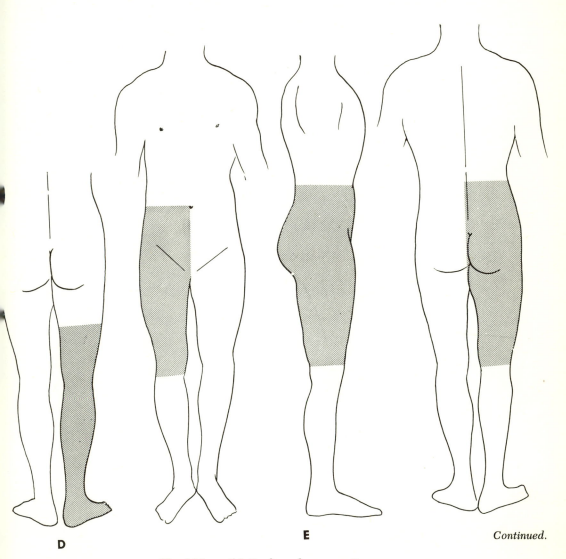

**D**

**E**

*Continued.*

**Fig. 4-12, cont'd.** For legend see opposite page.

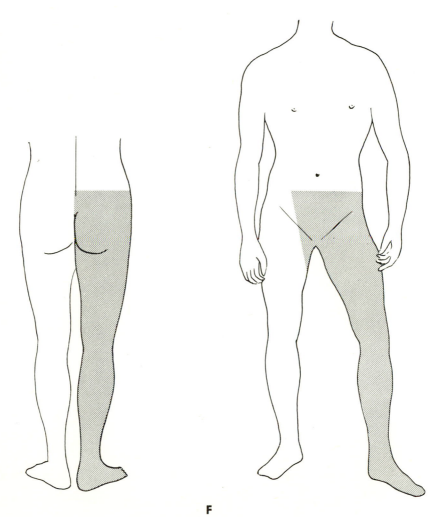

**F**

Fig. 4-12, cont'd. For legend see p. 70.

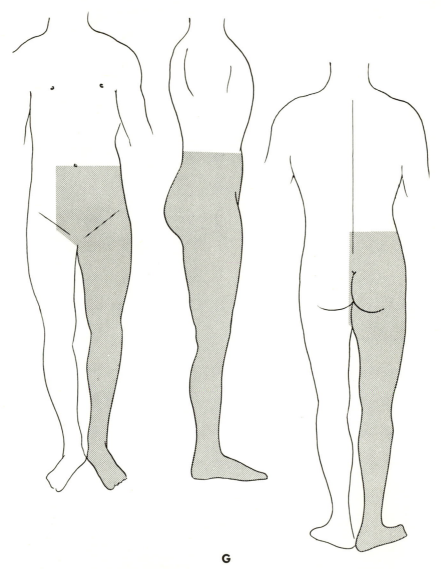

**G**

**Fig. 4-12, cont'd.** For legend see p. 70.

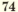

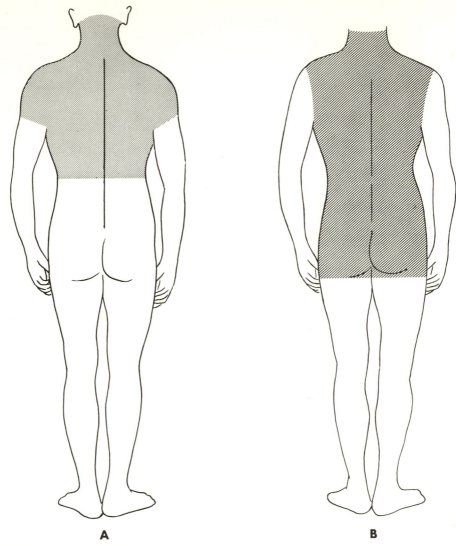

**A**                                                                 **B**

Fig. 4-13. **A,** Preparation for cervical laminectomy. **B,** For lumbar laminectomy. **C,** For sympathectomy—cervicothoracic, posterior approach. Preparation may include from hairline to fold of buttocks and to bedline laterally. (From Pate, M. O.: The preparation manual, Long Island City, N. Y., 1963, Edward Weck & Co., Inc.)

to the wound will not be a source of gross contamination during manipulation or draping. It also permits the incision to be safely extended if this becomes necessary. Adhesive dressings can readily be applied to the shaved area without the prospect of discomfort for the patient from pulled hair.

In head and neck surgery, for cosmetic and psychological reasons, preparation may be done in the operating room after the induction of anesthesia under the direction of the surgeon. It is rarely necessary to shave the face and neck of children or female patients or for most eye surgery. The eyebrows are never shaved. In nasal surgery the nares are swabbed out with a germicide prior to the application of a topical anesthetic. (See Chapters 8 and 9.) The head and neck are not generally prone

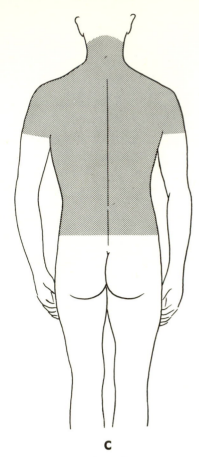

**c**

**Fig. 4-13, cont'd.** For legend see opposite page.

to wound infection in spite of the openings of the eyes, ears, nose, and mouth because of the generous blood supply to this area. Ordinary cleanliness usually provides a safe surgical field.

In *gynecology*, following the perineal wash and shave, the vagina is prepared by washing with a detergent and water and applying an antiseptic such as povidone-iodine with sponge forceps. A vaginal speculum may be used. The bladder is emptied by urethral catheterization. The surgeon may specify that the open urethral catheter be left in place during abdominal surgery. The surgeon may examine the vagina and insert packing. (See Chapter 18.)

In *orthopedic surgery* on the limbs the

entire extremity on the affected side may be prepared to facilitate manipulation and draping (Figs. 4-11 and 4-12). Generally, preparation includes one joint above and one joint below the involved area. Great care is exercised in the preparation for surgery on the bone, since wound infection resulting from improper cleansing may cause a stubborn condition leading to crippling, disfigurement, and permanent dysfunction. The skin may be difficult to clean if it has been affected by the application of casts, splints, or braces that interfere with normal skin care or cause skin damage. Daily soaking may help clean up badly soiled feet in preparation for surgery, just as daily washing is advisable in general elective surgery preparation.

Traumatic orthopedic wounds require special treatment with copious irrigation to flush out foreign matter. In first-aid treatment, the wound is covered with sterile dressings and immobilized. Preoperative cleansing and disinfecting is carried out with the patient under anesthesia. In cleansing the injured area the surrounding skin is first carefully washed with a detergent. The open wound is irrigated with an isotonic solution, and the area is treated with a disinfectant.

*Open wounds and body orifices* are potentially contaminated areas and as such are prepared after the surrounding unbroken skin is cleansed. This is in contrast to the principle of working from the line of the proposed incision into intact tissue to the periphery of the surgical field.

Sponges used to cleanse or disinfect a wound, sinus, ulcer, intestinal stoma, the anus, or the vagina are applied *once* to that area and are immediately discarded. Intestinal fistulas may be walled off after preparation of the area, using one of the plastic adhesive drapes.

## SURGICAL SCRUB
### General considerations

Hospital regulations will govern the proper attire, the selection of materials, and the methods used for the surgical

scrub. No person should scrub unless he feels well and is free of upper respiratory infection and skin lesions. Cuts, abrasion, pimples, or hangnails tend to ooze serum, which is a medium for prolific bacterial growth and can endanger the patient by increasing the hazards of infection.

Members of the operating team should be properly attired before beginning to scrub. A clean scrub suit or scrub dress, with sleeves ending well above the elbows, should be worn each day. The shirt should be tucked into the trousers, and the scrub dress should be formfitting or fastened to prevent brushing against sterile surfaces. Headgear should be adjusted to cover all hair, and a fresh mask should be carefully fitted at all edges to cover the nose and mouth completely. Conductive shoe coverings should be worn by those who do not have conductive shoes. (See Chapter 5.)

The selection of a brush and suitable dispenser for handscrubbing should be based on realistic considerations of long-range effectiveness and economy. A good surgical hand brush with nylon bristles should be easy to clean and maintain and durable enough to withstand repeated heat sterilization without bristles becoming soft or brittle. Bristles should be rounded and firm, yet resilient, for effective friction without harshness.

The backs of brushes, available in plastic and wood, should be of convenient size to fit the hand easily. Plastic backs may be grooved to permit nesting in containers or channeled to hold a clip-on nail cleaner. Channel-backed brushes have the disadvantage that they are difficult to clean, since soap scum has a tendency to accumulate on the inside. Wooden-backed brushes also have disadvantages, since wood is porous and absorbs foreign matter. The wood also softens from repeated exposure to steam, bristles loosen and fall out, and problems of litter and clogged drains are created. Brushes that have deteriorated should be discarded.

Brushes may be sterilized in metal dispensers that fit wall brackets or covered metal boxes that will fit on a shelf above the scrub sinks. The dispenser or metal box will permit the extraction of single brushes without contaminating the others. They may be assembled without nail cleaners or with nail cleaners in units and sterilized in covered Monel Metal cans. They are arranged to permit removal of one unit or brush without touching others in the container. Brushes may also be packaged in individual wrappers, but this is a relatively expensive and time-consuming method. All containers and packages have to be opened aseptically before the scrub is started.

The use of gauze or synthetic sponges in place of brushes has gained some acceptance where long and repeated scrubbing may be traumatic to the skin. The need for brushes in removing bacteria from the nails and other heavy soil on the hands continues.

A number of nail cleaners, metal files, or orangewood sticks may be sterilized in a separate container.

Soaps and detergents containing hexachlorophene and iodine-based antiseptics have gained acceptance as agents for the preparation of the skin. Many authors advocate a germicidal wash or rinse as the final step in skin preparation.

*The skin can never be rendered sterile*, but it can be made "surgically clean" by reducing the number of microorganisms present. A lengthy mechanical scrub, even with strong antiseptics, will fail to remove all microorganisms. Friction and rinsing will significantly decrease the number of bacteria on the epidermis, but their numbers are constantly replenished by the continuous secretory activity of the skin glands.

The scrub procedure carried out by the members of the operating team is done to remove as many bacteria as possible and the detritus of the normal epidermis before taking part in surgical procedures. This is accomplished by softening the detritus with soap and water and by removing it by friction and running water (Fig. 4-14).

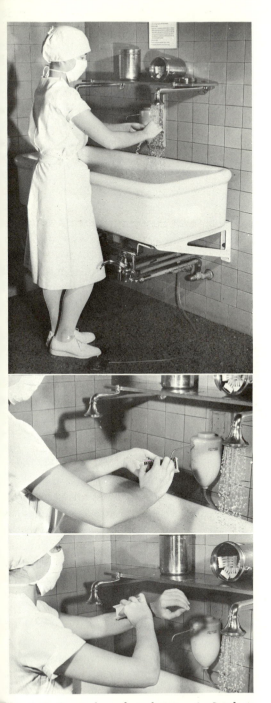

In washing, light friction is effective in removing the detritus of the epithelium. The friction will produce heat, dilatation of the blood vessels, and better circulation, which helps recondition the skin (Fig. 4-1).

Hard rubbing and harsh bristles tend to scrape away all the desquamatory epithelium, leaving a bleeding or weeping dermis. This is painful and predisposes to infection. It also may massage bacteria back into the deeper dermal layers.

An anatomical scrub using a prescribed amount of time or number of strokes plus friction is used to accomplish an effective cleansing of the skin. All surfaces of the hands and forearms must be treated, and, since the subungual spaces are the most difficult to clean, the nails should be short and neatly trimmed.

The prescribed amount of time for scrubbing with brushes is usually 7 to 10 minutes. Special attention should be placed on scrubbing the nails and hands, but all areas should receive a share of the time.

The prescribed number of strokes with a brush is usually thirty strokes to the nails and twenty strokes to each area of the skin.

The number of resident and deep flora is reduced by frequent scrubbing, but the number is increased when the surgical scrub is done only occasionally. A fully timed or stroke-counted scrub is recommended for persons scrubbing infrequently.

Shorter scrubs are occasionally permitted after the initial scrub of the day and between cases. Careful consideration should be given before proceeding with the shorter method, since inadvertent contamination of the gloved hand is always a danger and microorganisms proliferate rapidly under sterile gloves. Cultures taken from the cleansed skin on removal of sterile gloves show growth of microorganisms that populate the deep skin layers.

**Procedure**

Surgical scrub techniques that the staff must observe should be defined in writing. The major steps follow.

Fig. 4-14. Surgical scrub technique. **A,** Scrub-up facilities—splashproof sink, knee control for faucet, footpedal soap dispenser, and covered containers for brushes. **B,** Scrubbing nails. Hands held up and away from body and dress. **C,** Anatomical scrub. Brush held lengthwise along arm covers maximum area with each stroke.

1. Turn on the faucet and bring the water to a comfortable temperature. Most scrub sinks have knee controls for the faucets.

2. Wet the hands and forearms.

3. Using foot control, dispense a few drops of the cleansing agent into the palms.

4. Add small amounts of water and make a lather.

5. Wash the hands and forearms to a level well above the elbows. The amount of time needed will vary with the amount of soil and the effectiveness of the cleansing agent.

6. Clean the subungual spaces with a nail cleaner, metal file, or orangewood stick. Work the lather under the nail rims and rinse under running water.

7. Rinse hands and arms thoroughly, being careful to hold the hands higher than the elbows. Avoid splashing water onto the scrub suit or dress because this moisture will cause contamination to the sterile gown.

8. Apply a few drops of the cleansing agent to a moistened brush. Starting at the fingertips, vigorously scrub the nails while holding the brush perpendicular to them (Fig. 4-14). Scrub all sides of each digit, including the web spaces between them. Proceed to scrub the palm and back of the hand.

9. Repeat step 8 for the second hand.

10. Scrub each arm on all sides up to and including the elbows and antecubital spaces to a level well above the joint. The hands are held above the level of the elbows while scrubbing to allow the water and detritus to flow away from the first-scrubbed and cleanest areas. The hands and arms are also held away from the body. Add small amounts of water during the scrub to develop suds and remove detritus. Discard the brush into the proper receptacle.

11. Repeat step 7.

12. With a new brush, repeat steps 8, 9, and 10.

13. Again rinse hands and arms thoroughly.

14. Turn off the faucet using the knee control.

15. Rinse with germicidal solution if it is a hospital policy.

16. Keep hands up and in front of the body with elbows slightly flexed.

### Drying the cleansed skin areas

Moisture remaining on the cleansed skin after the scrub procedure must be dried with a sterile towel before a sterile gown and gloves are put on.

The towel must be used with care to avoid contamination to the cleansed skin. It should not be wadded or have a loose end that can become inadvertently contaminated against the unsterile attire or other objects.

The procedure for opening the sterile towel to dry the hands and forearms will vary, depending on the method used in folding the towel before sterilization. One method frequently used is to fold the towel to half its width and then to half its length. The two ends are then folded equally to the center, and the towel is again folded in half in the same direction.

Lift the towel straight up and away from its sterile field without dripping contaminated water or germicide from the skin onto the sterile area. Open the towel to half its length and width; then fold the two ends together. Lean forward slightly, with the hands and elbows above the waist and away from the body. Hold the towel securely in one hand and blot dry the opposite fingers and hand, making sure they are thoroughly dry before moving to the forearm (Fig. 4-15, *A*). To avoid contamination, use a rotating motion while moving up the arm to the elbow, and do *not* retrace an area (Fig. 4-15, *B*).

The second hand and arm are dried with the unused portion of the towel. To accomplish this, the used and unused parts of the towel must be reversed. Without touching the used part, tightly grasp the towel inside the last fold with the fingers and thumb of the dried hand. Move the moist hand away (Fig. 4-15, *C*). Carefully

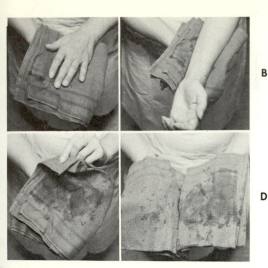

Fig. 4-15. Drying hands and forearms. **A,** Hold towel securely in one hand and blot dry the opposite fingers and hand. **B,** Use a rotating motion while moving up the arm to the elbow. Do not retrace. **C,** To turn the towel, grasp inside last fold with fingers and thumb of the dried hand. Move the moist hand away. **D,** Place moist hand under unused side of towel. Fold wet portion to the inside.

slide the moist hand under the unused side of the towel, folding the wet used part to the inside (Fig. 4-15, *D*). Proceed in the manner described while drying the second hand and forearm.

## GOWNING AND GLOVING PROCEDURES

Before the scrubbed personnel can touch sterile equipment or the sterile field, they must put on sterile gowns and sterile rubber gloves to prevent bacteria on their hands and clothing from being transferred to the patient's wound during surgery. The sterile gowns and gloves also protect the personnel's hands and clothing from bacteria present in the patient or in the atmosphere.

### Design and packaging of gown

The gown should be made of a good quality of cotton that provides for complete penetration of steam during the sterilization process. Sterile disposable paper gowns are now available. The shape and size of the gown, regardless of the material, should fit the wearer but not hamper him. To provide for extra protection, the gown's front (from the waist upward) may be made of two thicknesses of material. Each sleeve should be finished with a tight-fitting wristlet, which prevents the inner side of the sleeve from slipping down onto the outer side of the sterile glove. Cotton tapes or grip fasteners are attached to the back of the gown to hold it closed (Fig. 4-16).

A gown with a swing back or flap may be used to achieve better coverage of the back. The flap is triangular in shape, and the long side is sewn to the right side of the back from the neckline to the bottom of the gown. Tapes are sewn to the point of the triangle and right side of the gown, or grip fasteners are attached to the point and at various positions across the front of the gown at the level of the waist. The tapes or fasteners will allow for a comfortable fit and closure of the flap by the scrubbed person after gloving (Fig. 4-17).

Because the outer side of the front and sleeves of the gown will come within the sterile field during surgery, the gown must be folded so that the scrubbed person can put it on without touching the outer side with his bare hands. The gown is folded with the sleeves inside and the back edges together. It is then folded in half along the length of the gown with the center fold and back edges meeting and folded in half again in the same manner. The neckline and bottom are folded equally toward center, and the gown is again folded in half. Gowns with flaps are prepared in the same manner, with care taken to securely fasten the flap in place before folding. Place a folded towel on top of the gown. One or more gowns, each with a towel, are packaged in a double-thickness muslin wrapper and sterilized for 30 minutes in saturated steam at 250° F. (Chapter 3).

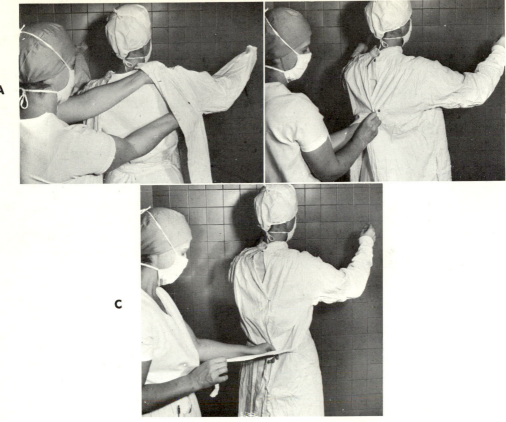

**Fig. 4-16.** Gowning procedure. **A,** Circulating person reaches under back flaps of gown to pull sleeves on scrubbed person. **B,** Circulating person fastens grippers at back of gown, always maintaining wide margin of safety, by touching only center back of gown. **C,** Circulating person grasps ends of tapes and ties them, restricting touch to center back.

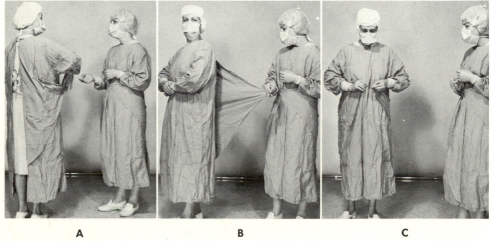

**Fig. 4-17.** Gowning procedure with extra flap back. **A,** Back of gown closed in conventional manner by circulating nurse. Extra flap released from the gripper or ties on the right side of the gown. **B,** While the wearer turns toward his left, the flap is held securely and brought across the back of the gown to cover the previously tied unsterile tapes. **C,** The wearer adjusts the fit and comfort by fastening the flap in front of him.

## Putting on the sterile gown

The outer side of the sterile gown must not touch any unsterile object. Before sterilization, the gown was prepared with the outer surface turned to the inside, and it may now be removed from the gowning table with scrubbed bare hands.

### Procedure

1. Pick up the sterile gown and step into an open area where the gown may be opened without contaminating it.
2. Open the first fold of the gown and grasp the neckband.
3. Hold the neckband in outstretched hands and allow the gown to unfold.
4. Continue unfolding the gown, keeping the outer side turned away from the body.
5. Slide both hands into the open armholes at the same time, keeping the hands at shoulder level and away from the body.
6. Push hands and forearms into the sleeves of the gown.

The circulating person pulls the gown over the shoulders, touching only the inner shoulder and arm seams. The neckband and back of the gown is adjusted and securely tied or snapped, avoiding unnecessary contamination. Gowns with tapes to close the back are now tied at the center back by the circulating person. The swing back or flap on the gowns is fixed into position after the scrubbed person has put on sterile gloves.

## Preparing gloves for surgical use
### Considerations

In the preparation of gloves, provision must be made for the scrubbed person to handle the glove on the inner side only. Although scrubbed, the skin is not sterile and must not come in contact with the outer surface of the glove that handles the instruments and other supplies on the sterile field.

To permit the scrubbed person to grasp the glove on the inside, a wide cuff is turned back on each glove. The cuffed gloves are placed right and left in either pocket of a wallet type of folder with the palms upward. To ensure sterilization of all surfaces, a wick of some material such as paper or gauze may be inserted into the palms to separate the layers of rubber. If powder is to be used as a hand lubricant, the small envelope containing it may be placed in the glove folder.

Each glove folder is wrapped in an outer cover for sterilization. Although muslin is the traditional material for glove folders and wrappers, manufacturers of disposable products for operating rooms now offer paper folders and wrappers. Studies of these new materials and the methods of gas sterilization indicate that wicking may not be necessary for these methods of preparing gloves.

### Use of glove lubricants

To prevent rubber surfaces from sticking together when autoclaved, it has been the practice to powder gloves. In the past, talcum powder was commonly used, but the particles of this substance were found to cause foreign body reactions in the tissues and to lead, in some cases, to the formation of granulomas. For this reason, starch powders such as Biosorb were developed, which are more benign. This powder is available in bulk for dusting the gloves and in envelopes for lubricating the hands to ease the donning of sterile rubber gloves.

The use of any form of powder adds to the dust hazard in an operating room where sterile goods and open wounds may be affected. Various efforts have been made to diminish or eliminate this hazard. Cream or liquid lubricants of various types have been developed and advocated, some of which contain antiseptic or bacteriostatic agents that assist in keeping the gloved hands relatively free of bacterial growth. Manufacturers of surgical gloves have also used silicone films to eliminate stickiness. Little or no lubrication of the hands is needed to don these gloves easily. In assessing these new products and practices, it is necessary to determine their

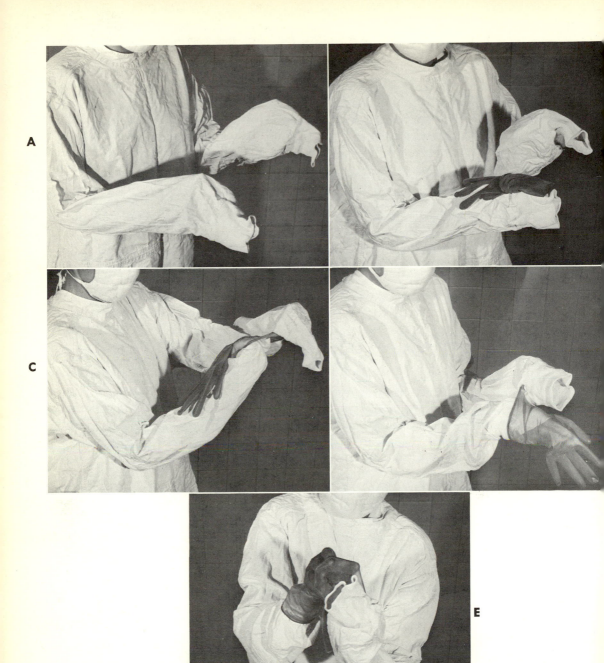

**Fig. 4-18.** Closed gloving procedure. **A,** The scrubbed person, in donning gown, does not slip hands through wristlets. Hands are not extended from sleeves. **B,** First glove is lifted by grasping it through fabric of sleeve. Gloves do not have to be cuffed for this method of gloving, but a cuff may be helpful in handling the glove more easily. Glove is placed palm down along the forearm of matching hand, with thumb and fingers pointing toward elbow. Glove cuff lies over gown wristlet. **C,** Glove cuff is held securely by hand on which it is placed, and, with other hand, cuff is stretched over opening of sleeve to cover gown wristlet entirely. **D,** As cuff is drawn back onto wrist, fingers are directed into their cots in glove, and glove is adjusted to hand. **E,** Gloved hand is then used to position remaining glove on opposite sleeve in same fashion. Glove cuff is placed around gown cuff. Second glove is drawn onto the hand and the cuff pulled into place.

effectiveness for the purpose and their harmlessness to the skin and other body tissues of both patients and personnel.

### Application of glove lubricant to hands

After they have finished drying their hands, some personnel may desire lubricant for them. Powder should be used before gowning; however, cream lubricants from sterile strip packages may be used either before or after gowning.

To lubricate the hands, each individual should grasp the protruding end of the envelope containing the lubricant, stand near the waste receptacle, open the envelope and pour or squeeze the lubricant carefully into the palms, discard the envelope in the waste receptacle, and apply the lubricant carefully over the surface of the hands.

### Putting on sterile gloves
#### Closed method

The closed method of gloving is easy for the novice. It has the advantage of prevent-

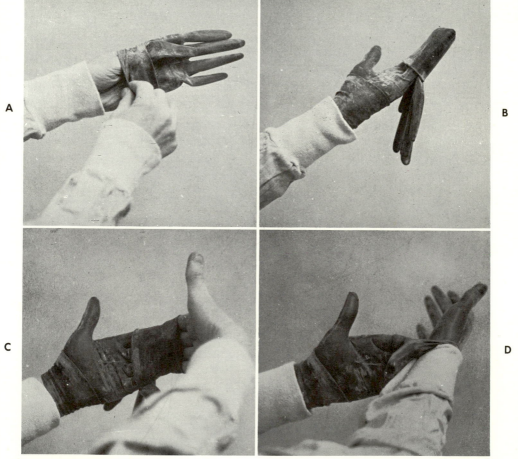

*Continued.*

Fig. 4-19. Putting on sterile gloves—seven steps. **A,** Gowned person takes one glove (right or left) from muslin envelope by placing fingers of opposite hand on fold of everted cuff at a point in line with glove's palm and pulls glove over hand, leaving cuff turned back. **B,** Gowned person takes second glove from muslin envelope by placing gloved fingers under the everted cuff. **C,** Gowned person, with arms extended and elbows flexed slightly, introduces the free hand into glove. **D,** Gowned person, with fingers under cuff of glove, draws it over cuff of gown and upper part of wristlet by slightly rotating arm externally and internally.

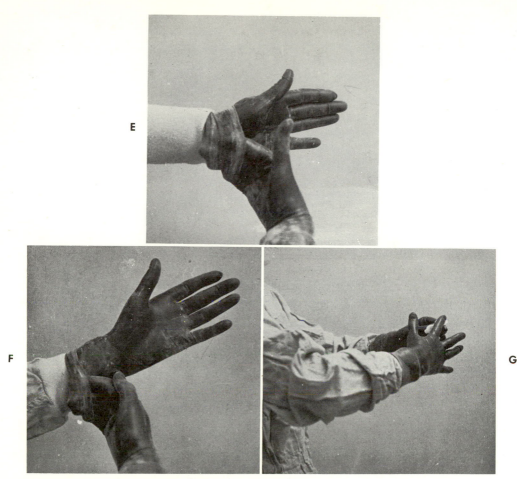

**Fig. 4-19, cont'd. E and F,** To bring turned-back cuff on other hand over wristlet of gown, the person repeats step shown in **D. G,** Gloved worker adjusts fingers of glove and removes excess powder, using wet gauze sponge.

ing the bare hands from coming in contact with the outside of the glove, which must remain sterile. The gloves are handled through the fabric of the gown sleeves. The hands are not extended from the sleeves and wristlets when the gown is put on. Instead, the hands are pushed through the cuff openings as the gloves are pulled in place.

The major steps to be carried out are described and demonstrated in Fig. 4-18.

### Open method

The everted cuff of each glove permits a gowned person to touch the glove's inner side with his ungloved fingers and to touch

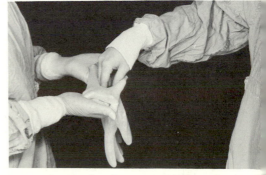

**Fig. 4-20.** Sterile gloves. Gowned and gloved person places fingers of each hand beneath the everted cuff, keeping thumbs turned outward and stretching cuff as gowned person slips his hand into sterile glove, using a firm downward thrust.

the glove's outer side with his gloved fingers. The gowned person should keep his hands in direct view, no lower than level with the waist, and flex his elbows. He should exert a light, even pull on the glove to bring it over the hands and, using a rotating movement, bring the cuff over the wristlet.

The major steps to be carried out are described and demonstrated in Fig. 4-19.

## Assisting others with gowning

A gowned and gloved person may assist another scrubbed individual in donning his sterile gown. The gown is opened in the manner previously described. The inner side with the open armholes is turned toward the individual who is to be gowned. A cuff is made of the neck and shoulder area of the gown to protect the gloved hands. The gown is held until the person has his hands and forearms in the sleeves of the gown. The circulating person will assist in pulling the gown onto the shoulders, adjusting the back, and tying the tapes. The swing back or flap on the gown is fixed into position after gloving is completed.

### Using sterile gown with extra flap

After the circulating nurse has secured the grippers or tapes at center back of the gown, the gowned and gloved nurse, using aseptic precautions, assists the other gowned person with the flap as described here and as shown in Fig. 4-17.

1. Release the extra flap from the gripper or ties on the right side of the gown.
2. Protect gloved hands and hold the flap securely while the wearer turns toward his left, which will bring the flap across his back and cover the unsterile previously tied tapes.
3. The wearer adjusts the fit and comfort of his gown by snapping the gripper or tying the tapes in front of him.

## Assisting others with gloving

A gowned and gloved person assists the gowned individual as follows and as shown in Fig. 4-20.

1. Grasp the glove under the everted cuff.
2. Turn the palm of the glove toward the other individual's hand.
3. Stretch the cuff to open the glove.
4. Exert a slight upward pressure on the cuff as the gowned individual inserts his hand into the glove.
5. Bring the cuff over the wristlet of the gown as the gowned individual slips his hand well into the glove.
6. Procedure is repeated to don the other glove.

## Removing soiled gown, gloves, and mask
### Procedure

To protect the forearms, hands, and clothing from contacting bacteria on the outer side of the used gown and gloves, the members of the scrubbed surgical team carry out the following steps:

1. Wipe off the gloves with a clean wet sponge.
2. Have the circulating person unfasten the gown.
3. Grasp the gown at one shoulder seam.
4. Bring the neck of the gown and sleeve forward, over and off the gloved hand, turning the gown inside out and everting the cuff of the glove.
5. Repeat for the other side, pulling the gown off completely.
6. Keeping the arms and soiled gown away from the body, fold the gown inside out and discard it carefully inside the linen hamper.

Used gloves are removed as follows:

1. Grasp the outer side of one glove with the gloved fingers of the other hand, being careful not to touch the skin with the soiled surface of either glove.
2. Pull off the glove and discard it in the appropriate receptacle.
3. Place the bare fingers on the ungloved hand under the everted inner cuff of the remaining glove to pull it off and discard it.

Proper technique for removing soiled gowns and gloves is demonstrated in Fig. 4-21.

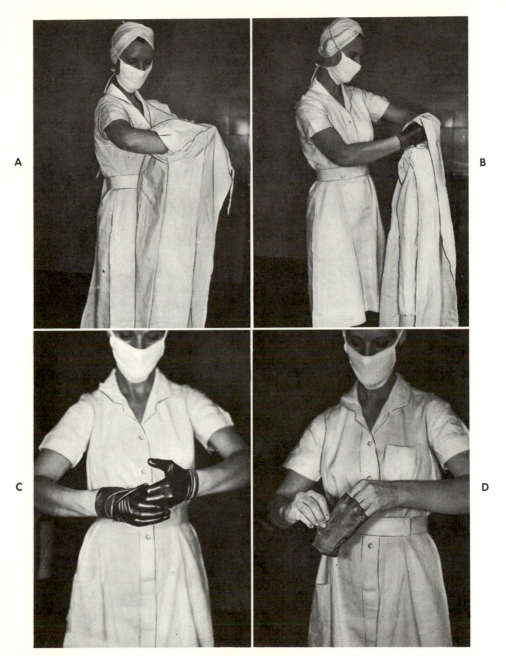

**Fig. 4-21.** Removing soiled gown and gloves—four steps. **A,** To protect uniform and arms from bacteria that are present on outer side of soiled gown, gowned and gloved person peels gown off one side of body, using opposite hand, and turns inner side of gown outward. **B,** Scrubbed person turns outer side of soiled gown away from body, keeping elbows flexed and arm away from body, so that soiled gown will not touch arms or uniform. **C,** To prevent outer side of soiled gloves from touching skin surfaces of hands, worker places gloved fingers of one hand on outer side of glove, then pulls it off hand and fingers. **D,** To prevent skin of ungloved hand from touching outer side of soiled glove, person grasps inner side of cuff and then pulls glove off.

Unfasten the face mask on leaving the operating area and discard it in the designated container.

Wash hands and forearms. When the individual is to scrub for another operation immediately, he dons a fresh mask and repeats the prescribed scrub procedure.

## REFERENCES

1. Altemeier, W. A.: Prevention and control of infections in hospitals, Hospitals **37**:62, May, 1963.
2. Becton, Dickinson & Co. Lectures: Antiseptics, 1957-1959.
3. Berry, E. C., and Kohn, M. L.: Introduction to operating room technique, New York, 1966, McGraw-Hill Book Co.
4. Brooks, H. L., and Rockwell, V. T.: Simple procedure for processing and donning surgical rubber gloves; closed glove method, O. R. Nurs. **2**:41, July-Aug., 1961.
5. Burrows, W.: Textbook of microbiology, ed. 18, Philadelphia, 1963, W. B. Saunders Co.
6. Colbeck, J. C.: Control of infections in hospitals, hospital monograph series, Chicago, 1962, American Hospital Association.
7. Cole, W. H.: Textbook of surgery, ed. 8, New York, 1963, Appleton-Century-Crofts.
8. Connell, J. F., Jr., and Rousselot, L. M.: Povidone-iodine: extensive surgical evaluation of a new antiseptic agent, Am. J. Surg. **108**:849, Dec., 1964.
9. Freeman, B. S., and Young, T. K., Jr.: Clinical study of the use of a synthetic detergent combined with hexachlorophene for disinfection of the skin, Surgery **25**:897, 1949.
10. Joress, S. M.: A study of disinfection of the skin: comparison of povidone-iodine with other agents used for surgical scrubs, Ann. Surg. **155**:296, 1962.
11. Meleny, F. L.: A comparison of the antiseptic value of certain surgical scrub-up preparations, Am. Surg. **30**:77, 1964.
12. Pate, M. O.: The preparation manual, Long Island City, N. Y., 1963, Edward Weck & Co., Inc.
13. Price, P. B.: Surgical scrubs and preoperative skin disinfection, J. Hosp. Res. **5**: Dec., 1967.
14. Reddish, G. F.: Antiseptics, disinfectants, fungicides, and chemical and physical sterilization, Philadelphia, 1957, Lea & Febiger.
15. Rockwell, V. T.: Surgical hand scrubbing, Am. J. Nurs. **63**:75, 1963.
16. Walters, C. W.: The aseptic treatment of wounds, New York, 1948, The Macmillan Co.
17. Walters, C. W.: Preoperative skin preparation, Hosp. Top. **31**:67, Jan., 1953; **34**:95, April, 1956; **30**:71, Oct., 1961.

# CHAPTER 5

# Standards for safe environment, equipment, and procedural policies

EILEEN MOEHRLE

Policies, regulations, and procedures are designed to ensure the safety of patients and personnel and to provide a setting in which all activities of the operating room staff fit together, resulting in an efficient course of action for the benefit of each patient.

A policy may be defined as a definite course of action or procedure approved by the controlling authorities as expedient and conforming to an accepted medical, nursing, or technological principle. Organizational structure, delegation of responsibilities, and authority of staff members are considered in Chapter 2.

## SAFE ENVIRONMENT

The design of a surgical suite in terms of systems, materials, and human needs has been described in Chapter 1. The design incorporates physical and mechanical means of reducing and controlling infection in the suite.

The cause and effect of infectious bacteria and basic principles of sterilization and disinfection are described in Chapter 3. Aseptic techniques concerning skin preparation are discussed in Chapter 4.

### Hospital administrative and medical staff control measures

The operating room nursing professional staff assists the hospital administrative and medical staffs in setting and maintaining standards, usually through scheduled conferences and the operating room committee (Chapter 2).

Each nurse should understand her professional legal and ethical responsibilities to each patient as established by the nursing practice act of the state and by the professional nursing organization, the American Nurses' Association.

### Records and forms

The operating room policy manual should contain directions to protect patients and personnel. Protection of patients' personal, moral, and legal rights begins at the time of admission. The course of action involves correct identification of the patient, safeguarding his right to privacy, and keeping confidential all records and reports. Condition of admission to the hospital and consent for treatment or operation are important records that protect both the patient and those persons who render him care.

The hospital administration provides appropriate forms that are legally acceptable. Personnel who obtain consents or witness them should be aware of the conditions that ensure their validity and their personal responsibility to appear in a court of law if necessary. It should be recognized that a signed consent must also be an informed consent, which implies adequate communication with the patient regarding the pro-

cedure for which the consent is being signed.

Special permits for specific operations such as sterilization, therapeutic abortion, disposal of severed members of the body, and autopsy provide additional safeguards for patient, staff, and hospital. In case of a death in the operating room or recovery room, the nursing service manual should state the course of action to be carried out in regard to informing the hospital authorities, notifying physicians and family, referring to the medical examiner, and so forth.

The Joint Commission on Accreditation of Hospitals requires that a record be kept of each operation, including the nature of the surgery performed, the preoperative and postoperative diagnoses, and the name of the personnel participating in the patient's care. The record should also indicate the results of the sponge count and, in some cases, the instrument count. The copying of these data onto a record ledger book may be delegated to a clerk or secretary. The operative and anesthesia records become a permanent part of the patient's chart.

## Admission of patient

The operating room manual should contain the admission procedure and delegation of responsibilities. The major facts of the admission procedure should include the following:

1. The operating room nurse should review the patient's identification and record. The band on the patient, the chart, and the tag on the carrier or bed should conform in name, spelling, location, and physician's name.

2. The history and physical and laboratory examination results should be complete. The controlling body of the institution informs the staff which examinations are mandatory as part of the patient's preoperative preparation. These usually include completed records for physical examination, health history, recent determination of blood and urine tests, and chest

x-ray examination. Administration shall provide a checklist of required medical admission records for reference of staff in the admission of patients. This tool aids in preventing oversights and omissions in routines designed to protect patients and staff. The checklist is also a helpful tool for intramural reporting when a patient is transferred from his room to the operating room department.

3. The patient should be examined for personal effects, including clothing, money, jewelry, wigs, religious symbols, and prostheses such as dentures, lenses, glass eyes, and hearing aids. The nurse is responsible for ensuring their proper disposition and safety.

4. The operating room nurse should review the orders and results concerning nutrition and elimination such as enema and amount of urine voided or catheterized. It is important to determine the condition of an infusion and whether or not preoperative dietary and fluid restrictions have been maintained. Aspiration of gastric contents during anesthesia induction is a danger. Every precaution should be taken to prevent such an accident by having the suctioning apparatus in operation and personnel present to assist the anesthetist.

5. The nurse should chart meticulously any fluids, blood, or plasma administered as ordered during the immediate preoperative period.

6. The nursing staff should apply side rails or restraint straps and use control devices on beds, carriers, and operating tables to prevent fall and injury of the patient during transportation, transfer, and positioning.

7. Peace of mind and reassurance are within the gift of nursing personnel in their care of and concern for the patient. By judicious use of *directions* and *self*, assuming a calm, confident manner and a quiet voice, using gentle, precise movements in execution of activities, and providing spiritual assistance on request, the nursing staff member can help the patient to face surgery with some equanimity.

## Safety control program

All operating room and recovery room personnel participate in the hospital safety program. A representative of the operating room department should be a member of the hospital safety program committee. Each worker should be prepared to carry out special duties in the care of patients in an emergency situation and in natural or man-made disasters. Periodic review of duties, fire drills, and other practice sessions should be initiated. All personnel should be aware of the daily hazards peculiar to operating room activities and working conditions.

### Explosion hazards

Specific preventive measures are taken to eliminate sources of ignition that could lead to fire or explosion. These measures include stated requirements such as high relative humidity, conductive flooring, explosion-proof switches, conductive or static electricity-free materials and textiles, and conductive footwear.

Static electricity is built up rapidly on nonconductors by the friction of one surface against another, resulting in an accumulation of free electrons that may be discharged on contact with a grounded body. Static electricity and sparks from an electrical apparatus have proved to be the major cause of explosions in operating and delivery rooms when a general anesthetic is administered. Anesthetic gases and vapors, with the exception of chloroform, trichloroethylene, and the newly developed halogens such as methoxyflurane and halothane, are inflammable and highly explosive when they are mixed with those concentrations of oxygen or nitrous oxide that are used during surgical procedures.

An explosion-proof electrical apparatus diminishes the hazard but does not completely eliminate all sources of igniting sparks. The *closed method* for administering a combustible anesthetic agent does not make the anesthetic safe from ignition by sparks because a small leak of gas or vapor is usually present. Although cautery, endo-

thermy, and electrical suction apparatus are all potential sources of sparks, static electricity is by far the most frequent hazard.

To reduce hazards of sparks from the discharge of static electricity, efforts are made to ensure a continuous drain off via conductive pathways to the ground. The program of control should support the most recent recommendations and reasonable measures for minimizing loss of life and property published by the National Fire Protection Association. Equipment must be explosion proof, and inspection and conversion of equipment outlets and switches must conform to national and state requirements.

General safety regulations should be approved by the operating room committee and hospital administration. Nursing service should be delegated the responsibility and authority to see that the regulations are put into effect by all operating room staff members.

General safety regulations and reports should be reviewed periodically by the operating room committee. The regulations may include the following:

1. The anesthesiologist-in-chief shall determine whether electrical apparatus, cameras, lights, and cauteries are safe for use in a given situation and shall be informed when the use of such apparatus is scheduled.

2. The use of any apparatus or device producing an open flame shall be prohibited within 10 feet of any area used for induction of anesthesia. The use of matches or alcohol spirit lamps shall not be permitted near anesthetizing areas or storage areas for anesthetic gases.

3. Signs indicating that an explosive anesthetic is in use should be posted prominently on the entrance door to the operating room, and all personnel in the room should be so informed.

4. Combustible anesthetic gases shall not be administered in the presence of cautery, endothermy, or radiographic equipment. Exceptions to this rule may

be made only with the consent of the chief of anesthesiology and if in the opinion of the operating surgeon the welfare of the patient requires the simultaneous use of a combustible anesthetic agent and the electrical device.

5. Nonexplosive anesthetic agents are recommended for use in the presence of electric drills, saws, diathermy, and other electric-powered apparatus.

6. A qualified electrician should make regular inspections of electrical outlets and equipment and file written reports with the director of the operating rooms.

### Transfer of patient

Patients shall not be moved from one carrier to another or from bed to stretcher or table during the administration of a combustible anesthetic.

### Smoking

No smoking or flame-producing devices shall be permitted in the restricted operating room area.

### Storage of anesthetic gases

Ether, ethylene, and cyclopropane shall be stored in a cool, dry room ventilated to the outside and separate from the room in which oxygen and nitrous oxide are stored. Cyclopropane shall not be stored in quantity greater than is needed in a 24-hour period.

### Volatile liquids

Ethyl oxide and other volatile liquids are prohibited for cleaning and incidental use in hazardous locations.

### Electrical equipment

All lights and other fixtures shall be switched on before the anesthetic equipment is used. Switching electricity on and off while combustible gases are in use is prohibited.

Contact with anesthetic machines is to be avoided by all persons other than the working anesthetist.

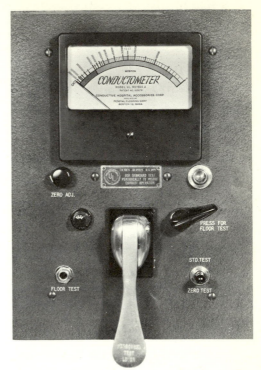

Fig. 5-1. Conductometer should be located in clean areas of suite for use of operating room personnel to test themselves for personal conductivity each time they enter a hazardous hospital operating space, where potentially explosive gases may be present. Conductometer is specially designed to test personnel, flooring, and equipment and is directly connected to 100- to 120-volt A.C. line. Elbow switch permits personnel testing under aseptic conditions, and indicator scale in color is easily read. (Courtesy Conductive Hospital Accessories Corp., Boston, Mass.)

No articles may be placed on the anesthetic machine while gases are being administered.

### Staff attire

Only outer clothing made of cotton or conductive materials and approved conductive footwear may be worn. Since the conductivity of footwear may change during use, it must be tested daily. Conductometers must be available for testing, and each individual is responsible for testing his own footwear (Fig. 5-1).

### Bed linen

Only cotton or paper sheets and cotton blankets are permitted. Materials must be adequately hydrated to reduce static electricity potential.

### Accessory equipment

Conductive casters and tips on chairs or metal furniture and conductive mattress covers, restraint straps, electrical cords, breathing tubes, anesthetic masks, and bags shall be used to establish conductive pathways.

### Test schedules for flooring and equipment

A regular schedule for testing conductive flooring and equipment shall be carried out with the assistance of the maintenance department. Reports of tests shall be kept on file.

### Prevention of accidents

All personnel should be instructed in the use of good body mechanics to avert common falls and strains when reaching, stretching, lifting, or moving heavy patients or articles. Good body mechanics and application of work simplification principles conserve human energy and protect the worker, thereby promoting good performance.

All personnel should be instructed and supervised in the proper use of equipment to avoid injury such as cuts from knife blades and glassware, burns from autoclaves and electrical equipment, and abrasions from contact with metal accessory levers and swinging doors.

All pieces of equipment should be tested periodically and prior to use for correct functioning. An item should not be used unless it is in good working order. The staff members should receive proper instructions before operating a machine or piece of apparatus.

The aftercare and regular inspection of complicated steam, electrical, vacuum, hydraulic, filtering, and pumping systems should be done periodically according to an established schedule agreed on by the hospital maintenance or engineering departments.

The maintenance and cleaning program should be clearly defined and understood by the nursing staff. Prompt attention to spillage, prompt drying of wet floors, use of warning signs in danger areas, and keeping the corridors and all traffic areas clear of obstacles are important housekeeping duties.

To prevent wound infection, there should be regulations for inspection, testing, and controlling of all traffic and portals of entry such as ventilation, plumbing, deliveries, visitors, and staff to ensure a safe environment.

Cleaning, disinfection, and sterilization of equipment, control of airborne contamination, and application of aseptic techniques are basic to an effective infection control program. Breaks in asepsis may also result from the intrusion of pests, vermin, insects, noxious substances, chemicals, gases, and infectious body fluids and wastes into the protected areas.

Effective disposal procedures for soiled materials and debris are essential to render the area safe for patients and personnel.

The professional nursing staff has a responsibility to work with the infection control committee in the establishment of regulations and the reporting of incidents.

## Decontamination practices for personnel

It is known that large quantities of bacteria are present in the nose and mouth, on the skin, and on the shoes and clothing of personnel who enter the protected areas of the operating room suite (Chapter 3). Proper design of facilities and regulations for use of operating attire are important ways to prevent transportation of microorganisms into operating rooms where they may infect the open wounds of patients.

### Changing areas for personnel

Decontamination locker and dressing areas for personnel and a special holding

unit for preoperative patients have been proposed to reduce contamination in the operating room. Areas are provided where workers may remove personal clothing, don operating room attire, and enter the clean operating suite directly without passing through a contaminated area.

### Health concepts

Daily body cleanliness and well-groomed, clean hair free of dandruff help prevent superficial wound infections. Hair is a fertile source of bacteria-bearing particles. The hair of the head and of other areas of the body may shed debris and dead cells that may be transported to an open wound.

The worker who is well rested and healthy is less subject to infectious diseases. Regulations should not permit workers who have infection of the nose or throat, are known to be carriers, or have open sores to enter the operating room.

### Operating room attire

The operating room apparel worn by personnel working in the *clean* areas of the operating room suite includes a one-piece or two-piece suit or a dress, special shoes and booties, headpiece, and face mask.

CLOTHING. The garment should be made of cotton or a material with similar qualities. Trousers, shirts, and dresses should be of good fit for comfort and appearance and should permit control around a sterile field. Loose, flapping folds or shirt-tails and baggy, drooping trousers are sources of possible contamination as the personnel move in performing their duties.

Each piece of clothing should be designed so that the personnel may don and remove it without passing it over the head, hair, or face. In some institutions, the women wear jumpsuits or suits similar to those worn by the men.

FOOTWEAR. Absorbent cotton socks or hose are helpful in maintaining healthy feet. The style of footwear should provide a well-fitting support for the feet. For easy, sanitary maintenance, footwear should be easy to clean.

To prevent explosive hazards, as previously discussed, conductive footwear is mandatory in anesthetizing locations and where anesthetic gases or electrical appliances are in use.

Because of the danger of static spark explosions, all personnel must test the conductivity of their own operating room footwear by means of a conductometer (Fig. 5-1).

The conductive elements may be integral parts of the shoe itself, being incorporated in soles and heel plates. Disposable adhesive conductive strips may be provided to add to regular types of footwear kept for operating room work.

Shoe covers that incorporate conductive strips in the soles are popular. Disposable shoe covers of an appropriate size must be moisture resistant, contain conductive elements, and meet sanitary and other safety measures for the worker.

HEADGEAR. Free hair may fall onto a sterile field, or the hair may shed contaminants. Within the clean and sterile operating room zones, all personnel are required to wear a headpiece that completely covers and controls the hair. Skullcaps that fail to cover the side hair above the ears and hair at the nape of the neck should not be worn in the operating room. Helmets that cover the long front hair, the side and back of the head, and the face provide the greatest degree of safety.

The head cover may be made of a loose-weave cotton or disposable material that provides for effective ventilation and comfort and yet is close enough in mesh or texture to prevent penetration of hair or escape of dandruff. Wide-gauged gauze, mesh net, or crinoline material should not be used. The outer edges of the headgear should fit snugly and securely by means of elastic or other type of fasteners or drawstring ties. Headgear should be laundered after each use.

Disposable headgear should be discarded in a designated receptacle imme-

diately after use. The headgear should not be worn outside the suite and should always be worn in those areas where equipment and supplies are processed and stored.

FACE MASKS. Until recently, the pre-shrunk, double-ply cotton mask has been the most acceptable mask. Surgical face masks are now made of disposable materials and the requirements of comfort, efficiency, cost, and durability have been met. The advent of new technological methods for isolating the patient's wound from airborne contamination may eliminate the need for face masks.

COTTON MASKS. Masks of this type are rectangular in shape, have horizontal tucks or pleats to fit the contours of the face, and cover the nose and mouth. Two pairs of twill tapes attached to the corners are used to fasten the mask around the head and neck. The cotton mask, consisting of six layers of gauze forty-four by forty-four threads per square inch, is estimated to filter about 77% of the pathogens from the breathed air. A mask that has too many thick gauze layers or one with a paper film insert forces the wearer to rebreathe expired air or to deflect the breathed air out around the edges of the mask. Any type of mask that becomes moist loses its efficiency rapidly as a filter.

The wearer who breathes through a face mask thickly inoculated with expired bacteria may expel a higher number of microorganisms into the atmosphere than does the individual who breathes normally and quietly without a mask. Forceful expulsion of the breath during talking, laughing, or sneezing propels large concentrations of microorganisms into the air. The mask should be changed frequently because it becomes relatively ineffective as a bacterial barrier after 30 minutes of wear. In removing a mask from the face, the wearer handles it carefully to prevent cross contamination.

A pliable metal strip should be inserted through the uppermost hem band of the cotton mask to provide a firm contour fit over the bridge of the nose. This strip also helps prevent fogging of eyeglasses.

DISPOSABLE MASKS. Some masks are made of synthetic materials designed as disposable products.

HANDLING OF MASKS. When cotton masks are laundered, they should receive a final rinse that contains a bacteriostatic agent such as quaternary ammonium. Old, frayed masks should be discarded. Clean cotton masks may be steam sterilized as an extra precautionary measure.

All clean masks, regardless of the type, should be stored in covered containers. Masks should not be kept in pockets or permitted to dangle around the neck.

To handle or don a mask of any design, the individual should first wash his hands to prevent contamination of the mask with microorganisms that later would be dispersed on the breath.

To remove a mask of any design, the wearer should handle only the tapes or band. The facepiece, which is highly contaminated with droplet nuclei, should not be touched. After use, the soiled mask should be discarded promptly in a designated receptacle.

If a metal strip has been used, it is removed and placed in a designated basin containing a germicidal solution. The strips may be collected, washed, steam sterilized, and reused. Bent strips are discarded.

After discarding the mask, the wearer must wash and dry his hands thoroughly. Storage mask receptacles must be thoroughly cleaned and sterilized at least once during each 8-hour period.

## Basic aseptic techniques

The basic principles of aseptic techniques are to prevent contamination of the open wound, isolate the operative site from the surrounding unsterile physical environment, and create or set up a sterile field in which surgery may be safely performed.

All materials in contact with the wound must be sterile. Sterile gloved hands and

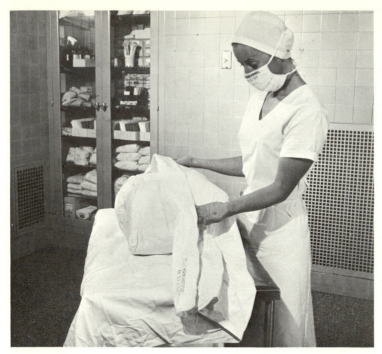

**Fig. 5-2.** Circulating person is shown opening outer cover of pack containing sterile linens for surgery. Cover is cuffed to provide protection for sterile contents. Worker avoids contact with sterile area by keeping all fingers under the cuff as cover is drawn back over table to expose inner pack.

sterilized instruments manipulate the tissues and organs in the wound.

Aseptic techniques to be followed in gowning, gloving, and skin preparation of the operative site are designed to preserve sterility of the operating field (Chapter 4). Instruments and attire of the operating team are rendered sterile by steam or gas sterilization (Chapter 3).

Certain basic conventions are observed many times during an operation to provide a well-defined margin of safety for the patient. They may be summarized as follows:

1. Certain areas of the gowns of the operating team are considered sterile: the area of each sleeve extending from the elbow to the wrist and the front part of the gown from below the axillary region to the waist, which can be observed directly by the wearer and protected from contamination.

2. Certain areas of the gowns of the operating team are considered unsterile:

the areas under the arms, neckline, and shoulders, which may become contaminated by perspiration or by collar and shoulder surfaces rubbing together during head and neck movements, and the back of the gown, since it cannot be observed by the wearer and protected from contamination.

3. When the circulator opens a sterile package, hand and arm motions are always from unsterile to unsterile objects. The hands are placed under the cuff to provide a protected wide margin of safety between the inside of the pack (sterile) and the hands (unsterile) (Fig. 5-2).

4. A wide area of separation must be preserved between the *sterile* field and the surrounding *unsterile* area. A worker is uncertain of sterility of the field he cannot personally observe. For this reason, one does not turn his back on a sterile field, since the back of the scrubbed worker's gown may brush against an unsterile object or surface.

5. The top surface is the only part of

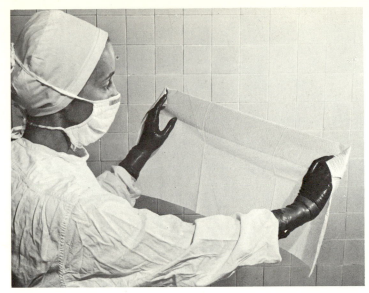

**Fig. 5-3.** To place towel on a surface, standard method of cuffing towel and rolling gloved fingers is used to protect gloved hands.

a draped table considered sterile. The scrubbed worker cannot see over the sides and behind the backs of tables. Supplies should not project or hang over the table because of risk of contamination.

6. The worker's motions should be from sterile to sterile areas and from unsterile to unsterile areas. For example, the gloved fingers are protected under a wide cuff of the drape as it is placed over a table or patient (Fig. 5-3). The underside of the surface of the drape should face the unsterile area, and the uppermost (sterile) surface must be in contact with the worker's gloved hands.

7. The gloved worker should have all parts of the suture or drape under positive control at all times during placement or transfer and should use precise and direct motions (Fig. 5-10). This means no dangling ends and no bunched masses may brush or contact an unsterile surface accidentally.

8. A towel, sheet, suture, or instrument cannot be moved from a nonsterile to a sterile field. When the object becomes contaminated, it must be discarded. A contaminated item must be lifted clear of the operative field without contacting the sterile surface and must be dropped with minimum handling to an unsterile person, area, or receptacle.

9. When a sterile gown or sheet is opened, it must not be flipped or shaken. Shaking of drapes creates air currents on which dust, lint, and droplet nuclei may migrate. Shaking of a drape also causes uncontrolled motion of the drape, which may cause it to come in contact with an unsterile surface or object. A drape should be carefully unfolded and allowed to fall gently by gravity into position. The low portion of a sheet that falls below the safe working level should never be raised or lifted back onto the sterile area.

10. The circulator maintains a wide margin of safety in pouring a solution into a sterile container, as well as in placing sterile materials in a sterile container or on a sterile surface (Figs. 5-4 and 5-5).

**Contaminants**

*Aftercare of operating room equipment*

CONSIDERATIONS. Experience with the virus of homologous serum jaundice (hepatitis) has resulted in a sharpened awareness

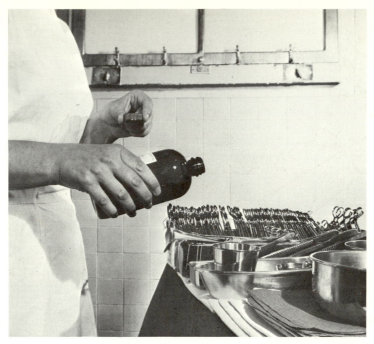

**Fig. 5-4.** Pouring antiseptic solution. Sterile cup on sterile field is placed near edge of instrument table, and solution is poured without reaching over sterile field.

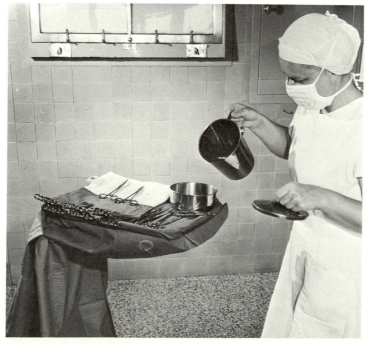

**Fig. 5-5.** Pouring antiseptic solution—cont'd. Circulating person avoids reaching over sterile field and maintains clear margin of safety. Note cover of pitcher is held with sterile inner surface downward to protect it from contamination. Outer surfaces of pitcher and lid are unsterile. Inner surfaces and pouring lip of pitcher are protected by sterile cover.

that blood and tissue fluids from any patient may contain organisms that are pathogenic to other persons (Chapter 3). As a result, operating room practices have been developed that provide complete isolation for each patient.

This is accomplished by considering every surgical wound to be a source of contamination. Establishment of procedures concerning the terminal disinfection or sterilization of all equipment and supplies used in each operation prevents the transfer of microorganisms and protects patients and staff alike.

METHOD. Instruments and reusable supplies are washed and sterilized immediately after use. Soiled linens are discarded in hampers. The outside of hampers must be kept clean for disposal in laundry chutes. This can be accomplished by careful disposal procedures and by use of waterproof liners and clean outer hamper covers.

Used disposable and expendable items are discarded in waterproof bags and placed in containers for incineration. Furniture and equipment are disinfected by thorough washing and wiping with disinfectant solution. Floors are mopped or wet vacuumed between cases with germicide solution. At end of schedule, a complete housekeeping and maintenance program is initiated.

The isolation procedures established by the hospital should be put into effect for patients who, in addition to a surgical wound, have a known communicable disease, and routine operating room procedures for the care of materials contaminated by the surgical wound should be observed. Isolation precautions usually involve use of gown and glove techniques by circulating workers and anesthetists. Care should be taken to prevent contamination of the patient's chart and anesthesia record. The operating team may use pencil to record data on the sheets and then sterilize the sheets after completion of the operation. The data are recopied on the patient's chart.

Spillage should be cleaned up immediately, and the affected area should be disinfected with the proper germicidal agent. For decontamination of rooms, agents in spray form should be considered.

## Preparation and handling of sterile supplies

To render supplies or instruments safe for the patient in surgery, the nursing personnel must follow safe methods in assembling, packaging, sterilizing, storing, and handling the items (Chapters 3 and 4).

### The wrapper

The material used to wrap sterile textiles and supplies, whether paper, plastic, or cotton, must be porous enough to permit penetration of the contents by the sterilizing agent (steam or gas). It must also be of a weave that is close enough or of a composition that will provide an effective physical barrier to dust and other minute particles that may convey bacteria to the contents. It should be strong, pliable, moisture resistant, and always free from detectable tears, holes, and weak spots. Reusable covers should be laundered after each use.

The double-thickness muslin wrapper should be made of a good quality bleached muslin of type 140 with thread counts of 68/72. Lightweight (2.85 yards per pound) jean cloth, cotton type 160 which has a close diagonal weave, 96 in warp and 64 in filling, may also be used. It is strong but less porous than regular weave materials. Muslin wrappers are made in suitable dimensions for the various items that must be packaged. Useful, adaptable sizes of wrappers are 9, 12, 18, 24, 36, and 54 inches square. Items that require a wrapper larger than 54 inches cannot be sterilized readily.

When the contents are wrapped, the wrappers should not be tightly folded about the contents, but it should be firm and sealed securely to prevent contamination in handling and storage (Fig. 5-6, A).

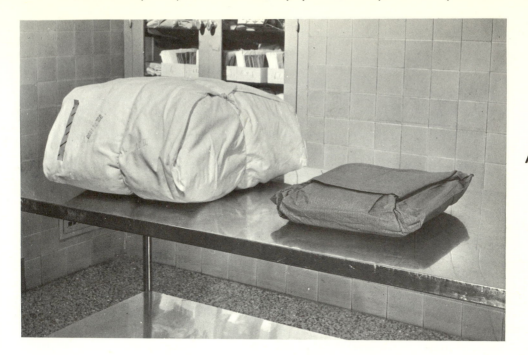

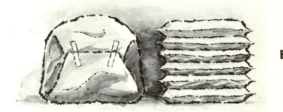

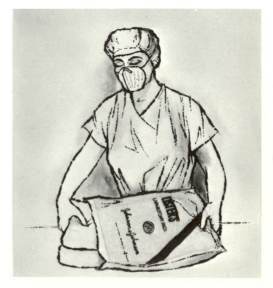

Fig. 5-6. **A,** Sterile standard cotton textile pack of drapes, including towels and sheets shown in light-colored pack with comparable pack of similar number of disposable drapes. **B,** Disposable sterile pack consists of sheets, towels, and drapes made of soft, moisture-resistant fabric. The components are functionally folded, packed in sequence of use for convenient aseptic handling. This type of flat pack conserves space in the operating room and storeroom. **C,** Sealed polyethylene bag protects pack during handling. Tear string of outer barrier bag guarantees sterility to pack's overwrap for nonsterile handling. **B** and **C** courtesy Johnson & Johnson, New Brunswick, N. J.) *Continued.*

D

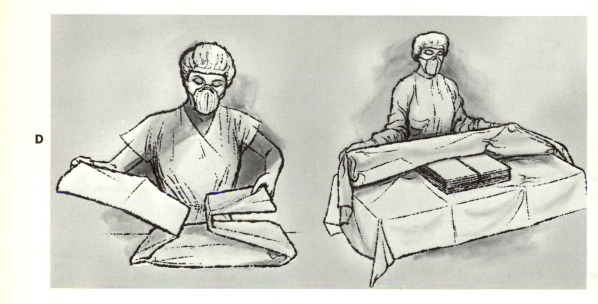

E

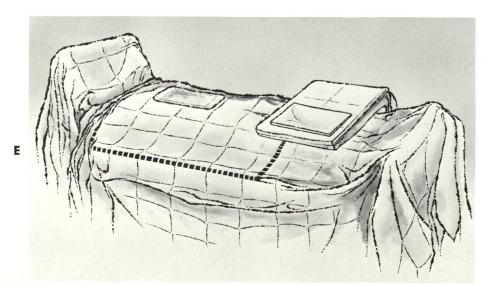

**Fig. 5-6, cont'd. D,** White overwrap is opened to become bottom layer of double table cover. Sterile, moisture-resistant drape protects pack until ready for use. Opens to become sterile surface of double table cover. **E,** Disposable, moisture-resistant laparotomy sheet covers anesthesia screen and foot of extended table. Large, double reinforcement around fenestration provides added moisture resistance. Drape is specially folded for easy aseptic application. Disposable cover for Mayo stand is specially folded and is tucked under tray for control, as shown. (Courtesy Johnson & Johnson, New Brunswick, N. J.)

The familiar envelope wrap is made by placing the articles diagonally in the center of the wrapper. The near corner should point toward the worker. It is brought up over the items, and the triangular tip is folded back to form a cuff. The two side flaps are folded to the center in like manner. The far corner of the wrapper is then folded on top of the other three and secured with autoclave indicator tape. The flap at the corners provides protection for the contents when the package is opened. The flaps are used to form a cuff over the worker's fingers and a safe barrier for the sterile goods. The items are placed in an appropriate place on the wrapper in relation to position on the sterile field, the sides are folded over, and the cuff and ends are brought over the previous folds.

Commercially prepared sterile disposable drapes, packs, and materials are sealed in a paper envelope, which is encased in a plastic sealed wrapper (Fig. 5-6, *B* and *C*).

### Dating of sterile packages

Dating of packages prepared in the hospital assists in inventory control and the rotation of older goods into early use. Supply standards should be planned to maintain adequate stock with prompt turnover. The longer an item is stored, the greater are the chances of eventual contamination. Ink stripes or letters on adhesive indicator tape that change color on exposure to the sterilizing agent should be used. Indicators for steam sterilization should be heat sensitive. Special tape sensitive to ethylene oxide gas is also available. Change in color indicators merely shows that the goods have been exposed to the sterilizing process. It does not guarantee sterility, although it provides a check on processing. The effectiveness of the process can only be assured by regular checks on the function of the equipment combined with control of the correct procedure for the use of the equipment.

Commercially packaged and sealed items

theoretically maintain sterility for indefinite periods; however, their sterility is dependent on their exposure during storage, the amount of handling, and the kind and condition of the wrapper (Fig. 5-6, *B* to *D*).

### Handling of sterile packages

Excessive handling, crowding, dropping, and pummeling of sterile packs tend to force particles through the mesh or matrix of the wrapping material, which might contaminate the contents. Sterile packages must be handled and stored with care. They must be kept in clean, dry, dustproof and verminproof areas. Shelving should be smooth and well spaced. There should be no splinters, nails, or sharp corners that might damage the wrappers. A dry humidity is required where sterile items are stored.

### Maintenance of sterilization equipment

All mechanical parts of sterilizers should be periodically checked by a competent engineer. Gauges, steam lines, and drains need attention. Temperature, humidity, and vacuum should be measured independently of the fixed gauges with control equipment (Chapter 3). Bacterial cultures of typical dry goods loads should be made regularly to ascertain that absolute sterility is achieved, and results of tests should be filed as a permanent record (Chapter 3).

Meshed or vented racks are useful for preventing condensation on steam sterilized packages and for aerating goods that have been gas sterilized.

## SELECTION AND MAINTENANCE OF SURGICAL INSTRUMENTS, OTHER EQUIPMENT, AND DRAPES
### Instruments and other equipment

There are many surgical instruments, each with variations in structure and design to meet a particular purpose, a specific requirement, and an individual surgeon's preference. Each manufacturer selects a name for his own particular design. There

is no standard nomenclature for instruments.

The manufacturers issue excellent catalogs that are most helpful in the selection of instruments for surgical specialties. By evaluating the surgeons' intentions and their methods of working and by understanding the objectives of surgical intervention, the nursing service supervisory staff provides invaluable assistance in helping directors to determine the appropriate instrument standards needed for the various clinical specialties, as well as for specific requests of individual physicians.

### Instrument control program

For an effective control program, the nursing staff must know the instrument inventory of the department, the routine instruments needed for each type of operation, the individual surgeon's preferences, the correct use and handling of instruments, the method of preparation, and the aftercare of the instruments.

Surgical instruments represent a major financial investment. They are precision tools and merit respect in handling and care. Instruments should be purchased from reputable manufacturers who have high standards concerning pattern, material, and workmanship.

Rules in relation to handling and caring for instruments may be summarized as follows:

1. Inspect each instrument before and after use to detect imperfections. An instrument or appliance should function perfectly to prevent needlessly endangering a patient's life and increasing the operative time because of failure of an instrument.

2. Set aside damaged instruments and send for repair or replacement.

3. Use instruments only for the purpose for which they are designed. Proper use prolongs their life. Fine clamps and dissecting scissors can be forced out of alignment, cracked, or broken if they are used on heavy tissues, gauze dressings, or drainage tubing.

4. Handle instruments gently at all times and avoid bunching, dropping, and weighing them down under heavy pieces of equipment.

5. Provide protection for cutting instruments, lensed instruments, and fine, delicate holding instruments that are unusually susceptible to damage by using specially designed metal racks and cases.

6. Clean instruments meticulously. Select soaps, detergents, and cleaning methods with care. Use washer-sterilizer and ultrasonic cleaner, both of which provide a thorough, easy method of cleaning. Protect the finish of instruments by not exposing them to chemicals, drugs, and acids that have oxidizing or corrosive properties or to water with a high mineral content. Make sure instruments are perfectly clean and dry before storage.

7. Keep oil away from instruments. Oil forms a bacterial protecting film that is difficult and time consuming to remove, and it also interferes with penetration of steam during the sterilization process (Chapter 3).

8. Store instruments safely. The use of locked cabinets or cupboards located in designated areas prevents pilferage and indiscriminate use. Cabinet shelving and hooks of cabinets should be adjustable and properly spaced for storage of various sizes and types of instruments. Attach labels and pictures in cabinets to assist personnel.

9. Give instruments regular maintenance such as sharpening, realignment, and setting of box locks. Select the instrument repair service carefully and use it effectively.

10. Keep inventory of fixed and movable equipment, appliances, and general items. Take inventory at periodic intervals during the year.

11. The central utility area for the processing of instruments should be properly designed and equipped to ensure safe, effective handling and care of all types of instruments (Chapter 1).

### Lensed instruments

To ensure long life of their optical system, the intricate, delicate, and expensive instruments used in internal manipulation and examination require the most thoughtful and meticulous care in cleaning, sterilizing, and storing.

Lensed instruments must be protected from breakage and distortion; each instrument must be kept straight at all times when not in use.

Flexible endoscopes such as the gastroscope should never be bent, except during introduction into a passage within the patient. The junction of the flexible and rigid portions of the scope is the most vulnerable point.

Only the instrument manufacturer should replace a part of the scope. When a telescopic scope is sent for repair, it must be packed in a padded instrument case and placed within a padded carton to protect the lens during transportation. A direct blow can break the objective window of modern telescopic endoscopes.

The unequal expansion and contraction of metal and glass parts due to temperature changes makes it impossible to autoclave lensed instruments without damage. Certain lens cements are affected by the solvents in disinfectants; therefore the substances used for cleaning and soaking lensed instruments must be selected with discrimination. Glass eyepieces must be protected from scratches and abrasives. Information and precise instructions should be sought from manufacturers regarding the specific care of their products.

*Electrical circuits and connections* must be maintained in watertight condition if the lighting systems are to work properly. Contacts must be kept clean and dry. Waxes provided for sealing the lamp bulbs against water are applied to the threads only and must not insulate the contacts. Lamps must not be handled with forceps or clamps. To change a cystoscope lamp, a rubber guard can be placed over the used lamp cap to remove it.

Each standard scope requires a lamp, light carrier, and cord. Duplicates of each should be available for use. The battery box or power supply unit should be tested periodically and also immediately before use.

The *metal and plastic parts of instruments* must be protected also, since they are introduced into body orifices. Sharp, uneven surfaces can damage tissues and complicate the procedure and the patient's course. Scratches on metal finishes become the sites of rust and corrosion that destroy the instrument for surgical use.

General precautions for the care of lensed equipment such as endoscopy and urological instruments are as follows:

1. Do not boil or autoclave instruments containing lamps or lenses.

2. Do not place lensed instruments in solvent solutions such as alcohol.

3. Do not place metal instruments in corrosive solutions such as those containing mercury, phenol (carbolic acid), or iodine.

Thorough cleaning in clear water and a selected bland soap or detergent is the first step toward disinfection and sterilization.

Endoscopes should always be held in a vertical position by the ocular end when they are cleaned. The flexible endoscope should never be held in a horizontal position unless the objective end is supported. The instrument is wiped downward repeatedly, using gauze sponges saturated with surgical soap and water. Special attention must be given to surface joints and crevices that may retain mucus. This process is repeated, using sponges saturated with a 70% alcohol solution. The scope is then dried thoroughly, using clean gauze sponges. For a gastroscope or a similar endoscope, several bulbfuls of air are blown through the scope to force out from under the sheath any fluid that may have worked its way into the air-egress holes.

The lumen of every hollow instrument requires special attention. Since it is impossible to see soil in these parts, gentle

hemolyzing solutions may be used to soak and flush out the lumen. Thorough rinsing immediately after use is the best precaution to prevent clotting and crusting of blood and body fluids in the instruments. Cotton swabs on stylets are used to wipe and dry the inner parts. If brushes are used, they should have soft bristles and should be handled gently. Abrasives should be avoided.

STERILIZATION. Ethylene oxide gas is the only sure method of sterilizing lensed instruments, which are damaged by high temperatures (Chapter 3). If a gas sterilizer is lacking, lensed instruments may be disinfected by soaking them in a chemical solution such as the quaternary ammonium compounds or glutaraldehydes (Cidex). The use of Formalin gas cabinets has been thoroughly discredited as a method of disinfection, although they may be used as storage areas.

Special trays with fitted holders for each piece of equipment can be made to safeguard instruments set up for sterilization. Fitted cases and custom-made racks also provide protection for instruments in storage.

### Nylon and silk catheters and bougies

Nylon and silk woven lacquered catheters and bougies require special care and handling. When they peel, crack, or become sticky and gummy because the coating has been damaged by cleaners and disinfectants, they must be discarded. Cleaning and sterilizing techniques that protect the instruments also protect the patient.

Washing and flushing catheters thoroughly with plain water or a nonionic detergent solution is recommended. Prolonged soaking should be avoided.

STERILIZATION. These articles may be autoclaved if special precautions are taken. They should not be soaked in water prior to sterilization. Although soaking prevents rubber from superheating at high temperatures, soaking will cause swelling and damage to woven catheters. Woven arti-

cles should be wrapped or covered and should be protected from coiling, kinking, and the pressure of other objects that distort them when they are autoclaved. Exposure to steam at 250° F. for 15 minutes is adequate for sterilization and will not damage the articles.

Woven catheters should be protected from alcohol, cresol, glycerines, strong alkalis, and acetone.

### Rubber and plastic goods

Rubber goods such as catheters, drains, drapes, bulbs, and bags can be cleaned by washing with mild soap or mild alkali cleanser. They should be thoroughly rinsed and are easier to clean if they are cared for immediately after use, when clotting and stubborn soil can be prevented.

STERILIZATION. All rubber items should be rinsed in water before they are autoclaved. The absorbed moisture will prevent superheating at autoclave temperatures. All tubes should have water in the lumen to ensure steam penetration and to evacuate air pockets.

Exposure to steam at 250° F. with 15 pounds pressure for 15 minutes will sterilize rubber goods effectively with minimal damage to the rubber.

Plastic goods, depending on their composition, may or may not withstand heat sterilization. Directions for disinfection by chemical, gas, or heat sterilization, appropriate to the item, should be obtained from the manufacturer who is acquainted with the chemical composition of the plastic item.

PROTECTIVE MEASURES. High temperatures are harmful to rubber, as is exposure to sunlight. Rubber goods must be stored in a cool, dry place and must be kept away from contact with the following substances, which cause deterioration.

1. Petroleum by-products and hydrocarbon solvents, including petrolatum, carbon tetrachloride, benzine, ether, and acetone
2. Vegetable oils
3. Alcohols

4. Sulfuric and hydrochloric acids
5. Copper and manganese metals
6. Compounds containing phenol (Lysol, cresol, carbolic acid, and the like)
7. Ammonium quaternary solutions, which will cause deterioration if the rubber is later heat sterilized
8. Formalin

### Instruments for specific uses
### Basic sets of instruments

The term *basic* refers to those instruments that are essential to accomplish a specific type of surgery. For example, a *basic major set* of instruments for general surgery should suffice to open and close the abdominal cavity, perform incision, excise, and repair gross defects in the major body musculature. A *basic minor set* of instruments for general surgery should include those items needed for simple superficial incision, excision, and suturing.

In this same way, basic instrument sets may be selected for opening other cavities such as the skull, chest, and pelvis.

### Classification of instruments
### in relation to function

Instruments are selected according to the size of the patient's body structures and the nature of the organs involved. Proper selection requires knowledge of anatomy, general understanding of surgical procedures and approaches, and knowledge of possible pathological conditions and the design and purpose of instruments.

For example, the nursing staff member needs to know that instruments for cutting and penetrating bone are different from those designed to cut soft tissues. Instruments designed for surgery on infants and of the eye, ear, blood vessels, nerves, brain, and facial structures are smaller, finer, and more delicate than those designed to handle thick fibrous tissues, cartilage, and bone.

Surgical instruments may be classified according to function. The nursing assistant should first understand the common basic maneuvers involved in every operation, which include the following.

When a body tissue is cut or divided in any way, bleeding or oozing of tissue fluids and of organ contents results. To control bleeding or oozing, clamps designed for hemostasis are applied. If these clamps are removed, hemostasis of a vessel or organ must be maintained by some other means such as ligature, suture (Chapter 6), or coagulation (Chapter 13).

When a ligature or suture is placed on the vessel, the excess free ends must be cut away with scissors of sufficient length to reach them (Chapter 6).

To view structures deep within the body, the superficial tissues must be either elevated or held apart. Retractors are designed to hold back and stabilize skin edges, muscle bodies, and major organs. There are instruments designed for holding the structures under manipulation.

The object of most surgical intervention is the removal, reconstruction, or repair of injured or diseased parts of the body. Diseased tissue is usually separated by cutting (sharp) or by blunt dissection.

When the purpose of intervention is accomplished, the surgical wound may be closed. Sewing (suturing) is the common method of holding the divided tissues together until healing takes place. Needles of various sizes and design, with or without special holders, are used to place the thread (suture material), and the excess suture is cut away (Chapter 6).

For each basic surgical maneuver, a definite class of instruments of suitable size, shape, and strength is needed. (See specific operations for illustrations.) The instruments may be classified as follows:

1. *Cutting* or *dissecting*. Included are such instruments as knives (scalpels), scissors, osteotomes, chisels, bone cutters, rongeurs, saws, drills, curettes, vein and fascia strippers, tenotomes, dermatomes, tonsillectomes, and adenotomes.

2. *Grasping* and *holding*. Included are tissue and dressing forceps, towel clamps, sponge forceps, tenacula, bone holders, rib

approximators, stone forceps, and tractors.

3. *Clamping* and *occluding*. Included are all hemostatic forceps and the clamps designed for particular organs and structures to prevent bleeding and spillage, such as the gallbladder forceps, stomach and intestinal clamps, blood vessel clamps, and kidney pedicle clamps.

4. *Exposing*. Included are all devices that enable the surgeon to approach and view the involved body parts, such as retractors, both self-retaining and manual, dilators, specula, and endoscopes.

5. *Suturing*. Included are all devices for closing the wound and holding tissues together for healing, such as needles and their holders, metal wound clips and applicators, and stapling devices.

6. *Accessory*. Included are all devices for manipulating other instruments and for facilitating a procedure, such as mallets, screwdrivers, plate benders, suction tubes and tubing, irrigating syringes, and the like.

When nursing team members can analyze the planned procedure and the approach, and can identify each instrument with its specific function, they are able to select instrument sets without omitting the necessary items and without including those which will not be used. This intelligent, understanding approach ensures economy of time and effort and protects instruments from abuse and unnecessary handling.

During the operation, the informed staff member becomes a more valuable assistant to the surgical staff.

### Hemostats

Hemostatic forceps are designed to occlude blood vessels. These are the instruments that make surgery possible by preventing excessive or fatal blood loss in the course of dissection. The well-designed modern instrument is styled for the lightness, balance, and security that yield maximum efficiency in closing the severed ends of each vessel with a minimum of tissue damage.

Hemostats are available in a wide range of sizes and shapes. The essential parts are the shanks, which incorporate the finger rings and ratchets for locking the instrument and maintaining the grip on the tissue and the jaws. The shanks cross at the locks, which maintain the alignment of the jaws. Most modern hemostats have the box lock, which is longer lasting and more securely balanced than is the old-fashioned screw lock, which works loose and permits the jaws to wobble or bend more easily.

The jaws of the hemostat may be straight or curved, may be serrated transversely or longitudinally, and may have smooth tips or end in teeth. The serrations and teeth must be cleanly cut and perfectly meshed to prevent the forceps from slipping from the tissue it must hold.

Special jaws are made for vascular clamps and have fine-meshed multiple rows of teeth longitudinally instead of the more transversely serrated jaws of most hemostats. The fine-meshed teeth of the hemostat prevent leakage and minimize trauma to the vessel walls when the severed vessels are anastomosed.

Toothed hemostats with coarse serrations are usually applied to heavy tissues, muscles, and wide organs. The fine, smooth-tipped designs are used for superficial blood vessels and fine anastomosis work on thin-walled organs.

Surgeons' preferences vary, and the surgical service usually selects one or the other of the toothed or smooth-tipped hemostat design in its varying sizes as a standard.

### Holding instruments

Tenacula and tissue-holding forceps may be equipped with multiple fine teeth like the Allis clamp or with fine serrations in specially shaped jaws. These jaws may be triangular, angular, straight, or T-shaped. The Babcock forceps is smooth and delicate, with rounded, fenestrated jaws.

Tissue forceps with smooth serrations and varying teeth combinations also belong

to the "holding" class of instruments and share variations common to other surgical forceps. They range from very small and fine to long and heavy.

Sponge-holding forceps, instruments of the cross action type, are available in 7- and 9-inch lengths with ring-shaped jaws, either serrated or smooth. A smooth sponge forceps may be used to handle tissue as a tractor.

Towel clamps are cross action instruments with ratchet- or spring-type closure. These clamps are available in lengths from 3 to 5½ inches and have sharp, needle-pointed, curved jaws that penetrate fabrics and tissue readily. They are unnecessarily traumatic when used to fix drapes to the skin, damaging both textiles and body tissues.

Modern methods of draping with adhesive fixation and sutures and new designs in drape holders are eliminating the need for these dangerous tools. Plastic clothes pegs are provided with some disposable drapes. The nonpenetrating disposable clamps for stabilizing sheets and towels represent refinements in technique.

### Needle holders

Needle holders are frequently used and are put through many different motions, even in a routine surgical operation. Since they must grasp metal rather than soft tissues or textiles, they are subject to greater damage. As a result, a fair number must be replaced regularly.

To be of service, needle holders must retain a firm grip on the needle. Many types of jaws have been designed to meet this need but all eventually become worn down and damaged beyond repair. Jaws may be flat, crosshatched in various designs, fenestrated, or grooved. Special steels of superior hardness are used to form jaw inlays that will give longer wear. The so-called diamond jaw needle holder has a tungsten carbide insert designed to prevent rotation of the needle. A shell of harder steel is provided on some needle holders.

A longitudinal groove or pit in the jaws of needle holders releases tension, prevents flattening the needle, and holds it firmly in needle holders of standard designs. The shanks of needle holders may have ratchets similar to those for locking ordinary hemostats, or they may be of a spring action and lock type. Some holders are designed with a scissors combination to save the surgeon exchanging instruments. Comparatively few use these regularly, since in most operations the first or second assistant takes responsibility for cutting the sutures as the surgeon continues to sew.

### Scissors

Scissors are designed in large, small, long, and short sizes and in various shapes for different purposes in cutting body tissues and surgical materials. Modern metallurgy provides steels that can withstand heavy usage and maintain a sharp cutting edge.

Styles of scissors range from heavy-duty to fine-duty types. Blades or shanks may be straight, curved, or angular in the desired degree and shape. Length may be obtained in the blades or in the shanks. The blades may have one sharp point and one blunt point, two sharp points, two blunt points, or tipped points.

Conventional scissors require two movements to use—one to open and another to close the jaws. Other scissors may have a spring action in the shank design that holds the jaws in an open position. A single movement pressing the spring together closes the jaws to cut. Scissors designed for delicate plastic and eye surgery are often of this latter type.

### Surgical drapes for various procedures

Draping materials that are made of natural or synthetic materials are employed in creating or setting up the sterile field in which surgery will be performed. Drapes take the form of towels, sheets, table covers, and gowns for the operating team.

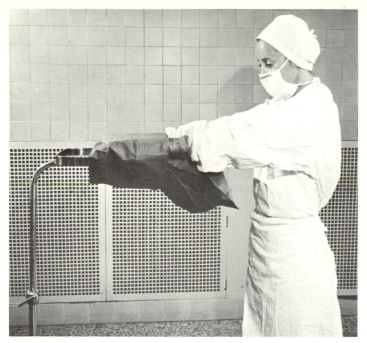

**Fig. 5-7.** Draping Mayo stand frame. Folded tray cover is slipped over frame. Worker's gloved hands are protected by cuff. Wide margin is maintained between cover and lower portion of worker's gown. Sleeves do not touch cover on stand. Cover is unfolded to extend over upright support of stand. Wide margin is maintained to ensure sterility of all working surfaces.

The draping materials are selected to provide an effective barrier between the surgical wound and the microorganisms in the surrounding unsterile environment.

### Purposes

A sterile field is created by placement of sterile sheets and towels in a specific position to maintain the sterility of surfaces on which sterile instruments and gloved hands may be placed. Objects draped include instrument tables, basin and Mayo stands, and trays. To provide for safe, easy handling and a wide margin of safety between the unsterile item and the scrubbed worker's gloved hands, the open end of the Mayo stand is folded back on itself (Fig. 5-7).

The patient and operating table are covered with sterile drapes in a manner that exposes the prepared site of incision and isolates the area of the surgical wound.

Draping procedures create an area of asepsis or a sterile field. All sterile items that come in contact with the wound are restricted within the defined area of safety to prevent transportation of microorganisms into the open wound.

### Cotton drapes

Cotton fabric, muslin with a thread count of 140 to 160 per square inch, bleached and preshrunk, is made into sheets with double-thickness specified for certain sizes or areas of the sheet. Good quality of cotton absorbs and retards fluid breakthrough for a short time. Cotton is penetrable by steam and gas under pressure for sterilization (Chapter 3). It must be carefully selected, folded, and wrapped. Cotton absorbs sound, conforms easily to body contours, and stays put.

Heavy twill, jean, and canvas materials inhibit steam penetration, are difficult to launder and handle, and retain heat on the patient; hence they should not be used for surgical drapes.

### Disposable synthetic drapes

Modern nonabsorbent synthetic disposable drapes are superior as bacterial barriers. These versatile materials can be manufactured to meet different specifications in both absorbent and nonabsorbent forms. The successful disposable drapes currently on the market are soft, lint free, lightweight, compact, readily sterilized, flame resistant and moisture resistant, nonirritating, and static free. These products are disposable and are available prepackaged and presterilized from commercial sources. White or colored drapes are available. The use of colored drapes depends on the surgeon's preferences and convictions concerning glare, eyestrain, and morale factors.

Lightness and compactness of synthetic drapes prevent heat retention by patients, contribute to ease in handling and storage, and conserve storage space and personnel's time. Because of the moisture-resistant properties of synthetic drapes, it is rarely necessary to reinforce them with additional multiple layers.

The disposable sheets are convenient for covering large surfaces such as instrument tables and operating tables used in conjunction with any adherent plastic incisional drape to cover the site of operation. Disposable drapes reduce the hazards of contamination in the presence of known infectious bacteria in body fluids and excreta and in situations in which laundering of grossly contaminated textiles is a problem.

The danger inherent in the use of synthetic drapes is that solvents, volatile liquids, and sharp instruments tend to penetrate the barrier. Manufacturers are continually improving disposable flat sheets, fenestrated drapes, and towels to permit easy handling and adaptability to the body.

### Plastic incisional drapes

Several types of plastic, impermeable polyvinyl sheeting are available in the form of sterile prepacked surgical drapes. These plastic drapes are useful adjuncts

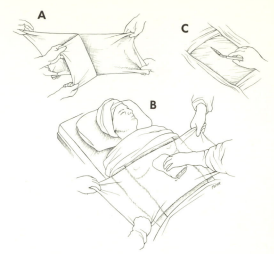

Fig. 5-8. Sterile plastic drape. For maximal sealing to prevent wound contamination, the prepared area must be dry and the drape applied carefully, avoiding wrinkles and air bubbles. **A,** Surgeon and assistant hold the plastic drape taut while another assistant peels off the back paper. **B,** Surgeon and assistant apply plastic drape to the operative site, and, using a towel, slight pressure is applied to eliminate air bubbles and wrinkles. **C,** Surgeon makes the incision through the plastic drape.

to the conventional draping procedure. They form a complete seal over the skin at the site of incision and prevent skin excretions and bacteria from coming in contact with the wound (Fig. 5-8). They obviate the need for skin towels and sponges to separate the surgeon's gloves from contact with the patient's skin. Skin color and anatomical landmarks are readily visible, and the incision is made directly through the adherent plastic drape. These materials facilitate draping of irregular body surfaces, such as neck and ear regions and extremities and joints. The draping procedure and surgical use of a commercial plastic drape are demonstrated in Fig. 5-8.

### Standard drapes

Careful planning by nursing and surgical departments helps determine the desired types and sizes of sheets and towels required for surgery. The variety of

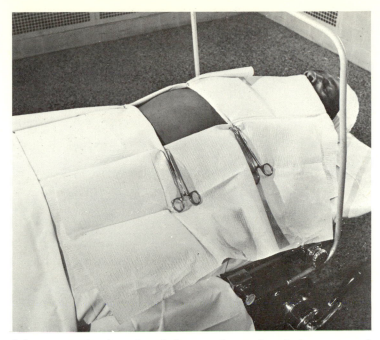

**Fig. 5-9.** Abdomen may be draped with four sterile towels, which are secured with towel forceps. Standard method of placement of disposable towels is used.

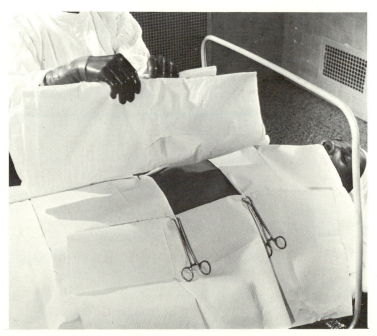

**Fig. 5-10.** Laparotomy drape. Placement of laparotomy (fenestrated, disposable) sheet. Scrubbed worker holds sheet by upper folds above prepared site of incision outlined by sterile towels. Worker stands away from operating table, protecting front of gown by wide margin from contact with unsterile surfaces.

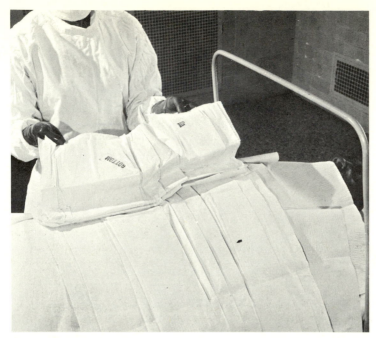

Fig. 5-11. Laparotomy drape—cont'd. Laparotomy sheet with fenestration in place is unfolded from side to side. Worker protects gloved hands under fanfolded upper edges as sheet is drawn out to drape patient and table.

drapes should be kept to a minimum. The most effective sheets and towels are simple and economical of time, body motions, and materials. Standard methods provide management control that ensures the safety of patients, simplifies teaching of staff, and conserves human and material resources.

A *whole*, or *plain, sheet* is needed to cover instrument tables, operating tables, and body regions. The sheet should be large enough to provide an adequate margin of safety between the surrounding physical environment and the prepared operative field. The sheet should meet requirements without waste. Usually two sizes of sheets suffice.

*Surgical towels* in one or two sizes should be available to drape the operative site. With the use of plastic incisional drapes, one to four surgical towels of cotton or synthetic material are usually sufficient (Fig. 5-9).

*Fenestrated*, or *slit, sheets* are used for draping patients, leaving exposed the operative site.

A typical fenestrated (laparotomy) sheet is large enough to cover the patient and operating table in any position and to extend over the anesthetist screen at the head of the table and over the foot of the table (Figs. 5-6 to 5-13). In some cases, it may incorporate the Mayo stand that has been placed over the patient.

The typical fenestrated laparotomy sheet usually can serve for most procedures on the abdomen, chest, flank, and back. This type of sheet for adults should measure 9 to 10 feet long and 6 feet wide. A rectangular slit 10 inches long by 4 inches wide beginning 4 feet from the uppermost end of the sheet at a point in the center line of the sheet is usually suitable for a routine laparotomy sheet. The fenestration area may be 9 to 10 inches in diameter. The top position of the laparotomy sheet should be identified by a suitable mark to assist workers in readily determining the short and long ends of the sheet (Figs. 5-10 and 5-11).

Other types of fenestrated sheets similar in length and width, but with smaller or

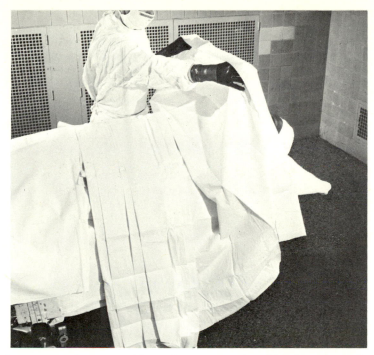

**Fig. 5-12.** Laparotomy drape—cont'd. Worker protects gloved hands under cuff of fanfolded disposable sheet and draws upper section above fenestration toward head of table, and then drapes it over anesthesia screen. Bottom portion of fanfolded sheet is then extended over foot of table in similar manner.

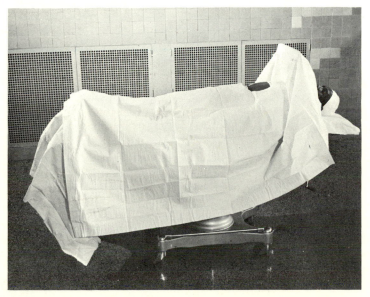

**Fig. 5-13.** Laparotomy drape completed. Fenestration provides exposure of prepared operative site.

split fenestration, may be used for the limbs, head, and neck with the patient in supine or prone position. The size of the fenestration is determined by the use for which the sheet is intended. It is fanfolded and handled as a typical laparotomy sheet.

A *perineal drape* is needed for operations on the perineum and genitalia with the patient in lithotomy position. A lithotomy drape consists of a fenestrated sheet and two triangularly shaped leggings. The leggings may be stitched to the sides of the sheet. The three-piece drape is less costly and is easier to handle and launder. A commercial, disposable lithotomy drape pack, including fenestration sheet with slit, two leggings, absorbent and nonabsorbent towels, and a small sheet, is suitable for delivery, cystoscopy, and hemorrhoidectomy and vaginal procedures.

### Assembling and folding drapes for use

The sheet should be folded so that the gowned and gloved members of the team can handle it with ease and safety. The larger, regular sheet is usually fanfolded from bottom to top. The bottom folds may be 4 inches wider than the upper ones. The small sheet is folded in half and then quartered, and the top corners of the sheet may be turned back or marked for easy identification.

Most fenestrated sheets are fanfolded to the opening from the top and the bottom, and then the folds are rolled or fanned toward the center of the opening. The edge of the top fold of the sheet is fanned so that it provides a cuff under which the worker may place his gloved hands. The top and lower sections should be identified by a marking to facilitate easy handling.

### Arrangement of instruments and other items on instrument tables

Standard arrangement of instruments, drapes, sutures, catheters, and other items on sterile tables for particular operations should be determined by the nursing service. Factors to be considered include the surgeon's method of working; ease in handling, preparing, and transporting items; and reduction in human energy. Methods of work are based on work simplification and aseptic principles.

The arrangement of the various setups should be clearly defined and understood by the personnel. Visual aids are excellent tools in teaching personnel proper procedural methods.

## ROUTINE PROCEDURES

The surgical committee of the medical staff, with the assistance of the operating room committee, is delegated by the governing board of the institution to define medical policies (Chapter 2) and rules and regulations.

### Administration of local anesthetics

Local anesthesia is anesthesia confined to one part of the body, and administration of the anesthetic agent is by topical application, local infiltration, subcutaneous injection, nerve block, or epidural or spinal injection. Local anesthesia may also be accomplished by refrigeration, which is the application of a low temperature (such as packing a limb in ice) to a part of the body to anesthetize it.

### Considerations

The topical agent may be cocaine hydrochloride, tetracaine (Pontocaine), or lidocaine applied to the mucous membranes of the nose, throat, or trachea, or it may be ethylene oxide sprayed onto a specific area of the skin. Procaine, 1%, and 0.5% to 2% lidocaine, with or without epinephrine, are the drugs commonly used for infiltration and injection anesthesia. For spinal anesthesia, the common drugs are procaine or tetracaine with 10% glucose solution.

Ampuls of drugs to be placed on a sterile field should be autoclaved. Because repeated heat sterilization of drugs may alter their properties, unused ampuls that have been autoclaved should be discarded. To conserve costs, the nurse should prepare

only the materials that will be used. Consultation with the anesthesiologist or the surgeon will provide information about drugs desired and technique to be followed.

Patients must be carefully observed for drug reactions, and emergency drugs, suction apparatus, and resuscitation equipment should be at hand. Symptoms to be observed include diaphoresis, complaints of nausea, palpitation, disturbed respiration, pallor or flushing, and convulsive movements.

### Setup

Disposable epidural or spinal sets complete with the drugs required are almost in universal use now. A sterile tray may include the following items:

    2 Luer-Lok syringes, 10 ml.
    1 Luer-Lok syringe, 2 ml.
    1 Needle set, as desired
        3 Infiltration needles: 25-gauge, ½ in.; 25-gauge, 1½ in.; 22-gauge, 2½ in.
        2 Tonsil needles, angular (optional)
        2 Spinal needles with stylets, 17 and 18 gauges, 3½ and 4 in.
    1 Medicine cup, graduated, 2 oz.
    1 Cup, metal, 6 oz.
    1 Basin, metal, 4 in. diameter
    2 Sponge-holding forceps
    4 Towel clamps (optional)
    4 Towels
    6 Sponges
    Anesthetic drugs as ordered

### Procedure

The patient should be attended by a registered nurse or an anesthesiologist when a local anesthetic is used. A general recommendation is that no more than 50 ml. of 1% solution or 100 ml. of 0.5% solution of an anesthetic drug such as lidocaine or procaine be injected per hour for local anesthesia.

POSITIONING AND PREPARATION OF THE PATIENT. Positioning and preparation of a patient will depend on the nature of the procedure. The local area is prepared, and the patient is draped in the routine manner for minor surgery.

For spinal anesthesia, the anesthetist may select a lateral recumbent position with the spine flexed for the patient, or he may have him sit up and flex the spine by bending forward. The patient needs support, protection, and assistance in maintaining these positions and in changing position after the spinal puncture and injection have been completed.

### Procedures for sponge and instrument counts

The legal liability of both the hospital and the physician has strong influence on the determination of sponge and instrument counts. The institution usually establishes a procedure that enables it to prove that due care has been exercised in the protection of patients.

#### Sponge counts

Radiopaque sponges should be used in surgery because they can be detected by x-ray examination within a wound if an incorrect count occurs.

A standard should be defined regarding the number of sponges in each package. Sponge counts are usually made whenever a body cavity is opened, as in laparotomy and chest operations; in major vaginal and perineal operations; in radical mastectomy; and in hip, shoulder, spinal, open kidney, ureter, and bladder operations.

Safety measures should be defined and observed in handling sponges during an operation. Each type and size of sponge should be kept separate from the other types. Sponges must be kept away from other supplies such as towels, sheets, and laparotomy packs to prevent a sponge from being carried inadvertently into the wound or misplaced.

When a body cavity is opened, free sponges must be removed from the operative field. From this point, free sponges should be handed to the surgeon only on specific request. Laparotomy packs with tapes or sponges on forceps are used within the open cavity.

It may be safer if the procedure calls for handing off all sponges and packs

from the field and wound as the first line of closure sutures is placed. This helps ensure that all sponges have been removed. It does little good to ascertain the number of sponges as the closure begins if a sponge that is being used to pack the wound is subsequently forgotten or is not removed before the final closure. After all sponges are discarded and counted, fresh ones are then supplied to complete wound closure.

Linen or waste containers should never be emptied nor their contents removed from the operating room until the counts have proved to be correct.

THE FOUR COUNTS. A count generally falls into four parts. The first count is performed by those who assemble the sponges in packages. Commercial suppliers provide prepackaged sterile sponges with verification of count for operating room use.

The second count is made by the scrubbed and circulating nurses or operating room technicians at the time the sponges are handed onto the sterile field.

The third count is made as the first line of closure sutures is placed. The fourth count is a recheck as the skin is closed.

When a hollow organ such as the uterus is opened, an additional check of the count is made as the organ is closed.

DUTIES OF CIRCULATING AND SCRUBBED NURSING TEAM. The circulating nurse opens the outside wrapper and transfers the sponges to the sterile field. The scrubbed nurse or operating room technician separates each sponge and counts audibly with the circulating nurse the number present. If the number is deficient according to the standard for the package, the entire package is discarded and returned to central service, and the discrepancy is noted on a slip.

The circulating nurse records on an appropriate form the number of sponges of each type on the sterile field and prepares a receptacle for soiled sponges by lining it with a moistened polyethylene conductive bag.

The scrubbed nurse or operating room technician places each type of sponge in a designated area on the table, keeping each sponge free of other items, attaches rings or disks to laparotomy packs if required, and attaches round sponges to serrated sponge-holding forceps.

DURING SURGERY. The scrubbed nursing team member discards soiled sponges and packs in a prepared kick bucket or receptacle without touching them or soiling her gloved hands.

The circulating nurse transfers and counts discarded sponges and places them in waterproof bags according to type and standard number previously recorded. When the prescribed number of discarded sponges per unit is reached and sealed in the bag, the number is checked off on a form.

At the beginning of the first line of closure sutures, all sponges are removed from the wound and operative field and discarded. The scrubbed nurse or operating room technician gives the count of all unused sponges according to type left on the sterile table.

The circulating nurse counts and totals all discarded sponges per unit bag and those in the kick bucket, adds the total number of discarded sponges to that number remaining on the sterile field, and subtracts this final number from the total number of sponges recorded on the form to determine if the two completely balance. If they do, she so informs the surgeon, stating, "First sponge count is correct."

*If the count does not balance,* the scrubbed nurse or operating room technician assists in finding the sponges and recounts the number of unused sponges on the field.

The circulating nurse opens the bags and recounts the discarded sponges. If a missing sponge cannot be found, an x-ray film may be taken to help establish whether or not the sponge is within the patient.

An incident form is made out by the circulating nurse and is signed by both scrubbed and circulating team members.

AT BEGINNING OF FIRST LINE OF SKIN CLO-
SURE. The scrubbed nurse or operating
room technician gives the count of all
sponges remaining on the sterile field.

The circulating nurse counts units of
sponges and discarded sponges in the
kick bucket, totals the numbers as in previous procedure for the first count, and
tells the surgeon, "Final count is complete."

The wound is closed when the correct
count has been ascertained. Sponges are
discarded in the routine manner.

### Instrument counts

The worker who assembles the tray
counts all items according to standard and
signs his own name on a designated slip
kept with the tray. The scrubbed nurse
or operating room technician rechecks the
count during arrangement of instruments
on the sterile field and again at the beginning of wound closure. The procedure
is performed as described for the sponge
count.

## Procedure for bone bank

The bone bank procedure consists of the
selection of bone for banking from persons
who have had a bone resection such as removal of a rib or an amputation. Bone is
not taken from patients who have a neoplastic or infectious disease.

### Setup

The setup for this procedure is the same
as that for an ostectomy and includes bone
saws, bone cutters, and rongeurs, plus the
following items:

Sterile jars with screw caps
Sterile dry test tubes with cotton stoppers
Labels
Laboratory culture slips
Ledger for recording bank contents

### Preparation of the bone

1. The surgeon takes the bone to be
saved and cleans it of all extraneous tissue,
cartilage, and periosteum.
2. The cortical bone is cut into strips

about 1 inch wide and 4 inches long. Cancellous bone is cut into pieces as desired.

3. The bone fragments are placed in
sterile jars of appropriate size, and the jars
are sealed with screw caps.

4. The jars are labeled with the donor's
name, numbered in sequence, and sent for
storage in a deep-freeze refrigerator.

### Bone culture

At the time the bone is obtained, a
small chip is removed from the specimen
and is placed in a dry culture tube that
is plugged with sterile cotton. The bacteriology laboratory makes a culture from
this chip of bone.

If the culture report is negative, which
indicates no bacterial growth, the bone is
considered ready for use. No further cultures of the banked specimen are taken
until the bone is used. If bone is rebanked, another specimen chip for culture
should be taken at the time of rebanking.

If the culture report is positive, which
indicates bacterial growth, the bone is
treated as if it were contaminated. It is removed from deep freeze, allowed to thaw,
and soaked for 1 hour in a germicide
such as 1:1000 solution of benzalkonium
chloride. Aseptic technique is used, the
bone is rinsed in normal saline solution,
and a new chip of bone is removed for
culture. Subsequent cultures are taken at
weekly intervals until three consecutive
negative reports have been obtained.

## Procedure for cartilage bank
### Collection

Cartilage is usually selected from patients between 17 and 45 years of age
and sometimes at the discretion of the
surgeon. Cartilage from patients younger
than 17 years of age is too small and is also
readily absorbed, and cartilage from patients over 45 years of age tends to be
yellow, brittle, or calcified.

Chest infection, positive serological
tests, contagious disease, bacteremia, and
malignancy are all contraindications to
taking cartilage from a patient.

The perichondrium is removed from the cartilage, and the cartilage is placed in a sterile jar. The jar is then sealed, labeled, and stored in the freezing unit of a refrigerator. Cartilage that has not been freed of perichondrium is placed in a sterile jar and stored in a freezing unit until the cleaning process can be done. It has proved unsatisfactory to preserve cartilage before the cleaning process has been done.

### Storage requirements

1. Prepared cartilage is kept in the refrigerator at 40° F.
2. Cartilage fresh from a patient, with the perichondrium removed, is placed in a sterile jar and covered with a germicide such as 1:1000 solution of thimerosal (merthiolate). The cartilage should be covered by at least 1 inch of solution.
3. The jar cap is sealed with adhesive and labeled, giving the patient's name and number, location of cartilage, date of procurement, and date of first culture.
4. At the time of procurement of cartilage, the first culture is taken. A small sliver of cartilage is cut from the main body to be stored and is placed in a sterile culture tube. These tubes, which should not contain broth or other culture media, should be specially prepared by the bacteriology laboratory and should have adequate cotton stoppers to prevent outside contamination of the tube and cotton. These articles are autoclaved with the sterile glass jar and cap and placed on the sterile field until the cartilage is properly prepared.
5. Culture slips should be made out in the routine manner and stamped to indicate that the cartilage is to be tested for sterility only. The labels attached to the culture tubes must also be filled out as for a routine culture.
6. Culture reports should be returned to the operating room nursing service where the records for the tissue banks are kept. Cartilage for which the first culture is positive should be cultured every week until three negative reports have been received.

7. Jars containing cartilage being held until three negative culture reports have been received should be stored in a refrigerator. After the three negative reports, the cartilage is ready to be used and can then be stored at room temperature in a sterile receptacle containing a 1:5000 solution of thimerosal in a designated area such as the plastic surgery division.
8. All cartilage should be cultured, and the preservative solution should be changed once every 6 to 8 weeks after the cartilage has been marked "ready for use."
9. If at any time the culture report of "ready" cartilage is positive, the procedure of storage in a germicidal solution is observed until three successive negative reports have been received. If two successive positive culture reports are received, the cartilage should be discarded.
10. Unused "ready" cartilage can be rebanked, but a specimen must again be cultured in the prescribed manner.

### Culture

The procedure is scheduled as a regular operation, and aseptic technique is maintained. The nursing staff sets up equipment and supplies, and the surgical staff carries out the sterile procedure. A separate setup is necessary for each jar of banked cartilage to be cultured.

#### Setup

The setup for each jar of cartilage should include the following items:

1 Culture tube
1 Sponge forceps or hemostat for removing cartilage from jar
1 Scalpel
1 Thumb forceps
1 Jar with screw cap
  Germicide, e.g., thimerosal (Merthiolate) solutions, 1:1000 and 1:5000
  Forms to accompany test tubes
  Labels for jars and tubes
  Ledgers for recording data on banked tissue, on culture reports, and on antiseptic storage solutions

#### Procedure

1. Individual sterile setups are prepared for each jar of cartilage to be cultured. The

surgeon scrubs, gowns, and gloves in the routine manner.

2. The circulating worker removes the top from the jar. The surgeon removes the cartilage from the jar with a sponge forceps or long hemostat, using instruments exclusively and avoiding contamination of his gloves or gown so that he may proceed from one jar to another without cross contamination.

3. The surgeon cuts a small piece of cartilage from the specimen, drops it into the culture tube, and stoppers the tube with cotton. He then hands the tube off to the circulating worker.

4. The surgeon drops the main cartilage specimen into a fresh jar. The worker covers this specimen to depth of 1 inch with the appropriate antiseptic solution. The surgeon screws on the sterile cap and hands the jar off. Each specimen is handled in the same manner.

5. The worker labels the culture tubes and the storage jars, keeping them in order and properly identified. The date of the culturing procedure is recorded in the ledger, and the results of all cultures are entered. Jars are labeled "ready for use" after the third successive negative report.

## Procedure for preparation of bone wax

Bone wax is sometimes used to control bleeding of bony structures such as in endaural, orthopedic, or neurological surgery.

The Horsley bone wax formula is as follows:

Beeswax, 87 parts
Olive oil, 12 parts
Salicylic acid, 1 part

Modifications of this formula have been used by suture manufacturers in preparation of sterile wax.

In the immediate preparation of sterile wax for use in surgery, the container of wax is placed in warm sterile water for a few seconds to soften it. The container is opened, and the wax is scooped out. The wax is broken into small pieces and

kneaded between the gloved hands to form small rounded pieces which are then placed on a small metal tray for the surgeon's use. The consistency of the wax must be pliable, yet firm. Hard wax will crumble, and very soft wax will not hold to tissue or bone.

## Procedure for preservation of skin

A skin graft is a temporary measure in which an excess piece of skin is used to cover a denuded area. The skin can be obtained from the patient on whom it is to be grafted or from a donor. Whatever the source, the skin must be preserved until it is used.

### Setup

The setup should include the skin specimen and the following items:

Sterile strip or square of gutta-percha or Dermatape large enough for stretched-out specimen
Sterile gauze compresses
Basin with normal saline solution
Sterile Vinylite of sufficient size to wrap specimen
Sterile jar with screw cap
Adhesive tape for sealing and labeling specimen jar

### Procedure

1. The skin should be kept on the instrument table until it is ready for storage.

2. The skin is gently flattened and smoothed out and is then placed on a piece of gutta-percha, with its external surface facing downward. If Dermatape is used. the skin is left adherent to the Dermatape. The mounted skin is wrapped in gauze sponges, saturated with saline solution, and then folded into a small packet so that it will fit into the jar.

3. The packet of skin is wrapped in a small square of Vinylite so that moisture will be retained.

4. The scrubbed nurse or operating room technician places the packet of skin in the sterile jar and screws on the cap.

5. The circulating nurse labels the jar with the patient's name and history num-

ber, location of donor site, date of operation, name of the operating surgeon, and date that skin is to be discarded, which is 3 weeks after removal of the skin from the body.

6. The preserved skin is stored in a refrigerator at 40° F. until it is used or discarded.

### Procedure for eye bank

See Chapter 9.

### Procedure for emergency signals

Every operating room suite must have an emergency system that can be activated from within each operating room proper. A light outside the door of the room involved should appear, and a buzzer or bell should sound in a central nursing or anesthesia area. The signals should remain on until the light is turned off at the source. All personnel should be familiar with the system and should know both how to send a signal and how to respond to it. Such a system, restricted to use in life-threatening emergencies, saves invaluable time in bringing additional assistance.

### Procedure for cardiopulmonary resuscitation

Cardiopulmonary resuscitation is the immediate restoration of circulatory and respiratory functions by means of manual and mechanical methods and administration of drugs to provide for ventilation and conversion of the heartbeat to normal sinus rhythm.

#### Considerations

Cardiac arrest, standstill, or fibrillation may occur in patients undergoing surgery because of the hazards of surgery such as blood loss and shock or unfavorable reaction to anesthesia such as hypoxia and poor ventilation.

For survival of the patient, all body organs and tissues must receive sufficient oxygen via the circulatory system. The circulating blood must carry the oxygen supplied by pulmonary ventilation. Ventilation may be reestablished by mouth-to-mouth breathing and by other manual and mechanical methods of artificial respiration, such as oxygen apparatus, face mask, and intubation (artificial airway and endotracheal tube). Cardiac compression by pressure on the closed chest, manual compression of the heart, or thoracotomy is directed toward reestablishment of circulation.

A cardiopulmonary arrest cart should be available for immediate use. Well-defined written instructions should be clearly understood by all personnel. Periodic practice sessions in relation to delegated duties should be scheduled as part of the safety program.

#### Setup

A movable emergency cart or table containing all the items that may be needed should be prepared and immediately available. The operating room committee and the surgical staff should determine the equipment needed and the plan of treatment to be initiated, stressing the hospital team approach.

The equipment should include the following items:

**Emergency thoracotomy kit**
- 1 Scalpel handle no. 4 with blade no. 20
- 1 Rib retractor, wedge retractor, or notched tube or
- 1 Finochietto or Harken self-retaining retractor

**Ventilation and resuscitation equipment**
- Resuscitubes
- Ambu resuscitator (air shields type), anesthesia machine, or Kreiselmann resuscitator
- Airways
- Endotracheal tubes
- Laryngoscope
- Suctioning apparatus

**Syringes (Luer control-type) and needles** (each hospital committee determines sizes needed)
- 5 Syringes, 2 ml.
- 1 Syringe, 10 ml.
- 2 Syringes, 20 ml.
- 1 Syringe, 50 ml.
- 5 Needles, 25-gauge, ⅝ in.
- 5 Needles, 20-gauge, 1½ in.
- 5 Needles, 18-gauge, 1½ in.

**Emergency drugs**

Sodium bicarbonate
Isoproterenol (Isuprel)
Calcium chloride or calcium gluconate
Epinephrine
Lanatoside C (Cedilanid)
Caffeine and sodium benzoate
Aminophylline
Procaine hydrochloride
Potassium hydrochloride
Procaine amide (Pronestyl)
Levarterenol (Levophed)

**Infusion equipment**

Fluids for intravenous injection
Phleboclysis set
Infusion tubing sets
Blood
Cutdown set and intracatheters

**Cardiac support equipment**

Defibrillator (pacemaker)
Cardiac monitoring equipment (electroenceph-
alograph and electrocardiograph)

OPEN CHEST SET. The items may include
the following:

**Cutting instruments**

1 Scapel handle no. 4 with blade no. 20
1 Mayo scissors, straight
1 Suture scissors

**Holding instruments**

2 Tissue forceps, 1 and 2 teeth, 5½ in.
1 Tissue forceps, 1 and 2 teeth, 8 in.
1 Foerster sponge forceps, 10 in.
4 Backhaus towel clamps, 5 in.
1 Rib approximator

**Clamping instruments**

6 Halsted hemostats, straight, 5½ in.
6 Crile hemostats, curved, 6¼ in.
2 Rochester-Ochsner hemostats, straight, 1 and
2 teeth, 8 in.

**Exposing instruments**

1 Pair Volkmann retractors, blunt, 4-pronged,
8½ in.

**Suturing instruments**

2 Mayo-Hegar needle holders, medium, 6 in.
3 Ferguson needles, medium
Prepackaged no. 3-0 silk on straight milliner
needles

**Accessory instruments**

1 Suction tubing and tube
1 Plastic chest drainage catheter
1 Rubber drainage tube, large, no. 28 or 32
Fr.

### Instructions for cardiac arrest

The instructions for cardiac arrest should
be printed on a laminated board and posted
in a designated area in each room. Instructions may read as follows:

**Respiratory measures**

1. Establish an airway.
2. Connect the airway to an oxygen supply.
3. Practice artificial ventilation.
4. Lower the patient's head.

**Cardiac measures**

1. Apply closed chest massage.
2. Apply open heart massage, as follows.
   a. Enter the left side of the chest through
      an incision extended from the sternal
      margin to the midaxillary line.
   b. Insert a rib wedge or chest retractor.
   c. Massage the heart to produce a palpa-
      ble peripheral pulse at a rate of 60 to
      70 beats per minute.

The instructions must be carried out by
a physician.

### Nursing service duties

1. Ring the emergency bell to alert the
operating room supervisor, surgeon, and
anesthesiologist. Note the exact time of
arrest and procure additional assistance as
required.

2. In the absence of an anesthetist or
resuscitative equipment, assist in ventilation of the patient by means of mouth-to-
mouth breathing or other artificial respiration.

3. Make a temporary thoracotomy cardiac arrest kit available to the surgeon.

4. Prepare and administer medications
as ordered.

5. Procure and prepare infusions or transfusions as ordered.

6. Procure cardiac defibrillator, pacemaker, and monitor, as required.

7. Prepare or procure open chest setup
for open massage as ordered.

8. Assist in chest closure.

9. Chart the care given.

10. Notify all hospital information and
administrative services, as the situation
requires. Included would be a request to
the service supplying religious rites and

notification to the proper services of the change in the patient's condition and the need to inform the patient's family.

Routine hospital emergency measures are started for cardiac arrest care. Resuscitation and fibrillation of the cardiac arrest patient is usually done in the cardiac care unit, with special monitoring and nursing services.

## REFERENCES

1. Beal, J. M., and Echenhoff, J. E., editors: Intensive and recovery room care, New York, 1969, The Macmillan Co.
2. Berry, E., and Kohn, M. L.: Introduction to operating-room technique, ed. 3, New York, 1966, McGraw-Hill Book Co.
3. Burgess, R. E.: Aseptic management of disposables, Hosp. Top. 48:95, Jan., 1970.
4. Crawford, M.: Infection control in the operating room, A.O.R.N. Journal 11:54, May, 1970.
5. Dineen, P.: Penetration of surgical draping material by bacteria, Hospitals 43:82, Oct. 1, 1969.
6. Evans, M. J.: Some contributions to prevention of infections, Nurs. Clin. North Am. 3: 641, Dec., 1968.
7. Guest, P. G., Sikora, V. W., and Lewis, B.: Static electricity in hospital operating suites, Washington, D. C., 1962, United States Bureau of Mines, bulletin no. 520.
8. Hayt, E., and Hayt, L. R.: Law of hospital, physician and patient, New York, 1962, Hospital Textbook Co.
9. Hershey, N.: Surgical intervention and the law. In Professional responsibility for nursing care of the surgical patient, New York, 1963, American Nurses' Association.
10. Litsky, B. Y.: Bacteriological housekeeping, A.O.R.N. Journal 9:37, May, 1969.
11. Malcolm, J. A.: Care of endoscopic instruments, Hosp. Top. 54:75, July, 1967.
12. National Fire Protection Association: Code for flammable anesthetics, Boston, 1968, The Association.
13. National Fire Protection Association: Recommended safe practice for hospital operating rooms, Boston, 1968, The Association.
14. Nicholes, P. S.: Comparative evaluation of a new surgical mask medium, Surg. Gynecol. Obstet. 118:579, 1964.
15. Pearsall, A. J.: Selection and handling of equipment. In Professional responsibility for nursing care of the surgical patient, New York, 1963, American Nurses' Association.
16. Perkins, E. W., and Cibula, M. E.: Aseptic techniques for operating room personnel, ed. 3, Philadelphia, 1964, W. B. Saunders Co.
17. Sister Mary Louise: The operating room technician, ed. 2, St. Louis, 1968, The C. V. Mosby Co.
18. Spivak, J., and Watt, D. S.: Disposable O. R. packs, Hospitals 44:105, July 1, 1970.
19. Thomas, G. J.: Fire and explosion hazards with flammable anesthetics and their control, J. Natl. Med. Assoc. 52:401, Nov., 1960.
20. Thompson, L. R.: Maintaining asepsis. In Professional responsibility for nursing care of the surgical patient, New York, 1963, American Nurses' Association.
21. Vallari, R.: Preventive maintenance program. In Professional responsibility for nursing care of the surgical patient, New York, 1963, American Nurses' Association.
22. Willingham, J.: Logic of operating room nursing, ed. 2, New York, 1967, Springer Publishing Co., Inc.

# CHAPTER 6

# Sutures, surgical needles, and suturing techniques

JACQUELYN C. TREYBAL

## HISTORY AND EVOLUTION OF SURGICAL SUTURES
### (2000 B.C. TO PRESENT)

The development of surgical sutures has been closely allied with the development of the art of surgery. Medical writings of ancient Egyptian and Assyrian cultures dating back to 2000 B.C. mention the various materials used, to a limited extent, for suturing and ligating. *Suture* is a generic term for all materials used to bring severed body tissue together and to hold these tissues in their normal position until healing takes place. A *ligature* is a strand of suture material used to "tie off" (seal) blood vessels to prevent hemorrhage and simple bleeding or to isolate a mass of tissue to be excised (cut out).

The concept of suturing and ligating is also recorded in the writings of the father of medicine, Hippocrates, born in 460 B.C. Gut of sheep intestines was first mentioned as a suture material in the writings of Galen around A.D. 200. The Arabian surgeon Rhazes is credited with first employing surgical gut, or *catgut*, in A.D. 900 for suturing abdominal wounds. The word *catgut* is a misnomer, however. The Arabic word *kit* means a dancing master's fiddle, but the word catgut has no relation to a cat.

In spite of these promising early beginnings, the science of surgery, including suturing and ligating, advanced and then regressed, with several cultures never advancing much beyond the rudimentary stages. The principal reasons surgery and its allied practices did not progress in early times were the critical problems of hemorrhage, pain, and infection. Even Ambroise Paré, the famous French army surgeon of the middle 1500's who developed the technique for ligating to replace cautery in treatment of traumatic war injuries, was confronted with the grim fact that severe pain and subsequent infection markedly curtailed advancements made possible by surgical repair and correction.

Surgery offered little promise of developing as a truly effective healing science until the nineteenth century when an American surgeon, Crawford W. Long of Georgia, demonstrated the use of ether as an anesthetic (1842) and Joseph Lister of England first used carbolic acid solution to attempt antiseptic surgery (1865). Lister also experimented with surgical gut as an absorbable suture material and recognized the need for sterile surgical sutures.

Progress in the development of surgical sutures was rapid after the middle 1800's. By 1901, catgut and kangaroo gut were available to the surgeon in sterile glass tubes. Since then, numerous materials have been employed as sutures and ligatures. Gold, silver, metallic wire, silkworm gut, silk, cotton, linen, tendon, and intestinal tissue from virtually every creature that walks, swims, or flies have been used at one

time or another during the evolution of surgery. During the twentieth century, surgical gut, silk, and cotton emerged as the most commonly used suture materials.

As late as the latter 1930's, the sterility of sutures commercially prepared and sterilized by manufacturers was subject to question. In addition, sutures varied considerably in their physical properties, such as diameter and strength. From the 1940's to the present, great strides have been made in the uniform preparation and sterilization of suture materials. Today the surgeon is assured of sterility, relatively uniform physical properties, and predictable performance in the sutures he receives in the operating room.

One further development in the history of surgical sutures is worthy of note. Since the early 1950's, a rapid trend toward individually packaged, presterilized needle and nonneedle sutures has resulted in operating rooms receiving more and more ligatures and sutures in a ready-to-use form. This trend relieves operating room nursing personnel of the time-consuming, and consequently expensive, tasks of preparing sutures and needles for sterilization and the actual sterilization process.

## KINDS OF SUTURE MATERIALS

Suture materials may be divided into two major categories: absorbable and nonabsorbable.

*Absorbable suture* is that which can be digested and assimilated by the tissues during the healing process. The United States Pharmacopeia defines an absorbable surgical suture as a "sterile strand prepared from collagen derived from healthy mammals. . . . It is capable of being absorbed by living mammalian tissue, but may be treated to modify its resistance to absorption. It may be impregnated with a suitable antimicrobial agent. It may be colored by a color additive approved by the federal Food and Drug Administration."*

---

*From The Pharmacopeia of the United States of America, eighteenth revision, September, 1970, p. 703.

Absorbable sutures vary in treatment, color, size, packaging, and resistance to absorption, according to their purpose. They may be either Type A suture or Type C suture. Both types consist of processed strands of collagen, but Type C suture is processed by physical or chemical means so as to provide greater resistance to absorption in living mammalian tissue.

Although they are not specifically recognized by the U.S.P., a Type B (mild treatment) and Type D (prolonged treatment) absorbable suture is supplied by some manufacturers.

*Nonabsorbable sutures* are strands of material that effectively resist enzymatic digestion in living animal tissue. A single strand may be composed of metal or of organic material. Each strand is of substantially uniform diameter throughout its length. It may be composed of a single filament or of filaments or fibers rendered into a thread by spinning, twisting, braiding, or by any combination thereof. It may be coated or uncoated. It may be untreated for reduction of capillarity and designated Type A, untreated and capillary, or it may be treated to reduce capillarity and designated Type B, treated and noncapillary. It may be uncolored, naturally colored, or dyed with a suitable dyestuff.

### Absorbable suture materials
#### Surgical gut

The sterility of absorbable surgical gut is now guaranteed. The elaborate processes of mechanical and chemical cleaning of the raw gut, sterilization with ethylene oxide gas or cobalt 60 irradiation, and storage in hermetically sealed packages all ensure sterility. Modern manufacturing processes also provide tensile strength, controlled absorption, and the predictable results desired by the surgeon performing modern surgery.

Proper chromicizing of gut ensures the integrity of the suture and maintenance of its strength during the early stages of wound healing. It enables the wound with slow healing power to gather sufficient

strength of its own before the suture is entirely absorbed. To chromicize the gut strands, the tanning process is applied either to the submucosal ribbons before they have been twisted into the strand or to the finished strand after it has been formed from the ribbons. The strength of the chrome content and the duration of the chromicizing process are accurately controlled and tested.

The absorption rate of surgical gut is also influenced by the type of body tissue it contacts and, to some extent, by the patient's general physical condition. Studies also show that surgical gut is absorbed faster in serous or mucous membranes than in muscular tissues. When fine chromic gut is properly buried in successive layers of the gastrointestinal tract, for example, it retains its strength for a sufficient length of time for primary union to take place.

### Tensile strength and size

To meet U.S.P. specifications, processed ribbons are spun into strands of various sizes ranging at present from the finest size no. 7-0 to the heaviest, no. 3. However, the U.S.P. identifies absorbable suture sizes from no. 9-0 to no. 5. Tensile strength is measured on the basis of knot-pull strength rather than on the basis of straight-pull strength. Minimum knot-pull strengths are specified for each size; minimum and maximum limits on diameter are also specified. For example, on size no. 6-0, diameter limits are 0.089 to 0.127 mm., with a minimum knot-pull strength of 0.18 kg. Size no. 1 has diameter limits of 0.526 to 0.584 mm., with a minimum knot-pull strength of 3.80 kg.

The smaller-sized sutures are in greater demand because the finer diameter provides better handling qualities and smaller knots. Improved suturing techniques are possible with sutures of finer diameter. Studies indicate that wounds heal more quickly and with less tissue reaction when sutures with a finer gauge are used. Because surgical gut is the most versatile of all suture material, it may be used in practically all tissue.

### Packaging and storage methods

Almost all suture materials are now supplied directly by manufacturers in some form of sterile package ready for immediate

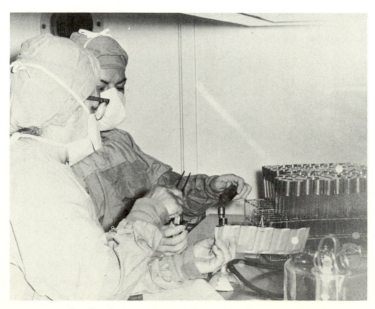

**Fig. 6-1.** Preparation of individual packages of suture. (Courtesy Ethicon, Inc., Somerville, N. J.)

use (Fig. 6-1). The U.S.P. specifies, "Preserve dry or in fluid, in containers so designed that sterility is maintained until the container is opened." The so-called *wet pack* method, now obsolete, consisted of sealing the sutures in glass tubes, foil or plastic packets, immersing these in a chemical solution, and storing them in glass jars or metal cans.

The current dry packaging method seals the suture material in a primary inner packet, which may or may not contain fluid, inside a dry outer overwrap strip packet. This unit is sterilized. This method permits self dispensing onto the sterile field. Various forms of foil, plastic, and special paper are used for both the inner and outer packets. Packages may be stored in any moistureproof and dustproof container.

Each primary suture packet is self-contained, and its sterility for each patient is assured as long as the integrity of the packet is maintained. Dispensing time and preparation time are reduced to a minimum. Unused and unopened primary packets may be returned to the manufacturer for repackaging and application of a new overwrap packet. The suture itself remains sterile in the sealed primary packet; only the outer surface of the primary packet and its overwrap packet require sterilization.

Absorbable surgical sutures are supplied by the manufacturer in sterile single- or multiple-strand packets, with or without a needle attached to the strand.

### Sterilization properties

The label *nonboilable* is used to indicate that the packaging method does not permit application of heat (boiling or autoclaving) for resterilization of the exterior of the packet without damage to the contents. Either the tubing fluid or the foil packet may be involved.

Nursing personnel should follow the precise recommendations of manufacturers for resterilization of their products if patients are to receive the benefits of the improved and safer suture materials now provided by modern manufacturing and packaging techniques. Once an absorbable suture strand is removed from the primary packet, it cannot be resterilized for future use.

### Restoring pliability

To provide maximal pliability of nonboilable surgical gut sutures, the gut should be used immediately after removal from the packet. When a gut suture is removed from its packet and is not used at once, the alcohol evaporates, which in turn causes the strand to lose it pliability. The strand's pliability may be restored just prior to use, by immersing it in sterile water or normal saline solution, preferably at 37° C. If the latter method is used, the gut strand should be immersed for only a few seconds.

### Other absorbable suture materials

*Fascia lata* is not true absorbable material, but sutures made of it become part of the tissue after the wound has healed. Fascia lata sutures are used to provide additional support to weakened fascial layers. This material is obtained from the fibrous tissue that covers the thigh muscles of beef cattle; it is prepared in strips (each 8 inches long and ¼ inch wide) and packaged in sterile containers. When an autogenous graft is used, the fascia lata may be taken from the patient, usually from the thigh.

*Bone wax*, although not a suture, is rubbed into bleeding stomas on the surface of bone to stop the bleeding. Modifications of the Horsley bone wax formula are used by suture manufacturers in preparing sterile bone wax. The handling of sterile wax for immediate use in a patient has been described in Chapter 5.

### Nonabsorbable suture materials

Nonabsorbable suture materials are not absorbed in tissues during the process of wound healing. Generally, the material remains encapsulated or walled off by the tissues around it. In suturing of skin, for which nonabsorbable materials are often the choice, the sutures are removed before healing is complete. Sometimes the

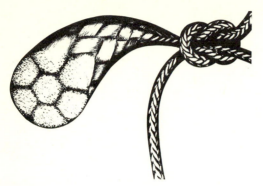

Fig. 6-2. Suture showing braiding of many strands into one. (Courtesy Ethicon, Inc., Somerville, N. J.)

skin edges are approximated with metal clips. The most common nonabsorbable materials are silk, nylon, polyester fiber, polypropylene, cotton, and stainless steel wire.

### Silk

Silk is the most widely used nonabsorbable suture material. It is prepared from thread spun by the silkworm larva in making its cocoon. Top-grade raw silk is processed to remove the natural waxes and gum, manufactured into threads, and dyed with a vegetable dye. The strands of silk are either twisted or braided to form the suture. The braided type is preferred because of its high tensile strength and better handling qualities (Fig. 6-2). Untreated silk has a capillary action through which body fluids may transmit infection along the length of the suture strand. For this reason, surgical silk is treated to render it *noncapillary* (able to withstand the action of body fluids and moisture). It is available in no. 9-0 to no. 5 sizes.

Braided surgical silk may be purchased on nonsterile spools or in packets or precut lengths, with or without swaged needles. The sterile, precut type relieves the nurse of having to expend time to prepare similar strands from spools.

Silk is considered to be an efficient suture when perfect aseptic techniques are applied and when the tissues are not infected. The commonly used Halsted silk technique includes placing fine-sized interrupted sutures, cutting the suture ends close to the knot, and carrying out strict aseptic measures.

### Cotton

Surgical cotton sutures are made from individual cotton fibers that are combed, aligned, and twisted to form a finished strand. They differ from other sutures in that twisted cotton gains 10% in tensile strength when wet; therefore they should be dampened when used. Fine cotton sutures, when buried in tissue, produce minimum tissue reaction. Ordinary sewing cotton, however, lacks the required tensile strength and smoothness throughout the strand and is difficult to handle. Methods of sterilization are described in Chapter 3.

### Synthetic materials
### Surgical nylon

Surgical nylon is a synthetic polyamide material. It is available in two forms: multifilament (braided) and monofilament strands. Multifilament nylon is relatively inert in tissues and has a high tensile strength. It is used in conditions similar to those in which silk and cotton are used. Because of its elasticity, the operator usually ties three knots in the small-sized sutures and a double square knot in the large-sized sutures. Monofilament nylon is a smooth noncapillary material used for closing skin edges and for tension sutures.

### Surgical polyester fiber

Surgical polyester fiber is available in two forms: a nontreated polyester fiber suture and a braided polyester fiber suture that has been specifically impregnated with Teflon. Polyester fiber is available in fine filaments that make it possible to braid multiple filaments into various suture sizes. They are closely braided to provide a smooth surface and good handling properties.

This material has many advantages over other nonabsorbable sutures. It has greater

tensile strength, minimal tissue reaction, maximum visibility, nonabsorbency, and no appreciable effect from repeated sterilization. The treated polyester fiber suture offers additional advantages of smooth passage through tissue and smooth tie-down on each throw of the knot.

Polyester fiber sutures are available in sterile packets of precut lengths, sizes no. 6-0 to no. 5, with or without swaged needles, or on nonsterile spools.

### Polypropylene

Polypropylene is a clear or pigmented polymer. This monofilament suture material is used for cardiovascular, general, and plastic surgery. Polypropylene is extremely inert in tissue, has high tensile strength, causes minimal tissue reaction, and holds knots well. Surgeons have indicated that polypropylene sutures can be tied into more secure knots than most other synthetic suture materials. Sizes available are no. 7-0 to no. 2, swaged to needles.

### Linen

Surgical linen is made of twisted linen thread that has sufficient tensile strength to be used as suture material. It may be impregnated with a nonpermeable material that makes it smooth and noncapillary. Linen is used almost exclusively in gastrointestinal surgery, sometimes as a pursestring suture around the stump of the appendix, or as a skin suture.

### Surgical stainless steel

Metallic suture materials have been used for centuries. The metal sutures of today are made of stainless steel. The history of the development of a truly surgical stainless steel dates back to the 1930's. W. W. Babcock of Temple University in Philadelphia wrote many papers on the economy of its use. Prompted by the Depression and hospital economics, the use of commerical stainless steel gained impetus. Commercial steel proved to be economical, but, unfortunately, it lacked uniformity in many of its characteristics.

Surgical stainless steel today, as supplied by suture manufacturers, is formulated to be compatible with stainless steel implants and prostheses. This formula, 316L (L for low carbon), assures absence of toxic elements, optimal strength, flexibility, and uniform size.

Surgical stainless steel, monofilament and multifilament, has an enviable reputation among nonabsorbable sutures for strength, inertness, and low tissue reaction. The stainless steel suturing technique is very exacting. Steel can pull or tear out of tissue, and necrosis can result from too tight a suture. Barbs on the end of steel can tear gloves, thus breaking sterile technique, or traumatize surrounding tissue. Kinks in the wire can render it practically useless. For this reason, packaging has played a unique part in the development of surgical stainless steel sutures.

Surgical stainless steel is available on spools or in packages of straight, precut, sterile lengths with or without a swaged needle. This packaging affords protection to the strands and delivery in straight unkinked lengths.

The application and use of surgical stainless steel today is widespread. Common areas of use include general closure, retention, skin suturing, neurosurgery, tendon repair, and orthopedic surgery.

Prior to surgical stainless steel's availability from suture manufacturers, it was purchased by weight, utilizing the Brown and Sharp (B&S) scale for diameter variations. Today the B&S gauge, along with U.S.P. size classifications, is used to distinguish diameter size ranges. (See comparisons in Table 1.)

*Metal Cushing* or *Frazier clips* are made of pieces of stainless steel or silver wire of small diameter and are heat sterilized. In neurosurgery and some orthopedic procedures, Frazier clips are applied to the ends of severed nerves and blood vessels by means of a forceps designed for the purpose.

*Wire skin clips* are also available to approximate wound edges and to secure

**TABLE 1.** Steel suture comparison

| Size | B&S gauge |
|------|-----------|
| 6-0 | 40 |
| 6-0 | 38 |
| 5-0 | 35 |
| 4-0 | 34 |
| 4-0 | 32 |
| 000 | 30 |
| 00 | 28 |
| 0 | 26 |
| 1 | 25 |
| 2 | 24 |
| 3 | 23 |
| 4 | 22 |
| 5 | 20 |
| 7 | 18 |

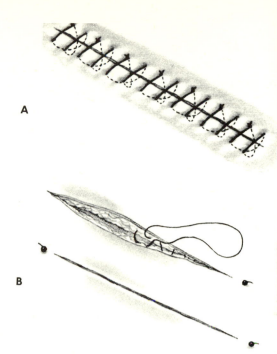

Fig. 6-3. Two types of skin closure. **A,** Interrupted figure-of-eight. **B,** Continuous subcuticular closure anchored with lead shot. (Courtesy Ethicon, Inc., Somerville, N. J.)

skin towels or stockinette to incised skin. Even though skin clips tend to produce scarring, they may be used when the wound is infected and when saving of time is important to the patient's physical welfare.

### Stapling instruments

The Auto Suture stapling set is a line of six instruments used to mechanically suture tissue. The instruments suture with tiny stainless steel staples that come preloaded and presterilized in double-wrapped packages ready for use.

The Auto Suture instruments are used in thoracic, abdominal, and gynecological surgery. One of the instruments, the Skin/Fascia stapler, is used to close fascia and skin, and it is also used in neurosurgery and orthopedic and plastic surgery. (See illustrations in Chapter 14.)

### SELECTION OF SUTURES

The operating room committee or surgical group who accept the responsibility for establishing standard suture sets for various operations should consult the current guides published by suture manufacturers. These guides, which list the specific suture materials recommended for various wounds, are based on current clinical practices and research.

To develop standards, nurses may use a collecting data sheet, which is divided into columns with the desired headings, such as sutures for subcutaneous use. A code or symbols may be used to identify the type and size. Suture cards may be obtained from some manufacturers.

### TYPES OF SUTURE LINES AND METHODS
#### For closure of wounds

The primary suture line refers to those sutures that hold the edges of the wound in approximation until the wound is fairly well healed. The secondary suture line refers to those sutures that supplement the primary suture line, obliterate dead space, and prevent serum from accumulating in the wound.

*Buried sutures* are those placed completely under the epidermal layer of the skin (Fig. 6-3).

A *ligature* is a strand used to encircle or close off the lumen of a vessel, effect

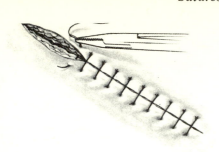

**Fig. 6-4.** Interrupted suture technique. (Courtesy Ethicon, Inc., Somerville, N. J.)

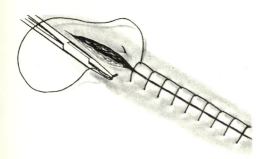

**Fig. 6-5.** Continuous suture technique. (Courtesy Ethicon, Inc., Somerville, N. J.)

hemostasis, close off a structure, and prevent leakage of materials.

A *suture ligature*, stick tie, or transfixion ligature is a strand of suture material threaded on a needle. The needle is used to prevent the ligature from slipping off the end of the vessel or structure. When two ligatures are used to ligate a large vessel, usually the free ligature is placed on the vessel and then the transfixion ligature is placed distal to the first ligature. To ligate a blood vessel situated in the deep tissues, the strand must be of sufficient strength and length to allow the surgeon to tighten the first knot.

Any one of several techniques can be used to apply the strand: (1) A hemostat is placed on the end of the structure; then the ligature secured in a forceps is placed over the vessel. The knot is tied and tightened by means of the surgeon's fingers or with the aid of forceps. (2) A slipknot is made, and its loop is placed over the involved structure by means of a forceps. (3) A forceps is applied to the structure; then the transfixion sutures are applied and tied. The preparation of ligatures and suture ligatures is discussed in a later section of this chapter.

An *interrupted suture* is inserted in tissues or vessels in such a way that each stitch is self-contained and tied. This type of suture is the most widely used and generally considered to be the most efficient (Fig. 6-4). Various techniques are used for the insertion of interrupted sutures in the tissue, resulting in a mattress suture, vertical, horizontal, or crossed in a figure-of-eight stitch. These techniques are designed to alter the angle of pull and the relationship of the wound's edges to each other. Such maneuvers cause the edges of the wound to either invert or evert; this, in turn, aids in wound healing, with fewer sutures used.

A *continuous suture* consists of a series of stitches, of which only the first and last ones are tied (Fig. 6-5). This type of suture is not widely used because a break at any point may mean a disruption of the entire suture line. It is used, however, to close a tissue layer such as the peritoneum, which does not have great strength but requires a tight closure to prevent the intestinal loops from protruding.

A *purse-string suture* is a continuous suture that is placed in such a way that it surrounds an opening in the structure and causes it to close. This type of suture may be placed around the appendix before its removal or may be placed in an organ such as the cecum, gallbladder, or urinary bladder prior to opening it, so that a drainage tube can be inserted.

A *retention* or *stay suture* provides a secondary suture line (Fig. 6-6). These sutures, which are placed at a distance from the primary suture line, relieve undue strain and help obliterate dead space. They are placed in the wound in such a way that they include most, if not all, of the layers of the wound. A simple interrupted

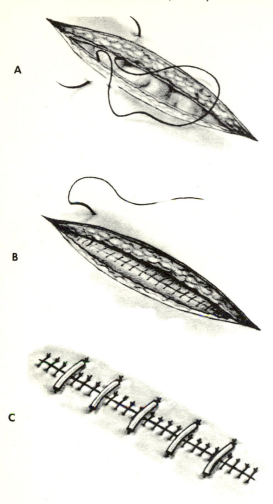

**Fig. 6-6.** Retention suture technique. **A,** Surgeons may place retention sutures from inside the peritoneal cavity through to the skin. **B,** Other surgeons prefer to close peritoneum first, then place retention sutures to penetrate only the layers from fascia to skin. **C,** To prevent heavy materials from cutting into skin, "bolsters" or "bumpers" are used with retention sutures. (Courtesy Ethicon, Inc., Somerville, N. J.)

or figure-of-eight stitch is used. Usually heavy, nonabsorbable suture materials such as silk, nylon, polyester fiber, or wire are used to close long vertical abdominal wounds and lacerated or infected wounds. To prevent the suture from cutting into the skin surface, a small piece of rubber tubing or other type of "bumper" is passed over or through the exposed portion of the suture.

### For holding a drain in place

If a drainage tube is inserted in the wound, the tube may be anchored to the skin with a nonabsorbable suture so that it will not slip in or out. If a tube is left in a hollow viscus, such as the gallbladder or common duct, it may be secured to the wall of that organ with an absorbable suture.

### Knot-tying technique

The successful use of the many varieties of suture material is, in the final analysis, dependent on the skill with which the surgeon ties the knot. The completed knot should be firm to prevent slipping and small, with ends cut short to minimize bulk of suture material in the wound. The suture may be weakened by excessive tension, sawing, friction between the strands, and inadvertent crushing with clamps or hemostats.

### SURGICAL NEEDLES

Surgical needles vary considerably in shape, size, point design, and wire diameter, dependent on the surgical procedure to be performed. Fig. 6-7 indicates the various types, shapes, and point designs available to the surgeon. The surgeon's selection of needle varies with the type of tissue to be sutured. Basically, cutting-edge needles are used on tough tissue (skin, eye tissues) and taper needles are used on soft tissue (bowel, subcutaneous tissue).

Surgical needles fall into three general categories: (1) eyed needles, in which the needle must be threaded with the suture strand, thus making it necessary to pull two strands of suture through the tissue, (2) spring or French eyed needles, in which the suture is forced through the spring, and (3) eyeless needles, a needle-suture combination in which a needle is swaged onto one or both ends of the suture material.

The most popular needle type is the swaged needle (Fig. 6-8). The surgeon draws a single strand of suture material through the tissue, thereby minimizing tis-

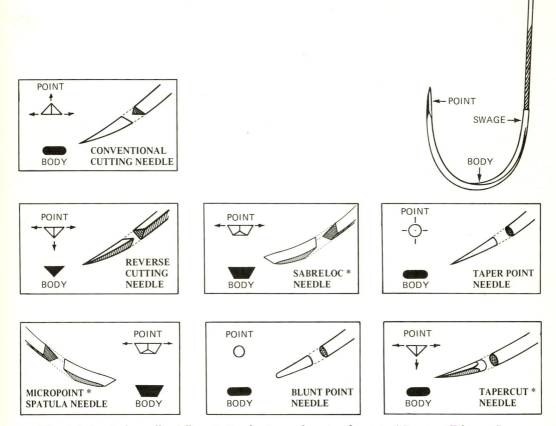

POINT

CONVENTIONAL CUTTING NEEDLE

BODY

POINT ← POINT

SWAGE →

BODY

POINT

REVERSE CUTTING NEEDLE

BODY

POINT

SABRELOC * NEEDLE

BODY

POINT

TAPER POINT NEEDLE

BODY

POINT

MICROPOINT * SPATULA NEEDLE     BODY

POINT

BLUNT POINT NEEDLE

BODY

POINT

TAPERCUT * NEEDLE

BODY

**Fig. 6-7.** Surgical needle differentiation by type, shape, and point. (Courtesy Ethicon, Inc., Somerville, N. J.)

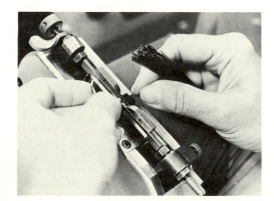

**Fig. 6-8.** Process of swaging needle to suture. (Courtesy Ethicon, Inc., Somerville, N. J.)

sue damage, and uses a new, sharp needle with every suture strand. Swaged needles also eliminate threading eyed needles before and during surgery. Studies indicate that swaged needles provide greater safety to patients and economic use of materials and time.

Surgical needles are made from either stainless steel or carbon steel. They must be strong, ductile, and able to withstand the stress imposed by tough tissue. Stainless steel is the most popular, not only because it provides these physical characteristics, but also because it is noncorrosive.

For certain types of delicate surgery, needles with exceptionally sharp points and cutting edges are produced. Microsurgery, ophthalmology, and plastic surgery require needles of this type; special honing wheels provide needles of precision-point quality for surgeons in these specialties.

Additionally, recent developments include the application of a microthin layer of plastic to the needle surface, providing for easier penetration and a reduction in drag of the needle through the tissue.

Most operating rooms have instituted standardization programs to reduce the variety of needle-suture combinations available for different types of surgical procedures. A continuing program should be developed for keeping needle counts and handling soiled needles. Such procedures should be described in the nursing procedure book (Chapter 2).

## SUTURING TECHNIQUES

In the preparation and use of sutures in surgery, every precaution must be taken to keep the sutures sterile and to prevent prolonged exposure and unnecessary handling. Before the nursing members of the team prepare the sutures for the patient, they should review the sutures listed in the card file for a particular procedure and surgeon. The scrubbed nursing team member should prepare only one of two sutures during the preliminary preparation,

but the circulating nurse should have an adequate supply of sutures available for immediate dispensing to the sterile instrument table. Use of suture materials in dry packages provides sterile sutures ready for use, reduces the length of time previously needed to prepare them, and decreases waste motion (Fig. 6-9).

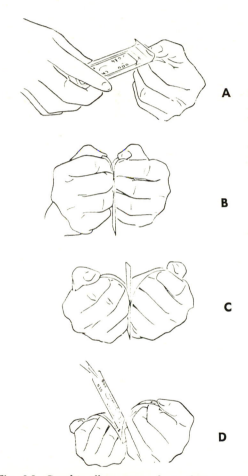

Fig. 6-9. Graphic illustration of circulating nurse dispensing sterile suture from dry strip pack. **A,** Grasp long foil flap with edge of thumb while holding pack in other hand. **B,** Fold back foil flap and grasp firmly between thumb and forefinger, exposing plastic flap, which extends automatically. **C,** Grasp plastic flap with thumb and forefinger of other hand, gripping packet between knuckles. **D,** Roll thumbs outward, separating flaps to expose sterile foil packet, keeping constant pressure between knuckles for best control. (From Instructional sheet on sterile-pack, dry handling technic, Somerville, N. J., Ethicon, Inc., Somerville, N. J.)

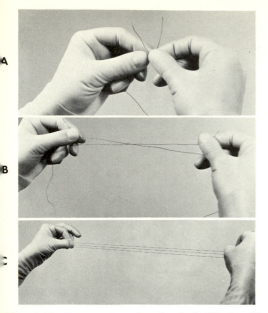

**Fig. 6-10.** Preparation of individual "freehand" ligatures. **A,** Free ends of ligature are grasped in each hand and gently pulled to remove kinks. **B,** Ligature is folded in equal parts of desired length. **C,** Ligatures are divided into individual pieces. (Courtesy Ethicon, Inc., Somerville, N. J.)

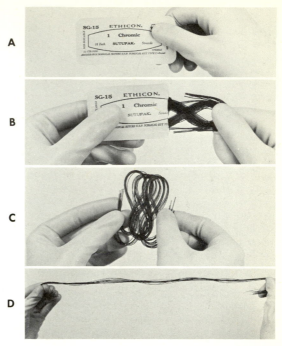

**Fig. 6-11.** Preparation of prepackaged individual ligatures. **A,** Sterile package. **B,** Remove suture strands from package as a unit. **C,** Grasp the strands at each end. **D,** Gently pull to remove kinks. (Courtesy Ethicon, Inc., Somerville, N. J.)

### Opening primary packets

The scrubbed nursing team member tears the foil packet across the notch near the hermetically sealed edge and removes the suture folder. Plastic packets may be torn or opened using suture scissors.

### Removal of sutures

Gut sutures should be removed from the suture folder immediately.

To remove a suture that does not have a needle, pull the loose end out with one hand while grasping the folder with the other hand. To straighten a long suture, grasp its free end (using the thumb and forefinger of the free hand), and remove the kinks by pulling it gently. Secure the free ends in one hand and the center loop in the other and then slowly abduct the arms slightly to straighten the strands.

Kinks should never be removed by running the fingers over the strand. The ten-

sile strength of a gut suture should not be tested before it is handed to the surgeon. Sudden pulls or jerks used to test the tensile strength of a suture may damage it so that it will break when in use.

To prepare single ligatures and sutures, the strand is folded in equal parts and held between the fingers; then the strand is divided (Fig. 6-10). Sutures are also provided in 12- to 18-inch precut lengths. (See Fig. 6-11.)

In some hospitals, spiral wound sutures are used. Long sutures (surgical gut, silk, or cotton) are wound on cylindrical or circular reels supplied by suture manufacturers (Fig. 6-12). The surgeon holds the reel in his hand as he ligates the bleeding vessels. This technique eliminates the need to rewind sutures on reels, saves nurses' time, and eliminates waste motion.

To remove a suture-needle combination, the scrubbed member grasps the needle

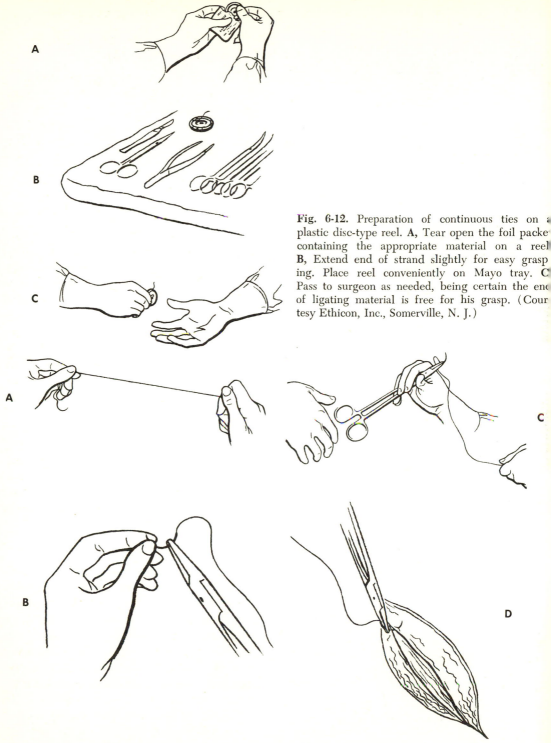

**Fig. 6-12.** Preparation of continuous ties on a plastic disc-type reel. **A,** Tear open the foil packet containing the appropriate material on a reel. **B,** Extend end of strand slightly for easy grasping. Place reel conveniently on Mayo tray. **C,** Pass to surgeon as needed, being certain the end of ligating material is free for his grasp. (Courtesy Ethicon, Inc., Somerville, N. J.)

**Fig. 6-13.** Preparation of swaged suture. **A,** If necessary to straighten grasp, strand 1 to 2 inches away from needle-suture junction and pull gently. **B,** Clamp needle holder about three fourths of distance from needle point. Do not clamp at swaged area. Place needle near tip of holder to facilitate suturing. **C,** Surgeon receives needle holder with needle point toward his thumb to prevent unnecessary wrist motion. Scrubbed team member controls free end of suture. **D,** Surgeon begins closing with swaged needle. (Courtesy Ethicon, Inc., Somerville, N. J.)

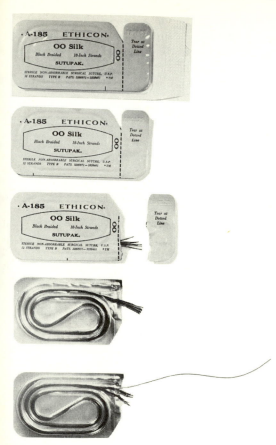

**Fig. 6-14.** Opening plastic packet, nonabsorbable sutures. **A,** Plastic packet enclosed in overwrap. **B,** Plastic packet as presented to scrubbed team member. **C,** Packet torn open along dotted line. **D,** Reverse of packet showing strand packaging. **E,** Individual strand removed from packet. (Courtesy Ethicon, Inc., Somerville, N. J.)

of the suture with her fingers or a needle holder and gently pulls the strand to remove and straighten it. The jaws of the needle holder are placed on the center of the flattened surface of the needle to prevent breakage and bending (Fig. 6-13).

### Nonabsorbable suture removal

The technique of removing the overwrap packet from nonabsorbable suture materials is identical to that shown in Fig. 6-9.

### Opening plastic packet, nonabsorbable sutures

The scrubbed nursing team member tears the packet along the dotted line and grasps the free ends with one hand. The sutures can be removed one at a time from some packets or all at once from others (Fig. 6-14). The sutures in or out of the packet may be placed under the towel with size markings showing.

### Cutting suture lengths

A suture or free ligature should not be too long or too short. A long suture is difficult to handle and increases the possibility of contamination because it may be dragged across the sterile field or fall below it. A short suture usually slips from the eye of the needle as it is being inserted and makes tying most difficult.

For general surgery, a continuous suture is usually about 24 inches long after threading, and its short end is 3 to 4 inches long. An interrupted suture is 12 to 14 inches long, with 2 or 3 inches threaded through the needle. To ligate a vessel in the epidermal and subcutaneous layers, the ligature may be 12 to 15 inches long. However, those vessels or structures deep in the wound are ligated with a suture 24 to 30 inches long.

### Threading surgical needles

The scrubbed nursing team member pulls the suture about 4 inches through the eye of the needle to prevent the suture from being pulled out of the eye during suturing. A curved needle is threaded from within its curvature so that the short end falls away from the outside curvature. This helps prevent easy pullout. To keep the needle secure in the jaws of the holder and to prevent damage to the eye of the needle, the needle holder is placed on the flattened surface of the needle, at least 1/8 inch from its eye.

**REFERENCES**

1. Bradford, R. T.: Use of mersilene in strabismus reoperations, Eye Ear Nose Throat Mon. **45**:54, 1966.

2. Britt, C. I., Miller, E. M., Felder, M. E., and Sirak, H. R.: Comparative reaction of mersilene and silk sutures implanted within the heart, Ann. Surg. **153:**52, 1961.

3. Dineen, P.: A suggested method for the control of staphylococcal infections in a large general hospital, Am. J. Surg. **100:**543, 1960.

4. Everett, W. G.: Suture materials in general surgery, Progr. Surg. **8:**14, 1970.

5. Haley, H. B., Jr., and Williamson, M. B.: Application of present knowledge of wound healing to clinical surgery, Surg. Clin. North Am. **42:**15, Feb., 1962.

6. Harvey, S. C.: History of hemostasis, New York, 1929, Harper & Row, Publishers.

7. Haxton, H.: The influence of suture materials and methods on the healing of abdominal wounds, Br. J. Surg. **52:**372, 1965.

8. Homsy, C. A., McDonald, K. E., Akers, W. W., et al.: Surgical suture—canine tissue interaction for six common suture types, J. Biomed. Mater. Res. **2:**215, 1968.

9. Lilly, G. E., Salem, J. E., Armstrong, J. H., et al.: Reaction of oral tissues to suture materials. III. Oral Surg. **28:**432, 1969.

10. Manual of operative procedures and surgical knots, Somerville, N. J., 1961, Ethicon, Inc.

11. McCallum, G. T., and Link, R. F.: The effect of closure techniques on abdominal disruption, Surg. Gynecol. Obstet. **119:**75, 1964.

12. McPherson, S. D., Crawford, R., Moore, L., and Michels, R.: Investigations of corneal suture material, Adv. Ophthalmol. **22:**49, 1970.

13. Mendoza, C. B., Jr., Watne, A. L., Grace, J. E., et al.: Wire versus silk: choice of surgical wound closure in patients with cancer, Am. J. Surg. **112:**839, 1966.

14. Miller, J. M., and Kimmel, L. E.: Clinical evaluation of monofilament polypropylene suture, Am. Surg. **33:**666, 1967.

15. Minckley, B.: A study of practices of handling and opening suture packets in the operating room, Nurs. Res. **18:**267, 1969.

16. Moloney, G. E.: The effect of human tissues on the tensile strength of implanted nylon sutures, Br. J. Surg. **48:**528, 1961.

17. Postlethwait, R. W.: Long-term comparative study of nonabsorbable sutures, Ann. Surg. **171:**892, 1970.

18. Postlethwait, R. W., Floyd, B. J., Dillon, M. L., and Stowe, D. G.: Tissue reaction to blood vessel sutures, Am. Surg. **28:**799, 1962.

19. Prostheses for surgery, bulletin no. 333, Murray Hill, N. J., 1965, C. R. Bard, Inc.

20. Shumacker, H. B., and Mandelbaum, I.: Clinical evaluation of Dacron suture material, Arch. Surg. **83:**647, 1961.

21. Smith, R. S., and Talboy, G. E.: Use of steel wire sutures for closure of abdominal wounds, Northwest Med. **62:**344, 1963.

22. Starr, A., and Edwards, M. L.: Mitral replacement, Ann. Surg. **154:**726, 1961.

23. Suture manual, Somerville, N. J., 1966, Ethicon, Inc.

24. The Pharmacopeia of the United States of America, eighteenth revision, September, 1970.

# CHAPTER 7

# Positioning the patient for surgery

JUDITH YVONNE JACOBS

The task of positioning the patient for surgery is one of the most important in which the operating room nurse participates, and it calls for knowledge and application of the principles of anatomy and physiology and for skill in using specific pieces of equipment. Positioning is accomplished with the guidance and direction of the anesthetist.

## MODERN OPERATING TABLES

Modern operating tables are specifically designed to meet the peculiar and highly specialized requirements of surgical therapy. Familiarity with this equipment is fundamental to its proper and effective use. Modern manufacture and design have done much to facilitate safe and effective positioning of the patient to meet the surgeon's need for accessibility to the body part to be treated. Judicious manipulation of the table obviates manipulation of the patient.

It is not feasible here to describe all the many types of operating tables now available. Nurses should be well versed in the use of those for specific situations. Nurses should keep abreast of new developments and evaluate their usefulness in actual practice.

## Types

In common surgical use are the major general operating table, the orthopedic table, the urology table, and the eye table. The modern general operating table (Fig. 7-1) is so versatile that the need

for specialty tables is declining. A table that is adapted to a wide range of uses is an economical investment and permits flexibility in the use of operating facilities (Fig. 7-2). The orthopedic table with its multiple movable and removable parts and suspension frames remains practically the only specialty table required (Fig. 7-3).

Modern general operating tables can be adjusted for height and length and can be tilted laterally to either side and horizontally at the head and foot. The table is divided into three or more sections that support the major body parts and permit their placement in flexion or extension. The head section is usually removable, and foot extensions may be added.

Controls and accessories maintain the patient in standard and modified supine, lithotomy, lateral, and prone positions. Headrests of various designs enable the general table to be used for cranial and eye surgery. Electric controls make table movements swift and smooth.

Perineal cutouts and drainage trays fitted to the lumbar section adapt the general operating table to the perineal approaches used in gynecological, urological, and proctological surgery. The newer tables are equipped with x-ray–penetrable tunnel tops that permit insertion of cassette holders at any position along the table.

Additional accessories for modern operating tables include pillows, pads, bolsters, and doughnut cushions of various sizes and shapes. They are made to fit the different anatomical structures of pa-

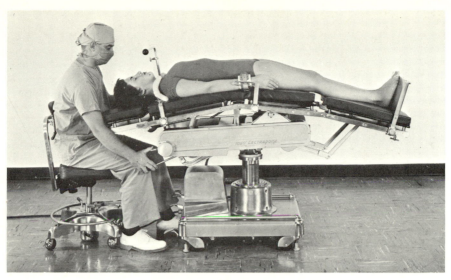

**Fig. 7-1.** Modern surgical operating table is equipped to meet surgeons' posturing needs. It has an x-ray–penetrable top, conductive rubber mattress pad that adheres to table without aid of snaps or tabs, adjustable anesthesia screen with ball joint that permits rotating or angling in any plane, padded rubber shoulder supports to relieve pressure on soft supraclavicular area, wristlets and other types of body restraints and supports such as footboard, which is used to support body weight when table is tilted or to extend length of table in horizontal position. Armboards, leg holders or stirrups, and other attachments are used to stabilize and protect patient in desired position. (Courtesy American Sterilizer Co., Erie, Pa.)

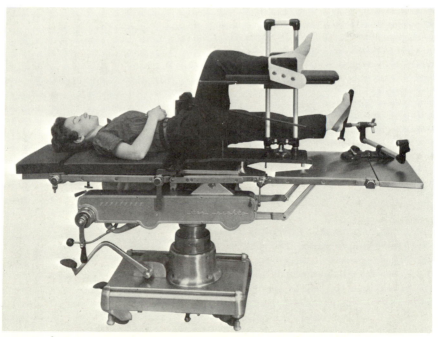

**Fig. 7-2.** Pelvic anchor sacral apparatus for general operating table. It permits accurate traction for fracture reduction and provides complete facilities for precision anatomical radiography. Pedestal leg support is located in midline, and patient is supported on either side of table with operative side free of table top, assuring improved surgical approach. (Courtesy American Sterilizer Co., Erie, Pa.)

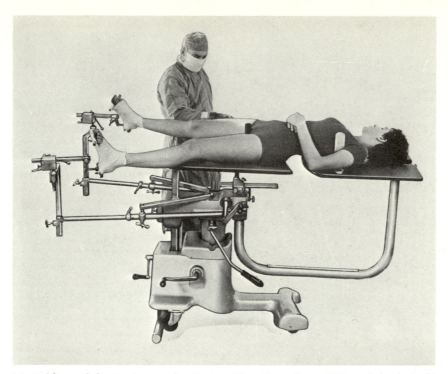

**Fig. 7-3.** Table used for treatment of patients with orthopedic conditions. It lends itself to all methods of spinal reductions. This table can be equipped with accessories vital for complete radiographic verification of any stage of any procedure. There are cassette holders for lateral positions (hips, femurs, and arms), cassette tunnel for anteroposterior positions only during hip nailing, and x-ray adapter, which allows x-ray head of appropriate type to be applied directly to table. Standard accessories also include elongated metal body seat, hand traction appliance, lateral body brace, strut for abduction bar, cervical yoke and headrest, and accessory panel. (Courtesy American Sterilizer Co., Erie, Pa.)

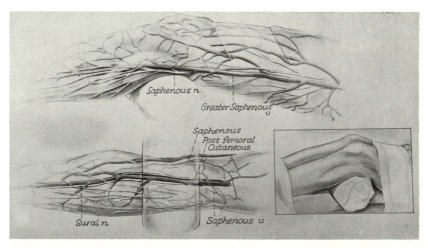

**Fig. 7-4.** Diagram of structures subject to injury in pressure areas as shown by compression of legs between hard knee roll and tight strap. (From Slocum, H. C., et al.: Surg. Gynecol. Obstet. **86:**729, 1948.)

tients and to suit preferences of surgeons. Some are soft and made of conductive foam rubber; others are firm, made of conductive rubber, and filled with kapok or fine sand.

### Anatomical and physiological factors

In making optimum use of equipment and accessories, the nurse must consider the anatomical and physiological factors that are involved in positioning the patient. The type of position is determined by the type of operation to be performed, the anesthetic to be given, the location of the injury or lesion, and the age, height, weight, and general condition of the patient, as well as by the surgical approach.

The *position* aims to provide the patient with good body alignment, free circulatory and respiratory movement, and protection from pressure, abrasion, and other injuries. Anomalies and physical defects, particularly those affecting joint motion, need special evaluation and consideration prior to induction of anesthesia.

### STANDARD POSITIONS AND PROTECTIVE MEASURES
### Supine position

The supine position is the most common position. It is the most natural position of the body at rest. The patient is usually anesthetized in this position, and modifications are made after induction of anesthesia.

The supine position is used to approach the anterior surfaces of the body and to enter the major body cavities.

The patient lies on his back with the arms at the sides and the legs extended, with the feet slightly separated. The position of the head should be in a straight line with the spine (Fig. 7-1). A small pad placed under the head allows the strap muscles to relax and prevents neck strain. Flexion or twisting may cause contractures in the neck and interfere with a clear airway.

To prevent postoperative discomfort such as backache and injury to the spine

from flexion contracture, the spine is kept in a straight line with the hips parallel, and the lumbar curve is supported with a small pad if necessary. To prevent hyperextension of the knees, the popliteal area may be elevated slightly (5 degrees), but heavy pressure is to be avoided to protect the perineal nerve and saphenous veins (Fig. 7-4). Heel prominences also need protection from prolonged pressure. A doughnut cushion or an ankle roll may be used.

The soles of the feet are supported on a firm foam rubber support or padded footboard that extends beyond the toes to prevent plantar flexion and to guard the toes from the weight and pressure of drapes. The legs are parallel and uncrossed to prevent nerve injury in the calf of the leg.

The skin surfaces of the body should not be in direct contact. Moisture from perspiration, antiseptic or irrigating solutions, and body fluids contribute to irritation and maceration of the skin.

On the high, relatively narrow operating table, the patient needs the protection of a restraint. Straps are usually placed above the knees of a supine patient and below the knees of a prone one. Straps must be secure enough to prevent a fall or shift in position but not tight enough to exert pressure. Straps are made of a conductive rubber material.

The arms should rest easily at the sides with the hands pronated (palms down). A broad lift sheet can be used to tuck around the arms to support the full length of the arm and prevent its slipping or coming to rest against the sharp edges of the metal table (Fig. 7-5). If the hands are placed under the buttocks, there is danger that the fingers will be compressed. When wristlets are used, there is danger of superficial pressure numbing the hand or damaging the skin and the nerves of the upper extremity (Fig. 7-6). The elbow may not be well enough supported and may slip over the side of the table to rest against hard metal. The superficial

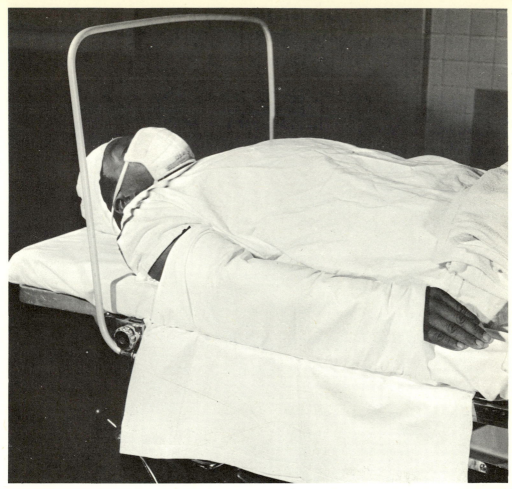

**Fig. 7-5.** Each flap of lift sheet should be of sufficient size to encase and support entire upper extremity. Palms should face downward, with fingers pronated and free at rest on table.

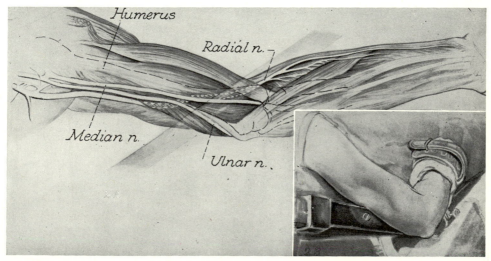

**Fig. 7-6.** Pressure may be exerted against median, ulnar, and radial nerves of arm when patient is improperly positioned on operating table. (From Slocum, H. C., et al.: Surg. Gynecol. Obstet. 86:729, 1948.)

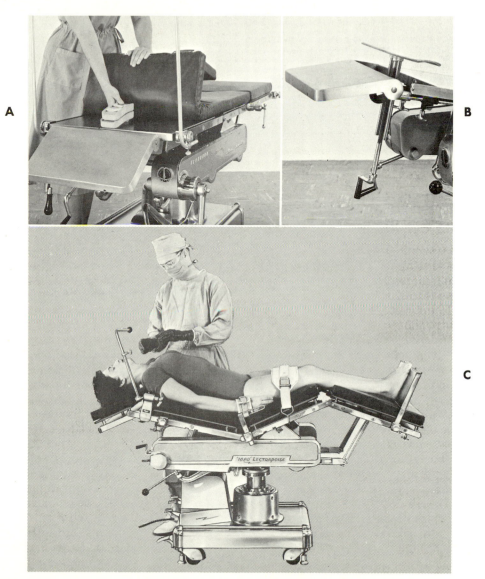

Fig. 7-7. **A,** Operations on thyroid and neck area. Head section of operating table may be lowered and sponge rubber shoulder pads placed directly under midline of shoulder area, thus carrying clavicles away from operative site. **B,** Shoulder bridge may be placed between head and back sections, replacing sponge rubber pads or sandbag. Bridge is raised and lowered by crank control. **C,** Neck area may be extended by lowering head section of table in approximately 10-degree increments below horizontal. At closure, anesthetist releases finger latch under section and raises it to level, where it automatically locks in place. In some cases, patient may be placed in Fowler's position to ensure comfort with table reflexed 20 degrees and lower foot section about 20 degrees. Slightly reflexed position with feet at approximately same height as head provides for better stabilization of blood pressure. (Courtesy American Sterilizer Co., Erie, Pa.)

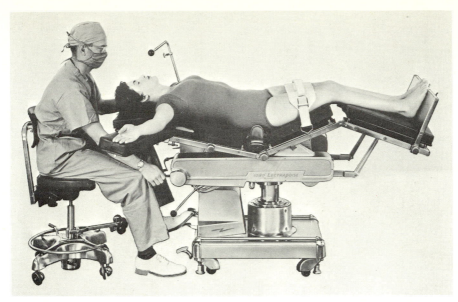

**Fig. 7-8.** Operation on breast and axillary area. To provide maximum patient comfort during operative procedure, table is placed in slight reflex 20 degrees and lateral tilt, head section 10 degrees, foot section relaxed, and arm on affected side raised laterally. It is important that neck, pelvis, and knees fall directly over appropriate area of tabletop as shown. Patient is stabilized by body support and body restraint strap. (Courtesy American Sterilizer Co., Erie, Pa.)

ulnar nerve over the epicondyle of the humerus is then subject to injury.

*Modifications*

When the position of the table is changed while the patient is on the dorsum, special precautions are necessary to protect him.

When the head is turned to one side or the other, it should be supported to keep the spine in alignment and secured in the desired position with a doughnut cushion, sandbag, or special headrest.

Pressure over bony prominences where nerves and blood vessels run superficially must be avoided. The eyes must be carefully guarded against pressure, and they must be protected as drapes are placed to prevent corneal irritation from textiles, solutions, and other foreign bodies.

For operations on the neck, the neck may be extended by placing a narrow support between the shoulder blades or by lowering the headpiece of the table.

There should be no gaps in the support of the neck in this position. A special screen that protects the face may be used in thyroid surgery (Fig. 7-7).

For anterolateral incisions and for surgery on the shoulder or the chest, the patient's affected side may be elevated on rolls or pads. To prevent twisting of the spine, the full length of the body needs support to keep the hips and shoulders in a plane. Body supports or straps in appropriate locations maintain the position and prevent rolling without interfering with the surgical approach (Figs. 7-8 and 7-16).

An armboard may be used to support the arm on the affected side. In some cases, both arms are supported on armboards. In a few cases the arm may be bandaged to the ether screen, using specific precautions against nerve and circulatory disturbances. In many procedures, one arm is usually extended on an armboard to administer intravenous therapy.

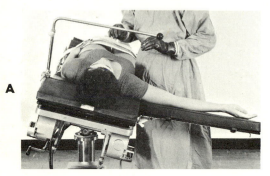
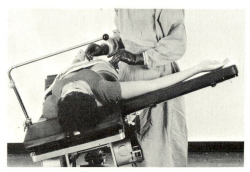

**Fig. 7-9. A,** Radical mastectomy. Lateral tilt toward surgeon and affected area during resection of medial flaps tends to carry excised tissue downward and away from incision by gravity. **B,** Tilt of table in opposite direction during progress of operation may be done without interference to surgeon during excision of lateral flaps and axillary dissection. Gravity retraction takes place. Lateral tilt away from affected area permits better viewing of wound in obese patients. (Courtesy American Sterilizer Co., Erie, Pa.)

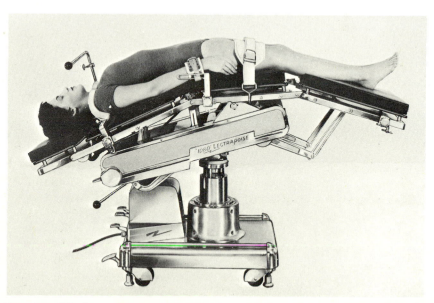

**Fig. 7-10.** Trendelenburg position for operations on lower abdominal organs. Slight flex and Trendelenburg position, with foot section lowered and patient maintained by body restraint strap and shoulder supports, provide optimum extension of operative site. Adustable sponge rubber shoulder supports are positioned directly under acromioclavicular joint to eliminate danger of brachial palsy. Anesthetist may operate head end controls to permit relaxation of abdominal tissues at closure. This control method outside sterile field eliminates unnecessary table movement during a procedure. (Courtesy American Sterilizer Co., Erie, Pa.)

One or both arms may be extended in radical mastectomy (Fig. 7-9) and other surgery on the upper extremity and chest regions.

The armboard is padded to protect the skin and superficial tissues from pressure. The arm is extended at an angle less than 90 degrees at the shoulder. The armboard is of the type that locks into position on the table to prevent inadvertent angle changes. Hyperabduction at the shoulder may cause both vascular and neural damage. Venous thrombosis may result when superficial veins are compressed by supports or straps or the weight of body structures. The subclavian or axillary arteries may be occluded in abduction (Fig. 7-9).

*Trendelenburg position* allows the abdominal viscera to fall away from the pelvis for good surgical exposure, but their weight on the diaphragm may decrease lung volume and inhibit adequate respiratory exchange (Fig. 7-10). Extreme Trendelenburg position or a steeper tilt of the table without flexing the knees may also be used to overcome shock by promoting circulation to the brain.

The nerve supply to the upper extremities, which comes from the spinal cord, gathers at the brachial plexus and emerges under the muscles in front at the root of the neck, where the neck and shoulder join. In this position, placement of well-padded braces at the outer aspect of the shoulders over the acromion and spinous process of the scapula prevents pressure on the brachial plexus (Fig. 7-10). Careful positioning of the knees over the break prevents pressure in the popliteal space and safeguards the perineal nerve. Breaking the table at the knees takes some of the body weight off the shoulder braces and reduces pressure there.

When the patient is returned to a horizontal position, the legs should be brought into a plane with the body before the body is tilted flat. This precaution overcomes circulatory stasis in the legs and

permits venous return, which is reduced when body parts are dependent.

Trendelenburg position presents certain advantages to the surgeon and disadvantages to the anesthetist because of the results of the force of gravity on the body organs.

The table is tilted at an angle of 45 degrees, lowering the head. The patient's body is prevented from slipping by use of shoulder braces and by breaking the foot section of the table to flex the knees.

The elbow should be slightly flexed, and the forearm and hand should be pronated. This prevents compression of the radial nerve due to abduction and external rotation of the arm. The fingers are separated and may be slightly flexed. The arm is secured to the board by a bandage encircling the forearm, wrist, or hand. Movement and shifting of the position are prevented, but tight pressure is avoided.

Pressure from shoulder braces placed too close to the neck may damage the brachial plexus. Compression of the vessels from hyperabduction and stretching may also cause ischemia, which results in nerve damage with loss of sensation and muscle control.

*Reverse Trendelenburg position* (Fig. 7-11) may be used for a reverse effect on the viscera; it may be called for in surgery on the biliary tract to bring the weight of the liver below the costal margin and to allow the intestines to fall away from the epigastrium. When the table is tilted toward the foot, the patient's body must be supported by the footboard, by body straps, and by a lift sheet around the arms, all of which must be securely in position. Lumbar and popliteal pads in place also tend to prevent the body from slipping.

Some surgeons make use of the elevator bridge of the operating table to expose the gallbladder. When this is anticipated, the patient must be positioned with the *costal margin at the level of the elevator.* If an elevator is lacking, the table may be flexed at this level, or a pad may be inserted to achieve the desired position.

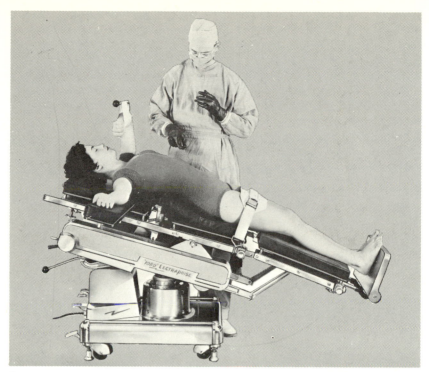

**Fig. 7-11.** Reverse Trendelenburg position for operations on gallbladder. Since gallbladder is located under rib cage, patient is positioned on table with twelfth thoracic vertebra over raised body elevator to provide maximum extension in thoracic vertebrae region, and the table is placed in reverse Trendelenburg position, thus utilizing gravity to keep unaffected organs away from the operative site. Usually one or both arms may be extended and supported on standard armboard. Or one arm may be supported from the anesthesia screen by means of soft dressing roll to minimize occlusion; otherwise both arms could be jeopardized at the brachium when elevator is raised. Head section may be removed and inserted at foot end to provide foot support at precisely the right extension. Body elevator is raised as needed, occasionally during exploration of common duct. Cassette and holder may be inserted from either head or foot ends or from either side. Cholangiograms are taken without repositioning patient. (Courtesy American Sterilizer Co., Erie, Pa.)

*Modified Fowler's and sitting position* may also be used for neurological surgery (Fig. 7-12). The position of the body in relation to the table breaks must be carefully adjusted to prevent abnormal pressures. The backrest is elevated, the knees are flexed, and the footboard is set in place. The more erect the patient's posture, the greater is the need to support the shoulders and torso. Such support requires adequate padding to protect the axilla and brachial plexus. Frequently a special headrest is used for cranial ventricular procedures and for posterior fossa craniotomy (Chapter 11).

The sitting position requires special attention to positioning of the arms. Depending on the surgery, the arms may be flexed across the abdomen and rest on a large pillow in the lap or may be placed in front of the patient on a padded stand. Hyperextension of the shoulder region must be prevented, and the arms must be secure from falling or pressing against hard surfaces.

**Lithotomy position**

The lithotomy position is really an extreme variation of the supine position. With the patient on his back, the legs are

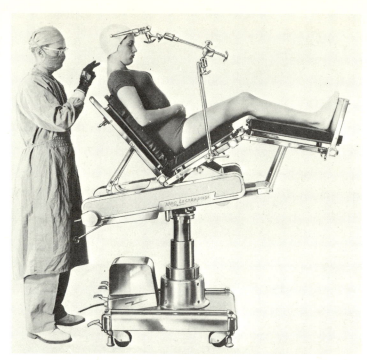

Fig. 7-12. Semiupright position for neurosurgical operations. It is used for exposure of suboccipital area. Surgeon may stand close to his patient and elevate or lower table himself by merely touching foot pedals. There are several neurosurgical attachments available for suboccipital and parietal approaches; attachments and headrest fit into mobile side rail sockets. Multipose headrest consists of a three-pin suspension, spring-loaded to hold skull itself rigid. Table is flexed, and footpiece is in position to ensure patient comfort and stability of position. (Courtesy American Sterilizer Co., Erie, Pa.)

raised and abducted to expose the perineal region in order to gain a surgical approach to the pelvic organs and genitalia (Fig. 7-13). This unnatural posture is fraught with danger and discomfort for the patient, and these hazards increase as the position is exaggerated for radical surgery. Extreme flexion of the thighs impairs respiratory function by increasing intraabdominal pressure. Gravity flow of blood from the elevated legs causes blood to pool in the splanchnic region.

Supports for the legs must be carefully chosen and applied. By placing the patient's anterior iliac spine on a line with the leg holder and the buttocks level and on a line with the edge of the table break, a good position can be achieved with a minimum of effort. The buttocks must not extend beyond the break or the rim of the table because when the legpiece is lowered, it will act as a fulcrum and increase arching of the back and strain the lumbosacral ligaments and muscles.

Modern leg holders provide secure support for the legs without the popliteal pressure of knee crutches and without undue external rotation and abduction, which stretch the abductor muscles and capsule of the hip joint.

The stirrups must be level. The height is adjusted to the length of the patient's legs. This prevents pressure at the knee and lumbar spine. The patient's position must be symmetrical: the perineum is in line with the longitudinal axis of the table, the pelvis is level, and the head and trunk are in a straight line (Fig. 7-14). This aids the surgeon in identifying anatomical landmarks. Support is provided for the

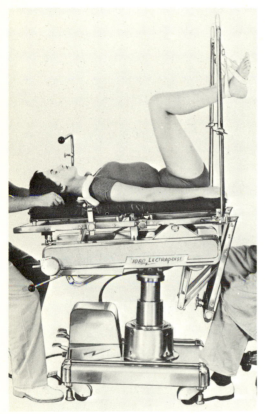

**Fig. 7-13.** Lithotomy position for vaginal and rectal operations. Lower section of mattress is removed, and foot section is fully lowered through a 105-degree arc, thus providing foot room under base. Standard lithotomy leg holders are easily adjustable and secured in clamp-on sockets. Large perineal cutout in foot section provides adequate space for instrumentation. Slight Trendelenburg position aligns perineal cavity with surgeon's line of vision. Shoulder braces are applied. Table is elevated approximately to 45-inch height range for perineal procedures. (Courtesy American Sterilizer Co., Erie, Pa.)

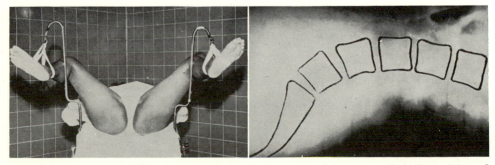

**Fig. 7-14.** Conventional lithotomy position with conventional stirrups and tracing of lateral x-ray film of lumbosacral spine of patient with this position. (From Hunter, R. G., et al.: Obstet. Gynecol. 4:344, 1954.)

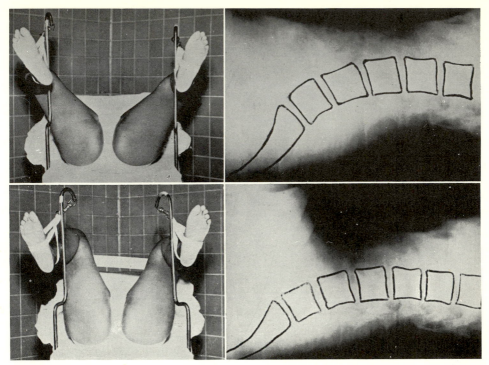

**Fig. 7-15.** Conventional stirrups rotated and raised, reducing abduction and extending of legs, and tracing of lateral x-ray films in this position. (From Hunter, R. G., et al.: Obstet. Gynecol. 4:344, 1954.)

head and neck if necessary. If the table is to be tilted headdown to raise the operative area, shoulder braces are used. All the cautions about the headdown position apply.

To position a patient in lithotomy position, the patient's leg is raised by grasping the sole of the foot in one hand and supporting the leg near the knee in the other. The leg is raised, and the knee is flexed slowly. The foot is secured in the holder at a right angle to the leg. One loop of the canvas sling is placed around the sole at the metatarsals and the other loop around the ankle. The lower leg should be free from pressure against the leg holders. Stirrups of modern design prevent this pressure (Fig. 7-15). Other stirrups may require foam rubber padding between the calves of the legs and the metal posts. Pressure against the soft tissues of the

leg may predispose to venous thrombosis. For high lithotomy position during extensive surgery or for patients with an ankylosed hip joint, the Bierhoff leg holders or Comper kneerest and footrest may be used.

The lower section of the table pad is removed, and the end of the table is lowered.

Arms require special care in lithotomy position. The hands should not extend along the sides since they will reach below the break of the foot section of the table and be in danger of injury from manipulation of the table parts. They may be folded loosely across the abdomen and supported by the folded gown or cover sheet. One arm may be extended on the armboard for infusion, and the other may be suspended from the anesthesia screen as previously described. Arms must not

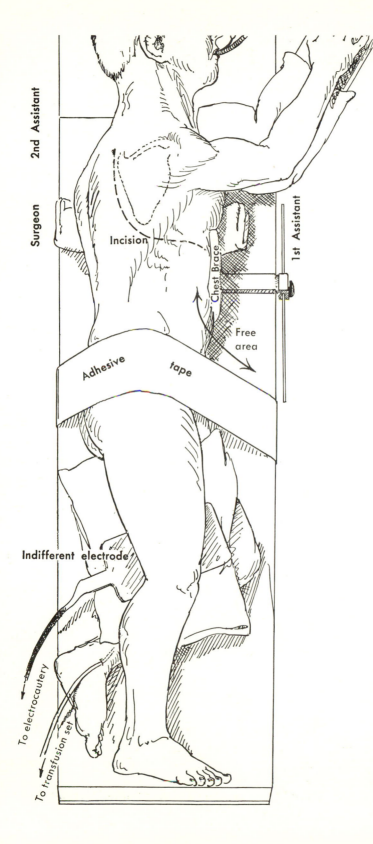

**Fig. 7-16.** Lateral position for chest surgery. Patient has been anesthetized, has endotracheal tube in place, and is in lateral position with padded chest brace at lower end of sternum. Brace is placed to avoid pressure against upper abdomen, which would restrict movement and interfere with ventilation. In order to assist spreading of intercostal spaces, three steps are taken: rolled towel is placed beneath dependent chest, top leg is put in straight position, and table is bent so that lower extremities as well as head are slightly below pleural space that is to be opened. Indifferent electrode is placed as indicated and supported by placement of pillow between knees. Pillow must be placed so that cannulated saphenous vein cannot become obstructed by pressure of top leg. Hip is anchored by adhesive tape to prevent patient's body from rolling backward or forward on table. Arms are extended forward on armrest supports and are accessible to anesthetist for venipuncture. Approximate length and location of incision are shown. Many operative difficulties begin with poorly positioned patient. (From Burch, B. H., and Miller, A. C.: The atlas of pulmonary resections, Springfield, Ill., 1965, Charles C Thomas, Publisher.)

impede chest movement and adequate respiratory excursion. The weight of the limbs on the chest, especially in infants and children, may tire the muscles of respiration and induce failure.

Adequate assistance must be available for placing the patient in lithotomy position and for releasing him from the position. Any change in body position affects hemodynamics. Movements must be slow and deliberate to allow gradual adjustment to the change. Muscles and joints must be protected from abnormal strain in their flaccid state. The legs should be raised simultaneously to place the feet in the loops of the canvas supports. They also should be lowered simultaneously, supporting the joints above and below to prevent strain on the lumbosacral musculature, which can stretch, tilt, and thereby place the pelvis and limbs in imbalance.

## Lateral position for chest procedures

The patient is placed on his side for surgical approach to the chest (Fig. 7-16). Full lateral position is also common for surgery on the kidney and upper ureter.

To place a patient in a lateral position, teamwork is necessary. After induction of anesthesia, the patient is turned so that the affected side is presented uppermost. This movement can be accomplished by two persons. The anesthetist supports the head and shoulders while the assistant moves the hips. From the head of the table, the anesthetist places his hand behind the patient's arm on the affected side. His other hand is placed on the opposite side of the patient's chest. The assistant places his arms under the hips from the patient's affected side. Together they raise the patient to tilt the affected side up. The anesthetist from his position supports the patient's head and neck along his forearm and elbow. The patient is maintained on his side by a pillow or support until the hips are stabilized.

The patient's hips are shifted back in line with the edge of the mattress, and the legs are positioned to give stability.

The under leg is flexed at the knee and the hip. The upper leg is straight. A long pillow or pad is placed between the legs. This position is secured by a strap at the level of the buttocks just below the iliac spine.

The shoulders are leveled with the hips. The head is supported on a pad or small pillow to keep the spine and neck in good alignment. The shoulders are stabilized by extending the arms on a well-padded double armboard.

The upper arm is flexed slightly at the shoulder and elbow. The lower arm is brought out from under the patient.

Well-padded body braces may be used to support the torso. Sandbags or body rolls may be substituted and secured by the lift sheet, since the braces tend to roll the mattress up to intrude on the operative area. A pad at the apex of the scapula in the axillary space will relieve pressure on the arm.

In chest surgery, infusion needles may be placed in the uppermost limb (arm or leg) or in the undermost limb (Fig. 7-16). Care must be taken to prevent compression, which can impede venous return. A body strap is placed at the hip region for additional stability.

With the patient in lateral position for chest surgery (Fig. 7-16), the intercostal muscles on the unaffected side are slightly narrowed, whereas those on the affected side are widened, thus providing a wider wound exposure. Slanting the upper section of the table downward at a 10-degree angle places the trachea and mouth at a level lower than the lungs. This encourages bronchial secretions and fluids to drain into the mouth and not to pass into the unaffected side of the chest and lessens the danger of air embolism to the cerebral vessels. The main disadvantage of this position is that the weight of the body must rest on the unaffected side, which makes it more difficult for the anesthetist to control the aspiration of secretions from this lung.

The lateral position restricts chest ex-

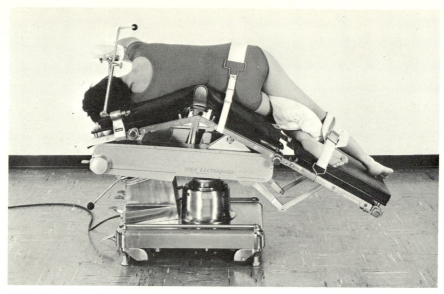

**Fig. 7-17.** Lateral position for kidney operations. Patient is positioned with iliocostal space (area between iliac crest and inferior costal margin) directly over break between seat and back sections. By flexing table in slight reverse Trendelenburg position, utilizing body supports positioned below lumbar vertebrae, entire side of patient is supported, minimizing physiological damage while providing excellent exposure of kidney area. Kraske arm support may be used to relieve pressure and provide complete support to independent arm. This arm may be used for administration of intravenous fluids. Body elevator may be raised to extend kidney area without using reverse Trendelenburg position; however, this concentrates all pressure in relatively vital area, and it may inhibit circulation and respiration. (Courtesy American Sterilizer Co., Erie, Pa.)

pansion. Flexing the table to lower the head and feet adds pressure on the diaphragm, and gravity pull tends to pool blood at both extremities. Extreme lateral flexion with the legs straight also strains the abdominal muscles. Padding under the scapula and upper chest relieves pressure on the lower arm. In females, the breasts must be protected from undue pressure of such padding. A pad may also be placed at the lumbar area for support and to provide freer respiratory excursion.

If the incision is to extend posteriorly, the upper arm is drawn forward and down to lift the scapula out of the way. When the arm support is not used, a foam rubber pad is placed under the arm. If the incision extends anteriorly in thoracoabdominal incisions, the position of the patient may be closer to supine than to lateral, with minimal tilting to the side.

**Lateral position for kidney procedures**

After the patient has been anesthetized, he is placed in a lateral position with the kidney region over the break between seat and back sections of the table, as described for chest surgery. The well-padded braces—the short one posterior and the long one anterior—are used to support and stabilize the patient (Fig. 7-17).

To render the kidney region readily accessible, the bridge of the table is raised so that the area between the twelfth rib and the iliac crest is elevated. Elevation is dependent on the cardiovascular physiological response of the body to the increased pressure created, especially on the inferior vena cava. The bridge of the table is slowly raised at the direction of the anesthetist until the patient's side presents a straight horizontal line from shoulder to hip. The table is flexed to lower the

head and legs. In this position, the upper arm may be suspended in well-padded wrapping from the anesthesia screen. The legs should be separated as usual with padding if they tend to overlie each other. Slight flexion will relieve strain on the abdominal muscles. The feet should be supported against foot drop, and the ankles or heels should be protected from undue pressure if necessary, as shown in Fig. 7-17.

To stabilize the body, a restraining strap or adhesive strips are placed across the hip area and secured to the tabletop.

At closure of the wound the strips are released, and the table is straightened to facilitate approximation of the suture line.

## Prone position

The patient lies on his abdomen for surgery on the back, spine, and rectal area. The hazards of the prone position include reduction in vital capacity due to pressure on the lower ribs and intra-abdominal pressure, which interferes with the action of the diaphragm. When the head is lowered, as in jackknife position, there may be increased venous and cerebrospinal fluid pressures that may interfere with arterial inflow. There may be venous stasis in the dependent legs.

After induction of anesthesia with the patient in the supine position, the patient is turned in two movements—first, to the lateral position as previously described and second, to the prone position by rotation. With one arm on the patient's chest and the hand under the axilla, the anesthetist holds the patient firmly as he is tilted and rotated. With the other hand supporting the back of the patient's neck and cradling the head on the forearm, the turn is completed as the assistant rolls the hips over. The patient's head is turned to the side with careful attention to protect the eyes. A flat pillow supports the head, keeping the neck on a level with the spine.

Body rolls extending from the shoulders to the iliac crests are placed on either side to raise the chest and permit the dia-

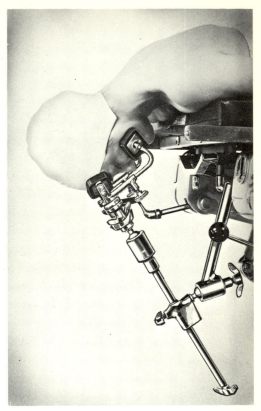

**Fig. 7-18.** Prone position with headrest. Patient is placed on table facedown with supports under thoracic cage to assure respiratory functioning and under legs to relieve strain and pressure. This padded headrest attached to table exposes occipital area and cervical vertebrae. There are padded headrests available to support head in supine, prone, unilateral, and upright positions. (Courtesy American Sterilizer Co., Erie, Pa.)

phragm to move freely and the lungs to expand. Supports must not press against the female breasts.

A cushion is placed under the ankles to prevent pressure on the toes and plantar flexion.

The arms may be extended at the sides, may be placed on armboards, or may be raised above the patient's head. Overextension of the shoulders is prevented if the elbows are slightly flexed and the palms are pronated.

The patient's weight must not rest on the elbows and displace the forearms. If the forearm hangs over the side of the

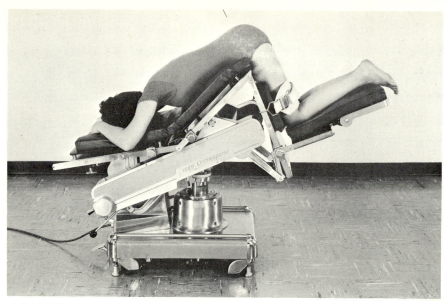

**Fig. 7-19.** Jackknife position for proctological procedures. Patient may be positioned with anterior superior spine and symphysis 1 to 2 inches above break between foot and seat sections. Mattress pad is reversed to cover perineal opening in seat section and provide patient support. Footpiece extension is attached to foot section. Table is fully reflexed and the foot section completely lowered with table in Trendelenburg position. This position increases gravitational effect in sigmoid flexure. Arms are placed over head to relieve pressure on chest. When patient is in proper angulation, head section simply slides out of its normal location and is inserted and locked into foot extension. (Courtesy American Sterilizer Co., Erie, Pa.)

table, the radial nerve may be compressed against the humerus and cause wristdrop.

Prone position may be modified for spinal operations to flex the affected spine over an arch attachment (Fig. 7-18). Modern tables permit the patient's hips to be flexed at one break and have a leg section that can be raised for the patient to kneel on. The surgeon will specify the position he prefers.

**Jackknife or Kraske position**

The jackknife position is a modification of the prone position. It is used for minor proctological procedures and for culdoscopy. The patient's hips are positioned over the central break in the table, and the table is flexed at a sharp angle of 90 degrees, raising the hips and lowering the head and feet to balance the body (Fig. 7-19). The patient's chest and arms need the usual support and restraint in this posi-

tion, and the feet must be protected from dangling off the table.

Leg straps should be applied. The buttocks may be separated with broad straps of adhesive tape secured firmly at the level of the anus a few inches from the midline on either side. These straps are pulled tight and fastened to the side of the operating table. The straps are released at the end of the procedure to facilitate the approximation of the wound edges.

**REFERENCES**

1. Berry, E. C., and Kohn, M. L.: Introduction to operating room technique, ed. 3, New York, 1966, McGraw-Hill Book Co.
2. Chodoff, P.: The influence of position on anesthetic management, J. Am. Assoc. Nurs. Anesth. **32**:307, Oct., 1964.
3. Coleman, C. C.: Positioning the patient for head and neck surgery, J. Am. Assoc. Nurs. Anesth. **35**:117, April, 1967.
4. Collins, V. J.: Positioning the patient for

surgery, A.O.R.N. Journal **4:**55, Nov.-Dec., 1966.

5. Collins, V. J.: Principles of anesthesiology, Philadelphia, 1966, Lea & Febiger.

6. Day, M.: Effects of positions on vital signs during anesthesia, J. Am. Nurs. Anesth. **23:** 178, Aug., 1955.

7. Dornette, W. H.: Anatomy for the anesthesiologist, Springfield, 1963, Charles C Thomas, Publisher.

8. Genereux, T. B.: Positioning patients in the operating room, Am. J. Nurs. **59:**1572, 1959.

9. Keating, V.: Anesthetic accidents, Chicago, 1961, Year Book Medical Publishers, Inc.

10. Minckley, B. B.: Physiologic hazards of position changes in the anesthetized patient, Am. J. Nurs. **69:**2606, 1969.

11. Nahum, L. H.: Improper positioning during surgery, Conn. Med. **28:**2, 1964.

12. Nicholson, M. J., and Eversole, U. H.: Nerve injuries incident to anesthesia and operation, A.O.R.N. Journal **2:**44, March-April, 1964.

# CHAPTER 8

# Operations on the ear, nose, and throat

**LINDSAY L. PRATT** and **MAXINE LOUCKS**

## Operations on the ear

The Latin word *audire* means to hear; thus the word auditory pertains to the sense of hearing. The physical nature of sound pertains to the pressure waves and moving molecules, whereas the sensations man feels lie in the ears, nerves, and brain. The study of the ear and its diseases is known as otology, derived from the Greek word *oto-*, meaning ear.

The ear is a complex mechanism that receives sound waves, discriminates their frequencies, and transmits auditory information into the central nervous system. When a person falls asleep, the sense of hearing is the last of the senses to disappear; when a person awakens, it is the first sense to respond. In man, the ear has an additional function in relation to the maintenance of body equilibrium.

### GENERAL ANATOMY AND PHYSIOLOGY OF THE EAR
#### Ear

The ear comprises three distinct divisions: the external ear (pinna, or auricle), the middle ear, and the inner ear (Fig. 8-1). The middle and inner ear structures are situated in the temporal bone cavity.

EXTERNAL EAR. The external ear consists of an auricle, or pinna, and an external auditory meatus (a tube that ends at the tympanic membrane, or drum, Fig. 8-2).

The auricle is almost lacking in function and is motionless in man. It is covered with skin and consists of a plate of elastic cartilage and some subcutaneous tissue, which form elevations and depressions. The skin on the outer side (front) of the auricle is tightly adherent to the underlying cartilage, whereas that on the posterior (back) surface is looser (Fig. 8-2). For this reason a skin graft is frequently taken from the posterior surface, thus resulting in less gross deformity and scarring.

The external ear has an abundant blood and lymphatic supply. The nerve supply to the external ear is chiefly derived from the trigeminal nerve (fifth cranial) and from the cervical nerves. A branch of the vagus nerve (tenth cranial) enters the posterior part of the ear canal. There is a good neural anastomosis between the external ear and middle ear. (See Fig. 8-1.)

The external auditory canal collects sound waves and serves as a protector and a pressure amplifier. This canal is a sinuous passageway about ½ inch long, directed inward and forward, lying between the concha and the tympanic membrane (Fig. 8-3). It terminates medially in a sulcus (depression) of the tympanic membrane. The walls of the outer third of the canal are fibrocartilaginous; those of the inner two thirds, bony. When the physician inspects the eardrum, the cartilag-

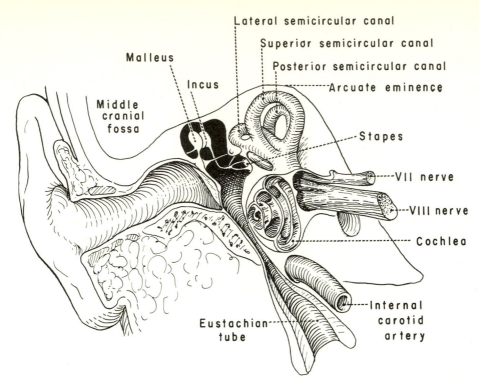

Fig. 8-1. Schematic drawing of external ear, middle ear, and internal ear. *Note:* It is not possible to show all structures in a single plane. Therefore there are distortions from actual anatomy in this schema. (From DeWeese, D. D., and Saunders, W. H.: Textbook of otolaryngology, ed. 3, St. Louis, 1968, The C. V. Mosby Co.)

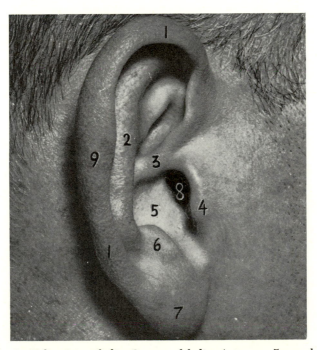

Fig. 8-2. Auricle. 1, Helix; 2, antihelix; 3, crus of helix; 4, tragus; 5, concha; 6, antitragus; 7, lobule; 8, external auditory meatus; 9, Darwin's tubercle. (From DeWeese, D. D., and Saunders, W. H.: Textbook of otolaryngology, ed. 3, St. Louis, 1968, The C. V. Mosby Co.)

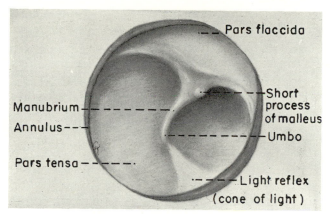

**Fig. 8-3.** Landmarks of right tympanic membrane. Size of pars flaccida is exaggerated in this drawing. (From DeWeese, D. D., and Saunders, W. H.: Textbook of otolaryngology, ed. 3, St. Louis, 1968, The C. V. Mosby Co.)

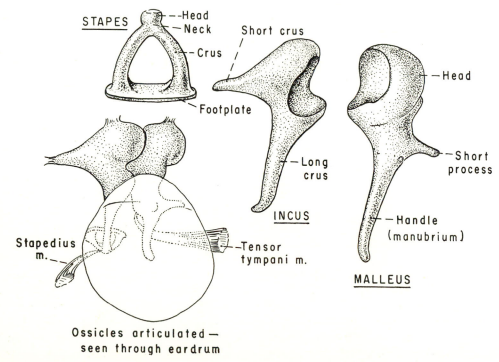

**Fig. 8-4.** Ossicles of middle ear—separate and articulated. Drawing of right ear showing articulated ossicles. (From DeWeese, D. D., and Saunders, W. H.: Textbook of otolaryngology, ed. 3, St. Louis, 1968, The C. V. Mosby Co.)

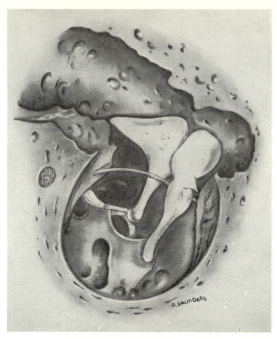

**Fig. 8-5.** Lateral view of right middle ear after drumhead has been removed. Chorda tympani nerve passes behind malleus but in front of long crus of incus. Stapedial tendon joins neck of stapes. (From DeWeese, D. D., and Saunders, W. H.: Textbook of otolaryngology, ed. 3, St. Louis, 1968, The C. V. Mosby Co.)

inous portion of the canal is straightened by drawing the auricle upward and backward with an aural speculum. Lying within the cartilaginous portion of the auricle are fine hairs, sebaceous glands, and special glands that produce cerumen. The tympanic membrane, or eardrum, is the so-called closing membrane. It stretches across the deepest part of the ear canal, thereby serving as a partition between the external canal and the tympanic cavity (Fig. 8-1).

**TYMPANIC MEMBRANE.** The tympanic membrane is composed of three layers: the external layer, which is continuous with the epidermal lining of the meatus; the middle fibrous layer; and the inner layer, which is a continuation of the mucous membrane of the middle ear. The small upper portion of the tympanic membrane is known as Shrapnell's membrane, or the pars flaccida (Fig. 8-3). The larger, vibrating part of the tympanic membrane, which has a fibrous layer, is called the

*pars tensa* (Fig. 8-3). The fibers of the tympanic membrane at its margins form a thickened incomplete band, called the *annulus*. It fits into the bony tympanic sulcus. The annulus breaks superiorly between the anterior and lateral ligaments of the malleus.

**MIDDLE EAR.** The middle ear is a narrow, irregular, oblong, air-conditioning cavity located in the tympanic portion of the temporal bone, which is directly behind the eardrum. In this air-filled space are three very small bones: the malleus, incus, and stapes (Figs. 8-1 and 8-4), as well as the facial nerve (seventh cranial) that controls movements of the face and the chorda tympani nerve that provides taste for most of the anterior portion of the tongue (Figs. 8-5 and 8-6). The temporal lobe of the brain and its meninges are in close association with the middle ear and mastoid (Fig. 8-6). This cavity communicates anteriorly, via the eustachian tube, with the nasopharynx and pos-

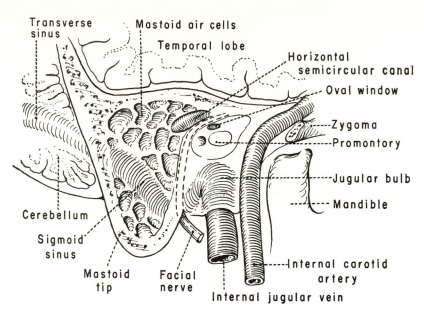

Fig. 8-6. Composite drawing of right ear showing relationship between middle ear, mastoid, and surrounding structures. (From DeWeese, D. D., and Saunders, W. H.: Textbook of otolaryngology, ed. 3, St. Louis, 1968, The C. V. Mosby Co.)

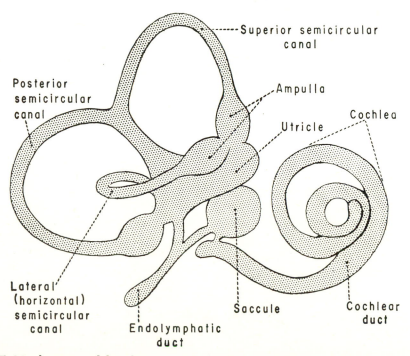

Fig. 8-7. Membranous endolymphatic system of right ear, lateral view. Note that endolymph of cochlea and labyrinth is continuous. Bony capsule of internal ear surrounds endolymphatic system and is separated from it by perilymphatic space. (From DeWeese, D. D., and Saunders, W. H.: Textbook of otolaryngology, ed. 3, St. Louis, 1968, The C. V. Mosby Co.)

teriorly, via the aditus, with the mastoid. The middle ear is lined with mucous membrane, which extends into the eustachian tube (Figs. 8-1 and 8-6).

The middle ear cavity is separated from the inner ear by the former's medial or inner wall. There is a so-called promontory on the medial wall that marks the first turn of the cochlea in the internal ear (Fig. 8-7). Above and slightly behind the promontory is an opening, called the *oval window*, with which the stapes is connected (Figs. 8-1 and 8-6). Below the promontory, covered by mucous membrane, is the round window.

The auditory ossicles in the middle ear cavity form a chain that conducts sound from the eardrum across the middle ear to the oval window, the opening in the inner ear (Fig. 8-6). The *malleus*, resembling a hammer, consists of a head, neck, handle, and long and short processes (Fig. 8-4). The handle and short process of the malleus are attached to the eardrum by very small muscles and join the second bone, the *incus*. Resembling an anvil, the incus consists of a body and long and short processes. The long crus of the incus is in contact with the third and innermost bone, the *stapes* (Figs. 8-4 and 8-5). Resembling a stirrup, the stapes consists of a head, neck, anterior and posterior crura, and footplate that fits in the oval window (Figs. 8-4 and 8-5). The tensor tympani muscle and stapedius muscle and their ligaments connect the ossicles together. The ligaments and muscles attached to the ossicles are essential to the latter's proper functioning. For example, the tensor tympani muscle acts to draw the drum inward to increase tension of the latter, whereas the stapedius muscle acts to draw the stapes away from the oval window to lessen tension of the drum. The middle ear and mastoid are supplied with blood from the branches of the internal maxillary artery, a branch of the external carotid system. Important vascular channels are closely associated with the middle

ear (Fig. 8-6). It has an abundant neural anastomosis.

Difficulties in hearing airborne sound may be corrected by a hearing aid, but proper bone conduction is essential to hearing one's own voice. When a bony growth is present in the ossicular chain, the ligaments and bones are unable to move mechanically as intended and thus interfere with the passage of sound waves to the inner ear.

INNER EAR. The inner ear is a complex structure located in the petrous portion of the temporal bone that has two distinct parts, each with specific functions that are delicately coordinated. One part (cochlea) is concerned with the special sense of hearing and the other part (vestibular labyrinth) with the maintenance of equilibrium (Fig. 8-7). The two major parts of the inner ear—the cochlea and the vestibular labyrinth—have various compartments.

The bony cochlea and vestibular labyrinth lie in the petrous portion of the temporal bone (Fig. 8-6). In the small channels of these two structures are two distinct fluids: the perilymph and endolymph. The perilymphatic fluid, lying in the bony canals, surrounds the membranous inner ear, thus serving as a protective cushion to the end organ receptors for hearing. The perilymphatic fluid is continuous with the subarachnoid space and its cerebrospinal fluid through the aqueduct of the cochlea (cochlear duct). The endolymph, which is contained in a fragile membranous tube, bathes and nourishes the sensory cells and their supporting structures. The endolymph in the cochlea and labyrinth is contained in a continuous closed system with no ducts (Fig. 8-7).

COCHLEA. The cochlea is a tubular formation that winds as a spiral around a central part, called the *modiolus*. Within the cochlea are three compartments (Fig. 8-8): the scala vestibuli, which is associated with the oval window; the scala tympani, which is associated with the

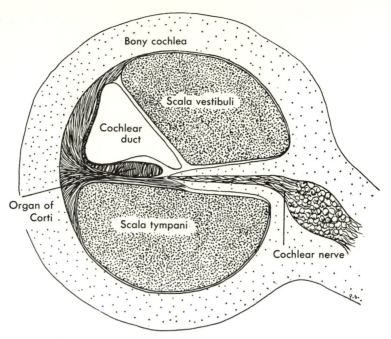

**Fig. 8-8.** Diagram of cross section of cochlea. (From DeWeese, D. D., and Saunders, W. H.: Textbook of otolaryngology, ed. 3, St. Louis, 1968, The C. V. Mosby Co.)

round window; and the cochlear duct. The scala vestibuli and scala tympani rest in perilymph, whereas the cochlear duct contains endolymph.

On the vestibular surface of the basilar membrane of the cochlea is the delicate neural end organ for hearing, called the *organ of Corti*. From its neuroepithelium project thousands of fragile *hair cells* that are set in motion by the sound waves on entrance into the cochlea (Fig. 8-8). The organ of Corti extends along the entire length of the cochlea, except at the apex of the modiolus (helicotrema), where the scala tympani and scala vestibuli join.

The cochlea transmits sound waves to the auditory nerve and also acts as a microphone through which the mechanical energy of vibrations is converted into electrochemical impulses, probably by means of the hair cells of the organ of Corti.

The inner ear is connected with the brain through the eighth cranial (acoustic) nerve, which enters the temporal cortex of the cerebrum, where the impulses are

interpreted as meaningful sound. This connecting fiber system (transverse gyri of Heschl) is located on both sides of the brain.

VESTIBULAR LABYRINTH. This part of the inner ear is composed of the utricle, saccule, and three semicircular canals (Fig. 8-7) that are known as lateral, superior, and posterior canals. In each ear, the canals are arranged at right angles to one another so that any movement of the head affects one or more of the semicircular canals. For example, when the head is in an erect position, the lateral (horizontal) canal is not quite horizontal. When a patient is turned quickly on the operating table, a current is set up in the endolymph by the neural cells in the vestibular labyrinth, thereby resulting in vertigo. Each canal is enlarged at a point near the utricle. This enlargement is called the *ampulla* of the canal, in which resides the specialized neuroepithelium (end organ of equilibrium).

The utricle of the vestibular labyrinth is concerned with static equilibrium and

regulation of the sense of position in space. Stimulation of the utricle results in compensatory eye positions. The neural fibers from the utricle and semicircular canals join to form the vestibular portion of the eighth cranial nerve.

The blood supply of the internal ear is derived from the internal auditory branch of the basilar artery and the stylomastoid branch of the posterior auricular artery. The internal auditory artery enters the internal meatus and divides into the cochlea and vestibular labyrinth branches. The veins from the cochlea and labyrinth unite at the bottom of the internal meatus with the veins from the semicircular canals to form the internal auditory veins.

## Temporal bone

The temporal bone is composed of five separate parts, which are joined together by suture lines (Fig. 8-6). Only the tympanic and petrous portions contain structures directly related to hearing. The *squamous* portion is a large piece of bone that is frequently pneumatized (Fig. 8-22). On its external surface is a groove for the middle temporal artery; on its internal surface, grooves for the middle meningeal vessels.

The *mastoid* portion of the temporal bone lies behind and below the squamous portion, attached to the sternocleidomastoid and digastric muscles. The internal surface of the mastoid process is in close association with important intracranial structures and with those of the middle ear (Fig. 8-6). The interior of the mastoid process is composed of a cortex that covers a system of intercommunicating air cells. The mastoid antrum is the largest of these air cells and connects directly with the middle ear through the aditus. The air cells are lined with a thin mucous membrane that is continuous with that of the middle ear.

The *petrous* portion of the temporal bone fuses with the base of the skull and contains the structures of the inner ear, in-cluding the sensory end organs of hearing and equilibrium. In the petrous portion are openings for the trigeminal ganglion, facial and auditory nerves, and internal auditory artery.

The *zygomatic* portion of the temporal bone extends anteriorly and joins the zygoma or malar bone of the cheek.

The *tympanic* portion of the temporal bone contains the middle ear and forms part of the ear canal.

## Hearing loss

The amplitude of the air waves that strike the tympanic membrane determines the loudness or intensity of the sound.

In dealing with hearing loss, the loudness is measured in decibels (db). It is a logarithmic method of dealing with large numbers: the decibel is a ratio, not an absolute value; it compares the relationship between two sound intensities and the smallest perceptible change in loudness that the human ear can hear. Hearing loss is expressed by recording auditory acuity for each frequency in decibels.

• • •

The physiology of hearing may be summarized as follows:

1. The sound waves collect in the auricle.

2. The vibrating air waves pass into the external canal and hit the eardrum.

3. The ossicles, arranged in a lever system, respond to the vibration, thus amplifying the sound. First the malleus moves, and then this movement is transmitted to the incus, which in turn transmits it to the stapes.

4. The small footplate of the stapes delivers the sound to the inner ear by rocking the oval window.

5. Sound pressure, delivered through the oval window into the cochlea, agitates the perilymph and endolymph.

6. Relief of pressure is provided by shielding of the round window from sound.

7. The receptors of hearing (hair cells) are distorted.

8. Mechanical sound is transformed into electrochemical impulse.

9. These impulses are sent via the acoustic nerve to the temporal cortex of the brain, where they are interpreted as meaningful sound.

## PREPARATION FOR OPERATIONS ON THE EAR AND ASSOCIATED STRUCTURES

With the introduction of antibiotics, the operating microscope, delicate instruments, and accurate understanding of the anatomical structures involved, the otological surgeon is now more able to improve the hearing of the patient, as well as control a disease process of the mastoid.

At present, new concepts and techniques are being introduced. Surgical treatment of hearing loss, including stapedectomy and stapes replacement, is aimed at correcting abnormalities of the conduction apparatus. Surgical treatment of sensory-neural hearing loss (Ménière's syndrome) is offered to selected patients suffering from a disabling vertigo or an intolerable tinnitus.

### Preparation of the patient for otological procedures

SKIN CLEANSING. Aseptic techniques are presented in Chapter 4. Prior to surgery, whenever possible, the male patients are requested to get a close haircut and the women a shampoo, since shampooing will not be permitted for about 2 weeks after surgery.

For most otological procedures, the hair is removed and skin shaved at least 1½ inches from the site of the proposed incision. The hair is removed mainly from the area above the ear for an endaural approach, from behind the ear for a postauricular approach. Long hair may be tied in small braids and petrolatum rubbed into the hair along the hairline; then it is brushed away from the operative field.

A solution of mild soap and water or 3% hexachlorophene (pHisoHex) and water is used to cleanse the exposed auricle and the periauricular skin (Chapter 4). The meatus is cleansed with the aid of cotton applicators. A small amount of acetone is applied around the ear to remove some of the soap fats and allow a disposable drape to adhere more securely to the skin.

### Positioning of the patient for otological procedures

Quietness and immobility of the patient is most important in otological surgery. In some procedures (myringotomy under local anesthesia) the attendant should hold the patient's head firmly in position. For other operations (stapedectomy) the patient's head may be mobilized and supported in a padded headpiece attached to the operating table. The comfort of the patient and proper body alignment are most important, especially in long procedures such as tympanoplasty. Principles of positioning are discussed in Chapter 7.

The patient is placed on the operating table in a dorsal recumbent position, his head resting on a firm pad or brace and turned to the side with the affected ear uppermost. The upper extremities should rest alongside the body and be secured in a flap-type restraint sheet. The arms and body of an infant may be wrapped in a mummy-type sheet. To relieve pressure on nerves and support muscles, firm padding of suitable shape and size should be used. In some cases the surgeon may prefer the patient to be in the prone position with a headpiece or firm pad.

To accomplish effective visualization, the head of the patient is turned with the affected ear uppermost; the surgeon stands or sits in a frontal position. With inclined oculars, he looks directly ahead to visualize the postcanal wall. The entire operating table is tilted laterally 20 degrees to bring the external canal into proper position.

### Draping the patient for otological procedures

In the presence of infectious organisms, disposable sheets and towels should be used. An opening can readily be made with scissors in the sterile disposable sheet or towel to expose the operative site. A standard ear pack is used.

The principles of draping the patient for surgery are discussed in Chapter 5. For major otological procedures the towels and sheets, preferably a disposable type, are placed on the patient as follows.

Three towels, folded lengthwise, are placed around the operative site. The first towel is placed horizontally above the ear, the second towel is placed diagonally on the outer prepared skin area surrounding the ear, and the third towel is placed vertically in front of the meatus, thereby creating a triangular operative field around the affected ear.

A folded fenestrated sheet is unfolded over the patient and table, with the operative site in view through the opening.

The draped tables with sterile instruments and the operating microscope are positioned around the patient. For example, if the operation involves the left

ear, the sterile instrument table is placed near the left side of the operating table. The scrubbed nurse or technician usually sits or stands near the instrument table and passes the instruments to the surgeon in such a manner that he does not have to turn away from the operative microscope.

All safeguards should be taken to prevent explosive hazards. This is most important because there are many electrical appliances in use during otological surgery. Safety standards are discussed in Chapter 5.

### Instruments and supplies for otological procedures

(Figs. 8-9 to 8-14)

#### Endaural mastoidectomy instruments

The endaural mastoidectomy setup includes the major ear pack, a head drape, a basin set, a skin preparation set, operating

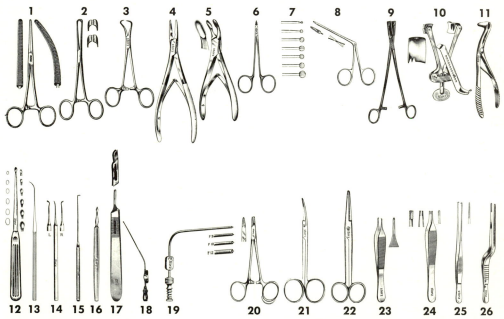

**Fig. 8-9.** Instrument arrangement of back table for mastoidectomy. **1,** Rochester-Pean forceps; **2,** Allis forceps; **3,** towel clamps; **4,** Lempert rongeur; **5,** Hartman rongeur; **6,** malleus nipper; **7,** assorted dental burrs; **8,** Littauer ear forceps; **9,** Proud fascia crusher; **10,** House endaural retractor; **11,** endaural speculum; **12,** assorted endaural curettes; **13,** straight pick; **14,** picks—right and left curved; **15,** incus hook; **16,** lancet knife; **17,** knife handle; **18,** ear suction tube; **19,** assorted Ferguson-Frazier suction tubes; **20,** malleus nipper; **21,** Mayo scissors, curved; **22,** Mayo scissors, straight; **23,** Adson forceps; **24,** Brown-Adson forceps; **25,** Walsh dressing forceps, with and without teeth; **26,** nasal dressing forceps. (Courtesy Storz Instrument Co., St. Louis, Mo.)

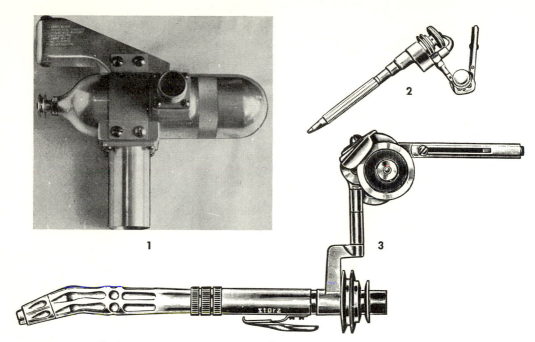

**Fig. 8-10.** Drills for ear operation. **1,** Storz-Jordan-Day bone engine; **2,** Chayes handpiece; **3,** Wullstein handpiece for use with Jordan-Day engine. (Courtesy Storz Instrument Co.; New York, N. Y.)

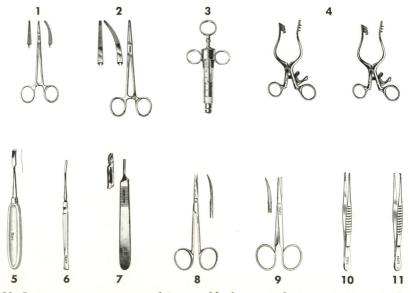

**Fig. 8-11.** Instrument arrangement of Mayo table for mastoidectomy. **1,** Mosquito hemostat; **2,** Crile hemostat; **3,** Sana-Lok syringe; **4,** Wullstein-Weitlaner retractors; **5,** Lempert elevator, heavy; **6,** Lempert elevator, angled; **7,** knife handle and no. 15 blade; **8,** small eye scissors, straight and curved; **9,** blunt scissors, straight and curved; **10,** dressing forceps, without teeth; **11,** dressing forceps, with teeth. (Courtesy Storz Instrument Co., St. Louis, Mo.)

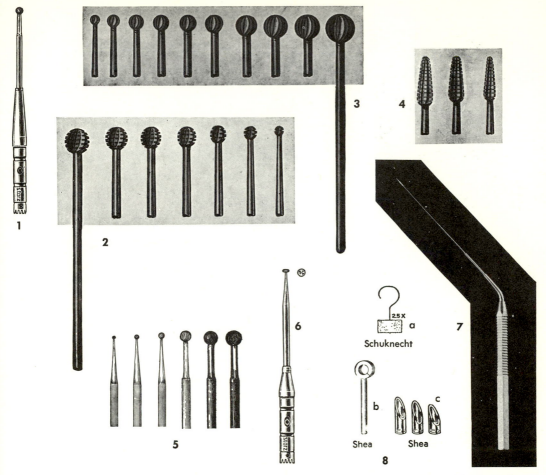

**Fig. 8-12.** Instruments for operations on middle and inner ear. **1,** Wullstein diamond burr, available in various sizes; **2,** crosscut burrs, sizes 6 to 2 mm.; **3,** cutting round burrs, sizes 2.3 to 8 mm.; **4,** perforating burrs, various sizes; **5,** polishing burrs, various sizes; **6,** Hough-Wullstein crurotomy saw burr; **7,** Goodhill strut introducer; **8,** prosthetic struts, various types and sizes— **a,** Schuknecht (Gelfoam and wire); **b,** Shea piston (Teflon); **c,** Shea (polyethylene). (Courtesy Storz Instrument Co., New York, N. Y.)

table appliances, sutures, and the following instruments:

**First group**

2 Lancet knives
1 Lempert flap knife
1 Myringotomy knife, curved
2 Knife handles no. 3 with no. 15 blades
2 Dental picks, nos. 11 and 12
1 Dental pick, curved
1 Small sharp curved scissors
1 Small blunt curved scissors
1 Small sharp straight scissors

1 House-Tragus hook
1 Mayo scissors, straight
1 Mayo scissors, curved
2 Joseph double hooks
1 Endaural speculum
3 Walsh hand retractors, assorted
6 Endaural curettes, nos. 5-0 through 1
1 Olivekrona rongeur
1 Malleus nipper
1 Heavy periosteal elevator
1 Light periosteal elevator
2 Metal applicators
1 Burr holder with assorted cutting burrs
2 Fine tissue forceps (with and without teeth)

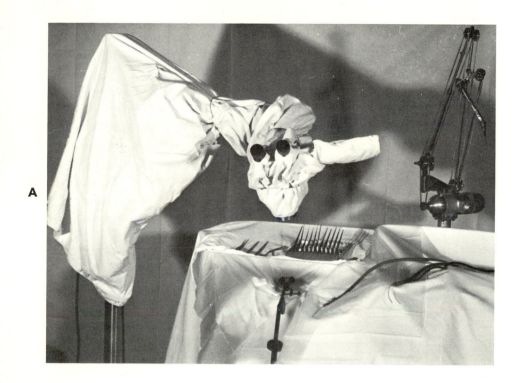

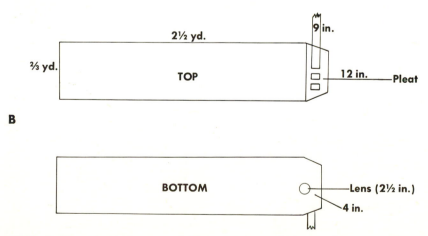

Fig. 8-13. **A,** Draped microscope and Mayo stand are shown in place over patient. Suction and tubing and Jordon-Day drill are assembled in position ready for use. Instruments in tray and self-retaining aural speculum holder are on stand. Microscope is draped with sterile tubular cover made of cotton. **B,** Diagrammatic drawing of microscopic drape. Microscope drape made of cotton material. This cover is 2½ × ⅔ yards; side observation tube cover is 9 × 4 inches with a 3-inch opening that is elastic bound; binocular cover is 2 × -½ inches with elastic-bound opening; and lens cover is 2½ inches in diameter and elastic bound.

2 Heavy tissue forceps (with and without teeth)
1 Bayonet tissue forceps
1 Adson tissue forceps
2 Needle holders
3 Straight mosquito forceps, 5 in.
6 Curved mosquito forceps, 5 in.
4 Towel clamps
1 Allis clamp, 6 in.
1 Rochester-Pean forceps, curved, 6¼ in.
1 Crile forceps, curved, 5½ in.
1 Self-retaining retractor with teeth
1 Self-retaining retractor without teeth
3 Temporal muscle retractors with blades
1 Littauer ear forceps
  Assorted endural specula
  Assorted sizes of Ferguson-Frazier suction tubes
2 Baron suction tubes, nos. 5 to 7 Fr.

### Second group

2 Large irrigating bulbs and plastic tips
1 Sana-Lok control syringe, 10 ml.
1 Suction tubing
1 Electrosurgical unit with electrodes
1 Operating microscope with sterile cover (Figs. 8-13 and 8-14)
1 Headlight
1 Tube antibiotic ointment
1 Gauze pack
1 Closure suture (silk no. 3-0 swaged to a cutting needle)
1 Jordan-Day drill set (sterile)

### Stapedectomy and mobilization instrument setup (Figs. 8-15 and 8-16)

The items include a head drape pack and basin set, a skin cleansing preparation set, an operating table side extension, a local anesthesia set, and the following instruments:

1 Guilford-Wright flap knife
1 House lancet knife
1 Myringotomy knife, curved
1 Walsh crurotomy knife
1 House elevator
1 House strut guide
1 Walsh footplate chisel
1 Hough pick, 45-degree angle
1 Hough pick, straight
1 House curette
1 House pick, 1 mm., 90-degree angle
1 Walsh footplate pick, 90-degree angle
1 Walsh footplate pick, 30-degree angle
1 Walsh pick, curved up
1 Shea oblique pick
1 Shea fenestra hook, 25-degree angle
1 Crimper forceps
2 House strut forceps
2 Fine serrated ear forceps
1 Littauer ear forceps
2 Bellucci scissors, left and right
1 Knife handle no. 3 with no. 15 blade

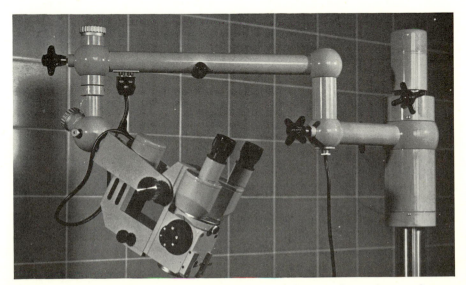

**Fig. 8-14.** Operating microscope used during stapes mobilization, fenestration, and tympanoplasty procedures. Lens system allows magnification change from 6 to 40 times without change in distance between microscope and ear. (From DeWeese, D. D., and Saunders, W. H.: Textbook of otolaryngology, ed. 3, St. Louis, 1968, The C. V. Mosby Co.)

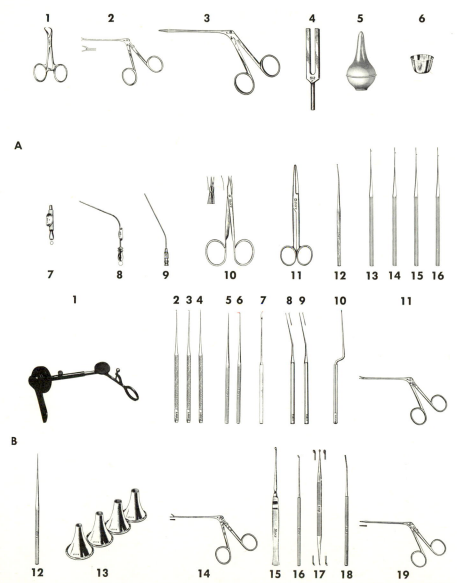

**Fig. 8-15. A,** Instrument arrangement of back table for stapedectomy. **1,** Towel clamps; **2,** McGee wire closure forceps; **3,** Noyes ear forceps; **4,** tuning fork; **5,** ear syringe; **6,** basin; **7,** suction adapter; **8,** Baron ear suction; **9,** Rosen suction tube; **10,** scissors, small sharp-pointed; **11,** Mayo scissors, straight; **12,** House strut guide; **13 to 16,** House strut calipers. **B,** Instrument arrangement of Mayo table for stapedectomy. **1,** Shea speculum holder; **2,** Shea fenestra hook, 90-degree; **3,** Shea fenestra hook, 90-degree, short; **4,** Shea pick; **5 and 6,** House picks; **7,** myringotomy knife; **8,** Hough pick, 45-degree; **9,** Hough pick, 90-degree; **10,** Walsh footplate chisel; **11,** Bellucci scissors; **12,** House straight pick; **13,** assorted ear specula; **14,** House alligator forceps; **15,** Lempert flap knife; **16,** House lancet knife; **17,** House curette; **18,** House elevator; **19,** House alligator and crimper forceps. (Courtesy Storz Instrument Co., St. Louis, Mo.)

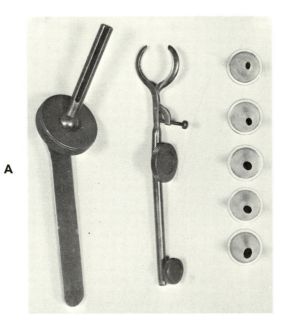

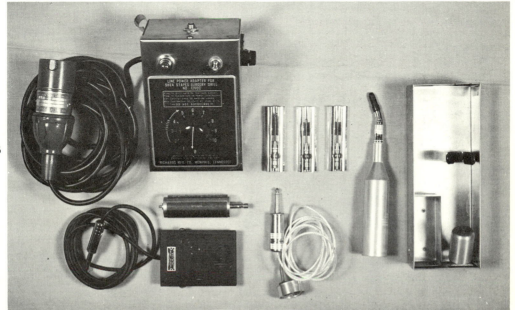

**Fig. 8-16.** **A,** Shea speculum holder. **B,** Battery cords, transformer, and drill and bits.

1 Small sharp straight scissors
2 House suction tubing adapters
6 Assorted Rosen suction tubes
2 Baron suction tubes, nos. 5 to 7 Fr.
1 Suction tubing
4 House strut calipers
1 Tuning fork
6 Assorted sizes of ear specula
1 Small bulb syringe
1 Shea speculum holder
8 Towel clamps, 3 in.
1 Needle, 28-gauge × 1½ in.
1 Sana-Lok control syringe, 5 ml.
  Prosthesis of choice
1 Microscope with sterile cover
1 Shea drill set with sterile handle and assorted burs
1 Wire bending die
1 Ruler
1 Schuknecht wire cutter
  Steel wire, 28-gauge

**For vein graft**

1 Minor plastic dissecting tray
1 Minor linen and gown pack
1 Eye sheet
1 Local anesthesia set

### Care and handling of instruments and supplies

Each piece of equipment must be kept in working order. Each surgeon has his own preferences regarding instruments. Standard instrument setup should be determined by the surgeons, with assistance of the operating room supervisory staff. Listings of items for the various types of operations and the individual surgeon's preference should be kept up-to-date in the operating room file (Chapter 2).

The basic principles of sterilization of instruments are discussed in Chapter 3. Care and handling of instruments is discussed in Chapter 5. Fine, delicate instruments for tympanoplasty and stapedectomy procedures should be kept in special rack-type instrument trays. This type of metal tray provides for the separation of instruments from each other, thereby protecting them from damage and facilitating easy handling during surgery. The instruments should be arranged in the rack from left to right or from right to left, in the order of use.

The arrangement of the setup on the instrument table and Mayo stand must be standardized for effective teamwork during the operation (Fig. 8-13).

OPERATING MICROSCOPE. Proper illumination of the operative site is provided by means of the microscope that illuminates and magnifies the small delicate anatomical structures encountered in otological surgery. Several kinds of operating microscopes (Figs. 8-13 and 8-14) are available, with different attachments. For operations through an ear speculum, the microscope provides direct light and permits the surgeon to work effectively at a distance, using his own vision and selected magnification of 6, 10, 16, 25, or 40 times.

The microscope is draped with a sterile cover (Fig. 8-13). The surgeon adjusts the microscope before it is draped in readiness for surgery and manipulates it during the procedure.

When the microscope is not in use, it should be kept in a storage area that is away from traffic, free of dust, and properly ventilated.

SPECULA. Varying sizes of specula are needed to fit the different sizes and shapes of the canals encountered.

NEEDLES AND SYRINGES FOR LOCAL INJECTION. Local anesthesia is preferred for some operations and obtained by block injection (Chapter 5).

For stapes surgery, the initial local anesthetic such as a solution of lidocaine-epinephrine (Xylocaine-Adrenalin) is injected, using a 28-gauge, 1½-inch needle attached to a 5 ml., double-ringed Luer-Lok syringe. For the secondary injection, a heavier-gauged needle (26-gauge, 1½-inch) is generally used. Metal or Pyrex glass medication cups, properly labeled, are necessary for storage of the solution.

KNIVES. For myringotomy, a sharp knife in perfect condition is needed. After one use, the myringotomy knife should be resharpened. For stapes surgery, the circumferential knives with blades facing to the right and others to the left are designed for various purposes: (1) to make the

primary incision, (2) to elevate the periosteum, (3) to enucleate the fibrous annulus, (4) to separate the incudostapedial joint, and (5) to dissect or resect the scar tissue or the stapedial tendon.

SCISSORS. Mayo scissors, curved and straight, are used for radical mastoidectomy approach and for cutting suture ends. Delicate scissors with angular blades (Bellucci type) are used in middle ear operations to incise and divide the stapedial tendon or incise this tendon and scar tissue bands (Figs. 8-9, 8-11, and 8-15, *B*).

ELECTRIC DRILL AND BURRS. The electrically driven dental drills and burrs are used to remove bone (Fig. 8-12). Cortical and hard cellular bone may be removed by means of an electric drill with a rotating-type burr. For stapes procedures, several microburrs are needed. Both cutting- and diamond-type burrs are used. These burrs may be attached to an angular Wullstein-type handpiece driven by a cable-drive engine or Shea drill set (Figs. 8-10 and 8-16). During surgery, the surgeon holds the handpiece as he would hold a pen and uses the sides of the burr as the cutting edge.

RONGEURS, PERIOSTEAL ELEVATORS, AND DISSECTORS (Figs. 8-9 and 8-11). To remove overhanging cortical bone, a Kerrison-type rongeur may be desired. To remove the thin bony plate, meatal wall, or bridge, a delicate narrow rongeur may be preferred. Fine dissectors of many variations are available.

For radical mastoidectomy or tympanoplasty procedures, fine narrow-angular periosteal elevators and dissectors are needed to free the periosteum from the bone (Figs. 8-9 and 8-11).

For stapes surgery, very fine hooks with 45-degree, 90-degree, and 180-degree angles are essential dissecting tools (Fig. 8-15, *B*).

BONE CURETTES. Various types of bone curettes are used to remove soft bone or substance on the dura, on the sinus wall, or in the vicinity of the facial nerve. Curettes must be sharp.

For stapes surgery, strong-shank curettes are needed to remove the annulus and posterior canal wall bone or bridge. Right and left curettes, each with large and small cups, are also needed (Fig. 8-15, *B*).

DRILLS AND BURRS. The use of many different types of drills, according to the surgeon's preference, has replaced the need for mallet, chisels, and gouges. The corresponding burrs come in many different types and sizes. Very tiny ones are available for stapes surgery.

DISSECTING FORCEPS. In radical mastoidectomy and tympanoplasty, several types of grasping and cutting alligator forceps are needed to manipulate within the canal and the middle ear (Fig. 8-9).

STAPES STRUT INTRODUCER, MALLEABLE PROBES, AND NEEDLES (Fig. 8-15). The malleable fine probes are used to determine the mobility of a footplate fragment, palpate other areas within the middle ear, or palpate the position of the facial nerve. The sharp needle probe is used to manipulate fragments of the tympanic membrane. The strut introducer is used to open the collar of the articulated polyethylene strut so that it may encircle and grasp the short process and create an effective articulated incus-strut union.

SUCTION TUBES. For mastoidectomy and tympanoplasty procedures, several patent suction cannulae are needed. Adequate suctioning must be available at all times.

For stapes surgery, the tips of the suction apparatus must be available in three gauges 18, 22, and 24—and equipped with cutoffs to vary the degree of suction (Fig. 8-15, *A*).

CAUTERIZATION OR COAGULATION TIPS. In radical mastoidectomy, tympanoplasty, and stapes procedures, electrical coagulation is desired to control oozing. In stapes surgery, an insulated suction tube may be used to cauterize small bleeding vessels at the margin of the incision. This tube is attached to the patient's cord of a delicate coagulating machine. The objective is to control oozing and prevent blood from entering the middle ear during suctioning.

CONTINUOUS IRRIGATION EQUIPMENT. Irrigation of the field is done frequently and quickly with sterile warm saline or Ringer's solution, suctioning apparatus, and bulb syringes to prevent clogging of the burr and remove bone dust in areas where osteogenesis is to be avoided.

SYNTHETIC MATERIALS TO CONTROL BLEEDING. Absorbable gelatin sponge (Gelfoam) plugs or pledgets may be placed against the bone. Bone wax may be used in some cases; however, since it is a foreign body, absorbing substances are preferred.

ANESTHESIA EQUIPMENT. For myringotomy in adults or children, a general anesthetic may be administered. Myringotomy in infants may be done without an anesthetic agent.

For procedures such as endaural radical mastoidectomy and tympanoplasty, a general anesthetic is used. Intubation of the trachea is usually done by means of the

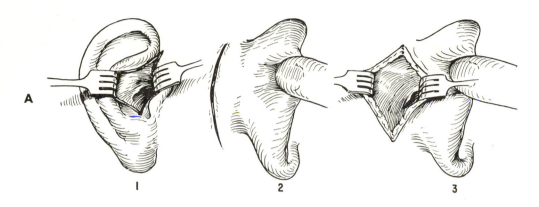

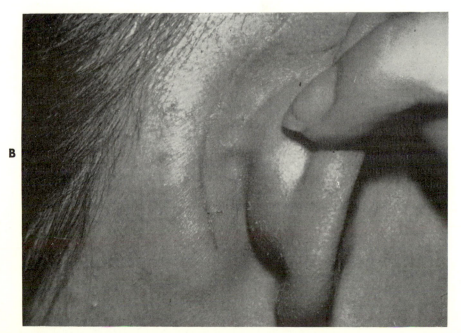

Fig. 8-17. A, Mastoidectomy incisions. 1, Endaural; 2, postaural; 3, postaural incision open. B, Postaural incision 10 days after operation. (From DeWeese, D. D., and Saunders, W. H.: Textbook of otolaryngology, ed. 3, St. Louis, 1968, The C. V. Mosby Co.)

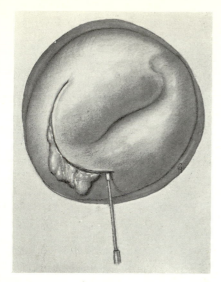

Fig. 8-18. Circumferential incision provides for visibility of eardrum without damage to ossicles and for removal of pus or fluid from middle ear. (From DeWeese, D. D., and Saunders, W. H.: Textbook of otolaryngology, ed. 3, St. Louis, 1968, The C. V. Mosby Co.)

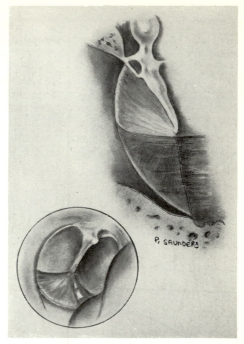

Fig. 8-19. Air-fluid level behind tympanic membrane. *Inset:* Typical appearance of retracted drumhead and meniscus. (From DeWeese, D. D., and Saunders, W. H.: Textbook of otolaryngology, ed. 3, St. Louis, 1968, The C. V. Mosby Co.)

oral route, then the endotracheal tube is connected to the anesthesia apparatus. An intravenous anesthetic agent may be administered in addition to nitrous oxide and oxygen.

For stapes surgery, a local block anesthetic such as a lidocaine-epinephrine mixture is administered. Moistened cotton on applicators may be used to massage the solution from the injection site medially toward the region of the annulus.

## OPERATIONS ON THE EAR AND ASSOCIATED STRUCTURES
### Incisional approaches for otological operations

The endaural (vertical) incision frequently is used for temporal operations, except for simple mastoidectomy. The first incision extends from the superior neatal wall, and the second extends directly upward to a point between the meatus and the upper edge of the auricle, where the two incisions join (Fig. 8-17).

The high posterior incision may be used in operations on infants or young children. The incision is placed at a higher posterior level than is the endural incision, thereby avoiding possible damage to the facial nerve.

The postaural incision may be used to expose the mastoid process. It follows the curve of the postaural fold, beginning at the upper attachment of the auricle and continuing behind the postaural fold downward to the tip of the mastoid process (Fig. 8-17).

For stapes surgery, a circumferential incision is made in the posterior half of the canal, starting at the inferior aspect of the annulus and ending posterior to the short process of the malleus.

For myringotomy, a circumferential (posteroinferior) incision is made. It provides for wide drainage and removal of pus or fluid under pressure from the middle ear (Fig. 8-18).

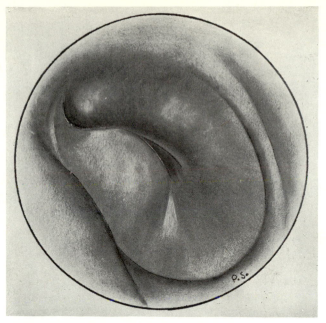

Fig. 8-20. In purulent otitis media, pus under pressure pushes eardrum outward, thus resulting in bulging tympanic membrane. (From DeWeese, D. D., and Saunders, W. H.: Textbook of otolaryngology, ed. 3, St. Louis, 1968, The C. V. Mosby Co.)

## Myringotomy

DEFINITION. Incising of the tympanic membrane under direct vision.

CONSIDERATIONS. Myringotomy is done to treat an acute otitis media, in the presence of an exudate, or, more commonly now, for the presence of fluid in the middle ear that produces a hearing loss. The patient has severe pain. There is a bulging of the membrane (Figs. 8-19 and 8-20). By releasing the pus or fluid, hearing is restored and the infection controlled. Frequently, tubes are inserted through the tympanic membrane.

SETUP AND PREPARATION OF THE PATIENT. Skin cleansing and positioning of the patient, as described previously. The instrument setup includes the following:

1 Myringotomy knife
2 Aural applicators, metal
1 Hartman aural forceps, delicate type
1 Aural speculum
1 Asepto syringe, 2 oz.
1 Tube gauze packing, ⅛ and ¼ in. width
1 Culture set
1 Square cotton, absorbent
1 Suction set
1 Minor ear pack

OPERATIVE PROCEDURE

1. Through microscopic visualization, the aural speculum is inserted in the canal; using a sharp myringotomy knife, a small curved incision is made in the posteroinferior quadrant or the pars tensa, and the thickened membrane is cut.

2. A culture is taken to determine the type of organisms present.

3. Pus and fluid are suctioned out.

4. A eustachian tube prosthesis is usually put into place.

## Radical mastoidectomy

DEFINITION. Removal of the mastoid air cells and the tympanic membrane, thereby converting the middle ear and mastoid into a single cavity, and removal of the involved malleus, incus, chorda tympani, and mucoperiosteal lining.

CONSIDERATIONS. A radical mastoidectomy is done to treat chronic otitis media

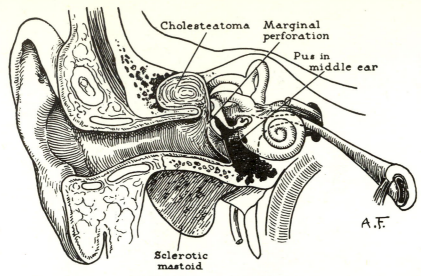

Fig. 8-21. Cholesteatoma of middle ear is mass of epidermoid cells arranged in concentric layers, intermingled with cholesterin crystals. Squamous epithelium grows through tympanic perforation to form pouch, which finally lines middle ear cavity and adjacent mastoid cells. Center of pouch tends to become necrotic and houses infectious bacteria. These lesions increase in size slowly at margins of tympanic membrane. (From Davis, H., and Fowler, E. P.: In Davis, H., and Silverman, S. R., editors: Hearing and deafness, rev. ed., New York, 1960, Holt, Rinehart & Winston, Inc.)

when it has involved the mastoid air cells. A cholesteatoma may be associated with a chronic otitis media (Fig. 8-21). In this condition, skin from the external auditory canal has grown into the middle ear, where it acts as a foreign body producing erosion and more serious complications. Cholesteatoma should be surgically removed.

Radical mastoidectomy may also be done to provide adequate exposure in the treatment of facial nerve decompression to drain an extradural abscess in the bony labyrinth.

**SETUP AND PREPARATION OF THE PATIENT.** The preparation, including skin cleansing and positioning of the patient in a dorsal recumbent position, has been discussed in Chapters 4 and 7. The endaural setup has been described earlier in this chapter.

**OPERATIVE PROCEDURE**

1. An endaural or postaural incision is made using a Bard-Parker knife. Bleeding vessels are clamped and ligated. With a second knife the periosteum is incised and freed to form a flap. The wound is retracted with a self-retaining retractor (Fig. 8-11).

2. The meatal flap is cut, exposing the mastoid area by means of a circumferential knife, narrow periosteal elevator, and curved scissors.

3. The mastoid antrum is exposed. By means of round cutting burrs attached to an electric drill, the bone of the outer cortex is removed. The osseous meatal walls are removed with rongeurs or burrs. The wound is irrigated and suctioned. Cotton pledgets are used for sponging the operative site.

4. The thin bridge of bone between the meatus and antrum is removed with angular dissectors and fine curettes (Fig. 8-22).

5. The tympanic membrane, malleus, incus, and mucoperiosteal lining of the middle ear cavity are excised by means of stapes instruments, as for a stapes operation (Figs. 8-5 and 8-21).

6. The tympanic cavity is cleaned. The wound is closed with sutures. A musculoplasty may be done by taking a strip of temporalis muscle from above the ear and

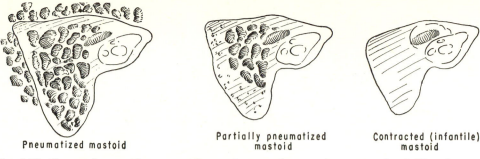

Pneumatized mastoid        Partially pneumatized        Contracted (infantile)
                                    mastoid                         mastoid

Fig. 8-22. Types of mastoid pneumatization. Otitis media in infancy or early childhood can arrest normal pneumatization at any stage. (From DeWeese, D. D., and Saunders, W. H.: Textbook of otolaryngology, ed. 3, St. Louis, 1968, The C. V. Mosby Co.)

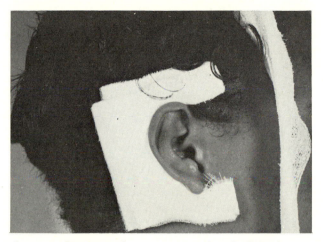

Fig. 8-23. Head dressing after mastoidectomy. Space directly behind ear is padded because ear, if pressed lightly against skull, becomes painful. Gauze strip of bandage will later be used to tie together the several windings of gauze. (From Saunders, W. H., Havener, W. H., Fair, C. J., and Hickey, J. T.: Nursing care in eye, ear, nose, and throat disorders, ed. 2, St. Louis, 1968, The C. V. Mosby Co.)

placing it in the mastoid cavity. In time, the skin grows over the muscle.

7. The mastoid cavity is usually packed with a strip of ½ × 8 inch gauze packing that has been impregnated with petrolatum or an antibiotic ointment. The wound is closed.

8. The ear dressing is applied, including a shaped ear pad (Fig. 8-23). Fluffed 8 × 4 inch gauze sponges are placed around and behind the affected ear and then flat compresses over the affected ear. A gauze bandage is applied in a particular manner to hold the dressings in place and avoid pressure (Fig. 8-24).

## Simple mastoidectomy

DEFINITION. Removal of the air cells of the mastoid process without disturbing the contents of the middle ear (Fig. 8-22).

CONSIDERATIONS. Simple mastoidectomy may be done occasionally to treat acute empyema of the mastoid. However, because of the effectiveness of antibiotics, this procedure is almost obsolete.

SETUP AND PREPARATION OF THE PATIENT. As described for radical mastoidectomy, omitting stapes instruments.

OPERATIVE PROCEDURE

1. A postaural or endaural incision is made. The steps of the procedure as de-

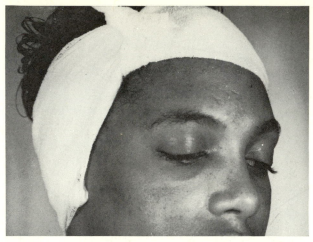

**Fig. 8-24.** Head dressing after mastoidectomy is completed. Several fluffed 8 × 4 inch dressings are placed over ear to absorb drainage before gauze is wrapped about head. Dressing is placed high enough so that it does not fall over eyes. Dressings should be actually in hair, not across forehead. (From Saunders, W. H., Havener, W. H., Fair, C. J., and Hickey, J. T.: Nursing care in eye, ear, nose, and throat disorders, ed. 2, St. Louis, 1968, The C. V. Mosby Co.)

scribed under radical mastoidectomy, steps 1 to 3 and 6 and 7, are carried out.

## Modified radical mastoidectomy (atticoantrotomy)

**DEFINITION.** A simple mastoidectomy plus the removal of the bony posterior external auditory canal wall. This exposes the mastoid cavity to the external auditory canal for drainage. The middle ear is not disturbed.

**CONSIDERATIONS.** This procedure may be done in the presence of a small tympanic perforation or in the presence of an attic and mastoid-antrum disease but does not involve the middle ear. It may also be done as a preliminary surgical exposure for a fenestration operation.

**SETUP AND PREPARATION OF THE PATIENT.** As described for radical mastoidectomy, omitting the stapes instruments.

**OPERATIVE PROCEDURE.** As described for radical mastoidectomy, steps 1 to 4 and 6 and 7. The middle ear structures and drum are preserved. The eardrum is left attached to the skin of the external auditory canal posteriorly. Both are used to seal the middle ear from the mastoid cavity.

## Tympanoplasty operations

**CONSIDERATIONS.** The term *tympanoplasty* refers to a group of operations selected to restore or improve hearing in patients with middle ear or conductive-type hearing loss, resulting from chronic otitis media.

Conductive deafness is caused by an obstruction in the external canal or middle ear, which impedes the passage of sound waves to the inner ear. The action of the round window and oval window has been reviewed previously.

The objectives of tympanoplasty are to restore two functions of the middle ear: the areal ratio and sound protection for the round window. The objective of the skin graft laid across the middle ear, touching the stapes and leaving an air pocket about the round window, is to improve hearing. The sound waves are transmitted through the graft to the stapes and the oval window. The sound waves striking the graft covering associated with the round window are reflected backward, thereby providing sound protection.

**TYPES OF TYMPANOPLASTY PROCEDURES** (Figs. 8-25 and 8-26). Many procedures are now in the developmental stage. Var-

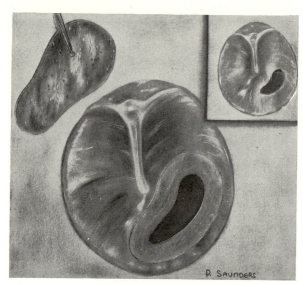

**Fig. 8-25.** Tympanoplasty—type I (myringoplasty). (From DeWeese, D. D., and Saunders, W. H.: Textbook of otolaryngology, ed. 3, St. Louis, 1968, The C. V. Mosby Co.)

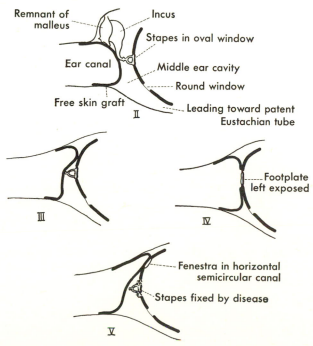

**Fig. 8-26.** Tympanoplasty—types II, III, IV, and V. (From DeWeese, D. D., and Saunders, W. H.: Textbook of otolaryngology, ed. 3, St. Louis, 1968, The C. V. Mosby Co.)

TABLE 2. Tympanoplastic procedures*

| Type | Damage to middle ear | Methods of repair |
|------|----------------------|-------------------|
| I | Perforated tympanic membrane with normal ossicular chain | Closure of perforation; type I same as myringoplasty |
| II | Perforation of tympanic membrane with erosion of malleus | Closure with graft against incus or remains of malleus |
| III | Destruction of tympanic membrane and ossicular chain *but with* intact and mobile stapes | Graft contacts normal stapes; also gives sound protection for round window |
| IV | Similar to type III, but head, neck, and crura of stapes missing; footplate mobile | Mobile footplate left exposed; air pocket between round window and graft provides sound protection for round window |
| V | Similar to type IV plus *fixed* footplate | Fenestra in horizontal semicircular canal; graft seals off middle ear to give sound protection for round window |

*From DeWeese, D. D., and Saunders, W. H.: Textbook of otolaryngology, ed. 3, St. Louis, 1968, The C. V. Mosby Co.

ous methods and materials are being introduced as a means of constructing a closed, air-contained middle ear cavity and restoring a sound-pressure transformer action.

In tympanoplasty types I, II, and III (Table 2), fresh tissue—either a vein or a piece of perichondrium, fascia, or skin from the inner third of the external auditory canal—is used to repair the tympanic membrane and close off a pocket of air in front of the round window. In some cases, a new areal ratio is created if there is a sufficient ossicular chain present.

Tympanoplasty types IV and V provide only sound protection for the round window, since the areal ratio cannot be restored. In tympanoplasty type IV, a new opening into the inner ear is established by placing a graft over the fenestra in the lateral canal (fenestration operation) (Fig. 8-27).

### Tympanoplasty type I (myringoplasty)

DEFINITION. Reconstruction of the tympanic membrane by means of a sliding graft fashioned from the inner part of the ear or by means of a vein graft (Fig. 8-25).

SETUP AND PREPARATION OF THE PATIENT. The setup as listed previously includes instruments for modified radical mastoidec-

tomy and for stapedectomy and vein graft.

The skin preparation, positioning, and draping of the patient have been described previously (Chapters 4, 5, and 7).

OPERATIVE PROCEDURE. Many different incisional approaches are used; however, an endaural approach is commonly preferred.

WULLSTEIN TECHNIQUE

1. The ear speculum is introduced and the microscope brought into place. An endaural incision is made either within the meatus, as for stapes mobilization, or extended upward from the meatus by means of a knife, sharp curettes, and fine cupped forceps.

2. The tympanic membrane is entered and a modified radical mastoidectomy may be done, depending on the extent of the disease.

3. The antrum is inspected, and a stapedial fossa tympanotomy is accomplished by means of burrs, dissectors, suction, and forceps (Fig. 8-25).

4. The graft is taken. The middle ear is reconstructed by placing the graft in position with smooth forceps, fine knives, and moist cotton pledgets. Small pledgets of Gelfoam or a similar substance may be inserted to lightly hold the graft in position. A cotton tampon is used to occlude the outer meatus.

5. The wound is closed with no. 4-0 silk sutures, and a mastoid dressing is applied (Figs. 8-23 and 8-24).

AUSTIN-SHEA TECHNIQUE

1. A segment of vein is taken from the antecubital fossa or forearm. The excessive connective tissue is trimmed from the adventitial surface. The vein graft is split or thinned, cut, converted into a quadrilateral graft, and stored in a sponge saturated with normal saline or Ringer's solution until needed.

2. The ear speculum is inserted, and an endaural incision is made. Tympanotomy is performed.

3. The ossicular chain or remnants are mobilized; diseased bone may be removed, using stapes instruments.

4A. Clearance of diseased mastoid cells is done. The middle ear is reconstructed by means of a vein graft, resulting in closure of the perforated membrane.

4B. Reconstruction of the middle ear may be done by other methods, depending on the condition of the structures encountered. A polyethylene prosthetic substitution may be used that becomes a strut from malleus to footplate, from incus to footplate, or from membrane to footplate, or the tympanic remnant and vein graft may be used to secure sound protection of the round window.

5. Bleeding is controlled, the skin flap and drum replaced to original position, and the incision closed with no. 4-0 silk sutures. Antibiotic solution is instilled in ear. A mastoid dressing is applied.

## Fenestration operation

DEFINITION. Reconstruction of the outer and middle parts of the ear by means of a new drum or skin flap or creation of a new window into the internal ear mechanism by a newly established drum or skin flap; also partial mastoidectomy.

CONSIDERATIONS. The Lempert endaural fenestration operation is done to restore hearing in persons who had bilateral conduction deafness because of otosclerosis of the tympanic membrane and ossicles (Figs. 8-27 to 8-29).

Otosclerosis is the most common cause of conductive hearing loss in people from 15 to 50 years of age. It is a hereditary defect of unknown cause, is more common in women than in men, and is not common in blacks.

In otosclerosis, the normal bone is absorbed and replaced by otosclerotic bone, which is vascular. It grows into the bony labyrinth, thus causing progressive fixation of the footplate of the stapes.

The objective of surgery is to restore the mechanical aspects of the middle ear and the external canal.

The objective of fenestration is to create a new permanent window through which sound waves can enter the inner ear when the oval window is fixed.

SETUP AND PREPARATION OF THE PATIENT. As described for endaural mastoidectomy and stapes surgery, including the following additional instruments:

3 Lempert excavators
2 Joseph hooks, double-ended
2 Iris hooks
2 Lillie hooks
1 Lempert elevator
1 Lempert knife

OPERATIVE PROCEDURE

1. An endaural incision is made inside the ear by means of an ear speculum, microscope, and small knife.

2. A modified radical mastoidectomy is done. The bridge is reduced, incus removed, head of malleus amputated, and ampulla and lateral semicircular canals identified by means of electric drill with burrs attached, Rosen knives, and Bellucci scissors. The operative field is irrigated with warm normal saline solution.

3. A fenestra is created by means of the microscope and diamond paste burrs (Fig. 8-29). The membranous labyrinth is left exposed by a thin dome or cupola of endosteal bone, which is removed. The edges of the fenestra are trimmed with fine picks.

4. A pedicle flap is made from the

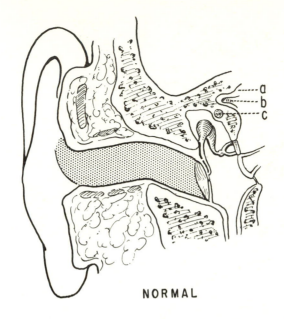

NORMAL

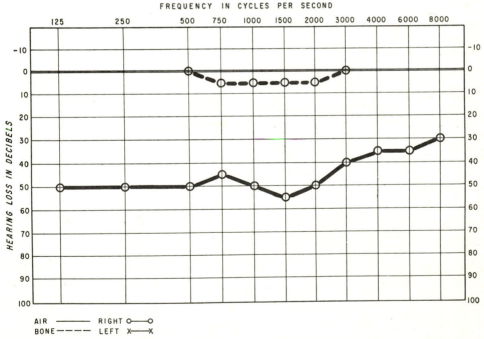

**Fig. 8-27.** Fenestration of labyrinth for otosclerosis. **a,** Perilymphatic space of horizontal semicircular canal. **b,** Membrane of semicircular canal with facial nerve. **c,** Audiogram with decibel and frequency scales indicates hearing by bone conduction and air conduction. When hearing loss is caused by defect in external or middle ear, audiogram indicates good hearing to inner ear by bone conduction and poor hearing by air conduction. When defect involves inner ear, bone conduction measurements are no better than air conduction measurements. (From De-Weese, D. D., and Saunders, W. H.: Textbook of otolaryngology, ed. 3, St. Louis, 1968, The C. V. Mosby Co.)

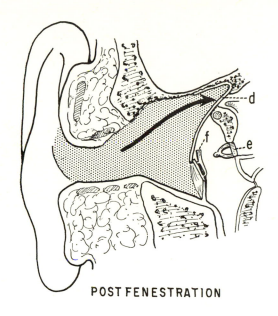

POST FENESTRATION

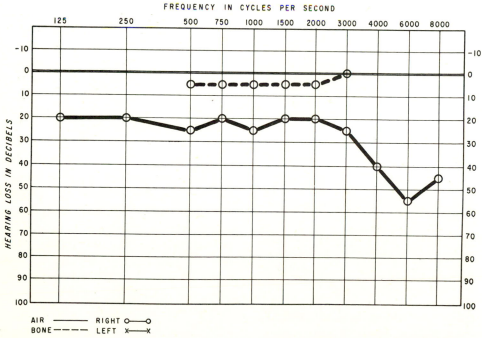

Fig. 8-28. After fenestration. **d,** Skin of ear is attached to eardrum and molded into cavity to cover fenestra made through bony wall of labyrinth. **e,** Stapes is still fixed in oval window. **f,** Neck of malleus. Audiogram indicates degree of conductive hearing loss due to diseases of external ear and middle ear, as well as hearing loss due to diseases of inner ear caused by nerve or perceptive hearing loss. (From DeWeese, D. D., and Saunders, W. H.: Textbook of otolaryngology, ed. 3, St. Louis, 1968, The C. V. Mosby Co.)

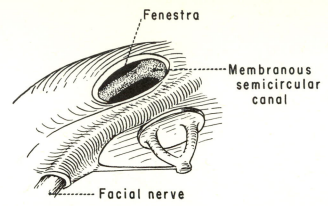

**Fig. 8-29.** Fenestration operation. Fenestra made in horizontal semicircular canal for otosclerosis. Incus is removed. Fenestra is ready to be covered by flap fashioned from eardrum and skin of external auditory canal. (From DeWeese, D. D., and Saunders, W. H.: Textbook of otolaryngology, ed. 3, St. Louis, 1968, The C. V. Mosby Co.)

skin and periosteum of the superior and posterior canal walls.

5. Endosteum and bone dust are removed by fine excavators. The graft is laid over the fenestra. The cavity may be lined by pledgets of synthetic sponge (Fig. 8-29).

6. The endaural incision is closed with fine silk sutures. The meatal opening is lightly packed with gauze saturated with an antibiotic solution. Mastoid dressing is applied (Figs. 8-23 and 8-24).

## Stapedectomy

DEFINITION. Removal of the stapes (the head, neck, and crura) and reestablishment of linkage between the incus and oval window by interposition of a vein graft, polyethylene tube, or other prosthetic material.

CONSIDERATIONS. Stapes surgery is done to restore hearing in patients with conductive deafness due to stapedial ankylosis, which causes a gradually progressive hearing loss.

If the stapes is fixed in the oval window, the stapes is either freed (stapes mobilization) or removed and replaced with an artificial bone (stapedectomy).

SETUP AND PREPARATION OF THE PATIENT. As described for stapes surgery, plus graft set (Figs. 8-12 to 8-15).

OPERATIVE PROCEDURE (Fig. 8-30)

1. With the aid of a microscope, knife, and suction needles, an incision is made in the posterior half of the osseous meatal wall about 5 mm. from the annulus. The posterior flap, consisting of skin and periosteum, is dissected from the bone with a large circumferential knife and wet cottonoid pledgets or applicators. The elevation is carried medially until the posterior margin of the annular sulcus is reached, using narrow or duckbill elevators, modified Kos or angular Rosen elevators, or right or left Shea elevators.

2. The delicate middle ear mucosa is separated, and the tympanic membrane is folded forward on itself to expose the contents of the middle ear, using delicate periosteal elevators. With a microscope, the middle ear is inspected for patency of the round window. The posterior superior bony canal rim is removed with a small, round, flat knife (Rosen, Shea, or Goodhill), spud, and curettes above the exit of the chorda tympani nerve to provide for exposure of the incudostapedial joint. The incus, the incudostapedial joint, and the head of the stapes are palpitated, using Rosen picks or a Derlacki mobilizer.

3. The crura are fractured from the

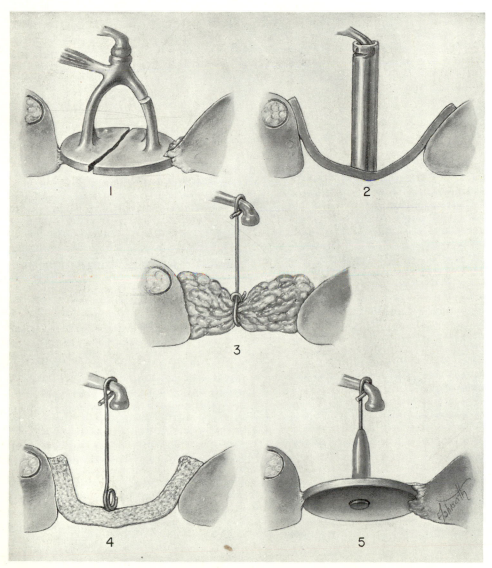

**Fig. 8-30.** Techniques of stapedectomy. **1,** Partial stapedectomy by cutting anterior crus and bisecting footplate. Posterior crus and remaining footplate are mobile (Hough procedure). **2,** Stapes removed and replaced with vein graft. Polyethylene strut provides continuity (Shea procedures). **3,** Wire-fat prosthesis replacing stapes (Schuknecht procedures). **4,** Oval window covered with Gelfoam. Preformed wire placed on Gelfoam (House procedure). **5,** Footplate not removed. Footplate drilled and preformed wire-Teflon piston placed through hole in footplate (Shea and Guilford procedures). Note otosclerotic fixation of anterior footplate margin is shown in **1** and **5.** (From DeWeese, D. D., and Saunders, W. H.: Textbook of otolaryngology, ed. 3, St. Louis, 1968, The C. V. Mosby Co.)

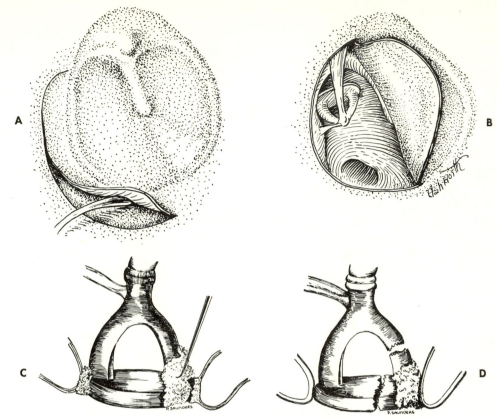

**Fig. 8-31.** Stapes mobilization. **A,** Incision in posterior ear canal wall. **B,** Operative field seen through aural speculum. **C,** Fracturing through otosclerotic focus. Earlier, surgeons applied pressure only to incus or head of stapes. **D,** Anterior crurotomy technique—otosclerotic focus is bypassed. (From DeWeese, D. D., and Saunders, W. H.: Textbook of otolaryngology, ed. 3, St. Louis, 1968, The C. V. Mosby Co.)

footplate, and the stapes superstructure is removed (Fig. 8-31).

4. Fragments of the footplate are removed. The opening into the vestibule is covered with a graft. The prosthesis is articulated with the long process of the incus by means of stapes forceps. Blood is gently suctioned from the tympanic cavity, and the tympanic membrane is replaced in its original position.

5. On completion of the lysis or the prosthetic procedure, audiometric status is determined by lightly striking a 256-cycle magnesium tuning fork. All blood is gently suctioned from the tympanic cavity, and the operative wound is closed. The tympanic membrane–posterior skin

flap is gently replaced in position, using Rosen or Shea picks and House alligator forceps.

6. The extraneous blood is suctioned from the canal. Part of the incision is covered with several gelatin sponges (Gelfoam) moistened in Adrenalin solution to keep the meatal skin in position and prevent bleeding into the middle ear. In some cases, several saline-soaked strips of rayon are placed over the skin incision area to line the bony external auditory canal.

## Stapes mobilization

**DEFINITION.** Creation of an opening into the vestibule of the labyrinth and rees-

tablishment of a functioning linkage between the incus and the inner ear (Fig. 8-31).

CONSIDERATIONS. Stapediolysis is remobilization of the entire middle ear mechanism. The term *stapediolysis* means removal or lysis of bony or fibrous adhesions around the stapes. Patients with conductive hearing loss resulting from fixation of the stapes are selected for stapes mobilization.

SETUP AND PREPARATION OF THE PATIENT. As described for stapes surgery.

OPERATIVE PROCEDURE. The major steps and items used are similar to stapedectomy (Fig. 8-31). The stapes is freed from the hardened otosclerotic membrane by means of fine probes, dissectors, and picks. The auditory canal is packed and mastoid dressing applied.

## Labyrinthectomy

DEFINITION. Opening of the labyrinth in order to destroy the inner ear.

CONSIDERATIONS. This operation is done to relieve the medically uncontrollable symptoms of unilateral Ménière's syndrome or to prevent the intracranial spread of infection from the labyrinth.

SETUP AND PREPARATION OF THE PATIENT. As described for tympanoplasty.

OPERATIVE PROCEDURES. These are dependent on the type of approach used. The transmeatal approach is performed as a stapedectomy. After the stapes is removed, the inner ear is suctioned to remove the membranous labyrinth. The round and oval windows are combined to make a single large window by the use of a burr. In the transmastoid approach a modified radical mastoidectomy is performed. The stapes is removed and the inner ear suctioned to remove the membranous labyrinth. The semicircular canals are opened.

# Operations on the nose

Surgery of the nose is performed to treat external injuries and malformations and provide for effective function of the respiratory system (Fig. 8-32).

## ANATOMY AND PHYSIOLOGY OF THE NOSE

The nose is divided into the prominent external nose and the internal nose known as the nasal cavity. The chief purpose of the nose is the preparation of air for use in the lungs.

The *external* nose projects from the face. The upper portion of the external nose is formed by the nasal bones and the frontal process of the maxillae, and the lower portion is formed by a group of nasal cartilages and connective tissue covered with skin. The nostrils and the tip of the nose are shaped by the major alar cartilages (Fig. 8-33). The nares are separated by the columella, which is formed by the lower margin of the septal cartilage, the medial parts of the major alar cartilages, and the anterior nasal spine, all of which are covered by skin.

The nasal septum is composed of three structures: the nasal cartilage, the vomer bone, and the perpendicular plate of the ethmoid bone (Fig. 8-33). The septum is covered by mucous membrane on either side. The deviated or fractured septum may be repaired surgically by mobilization of the fracture or removal of the deformed cartilage or bone.

The *internal* nose or nasal cavity is divided into two parts at its midline by the nasal septum. The nasal cavity communicates with the outside by its external openings, called the *anterior nares*. The nares open into the nasopharynx behind through the choanae. The nasal cavity is also associated with each ear by means of the eustachian tube and with the paranasal air sinuses (frontal, maxillary, ethmoid, and sphenoid) via their respective orifices (meatuses). The nasal cavity also communicates with the conjunctiva through the nasal duct. The nasal cavity is separated from the lingual cavity by the hard and soft palates (Figs. 8-32 and 8-33) and from the cranial cavity by the

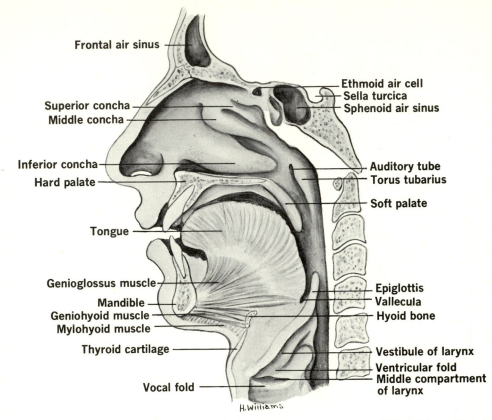

Fig. 8-32. Sagittal section of face and neck. (W.R.U. museum specimen C228.) (From Francis, C. C: Introduction to human anatomy, ed. 5, St. Louis, 1968, The C. V. Mosby Co.)

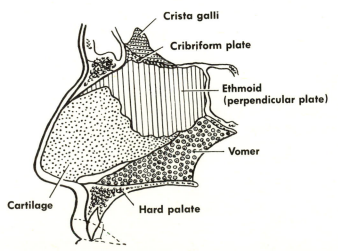

Fig. 8-33. Diagram showing formation of nasal septum by perpendicular plate of ethmoid, by vomer bone, and by cartilage. (From Anthony, C. P.: Textbook of anatomy and physiology, ed. 6, St. Louis, 1963, The C. V. Mosby Co.)

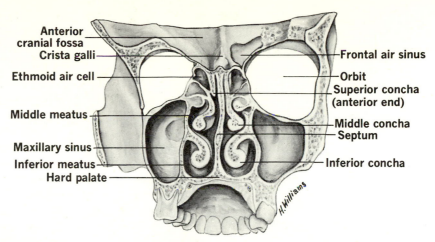

**Fig. 8-34.** Vertical section through nose. Plane of section passes slightly obliquely through left first molar tooth and behind second right premolar tooth. Posterior wall of right frontal sinus removed. (W.R.U. museum specimen.) (From Francis, C. C: Introduction to human anatomy, ed. 5, St. Louis, 1968, The C. V. Mosby Co.)

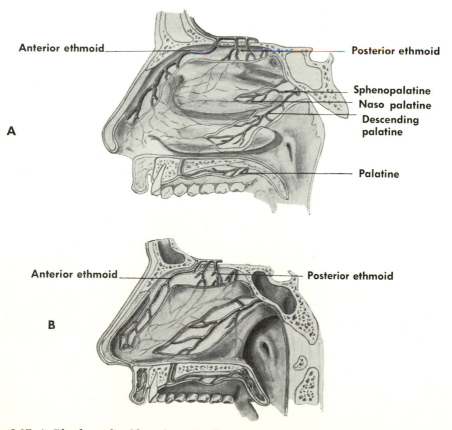

**Fig. 8-35. A,** Blood supply of lateral nasal wall. **B,** Arteries of nasal septum. (From Ryan, R. E., Ogura, J. H., Biller, H. F., and Pratt, L. L.: Synopsis of ear, nose, and throat diseases, ed. 3, St. Louis, 1970, The C. V. Mosby Co.)

ethmoid bone. The nasal cavity is held together by periosteal covering and by perichondrium, which extends over the cartilages.

The *turbinate bones* of the nasal structure are arranged one above the other, separated by grooves (the meatuses). These act as drainage passages of the accessory sinuses and are known as the sphenoethmoidal recesses and the superior, middle, and inferior meatus, respectively (Fig. 8-34).

The nasal sinuses serve as air spaces and communicate with the nasal cavity via the meatuses. Anteriorly, on each side of the skull, the frontal sinus, the anterior ethmoid cells, and the maxillary sinus (antrum of Highmore) drain into the middle meatus; posteriorly, the ethmoid cells and the sphenoid sinus drain into the superior meatus and the sphenoethmoidal recess. A passageway for the flow of air is provided by the irregular air spaces present between these structures. Because of their shape, the air is forced to flow in thin air waves.

The sensory nerve supply of the nasal cavity is derived from the trigeminal nerve.

The nose and sinuses receive their blood supply (Fig. 8-35) from the branches of the internal maxillary artery. There are masses of communicating veins below the epithelial layer of the turbinated bones, and those veins lying just beneath the skin anastomose freely. Dilatation of the superficial veins may cause the turbinated bones to swell, whereas contraction of these vessels may cause the bones to shrink.

## OPERATIONS ON THE EXTERNAL NOSE AND NASAL CAVITY
### Submucous resection of the septum

DEFINITION. Removal of either the cartilaginous or osseous portions of the septum that lie between the flaps of the mucous membrane and the perichondrium.

CONSIDERATIONS. When the nasal septum (Fig. 8-33) is deformed, fractured, or injured, normal respiratory function and nasal drainage may be impaired. Devia-

tions of the septum, involving cartilage, bony parts (spurs), or both, may block the meatus and compress the middle turbinate on that side, thereby resulting in an obstruction of the sinus opening. Septal deviations tend to produce sinus disease and nasal polyps.

The objective of a submucous resection is to establish an adequate partition between the left and right nasal cavities, thereby providing a clear airway of both the internal and external cavity and the parts of the nose.

SETUP AND PREPARATION OF THE PATIENT. Before the patient arrives, the room should be darkened. The surgeon's headlight, whether electrical or reflecting head mirror with lamp, suction apparatus, emergency tray, anesthetic setup, and other equipment should be available and in working order.

This operation is generally done with the patient under local anesthesia. Before the patient arrives, the operating table is made into a reclining chair by use of footpiece and pillows placed for protection of feet from pressure and relief of strain on vessels and tendons of the lower extremities. The reclining chair is adjusted to meet the physical characteristics and comfort of the patient. The table is raised or lowered to accommodate the surgeon. If the surgeon prefers to use the reflecting head mirror for his light source, the reflecting lamp is placed behind the head of the table on the opposite side from the surgeon. In some cases, the patient may be placed on the table in a dorsal recumbent position.

In some cases the hair of the nostrils may be clipped with fine, curved scissors. Sterile mineral oil drops or an antibiotic ointment may be put into the eyes of the patient to protect them from prepping solutions. The face is scrubbed with a mild soap and water. The face prep and draping of the patient is done prior to injection of the local anesthetic. The circulating nurse should observe changes in the vital signs of the patient. When cocaine or

another similar narcotic agent is used, a thiopental (Pentothal) sodium setup and oxygen equipment should be in the room. Topical medications that have changed color should not be used. The amount of the topical agent dispensed for the operation must be recorded on the anesthesia record and on the pharmacy narcotic form.

The patient is draped with sterile towels and sheets as follows:

1. Place the small sheet with two towels on top of it over the head of the table and under the head of the patient.

2. Bring the uppermost towel around the head, including the hairline.

3. Secure the ends of the uppermost towel with a towel forceps, and tuck the free ends under the patient's head.

4. Drape a large sheet over the patient, bringing its upper end up to the chin.

5. Place the tray with the instruments in position for the surgeon.

6. Connect the suction apparatus.

7. Adjust the lighting system.

8. Record the comfort and the vital signs of the patient.

9. Reassure the patient if awake. (See Chapter 5.)

Sterile instruments, supplies, and other items include the following:

### Topical anesthesia setup

Cocaine, 10%
Procaine, 2%
Epinephrine (Adrenalin), 1:1000
2 Luer-Lok syringes, 5 ml.
3 Needles, 25-gauge, ½ in.

### Supplies

One nasal pack, including the following items.
1 Small sheet and 2 towels
1 Large sheet
3 Towels
1 Mayo stand cover
1 Instrument table cover
1 Piece absorbent cotton
6 Cotton applicators
12 Submucous gauze sponges
6 Compresses, 4 × 4 in.

*Accessory items*

1 Tube petrolatum gauze packing, ½ in. wide
3 Medication cups, labeled

1 Minor basin set
1 Glove set
1 Gown pack

### Cutting instruments (Figs. 8-36 and 8-37)

1 Myles septum-cutting forceps
1 Knife handle no. 3 with blade no. 15
2 Ballenger swivel knives
1 Freer septum knife, rounded blade
1 Hartman septum forceps
1 Jansen-Middleton septum punch forceps
1 Luc nasal cutting forceps, curved sideways
1 Freer septum chisel
2 Douglas nasal snares with wires
1 Freer dissecting elevator
1 Ballenger nasal gouge
1 Pierce submucous dissector, double-ended, right or left

### Holding and clamping instruments (Figs. 8-38 and 8-39)

3 Applicators, serrated end
1 Allis forceps
3 Towel forceps
2 Kelly forceps, straight
1 Mayo hemostat, curved
1 Adson bayonet forceps
1 Adson tissue forceps

### Exposing instruments (Fig. 8-40)

1 Nasal self-retaining wire speculum
1 S-type retractor
2 Killian nasal specula
1 Bayonet forceps

### Suturing items (Chapters 5 and 6)

1 Needle holder, small
1 Septal suture, as desired, silk no. 3-0 on ½-circle, taper point needle

### Accessory items (Fig. 8-41)

2 Frazier nasal suction tubes and tubing
2 Antrum suction tubes
1 Metal wire for cleaning suction tube
1 Bulb syringe and saline solution
1 Mallet

The face of the patient is cleaned, a local anesthetic is injected, and the patient is draped with a sterile sheet and towels.

OPERATIVE PROCEDURE. The operative procedure will vary with the individual surgeon. A general review of most procedures is as follows:

1. The nostril is opened with a speculum. An incision is made through the mucoperichondrium and mucoperiosteum

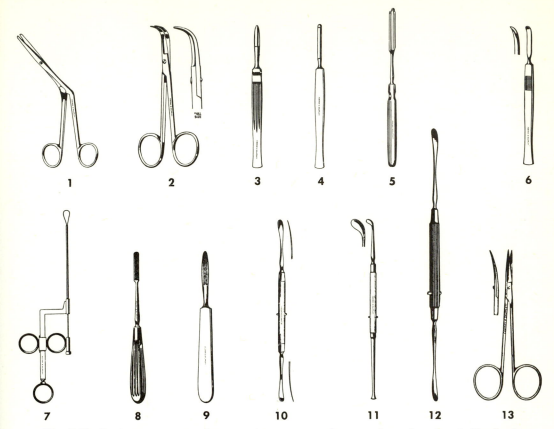

Fig. 8-36. Cutting instruments for operations on external nose and nasal cavity. **1,** Nasal scissors, angled; **2,** Fomon upper lateral scissors; **3,** cartilage knife, beveled blade; **4,** cartilage knife, straight; **5,** cartilage knife, swivel blade; **6,** cartilage nasal knife, curved; **7,** nasal snare; **8,** nasal rasp, narrow; **9,** nasal rasp; **10,** double-ended elevator; **11,** golf stick elevator-dissector; **12,** Freer dissecting elevator; **13,** iris scissors, straight and curved. (See Chapter 17 for basic instruments.) (Courtesy Codman & Shurtleff, Inc., Randolph, Mass.)

of the septum with a knife with blade no. 15. The tissues are separated and elevated, using a Freer knife. (Fig. 8-42.)

2. The cartilage is incised with a knife, and the mucous membrane is elevated with a Ballenger knife and a septal elevator; deviated cartilage and bony, thickened structures are removed with a septum punch and a nasal cutting forceps.

3. The mucous membrane is freed from the bony septal base by means of a chisel, gouge and mallet, or punch forceps. Bleeding is controlled by gauze sponges; suctioning is used to expose the field.

4. The perpendicular plate of the ethmoid may be removed, as well as the vomer, by means of the S-retractor, chisel and mallet, and a suitable septum-cutting forceps (Fig. 8-37).

5. The incision may or may not be sutured with silk no. 3-0 fused to a ½-circle taper point small needle on a Crile needle holder.

6. Nostrils are packed with petrolatum gauze in order to keep the septal flaps in a midline position. The face is cleansed with both moist and dry compresses.

## Corrective rhinoplasty

**DEFINITION.** Removal of the hump, narrowing and shortening of the nose, and reconstruction of the tip of the nose.

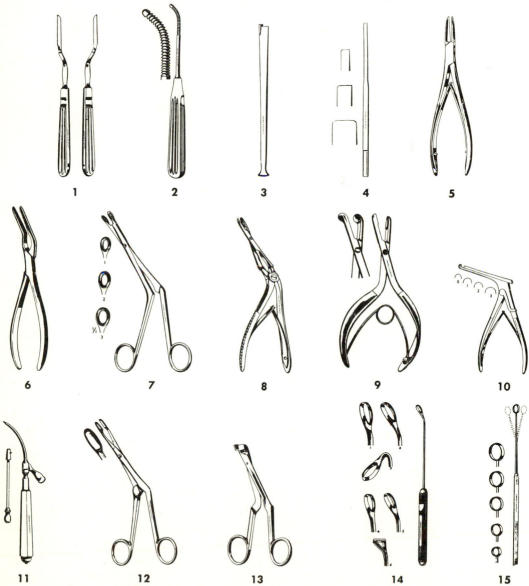

**Fig. 8-37.** Cutting instruments for operations on external nose and nasal cavity—cont'd. **1,** Freer nasal saws, right and left; **2,** reamer; **3,** nasal chisel with guard; **4,** osteotome, narrow widths; **5,** nasal bone cutter; **6,** nasal rongeur; **7,** Bruening septum forceps; **8,** double-action nasal rongeur; **9,** McCoy septum forceps; **10,** punch; **11,** antrum trocar and stylet; **12,** septum-cutting forceps; **13,** septum ridge-cutting forceps; **14,** Coakley ethmoid sinus curette; **15,** Myles antrum ring curettes. (See Chapter 17 for basic instruments.) (Courtesy Codman & Shurtleff, Inc., Randolph, Mass.)

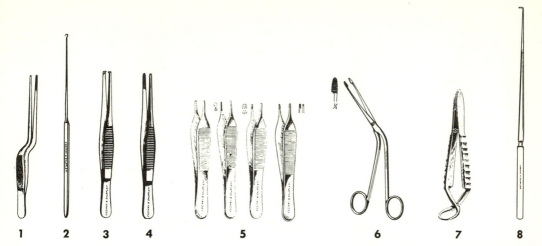

**Fig. 8-38.** Holding instruments for operations on external nose and nasal cavity. **1,** Adson bayonet dressing forceps; **2,** single hooks; **3,** Adson tissue forceps; **4,** dressing forceps; **5,** Adson dural forceps; **6,** Hartman forceps; **7,** Jones towel forceps; **8,** Dandy nerve hook. (See Chapter 17 for basic instruments.) (Courtesy Codman & Shurtleff, Inc., Randolph, Mass.)

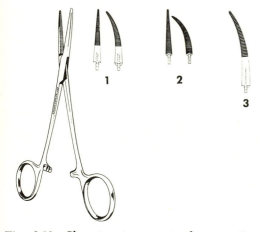

**Fig. 8-39.** Clamping instruments for operations on external nose and nasal cavity. **1,** Halsted hemostats, straight and curved; **2,** mosquito hemostats, straight and curved; **3,** Kelly hemostat, curved. (See Chapter 17 for basic instruments.) (Courtesy Codman & Shurtleff, Inc., Randolph, Mass.)

**CONSIDERATIONS.** Rhinoplasty may help in solving the patient's physiological, psychological, or economic problems.

**SETUP AND PREPARATION OF THE PATIENT.** The patient's face is prepared as described for submucous resection. The patient is usually placed in a dorsal recumbent position with his head stabilized be-

tween sandbags. The instruments and setup will depend on the preferences of the surgeon. The nasal and plastic setups are shown in Figs. 8-43 to 8-45.

**OPERATIVE PROCEDURE**

1. An incision is made through the skin of one nostril with a knife, blade no. 15; then a second incision is made in the other nostril and carried around the columella to join the first incision. A nasal speculum, sponges, and skin hooks are used.

2. The skin of the nose is undermined, using elevators, knives, and scissors; the periosteum and perichondrium are freed, using elevators, saws, and a periosteal dissector.

3. The nasal bone or upper lateral cartilage is fractured; the hump and possibly septal cartilage are removed by means of cutting forceps such as the Jansen-Middleton, osteotomes such as the Kazanjian action-type, mallet, plastic scissors, and Adson forceps (Fig. 8-45). The field is cleaned by suctioning tubes and sponges with bayonet forceps.

4. The edges of the cartilages are trimmed, using septum forceps and scissors (Fig. 8-45).

5. To prevent or control infection and the formation of a hematoma, the blood

*Text continued on p. 200.*

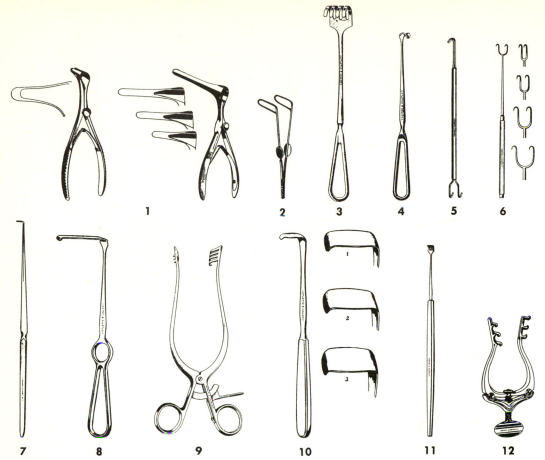

**Fig. 8-40.** Exposing instruments for operations on external nose, nasal cavity, and mastoid. 1, Vienna and Killian nasal specula; **2**, Bosworth nasal wire speculum; **3**, Volkmann rake retractor; **4**, Cushing vein retractor; **5**, 1- and 2-pronged retractor, double-ended; **6**, 2-pronged retractors, sharp, various sizes; **7**, Hoen nerve hook; **8**, Kocher retractor; **9**, Weitlaner self-retaining retractor; **10**, Langenbeck retractors, various sizes; **11**, delicate 4-pronged retractor; **12**, Jansen mastoid retractor. (See Chapter 5 for basic instruments.) (Courtesy Codman & Shurtleff, Inc., Randolph, Mass.)

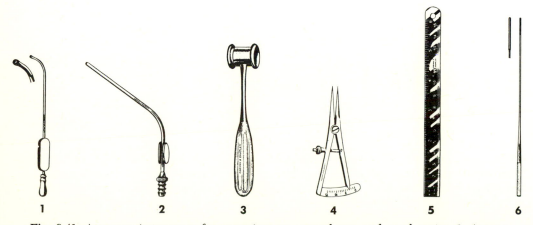

**Fig. 8-41.** Accessory instruments for operations on external nose and nasal cavity. **1**, Antrum suction tubes; **2**, Frazier suction tube; **3**, metal mallet; **4**, caliper; **5**, ruler; **6**, nasal applicators. (See Chapter 17 for basic instruments.) (Courtesy Codman & Shurtleff, Inc., Randolph, Mass.)

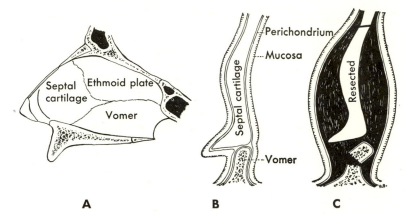

A    B    C

**Fig. 8-42. A,** Chief components of septum. Incision line is for Killian type of submucous resection. **B,** Septum with deviated cartilage and spur at junction of vomer and septal cartilage. **C,** Resection of obstructive parts after careful elevation of mucoperichondrium and mucoperiosteum. (From DeWeese, D. D., and Saunders, W. H.: Textbook of otolaryngology, ed. 3, St. Louis, 1968, The C. V. Mosby Co.)

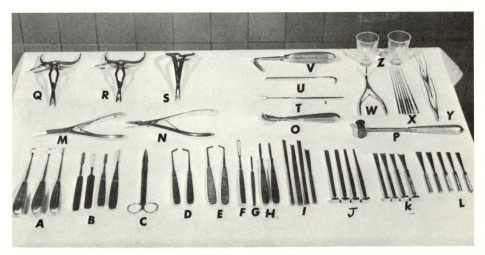

**Fig. 8-43.** Rhinoplasty instruments. **A,** Glabella rasps; **B,** Joseph rasps, assorted; **C,** Mayo scissors, serrated; **D,** pair of cartilage knives, angled; **E,** pair of button-ended knives, angled; **F,** swivel knife; **G,** button-ended knife, straight; **H,** pair of Joseph bayonet saws; **I,** guarded chisels; **J,** osteotomes, light, narrow; **K,** McIndoe chisels and osteotomes; **L,** French chisels and osteotomes; **M,** Kazanjian forceps, double-action; **N,** Kazanjian forceps, single-action; **O,** wire brush; **P,** mallet; **Q,** Jansen-Middleton septum-cutting forceps; **R,** Jansen-Middleton biting forceps; **S,** Hayes forceps; **T,** ball-ended retractor; **U,** dorsum nasal retractor; **V,** Aufricht retractor; **W,** nasal speculum; **X,** nasal applicators; **Y,** bayonet forceps; **Z,** medicine glasses.

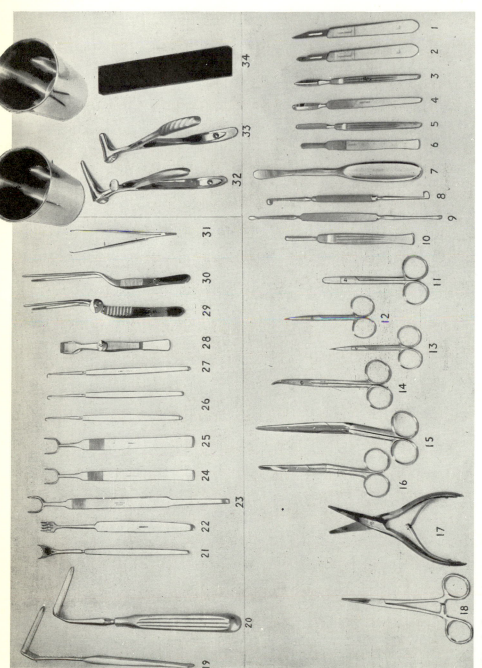

**Fig. 8-44.** Nasal and plastic setup used by Maurice H. Cottle, M.D. 1, Bard-Parker knife handle no. 3 with rib-back blade no. 11; 2, Bard-Parker knife handle no. 3 with rib-back blade no. 15; 3, Cottle knife, double-edged, straight; 4, Fomon knife, double-edged, curved; 5, Joseph buttonhole knife, straight; 6, Cottle knife, straight; 7, Cottle skin elevator, curved; 8, Pierce submucous dissector; 9, Cottle elevator, graduated; 10, MacKenty septum elevator; 11, Cottle bulldog scissors, 4½ in.; 12, Knapp strabismus scissors, curved; 13, Knapp iris scissors, curved, sharp-pointed; 14, Fomon upper lateral scissors, full curved; 15, Cottle angular scissors, 6½ in.; 16, Fomon angular scissors, light; 17, scissors, straight, spring-action; 18, Kelly artery forceps, straight; 19, Aufricht nasal speculum, fenestrated; 20, Aufricht nasal speculum, solid; 21, Cottle alar protector; 22, Cottle 4-pronged retractor, blunt; 23, Cottle-Neivert retractor, double-ended; 24, Cottle retractor, 2-pronged, small; 25, Cottle retractor, 2-pronged, large, sharp; 26, Straight tenaculum, single; 27, Cottle tenaculum, single; 28, Cottle columella clamp; 29, Cottle lower lateral forceps, bayonet; 30, Gruenwald nasal dressing forceps, 6¼ in.; 31, Cottle-Graefe *[...]*

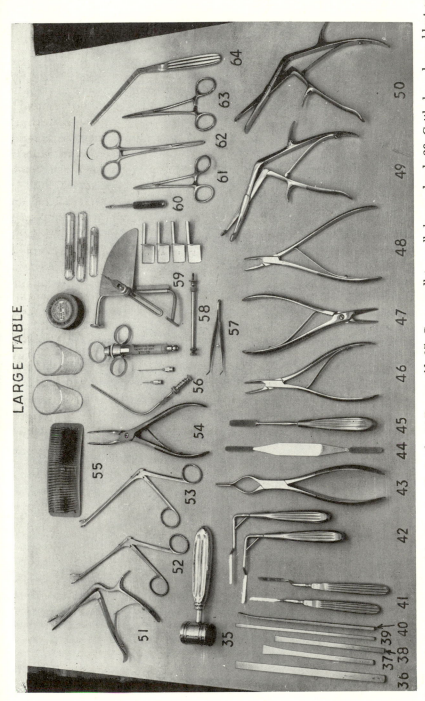

**LARGE TABLE**

**Fig. 8-45.** Nasal and plastic setup used by Maurice H. Cottle, M.D.—cont'd. **35,** Crane mallet, small, bronze head; **36,** Cottle bone lever, blunt end; **37** to **39,** Cottle chisels, thin blade, rounded corners, 12, 8, and 4 mm.; **40,** Cottle chisel, curved; **41,** Joseph bayonet saws, right and left; **42,** Joseph-Maltz angular saws, right and left; **43,** Cottle-Walsham septum straightener; **44,** Fomon rasp, double-ended; **45,** Cottle nasal rasp (Sweeper); **46,** Cottle-Kazanjian cutting forceps; **47,** Kazanjian nasal hump-cutting forceps; **48,** Cottle-Lempert rongeur forceps; **49** and **50,** Cottle septal ridge-cutting forceps; right and left; **51,** Kofler-Lillie septum forceps; **52,** Ferris-Smith fragment forceps; **53,** Bruening septum forceps, alligator jaws, 6.5 mm. wide; **54,** Cottle-Jansen rongeur forceps, angular jaws, with cupped portion of jaws straight; **55,** Turchiks instrument holder; **56,** Frazier nasal suction tube; **57,** Prince forceps, with teeth; **58,** Cottle cartilage holder; **59,** Cottle profilometer; **60,** Keyes cutaneous mucoperichondrium punch, 2 mm. diameter; **61,** Neivert needle holder; **62,** Allis tissue-holding forceps, 6 in.; **63,** Kelly artery forceps, straight; **64,** Joseph measuring instrument, angular; Dermalon suture no. 5-0; plain catgut sutures no. 3-0 and no. 2-0; braided black silk no. 2-0; cutting needle, curved, size 20; Luer-Lok control syringe, 5 ml.; hypodermic needles, 22-gauge, 2 in., and 25-gauge, ½ in.; medicine glasses for cod-liver oil and methylene blue. (From V. Mueller Armamentarium, no. 10, with permission of V. Mueller & Co., Chicago, Ill.)

is removed from the nose and the wound cleaned.

6. The cartilage and bones are molded into proper position. The columella is sutured back onto the septum with fine silk sutures. The membranous septal edges are closed; dressings with a pressure splint are applied and held in place with tape and a head bandage. A small gauze pad may be secured below the nares to absorb any bleeding. The head is elevated, and ice packs may be applied to the eyelids.

## Intranasal antrostomy (antral window)

DEFINITION. An opening made in the lateral wall of the nose under the middle turbinate and the removal of the anterior end of the inferior turbinate (Figs. 8-34 and 8-35).

CONSIDERATIONS. The patient suffers from headaches, edema, infection, or swelling of the lining membranes of the sinuses.

SETUP AND PREPARATION OF THE PATIENT. As described for submucous resection, plus the following items (Figs. 8-36 to 8-40):

Cutting instruments

2 Wilde ethmoid forceps
1 Hajek-Ballenger nasal V-shaped chisel
1 Myles antrum-cutting forceps
2 Antrum punch forceps
2 Nasal cutting forceps
2 Coakley antrum trocars
2 Coakley curettes, curved
1 Thornwald antrum perforator and irrigator
1 Kerrison cutting forceps

Exposing instruments

1 Mouth gag
1 Throat suction set

Accessory item

1 Postnasal plug or pack (Figs. 8-46 and 8-47)

OPERATIVE PROCEDURE

1. When the patient has been prepared, draped, and anesthetized, the postnasal plug is inserted (Fig. 8-47). The inferior turbinate is explored by means of bone-cutting forceps, elevators, and dissectors (Fig. 8-36).

2. An opening is made into the maxillary sinus (Fig. 8-34) beneath the inferior turbinate by means of a gouge, perforator, or antrum cannulae (Fig. 8-37). The opening is enlarged with cutting forceps and antrum punches. Accessory polyps and degenerate mucosa are removed with a snare, septum forceps, and suction (Figs. 8-36, 8-37, and 8-41).

3. The sinus is irrigated with saline solution by means of a Thornwald irrigator and suction apparatus; the sinus is packed with petrolatum gauze, and the face is cleaned and dried.

## Removal of nasal polyps

DEFINITION. Removal of polyps from the nasal cavity (Fig. 8-48).

CONSIDERATIONS. The tissues become edematous, resulting in the formation of polyps that obstruct the free passage of air and make breathing difficult.

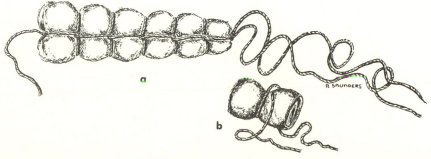

Fig. 8-46. Postnasal pack for hemorrhage. a, Three strings are needed. b, Pack can also be made from roller bandage or gauze; however, do not make pack *too large* for it may not only obstruct *both* choanae but also block eustachian tube. This pack should also have third string to dangle in nasopharynx to make removal easier. (From DeWeese, D. D., and Saunders, W. H.: Textbook of otolaryngology, ed. 3, St. Louis, 1968, The C. V. Mosby Co.)

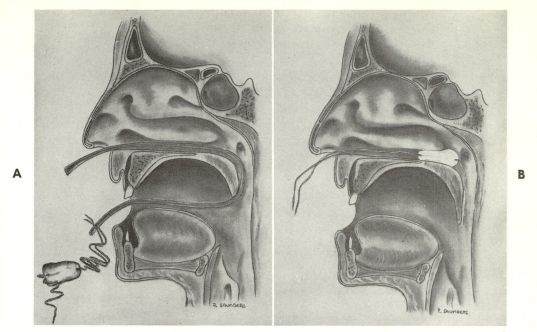

**A**       **B**

Fig. 8-47. Postnasal packing. **A,** First step. **B,** Second step. Anterior packing with ½-inch petrolatum gauze is then placed. (From DeWeese, D. D., and Saunders, W. H.: Textbook of otolaryngology, ed. 3, St. Louis, 1968, The C. V. Mosby Co.)

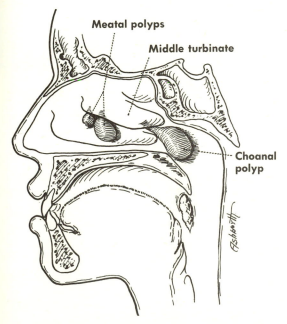

**Meatal polyps**

**Middle turbinate**

**Choanal polyp**

Fig. 8-48. Nasal polyps. Choanal polyp is usually single and originates in maxillary sinus. However, most polyps are found in middle meatus. (From DeWeese, D. D., and Saunders, W. H.: Textbook of otolaryngology, ed. 3, St. Louis, 1968, The C. V. Mosby Co.)

**SETUP AND PREPARATION OF THE PATIENT.** For polyps arising from the border of the middle turbinate, the instruments are as described for submucous resection. An intranasal setup is used if the polyps arise from above or from the hiatus semilunaris. In some cases, polyps are removed in conjunction with a Caldwell-Luc operation, ethmoidectomy, enlargement of the frontal sinus, or opening of the sphenoid.

**OPERATIVE PROCEDURE.** As described for intranasal antrostomy or other types of operations on the sinus with removal of the polyps and degenerated tissue.

### Radical antrostomy (Caldwell-Luc operation)

**DEFINITION.** Use of an incision into the canine fossa of the upper jaw and exposure of the antrum for removal of bony diseased portions of the antral wall and contents of the sinus, or establishment of drainage by means of a counteropening into the nose through the inferior meatus (Fig. 8-49).

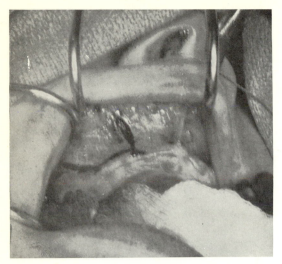

**Fig. 8-49.** Caldwell-Luc operation. Two separate openings are made, one in canine fossa to gain access to antrum and other in nasoantral wall. (From Thoma, K. H.: Oral surgery, ed. 5, St. Louis, 1969, The C. V. Mosby Co.)

**CONSIDERATIONS.** In the presence of pus in an acute sinus disease, the mucous membrane may become thickened and polyps may form, resulting in an obstruction of the nasal cavity and external passageway. In such cases, the patient suffers from nasal catarrh, headaches, and cough. Chronic sinusitis may be associated with asthma (Figs. 8-32 and 8-34).

The purpose of a radical antrostomy is to establish a large opening in the nasoantral wall of the inferior meatus, which will ensure adequate gravity drainage and aeration and permit removal, under direct vision, of all diseased tissue in the sinus.

**SETUP AND PREPARATION OF THE PATIENT.** As described for intranasal antrostomy, plus the following items:

**Holding instruments**
2 Adson tissue forceps (Fig. 8-38)

**Exposing instruments** (Fig. 8-44)
1 Lip retractor
1 Nasal pronged retractor

**Clamping instruments**
4 Kelly hemostats (Fig. 8-39)

**Accessory items**
12 Long gauze fluff sponges
1 Roll folded gauze packing, 2 in. wide, 18 in. long
1 Penrose tissue drain, ⅜ in. wide

**OPERATIVE PROCEDURE.** Steps are shown in Figs. 8-49 and 8-50.

1. The upper lip is elevated with a retractor, and a transverse incision is made in the gingivolabial sulcus just above the teeth; the incision is carried down to the underlying bone. Periosteum and soft tissue are elevated with dissectors and periosteal elevators.

2. The thin bony plate is perforated with a gouge, the antrum is entered, and its opening is enlarged with nasal rongeurs. The anterior angle of the sinus may be opened by enlarging the window with Jansen-Middleton septum-cutting forceps, double-action rongeurs, and Kerrison forceps (Fig. 8-37).

3. The mucous membrane of the antrum is removed with Coakley or Myles angled curettes (Fig. 8-37).

4. Nasoantral drainage may be established by removal of a portion of the nasoantral wall below the inferior turbinate by means of cutting forceps and rasps (Figs. 8-36 and 8-37).

5. Permanent communication between the oral cavity and the antrum may be established by removal of a portion of the hard palate and alveolar ridge, with chisel and mallet for resection. The edges of the palate are trimmed with a rongeur; the antrum is packed with petrolatum gauze.

6. The labial incision may or may not be sutured. The face of the patient is cleaned and dried.

### Frontal sinus operation (external approach)

**DEFINITION.** The making of an incision above the eyebrow of the affected side through the anterior wall and floor of the frontal sinus for removal of the diseased tissue, cleansing of the sinus cavity, and drainage.

**CONSIDERATIONS.** In an acute frontal

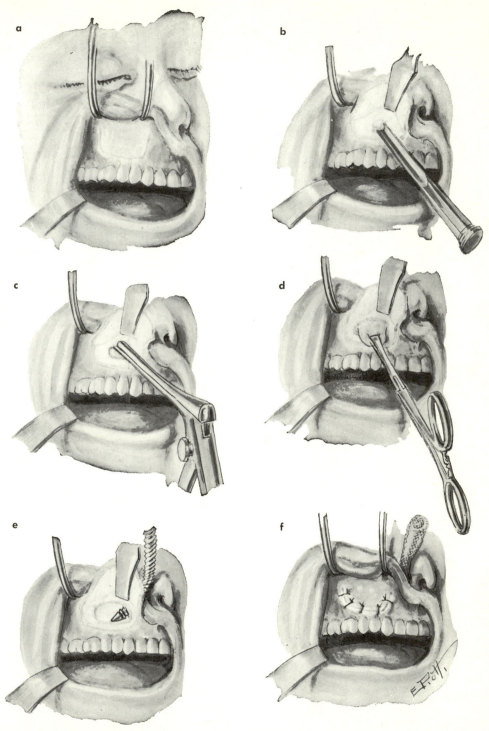

**Fig. 8-50.** Caldwell-Luc operation. **a,** Incision. **b,** Flap retracted and perforation made in canine fossa with gouge. **c,** Perforation enlarged with Kerrison forceps. **d,** Removal of diseased antral membrane. **e,** Trocar used to make nasoantral window. **f,** Incision closed. (From Thoma, K. H.: Oral surgery, ed. 5, St. Louis, 1969, The C. V. Mosby Co.)

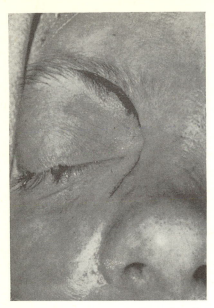

Fig. 8-51. Incision to expose ethmoid and frontal sinuses. Almost no visible scar results. (From De-Weese, D. D., and Saunders, W. H.: Textbook of otolaryngology, ed. 3, St. Louis, 1968, The C. V. Mosby Co.)

sinusitis in which the patient suffers from persistent headaches and edema of the upper lid, and in those cases in which medical therapy has failed, surgical treatment may be indicated. Drainage of the frontal sinus may be performed by a simple trephine opening through the floor of the sinus. In the presence of chronic suppuration with repeated acute attacks of frontal sinusitis, surgery may be done to remove the diseased lining of the sinus and to reconstruct the nasofrontal duct, thereby ensuring adequate drainage.

SETUP AND PREPARATION OF THE PATIENT. As described for intranasal antrostomy, plus the following items:

**Cutting instruments**
 1 Stryker saw with oscillating blade
 2 Brawley or Spratt frontal rasps

**Holding instruments**
 1 Potts or Cushing blunt hook
 2 Cushing straight fine forceps
 2 Adson tissue forceps

**Exposing instruments**
 1 Weitlaner self-retaining retractor (Fig. 8-40)

The patient is anesthetized and prepared as described for intranasal antrostomy.

OPERATIVE PROCEDURE

1. An incision is made over the affected frontal sinus, extending from the base of the nose through the eyebrow as far as the supraorbital notch (Fig. 8-51). A self-retaining retractor, hook retractor, knife, sponges, fine hemostats, fine ligatures, and suction set are needed.

2. Either the anterior wall of the frontal sinus or the floor of the sinus is opened by means of dental burrs, chisel, mallet, gouges, septum-cutting forceps, and curettes and nasal forceps. Drainage is established by either the nasofrontal duct or the insertion of drains.

3. An ethmoidal incision is made behind the nasal process of the superior maxillary bone with a chisel and mallet. The lacrimal duct is identified and preserved. Ethmoid cells are curetted.

4. A Penrose drain is introduced; the external wound is approximated with fine silk sutures and dressing applied. The patient's face is cleaned and dried.

### Ethmoidectomy

DEFINITION. Removal of the diseased portion of the middle turbinate, opening and removal of ethmoid cells, and removal of diseased tissue in the nasal fossa through a nasal approach or external approach.

CONSIDERATIONS. The purpose of an ethmoid operation is to reduce the many-celled ethmoid labyrinth into one large cavity to ensure adequate drainage and aeration (Fig. 8-32).

SETUP AND PREPARATION OF THE PATIENT. For the nasal approach, as described for intranasal antrostomy; for the external approach, as described for the frontal sinus operation.

OPERATIVE PROCEDURE. For the nasal route, the procedure is similar to intranasal antrostomy described previously. For the external route, the procedure is similar to the frontal sinus operation described previously (Fig. 8-51).

## Sphenoidectomy

**DEFINITION.** The making of an opening into one or both of the sphenoid sinuses by the intranasal or external ethmoidectomy approach.

**CONSIDERATIONS.** In surgical treatment of sinusitis of the sphenoid, it is difficult to visualize the cavity because of its depth. Surgery of the sphenoid sinus is usually done intranasally or through an external ethmoidectomy approach.

**SETUP AND PREPARATION OF THE PATIENT.** As described for intranasal antrostomy, with the addition of long sphenoid curettes, antrum rasps, and antrum punches (Figs. 8-36 and 8-37).

**OPERATIVE PROCEDURE.** As described for intranasal antrostomy.

## Turbinectomy

**DEFINITION.** (1) Anterior inferior turbinectomy—removal of the anterior end of the inferior turbinate. (2) Inferior turbinectomy—removal of the greater part of the lower border of the hypertrophied inferior turbinate. (3) Anterior middle turbinectomy—removal of the anterior end of the middle turbinate body. In all cases may include removal of polyps (Fig. 8-48).

**CONSIDERATIONS.** A turbinectomy is performed to provide for adequate ventilation and drainage and relieve pressure against the floor of the nose (Fig. 8-32).

**SETUP AND PREPARATION OF THE PATIENT.** As described for intranasal antrostomy.

**OPERATIVE PROCEDURE.** The nose is packed with petrolatum gauze on all sides of the turbinate. An incision is made, the affected turbinate amputated and removed, polyps removed, and cavity packed, as described for intranasal antrostomy.

## Fracture of the nose

**DEFINITION.** Manipulation and mobilization of nasal bones.

**CONSIDERATIONS.** When the nose is struck by a direct frontal blow, usually both nasal bones are fractured, displaced outward, and depressed into the ethmoid sinus (Fig. 8-34). The septal cartilage is usually broken or deviated, and lateral cartilages are displaced. Early reduction is done.

**SETUP AND PREPARATION OF THE PATIENT.** The patient is placed on the operating table in a dorsal recumbent position, and a topical anesthetic may be applied.

The setup includes a topical anesthesia set, plus a rubber-covered forceps or Ash septum-straightening forceps, a straight hemostat, petrolatum gauze packing, a plastic mold or aluminum splint, and adhesive tape.

**OPERATIVE PROCEDURE.** A rubber-covered narrow forceps is inserted into the nostril; the nasal bones are elevated and molded into place by external manipulation.

# Operations of the throat, tongue, and neck

## ANATOMY AND PHYSIOLOGY OF THE THROAT AND NECK

The word *throat* refers to those structures of the neck in front of the vertebral column, including the mouth, tongue, pharynx, tonsils, larynx, and trachea (Fig. 8-32).

The *mouth* extends from the lips to the anterior pillars of the fauces. The portion of the mouth outside the teeth is known as the buccal cavity and that on the inner side of the teeth as the lingual cavity. The tongue occupies a large portion of the floor of the mouth. The hard and soft palates form the upper and posterior boundaries of the oral cavity, separating it from the nasal cavity and the nasopharynx. The soft palate emerges from the posterior border of the hard palate to form the uvula, a fingerlike movable projection. On either side, the uvula joins the base of the tongue anteriorly and the pharynx posteriorly.

The *pharynx* serves as a channel for both the digestive and respiratory systems.

It is situated behind the nasal cavities, mouth, and larynx (Fig. 8-32). The food and air passages cross each other in the pharynx. The pharynx is a funnel-shaped structure, wide above and narrower below, about 12 cm. in length. It is composed of muscular and fibrous layers and lined with mucous membrane. It is associated above with the sphenoid and the basilar part of the occipital bone, and it joins the esophagus below. Seven cavities communicate with the pharynx: the two nasal cavities, the two tympanic cavities, the mouth, the larynx, and the esophagus. The cavity of the pharynx may be subdivided from above downward into three parts: nasal, oral, and laryngeal. Infection may spread from the pharynx to the middle ear via the auditory tube. This auditory tube can be catheterized through the nostril.

The nasopharynx communicates with the oropharynx through the pharyngeal isthmus, which is closed by muscular action during swallowing. The oropharynx and the laryngopharynx cannot be closed off from each other; both serve respiratory and digestive functions.

The pharynx comprises three groups of constrictor muscles (Fig. 8-52). Each muscle fits within the one below, and each inserts posteriorly in the median line with its mate from the opposite side. The constrictor muscles provide constriction of the pharynx for deglutition. Between the origins of the constrictor muscle groups, there are so-called intervals through which pass ligaments, nerves, and arteries (Fig. 8-52). The recurrent laryngeal nerve is closely associated with the lower portion of the pharynx.

The *tonsils* are situated one on each side of the oropharynx, lodged in a tonsillar fossa that is attached to folds of membrane containing muscle. One pair, the palatine tonsils, is the only lymphatic organ covered with stratified squamous epithelium. The lateral surface of each

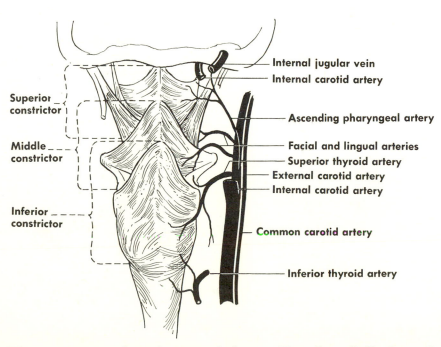

Fig. 8-52. Constrictor muscles and arteries of pharynx. (From Ryan, R. E., Ogura, J. H., Biller, H. F., and Pratt, L. L.: Synopsis of ear, nose, and throat diseases, ed. 3, St. Louis, 1970, The C. V. Mosby Co.)

tonsil is usually covered with a fibrous capsule. The anterior and posterior tonsillar pillars join to form a triangular fossa, with the posterior lateral aspects of the tongue at its base. The so-called lingual tonsils are lodged in each fossa. The adenoids or pharyngeal tonsil is suspended from the roof of the nasopharynx and consists of an accumulation of lymphoid tissue.

The arteries of the tonsils enter the upper and lower poles. The tonsils are supplied with blood by tonsillar branches of the ascending palatine branch of the facial artery (branches of the external carotid artery). The external carotid artery on each side lies behind and lateral to each tonsil. The nerves supplying the tonsils are derived from the middle and posterior palatine branches of the maxillary and glossopharyngeal nerves.

## Larynx and associated cartilages and muscles

LARYNX. The larynx is located at the upper end of the respiratory tract. It is situated between the trachea and the root of the tongue, at the upper front part of the neck (Figs. 8-32 and 8-67). The larynx has three main functions: (1) a passageway for air, (2) a valve for closing off air passages from the digestive system and the pharynx, and (3) a voice box on which sound and speech depend to a degree.

The larynx is a cartilaginous box situated in front of the fourth, fifth, and sixth cervical vertebrae. The upper portion of the larynx is continuous with the pharynx above, and its lower portion joins the trachea. The skeletal structure provides for patency of the enclosed airway. The complex muscle action and arrangement of tissues within the structure provides for closure of the lumen for protection against trauma and entrance of foreign bodies and for phonation.

CARTILAGES. The skeletal framework of the larynx consists of cartilages and membranes. There are nine separate cartilages —three of them single and six arranged in pairs. The main cartilages of the larynx include the thyroid, cricoid, epiglottis, two arytenoid, two corniculate, and two cuneiform. The thyroid cartilage (Adam's apple) forms the anterior portion of the voice box. The cricoid cartilage, which resembles a signet ring, rests beneath the thyroid cartilage and within the laryngotracheal space (Fig. 8-53). The epiglottis is a slightly curled, leaf-shaped, elastic fibrous membrane. It is prolonged below into a slender process, attached in the midline to the upper border of the thyroid cartilage. When the cricothyroid muscle contracts, it pulls the thyroid cartilage and the cricoid cartilage, thereby tightening the vocal cords and, if unopposed, closing the glottis. The arytenoid cartilages, which rest above the signet ring portion of the cricoid cartilage, support the posterior portion of the true vocal cords.

LARYNGEAL LIGAMENTS. The extrinsic ligaments of the larynx are those connecting the thyroid cartilage and epiglottis with the hyoid bone and the cricoid cartilage with the trachea. The intrinsic ligaments of the larynx are those connecting several cartilages of the organ to each other. They are considered the elastic membrane of the larynx (Fig. 8-53).

The mucous lining of the larynx blends with the fibrous tissue to form two folds on each side of the larynx. The upper set are known as the false cords. The lower set are called the *true vocal cords* because they are primarily concerned with the speaking voice and protection of the lower respiratory channels against the invasion of food and foreign bodies.

LARYNGEAL MUSCLES. The laryngeal muscles perform two distinct functions. There are muscles (extrinsic type) that open and close the glottis and those (intrinsic type) that regulate the degree of tension on the vocal cords (Fig. 8-54).

It should be noted that the spoken voice

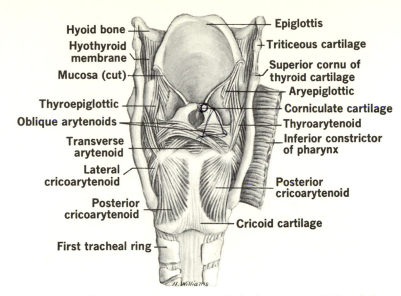

Hyoid bone
Hyothyroid membrane
Mucosa (cut)
Thyroepiglottic
Oblique arytenoids
Transverse arytenoid
Lateral cricoarytenoid
Posterior cricoarytenoid
First tracheal ring

Epiglottis
Triticeous cartilage
Superior cornu of thyroid cartilage
Aryepiglottic
Corniculate cartilage
Thyroarytenoid
Inferior constrictor of pharynx
Posterior cricoarytenoid
Cricoid cartilage

H. Williams

**Fig. 8-53.** Intrinsic muscles and general structure of the larynx, viewed from behind. (Dissection by Dr. L. D. Chapin: W.R.U. 2686, male, 65 years of age.) (From Francis, C. C: Introduction to human anatomy, ed. 5, St. Louis, 1968, The C. V. Mosby Co.)

also depends on the sphincter action of the soft palate, tongue, and lips. The muscle action of the larynx permits the glottis to close either voluntarily or involuntarily by reflex action. The closure of the inlet by this mechanism protects the respiratory passages. The closure of the glottis and the action of the vocal cords are precisely coordinated to produce the spoken voice.

Two branches of the vagus nerve supply the intrinsic muscles. The recurrent laryngeal nerve branch of the vagus nerve is the important motor nerve of the intrinsic muscles of the larynx. The sensory nerve, which is derived from the branches of the superior laryngeal nerve, supplies the mucous membrane of the larynx.

When both the recurrent laryngeal nerves become divided or paralyzed, the glottis remains closed so tightly that air cannot be drawn into the lungs. As a lifesaving measure, an endotracheal or tracheostomy tube is inserted immediately.

The larynx derives its blood supply from the branches of the external carotid and subclavian arteries.

## Trachea

The trachea, a cylindrical tube abou 15 cm. in length and from 2 to 2.5 cm. i diameter, begins in the neck and extend from the lower part of the larynx, on level with the sixth cervical vertebra, t the upper border of the fifth thoraci vertebra. The tube descends in front the esophagus, enters the superior me diastinum, and divides into right and le main bronchi (Chapter 14). The trache is composed of a series of incomplet rings of hyaline cartilage. The carina a ridge on the inside at the bifurcatio of the trachea. It is a landmark durin bronchoscopy and separates the uppe end of the right main branches from th upper end of the left main branches the bronchi. Branches given off from th arch of the aorta—the brachiocephalic (i nominate) and left common carotid arteri —are in close relation to the trachea. Th cervical portion of the trachea is relate anteriorly to the sternohyoid and stern thyroid muscles and to the isthmus of th thyroid gland.

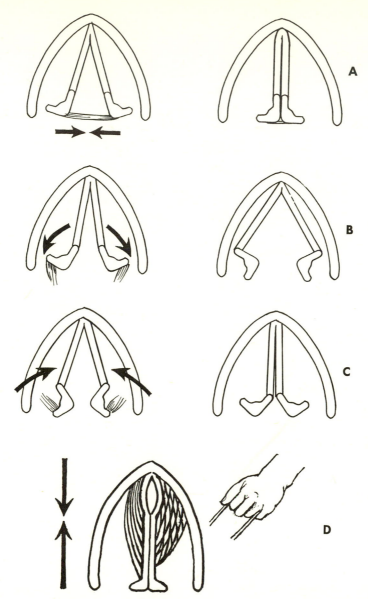

**Fig. 8-54. A,** Action of transverse arytenoid muscle. **B,** Action of posterior cricoarytenoid muscles. **C,** Action of lateral cricoarytenoid muscles. **D,** Action of thyroarytenoid or vocalis muscles. (From Ryan, R. E., Ogura, J. H., Biller, H. F., and Pratt, L. L.: Synopsis of ear, nose, and throat diseases, ed. 3, St. Louis, 1970, The C. V. Mosby Co.)

## Salivary glands

The salivary glands consist of three paired glands: the sublingual, submaxillary, and parotid. They communicate with the mouth and pour their secretions into cavities. The combined secretion of these glands is termed *saliva*. The salivary glands consist of tissue found in the mucosa of the cheek, tongue, palate, floor of the mouth, pharynx, lip, and paranasal sinuses. A tumor of a salivary gland may occur in any of these structures.

The external carotid artery supplies the salivary glands and divides into its terminal branches: the internal maxillary and superficial temporal. The superficial tem-

poral and internal maxillary veins unite to form the posterior facial vein.

The *sublingual* gland lies on the undersurface of the tongue beneath the mucous membrane of the floor of the mouth at the side of the frenulum linguae, in communication with the sublingual depression on the inner surface of the mandible.

The sublingual gland is supplied with blood from the submental arteries. Its nerves are derived from the sympathetic nerves. The many tiny ducts of each gland separately enter into the oral cavity on the sublingual fold.

The *submandibular* gland lies partly above and partly below the posterior half of the base of the mandible and on the mylohyoid and hyoglossus muscles. This gland is closely associated with the lingual veins and the lingual and hypoglossal nerves. The external maxillary artery lies on the posterior border of the gland. Its duct (Wharton's duct) enters the mouth at the frenulum of the tongue.

The *parotid* gland, the largest of the salivary glands, lies below the zygomatic arch in front of the mastoid process and behind the ramus of the mandible. This gland is enclosed in fascia, attached to surrounding muscles, and divided into two parts—a superficial and a deep portion—by means of the facial nerve. The parotid duct (Stensen's duct) pierces the buccal pad of fat and the buccinator muscle, finally opening into the oral cavity opposite the crown of the upper second molar tooth. The superficial temporal artery and small branches of the external carotid arise in the parotid gland behind the neck of the mandible (Fig. 8-65).

### General structures of the neck

The general topography of the organs lying in front of the prevertebral fascia has been described. A layer of deep cervical fascia surrounds the neck like a collar and is attached to the trapezius and sternocleidomastoideus (sternocleidomastoid) muscles. In front of the neck the deep fascial layer is attached to the lower border of the mandible.

The *pretracheal fascia* of the neck lies deep in the strap muscles (sternothyroid, sternohyoid, and omohyoid) and partially encloses the thyroid gland, trachea, and larynx. The pretracheal fascia is pierced by the thyroid vessels. It fuses with the front of the carotid sheath on the deep surface of the sternocleidomastoid. The carotid sheath consists of a network of areolar tissue surrounding the carotid arteries and vagus nerve.

Laterally, the carotid sheath is fused with the fascia on the deep surface of the sternocleidomastoideus; anteriorly, it is fused with the middle cervical fascia along the lateral border of the sternothyroideus muscle. Lying between the floor and roof of this triangular formation of muscles are the lymph glands and the accessory nerve. Arteries and nerves traverse and pierce this triangle.

### Lymphatic system of the neck

The lymph glands of the neck are closely associated with the salivary glands and the lymph plexus. The submaxillary nodes, located in the submaxillary triangle, drain the cheek, side of the nose, upper lip, side of the lower lip, gums, side of the tongue, and medial palpebral commissure. Lymph from the facial and submental nodes also drains to these glands. The superficial cervical nodes, following the external jugular vein, drain the ear and parotid area to the superior deep cervical nodes. The cervical nodes are in close contact with the larynx, thyroid gland, nasal cavities, ear, nasopharynx, palate, esophagus, and skin and muscles of the neck.

## OPERATIONS ON THE THROAT AND ASSOCIATED STRUCTURES
### Laryngoscopy

DEFINITION. Direct visual examination of the interior of the larynx by means of an electric-lighted speculum known as a laryngoscope (Fig. 8-55), in order to obtain a specimen of tissue or secretions for pathological examination or to instill a drug.

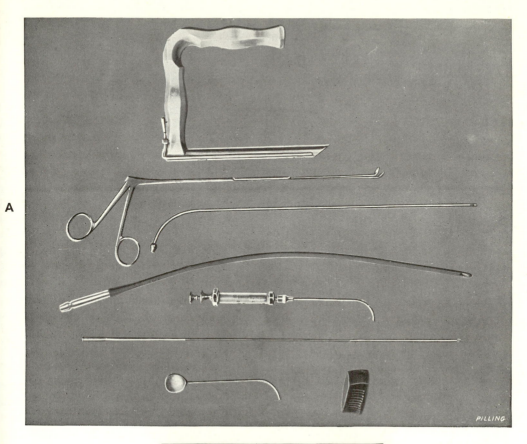

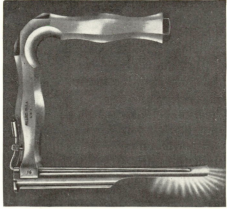

Fig. 8-55. **A,** Instruments for diagnostic laryngoscopy. From above downward: anterior commissure laryngoscope (C. L. Jackson model); tissue forceps (laryngeal grasping forceps should be included, similar to tissue forceps but with straight alligator jaws); aspirating tube, metallic; aspirating tube, silk-woven; laryngeal syringe (Lukens model); sponge carrier for secure holding of gauze sponges for swabbing, hemostasis, and obtaining smear specimens; mouth opener (C. L. Jackson model); bite block, suitable size. **B,** Laryngoscope for introduction of bronchoscope. Slide permits removal of this necessarily rather heavy displacing instrument in trachea for safe exploration of tracheobronchial tree and for passage of bronchoscope. (From Jackson, C., and Jackson, C. L.: Bronchoesophagology, Philadelphia, 1950, W. B. Saunders Co.)

**CONSIDERATIONS.** The patient has to be sufficiently relaxed to make examination easier. This is accomplished by both psychological and proper drug preparation. An oral sedative is usually given the night before and again at approximately 1 hour prior to the examination.

**SETUP AND PREPARATION OF THE PATIENT.** Very small infants usually do not require an anesthetic; children and adults who cannot relax are given a general anesthetic; adults who are well prepared do very well with the application of a local anesthetic of lidocaine (Xylocaine), tetracaine (Pontocaine), or cocaine. The instrument setup includes the following:

> Local anesthesia set
> 1 Bite block
> 1 Mouth opener
> 1 Laryngoscope (surgeon's choice)—size suitable to the patient (adult, child, or infant)
> 2 Aspirating tubes
> 1 Light carrier and extra bulb
> 2 Laryngeal biopsy forceps—straight and upbiting
> 2 Sponge carrier forceps with extra sponges
> Specimen jar or jars

The patient is placed in a supine position, and an assistant holds the patient's head in the proper position for good visualization of the vocal cords.

**OPERATIVE PROCEDURE**

1. The spatula end of the laryngoscope is introduced into the right side of the patient's mouth and directed toward the midline; then the dorsum of the tongue is elevated, exposing the epiglottis.

2. The patient's head is first tipped backward and then elevated and lifted upward as the laryngoscope is advanced into the larynx.

3. The larynx is examined, a biopsy is taken, secretions are aspirated, and bleeding is controlled.

4. The patient's face is cleansed. The patient is reassured and taken to his room or the recovery room.

## Tonsillectomy and adenoidectomy

**DEFINITION.** Complete removal of the tonsils and adenoids by either the sharp or blunt dissection method.

**CONSIDERATIONS.** Enlarged tonsils and adenoids are usually associated with difficulty in breathing, chronic colds, enlarged glands of the neck, and pressure on the eustachian tubes because of adenoiditis. Rheumatism, bronchitis, and deafness may be associated with diseased tonsils.

**SETUP AND PREPARATION OF THE PATIENT.** If a general anesthetic is to be administered, the patient is anesthetized first, then placed in a slight Trendelenburg position. The neck is hyperextended by placing a roll under the shoulders. If a local anesthetic is to be administered, the patient is placed in a sitting position.

The patient's face may be cleaned with a germicide. The patient is draped as follows: (1) An opened sheet with two opened towels on top is placed under the head of the patient. (2) The uppermost towel is wrapped around the head and secured by a forceps, and the free ends of the towel are tucked under the head. (3) A second sheet is placed over the patient.

The instruments and supplies required include the following (Figs. 8-56 and 8-57):

**Cutting instruments**
> 1 Knife handle no. 7 with blade no. 12
> 1 Tonsil knife, single-edged
> 1 Tonsil knife, double-edged, if desired
> 2 Eves snares with wires
> 2 LaForce or Sluder tonsil guillotines, if desired
> 1 Metzenbaum scissors, curved or flat, 7½ in.
> 1 Mayo scissors, straight
> 1 Tonsil curette
> 2 Adenoid curettes, suitable size
> 1 Adenoid punch, suitable size
> 1 LaForce adenatome, suitable size
> 1 Hurd dissector and pillar elevator

**Holding instruments**
> 2 Robb sponge-holding forceps
> 1 Towel forceps
> 1 Adson tissue forceps
> 2 Allis forceps
> 2 Pillar-grasping forceps
> 2 Tenacula for seizing tonsils

**Clamping instruments**
> 2 Boettcher tonsil hemostats
> 2 Mayo-Pean hemostats, curved, 6¼ in.
> 2 Dean hemostatic forceps

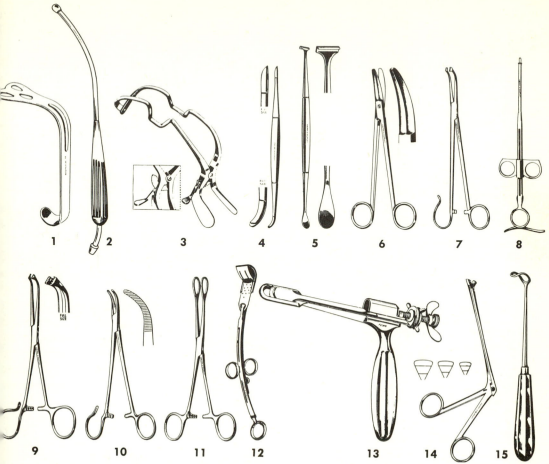

**Fig. 8-56.** Special instruments for tonsillectomy and adenoidectomy. **1,** Tongue depressor; **2,** Yankauer suction tube; **3,** Jennings mouth gag; **4,** tonsil knife; **5,** Hurd dissector and pillar retractor; **6,** Boettcher tonsil scissors; **7,** White tonsil-seizing forceps; **8,** Eves tonsil snare and wire; **9,** Allis-Coakley forceps, straight and curved; **10,** Dean hemostatic forceps; **11,** Ballenger sponge-holding forceps, serrated jaw; **12,** LaForce adenotome; **13,** Daniel tonsillectome; **14,** adenoid punch; **15,** Barnhill adenoid curette. (Courtesy Codman & Shurtleff, Inc., Randolph, Mass.)

**Exposing instruments**

1 Jennings mouth gag, suitable size
1 Uvula retractor
1 Tongue depressor

**Suturing instruments**

1 Needle holder, 7 in.
  Plain gut ligatures, nos. 0 and 2-0 (Chapter 6)
  Plain gut sutures, no. 2-0 swaged to ½-circle tonsil needle

**Accessory items**

2 Yankauer throat suction tubes with tubing
1 Pharyngeal tube
1 Tongue depressor

1 Vapor hook
  Minor throat pack, including tonsil sponges, gauze compresses, and tonsil tampons (Fig. 8-57)
  Minor neck drape pack
  Gowns and gloves (Chapter 4)

**OPERATIVE PROCEDURE**

1. When a general anesthetic is used, the mouth is retracted open with a self-retaining retractor, the tongue depressed with a blade retractor, and an anesthesia tube placed in the corner of the mouth. An efficient suction apparatus is most important. The metal suction tube is intro-

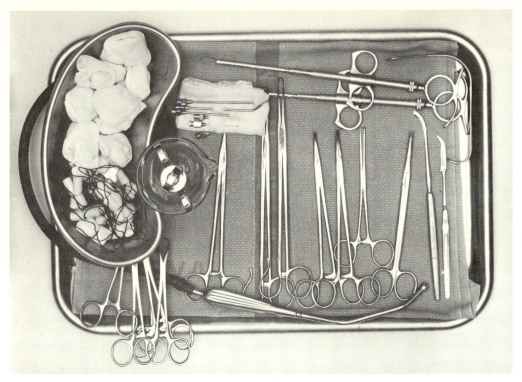

**Fig. 8-57.** Sterile tonsil tray setup ready for use. Sterile towels and sheet are placed on top of instruments.

duced gently and passed along the floor of the mouth, over the base of the tongue, and into the pharynx. During the procedure the suctioning ensures adequate exposure of the operative site and prevents blood from reaching the lungs.

2. The tonsil is grasped with a pair of tonsil-grasping forceps and the mucous membrane of the anterior pillar incised with a knife; the tonsil lobe is freed from its attachments to the pillars with a tonsil dissector, curved scissors, and gauze sponges on a holder. The tonsil is withdrawn with forceps (Fig. 8-58).

3. The posterior pillar is cut with scissors, and the tonsil is removed with a snare (Fig. 8-58). In some cases the La-Force or Sluder tonsil guillotine clamp may be used.

4. A tampon (cottonoid or gauze tied securely to silk) is placed in the fossa by means of a hemostat.

5. Bleeding vessels are clamped with tonsil forceps, tied with slipknot ligature of plain gut no. 0, and the free ligature ends are cut (Chapter 6).

6. The adenoids are removed with an adenotome or curette. Bleeding is controlled by pressure with sponges.

7. The fossa is carefully inspected, and any bleeding vessels are clamped and tied. Retractors are removed, the face of the patient is cleaned, and his head is turned to one side. The patient is kept in the semirecumbent (Fowler) position or on his side horizontally, to avoid aspiration of blood and venous engorgement.

### Surgery of the oral cavity

**DEFINITION.** The excision of benign or malignant lesions of the tongue, floor of the mouth, alveolar ridge, buccal mucosa, or tonsillar area.

**CONSIDERATIONS.** Benign or small malig-

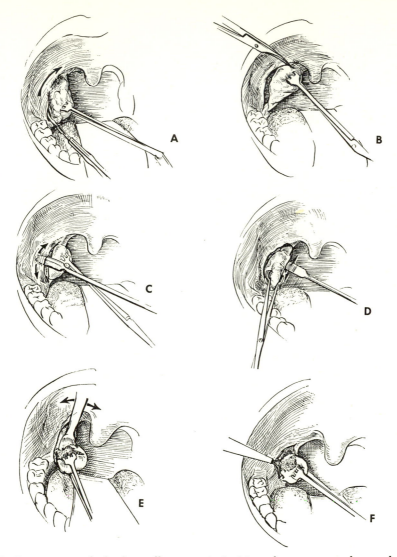

**Fig. 8-58.** Dissection method of tonsillectomy. **A,** Incision of mucous membrane along edge of anterior pillar. **B,** Extension of mucosal incision along its superior and posterior attachments. **C,** Separation of tonsil from anterior pillar. **D,** Separation of tonsil from posterior pillar. **E,** Completion of dissection along superior and lateral walls. **F,** Application of snare for removal of tonsil. (From Ryan, R. E., Ogura, J. H., Biller, H. F., and Pratt, L. L.: Synopsis of ear, nose, and throat diseases, ed. 3, St. Louis, 1970, The C. V. Mosby Co.)

nant tumors of the oral cavity may be excised without neck dissection. In the presence of tongue cancer without evidence of metastasis, a "prophylactic" neck dissection may be performed in an effort to control a cancerous growth in the upper jugular chain of the neck.

In the treatment of typical carcinoma of the floor of the mouth with involvement of

the mandible, a portion of the tongue is removed in the combined operation—a radical neck dissection and resection of both the mandible and the tongue. When the primary intraoral lesion is confined to the tongue, a neck dissection and a hemiglossectomy are performed without resection of the mandible.

In the presence of a lesion of the tonsil

or an extensive lesion at the base of the tongue with pharyngeal wall involvement, a resection of the ascending ramus of the mandible is necessary, and portions of the base of the tongue, pharyngeal wall, and the soft palate are removed to secure an adequate margin of normal tissue about the lesion.

SETUP AND PREPARATION OF THE PATIENT. The patient is placed in a dorsal recumbent position with shoulders elevated. Generally, endotracheal anesthesia is used, and a pharyngeal pack of moist gauze is inserted in the mouth. Instruments and supplies include the following items:

Cutting instruments

2 Knives nos. 3 and 7, blades nos. 10 and 15
1 Metzenbaum scissors, curved, 7¼ in.
1 Mayo scissors, straight
1 Mayo scissors, curved
1 Suture scissors
  Electrosurgical unit with coagulation and cutting electrodes

Holding instruments

4 Foerster or Ballenger sponge-holding forceps
6 Towel forceps
3 Tissue forceps, 2 and 3 teeth, 7 in.
2 Tissue forceps without teeth, 5½ in.
1 Tissue forceps without teeth, 7 in.
2 Nasal dressing forceps
4 Allis forceps, 3 and 4 teeth

Clamping instruments

6 Mayo-Pean hemostats, curved, 6½ in.
3 Mayo-Pean hemostats, curved, 6¼ in.
6 Crile hemostats, straight
2 Rochester-Carmalt hemostats, 8 in.
3 Tonsil artery forceps

Exposing instruments

1 Metal anesthesia tube
1 Mouth gag
2 McBurney retractors
3 Bosworth tongue depressors
1 Cheek retractor
2 Parker retractors
1 Cushing loop retractor
1 Nerve hook

Suturing instruments

1 Crile-Wood needle holder, 8 in.
1 Crile-Wood needle holder, 5½ in.
  Chromic gut, nos. 2-0 and 3-0, for ligatures (Chapter 6)
  Silk, no. 2-0, for traction suture

Silk, no. 4-0 for sewing, swaged to ⅜-circle, cutting-edge needles (surgeon's type)
Silk, no, 3-0 for sewing, swaged to ½-circle, taper point needles (Murphy type)

Accessory items

1 Catheter, whistle-tipped, with open end 14 Fr. (Chapter 12)
1 Roll folded gauze packing with petrolatum
1 Postnasal plug set (Figs. 8-46 and 8-47)
2 Yankauer suction tubes and rubber tubing
1 Tracheostomy set
1 Local anesthesia set for nerve block, if desired
1 Minor pack set, including gauze compresses, pads, and tonsil tampons
1 Minor neck drape pack, including towels and flat sheets (Chapter 5)

OPERATIVE PROCEDURE

Although the case may be scheduled as a local excision, frequently lesions of the oral cavity require more extensive excisions than planned preoperatively. The setup should be designed to include the instruments for a neck dissection, or to have them available.

In most tumors of the oral cavity a tracheostomy is performed to assure an airway postoperatively.

## Elective tracheostomy

DEFINITION. Opening of the trachea and insertion of a cannula through a midline incision in the neck, below the cricoid cartilage.

CONSIDERATIONS. Tracheostomy is used as an emergency procedure to treat upper respiratory tract obstruction and as a prophylactic measure in the presence of chronic lung disease in which an obstruction could occur. A prophylactic tracheostomy is performed at the time of surgery, thus providing for easy and frequent aspiration of the tracheobronchial tree and diminishing the dead space that exists from the opening of the mouth down to the supraclavicular region. The creation of a new clearance (tracheostomy) nearer to the functional areas in the lung provides for greater volume of air for the patient with a partly destroyed lung. Anesthesia may be maintained via a prophylactic tracheostomy.

SETUP AND PREPARATION OF THE PATIENT.
The patient is placed in a dorsal recumbent position, with the shoulders raised by a folded sheet to hyperextend the neck and head (Chapter 7). The neck is cleansed and sterile drapes applied (Chapters 4 and 5). Along with a basic minor pack, the following instruments should be included:

Cutting instruments
  2 Knife handles no. 3 with blades nos. 10 and 15
  1 Metzenbaum scissors, curved
  1 Mayo scissors, straight
  1 Suture scissors

Holding instruments
  2 Allis forceps, straight
  1 Needle holder
  2 Tissue forceps, fine teeth
  2 Tissue forceps without teeth
  4 Towel forceps
  2 Sponge-holding forceps

Clamping instruments
  4 Mosquito hemostats, straight
  4 Kelly hemostats, curved
  1 Mayo-Pean hemostat, curved
  2 Crile hemostats, curved

Exposing instruments
  2 Volkmann rake retractors
  2 Cushing loop retractors
  2 Frazier skin hooks
  1 Jackson tracheal retractor
  1 Cushing nerve hook
  2 Brophy tenaculum hooks

Suturing items
  Plain gut no. 3-0 sutures
  Chromic gut no. 4-0 sutures swaged to fine, ½-circle, taper point needle
  Silk no. 4-0 sutures swaged to ⅜-circle, cutting-edge needle

Accessory items
  2 Catheters, whistle-tipped, open-ended, 14 Fr.
  1 Throat suction tube
  1 Adson suction tube
  2 Pieces suction tubing, length to reach suction apparatus
  Tracheostomy tubes (Figs. 8-59 and 8-60), appropriate size (for adults, nos. 6 or 8, or 2 or 4); Martin extension on inner cannula, if desired, for use with bulky dressing
  Cardiac arrest setup, oxygen, and thiopental (Pentothal) sodium setup (Chapter 5)
  Local anesthesia set and anesthetic agents, as desired
  Minor pack set

OPERATIVE PROCEDURE

1. A vertical or transverse incision may be used. A vertical incision is made in the midline from approximately the cricoid cartilage to the suprasternal notch. When a transverse incision is made, it extends approximately one fingerbreadth above the suprasternal notch parallel to it and from the anterior border of one sternocleidomastoid muscle to the opposite side. Soft tissues and muscle are divided, and the isthmus of the thyroid gland that joins both lobes of the gland in the midline over the trachea is retracted in an upward

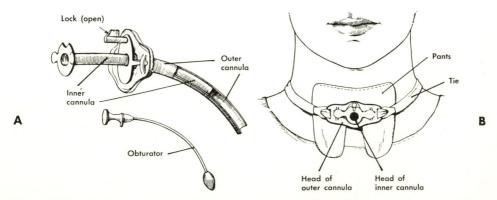

Fig. 8-59. **A,** Parts of metal tracheostomy tube. **B,** Tracheostomy ties and gauze pants in place. (From Work, W., and Smith, M. F. W.: Postgrad. Med. **34:**479, 1963.)

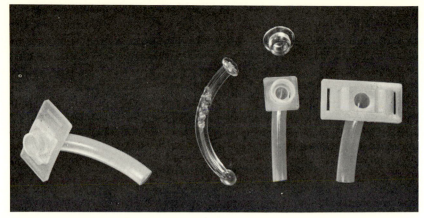

**Fig. 8-60.** Plastic tracheostomy tubes. Left to right: assembled tube, pilot to help introduce tube, inner tube, outer tube, and cork to plug tube to test airway. (From DeWeese, D. D., and Saunders, W. H.: Textbook of otolaryngology, ed. 3, St. Louis, 1968, The C. V. Mosby Co.)

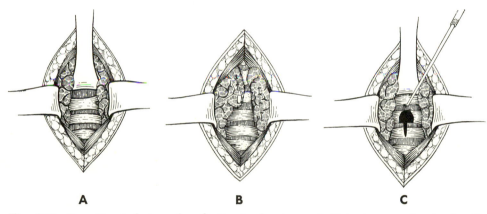

**A**   **B**   **C**

**Fig. 8-61.** Operative technique for elective tracheostomy. **A,** Retractor exposing trachea by drawing isthmus of thyroid upward. **B,** Alternate method to that shown in **A;** isthmus of thyroid is divided to expose trachea. **C,** Two tracheal rings are cut, and upper ring is partially resected. Tracheal hook pulls trachea from depth of wound nearer surface. (From DeWeese, D. D., and Saunders, W. H.: Textbook of otolaryngology, ed. 3, St. Louis, 1968, The C. V. Mosby Co.)

direction with Cushing retractors, thus resulting in exposure of the underlying tracheal rings, usually the third and fourth (Fig. 8-61). In some cases two curved clamps may be inserted through this incision across the isthmus and the isthmus transected (Fig. 8-61). The transected ends of the isthmus are secured with chromic gut sutures.

2. One to 2 ml. of 10% cocaine solution

may be injected with a 24-gauge, ½-inch hypodermic needle. Air is first drawn into the syringe to be sure that the needle point is located in the lumen. With a knife and no. 15 blade, a vertical incision is made in the trachea directly across the two tracheal rings. The cut ends of the cricoid cartilage are retracted with a hook (Fig. 8-61).

3. The previously prepared tracheostomy tube is inserted into the trachea, the ob-

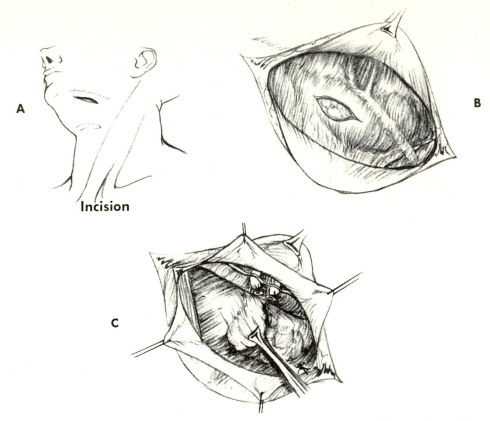

Incision

**Fig. 8-62.** Excision of submaxillary gland. **A,** Small incision is made below and parallel to mandible and extending forward beneath skin. **B,** Skin flaps and platysma are dissected and cervical fascia incised to expose gland. **C,** Gland is grasped, to be freed by blunt dissection. (From Wilder, J. R.: Atlas of general surgery, ed. 2, St. Louis, 1964, The C. V. Mosby Co.)

turator is quickly removed, and the trachea is suctioned with a catheter.

4. The wound edges are lightly approximated with silk sutures no. 4-0, or the wound edges are allowed to fall together around the tube. One or two skin sutures are inserted above the tube. The lower angle of the wound may be left open for drainage.

5. The tracheostomy tube is held in place with tapes tied with a square knot behind the neck. The inner tube is then inserted. A gauze dressing split around the tube is applied to the wound (Fig. 8-59, *B*).

### Excision of the submaxillary gland

**DEFINITION.** Removal of the gland and tumor through an incision made in the neck, just beneath the chin (Fig. 8-62).

**CONSIDERATIONS.** This operation is performed to remove mixed tumors and multiple calculi associated with extensive chronic inflammation.

**SETUP AND PREPARATION OF THE PATIENT.** The patient is placed on the table in a dorsal recumbent position, with the affected side uppermost, and prepared as for neck surgery (Chapters 4 and 7).

The instruments include a minor neck dissection setup with fine dissecting scissors and hemostatic clamps. A tracheostomy setup should be available.

**OPERATIVE PROCEDURE**

1. A small skin incision is made below and parallel to the mandible, extending forward to beneath the chin. The platysma is incised with scissors; the skin flaps and undersurface of the platysma and cervical

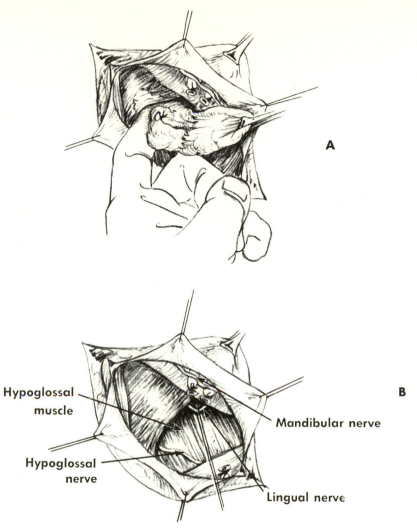

**A**

Hypoglossal
muscle

**B**

Mandibular nerve

Hypoglossal
nerve

Lingual nerve

**Fig. 8-63.** Excision of submaxillary gland—cont'd. **A,** Posterior lobe delivered. **B,** Dissection completed. (From Wilder, J. R.: Atlas of general surgery, ed. 2, St. Louis, 1964, The C. V. Mosby Co.)

fascia covering the gland are undermined, using fine hooks, tissue forceps, and Metzenbaum scissors (Fig. 8-62).

2. The mandibular branch of the facial nerve is retracted away with a small loop retractor.

3. The submaxillary gland is elevated from the mylohyoid muscle (Fig. 8-63). The edge of the muscle is retracted to expose the lingual veins and nerve and the hypoglossal nerve.

4. The gland is freed by blunt dissec-

tion, and the submaxillary (Wharton's) duct is clamped, ligated, and divided.

5. The external maxillary artery is clamped, ligated, and divided. The submaxillary gland is removed (Fig. 8-63).

6. The wound is closed with interrupted fine silk or chromic gut sutures. The skin edges are approximated with nylon sutures. A Penrose drain is inserted in the submaxillary bed and secured to the skin. Dressings are applied.

## Parotidectomy

**DEFINITION.** Removal of the tumor and gland through a curved incision in the upper neck and behind the lobe of the ear (Fig. 8-68) or through a Y-type incision in both sides of the ear and below the angle of the mandible (Fig. 8-64).

**CONSIDERATIONS.** The majority of benign tumors of the salivary glands occur in the parotid gland. These benign tumors are of the same types as are those found in soft tissues in other parts of the body. In the parotid gland, the closeness of the facial nerve makes it difficult to remove the entire tumor. Parotidectomy is indicated for removal of all benign and some malignant tumors, for inflammatory lesions, for vascular anomalies, and for metastatic cancer involving lymph nodes overlying the gland.

In the removal of malignant tumors involving adjacent structures such as the mandible or cheek, the operation may become a radical removal of the involved structures.

**SETUP AND PREPARATION OF THE PATIENT.** The patient is placed on the operating table in a dorsal recumbent position with the entire affected side of the face uppermost (Chapter 7). The entire side of the face, the mouth, the outer canthus of the eye, and the forehead are prepared and left exposed (Chapter 4).

The instrument setup includes the following items: minor dissecting tray with fine dissecting scissors, 2-pronged retractors, Kocher retractors, nerve hooks, fine tissue forceps and hemostats, suction apparatus, nasal periosteal elevator, and curettes. A nerve stimulator should be set up and ready for use should the surgeon request one.

**OPERATIVE PROCEDURE**

1. The incision may extend from the posterior angle of the zygoma downward in front of the tragus of the ear and behind the lobule of the ear backward over the mastoid process, then downward and forward on the neck parallel to and below the body of the mandible (Fig. 8-64).

(A chin incision may be used.) Bleeding vessels are controlled by hemostats and fine ligatures.

2. Using fine-toothed tissue forceps and scissors, the skin flaps are elevated as described for thyroidectomy. The skin wound edges are retracted away by means of silk sutures fastened to the clamps.

3. The upper portion of the sternocleidomastoid muscle is exposed and retracted, the auricular nerve is identified (Fig. 8-64), and the lower part of the parotid gland is elevated, using curved hemostats.

4. The superficial temporal artery and vein and external jugular vein are identified by means of blunt dissection.

5. The parotid tissue is dissected from the cartilage of the ear and the tympanic plate of the temporal bone. The temporal, zygomatic, and mandibular and cervical branches of the facial nerve are identified and preserved.

6A. The superficial portion of the parotid gland containing the tumor is removed. In some cases, the entire superficial portion is removed, followed by ligation and division of the parotid duct.

6B. When the deep portion of the parotid gland must be removed, the facial nerve is retracted upward and outward by nerve hooks; then the parotid tissue is removed from beneath the nerve. Kocher retractors are used to retract the mandible. The external carotid artery is identified. In many cases the internal maxillary and superficial temporal arteries are clamped, ligated, and divided.

7. The wound is closed in layers with fine silk sutures. A small Penrose drain is inserted, and a pressure dressing is applied (Fig. 8-65).

## Laryngofissure

**DEFINITION.** The opening of the larynx for exploratory, excisional, or reconstructive procedures.

**CONSIDERATIONS.** A laryngofissure is performed whenever access to the intrinsic larynx is necessary. The thyroid cartilages

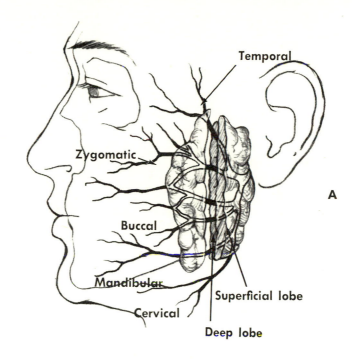

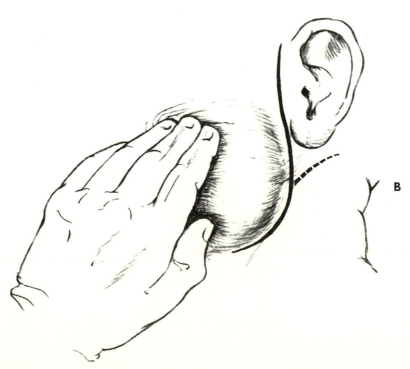

**Fig. 8-64.** Excision of parotid gland. **A,** Anatomy of facial nerve. **B,** Incision. (From Wilder, J. R.: Atlas of general surgery, ed. 2, St. Louis, 1964, The C. V. Mosby Co.)

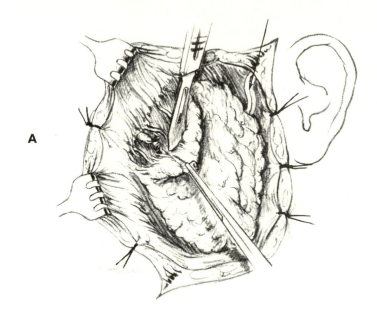

A

**Superficial temporal
artery and vein**

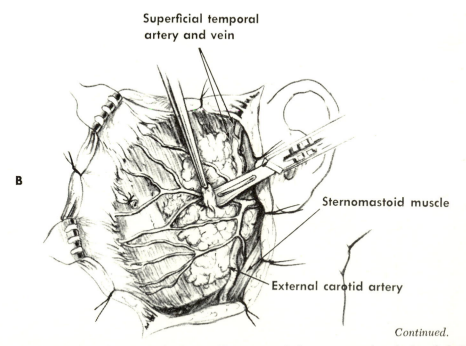

B

**Sternomastoid muscle**

**External carotid artery**

*Continued.*

**Fig. 8-65.** Excision of parotid gland—cont'd. **A,** Parotid duct is exposed and identified. By sharp and blunt dissections, duct is mobilized and ligated with fine gut suture and divided. **B,** Following anterior lobe mobilization and identification of facial nerve and vessels, posterior lobe is removed. **C,** Wound is cleansed, bleeding controlled, Penrose drain inserted, and wound closed. (From Wilder, J. R.: Atlas of general surgery, ed. 2, St. Louis, 1964, The C. V. Mosby Co.)

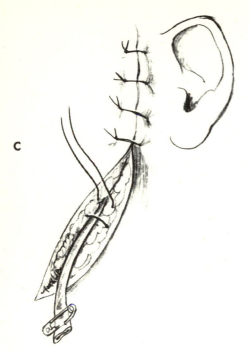

C

Fig. 8-65, cont'd. For legend see p. 223.

are split in the midline, and the true vocal cords and false vocal cords are incised at the midline anteriorly.

SETUP AND PREPARATION OF THE PATIENT. See partial laryngectomy.

OPERATIVE PROCEDURE

1. A tracheostomy is performed, and an endotracheal tube is inserted. A general anesthetic is administered. (This procedure can be done with the patient under local anesthesia.)

2. A transverse incision is made through the skin and first layer of the cervical fascia and platysma muscles, approximately 2 cm. above the sternoclavicular junction or in the normal skin crease by means of a knife handle no. 3 with a blade no. 10. The upper skin flap is undermined to the level of the cricoid cartilage; then the lower flap is undermined to the sternoclavicular joint.

3. Bleeding vessels are clamped with mosquito hemostats and ligated. The strap muscles are elevated and incised in the midline.

4. The thyroid cartilages are cut with

a Stryker saw, and the true vocal cords are visualized through an incision into the cricothyroid membrane. The true vocal cords are divided in the midline (anterior commissure), and the interior of the larynx is exposed.

5. The tracheostomy tube must be left in place postoperatively to ensure an airway.

### Partial laryngectomy

DEFINITION. The removal of a portion of the larynx.

CONSIDERATIONS. A partial laryngectomy is done to remove superficial neoplasms that are confined to one vocal cord or remove a tumor extending up into the ventricle on the anterior commissure or a short distance below the cord. Cancers confined to the intrinsic larynx (Figs. 8-53 and 8-66), are generally of a low grade of malignancy and tend to remain localized for long periods.

SETUP AND PREPARATION OF THE PATIENT. The patient is placed on the table in a dorsal recumbent position (Chapter 7). The operative site is prepared and the patient draped with sterile sheets, as described for thyroidectomy.

The setup for partial laryngectomy includes a basic neck tray, tracheostomy set, and the following additional items:

1 Bayonet forceps
1 Freer periosteal elevator
2 Frazier suction tubes
1 Beckman self-retaining retractor
2 Laryngectomy tubes, desired type and size, with extension
1 Ball-point laryngeal scissors
1 Stryker motor saw with oscillating circular blades of proper size
Topical anesthetic agent, as desired

OPERATIVE PROCEDURE

1. A tracheostomy is performed as previously described, and an endotracheal tube is inserted.

2. A vertical incision or a thyroid incision with elevation of a flap may be employed (Fig. 8-66).

3. The sternothyroid muscles are sep-

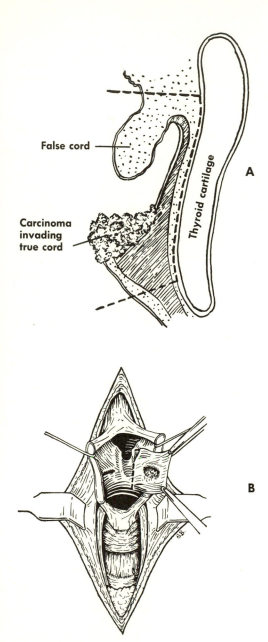

False cord

Carcinoma
invading
true cord

Thyroid cartilage

A

B

Fig. 8-66. Partial laryngectomy. **A,** Lesion suitable for removal. Dotted line indicates wide margin of normal tissue removed along with tumor. When limits of tumor are known, false cord may not be excised. **B,** Incision into larynx is from thyroid notch above to cricoid below. Drawing shows excision of lesion on true cord along with wide margin of normal tissue. (From DeWeese, D. D., and Saunders, W. H.: Textbook of otolaryngology, ed. 3, St. Louis, 1968, The C. V. Mosby Co.)

arated in the midline and retracted by means of loop retractors.

4. The fascial covering over the thyroid cartilage is incised with a knife, and the perichondrium is elevated from the cartilage on the side of the tumor with a Freer periosteal elevator.

5. The thyroid cartilage is divided longitudinally in midline by means of a Stryker power saw.

6. The cartilages are retracted with loop retractors. The cricothyroid membrane is incised with a knife. A blunt-nosed laryngeal scissors is introduced between the vocal cords to divide the mucosa of the anterior wall of the glottis.

7. The divided cartilages are retracted with Kocher retractors to expose the interior of the larynx. A small pack of moist gauze may be placed in the trachea to prevent aspiration of blood or mucus. A 10% solution of cocaine may be applied to the larynx to prevent laryngeal muscular spasm. The extent of the intrinsic laryngeal tumor is determined.

8. With a small periosteal elevator, the mucosa on the involved side of the larynx is freed; the false cord and mucosal layer of the region are lifted by means of a periosteal elevator and hooks. The involved cord is excised, using straight scissors (Fig. 8-66).

9. In some cases the thyroid cartilage may be removed with a knife and straight scissors. Bleeding is controlled with hemostats and fine chromic gut ligatures and sutures.

10. The gauze pack is removed from the trachea. The perichondrium is approximated with chromic gut no. 2-0 sutures. The strap muscles are approximated in the midline with chromic gut no. 2-0 sutures; then the platysma and the skin edges are approximated separately with fine silk sutures.

11. A tracheal-laryngeal tube is left in place. It is removed at a later date when the airway is adequate. Dressings are applied to the wound and around the tube.

## Supraglottic laryngectomy

DEFINITION. The supraglottic laryngectomy is the excision of the laryngeal structures above the true vocal cords.

CONSIDERATIONS. This surgery is indicated in cancer of the epiglottis and false vocal cords. It is designed to remove the cancer, yet preserve the phonatory, respiratory, and sphincteric functions of the larynx. A neck dissection is always performed.

SETUP AND PREPARATION OF THE PATIENT. Same as for total laryngectomy.

## Total laryngectomy

DEFINITION. Complete removal of the cartilaginous larynx, the hyoid bone, and the strap muscles connected to the larynx and possible removal of the pre-epiglottic space with the lesion.

CONSIDERATIONS. A wide-field laryngectomy is done when there is a loss of mobility of the cords and to treat cancer of the extrinsic larynx and hypopharynx. Malignant tumors of the extrinsic larynx are more anaplastic and tend to metastasize. When laryngeal carcinoma involves more than the true cords, a prophylactic (preventive) radical neck dissection is done to remove the lymphatics. In the presence of malignant tumors, the patient usually has no previous hoarseness, and the first symptom is the appearance of a lump in his neck.

Laryngectomy presents many psychological problems. The loss of voice that follows total laryngectomy is a most tragic event for the patient and family. The patient may be taught to talk either by using esophageal voice or with an artificial larynx. Esophageal voice is produced by the air contained in the esophagus rather than by that in the trachea. Speech requires a sounding air column. With instruction and practice, the patient is able to control the swallowing of air into the esophagus and reintroduction of this air into the mouth with phonation. The sounding air column is then transformed into speech by means of the lips, tongue, and teeth.

Because the stump of the trachea is brought out to the skin of the neck, all the patient's breathing is done directly into the trachea. This air is no longer moistened by the nose. Drying and crusting of the tracheal secretions occur. Humidification may be provided by covering the opening with a moist gauze compress.

SETUP AND PREPARATION OF THE PATIENT. The patient is placed on the table in a dorsal recumbent position with his neck extended and shoulders raised by a rubberized block or folded sheet. The table is slated downward to elevate the upper part of the body for the convenience of the surgeon (Chapter 7).

An endotracheal anesthetic is administered. An effective suction apparatus is most essential.

The proposed operative site, including the anterior neck region, lateral surfaces of the neck down to the outer aspects of the shoulders, and the upper anterior chest region, is cleansed in the usual manner.

The instrument setup includes the basic thyroidectomy set (Chapter 18), plus the following:

**Cutting instruments**

2 Curettes for paranasal sinuses
1 Stryker saw with oscillating blades
2 Osteotomes, narrow
1 Bone-cutting forceps
2 Periosteal elevators, slightly curved, 1 sharp, 1 blunt
1 Dissecting scissors, long, light

**Holding instruments**

4 Adair forceps
4 Cushing forceps
4 Potts-Jahnke bulldog clamps
2 Bayonet forceps

**Clamping instruments**

56 Mosquito hemostats, 36 curved and 20 straight
24 Kelly hemostats, curved
4 Mixter duct forceps

**Exposing instruments**

Mouth gag
Tongue depressor
Cheek retractor, if desired

**Accessory items**

1 Mallet, lightweight
1 Tracheostomy set with tubes nos. 6 and 8 for adults
2 Laryngectomy tubes nos. 8, 10, or 12
2 Frazier suction tubes
1 Yankauer suction tube
1 Abdominal suction tube
1 Bovie electrosurgical unit
2 Pieces Penrose tubing and folded gauze wicks
1 Nasal feeding catheter
2 Catheters, whistle-tipped, open-ended, 12 and 14 Fr.
2 Foley catheters, desired size
2 Asepto syringes with bulbs
1 Hemovac set, if desired (Fig. 8-68)

**OPERATIVE PROCEDURE**

1. A tracheostomy may be performed to control the airway.

2. A midline incision is made from the suprasternal notch to just above the hyoid bone. Skin flaps are undermined on each side. The sternothyroid, sternohyoid, and omohyoid muscles (strap muscles) on each side are divided by means of curved hemostats and a knife.

3. The suprahyoid muscles are severed from the portion of the hyoid to be divided. The hyoid bone is divided at the junction of its middle and lateral thirds with bone-cutting forceps. Bleeding vessels are clamped and ligated.

4. The superior laryngeal nerve and vessels are exposed and ligated on each side, using long curved fine hemostats and fine chromic gut or silk ligatures.

5. The isthmus of the thyroid gland is divided between hemostats. Each portion of the thyroid gland is dissected from the trachea, using fine dissection Stevens and Metzenbaum scissors and fine tissue forceps. The superior pole of the thyroid is retracted in a Greene retractor. The superior thyroid vessels are freed from the larynx by sharp dissection.

6. The larynx is rotated. The inferior pharyngeal constrictor muscle is severed from its attachment to the thyroid cartilage on each side (Fig. 8-52).

7. The endotracheal tube is removed. The trachea is transected just below the cricoid cartilage over a Kelly or Crile

hemostat previously inserted between the trachea and esophagus. The upper resected portion of the trachea and the cricoid cartilage are held upward with Lahey forceps (Fig. 8-67). A balloon-cuffed tube (endotracheal) or a Foley catheter is inserted in the distal trachea.

8. The larynx is freed from the cervical esophagus and attachments by sharp and blunt dissection. A moist pack is placed around the endotracheal tube to help prevent leakage of blood into the trachea.

9. The pharynx is entered. In most cancers of the intrinsic larynx, the pharynx is entered above the epiglottis. The mucosal membranous incision is extended along either side of the epiglottis; the remaining portion of the pharynx and cervical esophagus is dissected well away from the tumor by means of fine-toothed tissue forceps, Metzenbaum scissors, knife, suctioning, and fine hemostats. The specimen is removed en masse.

10. A nasal feeding tube is inserted through one naris into the esophagus; closure of the hypopharyngeal and esophageal defect is begun, using continuous inverting fine sutures of chromic gut no. 3-0. The nasal tube is guided down past the pharyngeal suture line.

11. The pharyngeal suture line is reinforced with interrupted sutures; the suprahyoid muscles are approximated to the cut edges of the inferior constrictor muscles.

12. The diameter of the tracheal stoma is increased by means of a knife and heavy straight scissors. The two portions of the thyroid behind the tracheal opening are approximated with interrupted silk sutures, thereby obliterating dead space posterior to the upper portion of the trachea (Fig. 8-67).

13. A small Penrose drain or catheter is inserted through two separate stab wounds on each side of the neck just below the pharyngeal suture line (Fig. 8-67). If a closed suction system is used, catheters connected to a suction apparatus are used (Fig. 8-68).

14. The edges of the deep cervical fascia

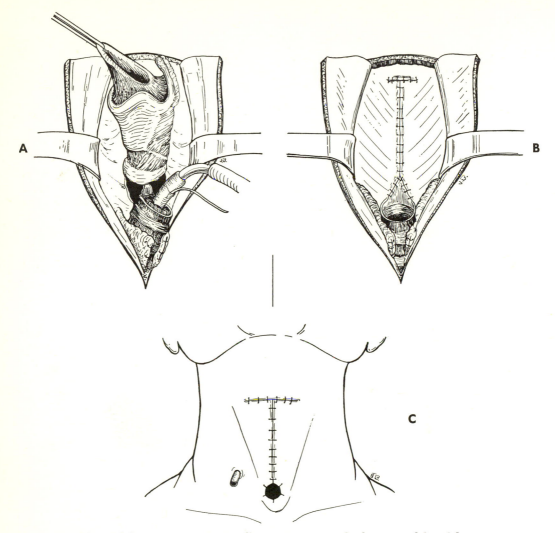

Fig. 8-67. Total laryngectomy. **A,** Usually one or two tracheal rings *and hyoid bone* are included with specimen. **B,** Mucous membrane and muscles of pharynx are closed in layers. **C,** Tracheostomy—trachea is sutured to skin. (From DeWeese, D. D., and Saunders, W. H.: Textbook of otolaryngology, ed. 3, St. Louis, 1968, The C. V. Mosby Co.)

and the platysma are closed separately with interrupted fine silk sutures. When a great amount of the fascia and platysma has been removed, the wound edges are approximated with silk sutures.

15. A laryngectomy tube, desired size, is inserted into the tracheal stoma; a pressure dressing is applied to the wound and neck.

## Radical neck dissection

**DEFINITION.** Removal of the tumor, surrounding structures, and lymph nodes en masse, through a Y-shaped or trifurcate incision in the affected side of the neck.

**CONSIDERATIONS.** Radical neck dissection is done to remove the tumor and metastatic cervical nodes present in malignant lesions and all nonvital structures of the neck. Metastasis occurs through the lymphatic channels via the bloodstream. Disease of the oral cavity, lips, and thyroid gland may spread slowly to the neck. Radical neck surgery is done in the presence of cervical node metastasis from a cancer of the head

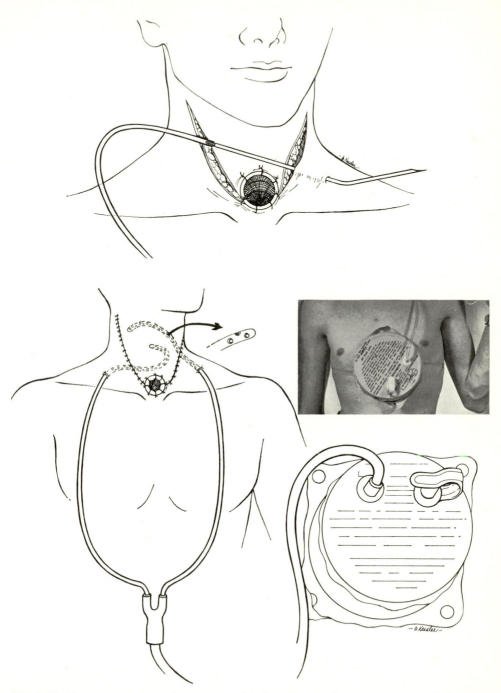

**Fig. 8-68.** Hemovac apparatus for constant closed suction. In this system of wound drainage, suction is maintained by plastic container with spring inside that tries to force apart lids and thereby produces suction, which is transmitted through plastic tubing. Neck skin is pulled down tight, and no external dressing is required. Container serves as both suction source and receptacle for blood. It is emptied as required, and drainage tubes are left in neck for 3 days. (From DeWeese, D. D., and Saunders, W. H.: Textbook of otolaryngology, ed. 3, St. Louis, 1968, The C. V. Mosby Co.)

and neck, which has a reasonable chance of being controlled.

A prophylactic neck dissection implies elective radical neck surgery when there is no clinical evidence of metastatic cervical cancer. This may be done in the presence of cancer of the tongue.

SETUP AND PREPARATION OF THE PATIENT. The patient is placed on the table in a dorsal recumbent position, with the head in moderate extension and the entire affected side of the face and neck facing uppermost. During surgery, the face of the patient is turned away from the surgeon.

The preoperative skin preparation is extensive (Chapter 4). The patient is draped with sterile towels and sheets, leaving a wide operative field (Chapter 5). Endotracheal anesthesia is used. The anesthetic is administered before the patient is positioned for surgery. During the operation, the anesthesiologist works behind the sterile barrier, away from the surgical team.

The instrument setup includes a total thyroidectomy setup and laryngectomy setup, plus the following:

**Cutting instruments**
2 Rongeurs, duckbill-type
2 Bone-cutting forceps, light
2 Gigli saws, 20 in., with handles, if desired
1 Dental elevator
1 Wire-cutting forceps
1 Metzenbaum scissors, long

**Holding instruments**
1 Dental forceps
4 Allis forceps

**Clamping instruments**
8 Rochester-Mayo hemostats, curved
Additional hemostats

**Accessory items**
Bulky neck dressings
Neck rolls
Catheters, 12 and 14 Fr.
Elastic bandage, if desired

OPERATIVE PROCEDURE

1. One of several types of incisions may be used, including the Y-shaped, H-shaped, or trifurcate incision (Fig. 8-69).

2. The upper curved incision is made through the skin and platysma, using a

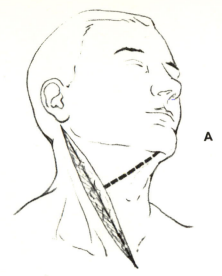

Fig. 8-69. Radical neck dissection. **A,** Incision. **B,** Developing skin flaps. **C,** Sternocleidomastoid muscle divided. (From Wilder, J. R.: Atlas of general surgery, ed. 2, St. Louis, 1964, The C. V. Mosby Co.)

knife, tissue forceps, and fine hemostats and ligatures for bleeding vessels. The upper flap is retracted; then the vertical portion of the incision is made and the skin flaps retracted anteriorly and posteriorly with retractors. The anterior margin of the trapezius muscle is exposed by means of curved scissors. The flaps are retracted to expose the entire lateral aspect of the neck (Fig. 8-70). Branches of the jugular veins are clamped, ligated, and divided.

3. The sternal and clavicular attachments of the sternocleidomastoid muscle are clamped with curved Rochester-Mayo clamps and then divided with a knife. The superficial layer of deep fascia is then incised. The omohyoid muscle is severed between clamps just above its scapular attachment (Fig. 8-69).

4. The internal jugular vein is isolated by blunt dissection and then doubly clamped, ligated with medium silk, and divided with Metzenbaum scissors (Fig. 8-70). A transfixion suture is placed on the lower end of the vein.

5. The common carotid artery and vagus nerve are identified. The fatty areolar

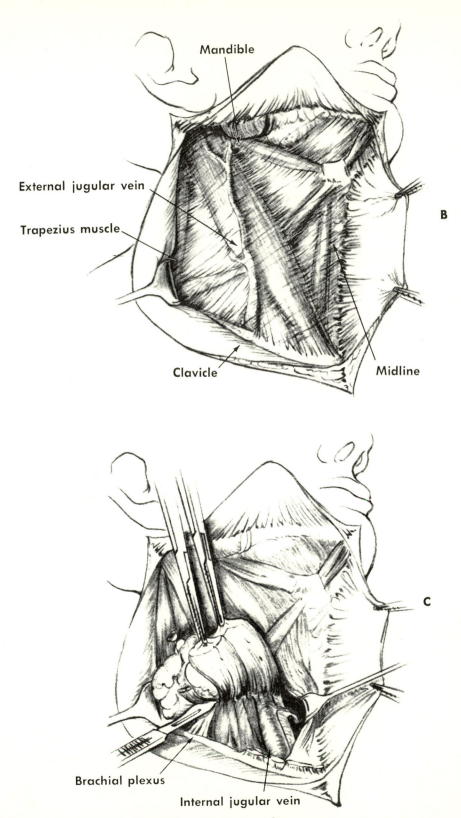

Mandible

External jugular vein

Trapezius muscle

Clavicle

Midline

B

Brachial plexus

Internal jugular vein

C

Fig. 8-69, cont'd. For legend see opposite page.

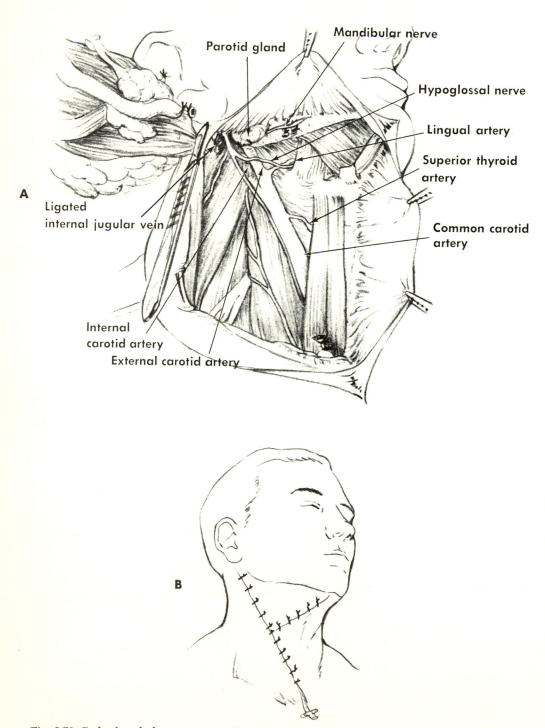

**Fig. 8-70.** Radical neck dissection—cont'd. **A,** Dissection completed. **B,** Closure. (From Wilder, J. R.: Atlas of general surgery, ed. 2, St. Louis, 1964, The C. V. Mosby Co.)

tissue and fascia are dissected away, using Metzenbaum scissors and fine tissue forceps. Branches of the thyrocervical artery are clamped, divided, and ligated.

6. The tissues and fascia of the posterior triangle are dissected, beginning at the anterior margin of the trapezius muscle, continuing near the brachial plexus and the levator scapulae and the scalene muscles. During the dissection, branches of the cervical and suprascapular arteries are clamped, ligated, and divided.

7. The anterior portion of the block dissection is completed. The omohyoid muscle is severed at its attachment to the hyoid bone. Bleeding is controlled. All hemostats are removed, and the operative site is covered with warm, moist laparotomy packs.

8. The sternocleidomastoid muscle is severed and retracted. The submental space is dissected free of fatty areolar tissue and lymph nodes from above downward.

9. The deep fascia on the lower free edge of the mandible is incised; the facial vessels are divided and ligated.

10. The submaxillary triangle is entered. The submaxillary duct is divided and ligated. The glands with surrounding fatty areolar tissue and lymph nodes is dissected toward the digastric muscle. The facial branch of the external carotid artery is divided. Portions of the digastric and stylohyoid muscles are severed from their attachments to the hyoid bone and on the mastoid. The upper end of the internal jugular vein is elevated and divided. The surgical specimen is removed (Fig. 8-70).

11. The entire field is examined for bleeding and then irrigated with warm saline solution. Penrose drains are placed in the wound and brought out through a stab wound, and no. 12 Fr. catheters may be used.

12. The flaps are then approximated with interrupted fine silk sutures (Fig. 8-70). A bulky pressure dressing is applied to the neck. Gauze dressings are applied to the wound edges and covered with sterile fluffed gauze to provide even pressure. A wide gauze roller bandage is wrapped snugly around the neck and in some cases encircles the head. The dressing may then be covered with elastic bandage that is wrapped around the neck and anchored to the chest wall.

## REFERENCES

1. Boies, L., Hilger, J. A., and Priest, R. E.: Fundamentals of otolaryngology, ed. 4, Philadelphia, 1964, W. B. Saunders Co.
2. Brantigan, O. C.: Clinical anatomy, New York, 1963, McGraw-Hill Book Co.
3. Davis, H., and Silverman, S. R., editors: Hearing and deafness, rev. ed., New York, 1960, Holt, Rinehart & Winston, Inc.
4. Davis, L.: Christopher's textbook of surgery, ed. 8, Philadelphia, 1964, W. B. Saunders Co.
5. DeWeese, D. D., and Saunders, W. H.: Textbook of otolaryngology, ed. 3, St. Louis, 1968, The C. V. Mosby Co.
6. Goodhill, V.: Stapes surgery for otosclerosis, New York, 1961, Harper & Row, Publishers.
7. Guyton, A. C.: Textbook of medical physiology, ed. 2, Philadelphia, 1961, W. B. Saunders Co.
8. Last, R. J.: Anatomy—regional and applied, ed. 4, Baltimore, 1967, The Williams & Wilkins Co.
9. Mawson, S. R.: Diseases of the ear, Baltimore, 1963, The Williams & Wilkins Co.
10. Ryan, R. E., Ogura, J. H., Biller, H. F., and Pratt, L. L.: Synopsis of ear, nose, and throat diseases, ed. 3, St. Louis, 1970, The C. V. Mosby Co.
11. Saunders, W. H., Havener, W. H., Fair, C. J., and Hickey, J. T.: Nursing care in eye, ear, nose, and throat disorders, ed. 2, St. Louis, 1968, The C. V. Mosby Co.
12. Schuknecht, H. F., editor: Otosclerosis, Henry Ford Hospital International Symposium, Boston, 1960, Little, Brown & Co.
13. Schuknecht, H. F., Chasin, W. D., and Kurkjian, J. M.: Stereoscopic atlas of mastoidotympanoplastic surgery, St. Louis, 1966, The C. V. Mosby Co.
14. Shambaugh, G. E.: Surgery of the ear, ed. 2, Philadelphia, 1967, W. B. Saunders Co.
15. Thoma, K. H.: Oral surgery, ed. 5, St. Louis, 1969, The C. V. Mosby Co.
16. Warren, R., et al.: Surgery, Philadelphia, 1963, W. B. Saunders Co.
17. Wilder, J. R.: Atlas of general surgery, ed. 2, St. Louis, 1964, The C. V. Mosby Co.
18. Wise, R. A., and Baker, H. W.: Surgery of the head and neck, ed. 2, Chicago, 1962, Year Book Medical Publishers, Inc.

# CHAPTER 9

# Ophthalmic surgery

RONALD M. BURDE and MAXINE LOUCKS

---

Sight is the most precious sensory possession of man. Aristotle said, "The eye is the chief organ through which objective reality is appreciated," and that "Sight is the most comprehensive of all the senses."

Ophthalmology is closely associated with general medicine because in the presence of many diseases the eyes are affected. Many ocular disorders are manifestations of systemic disease such as endocrine disturbances, diabetes, brain tumor, nephritis, and syphilis.

In the time of Hippocrates, surgery of the eye was confined to the eyelids. Because of the advent of asepsis and advances in ophthalmology and anesthesia, many eye disorders are now treated by surgery. The success of the surgeon's plan of treatment depends to a degree on the knowledge and skill of the members of the nursing team as they perform their functions before, during, and after surgery.

## ANATOMY AND PHYSIOLOGY OF THE EYE

General knowledge of the anatomical structures involved in an operation provides for understanding of the surgeon's plan of treatment and the need for specific instruments.

### Bony orbit

The two orbital cavities are situated on either side of the midvertical line of the skull between the cranium and the skeleton of the face. Above each orbit are found the anterior cranial fossa and the frontal sinus; medially, the nasal cavity; below, the maxillary sinus; and laterally, from behind forward, the middle cranial and temporal fossae (Figs. 9-1 and 9-2).

The seven bones that form the orbit are the maxilla, palatine, frontal, sphenoid, zygomatic, ethmoid, and lacrimal bones. The margins of the bony orbit may be subdivided into four continuous parts: supraorbital, lateral, infraorbital, and medial.

The orbit may be considered as a four-sided pyramid, its base directed forward, laterally, and slightly downward, with its apex facing posteriorly. The periosteum of the orbital walls is continuous with the dura mater.

The orbit is essentially a socket for the eyeball and the muscles, nerves, and vessels that are essential to proper functioning of the eye. The orbit also serves as a distribution center for the transmission of certain vessels and nerves that supply the areas of the face around the orbital aperture.

### The globe

The eyeball (globe) is delicately poised in the orbital cavity on a cushion of fat supported by fascia (Fig. 9-3). The eye occupies one third or less of the cavity of the orbit. The eyeball has three concentric layers: (1) the external, protective fibrous tunic, comprising the cornea and sclera; (2) the middle, vascular, pigmented tunic, comprising the iris, ciliary body, and choroid;

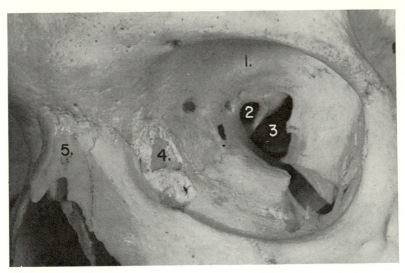

**Fig. 9-1.** Orbit. Bony orbital cavity, **1,** communicates with brain via optic foramen, **2,** which transmits optic nerve, and superior orbital fissure, **3,** which transmits most of other nerves and vessels entering orbit. Lacrimal fossa, **4,** contains lacrimal sac. **5** is nasal bone. (From Saunders, W. H., Havener, W. H., Fair, C. J., and Hickey, J. T.: Nursing care in eye, ear, nose, and throat disorders, ed. 2, St. Louis, 1968, The C. V. Mosby Co.)

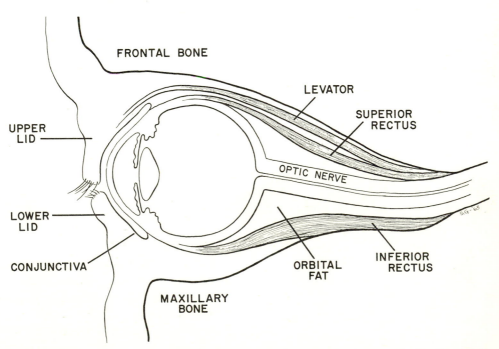

**Fig. 9-2.** Diagrammatic section of orbit. (From Saunders, W. H., Havener, W. H., Fair, C. J., and Hickey, J. T.: Nursing care in eye, ear, nose, and throat disorders, ed. 2, St. Louis, 1968, The C. V. Mosby Co.)

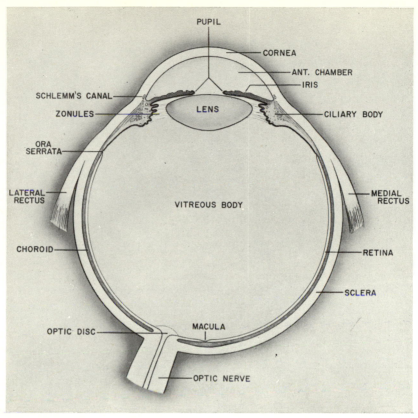

Fig. 9-3. Diagrammatic cross section of eye. (From Saunders, W. H., Havener, W. H., Fair, C. J., and Hickey, J. T.: Nursing care in eye, ear, nose, and throat disorders, ed. 2, St. Louis, 1968, The C. V. Mosby Co.)

and (3) internal tunic, called the *retina* (Fig. 9-3).

EXTERNAL TUNIC. The cornea is the anterior, transparent, avascular part of the external tunic and is, for the most part, continuous with the sclera. The cornea serves as a window through which light rays may pass to the retina. The branches of the ophthalmic division of the fifth cranial nerve supply the cornea.

The junction of the clear cornea and the opaque sclera is called the *limbus*.

The *sclera* is the posterior opaque part of the external tunic. A portion of the sclera can be seen through the conjunctiva as the white of the eye. The sclera consists of collagenous fibers loosely connected with fascia, which receives the tendons of the muscles of the globe. The sclera is

pierced by the ciliary arteries and nerves and posteriorly by the optic nerve (Fig. 9-3).

MIDDLE TUNIC. The middle covering of the eye comprises the choroid, ciliary body, and iris from behind forward. The choroid is a brownish colored coat, comprising three layers itself, which lines the greater part of the sclera. The choroid contains many blood vessels and is the main source of nourishment of the receptor cell and pigment epithelial layers of the retina.

The ciliary body consists of an extension of the choroidal blood vessels, a mass of muscle tissue, and an extension of the neuroepithelium of the retina. The ciliary muscle acts in effecting accommodation. The neuroepithelium becomes secretory in

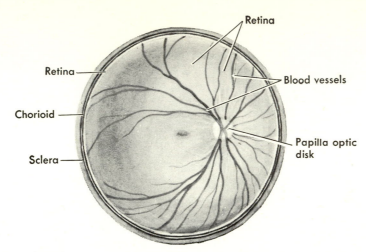

**Fig. 9-4.** Normal fundus of eye. This is view of eye seen through ophthalmoscope. (From Anthony, C. P.: Textbook of anatomy and physiology, ed. 6, St. Louis, 1963, The C. V. Mosby Co.)

nature and is responsible for the formation of the aqueous humor.

The iris, a thin membrane, is the anterior portion of the middle tunic and is situated in front of the lens. The peripheral border of the iris is attached to the ciliary body, whereas its central border is free. The iris aperture is located slightly nasal to its center, known as the *pupil* (Fig. 9-3). The iris divides the space between the cornea and the lens into an anterior and posterior chamber. Both chambers are filled with aqueous humor.

The iris with its many striations regulates the amount of light entering the eye and assists in obtaining clear images. The movement of the iris takes place by means of smooth muscle fibers situated within the connective tissue. The sphincter pupillae contract the pupil, and the dilatator pupillae dilate the pupil. As more light strikes the eye, the sphincter constricts the pupil.

INTERNAL TUNIC. The innermost tunic, sometimes called the *nervous covering*, is the retina. This thin network of nerve cells and fibers receives images of external objects and transfers the impression via the optic nerve, optic tracts, lateral geniculate body, and optic radiations to the occipital lobe of the cerebrum (Chapter 11). The retina lies at the back of the eyeball (Fig. 9-3). The nerve fibers from the retina converge to form the optic nerve, which pierces the eyeball almost at its posterior point, slightly to the inner side. This point is called the *optic disc* (Fig. 9-4). In field testing, this is the anatomical blind spot.

The retina is composed of many layers. The receptor cell layer, which consists of the rods and cones, contains the photosensitive pigments that respond to light energy and initiate the neural response, which is eventually interpreted in the occipital cortex. The point of highest resolution is the foveal pit, which exists in the center of the area that takes on a yellow hue after death (the macula lutea).

An inverted image of the object is focused on the retina. The nerve fibers leaving the retina by the way of the optic nerve travel to the lateral geniculate body of the thalamus. The fibers nasal to the foveal pit cross in the optic chiasm to go to the contralateral geniculate body. Thus all fibers composing the same half of the visual field project to the same geniculate body, from which fibers project to the ipsilateral occipital cortex for interpretation.

REFRACTIVE APPARATUS OF THE EYE. The

refractive apparatus comprises the cornea, the aqueous humor, the lens, and the vitreous body (Fig. 9-3).

The lens of the eye is biconvex and has a diameter of 1 cm. (Fig. 9-3). It is suspended behind the iris and connected to the ciliary body by means of zonular fibers. Its anterior and posterior surfaces are separated by a rounded border known as the *equator*. The lens hardens with age and therefore cannot respond to accommodative effort with an increase in power. This is why many older persons need bifocals. An opacity of the lens is termed *cataract*.

The vitreous body is a glasslike, transparent, gelatinous mass, of which 98.8% is water. It fills the posterior four fifths of the eyeball and is adherent to the margin of the retina.

The central components of a light wave enter the eyes perpendicularly and at the sides obliquely. For clear vision the oblique rays must converge and come to a focus with the central rays on the retina. Light rays from an object pass through the system of refractory devices—the cornea, aqueous humor, lens, and vitreous—and are refracted so that rays strike the macular area.

## Conjunctiva and lacrimal apparatus

The conjunctiva is a thin, transparent mucous membrane that lines the back surface of the eyelids and the front surface of the globe. The conjunctiva forms a sac (conjunctival sac) that is open in front. The opening is called the *palpebral fissure*. When the eye is closed, the fissure becomes a mere slit.

The conjunctiva is divided into a palpebral and bulbar part. The palpebral portion lines the back of the eyelids and contains the openings (puncta) of the lacrimal canaliculi, which establish a passageway between the conjunctival sac and the inferior meatus of the nose. The bulbar part of the conjunctiva is transparent, thereby allowing the sclera, termed the white of the eye, to show through. The central portion of the bulbar conjunctiva

is continuous at the limbus with the anterior epithelium of the cornea.

The lacrimal apparatus comprises the lacrimal gland and its ducts, the lacrimal passages, the lacrimal canaliculi and sac, and the nasal lacrimal duct. The lacrimal gland produces tears and secretes them through a series of ducts into the conjunctival sac. The tears then make their way inward to the puncta, from which they are conducted by the canaliculi to the lacrimal sac, to finally pass into the nasal duct. When the lacrimal glands secrete too profusely, this normal process becomes insufficient and overflow tearing results.

## Eyelids

The eyelids are two movable musculofibrous folds placed in front of each orbit to protect the globe and rest the eye from light.

The upper eyelid is more mobile and larger than the lower. The upper and lower lids meet at the medial and lateral angles (canthi) of the eye. The palpebral fissure, as previously mentioned, is located between the margins of the two eyelids. When the eye is closed, the cornea is completely covered by the upper eyelid. The eyelids are closed by the orbicular muscle of the eye, which is arranged in a circular fashion and acts as a sphincter. When the fibers contract, the eyes close. The upper lid is opened by the levator muscle, which is innervated by the third cranial nerve (also relaxation of the orbicular muscle).

The eyelid consists of several layers, moving from anterior backward. The lid consists of skin, subcutaneous tissue that contains lymphatics, and muscles. Dense fibrous tissue, called *tarsal cartilage*, forms the framework of the lids. The tarsus is anchored to the walls of the orbit by the medial and lateral palpebral ligaments.

The free margins of each eyelid possess two or three rows of hairs called *cilia*, or eyelashes. Posterior to the lashes is a row of glandular orifices of the meibomian glands. Near the medial ends, the free margin of

each eyelid presents an opening known as the *punctum lacrimale*. The eyelids serve to distribute all adnexal secretions, thereby keeping the cornea moist and washing away any dust.

## Muscles of the eye

The extrinsic ocular muscles of the eyeball are the four recti and two oblique muscles. These six striated muscles are inserted into the sclera by means of tendons. These muscles arise, except for the inferior oblique muscle, from the back of the orbit. All the muscles are supplied by cranial nerves (III oculomotor, IV trochlear, and VI abducent). All of the muscles work in pairs. Movements of the eyes are brought about by an increase in the tone of one set of muscles and a decrease in the tone of the antagonistic muscles. According to the position of the recti muscles in the eyes, they are referred to as the superior rectus, inferior rectus, medial rectus, and lateral rectus muscles. The oblique muscles insert on the back of the eye and are designated as the superior oblique and inferior oblique muscles.

## Nerves and arteries of the eye

The third cranial nerve is the chief motor nerve to all the recti muscles except for the lateral rectus, which is innervated by the sixth cranial nerve of the eye. The fourth cranial nerve innervates the superior oblique muscle, the so-called pulley muscle. The fifth cranial nerve is the sensory nerve to the orbit and globe. The optic nerve, or second cranial nerve, extends between the eyeball and the chiasma (Fig. 9-5).

The ophthalmic artery, the main arterial supply to the orbit and globe, is a branch of the internal carotid artery. It divides into branches supplying the globe, muscles, and eyelids.

## PREPARATION OF THE PATIENT FOR EYE SURGERY

For a successful operation, the physical, spiritual, and emotional needs of the person must be considered. Each member of

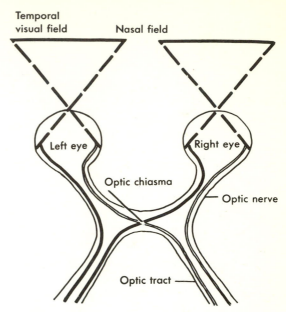

**Fig. 9-5.** Diagram to show why destruction of one optic nerve causes blindness in eye of affected side, but destruction of one optic tract causes blindness for temporal visual field on opposite side and for nasal visual field on affected side. Note that fibers from medial half of each retina cross to opposite optic tract. (From Anthony, C. P.: Textbook of anatomy and physiology, ed. 6, St. Louis, 1963, The C. V. Mosby Co.)

the staff should endeavor to meet the needs of each patient and help him to cope with his specific problems.

### Emotional factors

The loss of vision or any interference with the use of the eyes, even temporarily, has a severe emotional effect on any person. It means loss of mobility and ability to take care of or protect oneself. This tends frequently to make the patient nervous and sometimes depressed. Because the patient is often awake during the entire operation, one objective of all operating staff members should be to allay the fears of each patient. The emotional state of the patient is an important factor in a successful recovery.

A quiet environment and a calm, kindly, understanding voice creates confidence in the patient. The patient's comfort is

further enhanced by the use of an air-conditioned room, well-padded operating room table, soft lighting, proper room temperature, and freedom from noises such as telephones ringing or unnecessary talking and movements of personnel in the operating room (Chapter 5). When a patient is sedated, he is often unable to speak coherently but is usually conscious of noises, which become exaggerated in his mind.

## Preoperative sedation of the patient and dilatation of the pupil

To allay anxiety and reduce general muscle tone, the patient is usually given a barbiturate-narcotic combination on call to surgery. On arriving at the operating room suite, repeated instillation of topical anesthetic drops will produce relative anesthesia and somewhat allay the fear of a retrobulbar anesthetic.

TYPES OF DILATING DROPS USED PREOPERATIVELY. Dilating drops (mydriatics and cycloplegics) are used to dilate the pupil in order to examine the retinae objectively, refract the patient, or facilitate the removal of the lens. Mydriatic drugs dilate the pupil but permit the patient to focus his eyes. The most commonly used mydriatic is 10% phenylephrine (Neo-Synephrine).

A cycloplegic drug dilates the pupil and also prevents focusing of the eye. This type of drug is used to aid in refraction. Commonly used cycloplegics are 1% tropicamide (Mydriacyl), 1% atropine, and 1% cyclopentolate (Cyclogyl). Atropine has a long-lasting effect.

### Ophthalmic pharmacology

TYPES OF CONSTRICTING DROPS. Miotic drugs cause the pupil of the eye to contract. Commonly used miotics are 1% to 4% pilocarpine and 0.012% to 0.25% phospholine iodides. Miotics improve the ease with which the aqueous fluid escapes from the eye independent of their action on the pupil, thereby resulting in decrease of intraocular pressure. Miotics are used in the treatment of glaucoma. These drugs increase contraction of the sphincter of the iris, thus causing it to become smaller. Phospholine iodide is usually discontinued before intraocular surgery is performed.

CORTICOSTEROIDS. A great number of corticosteroid preparations exist. Corticosteroids are used to prevent the normal inflammatory response to noxious stimuli. Corticosteroids reduce the resistance of the eye to invasion by bacterial viruses and fungi. Presence of active infection is therefore an important contraindication to therapy with cortisone and its derivatives in the treatment of allergic eye conditions and chronic inflammations.

ANTIBIOTICS, ASTRINGENTS, LUBRICANTS, AND STAINS. Topical antibiotics are often used prophylactically to prevent infection. Antibiotic instillation may be given prior to intraocular surgery to help prevent wound infection.

Zinc sulfate, 0.25%, is used to reduce redness and swelling and to soothe tissue. It may be ordered in combination with a 0.125% preparation of phenylephrine. Zinc also is a necessary cofactor in wound healing.

Lubricating drops or ointments protect the cornea. Methylcellulose, 0.5%, is considered an excellent lubricant for use in dry eyes.

HYPEROSMOTIC AGENTS. This group of drugs increases the osmolarity of the serum and by the effect of the induced osmotic pressure gradient shrinks the vitreous body and reduces the intraocular pressure. These drugs are used routinely in the preoperative medication of patients about to undergo ophthalmic surgery, as well as therapeutically in cases of uncontrolled glaucoma (usually angle-closure glaucoma).

The commonly used agents may be divided into those given orally (glycerol and isosorbide) and those given parenterally (mannitol and urea). These drugs by their nature induce a diuresis; the nursing personnel must be aware of this and have

urinals available, as well as sterile urethral catheters.

IDENTIFICATION OF OPHTHALMIC DRUGS. To ensure the safety of the patient, all eye solutions should be packaged for individual use and clearly labeled. Ophthalmic solutions are usually supplied in prepackaged, disposable individual units. The more common drops are color coded, differentiating miotic agents and cycloplegic agents. The remaining medication in the bottle after the operation should be sent to the unit nurse. This system of packaging ensures freshness of solutions, prevents the possibility of cross contamination from one patient to another, and conserves cost.

## Admission, skin preparation, draping, and anesthesia

ADMISSION. Members of the nursing team have several important responsibilities in the admission of the patient and in the preparation of the room and the equipment (Chapters 2, 4, 5, and 7).

The factors relating to cross infection, safety, comfort, and the well-being of the patient before, during, and after surgery are evident in practice. The duties of the nursing team include the following:

1. Identify the patient by name if he is awake; seek to gain his cooperation and confidence by speaking softly, kindly, yet in a confident manner; and endeavor to keep the patient quiet and relaxed by staying with him, perhaps holding his hand.

2. Check the patient's name on his wristlet band with the name on the chart.

3. Review the surgeon's preoperative orders and nurses' notes to determine if the operative eye has been prepared properly and other procedures have been carried out according to hospital policies.

4. Reaffirm preoperative orders with the surgeon if necessary.

5. Prepare the operating table, making sure all the necessary attachments for the table are in proper readiness.

6. Attach a cardiac monitor.

PREPARATION OF THE PATIENT'S FACE. The preparation of the patient is done under aseptic conditions. Topical anesthetic drops are administered first if the patient is to be given a local anesthetic. A sterile preparation tray containing sterile normal saline solution, irrigation bulbs, basins, cotton, sponges, towels, and antibacterial skin disinfectant should be near the operating table (Chapter 4).

The clipping of eyelashes or shaving of eyebrows is not routinely done. When eyelashes are clipped, it is done prior to the skin preparation. A thin film of petrolatum is smoothed over the cutting surfaces of the curved eyelash scissors so that the free lashes will adhere to the blades. This prevents the free eyelashes from falling into the eyes or onto the face.

The preparation includes cleansing the eyelids of both eyes, lid margins, lashes, eyebrows, and surrounding skin with an antibacterial soap or disinfectant. To prevent the agent from entering the patient's ears, they may be temporarily plugged, using cotton pledgets. Care is taken to keep the agent out of the eyes. The preparation area is washed with warm sterile water, using soft-textured gauze or cotton sponges. The operative area is painted with an aqueous nonirritating skin antiseptic (Fig. 9-6).

When toxic chemicals or small particles of foreign matter must be removed, the eyes may be irrigated with tepid sterile normal saline solution. The conjunctival sac is thoroughly flushed, using an irrigating bulb or an Asepto syringe.

DRAPING THE PATIENT. In some cases the local anesthetic may be injected before completion of the draping procedure. The aseptic principles in draping a patient for surgery are discussed in Chapter 5.

For general eye surgery the basic draping procedure is shown in Fig. 9-7.

1. A large folded sheet is needed to cover the patient and operating table.

2. The head is draped with a double-thickness half sheet and two towels or appropriate disposable drapes.

3. A fenestrated eye sheet, 14 inches

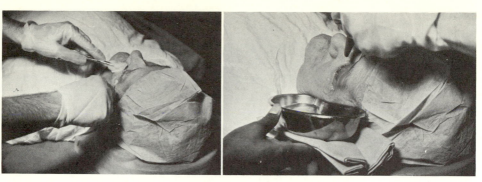

Fig. 9-6. Preparation of the operative site.

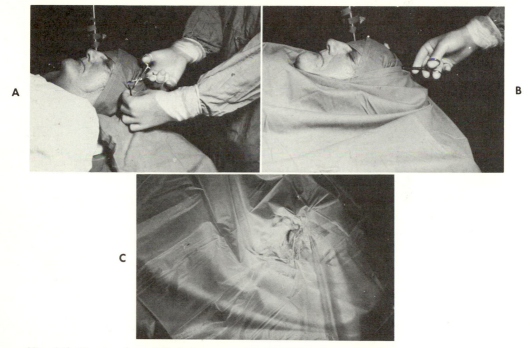

Fig. 9-7. Draping for ophthalmic surgery. A, Two sheets are placed under head; uppermost sheet is brought around head to cover eyebrows and nonoperative eye. B, Large body sheet is placed and secured over head drape. C, Disposable plastic drape sheet is placed over head and operative eye. Completely draped patient.

square, with a center opening of 2½ × 3 inches, is placed over the operative site. More recently, disposable plastic drapes have been used.

ANESTHESIA. Local anesthesia is frequently preferred and indicated for eye surgery in elderly individuals and in those with circulatory and other systemic diseases. A sedative is given the night before surgery and again 2 hours prior to surgery. An analgesic is administered 1 to 1½ hours before surgery, followed by topical tetracaine immediately prior to surgery.

The operating room staff assembles the sterile local anesthesia setup as ordered by the surgeon before the patient enters

the operating room and checks the bottles of drugs to make sure they are the correct medications and of the proper strength.

Suitable needles and syringes of proper size and gauge are necessary. For example, the following may be used:

Subcutaneous injection and infiltration—two Luer-Lok 2 ml. syringes and two 25-gauge needles, ½-inch length

Subconjunctival injection—two Luer-Lok 2 ml. syringes and two 26- or 27-gauge needles, 1- or 1½-inch length

Retrobulbar injection—two Luer-Lok 2 or 5 ml. syringes or one 10 ml. syringe and two 24-gauge needles, 1- or 1½-inch length

DRUGS FREQUENTLY USED. Tetracaine hydrochloride (Pontocaine hydrochloride) in a 2% solution may be instilled into the eye before operation. For local anesthesia in adults, 2% lidocaine (Xylocaine) with epinephrine hydrochloride in a 1:150,000 or 1:200,000 dilution is frequently used.

Hyaluronidase (Wydase, Alidase) is commonly mixed with the anesthetic solution (75 u./10 ml.). The enzyme increases the diffusion of the anesthetic through the tissue, thereby improving the effectiveness of the anesthetic nerve block. For cataract surgery, an effective retrobulbar injection reduces intraocular pressure by preventing positive muscle contraction, thus becoming a surgical safeguard against vitreous loss. Hyaluronidase is nontoxic and effective over a wide range of concentrations.

In cataract surgery, alpha chymotrypsin in a 1:5000 or 1:10,000 solution may be used to dissolve the zonular fibers that suspend the cataract within the eye. To produce eye muscle paralysis in intraocular surgery, tubocurarine chloride or succinylcholine chloride may be administered intravenously by the anesthesiologist.

Epinephrine in a 1:1000 solution may be applied topically to mucous membranes to decrease bleeding. Epinephrine in a 1:50,000 to 1:200,000 solution may be combined with injectable anesthetics to prolong the duration of anesthesia. Epinephrine in a 1:1000 solution is not used in local anesthetics because if it were used in such concentrations, the patient could succumb to cardiac arrhythmia.

METHODS USED FOR ADMINISTRATION OF LOCAL ANESTHETICS. The three methods of administration are instillation of eyedrops, infiltration, and block or regional anesthesia.

*Instillation of eyedrops* (Fig. 9-8). With the patient's face tilted upward, the first drop is placed in the lower cul-de-sac, and the following drops (number depends on the type of operation to be performed) may be placed from above, with the patient looking downward and the upper lid raised. However, the natural blinking of the lids distributes the drug evenly on the eye surface, regardless of where the drop is placed. When a toxic drug is instilled, the inner corner of the eyelids should be dried of excessive fluid with a tissue or clean cotton ball after each instillation drop, thereby minimizing systemic absorption of the drug. The tip of the applicator must not touch the patient's skin or any part of the eye.

*Infiltration method.* The surgeon injects the anesthetic solution beneath the skin, beneath the conjunctiva, or into Tenon's capsule, depending on the type of surgery.

Retrobulbar injection is usually performed 10 to 15 minutes before surgery to produce a temporary paralysis of the extraocular muscles.

*Block or regional anesthesia.* The solution is injected into the base of the eyelids at the level of the orbital margins or behind the eyeball to block the ciliary ganglion and nerves. For eyelid repairs, the solution is introduced through the lower lid. For operations on the lacrimal apparatus, the anesthetic is injected at the level of the anterior ethmoidal foramen in order to anesthetize the internal and external nasal nerves. In the Van Lint block method, procaine solution is injected into the orbicular muscle and reaches the ends of the facial nerve.

GENERAL ANESTHESIA. A general anesthetic, with or without intravenous injec-

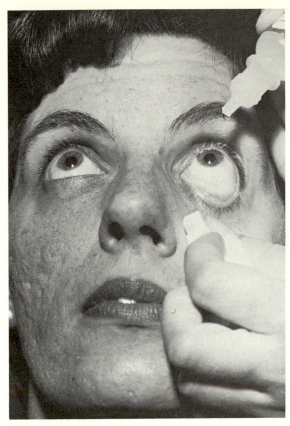

**Fig. 9-8.** Face of patient should be tilted upward to receive eyedrop. Note use of absorbent tissue to prevent excess drops and tears from flowing down patient's face. (From Saunders, W. H., Havener, W. H., Fair, C. J., and Hickey, J. T.: Nursing care in eye, ear, nose, and throat disorders, ed. 2, St. Louis, 1968, The C. V. Mosby Co.)

tion of thiopental sodium (Pentothal Sodium), is used when a patient is unable to cooperate because of youth, dementia, nervousness, or extensive operations of the orbit. Solutions of 20% mannitol (Osmitrol) or 5% glucose in water are given intravenously during surgery. A sedative is given the night before surgery, and a drying agent (atropine or scopolamine) and an analgesic are given 1 to 1½ hours prior to surgery. The patient must not eat or drink anything for 6 hours prior to induction.

**DURING THE OPERATION**

The duties of the nursing team are discussed in Chapters 2 and 5. The circulating and scrubbed team members assist the surgeons in accordance with delegated responsibilities.

This includes having necessary equipment ready, such as microscopes and indirect ophthalmoscopes, and maintaining decorum and quietness in the operating room at all times.

**AT COMPLETION OF THE OPERATION**

At completion of the operation the operative area is cleansed, using saline sponges.

Antibiotic ointment may be thinly spread over the skin and eyelashes to prevent adhesion of the bandage. This is frequently done after plastic procedures on the lids or lacrimal duct.

Dressings are applied to prevent palpebral movements, protect the operative wound from dust and external contami-

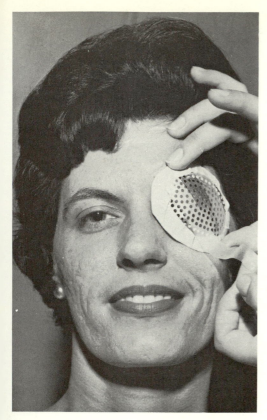

**Fig. 9-9.** Metal shield should protect eye with recent penetrating wound whether from surgery or injury. (From Saunders, W. H., Havener, W. H., Fair, C. J., and Hickey, J. T.: Nursing care in eye, ear, nose, and throat disorders, ed. 2, St. Louis, 1968, The C. V. Mosby Co.)

nants, and absorb any blood and tears that are produced.

The initial dressing usually consists of a piece of fine cotton. It is generally moistened in saline solution before it is applied to the operative site. An eye pad that is commercially prepared and sterilized is applied over the cotton splint.

The eye dressing may be held in place by means of adhesive or cellophane strips.

After intraocular operations, when external pressure on the eyes might be very harmful, the initial dressing is covered with a protector such as a wire gauze cap, perforated aluminum plate, convex perforated metal cup, convex flexible celluloid

plate, or another variety of shield (Fig. 9-9).

A pressure bandage may be used in some cases when a compression effect is desired. The gauze roller bandage is applied over the initial dressing, encircling the head.

Sterilization of instruments and disinfection methods have been discussed in Chapters 3 and 5. Clean, basic keratomes and knives can be kept submerged in an antibacterial disinfectant, but gas sterilization or dry heat sterilization is preferred.

*Testing all eye instruments to be sure they are in perfect condition is an important function of the nursing personnel.*

## BASIC INSTRUMENTS USED IN OPHTHALMIC SURGERY

The delicate, finely constructed eye instruments and supporting complex pieces of equipment must be handled with extreme care.

Forceps of recent design must be handled as sharp instruments. The precision grinding necessary to produce these instruments precludes the possibility of repair. Each instrument is designed to serve a particular purpose and to be used on specific tissues.

SUTURES. Sutures used in eye surgery are very fine, ranging in size from nos. 4-0 to 10-0. It is necessary, for increased visibility, to use a methylene blue dye on the fine white sutures. The needles used are very small and very sharp and are made especially for ophthalmic surgery. It is important that the scrubbed nursing team member handle ophthalmic needles in the same careful manner as he does the delicate knives.

BASIC EYE INSTRUMENT SETUP. Each ophthalmic operating room should have a sufficient number of basic standard eye surgery setups that can be supplemented to meet specific needs. Instruments routinely needed for a particular type of operation and each surgeon's personal preferences should be listed on cards and kept on file. (See Chapter 2.)

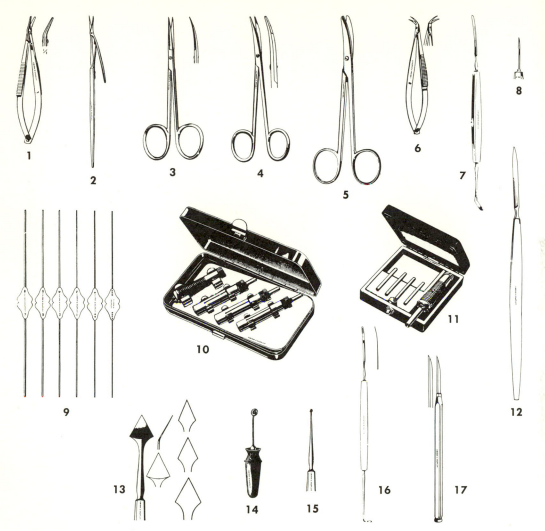

Fig. 9-10. Scissors, knives, and sharp dissectors (cutting instruments) for eye surgery. **1,** Aebli corneal scissors; **2,** Berens iridocapsulotomy scissors; **3,** iris scissors; **4,** Stevens tenotomy scissors; **5,** enucleation scissors; **6,** Castroviejo corneal section scissors, right and left; **7,** Castroviejo spatula; **8,** Ziegler knife needle; **9,** Williams lacrimal probes; **10,** corneal transplant trephines; **11,** Elliot corneal trephines; **12,** Von Graefe cataract knife; **13,** Jaeger keratomes; **14,** Bell erisiphake; **15,** curette; **16,** Knapp iris spatula and hooks; **17,** cataract knife. (Courtesy Codman & Shurtleff, Inc., Randolph, Mass.)

## SURGICAL PROCEDURES ON THE EYELIDS

The most common procedures performed on the eyelids are for treatment of chalazion, entropion, and ectropion and excisional biopsy and repair of traumatic injuries.

### Removal of chalazion

DEFINITION. A chalazion is a chronic granulomatous inflammation of one or more of the meibomian glands in the tarsal plate of the eyelid. Surgical treatment is by incision and curettage.

SETUP, PREPARATION OF THE PATIENT, AND ANESTHESIA. The following instruments should be available:

2 Chalazion clamps (large and small)
1 Lester fixation forceps
2 Chalazion curettes (medium and large)
1 Iris scissors
1 Bard-Parker knife with no. 15 blade

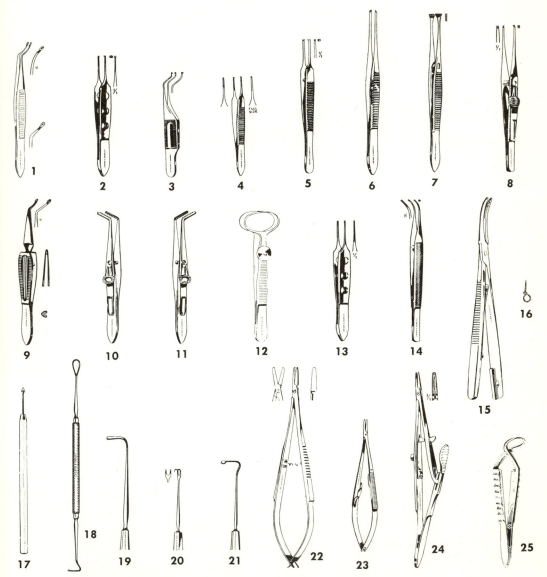

**Fig. 9-11.** Forceps and hooks (holding instruments) for eye surgery. **1,** Arruga capsule forceps; **2,** Bishop-Harmon iris forceps; **3,** Gill-Hess iris forceps; **4,** Von Graefe iris forceps; **5,** Lester fixation forceps; **6,** eye dressing forceps; **7,** Von Graefe fixation forceps; **8,** Kirby fixation forceps; **9,** Castroviejo capsule forceps; **10** and **11,** Jameson muscle recession forceps, left and right; **12,** Desmarres chalazion forceps; **13,** Bishop-Harmon eye dressing forceps; **14,** Kirby iris forceps; **15** and **16,** Pischel micropin introducing forceps and Pischel micropin; **17,** Kirby fixation hook; **18,** Kirby expressor hook and loop; **19,** Von Graefe strabismus hook; **20,** Guthrie fixation hook; **21,** Jameson strabismus hook; **22,** Castroviejo needle holder; **23,** Castroviejo needle holder, delicate; **24,** Castroviejo-Kalt needle holder; **25,** towel forceps. (Courtesy Codman & Shurtleff, Inc., Randolph, Mass.)

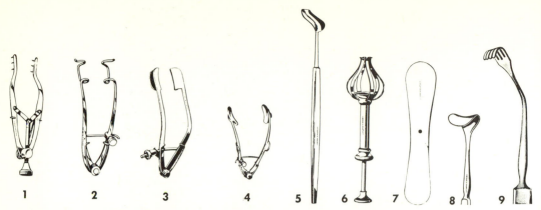

**Fig. 9-12.** Retractors (exposing instruments) for eye surgery. **1,** Stevenson lacrimal sac retractor; **2,** Knapp eye speculum; **3,** Lancaster eye speculum; **4,** Lester-Burch eye speculum; **5,** Arruga retractor; **6,** introducer and Carter holder for mule spheres in enucleation; **7,** Jaeger lid plate; **8,** Desmarres lid retractor; **9,** Fink retractor. (Courtesy Codman & Shurtleff, Inc., Randolph, Mass.)

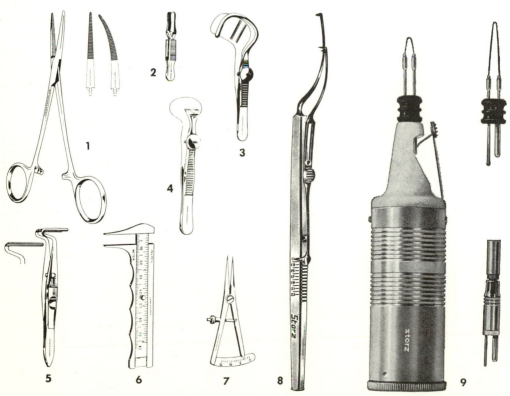

**Fig. 9-13.** Clamps and miscellaneous instruments for eye surgery. **1,** Mosquito hemostatic forceps, straight and curved; **2,** serrefine; **3,** Snellen entropion forceps; **4,** Erhardt lid clamp; **5,** Berke ptosis clamps; **6,** Jameson caliper; **7,** Castroviejo caliper; **8,** Gonnin-Amsler marker used in detached retinal procedure; **9,** Hildreth cautery with assorted electrodes and transilluminator used with Hildreth cautery handle. (Courtesy Codman & Shurtleff, Randolph, Mass., and Storz Instrument Co., New York, N. Y.)

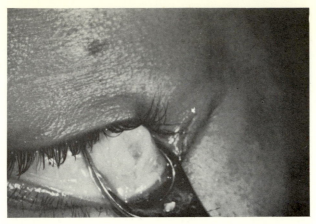

Fig. 9-14. Clamp everts eyelid during surgery for chalazion. Incision has been made on inner lid surface to avoid scarring. Viscous contents of chalazion will be removed with curette. (From Saunders, W. H., Havener, W. H., Fair, C. J., and Hickey, J. T.: Nursing care in eye, ear, nose, and throat disorders, ed. 2, St. Louis, 1968, The C. V. Mosby Co.)

The patient is prepared for surgery as described on p. 239. A local anesthesia setup is also needed.

**OPERATIVE PROCEDURE**

1. The affected lid is everted with a lid retractor to expose the chalazion.

2. A cruciate incision is made on the inner lid surface, using a sharp knife; corners of the tarsal plate are resected (Fig. 9-14).

The contents of the chalazion are removed with a curette. The affected eye is dressed and patched.

## Canthotomy

**DEFINITION.** A lengthening of the opening (slit) between the eyelids may be done prior to cataract surgery when exposure of the globe is inadequate or when necessary to correct ankyloblepharon or blepharochalasis.

**SETUP, PREPARATION OF THE PATIENT, AND ANESTHESIA** (pp. 241-244)

1 Straight hemostat
1 Small blunt scissors

**OPERATIVE PROCEDURE**

1. The hemostat is clamped over the full thickness of the outer canthus and left in place for 60 seconds.

2. The skin and conjunctiva are incised. For canthoplasty the adjacent bulbar conjunctiva is dissected, and its borders and those of the skin are sutured together with fine silk sutures.

3. The affected eye is dressed and patched.

## Surgery for positional defects of the eyelids

Several techniques are followed to treat faulty position of the eyelids. Plastic surgery is effective in the treatment of entropion, ectropion (Fig. 9-15), and blepharochalasis of the eyelids.

### Plastic repair of entropion

**DEFINITION.** Surgical correction of muscular fibers of the lid to evert the lid margins and eyelashes.

**CONSIDERATIONS.** Entropion (turning inward of the lid) usually affects the lower lid but may affect the upper lid. It seldom occurs in persons under 40 years of age. There are two types: the spastic and cicatricial. Spastic entropion results from degeneration of fascial attachments between the pretarsal muscle and the tarsus, which permits the former to override the lid margin on contraction. Cicatricial en-

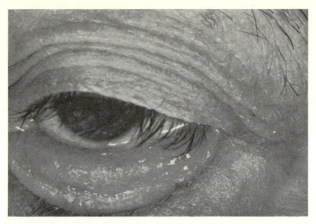

Fig. 9-15. Ectropion, or turning out of lid, is most commonly caused by senile relaxation of eyelid framework. (From Saunders, W. H., Havener, W. H., Fair, C. J., and Hickey, J. T.: Nursing care in eye, ear, nose, and throat disorders, ed. 2, St. Louis, 1968, The C. V. Mosby Co.)

tropion is a complication of spastic entropion resulting from scarring of either the upper or lower tarsus and its conjunctiva, turning in the lashes (trichiasis) so that they rub on the cornea.

**SETUP, PREPARATION OF THE PATIENT, AND ANESTHESIA.** The following plastic tray and local infiltration set are needed:

6 Hemostats
1 Large Kelly forceps
1 Razor blade breaker
2 Desmarres lid retractors
1 Von Graefe muscle hook
1 Double-pronged skin hook
2 Single-pronged skin hooks
1 Ruler
1 Conjunctival forceps with teeth
1 Serrated conjunctival forceps
1 Quevedo utility forceps
1 Lester fixation forceps
2 McCullough suture forceps
1 Adson forceps with teeth
1 Jeweler's forceps
1 Storz suturing forceps
1 Straight iris forceps
2 Bishop-Harmon iris forceps
2 Bard-Parker knives
1 Stevens scissors
1 Small iris scissors
1 Large iris scissors
1 Metzenbaum scissors
1 Kalt needle holder
1 "Plastic type" needle holder
2 Castroviejo needle holders
1 Nasal suction tube

1 Hildreth cautery with white tip
2 Senn retractors
1 Beaver knife handle
1 Rubber band
2 Richardson retractors
1 Rake retractor
1 Sharp Freer elevator
1 Metal bone plate
2 Sempken tissue forceps
1 Small double fixation hook
1 Ribbon retractor
1 Special bone plate with suture holder
1 Small rake retractor

**OPERATIVE PROCEDURE.** The treatment of these processes basically involves either removing a base down triangle of skin, muscle, and tarsus and suturing the edges together to evert the lid margin or exposing the orbicular muscle, dividing it, and suturing it to the lower border of the tarsus.

### Plastic repair of ectropion

**DEFINITION.** A plastic operation to shorten the lower lid in a horizontal direction (Figs. 9-15 and 9-16).

**CONSIDERATIONS.** Ectropion (sagging and eversion of the lower lid), which is usually bilateral, is common in older persons. Ectropion may be caused by the relaxation of the orbicular muscle. Symptoms are tearing, conjunctival infection, and irritation. Minor ectropion may be treated by elec-

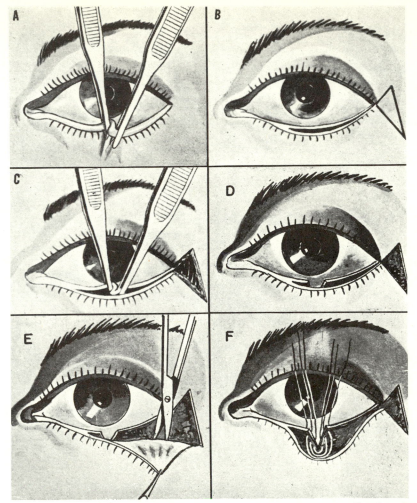

*Continued.*

Fig. 9-16. Kuhnt-Szymanowski operation for atonic ectropion. **A,** Lower lid is picked up with two smooth forceps and amount of lengthening gauged. **B,** Lateral skin triangle is marked out, and lid is split. **C,** Lateral triangle is resected, and amount of tarsoconjunctiva to be excised is gauged. **D,** Tarsoconjunctival triangle is receded. **E,** Skin-muscle lamina is dissected free. **F,** Tarsal wound is closed. **G,** Excess cilia are resected. **H,** Sutures are placed to form new canthus. **I,** Sutures are tied. **J,** Final closure is done. **K** and **L,** Senile ectropion of right lower lid and result of repair. (From Fox, S. A.: Ophthalmic plastic surgery, ed. 3, New York, 1963, Grune & Stratton, Inc.)

trocautery penetrations through the conjunctiva. Surgery is indicated when facial paralysis is permanent or when there is scarring following lacerations, lesions, or penetrating injuries and the cornea becomes exposed, resulting in ulceration and photophobia.

**SETUP, PREPARATION OF THE PATIENT, AND ANESTHESIA.** As described for entropion.

A pressure dressing and a local or general anesthesia setup should be prepared.

**OPERATIVE PROCEDURE.** Correction of cicatricial ectropion. Replacement after scarring and loss of tissue is done either by mobilization from the surrounding skin or by free grafting. Many procedures have been devised, such as the *Wharton Jones* V-Y *procedure,* free whole skin graft, or epi-

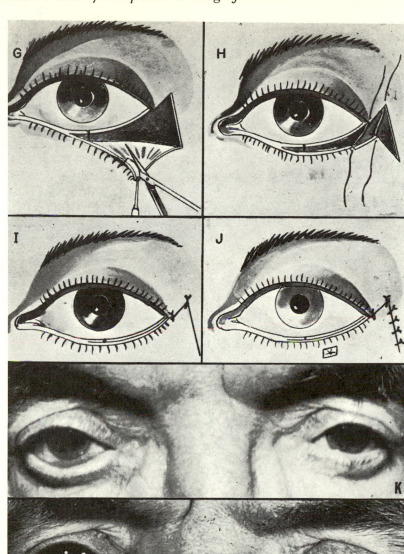

**Fig. 9-16, cont'd.** For legend see p. 251.

dermis graft. The operation includes removal of scar tissue and approximation of layers, small sliding grafts from the immediate area by means of Z-plasty or V-Y incision if loss is minimal, and free graft from upper lid for the lower lid by means of tarsorrhaphy.

The *Kuhnt-Szymanowski operation* is performed to treat senile or full-blown atonic ectropion. The external two thirds or the entire lid is split, the tarsoconjunctival triangle is resected, and the wound is closed by means of sutures in such a manner that a new canthus is formed (Fig. 9-16).

### Plastic repair for blepharochalasis

**DEFINITION.** Removal of redundancy of skin of the upper eyelids.

**CONSIDERATIONS.** Blepharochalasis causes the upper lids to hang down over the eyes,

sometimes obscuring vision. It may occur in older persons who have lost normal elasticity of the skin of the upper lids or in persons who have suffered from persistent angioneurotic edema with stretching of the skin of the eyelids.

SETUP, PREPARATION OF THE PATIENT, AND ANESTHESIA. As described for entropion.

OPERATIVE PROCEDURE. An elliptical segment of skin of the upper lid is removed by plastic surgical technique.

## Unilateral or bilateral ptosis

CONSIDERATIONS. Drooping of the upper lid is considered to be congenital, acquired, or senile. In congenital ptosis, there is frequently weakness of the superior rectus muscle. Acquired ptosis is generally caused by laceration of the third cranial nerve or the levator muscle, or both. Tumors may cause ptosis. Senile ptosis is the result of poor muscle tone of the levator.

The objective of ptosis surgery is to achieve a perfect cosmetic result by creating a good upper lid fold with elevation of the lid. The many surgical procedures that have been devised are based on the advancement of the levator muscle, the frontalis muscles, or the superior rectus muscle. These muscles are the elevating forces of the upper lids. Some of the techniques involve resection of the levator (Iliff method), utilization of the superior rectus muscle (Berke method), or modification of other methods such as the Motais or the Crawford frontalis collagen sling procedure.

### *Iliff method for ptosis (resection of the levator)*

DEFINITION. Creation of an effective upper lid by reapproximation of the conjunctiva and muscles in order to reestablish the correct relationship of the involved structures.

SETUP, PREPARATION OF THE PATIENT, AND ANESTHESIA. The plastic tray setup previously described is used. The patient is prepared as described previously for eye surgery. General anesthesia is preferred.

OPERATIVE PROCEDURE

1. The upper lid is everted over the lid clamp. With a sharp-pointed scissors, two buttonhole incisions are made through the conjunctiva medial and lateral to the superior edge of the tarsus.

2. Blunt scissors are directed through the buttonhole incisions and spread open to enlarge the incisional opening. As scissors are withdrawn, the angular, rubber-shod, jawed ptosis clamps are positioned to contain the conjunctiva, superior edge of tarsus, superior arcuate artery, aponeurosis of the levator, and orbital septum.

3. Another incision is made with scissors distal to the clamp and through all structures held by the clamp.

4. The orbital septum is freed from the clamp. Structures between the orbital septum and levator are dissected by means of blunt instruments.

5. Traction is applied to the clamp. Fine double-armed silk sutures no. 4-0 are inserted from the cut tarsal edge through all structures held within the clamp. The tissues distal to the suture line are excised.

6. The free end of each of the double-armed sutures is passed through the orbital septum, between the skin and tarsus, and brought out through the skin at the cilia margin.

7. Sutures are tied over a silicone strip or small beads. Redundant skin is invaginated with a peg to form a good lid fold.

8. The eye is closed by fastening a single suture that is passed through the skin of the lower lid to the forehead by means of an adhesive strip. Bland eye ointment is applied, and then eye pads are secured to the eyes by means of nonallergenic adhesive tape.

### *Silver-Hildreth Supramid suspension*

DEFINITION. Attachment of the lid by Supramid sutures anchored in periosteum to the frontalis muscle.

CONSIDERATIONS. This procedure may be done in the total absence of levator and superior rectus action.

SETUP, PREPARATION OF THE PATIENT, AND ANESTHESIA. Plastic tray, Wright fascia needle, and no. 4-0 Supramid suture.

**OPERATIVE PROCEDURE**

1. An incision is made in the lid fold exposing the tarsus. An incision is made over the eyebrow centrally to the frontalis muscle.

2. A double-armed Supramid suture is woven through the tarsus.

3. The needles are removed from the suture, and the suture is threaded on the fascia needle.

4. The fascia needle is passed under the skin of the lid through the periosteum of the orbital rim and out through the brow incision. This is repeated so that both ends of the suture are now in the brow incision.

5. The suture is tied as it lies on the frontalis muscle.

6. The skin is closed with a nylon subcuticular running suture no. 6-0.

7. The conjunctival sac is filled with antibiotic ointment. A double-armed silk suture no. 4-0 is passed through the center of the lower lid margin and fastened to the brow with adhesive tape, thus covering the exposed cornea. A pressure dressing is applied.

## Excisional biopsy

**DEFINITION.** Removal of lesions either neoplastic (benign or malignant) or viral in nature.

**CONSIDERATIONS.** Basal cell carcinomas account for 95% of neoplastic lesions of the lid; the treatment of choice is excisional biopsy. Viral lesions such as papilloma and molluscum contagiosum are also treated by excisional biopsy.

**SETUP, PREPARATION OF THE PATIENT, AND ANESTHESIA.** Plastic tray.

**OPERATIVE PROCEDURE.** Through-and-through excision of skin, muscle, tarsus, and conjunctiva, followed by careful structural closure of anatomical spaces.

## Surgery for traumatic injuries

**DEFINITION.** Repair of lacerations of the lids, including damage to the inferior canaliculus.

**CONSIDERATIONS.** Tantamount to success is the careful approximation of the borders of the lid margin and the ends of a torn canaliculus.

**SETUP, PREPARATION OF THE PATIENT, AND ANESTHESIA.** Plastic tray plus pigtail probe and Supramid suture.

**OPERATIVE PROCEDURE**

1. Lacerations of the lid margin are closed using a silk suture no. 5-0 to align the gray line of the lid that lies between the lash follicles and the orifices of the meibomian glands. Once this anatomical line has been approximated, all other sutures are placed, maintaining this relationship.

2. If the canaliculus has been lacerated, a pigtail probe is passed through the uninvolved punctum, through the sac, and carefully through the proximal and distal ends of the lacerated structure to emerge from the involved punctum. A Supramid suture no. 4-0 is hooked onto the probe and, by reversing the previous procedure, pulled out of the uninvolved punctum, thus establishing continuity of the system. Careful plastic closure of the lid defect is then carried out.

# SURGERY OF THE LACRIMAL GLAND AND APPARATUS

**CONSIDERATIONS.** Surgery of the lacrimal gland and apparatus is concerned generally with cure or diagnosis of tumors of the lacrimal fossa or with deficient drainage with overflow of tears. Chronic dacryocystitis in adults (Fig. 9-17) requires dacryocystorhinostomy because of resistant obstruction of the nasolacrimal duct. The dacryocystorhinostomy operation is done when the lower canaliculus is patent but the tear duct is blocked, thus causing epiphora, which cannot be tolerated. This deformity frequently follows malunited fracture of the medial wall of the orbit. Dacryocystorhinostomy creates a new large opening between the lacrimal sac and the nose.

## Surgery of the lacrimal fossa

**DEFINITION.** Involves biopsy of any structure in the lacrimal fossa and may involve

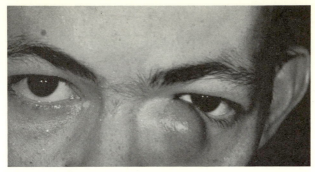

**Fig. 9-17.** Chronic infection of lacrimal sac (dacryocystitis) causes swelling of inner lower corner of eye socket. (From Saunders, W. H., Havener, W. H., Fair, C. J., and Hickey, J. T.: Nursing care in eye, ear, nose, and throat disorders, ed. 2, St. Louis, 1968, The C. V. Mosby Co.)

removal of the lacrimal gland (extirpation) for excess tearing.

**SETUP, PREPARATION OF THE PATIENT, AND ANESTHESIA.** Plastic tray.

**OPERATIVE PROCEDURE**

1. The lacrimal fossa, which is in the upper temporal quadrant of the orbit, may be approached directly through the lid or through the conjunctiva by everting the upper lid. The lacrimal gland is divided into a palpebral and orbital part by the orbital septum. All drainage ducts go through the palpebral portion; therefore surgery performed on this part alone will affect tearing, for although the orbital part will be intact, no access to the eye is available.

2. Routine surgical closure procedures are followed.

## Probing

**DEFINITION.** The opening of the lacrimal drainage system posterior and below the inferior nasal conchae is closed in approximately 35% of newborns. In most cases this closure opens spontaneously within the first 2 or 3 months of life. In those cases in which the lacrimal drainage system does not open spontaneously, an acute infectious process involving the lacrimal drainage system becomes obvious. The infectious process is treated with antibiotics, and then probing is carried out.

**SETUP, PREPARATION OF THE PATIENT, AND ANESTHESIA**

Plastic tray
Punctum dilators
Safety pins
Probe set
Lacrimal needles
Syringe

In a child under 6 months of age this procedure may be done with the infant under topical anesthesia with mummying. After this age the procedure is done with the patient under general anesthesia.

**OPERATIVE PROCEDURE**

1. Manipulation is done through the upper punctum and canaliculus in order to avoid trauma to the inferior part of the system, which carries 90% to 95% of the total amount of secretions.

2. The upper punctum is dilated first with a safety pin and then with a punctum dilator. A lacrimal probe is now passed through the upper punctum and canaliculus into the sac, at which time the resistance is met from the lacrimal bone. The probe is rotated 90 degrees, passed through the bony canal, and forced through the imperforate opening into the nose. A small amount of blood may regurgitate at this time. This may be repeated with a larger probe.

3. Using the blunt lacrimal needle, a

fluorescein solution is now irrigated to assure the patency of the system.

## Dacryocystorhinostomy

**DEFINITION.** The establishment of a new tear duct for drainage directly into the nasal cavity.

**SETUP, PREPARATION OF THE PATIENT, AND ANESTHESIA.** A basic eye surgery setup is needed, including the following:

Towel clamps
Mosquito hemostats
1 Kelly forceps
1 Allis forceps
1 Stevens scissors
1 Straight iris scissors
1 Von Graefe fixation forceps
2 McCullough suture forceps
2 Lester fixation forceps
2 Bayonet forceps
1 Adson forceps with teeth
1 Adson forceps without teeth

1 Quevedo utility forceps
2 Skin hooks—fine double-pronged
2 Skin hooks—fine single-pronged
1 Skin hook—medium double-pronged
2 Senn retractors
2 Desmarres lid retractors
1 Paul lacrimal retractor
1 Ballen-Alexander orbital retractor
3 Freer elevators (2 sharp, 1 blunt)
1 Jameson muscle hook
1 Small chisel
1 Periosteal elevator
2 Narrow malleable retractors
2 Small curettes
2 Gauges
1 Mallet
2 Angled suction tubes
1 Goldstein lacrimal retractor
2 Nasal speculums
  Assorted rongeurs
2 Sizes Kerrison punches
1 Cittelli punch, small
1 Alligator forceps
1 Kalt needle holder

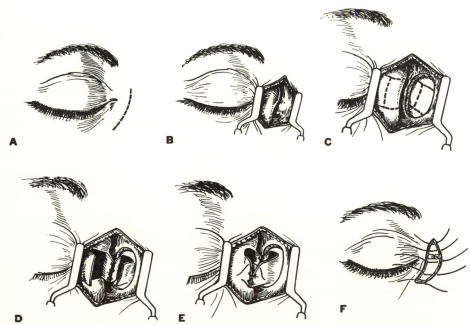

**Fig. 9-18.** Dacryocystorhinostomy. **A,** Skin incision for dacryocystorhinostomy or dacryocystectomy. **B,** Lacrimal sac and lacrimal bone exposed. **C,** Opening made in lacrimal bone and lacrimal crest, with dotted lines indicating incision to be made in wall of sac and in nasal periosteum and mucosa. **D,** Posterior flap of wall of sac sutured to posterior flap of nasal mucosa. **E,** Anterior flap of wall of sac sutured to anterior flap of nasal mucosa (drawing somewhat distorted for visualization of relative positions). **F,** Reattachment of medial canthal ligament and wire sutures in position for closure of skin incision. (From Allen, J. H., editor: May's manual of the diseases of the eye, ed. 23, Baltimore, 1963, The Williams & Wilkins Co.)

1 Castroviejo needle holder
2 Bard-Parker knife handles no. 9 with blade
   no. 15
1 Gold lacrimal needle
1 Silver lacrimal needle
   Set of assorted Bowman lacrimal probes
   Assorted Wilder dilators
   Stryker saw trephines
   Chromic gut no. 4-0 on ½-circle needle

The nasal cavity is anesthetized locally with cocaine just prior to surgery, and a general anesthetic is administered in the operating room. The patient is prepared as described for eye surgery.

OPERATIVE PROCEDURE (Fig. 9-18)

1. An incision is made on the nasal side of the orbital rim. With blunt-pointed, curved, or flat scissors, knife, retractors, and forceps, dissection is carried down to the periosteum, which is separated from the bone with elevators.

2. Through the lower canaliculus, the sac is probed, identified, and displaced laterally.

3. The anterior lacrimal crest is perforated by a Stryker saw or with a mallet and chisel. The hole is enlarged with rongeurs. During this time, the cornea is protected by a metal retractor or plastic contact lens.

4. Irregular fragments of bone and fibrous tissue are removed and hemostasis obtained with bone wax if necessary.

5. The lacrimal sac and nasal mucosa are incised with H incisions with the long line vertical.

6. The mucous membrane of the nose is sutured to that of the lacrimal sac with chromic gut sutures no. 4-0. A probe is passed through the nostril into the base of the wound to test the opening from the sac into the nose.

7. The interior flap of mucous membrane from nose and sac is sutured with interrupted chromic gut no. 4-0; skin margins are approximated and closed with silk sutures no. 6-0; interpalpebral sutures are placed to maintain position of the lids under the dressing. The wound is dressed.

## SURGERY FOR STRABISMUS

Strabismus (squint) is the inability to direct the two eyes at the same object because of lack of coordination of the extraocular muscles. Corrective surgery is performed in order to change the relative strength of individual muscles, therefore improving coordination (Fig. 9-2).

The deviation of the eye may be inward, outward, up, or down. The amount of deviation is a measurement of the angle formed by the visual axis of the two eyes. The lateral rectus muscle abducts the eye, the medial rectus muscle adducts the eye, and the other ocular muscles have both primary and secondary functions regarding elevation, depression, intorsion, and extorsion, according to the position of the eye.

Basically, there are two surgical approaches to the correction of strabismus: strengthening a muscle or weakening a

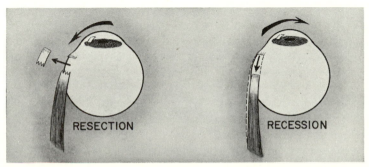

Fig. 9-19. In surgery for strabismus, resection of part of ocular muscle tendon rotates eye toward operated muscle, whereas recession moves muscle tendon backward on eye, permitting eye to rotate away from operated muscle. (From Havener, W. H.: Synopsis of ophthalmology, ed. 3, St. Louis, 1971, The C. V. Mosby Co.)

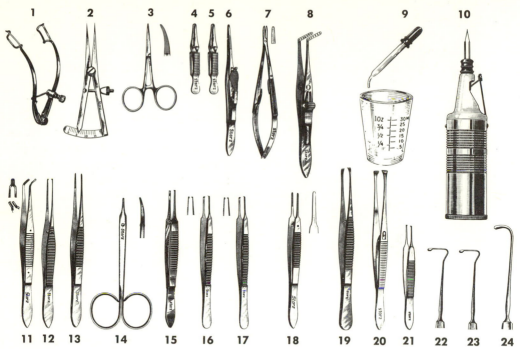

**Fig. 9-20.** Arrangement of instruments for eye muscle operations. **1**, Williams lid speculum; **2**, Castroviejo caliper; **3**, Hartman curved, short, delicate hemostat; **4** and **5**, small bulldog clamps (serrefine); **6**, Kalt needle holder; **7**, Castroviejo needle holder; **8**, Jameson muscle forceps; **9**, medicine glass with dropper; **10**, Hildreth cautery with white tip; **11**, Quevedo suturing and utility forceps; **12**, heavy serrated straight dressing forceps; **13**, heavy straight tissue forceps with mouse teeth; **14**, Stevens tenotomy scissors; **15**, McCullough suture tying forceps; **16**, Lester fixation forceps; **17**, Lester fixation forceps; **18**, Thorpe conjunctiva fixation forceps; **19**, Guist fixation forceps; **20**, Graefe fixation forceps; **21**, Graefe iris forceps; **22**, Jameson muscle hook; **23**, Jameson muscle hook; **24**, Von Graefe muscle hook. (Courtesy Storz Instrument Co., St. Louis, Mo.)

muscle. The strengthening operation is usually by resection procedure, and the weakening operation is usually by recession procedure. It may be necessary to operate on three or more muscles, in two stages. To some extent, the type of strabismus influences the type of surgery (Fig. 9-19).

## Operation for resection

**DEFINITION.** Removal of a portion of muscle and attachment of cut ends (Fig. 9-19).

**SETUP, PREPARATION OF THE PATIENT, AND ANESTHESIA.** The following muscle set is used (Fig. 9-20):

1 Williams lid speculum
1 Castroviejo caliper
1 Quevedo utility forceps
1 Delicate serrated conjunctival forceps
1 Delicate conjunctival forceps with teeth
1 Thorpe forceps
2 Lester fixation forceps
2 McCullough suture forceps
1 Guist fixation forceps
1 Von Graefe fixation forceps
2 Bulldog clamps (serrefine)
2 Jameson muscle forceps
1 Von Graefe muscle hook
1 Castroviejo needle holder
1 Kalt needle holder
1 Stevens scissors
1 Hildreth coagulator with tip

Suture material varies with the surgeon, but usually the suture is on a spatulate needle. The patient is prepared as described for eye surgery; local or general anesthesia is used.

## OPERATIVE PROCEDURE

1. A speculum is inserted, and the conjunctiva is incised at one border of the muscle to be resected.

2. The muscle insertion is hooked with a muscle hook, and the conjunctiva over the insertion is opened.

3. Double-armed sutures are passed through the muscle belly at the desired position of shortening, and the muscle is incised anterior to this suture.

4. The stump of the muscle is excised from the insertion, and the muscle is now sutured to the insertion using the double-armed suture.

5. The conjunctiva is closed with an absorbable suture.

## Operation for recession

DEFINITION. Severance of the muscle from its original insertion and its reattachment more posteriorly on the sclera (Fig. 9-19).

SETUP, PREPARATION OF THE PATIENT, AND ANESTHESIA. As described for strabismus resection operation.

OPERATIVE PROCEDURE

1. The insertion of the muscle is exposed as described previously.

2. Sutures are passed through the muscle tendon at its insertion into the globe, and the tendon is severed distal to the suture.

3. Using calipers, marks are made on the globe at the desired distance behind the insertion, and the muscle is anchored to the globe at that point.

4. The conjunctiva is closed with absorbable suture.

## Myectomy

DEFINITION. A myectomy is another method of weakening the action of the muscle. This may be done as a lengthening procedure such as a z marginal tenotomy or myectomy, an intersheath tenotomy of the superior oblique tendon, or as a complete severance of a muscle such as an inferior oblique myectomy procedure.

SETUP, PREPARATION OF THE PATIENT, AND ANESTHESIA. Muscle tray.

OPERATIVE PROCEDURE

1. The involved muscle is isolated as in the case of a z marginal tenotomy.

2. Cuts from opposite sides of the muscle are made through approximately three fourths of the width of the muscle, effectively lengthening the muscle.

3. In the case of the superior oblique muscle the tendon sheath is opened, and graded sections of tendon are excised according to the needs of the individual case.

4. Myectomy of the inferior oblique muscle is done in a graded fashion by placing two Kelly clamps across the muscle belly lateral to the inferior rectus muscle and excising the isolated strip of muscle. The ends of the muscle are cauterized with a Hildreth cautery and released. Because of the peculiar anatomy of this muscle, lateral discontinuity weakens the muscle and does not paralyze it.

## Tuck

DEFINITION. This is a method of shortening a muscle and thus strengthening it that is performed primarily on the superior oblique muscle.

SETUP, PREPARATION OF THE PATIENT, AND ANESTHESIA

Muscle set
Fink-Scobie hook
Fink tucker

OPERATIVE PROCEDURE

1. An incision is made in the conjunctiva medial to the superior rectus muscle. The Fink-Scobie hook is passed posteriorly into the orbit, and the superior oblique muscle is hooked and brought out into the incision. The Fink tucker is placed over the tendon, and a graded doubling of the tendon, like looping a rope, is completed. A double-armed Supramid suture is passed through the base of the loop, effectively shortening the muscle. The tip of the loop is sutured to the sclera. (The surgeon may often attempt to tuck the muscle lateral to the superior rectus muscle.)

2. The conjunctiva is closed with absorbable suture.

## SURGERY OF THE GLOBE AND ORBIT

CONSIDERATIONS. Rupture of the eyeball may be direct at the site of injury or,

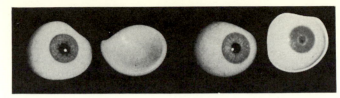

Fig. 9-21. Artificial eyes. Shell prosthesis is seen at right. (From Allen, J. H., editor: May's manual of the diseases of the eye, ed. 23, Baltimore, 1963, The Williams & Wilkins Co.)

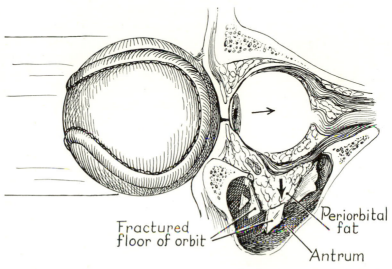

Fractured
floor of orbit

Periorbital
fat

Antrum

Fig. 9-22. Ball has struck rim of orbit and has pressed orbital contents backward, displacing fragments of bone into maxillary sinus. Inferior rectus muscle is incarcerated in fracture. At times, inferior oblique muscle may also be involved. (From Paton, R. T., and Katzin, H. M.: Atlas of eye surgery, ed. 2, New York, 1962, Blakiston Division, McGraw-Hill Book Co.)

more frequently, indirect from an increase in intraocular pressure, causing the wall of the eyeball to tear at weaker points such as the limbus. When the intraocular contents have become deranged so that useful function is prohibited, removal of the eye contents (evisceration procedure) or of the entire eyeball (enucleation) is indicated. If either procedure is required, implantation of an inert globe may be used as a space filler and to aid in the movement of a prosthesis (artificial eye) (Fig. 9-21).

Fractures of the walls of the orbit (Fig. 9-1) may be caused by direct blows or by extension of a fracture line from adjacent bones (Figs. 9-22 and 9-23). Isolated orbital floor or blowout fractures usually follow injury to the region of the eye by an object

the size of an apple or a man's fist. Orbital contents herniate into the maxillary sinus, and the inferior rectus or inferior oblique muscle may become incarcerated at the fracture site. A Caldwell-Luc antrostomy (Chapter 8) may be done with reduction of the fracture from below, or the fracture site may be approached directly through the lower lid along the orbital floor and the prolapsed tissue reduced, the orbital floor reduced, and the orbital floor defect bridged with a graft of bone, cartilage, or plastic material.

### Repair of laceration

The preferred method of closing corneal lacerations is the use of direct appositional suturing with the aid of an operating mi-

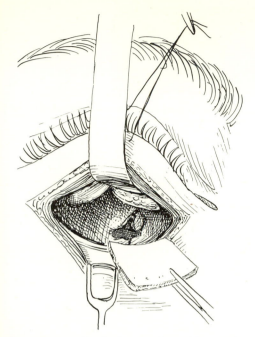

**Fig. 9-23.** Crosshatched area shows blowout fracture site. Autogenous graft from iliac crest is held by forceps ready to be placed over fractured site. The graft usually does not require suturing. (From Paton, R. T., and Katzin, H. M.: Atlas of eye surgery, ed. 2, New York, 1962, Blakiston Division, McGraw-Hill Book Co.)

croscope. The suture material used is generally no. 8-0 in gauge or finer.

Experimentally, tissue adhesives, that is, cyanoacrylate monomers, are being used. The tissue adhesive is applied to the well-dried tissue that has been properly oriented anatomically, and it polymerizes and seals the wound on contact with the tissue. The tissue adhesive is supplied in packaged sterile vials (Co-Apt).

## Enucleation

**DEFINITION.** Removal of the entire eyeball.

**SETUP, PREPARATION OF THE PATIENT, AND ANESTHESIA.** A muscle setup is needed, plus the following (Fig. 9-24):

1 Enucleation scissors
1 Enucleation snare

1 Eye sphere with introducer and holder
1 Implant as desired
1 Allis forceps
1 Large Kelly clamp
1 Weber canaliculus knife

**OPERATIVE PROCEDURE**

1. A speculum retractor is introduced into the palpebral fissure.

2. The conjunctiva is divided around the cornea, using a curved Weber canaliculus knife and forceps.

3. The medial, lateral, inferior, and superior recti muscles are divided, leaving a stump of medial rectus only. The globe is separated from Tenon's capsule with blunt-pointed curved scissors, retractors, hemostats, and forceps.

4. The eye is rotated laterally, using the stump of the medial rectus muscle.

5. A large curved hemostat is passed behind the globe, and the optic nerve is clamped for 60 seconds. The hemostat is removed, enucleation scissors are passed posteriorly, and the optic nerve is transected. The oblique muscles are severed as the eye is lifted out of the socket by the stump of the medial rectus muscle.

6. The muscle cone is packed with saline sponges to obtain hemostasis.

7. The muscle cone is filled with an implant, and careful closure of Tenon's capsule and conjunctiva is completed.

8. A socket conformer with ointment is placed in the cul-de-sac.

9. A pressure dressing, usually of the head roll type, is applied.

## Evisceration of the eye

**DEFINITION.** Removal of the contents of the eye, leaving the sclera intact and the muscles attached to the sclera.

**SETUP, PREPARATION OF THE PATIENT, AND ANESTHESIA.** Same as for enucleation (Fig. 9-24).

**OPERATIVE PROCEDURE**

1. The conjunctiva is not separated from the sclera as it is for enucleation. A sharp-pointed knife is inserted through the limbus anterior to the iris.

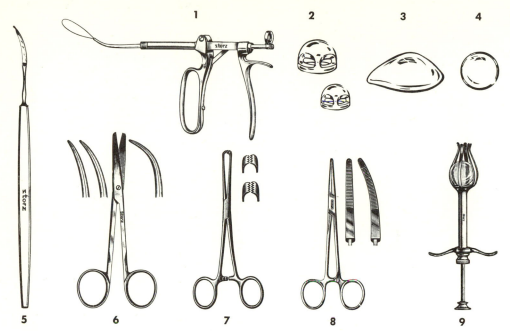

**Fig. 9-24.** Arrangement of special instruments for enucleation. **1,** Castroviejo enucleation snare; **2,** Allen implants, large and small; **3,** conformer; **4,** mule eye sphere; **5,** canaliculus knife; **6,** enucleation scissors; **7,** Allis forceps; **8,** Kelly forceps; **9,** Carter sphere introducer. (Courtesy Storz Instrument Co., St. Louis, Mo.)

2. The contents of the eye (iris, vitreous, lens) are removed.

3. The choroid adhering to the sclera is removed with curettes.

4. Bleeding is controlled with delicate hemostatic forceps, electrocoagulation, and sutures.

5. A plastic implant is now placed within the empty shell.

6. The conjunctival scleral edges are brought together with silk sutures no. 4-0 or 5-0, and a pressure bandage is applied.

### Repair of fracture of the orbit (blowout)

**DEFINITION.** Repair of the fractured orbit by means of graft or realignment of contents of the orbit (Fig. 9-23).

**SETUP, PREPARATION OF THE PATIENT, AND ANESTHESIA.** The setup is as for dacryocystorhinostomy, plus a graft set (for implantation of an autogenous graft or synthetic graft materials of various sizes and thicknesses) and a flexible, narrow-width retractor. The patient is prepared as de-

scribed for eye surgery. A general anesthetic is usually administered.

**OPERATIVE PROCEDURE**

1. The maximal ocular rotation is tested by exerting traction with a forceps on the tendon of the inferior rectus muscle to determine if the inferior muscle sling is trapped in the fracture.

2. To distribute tension over the lower lid and put the orbicular muscle on stretch, a traction suture is inserted through the lower lid margin.

3. Using a Bard-Parker knife handle no. 3 with blade no. 15, the lower lid is incised in the lid fold above the orbital rim.

4. The skin is separated from the orbicular muscle, and the orbital septum is identified by blunt dissection. Dissection is continued down to the periosteum of the orbital rim by means of scissors, loop retractors, elevators, and forceps.

5. The periosteum of the orbital rim is incised with a blade no. 15. Using periosteal elevators, the floor of the orbit is exposed

and explored. When the fracture site is identified, bone specules are removed, and the herniated contents are freed from the maxillary antrum. The contents of the orbit are elevated by means of narrow-width, flexible retractors, and a traction suture of black silk no. 4-0 is placed around the tendon of the inferior rectus muscle.

6. An autogenous graft is taken from the iliac crest, or an alloplastic material of proper size is used to repair the bony defect. The material may or may not be anchored to the orbital rim by wire sutures.

7. The periosteum is carefully closed with chromic gut sutures no. 4-0.

8. The skin is closed with black silk no. 6-0 and a pressure dressing applied.

## Exenteration of the eye

**DEFINITION.** The removal of the entire orbital contents, including periosteum for certain malignancies of the globe or orbit.

**SETUP, PREPARATION OF THE PATIENT, AND ANESTHESIA.** Same as for fracture of the orbit. Usually done with the patient under general anesthesia.

**OPERATIVE PROCEDURE**

1. This operation, depending on circumstances, may or may not include the removal of the lids. An incision is made down to the orbital rim, through the periosteum, and around the entire orbit.

2. Using periosteal elevators, the periosteum is freed from the orbital walls and the apex of the orbit.

3. The optic nerve is clamped, and the entire contents of the orbit are removed *en bloc.*

4. Hemostasis is obtained by the use of cautery and bone wax.

5. A skin graft or temporal muscle implant may be used to fill the orbital cavity, but this is not usually done.

6. Iodoform gauze is used to fill the cavity, a pressure dressing is put in place, and the cavity is allowed to granulate in.

## Corneal transplant (keratoplasty)

**DEFINITION.** Grafting of corneal tissue from one human eye to another (Figs. 9-25 and 9-26).

Keratoplasty may be classified as follows: (1) lamellar (partial-thickness) graft, (2) penetrating (whole-thickness) graft, (3) keratectomy (peeling of the cornea), and (4) tattooing (to simulate a pupil—rarely done).

**CONSIDERATIONS.** Corneal transplant is performed in the presence of corneal thickening and opacification. Impairment of the transparency of the cornea may be due to infection, thermal or chemical burns, and certain diseases of unknown etiology.

Corneal transplant is done to improve vision in those cases in which the basic visual structures of the eye, that is, the retina and the optic nerve, are properly functioning.

Corneas are obtained from recently deceased persons. Eye banks have helped to coordinate services for such operations (p. 267).

**SETUP, PREPARATION OF THE PATIENT, AND ANESTHESIA.** The basic cataract set plus special transplant instruments is used (Fig. 9-27).

1 No. 30 blunt needle
2 Katzin corneal transplant scissors (right and left)
1 Lahey suturing forceps
1 Paton double-ended spatula
1 Castroviejo double-ended spatula
1 Allis forceps
1 Castroviejo corneal trephine (surgeon will state size needed)
1 Corneal carrying case
1 Barraquer wire speculum
1 Double Flieringa-LeGrand fixation ring
1 Barraquer needle holder
1 Bonn forceps (0.2 mm. teeth)
2 Jeweler's forceps

**Lamellar transplant**

Castroviejo electrokeratome with shims
1 Gill corneal splitter
1 Paufique knife
1 Bard-Parker knife handle no. 3 with blade no. 15
1 Beaver handle with no. 64 blade

**OPERATIVE PROCEDURE**

**PENETRATING KERATOPLASTY (PERFORMED USING OPERATING MICROSCOPE)**

1. The eye speculum is put in place, and superior rectus and inferior rectus

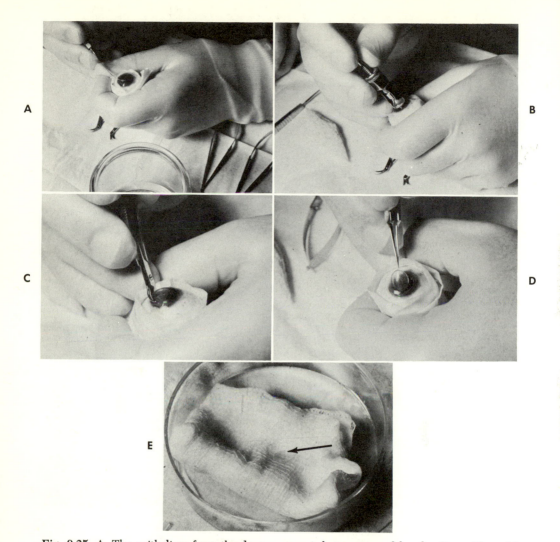

**Fig. 9-25. A,** The epithelium from the donor cornea is being removed by abrading with an iris spatula. The donor eye is wrapped in a smooth cloth dressing. **B,** The donor eye is firmly grasped in the left hand of the surgeon, and the corneal trephine is centered on the donor eye. By using a twisting motion, the cornea is cut through its entire thickness. **C,** Corneal scissors are used to cut any areas of corneal tissue that have not been penetrated by the trephine. **D,** The corneal button is removed with fine forceps, with care taken not to touch the endothelial surface. **E,** The donor corneal button (arrow) is stored on a moistened gauze pad, endothelial side up with a roof covering the Petri dish in order to preserve the moisture.

bridal sutures are put in place if a Flier-inga-LeGrand ring is not to be used. If a ring is used, it is sutured in place with four Dacron sutures no. 5-0.

2. The eye from the eyebank is removed from its container and washed in Neosporin solution.

3. The donor eye is then wrapped in surgical dressing for stabilization. The cornea is excised from the donor eye by means of a trephine cataract knife, corneal scissors, and forceps after the epithelium is removed with a sponge. The graft is placed, epithelial side down, in a Petri dish

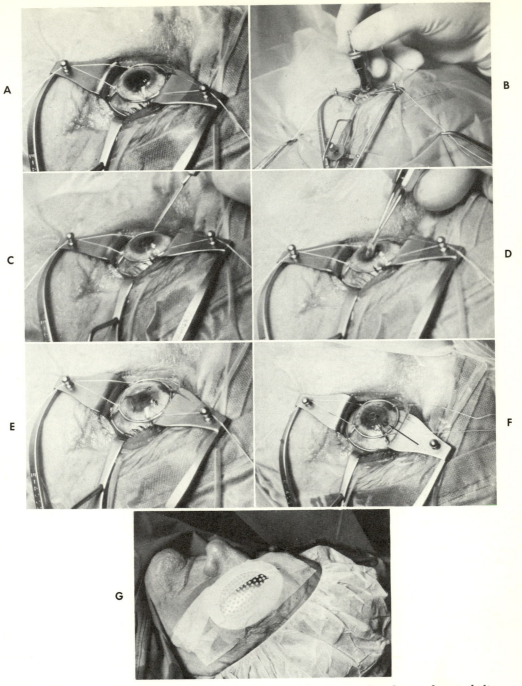

Fig. 9-26. A, This is the eye of a patient who will undergo a combined procedure including corneal transplantation and cataract extraction. A double Bonaccolto-Flieringa fixation ring is sutured in place with no. 5-0 Dacron sutures posted over the solid bladed eye speculum. B, The corneal trephine is placed on the recipient cornea, and a partial penetration approximately three fourths of the way through the stroma is made. C, The anterior chamber is entered through the groove with a Wheeler knife. The remainder of the button is excised with right and left micro-Katzin corneal scissors. D, Corneal button is removed. E, Demonstrates the donor button sutured in place with four no. 8-0 black silk sutures. F, Demonstrates the cornea in place with a running no. 10-0 suture (arrows) with air in the anterior chamber. G, The patient postoperatively with Fox shield properly applied on the bony margins.

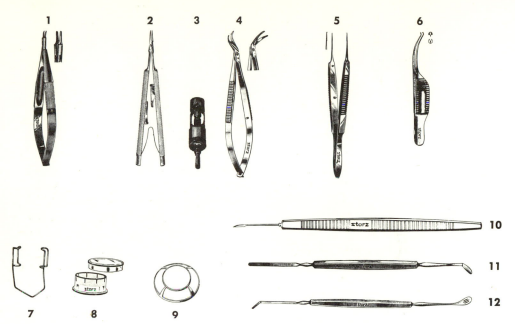

**Fig. 9-27.** Arrangement of special instruments for corneal transplant. **1,** Barraquer needle holder; **2,** Storz-Castroviejo needle holder; **3,** Castroviejo corneal transplant trephine; **4,** Katzin corneal transplant scissors; **5,** Bonn suturing forceps; **6,** Troutman (Colibri type) corneal forceps; **7,** Barraquer lid speculum; **8,** Fine corneal transplant carrying case; **9,** Flieringa-LeGrand fixation ring; **10,** Ziegler needle knife; **11,** Castroviejo double spatula; **12,** Paton double spatula. (Courtesy Storz Instrument Co., St. Louis, Mo.)

containing a saline-moistened gauze (Fig. 9-25). Some surgeons will preplace sutures in the graft.

4. The section of cornea removed from the recipient's eye is the same size as the graft taken from the donor's eye. A groove is made with the identical trephine used to obtain the donor button set at 0.3 to 0.4 mm. The anterior chamber is entered with one of the variety of cataract knives and the button excised with corneal scissors. (Care must be taken to close the guard on the trephine when the surgeon is finished to avoid damage to the cutting surface.)

5. Peripheral iridectomies or iridotomies may be performed at this time according to the surgeon's discretion, or a cataract extraction may be completed if the lens is opaque.

6. The graft is placed into the opening of the recipient's eye and anchored in place by means of four to eight single-armed black silk sutures no. 8-0 placed at the four

cardinal meridians, using an operating microscope. The graft is now sutured to the host with either running or interrupted nylon sutures no. 10-0 (Fig. 9-26).

7. Air may be injected into the anterior chamber of the recipient's eye to keep the iris from sticking to the suture line. Mydriatic or miotic solutions are used at the surgeon's discretion.

8. A subconjunctival injection of antibiotic solution or a topical application of antibiotic drops may be used at the completion of the procedure. A splint, eye patch, and metal guard are applied.

LAMELLAR KERATOPLASTY

1. The eye speculum is put in place, and superior rectus and inferior rectus bridal sutures are put in place.

2. The eye from the eye bank is removed from its container and washed in Neosporin solution.

3. The eye is wrapped in surgical dressing. A groove is made at the desired

depth in the cornea with the trephine. The Castroviejo keratome is now set at the desired depth, and the lamellar sheet of cornea is removed and placed in a Petri dish.

4. The recipient cornea is now grooved with the same trephine to the appropriate depth. Using the operating microscope, the surgeon performs a lamellar resection, that is, removes the anterior part of the cornea at a predetermined depth with a Gill knife, Beaver blade no. 66, or other corneal splitter.

5. The donor tissue is sutured in place with a continuous nylon suture no. 10-0.

6. A mydriatic agent and subconjunctival or topical antibiotics may then be used.

7. The eye is patched.

### Eye bank procedure

**DEFINITION.** Removal of eyes immediately after death in accordance with legal regulations.

**CONSIDERATIONS.** The bank may be a central community agency or may be maintained by the hospital. The containers for eyes and regulations for the procedure are generally obtained from the bank.

A special consent form is required and should be signed by the authorized next of kin and by the hospital administrative office.

**SETUP, PREPARATION OF THE DONOR, AND ANESTHESIA.** The instrument setup consists of a modified enucleation set, including the following:

**Cutting instruments**
1 Stevens scissors
1 Suture scissors
1 Enucleation scissors
1 Knife handle no. 3 with blade no. 15

**Holding instruments**
2 Lester forceps
2 Conjunctival forceps
2 Muscle hooks
1 Allis clamp, short
3 Towel clamps

**Exposing and clamping instruments**
2 Mosquito hemostats

**Extracting instrument**
1 Modified Guyton-Park speculum

**Accessory items**
1 Medicine glass
2 Eye specimen bottles

The eyes are washed and irrigated in the routine manner of preparation for eye surgery. The sterile field, drapes, and instruments are essentially the same as for an enucleation on a living patient, save that no anesthesia setup is required.

**OPERATIVE PROCEDURE**

1. Eye specimen bottles are labeled right and left eye. The speculum is inserted, and after routine enucleation the donated eye is placed in the sterile specimen bottle with the cornea up. The eye is supported on a sponge that has been soaked in saline solution. An antibiotic solution may be placed on the cornea. The eye sockets are packed with cotton and the lids closed.

2. Specimen bottles are sealed with tape and labeled with the donor's name, time and cause of death, time of enucleation, and date.

## Surgery of the lens (cataract operation)

**DEFINITION.** Extraction of the opaque lens from the interior of the eye.

**CONSIDERATIONS.** The lens consists of 64% to 65% water, 34% to 35% protein, and a trace of other body minerals. The disorders of the lens are opacification and dislocation, resulting in blurred vision without pain or inflammation.

Cataracts (opacification) vary in degree of density, size, and location and are usually caused by aging or trauma.

Various methods are used to remove the lens, basically intracapsular or extracapsular extraction.

The intracapsular method of cataract removal consists of removing the lens within its capsule.

In the extracapsular method the anterior portion of the capsule is first ruptured and removed, and the lens cortex and nucleus are expressed from the eye, leaving the posterior capsule behind. The in-

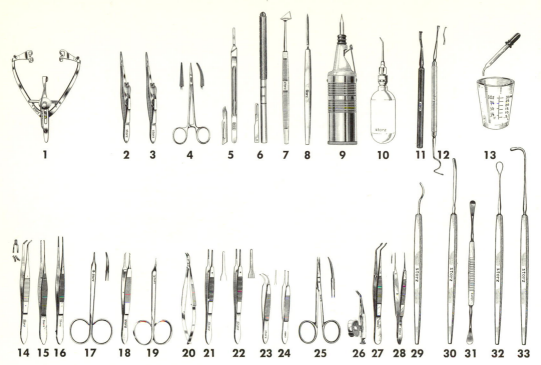

Fig. 9-28. Arrangement of instruments for cataract operation. 1, Guyton-Park lid speculum; 2, Kalt needle holder; 3, Kalt needle holder; 4, Halsted curved mosquito forceps; 5, no. 9 knife handle with no. 15 blade; 6, Beaver handle with no. 64 blade; 7, Jaeger keratome; 8, Von Graefe cataract knife; 9, Hildreth cautery and tip; 10, Bishop-Harmon anterior chamber irrigator; 11, Bronson-Turtz iris retractor; 12, Rizzuti iris retractor; 13, medicine glass with dropper; 14, Quevedo suturing and utility forceps; 15, delicate serrated straight dressing forceps; 16, delicate straight tissue forceps with mouse teeth; 17, Stevens tenotomy scissors; 18, Alvis fixation forceps; 19, McGuire corneal scissors; 20, Castroviejo small curved corneal scissors; 21 and 22, McCullough suture-tying forceps; 23, Von Graefe iris forceps, curved; 24, Von Graefe iris forceps, straight; 25, curved iris scissors; 26, Barraquer iris scissors; 27, Arruga capsule forceps; 28, Bonn suturing forceps; 29, Berens lens expressor; 30, iris spatula; 31, Green double spatula; 32, New Orleans eye and ear lens loop; 33, Von Graefe muscle hook. (Courtesy Storz Instrument Co., St. Louis, Mo.)

tracapsular method is the procedure of choice in most cases.

SETUP, PREPARATION OF THE PATIENT, AND ANESTHESIA. A basic setup for eye surgery is needed, including the following (Figs. 9-10, 9-11, and 9-28):

1 Guyton-Park lid speculum
1 Castroviejo corneal forceps
1 Quevedo utility forceps
1 Conjunctival forceps with teeth
1 Serrated conjunctival forceps
1 Alvis fixation forceps
1 Von Graefe iris forceps (curved, with teeth)
2 McCullough suture forceps
1 Arruga capsule forceps

1 Straight iris forceps
2 Kalt needle holders
1 Iris repositor
1 Spoon
1 Lens expressor
1 Von Graefe muscle hook
1 Lens loop
1 Hildreth coagulator with tips
1 Plastic anterior chamber irrigator with tip
1 Stevens scissors
1 Iris scissors
1 Corneal scissors
1 Von Graefe knife
1 Keratome knife
1 Bard-Parker knife handle with blade no. 15
1 Beaver knife handle with blade no. 64
1 Bonn forceps

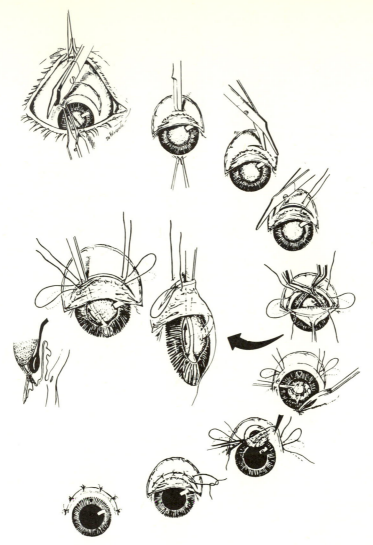

**Fig. 9-29.** Intracapsular lens extraction. (From Callahan, A.: Am. J. Ophthalmol. **63**:317, 1967.)

The patient is prepared as described for eye surgery.

**OPERATIVE PROCEDURE**

INTRACAPSULAR METHOD (Fig. 9-29)

1. A speculum is placed in the eye to hold the lids apart.

2. The globe is held by transfixion with a silk suture no. 4-0, which is inserted under the tendon of the superior rectus muscle and clamped to the drape. A conjunctival flap, either limbal or fornix based, may be prepared using scissors. Some surgeons will not dissect a flap.

3. Bleeding points are controlled by means of cautery. Partially penetrating incisions (grooves) are made at the limbus or in the cornea.

4. Corneal-scleral or corneal-corneal sutures are passed through the lips of the wounds. These sutures are then looped out the groove and set in an orderly fashion around the margins of the incision.

5. With the keratome or Von Graefe knife, the anterior chamber is entered and the limbal wound enlarged with corneal scissors.

6. A peripheral iridectomy or sector iridectomy is performed. The lens is grasped, in most cases with a cryoextractor, and pulled slowly from the eye.

7. The corneal-scleral sutures are tied, and the conjunctival flap is reapproximated with either absorbable or nonabsorbable sutures of the desired size.

8. Pilocarpine, 2%, or 1% atropine is topically administered. Antibiotics may be used topically or subconjunctivally. The eye is dressed and patched.

EXTRACAPSULAR METHOD

The procedure is essentially similar to an intracapsular extraction until the removal of the lens, when the capsule of the lens is opened by means of a cystotome or capsule forceps. The lens cortex is removed from the eye by irrigation, and the nucleus of the lens, if present, is removed by expression with a lens expressor and a lens loop. Cycloplegic agents are generally used. The remainder of the procedure is as just outlined for intracapsular extraction.

## Surgical procedures for glaucoma
### Iridectomy for glaucoma

DEFINITION. Removal of a section of iris tissue.

CONSIDERATIONS. Peripheral iridectomy is done in the treatment of acute, subacute, or chronic angle-closure glaucoma when extensive peripheral anterior synechiae have not formed. This operation is done to reestablish communication between the posterior and anterior chambers, thus relieving pupillary block and permitting the iris root to drop away from the trabecular meshwork in order to reestablish the outflow of aqueous through the canal of Schlemm.

SETUP, PREPARATION OF THE PATIENT, AND ANESTHESIA. A basic cataract setup is needed.

OPERATIVE PROCEDURE

1. The speculum is introduced. The globe is fixed with a black silk suture no. 4-0 passed under the superior rectus tendon with a fixation forceps and needle holder.

The suture is fastened to the drape with a hemostat.

2. A small peritomy is performed for approximately 2 hours of the clock at the superior limbus. The corneal scleral junction is scraped clean of epithelium. With a Beaver Knife handle and blade no. 64, a limbal groove is made down to Descemet's membrane. A preplaced suture, usually of black silk no. 7-0, is set in place.

3. The wound is spread apart using the preplaced sutures, and the anterior chamber is entered with a Bard-Parker blade no. 15. There is an attempt to make the incision into the anterior chamber as large as possible. Pressure is placed on the posterior lip of the wound, and the iris usually will spontaneously prolapse. The iris is grasped, and either peripheral or complete iridectomy can be performed. The iris will spontaneously retract into the anterior chamber without assistance, but gentle stroking of the corneal surface may be necessary.

4. The preplaced suture is passed through the conjunctiva and tied. Subconjunctival antibiotics may be administered and an eye dressing applied.

### Iridencleisis

DEFINITION. Creation of a tract lined with iris tissue to serve as a wick to accomplish filtration, thus reducing abnormal pressure in glaucoma.

CONSIDERATIONS. Iridencleisis is used in open-angle glaucoma and in chronic angle-closure glaucoma when extensive anterior synechiae have formed. The objective is to establish an artificial method of draining aqueous. By using the iris as a wick in a scleral opening, the surgeon permits the aqueous to drain into the subconjunctival space for reabsorption by the bloodstream.

SETUP, PREPARATION OF THE PATIENT, AND ANESTHESIA. The iridectomy setup is needed, plus scleral trephines, including interchangeable cutting blades. Routine instillation of drops to prevent excessive mydriasis and retrobulbar injection or general anesthesia may be used.

OPERATIVE PROCEDURE

1. A conjunctival flap is dissected from above the superior limbus.

2. A keratome is introduced into the anterior chamber through the superior limbus. An iris forceps is introduced in the chamber, and the iris is grasped and pulled outward.

3. After an iridectomy is performed, the iris is incarcerated in the wound. The operative site is covered by suturing the conjunctival flap.

4. Cycloplegic agents and an eye dressing are applied.

### Elliot trephination

DEFINITION. Formation of a drainage channel to the subconjunctival space in the treatment of chronic glaucoma.

CONSIDERATIONS. The object of this operation is to establish a route of aqueous drainage to subconjunctival space for absorption. The operation is similar to iridencleisis and is done primarily for open-angle glaucoma. Postoperatively, the aqueous escapes through the scleral hole into the subconjunctival space, where it is absorbed into the bloodstream.

SETUP, PREPARATION OF THE PATIENT, AND ANESTHESIA. As described for iridencleisis. The patient is prepared as described for eye surgery; a subconjunctival injection is carried out.

OPERATIVE PROCEDURE

1. A superior rectus bridal suture is set in place (black silk no. 4-0) and clamped to the drape.

2. A subtenon's injection of a solution consisting of 2 ml. of saline and one drop of 1:1000 epinephrine (Adrenalin) is injected superiorly in order to dissect a flap from the underlying sclerae.

3. The conjunctiva is incised to the sclera. The flap is dissected anteriorly into clear cornea.

4. With the conjunctival flap raised by means of forceps, the trephine is applied at the corneal limbus.

5. After completion of the trephining,

the scleral disc is cut at its hinge, if it is not free.

6. An iridectomy is performed with iris forceps and De Wecker scissors.

7. The operative area is cleansed of blood, and the conjunctival flap is resutured with a silk suture no. 6-0 or 7-0. Cycloplegic agents are administered. The eye is dressed with a splint, patch, and metal guard.

### Anterior and posterior lip sclerectomies

DEFINITION. Formation of a drainage channel to the subconjunctival space in the treatment of chronic glaucoma.

CONSIDERATIONS. Same as for iridencleisis and Elliot trephination.

SETUP, PREPARATION OF THE PATIENT, AND ANESTHESIA. As described for iridencleisis, adding 1 Holt or Goss punch to the set.

OPERATIVE PROCEDURE

1. Proceed as described for Elliot trephination through the dissection of the conjunctival flap (steps 1 to 3).

2a. *Thermal sclerectomy*—A scleral flap is made approximately 3 mm. from the limbus using a Beaver blade no. 64. The Hildreth cautery with a transilluminating head is used to outline the anterior chamber. The Hildreth cautery is used to apply heat energy to the posterior wound edge under the scleral flap. The anterior chamber is entered with a clean sweep of the cautery. The iris will usually spontaneously prolapse, or an iris forceps is used to grasp the iris, and a peripheral or radial iridectomy is performed.

2b. *Punch sclerectomy*—An incision is made into the anterior chamber either at the anterior or posterior margin of the limbus after the anterior chamber has been outlined with a transilluminator. A punch is introduced, and sections of either the anterior or posterior lip are removed, depending on which incision has been made. An iridectomy is performed.

3. A careful closure of conjunctivae and Tenon's capsule is accomplished with black silk suture no. 6-0, leaving both ends free.

4. Air is introduced under the flap with

a blunt 30-gauge needle on a 2 ml. syringe.

5. A delimiting suture is tied, using the free ends of the conjunctival suture. Atropine sulfate, 1%, is dropped onto the surface of the eye, and an eye dressing is put in place.

### Cyclodialysis

DEFINITION. Formation of a communication between the anterior chamber and the space located between the sclera and the choroid in order to reduce aqueous secretion and thus induce lower pressure.

CONSIDERATIONS. By means of this surgical procedure, aqueous secretion is reduced and absorption increased into the suprachoroidal space. This operation is usually reserved to treat glaucoma associated with peripheral anterior synechiae.

SETUP, PREPARATION OF THE PATIENT, AND ANESTHESIA. A basic cataract setup is needed. A local anesthetic is used.

OPERATIVE PROCEDURE

1. A superior rectus bridal suture is put in place (black silk no. 4-0) and clamped to the drape.

2. In one of the superior quadrants between the rectus muscles the conjunctiva is incised and dissected from the sclera. An incision is made through the sclera to the suprachoroidal space with the use of a Beaver blade no. 64.

3. A cyclodialysis spatula is introduced through the scleral opening, and the anterior chamber is entered in the neighborhood of the iris root; thus the ciliary body is detached from the sclera by means of the spatula. The scleral incision is closed.

4. The conjunctiva is closed with fine sutures. A dressing is applied.

## SURGERY FOR RETINAL DETACHMENT (SEPARATION)

Retinal detachment is actually a separation of the neural retinal layer from the pigment epithelium layer of the retina. Retinal detachment may occur because of the presence of intraocular neoplasms originating in the retina or choroid or, more commonly, secondary to retinal tears or holes associated with injury or degeneration.

This condition usually causes the sudden onset of the appearance of floating spots before the eye, due to freeing of pigment or blood cells into the vitreous. The vitreous humor of the eye is a gelatinous liquid possessing an ultrastructure of fine protein fibers in a network arrangement, with some attachments to the retina. Fluid from the vitreous cavity may seep through the retinal tears and separate the retinal components. This condition progresses as the liquid seeps behind the retina. The part of the retina that has become separated from its nutritional source becomes damaged and relatively nonseeing. Prompt treatment of retinal detachment is aimed at preventing permanent loss of central vision. Reattachment of the retina can be accomplished only by surgery. Repair is done from outside the globe. The principle involved in surgery is that of sealing off the area at which the tear or hole has been located with or without drainage of the subretinal fluid (Fig. 9-30).

Surgical procedures performed in the treatment of retinal detachment include scleral buckling with diathermy or cryotherapy, cryosurgery, light coagulation, or episcleral and intrascleral techniques.

CONSIDERATIONS. The purpose of surgery for retinal detachment is to cause an intrusion or push into the eye at the site of the pathological cause. Treatment by either diathermy or cryotherapy will cause an inflammatory reaction that leads to a permanent adhesion between the detached retina and underlying structures. In the treatment of retinal detachment the aim is to return the retina to its normal anatomical position.

SETUP, PREPARATION OF THE PATIENT, AND ANESTHESIA

1 Williams lid speculum
1 Cibis double muscle hook
4 Mosquito hemostats
1 Quevedo utility forceps
2 Serrated conjunctival forceps (heavy)
1 Thorpe forceps
3 Lester forceps

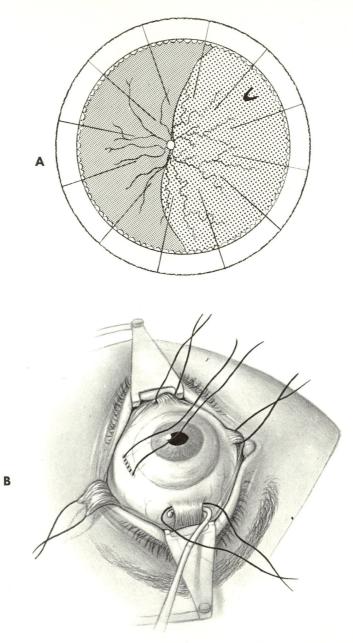

*Continued.*

**Fig. 9-30.** Scleral buckling operation for treatment of retinal detachment. **A,** Diagram of retina showing detachment of retina of temporal half of left eye, with retinal tear at equator of globe at 1:30 o'clock. **B,** Bulbar conjunctiva and Tenon's capsule are opened to explore sclera. Stay sutures are placed under involved rectus muscles so that eye may be rotated to expose area to be treated. In some cases, more than one rectus muscle is temporarily detached from globe to permit adequate exposure. (From Advancing with surgery, Somerville, N. J., 1963, Ethicon, Inc.)

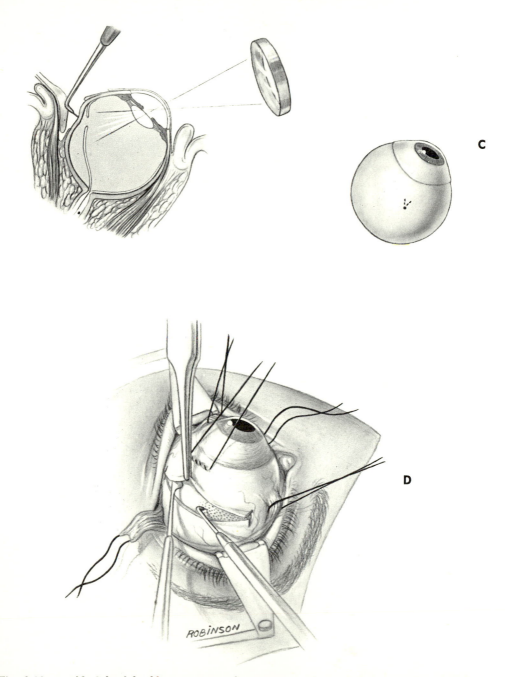

**Fig. 9-30, cont'd.** Scleral buckling operation for treatment of retinal detachment. **C**, Fundus is examined by means of ophthalmoscope and depression of sclera with diathermy electrode. Surgeon visualizes field and directs assistant in placement of electrode beneath retinal tear; burn mark is made on sclera at site of retinal tear with diathermy electrode. **D**, Cut or groove is made in sclera along equator of eye. Each edge of groove is undermined. (From Advancing with surgery, Somerville, N. J., 1963, Ethicon, Inc.)

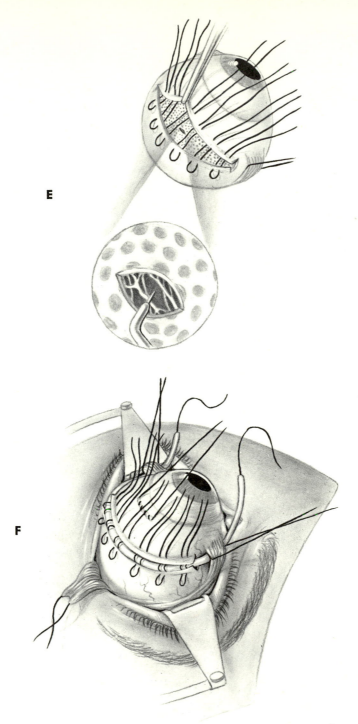

**E**

**F**

*Continued.*

**Fig. 9-30, cont'd.** Scleral buckling operation for treatment of retinal detachment. **E,** Mattress sutures of no. 4-0 or 3-0 braided silk or Mersilene are then placed across scleral groove. Small incision is then made through remaining layer of sclera down to choroid. Choroid is punctured with fine electrode to allow subretinal fluid to drain out. **F,** Polyethylene tube no. 90 is laid in bed of scleral groove under mattress sutures. (A no. 40 Silastic band is frequently used [see operative procedure, p. 276].) When retinal tears are large, a silicone strip may be placed under polyethylene tube. (From Advancing with surgery, Somerville, N. J., 1963, Ethicon, Inc.)

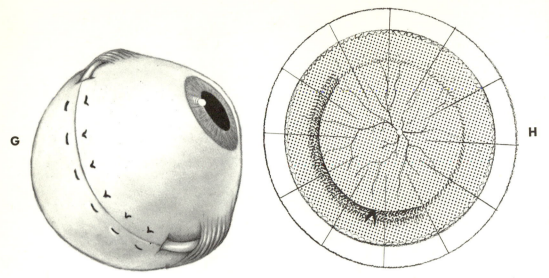

**Fig. 9-30, cont'd.** Scleral buckling operation for treatment of retinal detachment. **G,** Edges of scleral groove are closed over polyethylene tube and tube tied around eye by means of purse-string suture, a silk suture that is passed through lumen of free ends of tube. **H,** Diagram of fundus with retina in place and 1:30 o'clock retinal tear on buckle. Diathermy reaction is seen on buckle from 12 to 5:30 o'clock. (From Advancing with surgery, Somerville, N. J., 1963, Ethicon, Inc.)

1 McCullough suture forceps
1 Cyclodialysis spatula
2 Jameson muscle hooks
1 Von Graefe muscle hook
1 Von Graefe iris forceps (straight, with teeth)
1 Stevens scissors
2 Beaver knives no. 3 with blades no. 64
2 Bulldog clamps (serrefine)
1 Diatherm pencil and cord and electrodes
1 Watzke forceps
1 Caliper
1 Tonometer
1 No. 20 loop
1 Each 3, 5, and 7 mm. Silastic sponges
1 No. 40 Silastic band and sleeve
   Preserved sclera
   Indirect ophthalmoscope
   Diathermy unit
   Cryo unit
   Dacron suture no. 5-0
   Supramid sutures no. 4-0

The patient is prepared as described for eye surgery.

**OPERATIVE PROCEDURE.** A detailed drawing of the retina has been made before surgery and is displayed in the operating suite. On the basis of this drawing, the conjunctiva is opened to whatever extent has been previously determined, that is, 90 degrees for a simple horseshoe tear or 360 degrees for an aphakic detachment. Using the indirect ophthalmoscope, the abnormality is localized under direct visualization, and nonpenetrating diathermy marks are made over the site by indentation.

EPISCLERAL TECHNIQUE

1. Cryotherapy is applied to the pathological areas under direct visualization (an iceball will be seen to form in the proper areas until all of the lesion has been treated).

2. If a localized plombage (push) is to be used, Dacron sutures are set in the sclera surrounding the lesion and tied over Silastic sponges, causing the outer shell of the eye to be pushed toward the elevated retina. If an encircling band is to be used, belt loops will be made in the sclera in four quadrants with Beaver blades nos. 64 and 66. A Silastic band no. 40 will be passed 360 degrees around the eye through the belt loops, and a self-holding Watzke sleeve will be applied to the band

to maintain a predetermined circumference. This causes a 360-degree constriction of the outer coats into the eye.

3. If drainage of subretinal fluid is desired, an area is chosen under direct visualization, where a significant fluid level exists under the retina, and a diathermy mark is made on the sclera. The sclera is split to the choroid, and a preplaced suture is put in place. A small amount of diathermy is applied to the choroid bed. A needle is then used to puncture the choroid into the subretinal space with subsequent drainage of fluid. The preplaced suture is tied.

SCLERAL RESECTION

An incision is made into the sclera, and a scleral flap is dissected both anteriorly and posteriorly from the original incision. Diathermy can be used in this bed or cryotherapy placed under direct visualization. Preserved eye bank sclera or a groove piece no. 20 may be sutured into the bed using a Supramid suture no. 4-0 or Dacron sutures no. 5-0 with or without an encircling band as previously described. Drainage of subretinal fluid may be accomplished as previously described.

A culture is taken at the end of surgery, and a subconjunctival injection of penicillin and gentamycin is given routinely unless contraindicated. The conjunctiva is closed with a selected suture material, and the eye is patched.

## Photocoagulation, laser, and cryotherapy treatments

CONSIDERATIONS. Certain localized detachments, sites of potential pathological conditions, tumors, and some vascular proliferative diseases, for example, diabetic retinopathy, can be treated without opening the conjunctiva. The mode of therapy is selected by the surgeon according to the location and type of lesion he is attempting to treat. The patient's pupil is dilated preoperatively, and a retrobulbar anesthetic is used. The purpose is to form an adhesion between the retina and pigment epithelium or to destroy proliferating blood vessels or tumors.

## SURGERY OF THE CONJUNCTIVA

CONSIDERATIONS. The conjunctiva of the eye is elastic, and there is an abundance of it. Traumatic lacerations caused by injury and deficits due to excision of tumors, cysts, nevi, or pterygium can usually be repaired by simple undermining and suture.

## Pterygium excision

DEFINITION. A pterygium is a fleshy, triangular encroachment onto the cornea, which occurs nasally and tends to be bilateral. When the pterygium encroaches on the visual axis, it is removed surgically (Fig. 9-31).

SETUP, PREPARATION OF THE PATIENT, AND ANESTHESIA

1 Williams lid speculum
1 Mosquito hemostat
1 Quevedo utility forceps
1 Fine conjunctival forceps with teeth
1 Lester forceps
1 Bard-Parker knife handle no. 3 with blade no. 15
1 Beaver knife handle with blade no. 64
1 Stevens scissors
1 Kalt needle holder
1 Hildreth cautery with white (hot) tip

OPERATIVE PROCEDURE. The major steps in the McReynolds technique are described in Fig. 9-31.

Pterygium can also be excised totally and the limbus treated with a cautery. The conjunctiva can then be closed, or the sclera can be left bare.

## Excisional biopsies

Any suspicious lesion of the conjunctiva can be removed by simple elliptical excision for pathological examination. The conjunctiva may or may not be closed, depending on the surgeon's particular technique.

## Reformation of cul-de-sacs (mucous membrane graft)

CONSIDERATIONS. In cases of infections, for example, trachoma, or chemical burns, there may be severe scarring and contractures of the conjunctiva and underlying

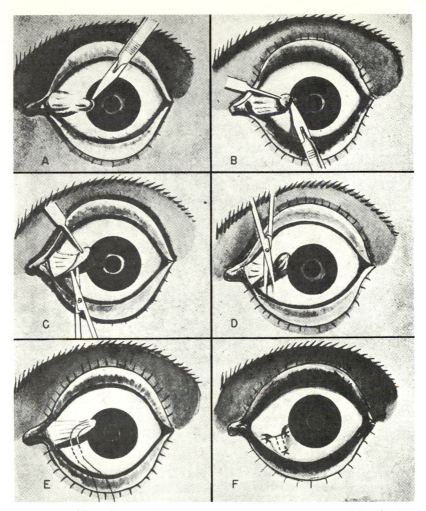

**Fig. 9-31.** McReynolds technique for pterygium repair. **A,** Cornea around head of pterygium is incised. **B,** Pterygium is dissected up, leaving clear cornea. **C,** Lower margin of pterygium is dissected up, and whole pterygium freed from sclera. **D,** Pocket is created in lower cul-de-sac. **E,** Double-armed suture is passed through head of pterygium, and sutures are passed down deep into fornix, to emerge above conjunctiva. **F,** Pterygium is drawn down into tunnel and conjunctiva closed. (From Fox, S. A.: Ophthalmic plastic surgery, ed. 3, New York, 1963, Grune & Stratton, Inc.)

tissues leading to motility problems, exposure problems, etc. Simple dissection is usually not satisfactory, and extra mucous membrane is required. This may be obtained from excess conjunctiva from the opposite eye, if available, or a mucous membrane graft may be obtained from the oral cavity.

**SETUP, PREPARATION OF THE PATIENT, AND ANESTHESIA.** A basic pterygium set is needed, plus a plastic tray for taking the mucous membrane graft.

A local or general anesthetic is used.

**OPERATIVE PROCEDURE**

1. An anesthetic solution is injected into the mucous membrane of the lower lip or the lateral wall of the mouth with a separate set of instruments. An elliptical incision is made with a blade no. 15, (if the incision is made into the lateral wall, the opening of the parotid duct must be avoided) and a thin, full-thickness layer of mucous membrane is removed by sharp

dissection. The wound is approximated with black silk suture no. 4-0.

A second method is the use of an electric Castroviejo dermatome. The mucous membrane is then always obtained from the lower lip.

2. The mucous membrane graft is placed in a Neosporin solution, the surgeon is re-gowned in a sterile gown, and another set of sterile instruments is used for reconstruction of the cul-de-sac.

### REFERENCES

1. Becker, S.: Cryosurgery of cataract. In Becker, B., and Burde, R. M.: Current concepts in ophthalmology, ed. 2, St. Louis, 1969, The C. V. Mosby Co.
2. Havener, W. H.: Ocular pharmacology, ed. 2, St. Louis, 1970, The C. V. Mosby Co.
3. Hogan, M. S., and Zimmerman, L. E.: Ophthalmic pathology, Philadelphia, 1962, W. B. Saunders Co.
4. Johnston, G. P., and Okun, E.: Evaluation of cryotherapy in retina surgery. In Becker, B., and Burde, R. M.: Current concepts in ophthalmology, ed. 2, St. Louis, 1969, The C. V. Mosby Co.
5. Last, R. J.: Wolff's anatomy of the eye and orbit, Philadelphia, 1968, W. B. Saunders Co.
6. Stallard, H. B.: Eye surgery, ed. 3, Baltimore, 1958, The Williams & Wilkins Co.

CHAPTER **10**

# Reconstructive plastic surgery

PAUL M. WEEKS and JUNE MUSTERMAN

## SCOPE

The specialty of plastic surgery is not limited to a single anatomical area or biological system. The specialty includes repair of a broad spectrum of congenital and acquired deformities, that is, resurfacing of burns, repair of cleft lip and palate, excision of neoplasms, reconstructive surgery of operative defects, cosmetic procedures, and functional reconstruction as in the hand.

The major portion of a plastic surgeon's practice deals with the correction of congenital defects such as cleft lip and cleft palate, ear deformities (for example, "lop" ears and microtia), syndactyly, hypospadias, hemangiomas, and hairy nevi.

In most medical centers today the plastic surgeon plays a major role in the treatment of the burn patient, helping to prevent many postburn complications that were seen frequently in previous years. The technique of transplanting tissues (skin, fascia, cartilage, bone, tendons, etc.) has been developed and advanced by the plastic surgeon.

Facial disfigurement from whatever cause is of primary concern to the plastic surgeon. Corrective operative procedures are considered both "reconstructive" and "esthetic." The practice of plastic surgery requires imagination, art, and skill. There is need for bold planning—such plans being executed with attention to detail and utmost concern for and gentle handling of tissues. The effectiveness of any recon-

struction depends on attention to myriad small operative details and can be maintained only by carefully applied dressings and conscientious postoperative care by the surgeon. Any other philosophy may result in failure of even the best planned procedure.

The techniques of plastic surgery require particular attention to the skin and soft tissues, relating to the excision of skin lesions, closure of skin wounds, skin grafts and flaps, and Z-plasty. The basic principles of plastic surgical techniques are (1) atraumatic handling of tissues, (2) placement of incisions in or parallel to the natural lines and folds of the skin, and (3) closure of the wound by measures appropriate to desired result.

Examples of representative cases will be presented in this chapter. Since anatomy and physiology of the various parts of the body have been included in other chapters, they will not be repeated here.

## PSYCHOLOGICAL APPROACH TO DEFORMITIES

Physical attractiveness is a dominant cultural value in the world today. This is a tremendous disadvantage to the disfigured. Physical deformity, particularly of the face and hands, may evoke negative reactions from others. These areas are the "contact" points in our daily relationships with one another. The differential treatment and devaluation of those who look different may

produce far more serious social and psychological consequences than the physical defect itself. Dr. Mayo has said, "Every human being has the divine right to look human and to resemble his fellow man." The rehabilitation of patients who have acquired disfigurements from trauma or disease depends not only on the reconstructive surgery but also on the degree of sensitivity displayed by those administering care to the psychological and emotional needs of the patient. The nurse is in a strategic position to reassure the patient with an attitude of matter-of-fact acceptance. Indeed, nowhere in medicine is the nurse more important in understanding and helping the patient than in the plastic surgery field. Such nursing care begins with admission to the hospital.

The surgeon must be aware that sympathetic understanding of the patient's psychological makeup contributes materially to the ultimate success of the surgical procedure. It is important that it be made clear to the patient what may or may not be anticipated from each operation, since hopes are high and the expected results are necessarily less than those for which the patient or surgeon hopes. Understanding avoids future disappointments. Since the normal person wants to look as good as possible, this is the aim of plastic surgery.

## GENERAL NURSING CONSIDERATIONS

**PREOPERATIVE PREPARATION OF THE PATIENT.** Cleanliness is essential for success in this type of surgery and should never be taken for granted. In nearly all operations, it is desirable for the operative site and adjacent areas to be washed with soap and water the night before (with brush if hand or foot, followed by manicure or pedicure). The hair should be shampooed if incisions are to be made in or near the hairline or if the hair is to be included in postoperative bandages. Men should come to the operating room recently shaved and women without cosmetics. Outpatients should be so advised.

Ordinarily, all areas that will be exposed at the time of operation and require shaving should be shaved. This is true of donor areas except when the graft is to be applied to the face, inside the mouth, or inside the orbit to be sure that hair-bearing skin is not transferred to these places. Shaving of scalp areas should be done by the surgeon himself. Eyebrows are NEVER shaved.

Particular attention should be given to oral hygiene in patients having general anesthesia and all patients having operations in or near the mouth. In operations in which the contour of the mouth and lips is important, the surgeon may want the patient to keep dentures in the mouth.

For general anesthesia, it is necessary that the patient be in a fasting condition. This is seldom necessary for administration of local anesthetics.

The preoperative medication should be administered at the proper time so that the patient gets the optimum results.

The local anesthetic is supplied by the scrubbed nursing team member from her supply table to the individual Mayo stand for administration by the surgeon.

**POSITIONING AND DRAPING OF PATIENTS.** The supine position is best for major operations and for patients under general anesthesia and is preferred for all work unless the operative site otherwise requires. Comfort and safety of the patient is attended to as carefully as in any other surgery (Chapter 7). The prepping and draping procedures are more extensive than in most other types of surgery because it may be necessary to expose important related features to permit wide undermining of the incisions and to avoid cumbersome drapes sewed to the skin, allowing freedom of movement while maintaining the sterile field.

For operations about the face and neck, both areas are completely painted with antiseptic of choice, being careful to keep it out of the patient's eyes. The prep solution is supplied from the nurse's table on a clamped sponge. Two sterile towels are placed under the head, the lower one to

cover the headrest, and the upper to wrap around the hair. An additional moisture barrier towel is used under the lower towel for cases in which drainage may be extensive. Additional towels are placed laterally along either side of the neck and the main sheet covers from the clavicles to the feet.

For draping of extremities, see specific cases.

A good suction apparatus is a necessary requisite for most work. Indeed, it may be vital in maintaining an airway in some cases; additional tubing is always available in case of malfunction. The sterile suction tubing with tip is clamped to the main sterile sheet, with the distal end connected to the vacuum source immediately after draping. Lights are then focused for optimum efficiency. "Surgery is vision."

CARE OF SPECIMENS. The importance of careful handling and accurate labeling of specimens and tissue biopsies cannot be overemphasized. The surgical outcome for many patients is dependent on the laboratory report. Procedure policies of the hospital must be familiar to the personnel entrusted with specimen care and conscientiously adhered to.

DRESSINGS. Dressings are of more importance to the plastic surgical operation than to any other type of surgery. The results hoped for *depend* on the skillful application of dressings. The type used depends on the results desired. In general, a dressing should accomplish fixation of the affected part and even, gentle pressure over the wound and allow for drainage and comfort to the patient. Dressings are applied only after complete hemostasis and cleansing of the surrounding area to minimize infection. A lubricating or nonadherent material is placed on the wound to prevent sticking of the dressing on removal, followed by sufficient bulky material to evenly distribute moderate pressure over a wide area (to prevent excessive swelling and discomfort) applied in such a fashion as to immobilize. To be done correctly, the dressing should be applied while the patient is still under anesthesia. Therefore an abundant supply

of dressing materials should be readily available on the nurse's sterile supply table. However, no attempt should be made to save time at this stage of treatment, since the operation and the surgical dressing are intimately and indispensably associated in plastic surgery.

Materials for compressive dressings include plain fine-mesh gauze, fine-mesh grease gauze rolls, Kling and Kerlix rolls, mechanic's waste, acrylic fiber, cotton, abdominal pads, eye pads, and sterile tape.

It is the nurse's responsibility to see that an adequate shelf count is maintained for all sterile supplies. These may include the following:

> Fine-mesh grease gauze rolls with 5% bismuth tribromophenate (Xeroform) and 5% scarlet red ointment
> Unexposed x-ray film for patterns
> Sterile tape, ½ in. and 1 in.
> Dermatome blades and tapes
> Buttons and lead shot
> Drill bits and Bovie tips
> Penrose-type drains and catheters
> Packing
> Ointments and medications
> Oxidized cellulose (Oxycel), Surgicel absorbable hemostat, and Gelfoam

It is also the nurse's responsibility to see that all sharp instruments are *sharp* when used by the surgeon. It is preferable to use a suitable solution for soaking of scissors and delicate sharp instruments between cases rather than repeated autoclaving.

SPECIAL MECHANICAL DEVICES. Frequent use is made of special mechanical devices such as drills and dermatomes. The scrubbed nursing team member should inquire ahead of time to determine need during a specific case. The device should be sterilized in the appropriate manner, and it must be in working order. The manufacturer's instructions on special care should be followed after each use. The following types of mechanical devices are used:

> Hand drill
> Motor drill
> Pneumatic drill (used with nitrogen supply tank)

Hand-operated dermatomes ("freehand" Ferris-Smith knife, Padgett and Reese dermatomes)

Motor driven (Brown electric) dermatome

Pneumatic dermatome

Hand-operated mesh-graft dermatome

Dermabrader, pneumatic

Dermatattoo, pneumatic

ALLOPLASTIC MATERIALS. The capabilities of the plastic reconstructive surgeon have been enhanced in recent years by the development of alloplastic materials. To be acceptable, such materials had to meet certain criteria: the prosthesis should (1) cause minimal reaction, (2) be noncarcinogenic, and (3) have physical properties similar to the tissue it is replacing.

The most popular material in present-day surgical use is silicone. Several types are used in plastic reconstructive surgery: silicone rubber or Silastic, silicone sponge, silicone sheeting, and blocks of varying hardness. Silicone is also made into a variety of preformed prostheses, such as the breast, ear, nose, and chin units. The units come in various sizes and may be supplied in a nonsterile state requiring autoclaving prior to use. Silicone may be sterilized a number of times without any change in physical properties.

It must be emphasized here that in the handling of silicone—and all plastic materials—care must be taken to avoid touching the prosthesis with the bare hand at any time. Persons handling the unit should wear gloves (without powder) or use instruments to eliminate transfer of skin oils that may contaminate the prosthesis and result in marked increase of tissue reaction. Silicone tends to develop a static charge on its surface, and it can attract and hold lint, dust, etc. Should the prosthesis become contaminated, it should be scrubbed with a hot water and soap solution (Ivory or pHisoHex). (Do not use oil-based soaps or detergents: see manufacturer's instructions.) Rinse copiously in tap water. Then sterilize by autoclaving under standard conditions. The sterile prosthesis is placed on the scrubbed nursing team member's supply table and covered with a sterile towel until use.

## BASIC SETUP

The basic sterile supply table setup used at Barnes Hospital for many years evolved through the teaching of Dr. Blair, Dr. Brown, and others, with the help of the nursing staff under Miss Everil McDavitt. It involves the use of two sterile supply tables.

To have the scrubbed nursing team member remain sterile throughout the schedule is a saving of time and materials. All the sterile supplies and instruments for the day's schedule are kept on the two large tables, which the scrubbed nursing team member alone touches. Individual Mayo tables with instruments and sterile supplies for the use of the surgeon for each operation are set up from the supply tables as they are needed. No operating team member may come into contact with the scrubbed nursing team member or the tables at any time. The scrubbed nursing team member is not to touch any part of the operative field, other members of the team, or the Mayo tables.

Additional instruments and sutures are to be dropped on the Mayo table by her or handed directly to a member of the operative team with Ochsner transfer forceps. By means of this forceps, which is left clamped to a corner of the Mayo table, she can keep the Mayo table neat and clean as necessary unless an additional scrubbed nursing team member is provided. The surgeon occasionally requests that an individual scrubbed nursing team member be provided for major operations.

This setup eliminates a great deal of waiting between operations, makes it possible to accommodate two operations at the same time, and, in addition, provides a large supply of sterile instruments and materials so that the surgeon does not have to wait if an unanticipated instrument is needed or if one is contaminated during the course of the operation. Without the constant interruptions of supplying the scrubbed nursing team member, the circulating nurses are free to efficiently carry out other duties such as tending the pa-

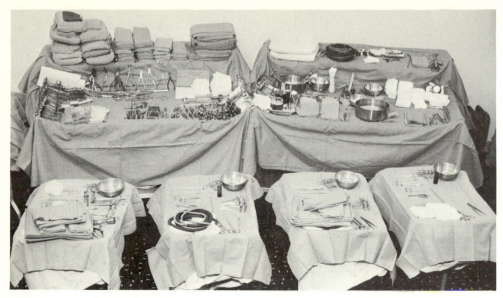

**Fig. 10-1.** Sterile supply table setup. The two sterile back tables contain instruments and supplies for the day's schedule; Mayo tables are set up for the first four procedures before the cases begin and are covered with sterile drapes until needed. (Courtesy K. Cramer Lewis, Washington University Department of Illustrations, St. Louis, Mo.)

tients, getting patients in and out promptly, etc. At the end of each operation the instruments from the Mayo tables are washed, resterilized, and returned to the scrubbed nursing team member to be ready for subsequent procedures. Instruments should be cooled and dry before being returned to the Mayo table for the surgeon's use.

Because of the type of surgery, vascularity of tissues involved, and careful technique by nursing team members, cross infection between patients is not a problem.

Careful technique should be a requisite of all types of surgery but cannot be over-emphasized in plastic surgery. It is to be expected that all personnel are adequately oriented and trained in the routine of the plastic surgery suite. Each should thoroughly understand the setup and what is expected of her. Good housekeeping techniques are as essential as good surgical techniques. Supplies on the sterile back tables include the following (Fig. 10-1):

**Linens and surgical drapes**

Sheets
Towels
Moisture-barrier drapes
Mayo table covers
Gowns and gloves
Stockinette rolls for extremities

**Sponges and dressing materials**

Large and small sponges
Abdominal pads (ABD's)
Pressure media such as mechanic's waste, acrylic (Acrilan) fiber, and cotton
Fine-mesh grease gauze according to surgeon's preference
Sterile tape
Packing (nasal)

**Suture material**

Various suture packs according to surgeons' routines

**Basin sets and solutions**

*Containers for stock skin prep solutions*
70% alcohol
About 3.5% tincture of iodine diluted with alcohol to the color of weak tea
Aqueous benzalkonium chloride (Zephiran), 1:5000, for mucous membrane
*Containers for local anesthetics*
Jar for stock supply of agent—2% procaine
Medicine glasses to supply anesthetic agent to individual Mayo table
Medicine glass for epinephrine, 1:1000, with medicine dropper

Basin of "weak epinephrine" (1:4 from above) for moistening folded sponges

Container for dyeing agent: alcoholic solution of 5% methylene blue and a number of bottles for use on individual Mayo tables

Large basin of normal saline solution and a number of small basins for individual Mayo tables

Instruments include a variety of the standard categories such as cutting, holding, clamping, and exposing (Chapter 5). Most are small scale for use on the delicate tissues usually involved. Additions include the following:

### Accessory instruments

Marking pens

Injection syringes, 3 ml. Luer-Lok, and 25-, 23-, and 19-gauge needles

Irrigating syringes (small Asepto)

Suction tubing and tubes ("pencil" or mastoid, neuro, antral)

Bovie cord, if needed

Probes, with eye and graduated, double-ended duct probes

### Special instruments for specific cases

Palate elevators and knife

Lip clamps

Rulers and caliper

Nasal and septal knives, saws, and rasps

Universal tooth extractors

Small bone cutters and rongeurs

Wire cutters

Drills

Dermatomes and blades

### Miscellaneous instruments

Applicator sticks

Tongue blades

Needle tray

Knife blades nos. 10, 11, 12, 15

Penrose-type drains

Catheters, red rubber Fr. no. 8-16

### Basic plastic Mayo setup (Fig. 10-2)

Knife handle with blade no. 15

Iris scissors

Schulte dissecting scissors

Brown-Adson forceps

Single skin hook

Double skin hook

6 Towel clamps, 3 in.

6 Mosquito hemostats, curved

6 Baby Ochsner forceps

Tissue forceps without teeth

Halsted clamp

Suture scissors

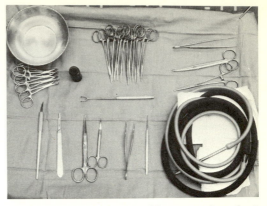

**Fig. 10-2.** Basic Mayo table setup for plastic surgery. (Courtesy K. Cramer Lewis, Washington University Department of Illustrations, St. Louis, Mo.)

Saline basin

Gauze sponges

Suction tubing and tip

Drape towels and sheet

Local anesthetic in medicine glass with syringe and needle (if required)

Marking pen and point, with dye (if needed)

Prep forceps and needle holders from nurse, as needed

## OPERATIONS
### Rhinoplasty

**DEFINITION.** Rhinoplasty might be considered the surgical answer to a psychological problem, with an excellent percentage of recovery. The operation may include any combination or all of the following stages: removal of the nasal hump, narrowing of the nose, adjusting the length of the nose, and remodeling of the nasal tip.

**CONSIDERATIONS.** Although the nose encloses the airways and is used to breathe and for sinus drainage, it is also the most prominent feature of the face. Deviations from normal (arising from trauma, racial or familial deformity, or other causes) may have to be restored to normal contour anatomy for the best function of the patient as a whole. Interference with normal expression, as in smiling, lip distortion, or aquilinity (especially in females) presents valid reasons for corrective rhinoplasty. Dramatic economic and career advantages have developed after nasal corrections, and rhinoplasty can generally be considered as

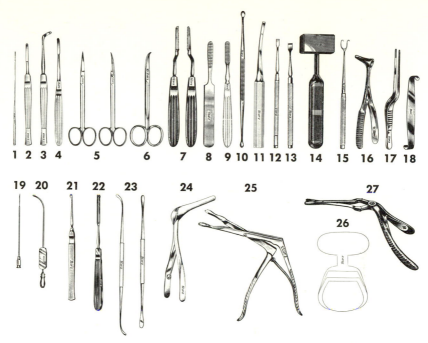

Fig. 10-3. Special instruments for rhinoplasty. **1,** Metal applicator; **2,** Joseph knife; **3,** Joseph knife, angled; **4,** Joseph elevator; **5,** Joseph scissors, straight and curved; **6,** Fomon lower lateral scissors; **7,** Brown-Joseph nasal saws, right and left; **8,** Brown rasp, upward stroke; **9,** Maltz rasp, downward stroke; **10,** curette; **11,** Blair chisel; **12,** Freer chisel; **13,** periosteotome; **14,** mallet; **15,** double skin hook; **16,** nasal speculum; **17,** bayonet forceps; **18,** S retractor. Additional instruments for septal resection. **19,** Tonsil needle; **20,** antral suction tube; **21,** Freer septum knife; **22,** Ballenger swivel knife; **23,** Freer elevators; **24,** septal speculum; **25,** Kofler septum forceps; **26,** assorted nasal splints; **27,** Jansen-Middleton septum forceps. (Courtesy Storz Surgical Instruments, St. Louis, Mo.)

giving new hope and status to persons burdened with deformed features.

**SETUP AND PREPARATION OF THE PATIENT.** Surgery is usually performed with the patient under local anesthesia, sometimes including topical 2% tetracaine (Pontocaine) on applicators. The routine head drape is used. Instruments used include the following:

**Basic plastic Mayo setup with local anesthetic**

2% procaine with 1:200,000 concentration of epinephrine in medicine glass

Syringe and 2 needles, 25- and 23-gauge (or according to surgeon's preference)

**Additions** (Fig. 10-3)

Metal applicators to introduce topical anesthetic

Nasal speculum

Nasal retractor, S-shaped

Freer knife, straight and angled

Joseph elevator

Double-ended Freer elevator

Nasal saws, right and left

Nasal rasps, "pusher" and "puller"

Bayonet forceps

Fomon right-angle scissors, 6½ in.

Nasal chisels, osteotomes and mallet

Sutures, silk or Ethiflex no. 5-0

Dressings, grease packing (Adaptic, 1 in., or Carbozine, ½ in.), sterile tape, aluminum splint

**Additional instruments for septal resection**

Septal speculum

Septal rongeurs and biters

Antral suction tip

Freer septal and Ballenger swivel knives

Tonsil needle for local anesthetic

Suture, chromic no. 4-0 or 5-0

**OPERATIVE PROCEDURE** (Fig. 10-4)

1. All incisions are made within the nose. The incisions are begun between the upper

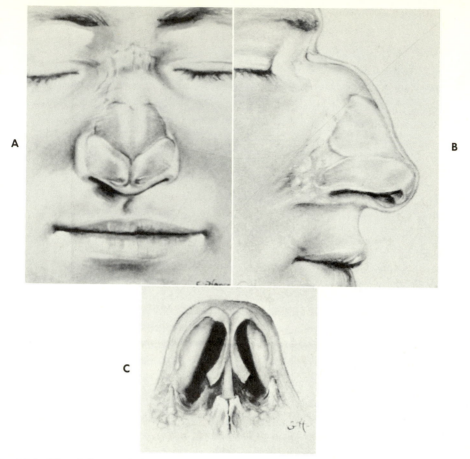

**Fig. 10-4.** The skeleton of the nose with soft tissues superimposed. (From Brown, J. B., and McDowell, F.: Plastic surgery of the nose, ed. 2, Springfield, Ill., 1965, Charles C Thomas, Publisher.)

and lower lateral cartilages and brought forward toward the tip of the septum and then pushed through the membranous septum to the opposite side of the nose to separate the columella and septum. A similar incision is made on the opposite side. Scissors are inserted through the incisions to elevate the skin of the nose to the level of the nasal bones. A Joseph elevator is inserted, and the periosteum and overlying nasal skin is elevated from the nasal bones over the entire nose.

2. Removal of the nasal hump is accomplished with a Joseph bayonet nasal saw (Fig. 10-5). The detached hump is removed as one section. Rasps are used to smooth bony edges.

3. Narrowing of the nose is accomplished after detaching the nasal bones from the septum in the midline and the maxilla laterally. The bones are outfractured and mobilized medially to narrow the nose.

4. Shortening of the nose is accomplished by a triangular resection of the nasal septum.

5. Reconstruction of the nasal tip is accomplished by trimming the upper and lower lateral cartilages through a second incision just within the nasal rim (Fig. 10-6).

6. All blood clots are removed from beneath the skin, and pressure is applied to the nose.

7. Skin edges are approximated and su-

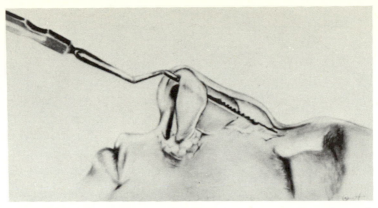

Fig. 10-5. Dorsal hump is removed with nasal saw. (From Brown, J. B., and McDowell, F.: Plastic surgery of the nose, ed. 2, Springfield, Ill., 1965, Charles C Thomas, Publisher.)

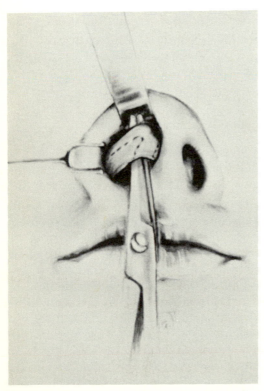

Fig. 10-6. Dotted line indicates the single hockey stick piece that can be excised to remove height, width, and length from the alar cartilage. (The large scissors are used merely for retraction.) (From Brown, J. B., and McDowell, F.: Plastic surgery of the nose, ed. 2, Springfield, Ill., 1965, Charles C Thomas, Publisher.)

tured with no. 5-0 silk. Dressings include nasal packs and an external nasal splint. (Postoperatively, the head is maintained in an elevated position, and ice packs may be applied to the face.)

### Cleft lip repair

CONSIDERATIONS. Satisfactory feeding is an immediate problem to the baby with a cleft lip. Since the psychic trauma to the parents and the feeding problem are lessened after closure, corrective surgery is done as early as possible. (A single cleft lip can be surgically corrected several days after birth.) However, this is not emergency surgery and is not done except under ideal conditions, with complete equipment and assistance available and the baby in good general health; the optimum time is about 3 months of age. The repair should be done with the greatest skill and accuracy, since it will markedly affect the patient's appearance throughout his entire life.

Repair of the cleft lip is directed toward reconstructing the upper lip so that the cleft side will equal the uncleft side in length and appearance (Fig. 10-7). Many operative procedures have been devised, using triangular, quadrangular, or other tissue flaps to repair the cleft. The procedure

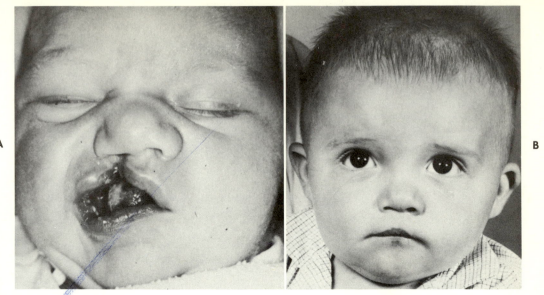

**Fig. 10-7. A,** Infant with complete unilateral cleft of the lip. **B,** Repair, 1 year later.

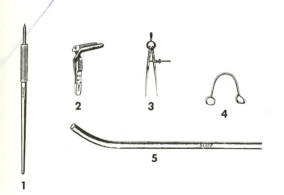

**Fig. 10-8.** Special instruments for cleft lip repair. **1,** Marking pen; **2,** lip clamp, right and left (used in pairs for hemostasis); **3,** caliper; **4,** Logan bow; **5,** ether insufflator (sometimes used to insufflate anesthetics in infants). (Courtesy Storz Surgical Instruments, St. Louis, Mo.)

described is the rotational advancement method of Millard.

**SETUP AND PREPARATION OF THE PATIENT.** The baby is usually "mummied" in a small sheet, his face prepped with alcohol, and a routine head drape used. The head and table pad are lowered slightly into the surgeon's lap as he sits at the head of the table facing the baby, who is upside down. The surgeon's hands are at rest, steadied on the baby's head. The availability of suction is of primary importance.

Supplies and instruments are as follows:

Basic plastic Mayo setup

**Additions** (Fig. 10-8)
Local anesthesia setup as desired for infiltration hemostasis
Knife handle no. 3 with blade no. 11
Dyeing agent and/or marking pen or no. 25 injection needle
Iris forceps
Bayonet forceps
Joseph elevator
Caliper
Lip clamps, right and left
Red rubber catheter no. 12 Fr. for use with suction tip
Small folded sponges moistened with weak epinephrine solution

**Optional supplies**
Logan bow
Silicone ointment for suture line dressing
Tongue stitch of heavy silk no. 2-0 on large palate needle
Ether insufflator if surgeon desires insufflation anesthesia

**OPERATIVE PROCEDURE** (Fig. 10-9)
1. The vestige of the cupid's bow and the philtrum dimple is identified. Starting

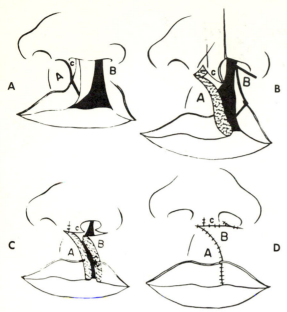

**Fig. 10-9.** Rotation-advancement method. Complete unilateral cleft of the lip. **A,** Rotation incision marked so that cupid's bow-dimple component A will rotate down into normal position; flap c will advance into columella and then form nostril sill. **B,** Flap A has dropped down, flap c has advanced into the columella, and flap B has been marked. **C,** Flap B is being advanced into the rotation gap; the white skin roll flap is interdigitated at the mucocutaneous junction line. **D,** Scar is maneuvered into strategic position where it is hidden at the nasal base and floor, philtrum column, and interdigitated at the mucocutaneous junction. (From Millard, D. R. In Grabb, W. C., and Smith, J. W., editors: Plastic surgery, a concise guide to clinical practice, Boston, Mass., 1968, Little, Brown & Co.)

at the peak of the cupid's bow on the non-cleft side, a line is measured to the midline and these points marked on the mucocutaneous junction with methylene blue. The distance between these points will determine the third point along the mucocutaneous junction line, which indicates the future cupid's bow peak on the cleft side.

2. An incision curves from this third point along the mucocutaneous junction to beneath the columella.

3. A flap is developed on the cleft side of the lip to be incorporated into the repair.

4. The muscles are approximated, and the skin and mucosa are sutured.

5. A Logan bow is applied with adhesive strips to the cheeks to minimize tension on the repair.

### Cleft palate repair

CONSIDERATIONS. Repair of the cleft palate is done to gain closure of the palate and provide adequate length to the palate to permit velopharyngeal closure.

The primary motive for surgical reconstruction is the desire to improve faulty speech commonly resulting from this deformity. Obvious benefits are improved hygiene of the mouth, nose, and middle ear and later the facilitation of dental prosthetics. It is important to emphasize that proper operative closure is necessary to avoid further hampering the already deficient muscle power of the existing palate. The operation is performed when the child is about 18 months old.

SETUP AND PREPARATION OF THE PATIENT. The operation is done with the surgeon sitting at the head of the table facing the child, who is placed upside down. The child's head is positioned at the end of the table with his neck hyperextended and his body elevated by a pad under his trunk so that blood will run into the nasopharynx rather than into the trachea. The tongue is retracted forward with a tongue suture held by the first assistant, who also employs suction to keep the airway clear and the field visible. It is important for all members of the team to develop constant awareness of breath sounds and to correct instantly any obstruction. (The circulating nurse must ensure that the suction equipment is operating efficiently and that the lighting is adequate.) Endotracheal anesthesia is generally used. Skin and endotracheal tubes are given an antiseptic prep before the routine head drape. Eyes are protected from corneal injury. A benzalkonium chloride (Zephiran) prep may be used in the oral cavity.

Supplies and instruments are as follows:

Basic plastic Mayo setup

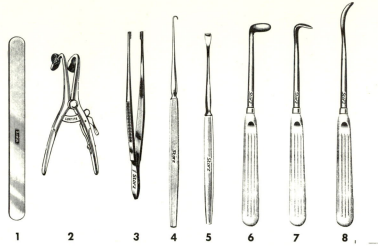

**Fig. 10-10.** Special instruments for cleft palate repair. **1,** Malleable retractor (for controlling the tongue); **2,** Denhart mouth gag; **3,** Brown forceps, 6 in.; **4,** palate hook; **5,** palate knife; **6 to 8,** palate elevators. (Courtesy Storz Surgical Instruments, St. Louis, Mo.)

**Additions** (Fig. 10-10)

Palate elevators, straight and right-angled
Palate retractor
Palate hook
Palate knife
Medium Brown forceps
Malleable metal spatula
Mouth gag—Dingman or Denhardt
Tongue retention suture, silk no. 2-0 on heavy palate needle
Red rubber catheter no. 14 Fr. for use with suction tip
Small folded sponges moistened with weak epinephrine solution

**Sutures**

Silk or Ethiflex no. 4-0
Chromic catgut no. 3-0

**OPERATIVE PROCEDURE** (Fig. 10-11)

1. Incisions are made in the form of a W, with the peak of the W at the most proximal extent of the cleft.

2. Through the skin incisions the mucoperiosteum of the palate is elevated with a palatal elevator. Bleeding is controlled with sponges soaked in weak epinephrine (1:100,000).

3. As the periosteum is elevated, the palatine vessels are identified emerging from the palatine foramen posteriorly. These are preserved.

4. The edges of the cleft are excised, and the muscle bellies of the soft palate are exposed.

5. The hook of the pterygoid process is palpated and infractured to release the tension in the tensor muscle of the palatine velum to permit closure.

6. Muscle closure is accomplished with no. 5-0 suture. The palate is closed posteriorly with black silk and catgut to prevent irritation of the posterior pharynx.

7. Anteriorly, vertical mattress sutures permit closure of the mucoperiosteal flaps.

## Surgery for prominent ears

**DEFINITION.** Surgical correction of prominent or "lop" ears. This involves some mechanical method of holding the ears back into the desired position, with or without incising the cartilage, until healing fixes the ears as desired.

**CONSIDERATIONS.** The deformity of protuberant ears (or promenauries) may be the cause of much grief and embarrassment to the patient. Proper diagnosis and correction is as important here as in other deformities. Surgical correction is usually done when the child is 4 to 5 years of age, before he enters school to minimize any

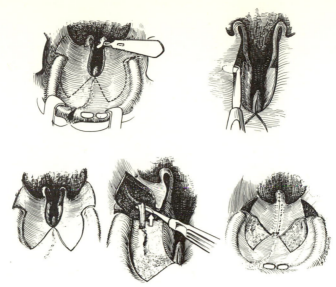

**Fig. 10-11.** Closure of the soft palate combined with a lengthening operation. Mucosal flaps are also raised from the floor of the nostrils to provide coverage for that part of the palatal flaps left raw by the lengthening operation. An additional incision is shown in the midportion of the soft palate on the nasal side parallel to the fibers of the levator muscle (upper right). The apices of these incisions are approximated so as to constrict the diameter of the naso-pharynx at the level of the levator eminence. The major palatine vessels are preserved and lengthened by stretching them out of their canals (lower center). (From Randall, P. In Grabb, W. C., and Smith, J. W., editors: Plastic surgery, a concise guide to clinical practice, Boston, Mass., 1968, Little, Brown & Co.)

psychological effect of the deformity. Requests for the operation by adults are not uncommon. Anesthesia may be either local or general.

**SETUP AND PREPARATION OF THE PATIENT.** The patient is placed in the supine position. In some cases, shaving the postauricular hair may be indicated, followed by the routine skin prep. The outer canal is cleaned with cotton applicators moistened with the prep solution. The routine head drape is used with the ears well exposed. The patient's head is turned with the affected ear up, with the lower one padded to avoid a pressure injury.

The basic plastic Mayo setup with marking pen is used. Additional instruments include the following:

Caliper
Ruler
Joseph elevator
Sutures (surgeon's preference)

**Dressings**

Bismuth tribromophenate (Xeroform) gauze
Cotton for ample padding
Acrylic fiber or mechanic's waste
3 in. Kling roll

**OPERATIVE PROCEDURE** (Fig. 10-12)

1. An elliptical incision behind the ears allows removal of excessive skin and permits exposure of the cartilage.

2. The auricular cartilage at its antihelical rim is either scored or cut, or sutures are placed into it to re-create the contours of the normal ears.

3. This can be followed in certain cases by approximating the concha to the mastoid process to hold the total ear back.

4. On completion of the second side, moderate compression dressings are applied.

## Surgery for microtia

**DEFINITION.** Surgical reconstruction of absent portions of the ear.

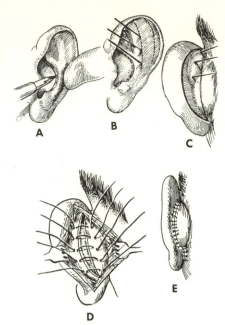

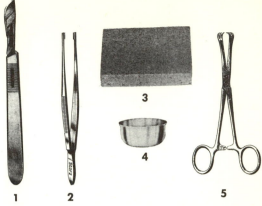

Fig. 10-13. Separate sterile table setup for preparation of implant. 1, Knife handle with no. 10 blade (for carving silicone block or cartilage); 2, Brown forceps; 3, cutting board; 4, basin with saline; 5, Lahey thyroid traction forceps (for firm grasping of the implant material). (Courtesy Storz Surgical Instruments, St. Louis, Mo.)

Fig. 10-12. A, Pressure applied over the body of the antihelix to throw the antihelix into prominence for marking by pen and ink. B, Lines of incision outlined on the lateral aspect of the ear and straight needles passed through the ear to serve as a guide for incision on the posterior aspect. C, Skin excised and raised from the scalp aspect of the ear, with the lines of incision guided by the needles. D, Crescent of cartilage removed following the proposed line of the superior crus. E, The completed postauricular incision. (Redrawn from Wood-Smith, D., and Porowski, P., editors: Nursing care of the plastic surgery patient, St. Louis, 1967, The C. V. Mosby Co., and Converse, J. M., editor: Reconstructive plastic surgery, vol. 3, Philadelphia, 1964, W. B. Saunders Co.)

**CONSIDERATIONS.** Microtias come in all varieties in that there may be just portions of the ear missing or the entire ear may be missing. This is a difficult problem to deal with in that the tissues involved in an ear (that is, cartilage, skin, subcutaneous tissue, etc.) are of a thin and delicate quality. The absence of an ear is an especially noticeable deformity in males—thus the best reconstruction possible is well worthwhile.

**SETUP AND PREPARATION OF THE PATIENT.** The same procedure is followed as outlined for prominent ears. A separate Mayo setup

used for preparation of the implant material, if needed, includes the following (Fig. 10-13):

No. 10 knife blade on no. 3 handle
Medium Brown forceps
Lahey thyroid traction forceps
Cutting board
Basin of saline solution

If the surgeon plans to use the patient's costal cartilage, a separate Mayo setup is used for this procedure and includes the following:

  Basic plastic Mayo setup
  No. 10 knife blade
2 Rake retractors
1 Key elevator
1 Duckbill rongeur
  Doyen rib raspatorys, right and left
1 Plenk-Matson rib raspatory
1 Alexander costal periosteotome
1 Small rib shears
1 Liston bone-cutting forceps

**OPERATIVE PROCEDURE.** The most commonly employed technique, requiring multiple-stage procedures, has been described by Tanzer. At the first stage the ear remnants are repositioned to properly orient the ear.

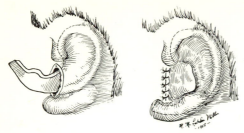

Fig. 10-14. Embedment of cartilage implant under mastoid skin after excision of previous scar. (From Tanzer, R. C., and Rueckert, F. In Grabb, W. C., and Smith J. W., editors: Plastic surgery, a concise guide to clinical practice, Boston, Mass, 1968, Little, Brown & Co.)

Simultaneously, or at a later date, the cartilaginous framework may be inserted. This framework may be carved using the patient's costal cartilages, or a silicone implant may be utilized (Fig. 10-14). Many months later, subsequent procedures are directed to elevating the ear from the side of the head. The reconstructed ear is elevated from the retroauricular area, and a split-thickness skin graft is placed in the raw defect. This is the major portion of the reconstructive procedure, yet small adjustments are needed and can be accomplished as indicated.

## Blepharoplasty

DEFINITION. Excision of redundant skin of eyelid and excessive periorbital fat.

CONSIDERATIONS. This procedure may be done alone or in combination with a rhytidectomy. In the latter procedure the blepharoplasty is performed first.

SETUP AND PREPARATION OF THE PATIENT. The patient is placed in the supine position and the routine prep and drapes are used.

The instruments used are as follows:

Basic plastic Mayo setup with addition of eyelid forceps with multiple nonpenetrating teeth
Sutures as desired by surgeon

**Dressings, when used**

Ophthalmic ointment to cornea
Grease gauze
Eye pads

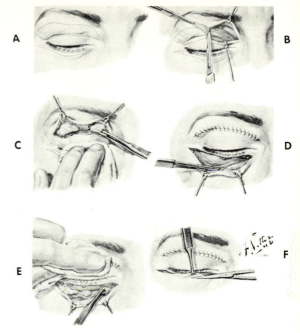

Fig. 10-15. Blepharoplasty for baggy eyelids. A, Areas of proposed skin excision marked out with methylene blue or marking pen. B, Strip of skin excised from upper lid; fat pad shining through orbital fascia and orbicular muscle of the eye. C, Orbital fascia opened in two places (medially and laterally). Pressure on eyeball causes fat pads to bulge. They are teased out meticulously. D, Upper lid incision sutured with no. 6-0 silk and continuous stitches. Orbicular muscle fibers are being separated from skin. E, Orbital fascia opened; fat pads bulge due to digital pressure and are teased out meticulously. F, Skin tailored to fit and sutured. (Copyright 1967 CIBA-GEIGY CORPORATION. Reproduced with permission from CLINICAL SYMPOSIA, illustrated by Frank H. Netter, M.D. All rights reserved.)

OPERATIVE PROCEDURE (Fig. 10-15)

1. An elliptical incision in the upper lid permits excision of excessive skin and exposure of underlying muscle.

2. An incision is made into the orbicular muscle, and, with pressure on the lower lid, the excessive fat is expressed into the wound.

3. The fat is clamped, ligated, and excised. No muscle suturing is done.

4. The skin is closed with fine multiple sutures.

5. An incision is made just beneath the last line on the lower lid.

6. The skin is elevated from the orbicular muscle.

7. An incision is made in the orbicular muscle and the herniated fat exposed by pressing on the upper lid.

8. The fat lobules are caught, ligated, and divided.

9. Skin closure is accomplished with interrupted fine sutures after discarding a minimum of tissue from the lower lid.

## Rhytidectomy

**DEFINITION.** Excision of excessively wrinkled skin of the face and chin by elevating the skin of the face and chin through incisions made virtually unnoticeable by their positioning in front of and behind the ear and neck.

**CONSIDERATIONS.** Redundant skin of the face and neck is usually associated with the aging process, and frequently a blepharoplasty is done at the same time.

**SETUP AND PREPARATION OF THE PATIENT.** The patient is placed on the operating table in the supine position with particular attention to comfort because the procedure is time consuming (Chapter 7). General anesthesia is tolerated best by most patients, but local anesthesia provides better hemostasis. A small braid is made from about a 1-inch section of hair in the temporal region, and the braids from each side are tied together and taped down. The face and neck are given the routine iodine and alcohol prep, including the ears. The head drapes are clipped or sewn in place (with ears and hairline exposed) so that there will be no slipping or movement with turning of the head. None of the hair is shaved preoperatively.

The basic plastic Mayo setup (including marking pen) is used, with these additions:

Rhytidectomy scissors
Additional small towel clamps
Long tissue forceps
Sutures as desired by the surgeon

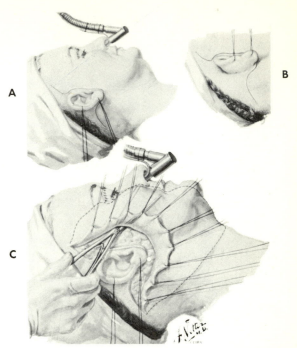

**Fig. 10-16.** Rhytidectomy: line of incision and undermining. **A,** Traction sutures of no. 4-0 silk placed in auricle; temporal incision curved posteriorly to better support upward pull. **B,** Incision carried under the earlobe, then curved posteriorly upward and then caudad toward the midline. **C,** Skin undermined almost to the nasolabial fold, the area of the mental foramen, and to the midline of the neck as far down as the thyroid cartilage. Care is taken to avoid injury to submandibular branches of facial nerve and facial artery. (Copyright 1967 CIBA-GEIGY CORPORATION. Reproduced with permission from CLINICAL SYMPOSIA, illustrated by Frank H. Netter, M.D. All rights reserved.)

Dressings needed at the close of the case include the following:

Grease gauze
Acrylic (Acrilan) fiber and cotton
Gauze sponges
Kling or Kerlix rolls

**OPERATIVE PROCEDURE** (Figs. 10-16 and 10-17)

1. The incisions are planned so as to extend from within the hairline in the temporal area down in front of the ear within a vertical fold and then continued around the lobule of the ear along the hairline of the neck posteriorly.

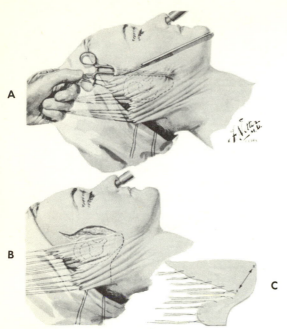

**Fig. 10-17.** Rhytidectomy: removal of superfluous skin. **A,** Skin drawn upward to proper degree of tension and incision made along posterior margin of clamp. **B,** Incision continued upward around posterior margin of auricle and then backward to excise specimen. **C,** Specimen: distance x to x' usually measures 1 to 2 inches. (Copyright 1967 CIBA-GEIGY CORPORATION. Reproduced with permission from CLINICAL SYMPOSIA, illustrated by Frank H. Netter, M.D. All rights reserved.)

2. The skin of the face is completely undermined almost to the nasolabial fold through the incision described.

3. Traction upward and posteriorly lifts the skin into its new position.

4. Excessive skin is excised.

5. Careful closure of the skin edges with fine subcutaneous and skin sutures is obtained.

6. A compressive dressing is applied.

### Surgical treatment of facial fractures

GENERAL CONSIDERATIONS. Facial bone fractures may be accompanied by soft tissue lacerations or actual tissue loss. Associated injuries can include skull fracture, brain and spinal cord damage, or damage to the orbit and the eye itself. The most immediate concern in emergency treatment is an adequate airway for the patient. Airway obstruction may be caused by bone displacement, blood clots, or foreign bodies. These must be removed immediately. A tracheostomy (see Chapter 8 for procedure) may be indicated not only because of obstruction but also because of concomitant cranial or chest injury. Of almost equal concern is control of hemorrhage. Moderate local pressure may be sufficient, or ligatures and packing may be necessary. After establishment of a patent airway and control of hemorrhage a careful diagnosis of other injuries is made, and, if advisable, the treatment of the facial injuries is delayed until the patient's general condition warrants. Rarely should the fractures be permitted to heal in malposition, however. The extent of the fractures is determined by palpation of the facial bones and by roentgenographic examination. When diagnosis is completed, the plan of treatment is established. Reduction and immobilization are the two basic principles used by the plastic surgeon in the treatment of facial fractures. Methods vary and often are accomplished with the assistance of the oral surgeon. Appropriate repair of overlying soft tissues after careful cleansing and debridement is mandatory.

### Surgical treatment of fractured mandible and maxilla

CONSIDERATIONS (Fig. 10-18). In treating fractures of the mandible or the maxilla there are two important considerations: (1) to restore the proper occlusion of the teeth and (2) to restore the esthetic contours of the face. Reduction and fixation is usually accomplished by exposing the fracture and direct wiring. Immobilization is usually accomplished by wiring the teeth together for a period of approximately 6 weeks. In surgical treatment of facial fractures as with any surgery involving the mouth, one is working in a contaminated field. Two separate setups are used: one for working in the mouth and the other

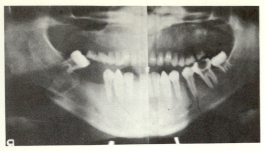

Fig. 10-18. Pantorex x-ray view reveals bilateral mandibular fractures.

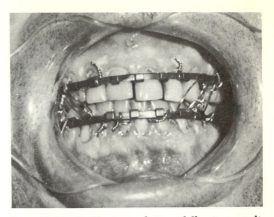

Fig. 10-19. Teeth in occlusion following application of dental arch bars and interdental wiring. Small hooks on arch bars will accept small latex bands that will hold the teeth in occlusion.

for the open reduction of the bony fractures, with complete change of gown, gloves, and drapes after intraoral procedures.

SETUP AND PREPARATION OF THE PATIENT. The patient is placed on the operating table in the supine position, and general anesthesia is induced. The routine prepping and draping procedures are carried out as for head and neck surgery. The basic plastic Mayo setup is used, with the following additions:

Bone drill and K-wire driver with appropriate accessories
Assorted K-wires
Wire cutter
Wire passing needles
Corks
Joseph elevator
Periosteal elevator
Flat palate elevator
Mouth gag
Appendix and malleable retractors
Tongue depressors
Wire pliers
Nasal and septal speculi
26-gauge stainless steel wire and cutter

Interdental wiring setup
Long needle holder
2 curved hemostats
Arch bars
Heavy wire cutters
Dental periosteal elevator
24- and 26-gauge stainless steel wire and wire cutter
Cheek retractors
Latex rubber bands

OPERATIVE PROCEDURE (Fig. 10-19). Arch bars are ligated to each individual tooth, the maxilla, and mandible with 26-gauge stainless steel wire. When the patient does not have natural teeth, the dentures may be wired to the maxilla and mandible. This is done by circummandibular wiring of the mandibular denture to the mandible and suspending the maxillary denture from the zygomatic arches. Wiring the arch bars or dentures in place may be adequate treatment for some fractures of the mandible and minor fractures of the maxilla. In more severe fractures of the maxilla the maxillary arch bar may have to be suspended from the zygomatic arches just as the maxillary denture is suspended. After the intraoral procedures have been completed, the surgeons are regowned and regloved, the patient is reprepped and draped, and a separate instrument setup is used for the direct reduction of the fracture sites.

1. The line of the appropriate incision is marked on the inferior surface of the mandible with a marking pen, and local anesthetic solution with 1:100,000 epinephrine is infiltrated in the area of the mark.

2. The skin is incised, and the inferior border of the mandible is exposed with sharp and blunt dissection.

3. The periosteum is incised and reflected.

4. After the bony fragments have been manually reduced, holes are drilled in each side of the fracture with a Hall drill.

5. Stainless steel wire, 24-gauge, is inserted through the holes and twisted tightly, securing the fractures in proper anatomical reduction.

6. A small Penrose drain is placed, and the wound is closed in layers.

7. A moderate compression dressing is applied. After the patient is fully reactive, which is usually the next day, small rubber bands are placed over the hooks on the upper and lower arch bars holding the jaws securely closed and the bones in proper position until they have healed.

### Reduction of nasal fractures

**DEFINITION.** Reduction of fractured nasal bones and cartilage by digital and instrumental manipulation.

**CONSIDERATIONS.** Fractures of the nose may be reduced with moderate ease in the absence of edema and ecchymosis of surrounding tissues. When edema is considerable, as after several hours, it may be desirable to wait until it subsides to allow for more accurate reduction. Nasal fractures beyond 1 to 2 weeks old may require reduction by osteotomy or rhinoplasty procedures.

**SETUP AND PREPARATION OF THE PATIENT.** Routine procedures for positioning, prepping, and draping the patient are carried out. In addition, the nares are prepped with applicators, and a topical anesthetic (10% cocaine) may be used. A local anesthetic setup is supplied on the Mayo tables with the following additional instruments:

Nasal speculum
Rubber-shod Kelly or Asch forceps
Joseph elevator
S-retractor
Bayonet forceps

**Accessory items**
Intranasal packing
Nasal splint
Sterile ½ in. tape

**OPERATIVE PROCEDURE**

1. Topical anesthesia of the nasal mucosa is accomplished by the use of 10% cocaine. Lidocaine (Xylocaine) is used for regional blocks of the infraorbital, infratrochlear, and anterior palatine nerves.

2. Asch or rubber-shod Kelly forceps are introduced intranasally to elevate the bony fracture.

3. Intranasal packing accomplishes internal splinting for 4 to 5 days.

4. An external nasal splint is applied and remains for 1 week.

### Reduction of fractures of the zygoma and orbit

**DEFINITION.** Elevation of depressed bony fragments and fixation in reduced position.

**CONSIDERATIONS.** A fracture of the zygoma usually causes a depression of the malar eminence. Also, the inferior rectus muscle of the eye may become trapped in the fracture line, where the frontal process of the maxilla joins the zygoma. The patient may complain of diplopia and anesthesia of the upper lip on the involved side. The objectives of treatment are to restore symmetry to the face, release extraocular muscles from the fracture line, and stabilize the bony fragments in their proper relationships.

In those cases in which there are no eye findings, adequate reductions can sometimes be done with just a bone hook. When stabilization is not affected with reduction, insertion of a transmolar Kirschner wire may be necessary.

**SETUP AND PREPARATION OF THE PATIENT.** Routine positioning, prepping, and draping procedures are carried out. For a simple closed reduction a local anesthetic setup and a jaw hook may be all that is needed. For more severe fractures and open reduction the basic plastic Mayo setup is used, with the following additions:

Bone drill and K-wire driver with appropriate
    accessories
Assorted K-wires and heavy wire cutter
Stainless steel wire, 24-, 26-, and 28-gauge, and
    cutter
Flat palate elevator
Joseph elevator
Towel clamp
Knavel retractors
Sutures of surgeon's choice

**OPERATIVE PROCEDURE**

1. An incision is made over the fracture line on the inferior orbital rim.

2. Bony fragments are visualized and reduced by instrumentation (bone hook, elevator, or towel clamp).

3. If there is a defect in the orbital floor, a piece of Silastic sheeting is used to cover the defect and prevent herniation of orbital structures.

4. To accomplish anatomical reconstruction, small holes are drilled in the fragments of bone.

5. Stainless steel wire is threaded through the holes and ligated to effect normal proximation. The steps just described may be repeated for fracture of the superior orbital rim if present.

6. Wounds are closed in layers.

7. A light dressing is applied, and it is important that the patient not be permitted to lie on the affected side.

## Mammoplasty

### Augmentation mammoplasty

**DEFINITION.** Plastic reconstruction of the breast by insertion of a prosthesis to augment the breast size and contour.

**CONSIDERATIONS.** The operation is performed at the request of the patient to fill a psychological or professional need due to the increased stress on physical appearance in today's society. A psychiatric consultant is helpful in selection of patients. The surgeon determines the size of the mammary prosthesis that he intends to insert. These prostheses are supplied in a sterile state. However, if they must be sterilized prior to use, follow the manufacturer's instructions for sterilization and keep them on the nurse's supply table covered with a sterile towel (Fig. 10-20).

**SETUP AND PREPARATION OF THE PATIENT.** The patient is positioned as the surgeon desires, supine or elevated to a 30-degree angle, arms at sides or outstretched on armboards. General anesthesia is induced, and a wide skin prep is done with iodine and

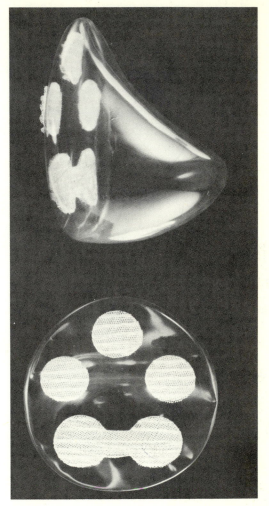

Fig. 10-20. Silastic mammary prostheses. Dacron net patches provide firm fixation to chest wall. (From Dow Corning Corporation, Medical Products Division, Bulletin 51-024A, September, 1971, Midland, Mich.)

alcohol (Chapter 4), followed by routine draping.

The basic plastic Mayo setup is used, with the possible addition of other clamping and retracting instruments.

**OPERATIVE PROCEDURE** (Fig. 10-21)

1. An incision is made along the inframammary fold to expose the pectoral fascia.

2. A pocket is developed between the breast tissue and the pectoral fascia.

3. All bleeding must be controlled.

4. The prosthesis is inserted and posi-

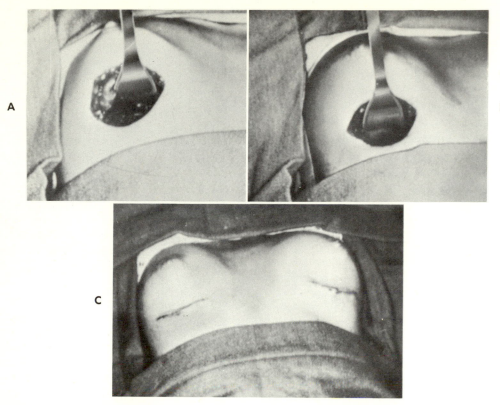

Fig. 10-21. A, Submammary incision with all available breast tissues and fat elevated from the underlying fascia. B, Mammary prosthesis in place with Dacron backing against muscle fascia for prosthesis fixation. C, Incision closed in layers with prosthesis in place. (From Dow Corning Corporation, Medical Products Division, Bulletin 14-157, March, 1967, Midland, Mich.)

tioned to provide a natural contour to the breast.

5. The wounds are closed with sub-cutaneous chromic catgut and the skin with nylon sutures.

6. A firm supportive dressing is applied and left undisturbed for 5 to 7 days.

### Reduction mammoplasty

DEFINITION. Surgical reduction in size and reestablishment of normal contours to the breast.

CONSIDERATIONS. The operation is performed in cases of overdevelopment or ptosis that is causing physical, mental, and social discomfort to the patient. The operative procedure is planned and marked with the patient in a sitting position. The operative procedure may be either a nipple trans-position or transplantation. Larger breasts require nipple transplantation, smaller, transposition.

SETUP AND PREPARATION OF THE PATIENT. The patient is positioned, prepped, and draped as for augmentation mammoplasty. Instruments, in addition to basic plastic Mayo setup, include the following:

Additional clamping and retracting instruments
Sterile tape measure
Caliper

OPERATIVE PROCEDURE. The operative procedure usually involves either transposition of the nipple to the desired position on a pedicle or transplantation of the nipple as a free graft. The operative procedures are basically the same.

1. In nipple transposition the excessive

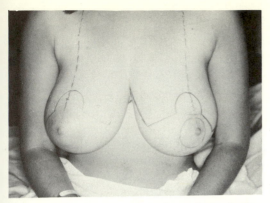

**Fig. 10-22.** Preoperative marking for reduction mammoplasty (Strombeck technique). Lines indicate areas of excision for reduction of breast size and transposition of nipple.

tissue is excised according to the method of Strombeck (Fig. 10-22).

2. The nipple and areola are transposed on a bipedicle flap. Similar incisions are utilized for nipple transplantation except that the nipple is taken as a free graft and the recipient site prepared as a dermal bed. Resection of breast tissue may be associated with significant blood loss.

3. Positioning of the remaining breast tissue is accomplished to provide form to the breast with the nipple and areola properly positioned.

4. After skin closure with no. 4-0 nylon, a supportive dressing fashioned from Elastoplast strips is applied.

### Plastic surgery of the hand

GENERAL CONSIDERATIONS. The ultimate goal in surgery of the injured hand is the restoration of function. This is most readily accomplished through a systematic approach to the restoration of the damaged units. Surgical management is directed toward the replacement of lost tissues, the restoration of bony architecture, the repair of severed nerves, and finally the restoration of the motor unit continuity either by tendon graft or tendon repair. The management of joints is of utmost importance during the entire restorative process. Restoration of each basic unit in the management of the injured hand will be illustrated.

SETUP AND PREPARATION OF THE PATIENT. The patient is placed on the operating table in the supine position with the affected arm extended and supported on a hand table (usually of special design as preferred by the surgeon). Application of a pneumatic tourniquet is usually required (Chapter 13). Proper draping of the upper extremity is most important: the hand, forearm, and upper arm are prepped in a standard fashion, using either iodine and alcohol or Betadine, up to at least halfway between the elbow and the axilla. A moisture-barrier drape and a half sheet are placed over the hand table or armboard. Underneath the arm is placed a full sheet, which is folded once down and once up to provide a cuff. A 4-inch stockinette is used over the hand, forearm, and to above the elbow. The arm is placed on the sterile field, and another sheet is placed over the ether screen and across the abdomen. This sheet is folded once down, again to provide a cuff. The cuffs of the lower sheet, the stockinette, and the upper sheet are then clipped to each other using a small towel clamp. A drape holder is placed between the upper part of the arm and the anesthesiologist, and sheets are used to cover the lower portion of the patient and operating table. This method provides at least two layers between the arm and the table and also provides a sterile cuff with four layers that are clipped together to maintain a sterile operating field even with movement of the arm.

The basic plastic surgery hand set should include the following:

**Cutting instruments**

   3 No. 3 knife handles with no. 15 blades
   1 Small Metzenbaum scissors
   1 Tenotomy scissors
   1 Suture scissors
   1 Wire cutter
   1 Small bone cutter (5-S rongeur)

**Holding instruments**

   4 Large Kelly hemostats for prep sponges
   8 Small towel clamps
   2 Large towel clamps
   2 Adson forceps with teeth

2 Adson forceps without teeth
1 5 in. forceps with teeth
2 Brown-Adson forceps
2 Nerve forceps with teeth
2 Nerve forceps without teeth
2 Allis clamps
2 Single skin hooks
2 Double skin hooks

**Clamping instruments**

12 Curved mosquito hemostats
4 Straight mosquito hemostats
6 Curved hemostats
2 Straight hemostats
2 Ochsner clamps

**Exposing instruments**

2 Senn (Knavel) retractors
2 S retractors
2 Army-Navy retractors
2 Rake retractors

**Suturing instruments**

2 Webster needle holders
2 Brown needle holders
Sutures according to the surgeon's preference

**Accessory instruments**

1 Joseph elevator
1 Langenbeck periosteal elevator
1 Small mallet
2 Small chisels
1 Hand drill with suitable bits (Bunnell)
Assorted Kirschner wires and suitable cutter
1 Kazanjian rongeur
1 Kazanjian bone cutter
1 Beyer rongeur
1 Needle-nose pliers
1 Nos. 4 and 3 neuro suction tips
Stryker saw and K-wire driver with attachments

**Instruments for special cases**

*Tendon*
  1 Tendon clamp
  Brand tendon stripper
  1 silver probe
  1 6 in. probe with eye
  Small buttons
  28-gauge wire
*Nerve*
  Razor blade
  Tongue blades
Skin grafting equipment as required

**Dressings**

Bismuth tribromophenate (Xeroform) gauze
Small and large sponges
Acrylic (Acrilan) fiber

Mechanic's waste
Abdominal pads (ABD's)
Splints
Casting equipment (plaster) (Chapter 13)

### Replacement of lost tissue

**DEFINITION.** Utilization of free skin grafts (split-thickness or full-thickness) or pedicle flaps to restore tissue losses.

**CONSIDERATIONS.** Free grafts are used when muscle, subcutaneous tissue, or granulation tissue forms the wound. Pedicle flaps are used when skin, bone, nerve, tendon, or joints are exposed.

**SETUP AND PREPARATION OF THE PATIENT.** Routine positioning, prepping, and draping procedures are carried out as just described. The instrument setup is the same as for skin grafts (p. 313).

**OPERATIVE PROCEDURE**

FREE GRAFTS

1. A skin graft is obtained as described on p. 310.

2. After thorough debridement and irrigation, the hand is fixed to a splint in the position of function with sterile tape.

3. If a tourniquet has been utilized during the steps just listed, it is released and all bleeding completely controlled before the graft is applied.

4. The graft is applied to the deficient area of the hand and sutured in place. The sutures are left long to permit the application of a stent dressing (Fig. 10-39).

5. A large bulky dressing is then applied to the hand, and the hand is maintained in an elevated position during the healing period.

PEDICLE FLAPS (Fig. 10-23)

The abdomen or upper thorax may be utilized for procurement of a pedicle flap. Position of the arm is carefully determined to ensure as much comfort as possible, since it will have to be maintained in the selected position for 3 weeks (to develop an adequate circulation from the recipient site).

1. The defect on the hand is outlined on clear x-ray film (or other suitable pattern material) and transferred to the donor site.

2. A flap (including epidermis, dermis,

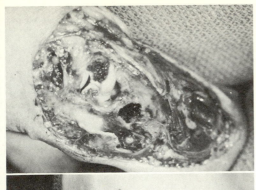

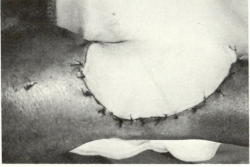

**Fig. 10-23. A,** Avulsion of dorsum of wrist, exposing carpal bones and wrist joint. **B,** Abdominal flap has been elevated and sutured into wrist defect.

and underlying subcutaneous tissue) is incised and elevated directly.

3. The donor area may be covered with a split-thickness graft taken from the thigh and sutured in place with a stent dressing.

4. The hand is placed beneath the pedicle flap, which is sutured into the defect on the hand.

5. Mechanic's waste and abdominal pads are used to fill the space between the arm and chest to allow proper immobilization and comfort.

6. After the dressing is applied, it is held in place with strips of 3-inch tape that encircle the chest and arm.

DETACHMENT OF THE PEDICLE FLAP. After the pedicle flap has secured its blood supply from the hand, it is detached from the donor area.

1. This is accomplished by cutting the base of the pedicle free from the abdominal or chest wall and closing the incision directly.

2. The pedicle flap is trimmed and set into the remaining defect in the hand.

3. A bulky dressing is applied to the hand to maintain optimum position.

### Management of bony fractures

CONSIDERATIONS. The operative procedure is designed to accomplish the following: reduction and fixation of the fracture, maintenance of digital length, and prevention of rotation of the digit.

Fixation may be accomplished with either external (plaster cast) or internal (direct wiring, use of pins, plates, etc.) splinting. Open reduction provides the most accurate means of obtaining reduction and fixation of a fracture. Crushing fractures are usually not amenable to surgery because of the inability to stabilize the many small fragments. Transverse or oblique fractures are more suitable because accurate reduction and fixation can be obtained to permit movement of juxtapositioned joints.

SETUP AND PREPARATION OF THE PATIENT. The patient is positioned, prepped, and draped using the routine procedures for hand surgery. The instrument setup includes the following:

Hand drill
Kirschner wires and wire cutter
Corks or tape for covering wire ends

OPERATIVE PROCEDURE. Fixation of metacarpal-phalangeal fractures is usually obtained by drilling K-wires in a crossing manner to extend from the proximal segment of a phalanx across the fracture site and out the distal segment of the same phalanx (Fig. 10-24). Care is taken to avoid impaling the tendons or juxtaposition joints with the Kirschner wires. The wires are usually left extending beyond the surface of the skin to allow ready removal after the fractures have healed.

### Peripheral nerve repairs

CONSIDERATIONS. The goal of the operative procedure is to accurately reapproximate the individual nerve bundles (after excision of any scar tissue within the dam-

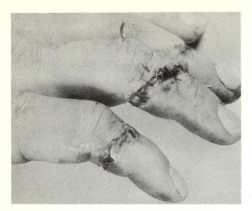

**Fig. 10-24.** Phalangeal fractures have beeen stabilized with crossing Kirschner wires.

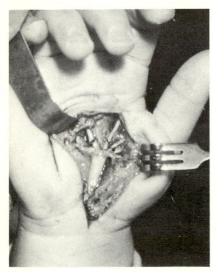

**Fig. 10-25.** Severed branches of median nerve have been reapproximated with fine sutures.

aged nerve ends) to ensure return of sensation and motor function.

SETUP AND PREPARATION OF THE PATIENT. The patient is positioned and the hand prepped and draped in the usual manner. A tourniquet is applied to obtain a bloodless field. The basic plastic surgery hand setup with delicate nerve instruments is used.

OPERATIVE PROCEDURE

1. The damaged nerve ends are exposed, and the proximal neuroma is excised with a fine razor blade back to the level of normal nerve.

2. The distal glioma is excised.

3. An operative microscope or other optical magnification devices are utilized to aid in identifying the individual nerve bundles.

4. A single suture (no. 8-0 silk) is utilized to approximate each nerve bundle.

5. The external covering of the nerve, the perineurium, is closed with a running stitch (Fig. 10-25).

6. The skin edges are closed with fine sutures.

7. The hand is immobilized with a large bulky dressing for 3 to 4 weeks to prevent tension at the line of nerve anastomosis.

### Flexor tendon grafts

DEFINITION. The restoration of motor function by insertion of a free tendon graft from the fingertip to the motor unit, either within the palm or distal forearm.

CONSIDERATIONS. Because function of the hand depends on the mobility of its small joints through proper balance and excursion of the tendons, the objective of surgery is to preserve the smooth, gliding articular surfaces of structures in the sheath.

SETUP AND PREPARATION OF THE PATIENT. The hand is positioned, prepped, and draped in the usual manner with utilization of a pneumatic tourniquet. The basic plastic surgery hand setup is used. The Brand tendon strippers are set up on a separate sterile table.

OPERATIVE PROCEDURE

1. A serpentine incision is made in the palm and extended out on the involved finger to expose the fibro-osseous tunnels from the distal palmar crease to the fingertip and the proximal muscle unit in the palm or the forearm.

2. If the digital sheath has been injured, it is completely excised except for "pulleys" that are left in the midportion of the proximal phalanx and the midportion of the middle phalanx.

3. All accompanying scar is excised.

4. Scar tissue about the proximal tendon is excised.

5. The tendon graft is procured utilizing

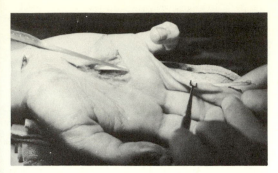

**Fig. 10-26.** The plantar tendon has been threaded through the palmar incision into the fibro-osseous tunnels and sutured to the distal bony phalanx. After release of tourniquet and relaxation of the muscle bellies, the proximal anastomosis will be accomplished.

either the long palmar tendon in the forearm or the plantar tendon in the leg. A Brand stripper allows procurement of either of these grafts through a single small incision either at the wrist or medially behind the medial malleolus.

6. As soon as the graft is procured, it is threaded through the palm beneath the pulleys and out to the fingertip (Fig. 10-26).

7. Proximal anastomosis is accomplished with no. 5-0 Ethiflex sutures and a distal anastomosis with no. 3-0 Ethiflex sutures passed through a drill hole in the distal phalanx and tied over a button on the nailbed.

8. The tension in the anastomosis is adjusted only after the tourniquet has been released for 15 minutes and the bleeding has been controlled by elevation and pressure.

9. All wounds are closed, and a large bulky dressing is applied to immobilize the hand for 3 weeks.

### Surgical correction of Dupuytren's contracture

**DEFINITION.** Surgical removal of fibrosed palmar aponeurosis.

**CONSIDERATIONS.** Dupuytren's contracture is a disorder producing a flexion deformity of the hand. Tissue changes localized to the aponeurosis cause the deformity. Removal

is restricted to the aponeurosis, including diseased portions of the interdigital ligaments. Interference with adjacent systems and fatty tissue is avoided. Early excision is indicated, since the disorder interferes with nutrition of the skin because of partial obliteration of blood vessels. The patient usually prefers surgery to one hand at a time.

**SETUP AND PREPARATION OF THE PATIENT.** The patient is positioned, prepped, and draped using the routine procedures for hand surgery. The operation is done with the patient under general anesthesia. A pneumatic tourniquet is applied in the proper manner to the upper arm of the affected hand. The basic plastic Mayo setup is used with the addition of small rake retractors (Senn-Knavel).

**OPERATIVE PROCEDURE** (Fig. 10-27)

1. A transverse incision is made across the palm of the hand, exposing the fibrosed palmar fascia.

2. Incisions are made along the side of the fingers as indicated for complete removal of diseased tissue.

3. Digital nerve slips are identified so that they may be preserved.

4. Palmar fascia is removed beneath carefully elevated flaps, and injury to nerves in the palm and fingers is avoided.

5. Removal is continued back to the heel of the palm, which is the fan of the palmar fascia.

6. The tourniquet is released, and when the wound is dry, the incisions are closed with no. 5-0 Ethiflex sutures.

7. A stabilizing dressing, comfortable to the patient, is applied.

### Surgery for syndactyly

**DEFINITION.** Surgical separation of webbed digits with adequate coverage to denuded areas.

**CONSIDERATIONS.** The most common form of syndactyly is symmetrical webbing in two normal hands, although it may be associated with an abnormal number of fingers (polydactyly) and can commonly involve the feet as well. Careful x-ray and

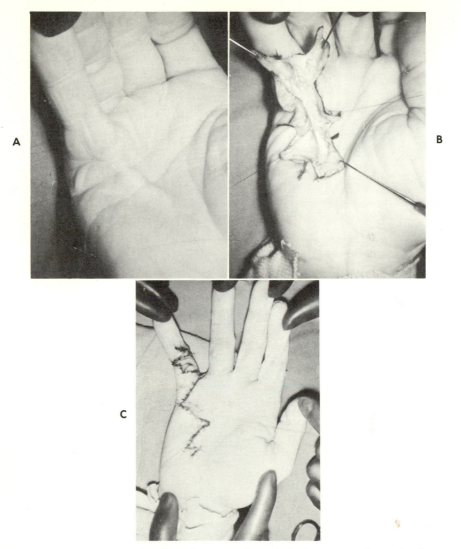

Fig. 10-27. A, Contracture of palmar fascia involving little finger. B, Fibrous band exposed throughout its extent. C, Wound closure by multiple Z-plasties.

functional studies are necessary, and the plan of treatment is individualized in each instance. The surgical correction is usually done when the patient is 3 to 5 years of age.

SETUP AND PREPARATION OF THE PATIENT. The patient is positioned, prepped, and draped using the routine procedures for hand surgery and skin grafts. The basic plastic Mayo setup is used. A separate sterile table is needed for the skin grafting equipment. The device will be chosen by the surgeon. For polydactyly, bone-cutting instruments may be added as needed from the nurse's instrument supply table.

OPERATIVE PROCEDURE. In this anomaly, there is a deficiency of tissue, and new tissue must be added in the form of free grafts or pedicle grafts (Fig. 10-28).

1. The incisions are planned to permit reconstruction of the digital web with local flaps.

2. The lateral skin defects are closed with full-thickness free grafts.

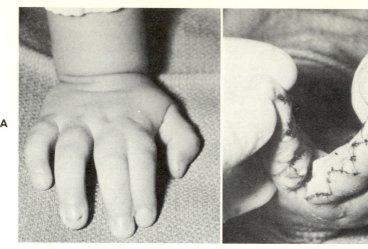

Fig. 10-28. A, Skin syndactyly involving long and index fingers. B, Syndactylism released and repair accomplished with skin grafts.

3. These grafts are inserted so as to avoid straight-line contractures.

4. The grafts are "stented" (Fig. 10-39).

5. The entire hand is immobilized with the dressing.

## Surgical correction for hypospadias

**DEFINITION.** Removal of the ventral chordee to lengthen and straighten the penis; reconstruction of the urethra to extend to the distal end of the penis.

**CONSIDERATIONS.** In this deformity the urethral opening of the penis does not extend to the terminal end of the organ. The position of the urethral opening may be located anywhere along the penile shaft, at the penoscrotal junction, or in the perineum. The chordee are always present, varying in degree. The goal of this procedure is correction of the ventral curvature by excision of the chordee and reconstruction of the urethra to extend to the tip of the penis. Accomplishment of these two goals allows function and recovery with a normal urinary stream and sexual function. The repair is best completed prior to school age.

**SETUP AND PREPARATION OF THE PATIENT.** The patient is placed in a supine position, with his hips elevated slightly by means of a folded sheet and the legs stabilized in a frog-leg position. After the induction of

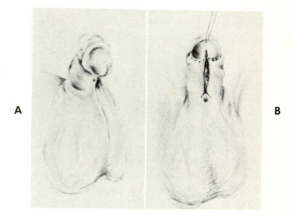

Fig. 10-29. A, Partial hypospadias with 90-degree flexion of glans. The prepuce is markedly redundant. B, Initial incision of first stage has removed remnants of mucous membrane or any other surface irregularities that might interfere with urethral reconstruction at later operation. Dotted line indicates next incision. (From Byars, L. T.: Functional restoration of hypospadias deformities. In Surgery, gynecology, and obstetrics, vol. 92, Chicago, 1951, F. H. Martin Memorial Foundation, Publisher.)

general anesthesia the genital area is scrubbed with soap and water and blotted dry with a sterile towel. The iodine and alcohol prep includes the lower part of the abdomen, genitalia, and thighs. The patient is draped, exposing the penis and perineum.

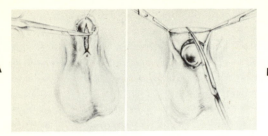

**A**    **B**

Fig. 10-30. **A,** Second incision of first-stage operation to relax ventral bend and mobilize preputial flaps. **B,** Dorsal slit that, with incision indicated in **A,** mobilizes two pedicle flaps of preputial skin. (From Byars, L. T.: Functional restoration of hypospadias deformities. In Surgery, gynecology, and obstetrics, vol. 92, Chicago, 1951, F. H. Martin Memorial Foundation, Publisher.)

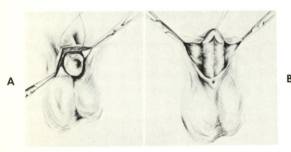

**A**    **B**

Fig. 10-31. **A,** Pedicle flaps from prepuce having been mobilized at first-stage operation by dorsal slit, midline suture is placed to stabilize known points. **B,** Retraction of skin reveals ventral half of circumference of shaft of penis from which all fibrous tissue limiting extension has been dissected. Double fold of skin forming prepuce separated so that the two preputial flaps can be brought to ventral surface of penis to replace skin deficiency. (From Byars, L. T.: Functional restoration of hypospadias deformities. In Surgery, gynecology and obstetrics, vol. 92, Chicago, 1951, F. H. Martin Memorial Foundation, Publisher.)

The basic plastic Mayo set-up is used, with the following additions:

    Urethral sounds, 8-12 Fr.
    Urethral catheters (red rubber 8-12 Fr.) and
        guide or stylet
    Metal cup containing glycerin for lubricating
        catheter
    Asepto syringe and basin
    Golf tee
    No. 4-0 silk traction suture
    Skin hooks

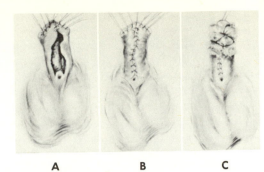

**A**    **B**    **C**

Fig. 10-32. **A,** Ventral raw surface of glans enlarged by traction on sutures as two pedicle flaps of preputial tissue are sutured into wound to supply excess skin in this region. Sutures in glans left long for use in securing dressing. **B,** Completion of closure of wound and of first-stage operation. Ventral bending of penis has been released, preputial flaps have been shifted to ventral surface to provide adequate skin in this deficient area. Sutures in glans left long to aid in enlarging defect in glans to accommodate an excess of skin at this point. **C,** An important step is proper dressing of penis applied at completion of first-stage operation: one layer of nonadherent gauze covers the wound, and over this is placed a wad of mechanic's waste (Acrilan fiber) secured by tying the long ends of sutures over it. The entire shaft of the penis is then snugly encased by bandaging with inch wide strips of Elastoplast. (From Byars, L. T.: Functional restoration of hypospadias deformities. In Surgery, gynecology and obstetrics, vol. 92, Chicago, 1951, F. H. Martin Memorial Foundation, Publisher.)

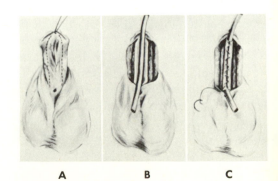

**A**    **B**    **C**

Fig. 10-33. **A,** Second stage of operation, outlining of skin incisions for formation of urethra (perineal urethrostomy has been done). **B,** Incisions completed and catheter temporarily placed. **C,** Skin-lined urethra sutured with inverting running suture. (From Byars, L. T.: Functional restoration of hypospadias deformities. In Surgery, gynecology and obstetrics, vol. 92, Chicago, 1951, F. H. Martin Memorial Foundation, Publisher.)

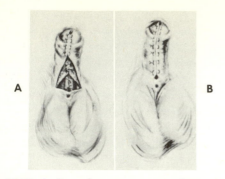

**Fig. 10-34. A,** Second-stage operation showing inverting suture of skin-lined urethra and closure of subcutaneous tissues (sutured with multiple superimposed tiers of stitches) and skin. **B,** Completed second-stage operation with formation of urethra that is connected with normal urethra. The catheter is withdrawn and reinserted into the bladder through the urethrostomy incision. (From Byars, L. T.: Functional restoration of hypospadias deformities. In Surgery, gynecology and obstetrics, vol. 92, Chicago, 1951, F. H. Martin Memorial Foundation, Publisher.)

OPERATIVE PROCEDURE (Figs. 10-29 to 10-34). The procedure described by Byars has stood the test of time. At the first stage the chordee is resected, and the resulting ventral skin defect is covered with the redundant "hood" of the foreskin. The urethra is reconstructed at a second stage by forming a tube with the excess dorsal skin to place the urethral meatus distally.

FIRST STAGE

1. An indwelling catheter is placed into the bladder through the existing urethral orifice.

2. A traction stitch of no. 4-0 silk is placed through the glans penis.

3. The chordee from the urethral opening to the tip of the glans is removed.

4. The prepuce on the dorsal aspect of the penis is incised in the midline from its free edge to the corona. An incision encircling the corona produces two folded flaps, which are unfolded. These skin flaps are rotated to the ventral defect and interdigitated with no. 5-0 chromic catgut.

5. A dressing of nonadherent gauze and acrylic fiber held in place with 1-inch strips of Elastoplast is applied.

6. The catheter is sutured in place and taped to the patient's thigh, and open drainage is maintained. This is facilitated with the use of ABD's and a Montgomery-type dressing on the thigh.

SECOND STAGE

1. A no. 12 Fr. catheter is inserted into the bladder with a urethral sound in the lumen. The sound is rotated to permit palpation of the tip in the perineum. Cutting directly down on this sound permits extraction of the flared end of the catheter through the perineal urethrostomy.

2. Traction suture is placed as in step 2 of the first stage.

3. A rectangular area is outlined in the area of the urethral defect. The edges are enfolded to form a tube. The surrounding excess skin is undermined and transferred over the new urethra and sutured into position.

4. A dressing is applied as in steps 5 and 6 of the first stage.

## Management of the burn patient

Burns are classified as first, second, or third degree. A first-degree burn indicates superficial blistering as seen in a sunburn. In the second-degree burn a portion of the dermis is lost but not the full thickness of the skin. A third-degree burn indicates a full-thickness skin loss extending into the subcutaneous tissue. This means that the entire layers of the skin are burned through and that covering has to be obtained by grafting. Obvious third-degree burn areas are anesthetic, white, and charred, with thrombosed veins visible in the eschar.

Care of the burn patient may be divided into two phases: (1) fluid and electrolyte balance and (2) burn wound management.

### *Fluid and electrolyte balance*

Increased capillary permeability associated with the burn injury results in the accumulation of fluid in the extravascular spaces. This fluid, containing protein and electrolytes, is unavailable for participation in the intravascular circulation. Replacement therapy must take into account the

fluid collection, the fluid loss from the burn wound surface, normal pulmonary loss, and the amount required for satisfactory urine output. Intravenous Ringer's lactate has become particularly useful in early burn therapy.

### Burn wound management

Coverage of the burn wound may be obtained as follows: The eschar may be immediately excised and the exposed area grafted, or the eschar may be allowed to separate spontaneously and the underlying granulation tissue covered with free grafts. Immediate excision of a local burn is managed as described in the section on management of tissue losses in the hand and subsequently in the section on skin grafting. In the burn treated conservatively, the eschar may be removed on the ward or as a separate procedure in the operating room. Once an adequate base has been obtained, the goal of the operative procedure is to provide complete coverage of the exposed areas with free skin grafts.

### Surgical treatment of burn wounds

DEFINITION. Procurement of skin grafts, meshing of grafts as indicated, application of grafts to open wounds, and immobilization either by external dressings or by skeletal support.

SETUP AND PREPARATION OF THE PATIENT. The position of the patient depends on the body areas to be debrided or grafted. After induction of anesthesia, dressings are carefully removed. The areas are scrubbed with soap and water and irrigated with saline solution. Donor sites are prepped with an antibacterial agent and draped. Although the use of ether is discouraged, it remains unexcelled in preparation of the donor site for maximum adherence of the dermatome adhesive to the skin and on the recipient site to eliminate serous accumulation that might prevent the graft from "taking" to its new bed. It is necessary to have a large number and variety of dressing materials assembled so that the patient will not be exposed to delay. A special burn pack may be

advisable. A tissue forceps and scissors will be needed for each member of the team for debridement. Occasionally, a freehand skin graft knife is additionally required.

Skin grafting devices, as the surgeon requires, are set up on a separate table.

OPERATIVE PROCEDURE

1. Split-thickness skin grafts, 8/1000 inch in thickness, are obtained with a Reese dermatome or other preferred devices.

2. These grafts are then removed from the dermatome tapes and placed on the tapes provided for the mesher.

3. The graft is passed through the mesher. This permits expansion of the skin graft to cover a much larger area than an unmeshed graft.

4. The mesh graft is then applied to the wounds.

5. The grafts may be immobilized either with packing, sutures, or dressings.

6. Skeletal support of the lower extremity is obtained with Steinman pins passed through the calcaneus and tibia. This allows elevation of the lower extremities from the bedclothing and prevents trauma to the freshly applied skin grafts. The upper extremity can be supported by a Steinman pin placed through the radius or ulna. The donor sites are covered with a single layer of fine-mesh gauze, and a moist pad is applied to provoke hemostasis.

### Skin grafting and pedicle flaps
#### Free grafts

DEFINITION. A free graft of skin is one of a given thickness and area that has been completely detached from its bed (the donor site) and transferred to another part of the body (the recipient site).

CONSIDERATIONS. Skin grafting is done to fill or cover defects from loss of tissue as soon as conditions are suitable, thereby preventing infection, fibrosis, and loss of muscle and joint function (Fig. 10-35).

Preparation of the recipient site for grafting should include measures to ensure freedom from infection and a well-vascularized bed of new granulation tissue. Measures such as frequent changes of dressing

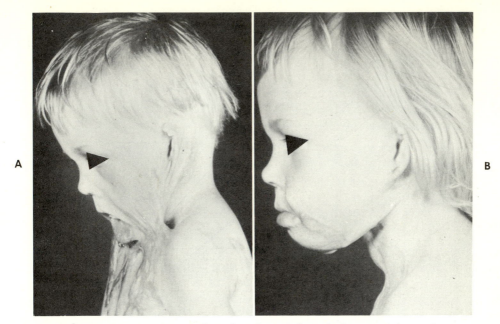

Fig. 10-35. **A,** Burn contracture involving lip, chin, neck, and chest. **B,** Release of contracture and coverage with split-thickness skin graft in one stage.

and debridement and moderate pressure to prevent overgrowth of granulation tissue are fundamental, as are the obvious ones of supporting the patient's general condition.

Selection of donor sites will be influenced by the availability of skin, its cosmetic suitability, and other factors such as presence or absence of hair follicles.

There are many classifications of free grafts, dependent on the varying thicknesses. The two main types are the *split-thickness graft,* in which all the epidermis but only a portion of the dermis is removed, and the *full-thickness graft,* in which the entire dermis is removed (Fig. 10-36).

The advantages of full-thickness grafts are that they retain more properties of normal skin. They are used whenever it is desirable to retain the full thickness of the skin and avoid depressions, that is, for the nose, face, etc. A full-thickness graft also maintains the functional capacity of normal skin, and this type of graft would be used where motion is desired, as on the hand and fingers.

To cover defects of the face with full-thickness grafts, the donor sites are usually the supraclavicular or postauricular area. The color match between these areas and the face is better than that between any other parts of the body and the face. Full-thickness grafts for the hand and functional areas are usually taken from the inguinal fold. Full-thickness skin can be obtained without causing an additional obvious deformity, since there is significant skin in these areas to close primarily without requiring overgrafting.

Split-thickness grafts of various thicknesses can be taken from the thigh, buttocks, or other areas (Fig. 10-37) either by hand or mechanical means. The thicker the graft, the more the properties of normal skin are retained, and, conversely, the thinner the graft, the less the properties of normal skin are retained. It should also be noted that the thicker the graft, the harder it is to get a "take" of the graft; conversely, the thinner the graft, the easier it is to get a "take," or healing, of the graft. In this type of graft, the exposed dermis of the donor site is covered again with epidermis

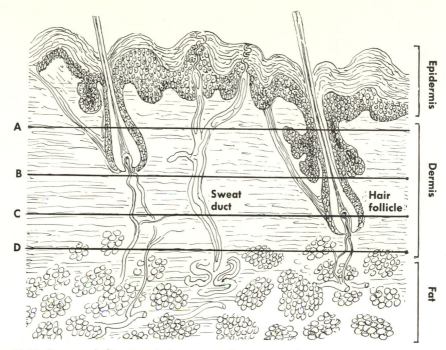

**Fig. 10-36.** Layers of skin. Level **A** corresponds to a superficial or thin split-thickness graft and level **D** to a full-thickness graft, with levels **B** and **C** representing intermediate-thickness split grafts. (From Wood-Smith, D., and Porowski, P., editors: Nursing care of the plastic surgery patient, St. Louis, 1967, The C. V. Mosby Co.)

by the proliferation of the epidermis from the lining of the hair follicles and sebaceous glands, which penetrate deep into the dermis, carrying their epidermal lining with them.

### Means of obtaining split-thickness skin grafts

FREEHAND METHOD. A freehand graft is usually taken with the Ferris-Smith knife (or modifications such as the Blair knife, Humbe knife, etc.). A well-trained operator will use a long, sharp blade on a handle in order to obtain split-thickness skin of desired thickness. The advantages of this method are: (1) it is faster and (2) a larger piece of skin can be obtained than by mechanical means.

MECHANICAL DEVICES

1. Reese dermatome. A precise thickness of skin can be obtained by use of a shim that is placed into the Reese dermatome underneath the blade. The drum of the dermatome is covered with a Reese dermatape. The skin is adhered to the tape by means of an adhesive, and the graft is taken by a to-and-fro motion of the knife itself. An exact thickness of skin can be obtained. The amount of skin that can be taken with each passage is limited by the size of the drum (4 x 8 inches) (Fig. 10-38).

2. Padgett dermatome. The Padgett dermatome is similar to the Reese dermatome. There is no shim or tape, and the thickness of the skin is obtained by setting the desired thickness on a gauge or by sight.

3. Brown dermatome. The Brown dermatome is an electrical, motor-driven dermatome that does not give as accurate a thickness of skin as the Reese or the Padgett instruments. However, longer strips of skin can be obtained, and this type of instrument is particularly useful in covering large burned areas.

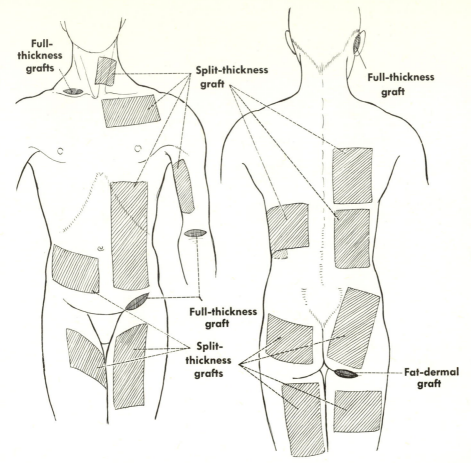

Fig. 10-37. Commonly employed sites for donor areas of skin grafts. (From Wood-Smith D., and Porowski, P., editors: Nursing care of the plastic surgery patient, St. Louis, 1967, The C. V. Mosby Co.)

**SETUP AND PREPARATION OF THE PATIENT.** The patient is placed on the operating table in a position that provides exposure of the wound and the donor site (Chapter 7). Both sites are prepped as the surgeon desires and are draped for adequate exposure and mobility as required. The reserve supply tables and the basic plastic Mayo setup will include most supplies needed. Additional items that may be necessary are as follows:

Local anesthesia set with no. 22 long needle for infiltration of donor site
Separate flat-top sterile draped table for setting up the grafting device preferred by the surgeon

**Freehand method**

Ferris-Smith handle and blade
Retracting board (tongue blades and soap dish)
Lubricating medium (sterile mineral oil or petrolatum)

**Mechanical method**

Reese or Padgett dermatome as specified
Suitable blades, tapes, adhesive, sponge sticks, sponges, and tongue blades
No. 10 knife blade and handle
Tissue forceps
Ether
Suture materials as the surgeon prefers, adequate for "stent"-type closure if required

**Dressings**

Scarlet red gauze
Nonadherent gauze

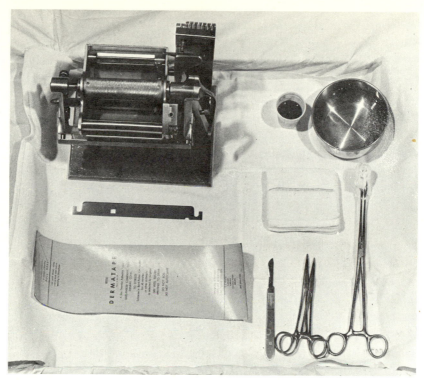

**Fig. 10-38.** Reese dermatome set. Setup arrangement for skin graft procedure. Clockwise from upper left: Reese dermatome drum on rack with shims; cup with glue; solution basin with ether sponges and holder; hemostats; scalpel; Dermatape; blade for dermatome.

Fine-mesh gauze
Sponges, large and small
ABD's, large and small
Kling and Kerlix rolls
Roller gauze
Tape
Elastic adhesive strips
Plaster casting supplies (Chapter 13)

**OPERATIVE PROCEDURE**

1. The recipient area is prepared by removing excessive granulation tissue to provide a smooth vascular bed for the graft and measured.

2. The donor site is further prepped with ether or alcohol. The dermatome is set at the desired thickness. The drum and donor site are painted with glue and allowed to dry sufficiently (5 minutes). The drum (or tape) is adhered to the glue on the donor site and the graft taken by a to-and-fro motion of the knife.

3. The graft is then rolled free from the tape (or left in place until needed), flattened out on a firm surface, and kept moist with saline sponges until transferred to the recipient bed.

4. The graft is sutured in place after bleeding has been controlled. Sutures may be left long to permit tying over a compressive dressing (Fig. 10-39).

5. A suitable dressing is applied, depending on compression and mobilization desired.

6. The donor site is dressed to provide hemostasis and a minimum amount of pain and discomfort to the patient.

*Full-thickness skin graft operation*

**DEFINITION.** Transplantation of a full depth of skin without any attached fat from a donor site to a recipient site to re-

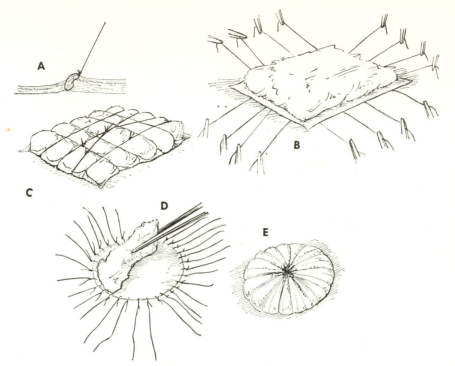

Fig. 10-39. **A,** Method of fixation of the skin graft to the edges of the wound. **B,** Nonadherent dressing is applied over the skin graft, and on this a generous pad of acrylic fiber. **C,** Long ends of the suture are tied over the fiber to produce an area of pressure between the graft and the base. **D,** Similar dressing is applied to a circular graft. **E,** Long suture ends are tied over the circular graft (often called a "stent" dressing). (From Wood-Smith, D.; and Porowski, P., editors: Nursing care of the plastic surgery patient, St. Louis, 1967, The C. V. Mosby Co.)

surface freshly opened wounds of the face and hands or small areas where the graft will be under pressure and wear.

**SETUP AND PREPARATION OF THE PATIENT.** The position of the patient will depend on the sites selected. Routine skin prepping and draping are carried out. The basic plastic Mayo setup is used, including a local anesthesia setup, a marking pen, and a small piece of sterile unexposed x-ray film.

**OPERATIVE PROCEDURE**

1. The scar tissue or lesion on the recipient site is excised.

2. The defect is measured with x-ray film and a pattern drawn in with a marking pen.

3. The pattern is cut and transferred to the donor site, whether it be the inguinal fold or the subclavicular or postauricular area, and is outlined on the skin with ink.

4. The periphery of the projected graft is incised just through the dermis.

5. By very careful technique (Fig. 10-40) the full-thickness graft of epidermis and dermis is dissected from its bed using a no. 15 blade, care being taken not to handle the graft except with skin hooks.

6. It is important that all fat be removed from the underside of the graft with sharp scissors (Fig. 10-40) because the presence of fat will cause difficulties in healing.

7. The graft is positioned on the recipient site and sutured in position with interrupted fine silk or nylon sutures.

8. Pressure over the graft, to keep it snugly applied to the underlying base, is maintained by use of a stent-type dressing (Fig. 10-39).

9. The donor site can usually be closed directly. If it is too large to close direct-

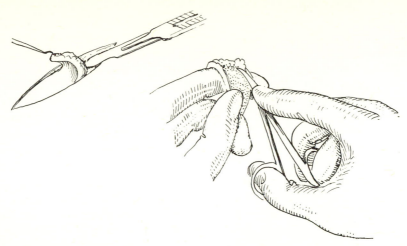

**Fig. 10-40.** Full-thickness skin graft is removed, using a hook to handle the graft. The graft is defatted, using a small sharp scissors and removing the major amount of the visible fat from its deep aspect. (From Wood-Smith, D., and Porowski, P., editors: Nursing care of the plastic surgery patient, St. Louis, 1967, The C. V. Mosby Co.)

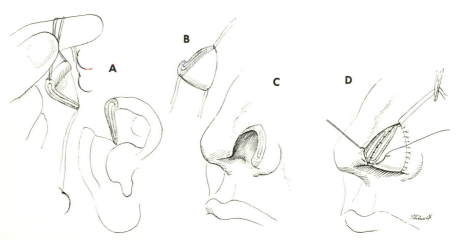

**Fig. 10-41.** Technique of composite auricular graft to repair a nasal defect. **A** and **B**, Composite chondrocutaneous graft removed from the auricle. **C**, Nasal defect. **D**, Composite graft inserted into nasal defect and sutured. (From Wood-Smith, D., and Porowski, P., editors: Nursing care of the plastic surgery patient, St. Louis, 1967, The C. V. Mosby Co.)

ly, it may be overgrafted with a split-thickness graft from another donor site.

### Composite grafts

A composite graft consists of more than one element, for example, skin, fat, and cartilage. Such a graft is often indicated to replace a segment of the alar border of the nose after excision. The auricle of the ear is a common donor site. The composite graft should not be traumatized by handling with instruments.

SETUP AND PREPARATION OF THE PATIENT. Routine procedures are carried out for preparation of the patient. The basic plastic Mayo setup is used, with the addition of a nasal speculum, an S-shaped retractor, and the pattern-making items.

OPERATIVE PROCEDURE (Fig. 10-41)

1. The nasal defect is prepared by cleanly excising the edges.

2. A pattern of the defect is prepared.

3. The ear is flattened against the head, and an area with approximately the same curvature as the missing portion of the nostril is located.

4. The pattern is traced on the rim of the ear and this portion excised with a sawing motion, using a stab blade (no. 11) knife.

5. The graft is sutured accurately into the nasal defect using the anterior surface of the ear for the lining and the posterior surface for covering.

6. Pressure is applied with internal nasal packing and an external aluminum nasal splint.

7. The resulting defect of the ear may often be closed directly, or, if it is too large, the raw edges are buried under the postauricular skin for 2 weeks. Then it is detached with a flap of this skin attached to it so that the flap may be rolled into a little tube to replace the missing portion.

### Pedicle flap operations

DEFINITION. A full-thickness area of skin and subcutaneous tissue raised from its bed but left attached to one or both ends until a sufficient blood supply has developed through the pedicle.

CONSIDERATIONS. Pedicle flaps are used principally for restoring contour and bulk in contrast with free skin grafts, which are used for surfacing. Flaps are often a necessity in restoring full-thickness tissue loss if vulnerable structures are exposed, as in the hand (Fig. 10-23), or if restoration of lost facial features is required.

Flaps may be classified as *direct flaps,* which are applied at the same time that they are raised, and *delayed flaps,* which are raised in stages to improve the blood supply before permanent application to the defect. Pedicle flaps used in the region from which they are raised may be called *local flaps,* whereas those transferred to another area of the body may be referred to as *distant flaps.*

The *tubed* pedicle flap is a delayed rectangular flap in which the two long edges are raised, undermined, and sutured together to form a tube. The donor defect may be closed directly or with a surfacing skin graft.

SETUP AND PREPARATION OF THE PATIENT. The position of the patient on the operating table depends on the area of the defect to be covered and the carefully selected donor site. Much the same setup as for a full-thickness graft would be used, with additional hemostats and suture material to suit the extent of the flap. Skin grafting devices should be available if required.

OPERATIVE PROCEDURE. See pedicle flap to the hand, p. 302.

### Neoplasms and congenital deformities of the skin

GENERAL CONSIDERATIONS. The objectives in removing carcinomas or birth defects of the skin are (1) to cure the patient and (2) to minimize the residual deformity.

Benign lesions that should be considered for removal because of troublesome or disfiguring location include nevi, warts, papillomas, keratoses, sebaceous cysts, some congenital hemangiomas, and hairy nevi. Most nevi are benign and are removed for cosmetic reasons.

Port-wine stains usually present as a red-staining discoloration on one side of the face. Excision and skin grafting, if necessary, may be done at any stage in life. However, when excision is not feasible, tattooing may be considered.

The cavernous hemangioma, however, may propose a threat to life, because with formation of arteriovenous fistulas, the heart decompensates, and the patient develops congestive heart failure. Therefore these must be attacked vigorously, and the hemangioma must be removed in its entirety, even if it involves bone. Complete surgical excision, whenever possible, is the best treatment for this type of hemangioma. Some may be treated with radiation, multiple suture ligations, or staged excision. A combination of methods may be required.

A plastic surgeon's treatment of carcinoma is not hampered by concern for wound closure or reconstruction. This is part of a paradox in the treatment of neoplasms; that is, the surgeon who resects the least amount of tissue appears conservative to the uninformed. In reality, he is the most radical because his patients have a high incidence of recurrence with a much worse prognosis. A surgeon who resects widely appears radical; however, his patients have a better chance for cure, and he is therefore more conservative with the patient's life.

The proper approach includes a tissue diagnosis of the tumor type. Surgery is planned to encompass a margin of normal tissue; the extent of resection is determined by the type of neoplasm. Resection of distant pathways of drainage (for example, the cervical lymph nodes) is determined by the biological character of the tumor.

Low-grade tumors, for example, basal cell carcinomas, can be adequately removed with a 4 to 5 mm. strip of surrounding tissue. To preserve cosmesis the incisions are placed in such a way as to conform to the lines or wrinkles in the face to minimize the scars.

NURSING CONSIDERATIONS. Surgical excision of skin tumors is often done on an outpatient basis with the patient under local anesthesia. Adequate facilities for outpatients should be provided. The same careful attention should be given to the care of specimens and records. Most patients appreciate reassurance from the attending nursing team. The nurse should be alert for any postoperative reaction and also make sure the patient understands postoperative instructions given by the surgeon.

### Surgical resection of carcinoma of the lip

CONSIDERATIONS. This typically may be a sun-induced carcinoma often associated with other premalignant changes in lip vermilion. The goal is complete excision and reconstruction in one stage.

SETUP AND PREPARATION OF THE PATIENT. The routine procedures for positioning, prepping, and draping of head and neck operations are carried out. The basic plastic Mayo setup, including the local anesthesia setup, is used. Lip clamps may be requested by the surgeon.

OPERATIVE PROCEDURE (Fig. 10-42)

1. The lesion is outlined with a marking pencil, and a 0.5 to 1 cm. margin is outlined with marker around this.

2. The nerves supplying the area are blocked with a local anesthetic.

3. The lesion is excised.

4. The circumoral labial artery must be clamped and ligated.

5. The specimen is oriented for later pathological examination. If there is any question about tumor extending to the margins, the wound is closed and the operation terminated to await permanent section. Otherwise, reconstruction is planned. Commonly, this will involve simple layered closure, since skin (particularly in older patients) can be mobilized for closure with minimal residual deformity.

6. The muscular layer is repaired, and then the mucosa and skin; care is taken to match the vermilion border precisely.

7. If more extensive reconstruction is necessary, a flap may be obtained from the upper lip with its blood supply coming into the pedicle from the labial artery. This flap is sutured into position. Division of the pedicle is delayed for 10 to 14 days until a new blood supply in the transpositioned tissue has adequately invaded from the surrounding tissue.

### Surgical resection of carcinoma of the tongue

CONSIDERATIONS. Tongue carcinoma less than 0.5 cm. in diameter does not often metastasize to cervical lymph nodes. Larger lesions may necessitate a radical neck dissection during the same operation. Lesions of the anterior and middle tongue may be treated by a wide resection of normal tissue surrounding the tumor. Commonly, a hemiglossectomy is performed for a lesion on the lateral margin of the

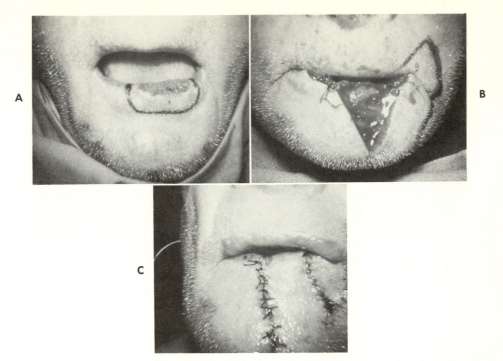

Fig. 10-42. **A,** Squamous cell carcinoma of the lower lip. **B,** Lesion excised and rotation flap outlined. **C,** Rotation flap sutured in place.

tongue. Carcinomas of the base of the tongue are usually detected later (after metastasis) and appear to be more aggressive in their behavior.

SETUP AND PREPARATION OF THE PATIENT. Routine procedures for prepping and draping the patient are carried out. The basic plastic Mayo setup is used. Additions include the following:

Denhardt mouth gag
Appendix retractor
Malleable retractor
Wooden tongue blades
Large towel clamp or heavy silk suture for retraction of the tongue
Several Ochsner clamps
Bovie cord if the surgeon desires

OPERATIVE PROCEDURE

1. A self-retaining mouth gag is inserted, and the tongue is grasped with a towel clamp.

2. A margin of normal tissue is outlined 2 cm. around the observable and palpable tumor.

3. The incision for a hemiglossectomy begins in the midline of the tongue and extends posteriorly and then laterally across the posterior margin.

4. The appropriate margin underneath the tongue is incised. Repeated palpation is helpful to indicate tumor depth and distance from the resection margin.

5. Bleeders are ligated with appropriate sutures.

6. The tongue is repaired with heavy chromic catgut, taking the tip from the other side and sewing it to the raw defect in the posterior edge of the wound, thus folding the tongue on itself. This is done because a long narrow tongue is more difficult to use for food manipulation than a short wide tongue.

### Radical neck dissection

DEFINITION. Excision of the superficial and deep cervical nodes to which a tumor may have spread from a primary lesion such as an intraoral lesion.

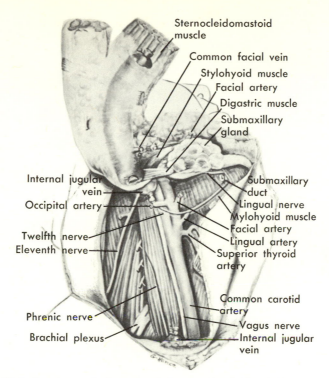

Sternocleidomastoid muscle

Common facial vein

Stylohyoid muscle

Facial artery

Digastric muscle

Submaxillary gland

Internal jugular vein

Occipital artery

Twelfth nerve

Eleventh nerve

Submaxillary duct

Lingual nerve

Mylohyoid muscle

Facial artery

Lingual artery

Superior thyroid artery

Phrenic nerve

Brachial plexus

Common carotid artery

Vagus nerve

Internal jugular vein

**Fig. 10-43.** High ligation and division of the jugular bulb. (The upper end is close to the skull and usually retracts upward out of view.) Submaxillary duct is ligated. Upper carotid sheath dissected free and included with the block. (From Brown, J. B., and McDowell, F.: Neck dissections, ed. 2, Springfield, Ill., 1957, Charles C Thomas, Publisher.)

**CONSIDERATIONS.** Radical neck dissection is indicated for removal of cancer that has spread to the neck lymph nodes. A tracheostomy may be necessary in combined resections (see Chapter 8 for tracheostomy procedure). Resection of a portion of the mandible is indicated if involved in the tumor.

**SETUP AND PREPARATION OF THE PATIENT.** After induction of general anesthesia, the patient's head is placed in extension with the affected side of the face and neck uppermost. The preoperative skin preparation is extensive, including the ear. The patient is draped with sterile head towels, side towels, and covering sheet. The instrument setup includes the basic plastic Mayo setup, with the addition of several dozen hemostats and one dozen Ochsner clamps. If a jaw resection is to be done in conjunction with dissection, additional instruments include the following:

2 Gigli saws, 20 in., with handles
1 Bone cutter
2 Bone-holding forceps or large towel clamps
   Kirschner wires and cutter
2 Pliers or wire benders

Accessory items
   Adequate supplies for bulky neck dressing as the surgeon desires
   Adequate supplies of catgut and silk ties and sutures as the surgeon's routine requires
Penrose drains

**OPERATIVE PROCEDURE** (Fig. 10-43). A variety of transverse incisions may be used to gain exposure of the neck. A submandibular incision combined with a vertical incision to the clavicle is the classic incision used. Parallel incisions, one above the clavicle and one below the mandible, have become more popular.

1. Skin flaps are developed posteriorly, anteriorly, and superiorly, preserving the mandibular branch of the facial nerve beneath the superior flap.

2. The sternocleidomastoid muscle is detached at the clavicle.

3. Dissection continues across the lower neck, dividing the fascia layers and the omohyoid muscle.

4. As the muscles are reflected cephalad, the internal jugular vein is identified, ligated, and divided.

5. The entire mass is now dissected superiorly by incising the fascia medially from the strap muscles and laterally from the trapezius muscle.

6. As the dissection continues upward, the carotid artery, vagus nerve, and phrenic nerve are identified and preserved. The accessory nerve is usually sacrificed.

7. With continued dissection superiorly, the hypoglossal nerve is identified at the bifurcation of the common carotid.

8. Superiorly, the digastric muscles and stylohyoid muscle are detached from the hyoid bone, and the hypoglossal nerve is preserved.

9. With the mandibular branch of the facial nerve retracted superiorly, a transverse incision at the level of the mandible extending through the parotid exposes the superior limits for division of the internal jugular vein.

10. After this is accomplished, the sternocleidomastoid muscle is detached from the mastoid process, completely removing the tumor-bearing lymph nodes of the neck.

11. All bleeding is meticulously controlled.

12. The skin flaps are sutured in place.

13. If suction catheters have been placed inferiorly and superiorly, no dressing is used on the neck. The surgeon may use Penrose drains and apply a compressive dressing.

## REFERENCES

1. Boyes, J. H.: Bunnell's surgery of the hand, ed. 4, Philadelphia, 1964, J. B. Lippincott Co.
2. Brown, J. B., Byars, L. T., McDowell, F., and Fryer, M. P.: Plastic surgery routine for surgical house staffs, Plast. Reconstr. Surg. 3:385, July, 1948.
3. Brown, J. B., and McDowell, F.: Neck dissections, ed. 2, Springfield, Ill., 1957, Charles C Thomas, Publisher.
4. Brown, J. B., and McDowell, F.: Skin grafting, ed. 3, Philadelphia, 1958, J. B. Lippincott Co.
5. Brown, J. B., and McDowell, F.: Plastic surgery of the nose, rev. ed., Springfield, Ill., 1965, Charles C Thomas, Publisher.
6. Byars, L. T.: Functional restoration of hypospadias deformities, Surg. Gynecol. Obstet. 92:149, 1951.
7. Converse, J., editor: Reconstructive plastic surgery, Surg. Clin. North Am. 47:261, April, 1967.
8. Grabb, W. C., and Smith, J. W., editors: Plastic surgery—a concise guide to clinical practice, Boston, 1968, Little, Brown & Co.
9. Kazanjian, V. H., and Converse, J. M.: The surgical treatment of facial injuries, ed. 2, Baltimore, 1959, The Williams & Wilkins Co.
10. Lampe, E. W.: Surgical anatomy of the hand, Clin. Symp. 21:66, July, 1969.
11. MacGregor, I. A., and Reid, W. H.: Plastic surgery for nurses, Edinburgh, 1966, E. & S. Livingstone Ltd.
12. McDowell, F., Brown, J. B., and Fryer, M. P.: Surgery of face, mouth and jaws, St. Louis, 1954, The C. V. Mosby Co.
13. Pickrell, K.: Reconstructive plastic surgery of the face, Clin. Symp. 19:71, July, 1967.
14. Skoog, T.: Reconstructive plastic surgery, Surg. Clin. North Am. 47:433, April, 1967.
15. Stark, R.: Plastic surgery, New York, 1962, Harper & Row, Publishers.
16. Struthers, A. M.: Principles of plastic surgery for nurses, Syracuse, N. Y., 1959, Syracuse University Press.
17. Wood-Smith, D., and Porowski, P. C., editors: Nursing care of the plastic surgery patient, St. Louis, 1967, The C. V. Mosby Co.

# CHAPTER 11

# Neurosurgery

PATRICIA TIPPETT

Functioning as a member of the neurosurgical operating team, the nurse must have a clear knowledge of the anatomy and some of the physiology of the central nervous system, its coverings, vasculature, and cerebrospinal fluid circulation. This knowledge should include an understanding of the peripheral and the autonomic nervous systems as well. The nurse must also be aware of the psychological and physical problems of neurosurgical patients. Only after appreciating problems such as paralysis, aphasia, and confusion will she be able to efficiently communicate and reassure the patient prior to induction of anesthesia. Also essential is a detailed knowledge of the care and functions of the increasingly complex instruments and equipment available to the neurosurgeon. Because of the duties she is expected to perform, the operating room nurse must be familiar with the procedures demanding the use of this equipment and these instruments.

## ANATOMY AND PHYSIOLOGY OF THE NERVOUS SYSTEM

The nervous system is divided into two parts: (1) the central nervous system, consisting of the brain and the spinal cord, and (2) the peripheral nervous system, comprising the cranial and spinal nerves and the peripheral portions of the autonomic nervous system. This mechanism, as a whole, is responsible for coordinating body activities in response to both external and internal stimuli.

The brain and the spinal cord are so well protected by massive bony and soft tissue structures that their exposure is

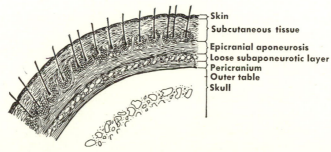

Fig. 11-1. Scalp is composed of following layers: skin, subcutaneous tissue, which contains blood vessels and nerves; aponeurotic layer (galea aponeurotica, or epicranial aponeurosis), which is the aponeurosis of occipitofrontal muscle; loose subaponeurotic layer; and pericranium. Outer three layers are adherent to each other. (From Berman, J. K.: Principles and practice of surgery, St. Louis, 1950, The C. V. Mosby Co.)

tedious and time consuming. Because the clamp and ligature technique for control of hemorrhage is inapplicable to delicate nervous tissue, specialized techniques are necessary to carry out modern neurosurgical procedures. These techniques will be considered as they relate to specific structures that are encountered during surgery.

### Extracranial structures

The scalp (Fig. 11-1) consists of several layers—the skin, the subcutaneous tissue, and the epicranial aponeurosis with its occipitofrontal musculature. The skin is thick, and the subcutaneous tissue, which is exceptionally dense, tough, and vascular, is firmly attached to the epicranial aponeurosis. Since most of the blood vessels lie superficial to the aponeurosis, bleeding from the scalp is best controlled by local pressure and skin clips or by everting hemostats that are applied to the aponeurosis. Scalp wounds or incisions are closed by placing interrupted sutures individually in both the aponeurosis and the skin. The subgaleal space contains loose areolar tissue, which permits mobility of the scalp and is a favorite site for abscess formation. Deep to the scalp is a layer of tissue that covers the cranium known as the pericranium, or outer periosteum of the skull. The surgeon may lift the scalp off the periosteum (osteoplastic craniotomy) or strip the periosteum off the skull (osteoclastic craniotomy) when turning down a scalp flap in preparation for a craniotomy.

The arterial supply of the scalp is derived from the external carotid artery through the superficial temporal, posterior auricular, occipital, frontal, and supraorbital branches. Scalp incisions are planned with this arterial supply in mind. Most veins roughly follow the course of the arteries, except those few that drain directly through the skull into the intracranial venous sinuses (emissary veins). The scalp, the extracranial arteries, and portions of the dura mater are the only pain-sensitive structures that cover the brain, which itself is insensitive. For this reason a local anesthetic

agent may be sufficient for many procedures, especially when small doses of some of the newer intravenous narcotic and neuroleptic agents are given in conjunction with the local medication. This is seldom done for most intracranial procedures. Most patients receive a general anesthetic, and a local anesthetic is injected into the proposed incision in order to reduce the amount of general anesthetic required.

### The skull

The bony structures of the head and face, twenty-four in all, form the skull. These are joined by serrated bony seams called *sutures*. In the infant, these sutures are not firm and so allow for considerable molding during childbirth.

At the top of the skull in front of and behind the parietal bones are the anterior and posterior fontanels, which are open at birth. In the baby, the subdural spaces or lateral ventricles can be easily reached through the anterior fontanel with an aspirating needle, without making burr holes in the skull. If the suture lines close prematurely, the skull cannot expand as the brain grows. This condition, which is called *craniosynostosis*, demands early opening of the fused sutures.

The skull, which as a whole is oval shaped, is wider in back than it is in front; it is composed of flattened or irregular bones that consist of two tables of compact substances that enclose a layer of spongy bone, known as *diploe*. The sides and roof of the skull are formed by the frontal, parietal, temporal, and occipital bones.

The interior of the skull at its base is anatomically divided into three cranial fossae: anterior, middle, and posterior (Fig. 11-2). The anterior fossa is limited posteriorly by the sphenoid ridge, along which pituitary tumors and aneurysms of the circle of Willis are generally approached. The frontal lobes and olfactory bulbs and tracts lie in the anterior fossa. The temporal lobes lie in the middle fossa, which is shaped like a butterfly. The sella turcica,

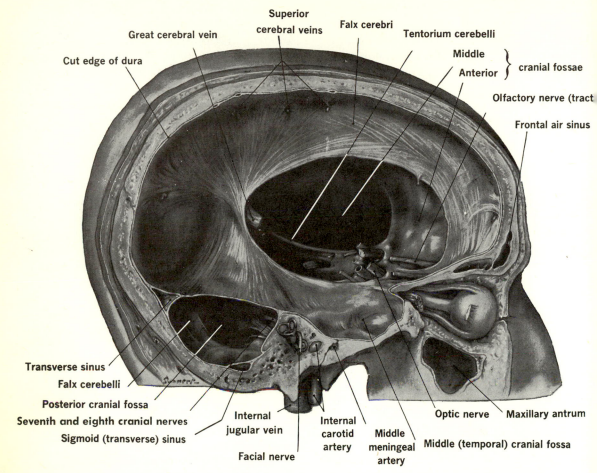

**Fig. 11-2.** Intracranial dura mater showing falx cerebri and tentorium cerebelli fanning out laterally, dividing posterior cranial fossa from middle and anterior fossae. (From Mettler, F. A.: Neuroanatomy, ed. 2, St. Louis, The C. V. Mosby Co.)

formed by the sphenoid bones, is the most central part of the middle fossa and houses the pituitary gland. The floor and lateral walls of the middle fossa are shaped from the greater wing of the sphenoid bone and parts of the temporal bone. The posterior fossa, which is the largest and deepest fossa, is formed by the occipital, sphenoid, and petrous portions of the temporal bones; the cerebellum, pons, and medulla lie here, along with many of the cranial nerves. The foramen magnum, which is the largest opening in the skull, transmits the spinal cord as it joins the brainstem in the posterior fossa. There are numerous other openings in the base of the skull for passage of arteries, veins, and cranial nerves.

## Meninges

Lying between the skull and brain are the meninges, which comprise three covering membranes, known as the *dura mater, arachnoid,* and *pia mater* (Fig. 11-3).

The dura mater is a tough, shiny, fibrous membrane that is closely applied to the inner surface of the skull and which, by several folds, separates the cranial cavity into adjoining compartments. The largest fold is the falx cerebri, which is an arch-shaped, vertically placed, midline structure that separates the right and left cerebral hemispheres from each other. A smaller fold of dura, known as the falx cerebelli, separates the cerebellar hemi-

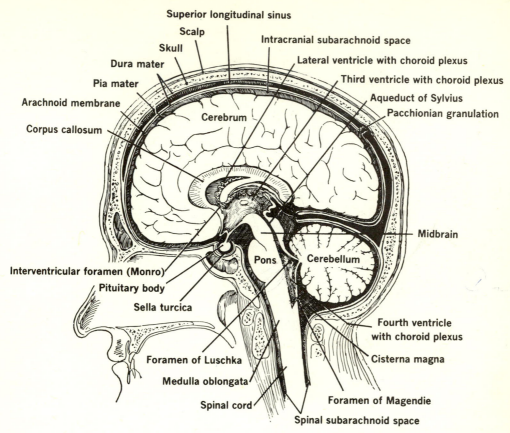

**Fig. 11-3.** Diagram of sagittal section of head showing cerebrospinal fluid spaces and their relationship to venous circulation and principal subdivisions of brain and its coverings. (From Carini, E., and Owens, G.: Neurological and neurosurgical nursing, ed. 5, St. Louis, 1970, The C. V. Mosby Co.)

spheres vertically. Another fold that is transversely situated, known as the tentorium cerebelli, forms the roof of the posterior fossa, on which rest the occipital lobes of the cerebral hemispheres. Below the tentorium lie the cerebellum and brainstem (Figs. 11-2 and 11-3).

At the margins of these dural folds lie large venous sinuses that drain blood from the intracranial structures into the jugular veins. Several arteries also lie within the layers of the dura, the largest of which, the middle meningeal, may give rise to serious hemorrhage if it is torn by an overlying fracture of the skull.

Beneath the dura mater is a fine membrane, the arachnoid. The outer layer of this membrane closely approximates the dura, whereas the inner layer gives off innumerable spidery filaments that bridge to the surface of the brain (Fig. 11-2). Whereas the outer surface of the arachnoid is closely applied to the dura with no space normally present between these two membranes, the inner surface of the arachnoid is separated from the pial membrane beneath it by a space. This is the subarachnoid space, which is filled with cerebrospinal fluid that constantly bathes the brain. In places, particularly around the base of the brain, this space becomes enlarged to form cisterns. Its function is more fully described in connection with the cerebrospinal fluid pathways.

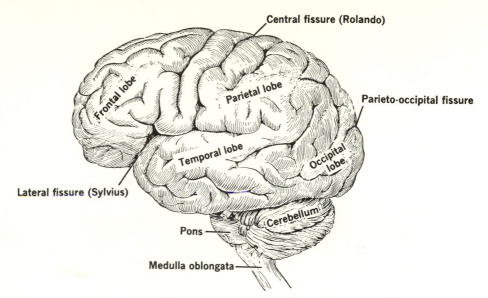

**Fig. 11-4.** Lateral view of cerebral hemisphere (showing lobes and principal fissures), cerebellum, pons, and medulla oblongata. (From Carini, E., and Owens, G.: Neurological and neurosurgical nursing, ed. 5, St. Louis, 1970, The C. V. Mosby Co.)

The pia mater, the innermost membrane, is gossamer-like and covers the brain intimately, dipping deep into each of the sulci. Directly below the pia mater is a rich, superficial vascular network.

**The brain**

The brain is surrounded by the three protective membranes (meninges) and is enclosed within the cranial cavity of the skull. It is divided into the cerebral cortex, basal ganglia, hypothalamus, midbrain, brainstem, and cerebellum.

The right and left cerebral hemispheres are the largest parts of the brain. Each hemisphere is composed of cerebral cortex comprising the frontal, parietal, occipital, and temporal lobes, as well as the insula, rhinencephalon, basal ganglia, and hypothalamus. The two hemispheres are joined underneath the falx by a huge transverse bundle of nerve fibers known as the corpus callosum. Among its other functions, each of the cerebral hemispheres controls motor activity and receives sensory stimuli from the opposite half of the body.

The surfaces of the hemispheres are thrown into folds, which are called *gyri*, or convolutions; between these gyri lie the fissures, or sulci of the brain. The two sulci of great anatomical importance to the surgeon are the central sulcus of Rolando, which separates the motor from the sensory cortex, and the fissure of Sylvius, which marks off the temporal lobe (Fig. 11-4). The insula (island of Reil) lies deep within the fissure of Sylvius and can be exposed by separating the upper and lower lips of the fissure. The part of the hemisphere that is anterior to the fissure of Rolando is the frontal lobe. To a considerable degree, it controls the higher functions of intellect and abstract reasoning. Within the frontal lobe, just in front of the rolandic fissure, is the motor cortex, destruction of which leads to loss of voluntary motor function on the opposite side (Fig. 11-5) of the body (hemiplegia). Behind the central sulcus is the parietal lobe, extending back to the parieto-occipital fissure. This area contains the final receiving and integrating station for sensory impulses from the contralateral

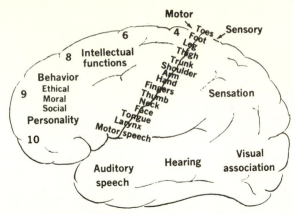

**Fig. 11-5.** Principal functional subdivisions of cerebral hemispheres. Note numbered areas (Brodmann) generally used to designate specific anatomical and physiological components. (From Carini, E., and Owens, G.: Neurological and neurosurgical nursing, ed. 5, St. Louis, 1970, The C. V. Mosby Co.)

side of the body. Most posterior is the occipital lobe, the function of which is to receive and integrate visual impulses and register them as meaningful images (Figs. 11-4 and 11-5). Inferior to the fissure of Sylvius, in the middle fossa of the skull, lies the temporal lobe. Lesions of the left temporal lobe in right-handed individuals, as well as in many but not all left-handed persons, often affect the comprehension and the verbalization of words; the result is aphasia. Rhinencephalic structures such as the anterior limbic area and the orbital surface may exert an inhibitory effect on brain mechanisms concerned in the expression of emotions such as anger. Restlessness and hyperactivity may result from lesions of this area. The rhinencephalon has many connections with the hypothalamus. It may affect sexual behavior, emotions, and motivation. Loss of recent memory may point to a lesion of this area.

The *cerebral hemispheres* are covered by a layer of gray matter, the cerebral cortex, which contains the cell bodies of the many nerve pathways of the brain. The underlying white matter consists of millions of myelinated nerve axons and is relatively avascular compared to the cortex. The nerve pathways are of three main types: (1) the transverse or commissural fibers, which pass from one cerebral hemisphere to the other; (2) the association fibers, which connect various portions of the cerebral hemisphere longitudinally; and (3) the projection fibers, including the great motor and sensory systems, which run vertically to connect the cortical regions with other portions of the central nervous system.

In prefrontal lobotomy the association fibers from the frontal lobe are divided, thus effecting changes in personality of the individual which may be of benefit in combating certain psychiatric disorders. More recently, another operation called *cingulotomy,* in which the cingulum is interrupted, has also been done for these disorders.

Deep in the brain are several important large cell stations. For example, the basal ganglia are collections of nuclei of the extrapyramidal system concerned with smoothing out motor activities. Lesions here cause rigidity of the skeletal muscles and various types of spontaneous tremor. The basal ganglia, including the thalamus, have been attacked surgically in an effort to relieve the tremors and rigidity associated with multiple sclerosis, Parkinson's disease, various forms of cerebellar degeneration, and late effects of severe brain trauma. The thalamus is the great receiving station of incoming sensory stimuli.

Many of these are subsequently relayed to a final destination in the parietal cortex. Because of its central role in perception of body sensations, surgical lesions have been made in the thalamus in an attempt to alleviate pain.

Along the floor of the third ventricle is the hypothalamus, which is principally concerned with the autonomic regulation of the body's internal environment and which is intimately connected with the pituitary gland.

The short, stocky portion of the brain, between the cerebral hemispheres and pons, is called the *midbrain* (Fig. 11-3). It is made up of the cerebral peduncles and numerous other nerve tracts and contains the nuclei and association centers that control the majority of eye movements. The hindbrain, or so-called brainstem, which is immediately below the midbrain, consists of the pons and medulla oblongata (Fig. 11-4). These form the floor of the fourth ventricle in the posterior fossa of the skull and contain many large efferent and afferent tracts, besides nuclei of most cranial nerves. This region of the brain controls respiration and influences the pulse and blood pressure. Since many vital structures are crowded together in this region, direct surgery is fraught with great danger.

The cerebellum (Fig. 11-4), which occupies most of the posterior fossa, forms the roof of the fourth ventricle. It has two lateral lobes and a medial portion, called the *vermis*. The fissures of the cerebellum are small and run transversely, giving it a laminated appearance. The cerebellum is principally concerned with balance and coordination of movement. It has many complex connections with higher and lower centers and exerts its influence homolaterally, in contrast to the cerebral hemispheres, which act contralaterally. At least half the brain tumors in children originate in the cerebellum. In adults and children the commonest surgical lesions that are operated on in this area are tumors and abscesses. By splitting the vermis in the exact midline, a satisfactory exposure of tumors that lie in the fourth ventricle is obtained without sacrificing the important cerebellar functions.

### Ventricles of the brain and cerebrospinal fluid circulation

Within the substance of the brain are four communicating cavities, called *ventricles*, which are filled with cerebrospinal fluid. In the lower medial portion of each cerebral hemisphere lies the large lateral ventricle, which resembles a wishbone and is separated anteriorly from its counterpart by a thin layer, the pellucid septum (Fig. 11-6). Each lateral ventricle consists of a body and three horns—frontal, occipital, and temporal. Below the bodies of the lateral ventricles is a centrally placed cleft, designated as the third ventricle. It communicates anteriorly with the lateral ventricles through the foramina of Monro and posteriorly with the fourth ventricle through the aqueduct of Sylvius, a long narrow channel passing through the midbrain. The fourth ventricle is a rhomboid-shaped cavity in the posterior fossa, between the cerebellum and the brainstem. In the roof of the fourth ventricle is an opening into the cisterna magna, known as the foramen of Magendie; at the lateral margins are the two foramina of Luschka.

Much of the cerebrospinal fluid originates in the choroid plexuses of the ventricles. These are tufted, vascular structures, which allow certain fluid elements of the blood to pass through their ependymal linings. A choroid plexus is found in each lateral ventricle along its floor, on the roof of the third ventricle, and in the posterior portion of the fourth ventricle. Most of the fluid is elaborated in the lateral ventricles, whence it flows through the interventricular foramina of Monro to the third ventricle. From there it traverses the aqueduct of Sylvius to reach the fourth ventricle, and from there it escapes into the subarachnoid space of the basal cis-

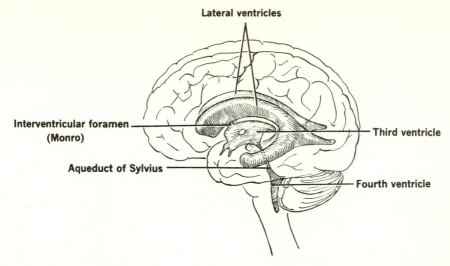

Lateral ventricles

Interventricular foramen (Monro)

Aqueduct of Sylvius

Third ventricle

Fourth ventricle

**Fig. 11-6.** Diagram of ventricular system showing its relationship to various parts of brain. (From Carini, E., and Owens, G.: Neurological and neurosurgical nursing, ed. 5, St. Louis, 1970, The C. V. Mosby Co.)

terns via the foramina of Magendie and Luschka. From the basal cisterns the fluid is directed down around the spinal cord, up over the cerebellar lobes or around the medulla, the base of the brain, and up over the cerebral hemispheres in the cranial subarachnoid space. The fluid returns to the bloodstream through little projections of the arachnoid (pacchionian granulations) into the great dural venous sinuses, particularly the superior sagittal sinus, and by diffusion through perivascular, perineural, and periradicular channels.

The total content of circulating cerebrospinal fluid averages 125 to 150 ml. in the adult. Each lateral ventricle contains 10 to 15 ml.; the rest of the ventricular system contains 5 ml.; the cranial subarachnoid space averages about 25 ml., whereas the spinal subarachnoid space contains about 75 ml. The ventricular fluid normally has 5 to 15 mg./100 ml. protein content, whereas the spinal fluid values are 25 to 45 mg./100 ml. These values may be considerably elevated in various lesions of the central nervous system.

The function of the cerebrospinal fluid is mainly mechanical. It bathes the brain and spinal cord, helps support the weight of the brain, and acts as a cushion for it and the spinal cord by absorbing some of the force of external trauma. By variation in its volume, it aids in keeping intracranial pressure relatively constant. If there is atrophy of the brain, it increases in amount to take up the dead space; if the brain swells due to trauma or a tumor, thus increasing the intracranial contents, the cerebrospinal fluid decreases in amount. The fluid is useful in carrying certain drugs to diseased parts of the brain. It does not, however, play a significant role in supplying nutrition to the structures that it bathes.

The rate of formation and absorption of cerebrospinal fluid is related to the osmotic and hydrostatic pressure of the blood. Frequently, some use is made of this fact. In instances of increased intracranial pressure, an intravenous injection of hypertonic mannitol or urea or a nonosmotic diuretic is employed to dehydrate the blood and thus draw off the cerebrospinal fluid.

Cerebrospinal fluid pressure may be elevated for a number of reasons: (1) an expanding mass lesion within the skull, such as a tumor, hemorrhage, or cerebral edema; (2) an increased formation of fluid, as in meningitis, encephalitis, and other febrile conditions; (3) an increase

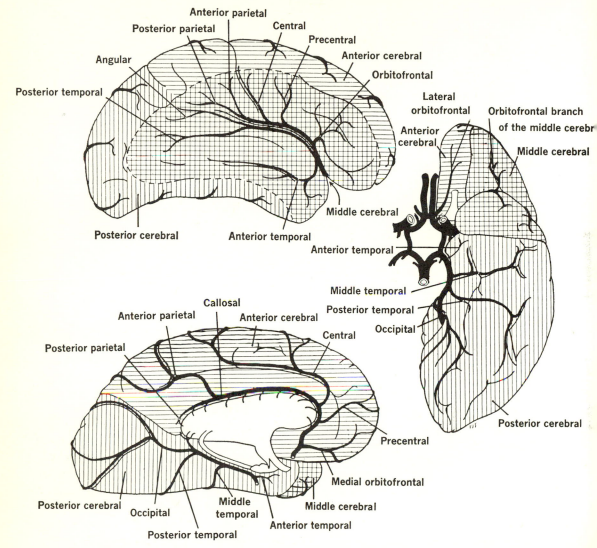

**Fig. 11-7.** Diagram of areas of distribution of anterior, middle, and posterior cerebral arteries. (From Mettler, F. A.: Neuroanatomy, ed. 2, St. Louis, The C. V. Mosby Co.)

in venous pressure within the skull from an obstruction to normal venous drainage; (4) a blockage of absorption by inflammatory conditions of the arachnoid and perivascular spaces; and (5) any mechanical obstruction of the ventricular or subarachnoid fluid pathways.

The neurosurgeon is vitally interested in the cerebrospinal fluid pressure, since many of the lesions that cause an increased pressure may be treated by modern neurosurgery.

### Vascular supply

The arterial supply of the brain is derived from the internal carotid arteries anteriorly and the vertebral arteries that join to form the basilar arteries posteriorly. Communications between these make up the arterial circle of Willis, which is situated at the base of the brain. The branches of the circle are of two types: (1) the small central terminal arteries, which dip perpendicularly into the brain and do not anastomose with one another, and (2) the

Anterior communicating

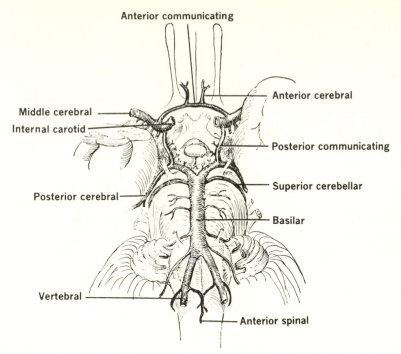

Middle cerebral

Internal carotid

Anterior cerebral

Posterior communicating

Superior cerebellar

Posterior cerebral

Basilar

Vertebral

Anterior spinal

**Fig. 11-8.** Diagram of the principal cerebral arteries and the circle of Willis. (From Carini, E., and Owens, G.: Neurological and neurosurgical nursing, ed. 5, St. Louis, 1970, The C. V. Mosby Co.)

three large cortical branches on either side, named the anterior, middle, and posterior cerebral arteries, respectively (Fig. 11-7). The latter have a fairly free communication with each other peripherally, so that occlusion of one may be partly compensated by its neighbor. They do not, however, anastomose with their counterparts, except through the often inefficient communicating branches of the circle of Willis. (See Fig. 11-8.)

The cerebral veins do not parallel the arteries as do the veins in most other parts of the body. The external cortical veins anastomose freely in the pia mater, forming larger cerebral veins, and as such they pierce the arachnoid space, cross the subdural space, and empty into the great dural venous sinuses, which have been described in conjunction with the meninges. A subdural hemorrhage that occurs following head trauma may arise from disruption of these bridging vessels, whereas extradural hemorrhage often results from

lacerations of the middle meningeal artery, a branch of the external carotid artery that supplies the dura mater. The deep cerebral veins that drain the interior of the hemispheres empty principally into the great vein of Galen and the inferior sagittal sinus.

The blood transports oxygen, nutrients, and other substances necessary for the proper functioning of living tissue. The needs of the brain are critical. The brain can store only very limited amounts of oxygen and energy-producing nutrients. Therefore constant flow of blood to the brain must be maintained.

The brain uses oxygen carried by the bloodstream for the oxidation of glucose. Metabolism of glucose in the brain is a chief source of energy. Protein and fat metabolism play little part in energy production. In the face of oxygen deficit, the survival time of the central nervous system tissue is very short. In the face of low blood sugar, central nervous system function is

compromised, and unconsciousness results.

Generally, all factors that affect the systemic blood pressure indirectly affect the cerebral circulation. However, only when systemic blood pressure falls to much below the patient's normal level is there usually any significant drop in cerebral blood flow. Thus controlled hypotension many be safely used in aneurysm surgery.

The blood-brain barrier prevents many substances in the blood from reaching the brain. It may influence brain function by determining composition of brain fluids. Some types of abnormal brain function could conceivably result from an abnormal blood-brain barrier.

### Cranial nerves

There are twelve pairs of cranial nerves, several of which are of considerable neurosurgical importance. It is appropriate to consider their anatomy, function, and surgery together.

CRANIAL NERVE I. The olfactory nerve, which actually is a fiber tract of the brain, is located under the frontal lobe on the cribriform plate of the ethmoid bone. This nerve governs the sense of smell. Frontal lobe tumors, fractures of the anterior fossa of the skull, and lesions of the nasal cavity frequently affect the olfactory nerve.

CRANIAL NERVE II. The optic nerve is actually a fiber tract of the brain. It originates in the ganglion cells of the retina and passes through the optic foramen in the apex of the orbit to reach the optic chiasm, where a partial crossing of the fibers occurs, so that those fibers from the nasal half of each retina pass to the opposite side. Posterior to the chiasm the visual pathway is called the *optic tract;* still further back, it becomes the optic radiation. Lesions in various parts of this pathway produce characteristic defects in the visual fields. For example, a lesion of the chiasm usually destroys the temporal vision of each eye (bitemporal hemianopsia), whereas a lesion of the occipital lobe will produce impairment of vision (homonymous hemianopsia) affecting the right or left halves of the visual fields of both eyes.

The lesions that affect the optic nerve and are treated by neurosurgery include primary gliomas of the nerve, pituitary tumors that press on the optic chiasm, and occasionally meningiomas in the region of the sella turcica and olfactory groove. The optic nerves and chiasm are best exposed through a frontal craniotomy, along the floor of the anterior fossa, or through a frontotemporal approach along the sphenoid ridge.

In malignant exophthalmos associated with hyperthyroidism, it is sometimes necessary to unroof the orbit and decompress its edematous contents to preserve vision. The widest decompression can be performed by an intracranial, extradural operation. This approach is also useful in exposing deep intraorbital tumors.

CRANIAL NERVES III, IV, AND VI. These three pairs of nerves are conveniently considered together, since they are the motor nerves to the muscles of the eye. They are the oculomotor, the trochlear, and the abducent, respectively. They are affected by many toxic, inflammatory, vascular, or neoplastic lesions. The third nerve may be affected by aneurysms of the internal carotid artery, and pressure against this nerve accounts for pupillary dilatation in cases with temporal lobe herniation due to increased intracranial pressure.

CRANIAL NERVE V. The trigeminal nerve has two functions: (1) the sensory supply of the forehead, eyes, meninges, face, jaw, teeth, hard palate, buccal mucosa, and tongue and (2) the motor innervation of the muscles of mastication. The sensory fibers that arise from cells in the gasserian ganglion travel along the medial wall of the middle cranial fossa and then extend peripherally in three divisions—ophthalmic, maxillary, and mandibular. Behind the ganglion, the fibers enter the brainstem via the sensory root. The motor root, which originates from cells in the

brainstem, follows the course of the larger sensory component.

The trigeminal nerve transmits a distressing neuralgia, tic douloureux, which is characterized by excruciating, piercing pains of brief duration affecting one or more of the major peripheral divisions. The recurrent attacks are usually brought on by stimulation of trigger zones present about the face, nares, lips, or teeth. This affliction, which is of unknown etiology, tends to occur unilaterally and mainly in older persons. Medical treatment is frequently unsuccessful, and a great variety of neurosurgical procedures have been proposed for its control. Peripheral neurectomies of the supraorbital or infraorbital nerves may easily be performed with the patient under local anesthesia in appropriate cases, but the effect is temporary because the nerves regenerate. The most certain method of relief is retrogasserian neurectomy. When the nerve root is divided behind the ganglion, no regeneration can occur, and the pain is permanently obliterated. However, some patients complain about the postoperative numbness of the face, and a few are disturbed by annoying paresthesia. Anesthesia of the cornea may rarely lead to serious keratitis. Differential section of the root has been sufficiently perfected to preserve a few sensory fibers to the cornea and prevent this complication in patients. In most cases, the motor root can be saved.

Retrogasserian neurectomy may be performed through a temporal approach along the floor of the middle fossa or via a posterior fossa exposure, in which case the nerve root is sectioned in the cerebellopontine angle where it emerges from the pons. By the posterior fossa approach the surgeon can more easily spare the motor root, but this advantage is countered by slightly greater morbidity than the temporal operation.

CRANIAL NERVE VII. The facial nerve supplies the musculature of the face and taste to the anterior two thirds of the tongue. It originates in the brainstem, passes through the skull with the eighth nerve via the internal acoustic meatus, continues along the facial canal, and exits just posterior to the parotid gland. The nerve may be damaged by acoustic neurinomas, fractures at the base of the skull, mastoid infections, or surgical procedures in the vicinity of the parotid gland. When permanent interruption occurs, useful operations for restoration of function include spinofacial or hypoglossofacial anastomosis (cranial nerves XI to VII and cranial nerves XII to VII, respectively). These operations are performed high in the neck behind the parotid gland.

CRANIAL NERVE VIII. The acoustic nerve has two parts, both sensory—the cochlear for hearing and the vestibular for balance. The former receives stimuli from the organ of Corti, the latter from the semicircular canals of the inner ear. The major surgical lesion of the eighth nerve is the acoustic neurinoma, which is a benign tumor growing from the nerve sheath at its entrance into the internal auditory meatus. This tumor arises deep in the angle between the cerebellum and pons. Symptoms may include unilateral deafness, tinnitus, unilateral impairment of cerebellar function, occasionally numbness of the face from involvement of the fifth cranial nerve, and, late in the course, papilledema caused by pressure on the pons. The operative approach is usually via a unilateral suboccipital craniectomy. Great care must be taken to avoid injury to the pons, and an attempt is made to preserve the facial nerve.

Ménière's disease is an eighth nerve affliction characterized by deafness and tinnitus, with episodic attacks of severe vertigo and vomiting. These episodes may pitch the patient violently to the floor without warning and even commit him to bed for days at a time. When simple medical measures fail to alleviate the problem, section of the eighth nerve intracranially may be performed with consistently excellent results.

CRANIAL NERVE IX. The glossopharyngeal

nerve supplies the sense of taste to the posterior one third of the tongue and sensation to the tonsils and pharyngeal region and partially innervates the pharyngeal muscles. Rarely, it is involved in a painful tic similar to trigeminal tic. There may be occasion to section its sensory component for this reason, to treat a hypersensitive carotid sinus, or, along with the fifth nerve, to treat painful malignancies of the face, mouth, and pharynx. It lies near the eighth nerve in the posterior fossa and is exposed in a similar fashion.

CRANIAL NERVE X. The vagus nerve has many functions, chief among which are innervation of pharyngeal and laryngeal musculature, control of heart rate, and acid secretion of the stomach. In neck surgery, the surgeon carefully avoids the recurrent laryngeal branch; in gastric surgery, he severs the nerve at the lower end of the esophagus to treat a peptic ulcer. The neurosurgeon is mainly concerned with avoiding damage to the vagus nerve during posterior fossa surgery.

CRANIAL NERVE XI. The spinal accessory nerve is a motor nerve to the sternocleidomastoid and trapezius muscles. To restore mobility to the face, it may be anastomosed to the peripheral end of a damaged facial nerve.

CRANIAL NERVE XII. The hypoglossal nerve innervates the musculature of the tongue. Its neurosurgical interest is similar to that of the spinal accessory nerve.

### Brain tumors

Of the brain lesions that are treated surgically, tumors are of great importance. They are not as rare nor is their prognosis as poor as the layman is often wont to believe. If the diagnosis is made early, the surgical treatment may be greatly simplified because increased intracranial pressure and severe neurological changes are not usually present.

Brain tumors may be considered malignant or benign, depending on the cell type. Primary tumors generally do not resemble the carcinomas and the sarcomas found

outside the central nervous system and rarely metastasize outside the central nervous system. Metastases from carcinomas or sarcomas growing elsewhere in the body grow well in the central nervous system.

If one includes all tumors, both primary and metastatic, of the brain and its covering membranes in the term *intracranial tumors*, such tumors may be conveniently classified as congenital, mesodermal, ectodermal, metastatic, and miscellaneous tumors. This pathological classification is as follows:

A. Congenital tumors
   1. Epidermoid
   2. Dermoid
   3. Teratoma
   4. Chordoma
   5. Craniopharyngioma occurs in children and adults and arises from the region of the pituitary stalk. It is usually cystic, and calcification above the sella turcica is often seen on x-ray films. Diabetes insipidus and visual field changes are common.
B. Mesodermal tumors
   1. Meningioma usually is encapsulated and easily separated from nervous tissue. It may be adherent to the dural venous sinuses or major arteries.
   2. Neurinoma usually arises from neurilemma sheath cells of the vestibular portion of the eighth cranial nerve within the auditory meatus. It grows to fill the cerebellopontine angle and may indent the brainstem.
   3. Vascular tumors
      a. Angioma is regarded by most writers as a malformation. Most of these are arteriovenous malformations ("AVM's").
      b. Hemangioblastoma is usually cystic and likely to occur in the cerebellar hemispheres. It is sometimes present in association with angiomas of the retina and other organs.
      c. Aneurysm is a saccular dilatation or outpouching of the cerebral arteries. It may rupture, producing subarachnoid hemorrhage.
C. Ectodermal tumors
   1. Gliomas
      a. Glioblastoma multiforme is an infiltrative, rapidly growing, rapidly recurring cerebral tumor that occurs most frequently in middle age. It may invade both cerebral hemispheres by crossing in the corpus callosum. Areas of necrosis are characteristic. Astrocytomas, astroblasto-

mas, and oligodendrogliomas may transform into this very malignant tumor with time.

b. Medulloblastoma is a rapidly growing, rapidly recurring tumor of the vermis of the cerebellum and fourth ventricle that usually occurs in young children. It characteristically metastasizes in the subarachnoid spaces, usually spreading to the base of the brain by this route.

c. Ependymoma occurs most frequently in children and is likely to arise in or near the ventricular walls. It commonly occurs in the fourth ventricle, where it abuts against or involves vital medullary centers. It also frequently metastasizes in the subarachnoid spaces.

d. Astrocytoma usually occurs in the cerebellum of children and the cerebrum of adults. It is often cystic and discrete in children, infiltrating and ill defined in adults.

e. Oligodendroglioma is usually found in the cerebral hemispheres and is infiltrating but occasionally moderately well defined.

f. Astroblastoma is a rare glioma occurring in the cerebral hemisphere of middle-aged adults. It may share the growth characteristics of astrocytoma and glioblastoma multiforme.

g. Spongioblastoma occurs predominantly in the optic chiasm and nerves of children and in the pons. This lesion grows in vital structures and is rarely amenable to even partial removal.

2. Pituitary tumors

a. Chromophobe tumor is relatively common in the anterior pituitary glands of adults. It causes compression of the pituitary, adjacent optic chiasm, and hypothalamus. The latter may lead to diabetes insipidus.

b. Chromophile tumor is often secreting (as are occasional chromophobe tumors). Acromegaly or, less commonly, Cushing's syndrome may occur and cause the patient to seek help long before the tumor has expanded sufficiently to compromise the optic chiasm.

D. Metastatic tumors usually arise from carcinoma, more rarely from sarcoma, and occasionally from melanomas and retinal tumors. The most common sources are bronchogenic carcinoma and carcinoma of the breast.

Tumors not discussed here are eosinophilic granuloma, tuberculomas and other granulomas, brain abscesses, pinealomas, colloid cysts, choroid plexus papillomas, microgliomas, fibrous dysplasia, and lymphomas.

A brain tumor is diagnosed by recognizing the symptoms and their evolution and then applying certain tests for more accurate localization. The neurosurgeon's diagnostic ability depends on a thorough knowledge of neuroanatomy and neurophysiology, plus an understanding of the behavior of various kinds of brain tumors. The manifestations of an intracranial tumor fall into two classes: those resulting from impairment or irritation of function in specific areas of the brain directly affected by the tumor and those resulting from diffuse increased intracranial pressure.

For example, lesions that are situated in the left frontotemporal region where motor speech originates lead to aphasia, occipital tumors produce hemianoptic visual defects, and large frontal lobe tumors may cause striking personality changes. Cortical tumors frequently produce focal seizures of diagnostic value. The onset of epileptiform seizures in the adult is often associated with an intracranial neoplasm. Pituitary tumors characteristically press on the optic chiasm and so impair temporal vision of each eye. They disturb pituitary glandular function, resulting in hypopituitary states, pituitary dwarfism, or acromegaly, as the case may be. The posterior fossa tumors more often manifest their presence by blocking the cerebrospinal fluid circulation, but they may also destroy cerebellar function, resulting in incoordination, ataxia, and scanning speech.

The commonest symptom of increased intracranial pressure is headache, but it does not always accompany increased pressure. The characteristics and location of the pain may vary and are seldom of specific diagnostic value. Vomiting is also a frequent sign of increased pressure and often is not associated with nausea. This is particularly true of tumors in the posterior fossa in children. Chronic increased pressure causes papilledema and not infrequently diplopia due to a sixth nerve

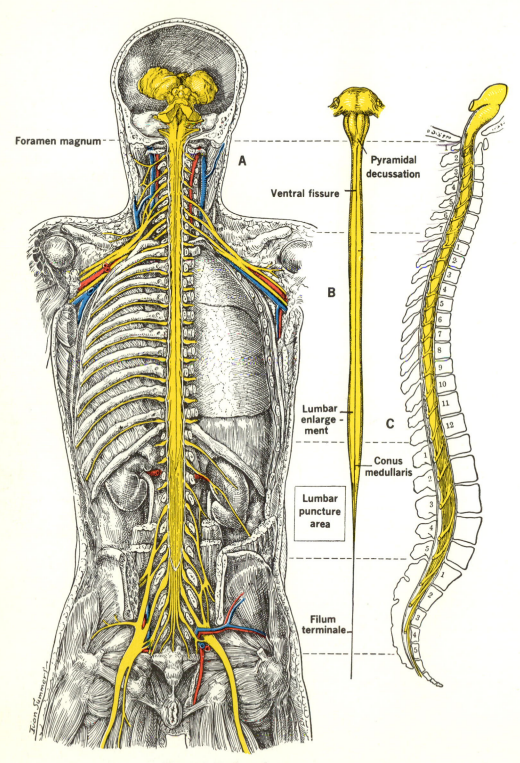

Foramen magnum

A

Pyramidal decussation

Ventral fissure

B

Lumbar enlarge-ment

C

Conus medullaris

Lumbar puncture area

Filum terminale

Fig. 11-9. For legend see opposite page.

palsy. Eventually mental dullness, unconsciousness, and coma occur. More acute rises in intracranial pressure produce dilatation of one or both pupils, decerebration, respiratory irregularities, slowing of the pulse, and elevation of blood pressure.

A careful historical account of the patient's symptoms and a thorough neurological evaluation are the most important aspects of diagnosis. Special methods of examination are also necessary in most instances; these include x-ray examination of the skull, electroencephalography, cerebral angiography, and, when there is no evidence of increased pressure, a study of the cerebrospinal fluid. In recent years brain scanning with various radioactive isotope techniques has been helpful in accurately localizing tumors of the cerebral hemispheres.

Finally, visualization of the position of the cerebral ventricles with air studies is often used to determine the exact position of the tumor for the neurosurgeon's attack.

### Spinal column, spinal cord, and peripheral nerves

The spinal column consists of thirty-three vertebrae: seven cervical, twelve thoracic, five lumbar, five sacral (fused as one), and one coccygeal, a fusion of four small vertebrae (Fig. 11-9).

The first cervical vertebra or atlas serves as a support for the skull and is distinguished by absence of a body and spinous process. The second cervical vertebra or axis is notable for its odontoid process, a vertical projection extending into the spinal canal of the atlas like a stick in a hoop. Strong ligaments hold the two together but allow for considerable rotational movement. When these ligaments are torn, as in a hanging, or when the odontoid is fractured by trauma, the atlas may slip on the axis and crush the cord, resulting in immediate death.

The remainder of the cervical, thoracic, and lumbar vertebrae have certain important anatomical points in common. Each has a body that is an oval block of spongy bone situated anteriorly and is separated from its neighbor by an intervertebral disc, a fibrocartilaginous elastic cushion (Figs. 11-10 and 11-11). Just posterior to the body in the midline lies the spinal cord in its canal (Fig. 11-10). This canal is formed by the body anteriorly, the pedicles laterally, and the laminae posteriorly, making up a complete arch. Articular surfaces projecting from the pedicles are called *facets* and form joints with the facets of the vertebrae above and below. Extending laterally from the arch are the transverse processes, which serve as hitching posts for muscles and ligaments. Posteriorly, the arch gives off a spinous process that may be palpated in all persons but the excessively obese (Fig. 11-10). The vertebrae are held together by multiple ligaments and muscles. Motion of the spine

---

Fig. 11-9. Posterior view of brainstem and spinal cord. **A,** Torso (His-Steger cast), dissected from back, is shown. Dura has been opened and cord exposed. Levels concerned can be easily determined by referring to ribs on left side of thorax. Cord proper terminates opposite body of second vertebra (see **B**) as conus medullaris. **B,** Ventral surface of cord stripped of dura and arachnoid. It is symmetrical structure, two halves of which are separated by ventral fissure. This fissure stops at levels of foramen magnum. Caudally, pia leaves conus medullaris as round, thin, glistening thread, filum terminale. **C,** Cord is exposed from lateral side. Dura has been opened. Since cord is shorter than canal that contains it and since spinal nerves leave through intervertebral foramina, one at a time, lowest portion of vertebral canal is occupied not by cord but by bundlelike accumulation of nerve roots, cauda equina. Caudal end of dural sac, which encloses spinal cord and cauda equina, lies somewhere between level of middle of bodies of first and third sacral vertebrae. Size and position of three views correspond, and delimitation of major vertebral levels is indicated by transverse lines for all three figures. (From Mettler, F. A.: Neuroanatomy, ed. 2, St. Louis, The C. V. Mosby Co.)

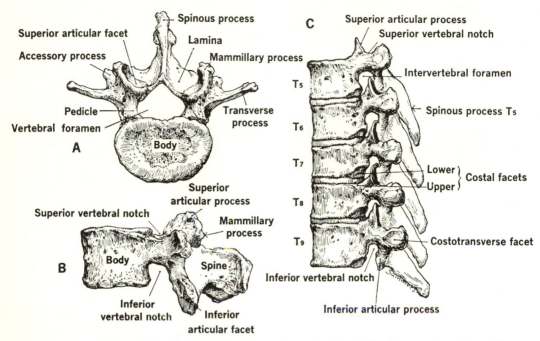

Fig. 11-10. **A,** Fourth lumbar vertebra from above. **B,** Fourth lumbar vertebra from side. **C,** Fifth to ninth thoracic vertebrae showing relationships of various parts. (From Mettler, F. A.: Neuroanatomy, ed. 2, St. Louis, The C. V. Mosby Co.)

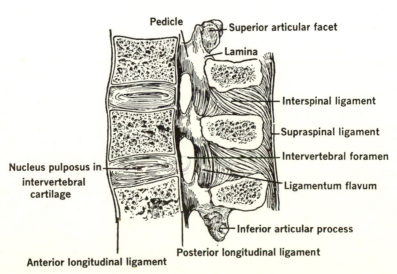

Fig. 11-11. Median section through three lumbar vertebrae showing intervertebral discs (nuclei pulposi). (From Mettler, F. A.: Neuroanatomy, ed. 2, St. Louis, The C. V. Mosby Co.)

occurs at the articular facets and through the elastic intervertebral discs (Fig. 11-11).

The spinal cord is thus enclosed in a heavy protective framework (Fig. 11-9). The dura is not firmly attached to its bony surroundings as the cranial dura is to the skull but is buffered with a layer of epidural fat. Beneath the dura mater is the arachnoid, which is a continuation of the same structure within the cranium. The subarachnoid space contains spinal fluid, and a thin layer of pia mater intimately covers the cord.

The spinal cord is a downward prolongation of the brainstem, starting at the upper border of the atlas and ending at the upper border of the second lumbar vertebra. The cord is oval in cross section, since it is slightly flattened in the anteroposterior diameter. A cross section looks like a gray letter H surrounded by a white mantle split in the midline anteriorly and posteriorly by sulci.

The peripheral white matter carries the long myelinated motor and sensory tracts, whereas the central gray matter consists of nerve cell bodies and short unmyelinated fibers (Fig. 11-9). The principal long pathways are the laterally placed pyramidal tracts carrying impulses down from the cerebral cortex to the motor neurons of the cord, the dorsal ascending columns mediating sensations of touch and proprioception, and the anterolaterally placed spinothalamic tracts carrying pain and temperature sensations to the thalamus, the great sensory receiving station of the brain.

At each vertebral level a pair of spinal nerves emerges from the cord. Each is formed by two roots, an anterior or motor root, the cell bodies of which lie in the anterior horn of the spinal gray matter, and a posterior root, the cell bodies of which lie in the spinal ganglia in the intervertebral foramina, through which the nerves exit from the spinal canal. The cervical nerves pass out horizontally, but at each lower level they take on an increasingly oblique and downward direction. In the lumbar region the course of the nerves is nearly vertical, and they form the cauda equina. This phenomenon is explained by the fact that the spinal cord, which fills the entire spinal canal in the fetus, grows at a slower rate than the bony spine, thus leaving the lower nerves a progressively longer course to their exit.

In the cervical and lumbosacral regions the spinal nerves regroup in a plexiform manner before they form the peripheral nerves of the upper and lower extremities, respectively, whereas those in the thoracic region become the intercostal nerves. The principal nerves of the upper or brachial plexus are the musculocutaneous, median, ulnar, and radial and those of the lumbosacral plexus, the obturator, femoral, and sciatic. Their branches and specific functions are detailed in anatomical texts and in works on peripheral nerve surgery.

SURGERY OF THE SPINAL CORD AND ITS ADJACENT STRUCTURES. Operations are directed toward the following conditions: congenital malformations, injuries, tumors, herniated intervertebral discs, and infections. Various operative procedures for the relief of intractable pain are also carried out on the spinal cord or its nerve roots.

The commonest congenital lesion encountered is a *meningocele* or *meningomyelocele* of the lumbar region due to failure of union of the vertebral arches in intrauterine life. This appears to be a fluid-filled, thin-walled sac that often contains neural elements. Surgical correction is necessary when the sac lining is precariously thin or there is a cerebrospinal fluid leak. The operation consists of excising the sac wall with great care to preserve any adhering nerves (the neurosurgical stimulator is most useful here), closing the dura, and reinforcing the closure with fascial flaps swung from the paraspinal muscles. Skin closure without tension is a prerequisite to primary healing. Large skin and subcutaneous flaps must occasionally be fashioned to attain this end.

Injuries to the spinal cord are of serious import, since no regeneration of destroyed

or divided nerve tracts occurs. Recovery, however, may take place with lesser degrees of injury, such as from contusion or compression. Surgery can only be of value in preventing further damage by debridement of penetrating wounds, removal of foreign bodies, relief of pressure on the cord or roots, open reduction of certain dislocations and fractures, and measures aimed at stabilizing the spine. In cervical injuries, skeletal traction by means of Crutchfield tongs applied directly to the skull is distinctly useful in many cases.

*Spinal cord tumors* are classified according to location as extradural (outside the dura mater) or intradural (within the dura mater). Intradural tumors may be either extramedullary (outside the cord) or intramedullary (within the cord). Extradural tumors include sarcomas and carcinomas either metastatic from a distal source or extending from adjacent involved structures in or about the vertebrae. Also found extradurally are Hodgkin's disease, lipomas, occasional neurofibromas, chondromas, angiomas, abscesses, and granulomas.

Intradural tumors include extramedullary tumors, which are usually benign and originate from the dura-arachnoid surrounding the cord and from the root sheaths of spinal nerves. Neurinomas are especially common in the thoracocervical area and may be part of generalized neurofibromatosis. Meningiomas also commonly occur in intradural extramedullary locations. Less commonly, lipomas or other types of tumors are found. Gliomas are the most common intramedullary tumors and have a less favorable prognosis. These tumors infiltrate the cord tissue and are much more difficult to remove than extramedullary tumors.

The majority of the intradural tumors are extramedullary and benign and, if diagnosed early before severe neurological deficits occur, offer an excellent prognosis. They manifest their presence by pain of a radicular nature and various motor and sensory disabilities below their segmental location. Cord tumors frequently produce spinal fluid block and can be pinpointed accurately by intraspinal injection of a radiopaque oil (myelography). A standard laminectomy is used for exposure and removal.

The rare surgical infections of the spinal cord take the form of extradural abscesses and granulomas. Treatment consists of a combination of excision, drainage, chemotherapy, and occasionally spinal fusion.

The most frequently encountered neurosurgical problem is the herniated intervertebral disc. Because of weakness or rupture of the circular ligament (annulus fibrosus), which confines the soft center of the disc (nucleus pulposus), herniation of the latter may occur and give rise to sciatic pain from nerve root compression. When pain is severe or nerve damage excessive, surgical excision of the offending disc offers the most satisfactory relief. The procedure entails an interlaminar exposure and piecemeal removal of the displaced nucleus. If the spine is unstable or there are other incontrovertible reasons for operative stabilization of the bony spine, a fusion of one type or another may be combined with the disc surgery (Chapter 13).

Certain painful lesions, usually of a malignant nature, are best controlled by dividing the pain fibers supplying the affected area. This may be accomplished by sectioning the sensory roots intraspinally (posterior rhizotomy) or by incising the spinothalamic tracts (anterolateral cordotomy) that carry pain and temperature impulses. A laminectomy is necessary for exposure.

### Autonomic nervous system

The autonomic (involuntary or vegetative) nervous system comprises all the efferent nerves through which the cardiovascular apparatus, viscera, glands of internal secretion, and peripheral involuntary muscles are innervated (Fig. 11-12). A major anatomical difference between the somatic and autonomic nervous sys-

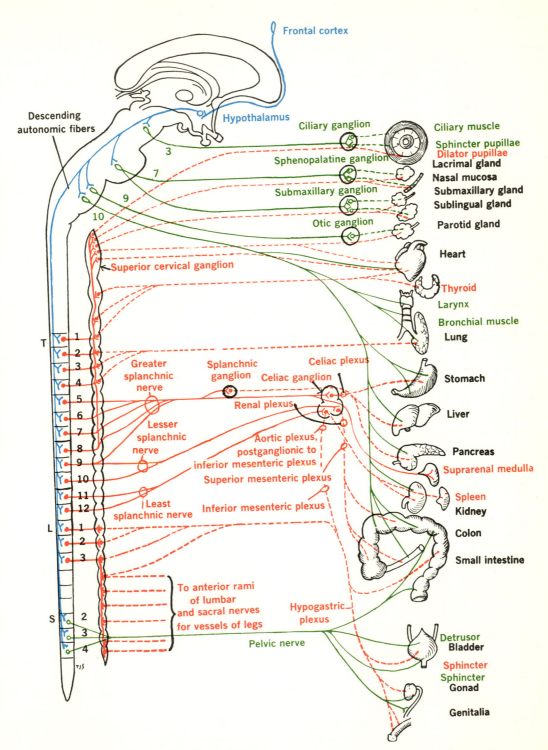

**Fig. 11-12.** Diagram of autonomic nervous system. (From Mettler, F. A.: Neuroanatomy, ed. 2, St. Louis, The C. V. Mosby Co.)

tems is that in the former an impulse from the brainstem or spinal cord reaches the end organ via a single neuron, whereas in the latter it traverses two neurons, the first ending in an autonomic ganglion, the second running from the ganglion to the end organ. Some of these ganglia lie along the side of the vertebral column to form the sympathetic trunks or chains, whereas others are closely associated with the end organs.

The preganglionic neurons from the brainstem, which go out along the cranial nerves, and those from the second, third, and fourth sacral segments to the pelvic viscera end in ganglia in proximity to their end organs; thus their postganglionic fibers are very short. This is known as the parasympathetic or craniosacral division of the autonomic nervous system. The preganglionic fibers from the thoracic and lumbar spinal cord end in the paravertebral ganglia, making up the sympathetic chain, and their postganglionic fibers are relatively long. This is termed the *sympathetic*, or thoracolumbar, division of the autonomic nervous system.

The two divisions are distinct anatomically and physiologically. The chemical substance mediating transmission of impulses at most sympathetic nerve endings is adrenaline, and at most parasympathetic endings is acetylcholine.

The majority of organs have a dual innervation, part from the craniosacral and part from the thoracolumbar divisions. The functions of these two systems are antagonistic. Together they preserve our body homeostasis, or *milieu interieur,* as Claude Bernard called it in 1878. In general, the thoracolumbar division functions as an emergency protective mechanism always ready to liberate an extraordinary amount of body energy to combat any variety of stressful or adverse circumstance. The craniosacral division functions to conserve energy in periods of rest.

Stimuli arising from internal organs or from the outside traverse visceral and somatic afferent nerve fibers to make reflex connections with preganglionic autonomic neurons in the brainstem and spinal cord. Such stimuli thereby call these involuntary systems automatically into appropriate activity. When these automatic mechanisms break down or overact, surgery may be indicated. For example, thoracolumbar sympathectomy was once performed in hypertension in order to lower blood vessel tone and therefore the blood pressure. Vagotomy is done to decrease acid secretion of the stomach in peptic ulcer patients, whereas lumbar sympathectomy is used to relieve vasospastic disorders of the legs. Herein lies the basis for the various forms of surgical sympathectomy.

## DIAGNOSTIC PROCEDURES

Most diagnostic procedures today are performed in the radiology department. Some of these include myelography (the injection of dye into the spinal subarachnoid space), pneumoencephalography (the injection of air into the subarachnoid space to outline the ventricular system and the cranial subarachnoid space), ventriculography (the injection of air, as a contrast medium, directly into the lateral ventricles), brain scans (the injection of radioactive substance intravenously with films made to demonstrate possible lesions), and angiography (the injection of radiopaque substance into the carotid, brachial, or vertebral arteries to study the intracranial blood vessels in order to demonstrate their size, location, or configuration in cases of suspected space-occupying lesions or pathological changes in the cerebrovascular system). Angiography may someday be used regularly in the operating room when vascular lesions are being corrected or removed.

## ANESTHETIC MANAGEMENT IN NEUROSURGERY

Anesthesia for neurological surgery differs from anesthesia for general surgery in several important ways. The vital functions of respiration and circulation in the patient with intracranial disease are usually more easily depressed than are those of most patients undergoing elective gen-

eral surgery. An open airway must be maintained at all times. Profound muscle relaxation is not required. Induced hypotension or hypothermia may be used. Early return of reflexes and consciousness is desirable.

## PHYSICAL FACILITIES AND SETUPS

The facilities needed for neurosurgical procedures are similar to those needed to perform other major surgery. The neurosurgical unit should be of sufficient size to accommodate extra equipment, machines, and supplies. It requires numerous electrical outlets, as well as mobile overhead operating room lights. Multiple view boxes must be included for adequate x-ray viewing. The special equipment for a neurosurgical unit includes a standard operating table with appropriate attachments and various neurosurgical headrests. In some hospitals the neurosurgeons use an overhead table attached to the standard operating table or a special neurosurgical Mayo table such as the Mayfield-Larsen table. Of importance are a large instrument table, preferably taller than the usual; a selection of footstools of various dimensions (enabling personnel to safely maintain sterility of the field and to participate effectively); two regulation Mayo tables; one small utility table for skin preparation or special equipment, two or three suction machines or outlets capable of high negative pressure; an electrosurgical unit; and a spotlight. An electrocardiograph monitor, a regulated blanket warmer with thermometer attachment (especially for the pediatric patient), and blood and fluid warmers are also necessary.

Special equipment may include a bipolar coagulation unit, surgical microscope, fiberoptic light source, headlight, and nerve stimulator.

## TECHNIQUES OF HEMOSTASIS AND OTHER BASIC NEUROSURGICAL MANEUVERS

Scientific advances that enable all surgeons to control more perfectly the age-old hazards of surgery—pain, hemorrhage, and infection—have contributed largely to the neurosurgeon's ability to deal with disease of the nervous system. The extent of a modern neurosurgical operation may be determined not so much by the physiological hazards involved as by the degree of neurological disability that may be expected after surgery.

Since the skull represents a rigid, nonexpansile box enclosing the brain, hemorrhage and swelling are doubly serious in this area where pressure on the tissue, however slight, may cause irreparable damage and destruction.

For this reason meticulous methods of hemostasis are of particular importance in neurosurgical technique. The first consideration is control of hemorrhage from the scalp. Simple compression of the edges of the wound with gauze sponges and fingers during the initial incision is followed by application of hemostatic clips and clamps. When clips are used, they are applied so that they include the epicranial aponeurosis and skin edge, whereas clamps are attached directly to the aponeurosis and then everted.

Bone wax, which is an essential hemostatic material, must be prepared for all cranial and spinal cord operations, as described in Chapter 5. The surgeon firmly rubs the wax into the bleeding surface of the bone after all periosteum has been scraped off. When the skull flap has been elevated, bone wax is also rubbed into the diploe to control bleeding from the bone edge. During spinal surgery, bone wax is used on the cut edges of the laminae in similar fashion.

Electrocoagulation has become an essential part of the neurosurgical setup. Nursing personnel must understand the switches, dials, plugs, and outlets of the electrosurgical unit before attempting to regulate it. They must be familiar with the proper safety measures for its use. Electrocoagulation may be used to stop bleeding in the epicranial aponeurosis and the periosteum, on the surface of the dura, on the spinal cord, and in the brain. The coagulation current is used for sealing the blood

vessels. The electric current is applied to the forceps, a metal suction tip, or other instrument, which acts as a conducting tool. To get results, the cauterizing current must contact the vessel in a dry field. For this reason, suctioning is necessary to remove the blood as the contact is made between the instrument carrying the current and the bleeding point. Except when bipolar coagulation units are being used, it is essential to have a large metal plate well covered with an electrolyte gel in broad contact with some portion of the patient's body. A broad area of contact is necessary to prevent burns. A Malis bipolar coagulator is used with the bipolar forceps. It provides a completely isolated output with negligible leakage of current from between the tips of the forceps. This permits the use of the coagulating current in close proximity to structures where ordinary unipolar coagulation would be impossible. Ringer's irrigation is used during bipolar coagulation, thereby minimizing tissue heating, shrinkage, drying, and sticking to the forceps (Fig. 11-13). Coagulation occurs only between the tips of the forceps so that

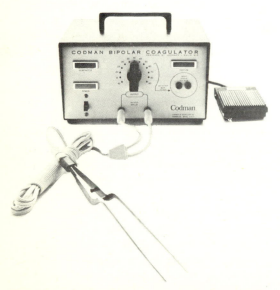

**Fig. 11-13.** Malis bipolar coagulation unit with forceps. (Courtesy Codman & Shurtleff, Inc., Randolph, Mass.)

they are particularly effective in handling vessels in areas where unipolar coagulation would be hazardous. Other advantages include lack of current spread or tissue heating; the ability to coagulate under irrigation so as to minimize tissue shrinkage, drying, and sticking; and the elimination of need for a ground plate.

The use of the bipolar coagulation technique allows hemostasis of almost any size vessel encountered. Vessels as large as the superficial temporal artery, as well as those too small for suture or clip ligation, may be coagulated.

Although electrocautery is principally used to control bleeding, it is also used for cutting. In this case a lower frequency current is employed. When the surgeon is using an electroknife or electrode to cut and remove a tumor of the brain, the circulating nurse should stand by the machine to adjust the current as he desires. As the surgeon uses the cutting electrode, an assistant holds a suction tip up and to one side of the area of dissection so as to suck up smoke as it arises.

Gauze compresses are used to control bleeding prior to entering the skull or spinal canal, as in any general surgical procedure. Wet compressed rayon cotton pledgets or strips ("cottonoid") are used in place of gauze sponges to control bleeding beneath the skull and around the spinal cord. Because coarse cotton mesh will injure fragile tissues, the compressed cotton should be of the finest quality but not so compressed that it has lost its absorbent property. Compressed cotton sheets are cut in various sizes. Each hospital has several standard sizes suitable to its specific needs, but, in general, the strips are usually three or four times longer than they are wide. A silk thread may be attached to some strips or pledgets, which are packaged according to size and then autoclaved.

During the operation, the nurse moistens cotton strips and pledgets in Ringer's solution and stores them in a basin or on a piece of metal within reach of the surgeon

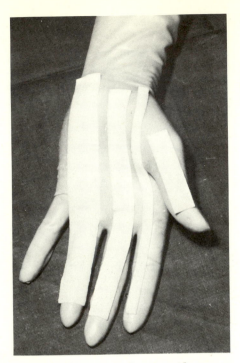

**Fig. 11-14.** Placement of cottonoid on nurse's hand. (Courtesy K. Cramer Lewis, Department of Illustrations, Washington University School of Medicine, St. Louis, Mo.)

to preserve their moisture. Assorted cotton strips may also be handed to the surgeon from a position on the scrub nurse's hand (Fig. 11-14). The various sizes are placed in order on the fingers and palm. In this way, once the surgeon has grasped the near end in a forceps, the nurse may hold the far end of the strip so as to assist the surgeon in placing the cottonoid with accuracy and without dragging it across the sutures, brain, or other tissues. The surgeon applies suction over the cotton strip after it is placed over an area of bleeding so as to remove the blood without further disturbing the bleeding vessels and to achieve better tamponade through close contact of the tip of the cotton strip with the bleeding point.

Occasionally, loose wet cotton balls are temporarily used to pack the bleeding cavity after a tumor has been removed. Gentle pressure of this kind will often stop troublesome venous ooze.

Silver clips are always included in each setup. The McKenzie clips are made of pieces of flat ribbon wire that are bent in the shape of an open V. Weck Hemoclips in small and medium sizes are commonly used today. Both McKenzie clips and Weck Hemoclips are stored on a sliding metal rack. The nurse secures the clip in the jaws of a special applier, which the surgeon uses to place the clip on the bleeding vessel. These clips are used if electrocoagulation is insufficient or dangerous because of its thermal effect on neighboring structures or if a silk ligature would be either difficult to place or unsuitable to use on a vessel. Olivecrona, Mayfield, or other clips are sometimes used in trapping or clipping the neck of large aneurysms (Figs. 11-32 and 11-33).

In some situations when electrocoagulation is ineffective, a hemostatic substance or solution may be used. After removal of certain tumors, compressed cotton strips saturated with thrombin may be placed in the tumor bed.

A hemostatic substance such as gelatin sponge (Gelfoam), absorbable hemostatic gauze or cotton (Surgicel absorbable hemostat), or oxidized cellulose (Oxycel) is used to stop hemorrhage from large blood vessels or sinuses or from an oozing surface in a tumor bed. The nurse cuts the dry hemostatic material into pieces of suitable shape and size and hands the surgeon a moist, compressed cotton strip, which he places over the hemostatic material. The surgeon holds the material and cotton strip against the bleeding area for several minutes by means of a forceps or suction tip; then he removes the cotton strip, leaving the hemostatic material adherent to the bleeding area. Small patches cut from fresh muscle tissue are often effective in controlling stubborn bleeding.

Silk sutures no. 4-0 or 5-0 on curved, taper point needles are needed to ligate bleeding vessels and to retract or close the dura membrane. Silk sutures no. 3-0 are used to close galeal and skin layers; silk no. 2-0 is used for approximating

heavier tissues such as the paraspinal muscles (Chapter 6).

Because washing the wound with warm lactated Ringer's solution is an effective hemostatic measure, the nurse should always have an Asepto syringe and suction set within reach of the surgeon. The suction apparatus is the best tool for keeping the wound dry and permitting control of hemorrhage. Although Cushing used a glass tube for suctioning blood and secretions from the wound, today metal tubes—the Adson, Bucy, Frazier, and Sachs types—are often used. The metal tubes are also used to conduct the coagulation current to the bleeding vessel.

Suctioning is used to (1) keep the wound clean and dry in order to identify the active bleeding source, (2) remove irrigating fluid rapidly, (3) suck out necrotic or traumatized brain tissue or soft brain tumors, (4) empty an abscessed cavity, (5) evacuate cerebrospinal fluid from a ventricle or subarachnoid space, (6) hold a tumor during its removal, (7) compress a bleeding vessel, and (8) conduct the electrocautery spark to a bleeding area via the metal sucker.

Blood loss is replaced with whole blood and intravenous solutions of Ringer's lactate with glucose at various rates of flow according to the surgeon's or anesthetist's order.

In the case of cerebral aneurysm the blood pressure is lowered by drugs to reduce the danger of hemorrhage, as well as to relax the aneurysm wall during its ligation.

## NEUROSURGICAL EQUIPMENT AND INSTRUMENTS

In descriptions of equipment and instruments throughout this chapter, specific items are listed. In most instances, other equivalent items are available and will prove equally satisfactory.

The advances in modern neurosurgery have required the design and development of special equipment and instruments assuring more rapid and safer surgical procedures, as well as permitting new neurosurgical procedures. These instruments and equipment include the following.

**HALL II AIR DRILL.** This air-powered instrument is used for precision cutting, shaping, and repair of bone. It was designed and developed specifically to reduce time and trauma, make possible new surgical procedures, minimize anesthesia, and remove from the operating room an electrical hazard (Fig. 11-15). The pneumatic power source is provided by the use of water-pumped, compressed dry nitrogen. This is an inert nonflammable liquid that can be conducted or supplied from a wall source or portable tanks. It is often used in performing anterior cervical fusions to widen the graft area and in eighth cranial nerve surgery to unroof the auditory canal. The drill is also available with a 20-degree angle, which can be used in less accessible areas.

**HALL NEURAIRTOME.** This is a heavier instrument. It accommodates certain types of burrs and perforators, including the Smith perforator ordinarily used with the Smith drill (Fig. 11-16). Some of the advantages, in addition to power and ease of handling, are that fewer burr holes are needed for craniotomy than when using the Gigli saws; osseous bleeding is reduced because of the rotary action of the blades, which packs bony particles on the bleeding surfaces; it withstands steam sterilization; and it is shock and explosion proof.

It may be used for burr holes, craniotomies, craniectomies, cranioplasties, craniostenosis, Cloward procedures, and laminectomies. In the cranioplasty procedure, it can be used to make a shelf for the plate and to drill suture holes in both skull and plate. The carborundum grinding wheel is used to smooth the edges.

The source of power is the same as for the Hall II air drill. The instrument, its case, and all the attachments are autoclavable. If it is necessary to cool the instrument, run cool by connecting nitrogen. It must never be immersed.

**SMITH AUTOMATIC PERFORATOR DRILL.** An

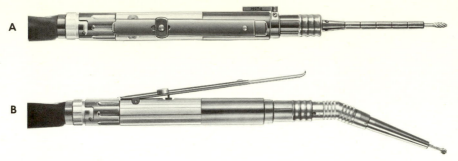

**Fig. 11-15.** Hall II Air Drill. **A,** With Cloward extra long burr guard. **B,** With 20-degree angle with long burr. (Courtesy Hall Surgical Systems, Inc., Santa Barbara, Calif.)

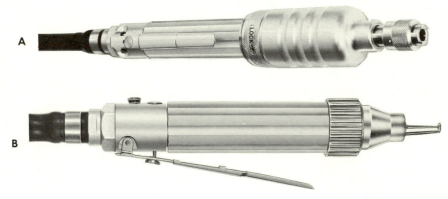

**Fig. 11-16. A,** Hall Neurairtome with 1000 r.p.m. drive. To be used with Smith perforator. **B,** Neurairtome with Duraguard and Neuroblade. (Courtesy Hall Surgical Systems, Inc., Santa Barbara, Calif.)

electrically powered instrument designed to disengage at the completion of the burr hole when the point breaks through the skull plate. It can be used in place of the Hall Neurairtome if just burr holes are needed or for posterior fossa craniotomy when several holes are needed.

FIBEROPTIC INSTRUMENTS. Fiberoptic cords can be attached to bayonet forceps, suction tips, or brain retractors. They may be built into the latter.

EDINBOROUGH, DEMARTEL, AND YASARGIL RETRACTORS. These are self-retaining bladed retractors anchored to the skull by means of a screw connector (Figs. 11-17 and 11-19).

SURGICAL MICROSCOPE AND CAMERA (see microsurgery, p. 380). The House-Urban vacuum rotary dissector is a combination of rotating cutter blades and sucker that makes it possible to vary its results from predominate suction to tissue resection (Fig. 11-18).

## OPERATIVE PROCEDURES

Procedures with similar approaches are grouped together in sections in this chapter, and care should be taken to refer to the earliest procedure described in each section for details of the basic procedure and instruments used.

Different operations performed for the same conditions are listed in separate sections of the chapter according to the type of operative approach. Whenever this

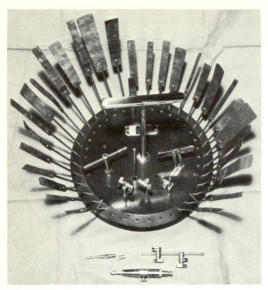

**Fig. 11-17.** Edinborough retractor with blades, poles, screws, and adapters. (Courtesy V. Mueller Surgical Instruments and Hospital Equipment, Chicago, Ill.)

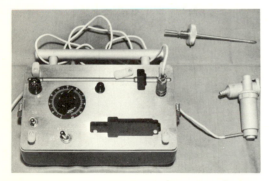

**Fig. 11-18.** House-Urban vacuum rotary dissector. (Courtesy Urban Engineering Co., Inc., Burbank, Calif.)

occurs, mention of the alternative procedure is made at the conclusion of the first procedure described for that condition.

**Burr holes**

Burr holes are placed in order to gain limited access to the surface of the brain. This may be useful where a localized fluid collection exists beneath the dura. If this is not composed of clot, it can be easily evacuated through a burr hole. Burr holes

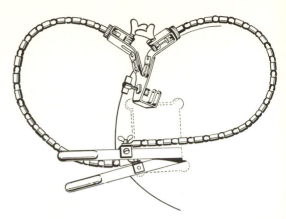

**Fig. 11-19.** Leyla-Yasargil self-retaining retractor. (Courtesy Holco Instrument Corp., New York, N. Y.)

also permit access to the brain so that it can be tapped with a needle. This is useful when ventriculography must be performed. This approach is also used by many surgeons when treating brain abscess. In this manner the abscess may be aspirated and antibiotics instilled. Other surgeons prefer to treat abscess by total excision. In this case, a craniotomy is necessary. Occasionally, burr holes are used to locate or drain subdural hematomas. However, a craniectomy is usually necessary to gain adequate exposure in these cases.

**Ventriculography**

PURPOSE. Variations from the normal in the size, shape, and position of the ventricles may assist the surgeon to diagnose and locate the cause of increased intracranial pressure due to tumor, obstruction, or other pathological conditions.

CONSIDERATIONS. In infants, needles may be placed into the ventricles via the open anterior fontanel instead of via holes through the skull.

SETUP AND PREPARATION OF THE PATIENT. The following basic minor neurosurgical instrument set is used for parieto-occipital burr holes for ventriculography (Figs. 11-19 to 11-21):

**Cutting instruments**

2 Scalpels no. 4 with no. 20 blades
2 Scalpels no. 3 with no. 11 blades

1 Scalpel no. 3 with no. 15 blade
2 Mayo scissors, curved
2 Metzenbaum dissecting scissors, curved
1 Strabismus scissors (light curved), 4 in.
1 Curved vascular scissors
1 Small bone curette (size 0)
2 Hudson braces
2 Cushing perforators and burrs
2 D'Errico perforator drill points
1 Schwartz-Kerrison rongeur
1 Cloward cervical punch (fine-tipped)
1 Stille double-action angular bone rongeur, 9 in. (duckbill)

**Holding instruments**

24 Backhaus towel clamps, 3½ in.
2 Tissue forceps, toothed, 6¼ in.
4 Adson dura forceps, 5 in., 2 fine-toothed, 2 heavy-toothed
4 Lucae or Gruenwald bayonet forceps, 5¾ in.
4 Bayonet forceps, 7½ in.
2 Dura hooks, 6 in.

**Clamping instruments**

12 Mosquito hemostatic forceps, 6 curved, 6 straight
12 Halsted hemostatic forceps, straight, 5½ in.

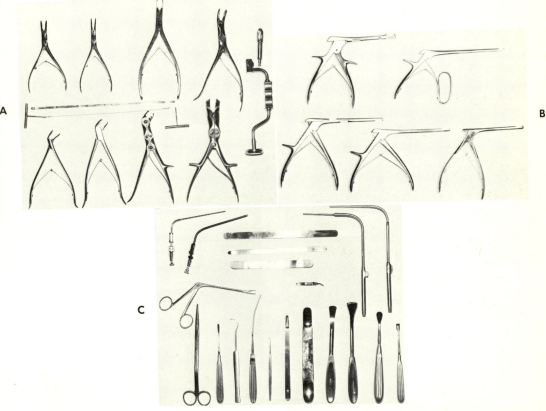

**Fig. 11-20.** Types of neurosurgical instruments. **A,** Top: Zaufal-Jansen rongeur, Beyer rongeur, Smith-Petersen rongeur, Leksell laminectomy rongeur, Hudson brace, D'Errico burr; center: Gigli saw guide, Gigli saw handle attached to saw, Gigli saw handle; bottom: Stookey rongeur, Bacon single-action rongeur, double-action rongeur (duckbill), Horsley bone-cutting forceps. **B,** Raney lamina punch, Cloward-Harper punch, Spurling-Kerrison rongeur (downbiting), Schlesinger punch, Schwartz-Kerrison rongeur. **C,** Top: Bucy suction tube, stainless steel brain retractor, Cushing spatula with lip, silver brain retractor, Sachs thin-tip suction, Sachs regular-tip suction tube; center: pituitary rongeur, notched bulldog towel clip; bottom: angled long scissors, Adson elevator (joker), aneurysm needle, staphylorrhaphy, dura hook, brain spoon (small and large), Cushing periosteal elevator, Campbell angled periosteal elevator, Lewin elevator, Adson elevator with sharp edge. (Courtesy K. Cramer Lewis, Department of Illustrations, Washington University School of Medicine, St. Louis, Mo.)

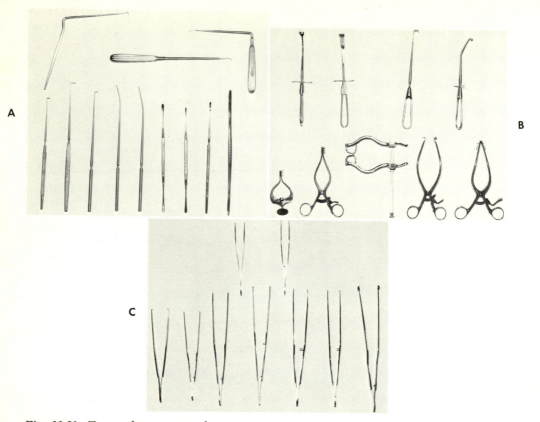

**Fig. 11-21.** Types of neurosurgical instruments. **A,** Top: Love nerve root retractor, straight Scoville nerve root retractor, angled Scoville nerve root retractor; bottom: Weary nerve hook, aneurysm needle (hook), Dandy nerve hooks, straight, angled, Sachs-Freer dural separator, double-tip regular ends, Sachs-Freer dural separator, double-tip (fine and regular), Sachs nerve separator, copper nerve root retractor. **B,** Top: Cushing decompression retractor, Sachs vein retractor (4-prong), Sachs vein retractor (smooth, straight), Sachs vein retractor (angled, smooth); bottom: Jansen mastoid retractor, Weitlaner retractor, Klemme self-retaining retractor, Schwartz lamina retractor for cervical cordotomy, Adson cerebellar retractor. **C,** Top: Adson tissue forceps with teeth, Adson dura tissue forceps with teeth; bottom: heavy tissue forceps with teeth, 7 in., Lucae bayonet forceps, 5¾ in., Lucae bayonet forceps, 7¼ in., Cushing bayonet forceps with teeth, 7¾ in., Gerald bayonet forceps without teeth, 7½ in., Gerald bayonet forceps with teeth, hypophyseal bayonet cup forceps without teeth, 7¼ in. (Courtesy K. Cramer Lewis, Department of Illustrations, Washington University School of Medicine, St. Louis, Mo.)

6 Rochester-Pean hemostatic forceps
4 Michel clip applicators and clips
3 Rubber-shod mosquito hemostatic forceps

**Exposing instruments**

2 Jansen mastoid or scalp retractors, self-retaining
1 Smith-Petersen periosteal elevator (wide)
1 Adson elevator, joker
3 Dural Sachs-Freer elevators, double-ended, curved tips, 1 regular, 1 fine-tip, and 2 with regular tips at both ends

1 Staphylorrhaphy elevator (Sachs dura separator)
1 Weitlaner self-retaining retractor, 8 in.
5 Sachs suction tips, 3 small, 2 extra small
2 Suction tubing
4 Vein retractors, 2 angled Sachs, smooth; 2 straight smooth

**Suturing instruments**

2 Sarot needle holders, 6 in.
2 Mayo-Hegar, needle holders, 7⅛ in.

2 McKenzie clip applying forceps, curved, 6 in., with clips (1 rack)
1 Needle set (Neurological)
4 No. 12 spring-eye cutting needles (for drapes)
4 No. 16 spring-eye cutting needles (for skin closure)
4 No. 4 Kelly spring-eye needles (for muscle and fascial closure)
6 No. 3 Kelly spring-eye needles (for periosteal and galeal closure)
6 Ophthalmic needles, ⅝ in. (for dural closure)
1 Keith needle, 2½ in. (for central dural stay suture)

**Accessory equipment and supplies**

2 Medicine glasses
3 Asepto syringes (½ oz.)
2 Luer-Lok syringes, 10 ml.
2 Plain tip syringes, 10 ml.
2 Cone ventricular needles, 2 hole, 3½ in. with obturator
2 Trupp ventricular needles with three way stopcock, 8 Fr. with obturator
1 Electrode cord and handle with spatulate tip
1 Suction tubing
3 Scott rubber ventricular cannulas (6, 8, 10 cm.) with obturator
Culture tubes
Bone wax
Fine-mesh gauze
4 × 4 in. gauze sponges without x-ray marking
4 In. wide, soft gauze roll (Kerlix)
3 In. wide, firm, pliable gauze roll (Kling)
1 In. adhesive tape

The patient is placed in a supine position on the operating table, with his head elevated and with the footboard and knee strap in place, or in an encephalographic chair. His arms are secured with the lift sheet or wristlets. The table is placed in a slight reverse Trendelenburg position (Chapter 7). The posterior aspect of the head is shaved, and the operative area is disinfected with an antiseptic (Chapter 4). The instruments to be used may be set up on a regular Mayo stand, or the nurse may set up her instrument table in the order the instruments are to be used.

OPERATIVE PROCEDURE

1. A towel is placed under the patient's head, and the incision site and towel clamp areas are injected with a local anesthetic agent.

2. Incision lines are marked with a no. 20 blade on a no. 4 scalpel handle, and the head is draped.

3. The surgeon and his assistant exert pressure on gauze sponges on either side of the incision line. With a no. 11 blade on a no. 3 scalpel handle, a short incision is carried down to the periosteum. Five or six Michel clips may be used on the scalp edges for hemostasis.

4. The periosteum is elevated, and the self-retaining mastoid or Weitlaner retractor is inserted. The procedure is repeated on the opposite side (Fig. 11-22).

5. Using the Hudson brace with the D'Errico perforator drill point, a burr hole is made in each incision (Fig. 11-23). A slow, continuous drip of warm Ringer's solution is used as an irrigant to help remove bony particles with the suction. The burr holes may be enlarged or trimmed using a rongeur, and the dura is separated from residual bone at the bottom of the burr hole with a dural elevator or Adson elevator (small joker).

6. The dura mater is coagulated using bayonet forceps. The dura is elevated with a dural hook and incised with a no. 15 blade on a no. 3 scalpel handle. The dural elevator is then used to guide further extensions of this incision.

7. Bleeding is controlled with cotton strips (1/16 inch) and suction or with the cautery. The cortical surface is coagulated and incised with a no. 11 blade.

8. Ventricular needles are tested for patency. A needle with a threeway stopcock is then inserted through the cortical incision into one ventricle. Occasionally both ventricles are tapped. Fluid is allowed to escape from the ventricle and is collected in a medicine glass for laboratory testing. An amount of air slightly less than the amount of fluid removed is injected into one ventricle with the 10 ml. syringe. The needle is then withdrawn.

9. The dura is checked for bleeding, and the mastoid retractors are removed. The galea is closed with no. 3-0 or 4-0 silk sutures on small needles. The skin

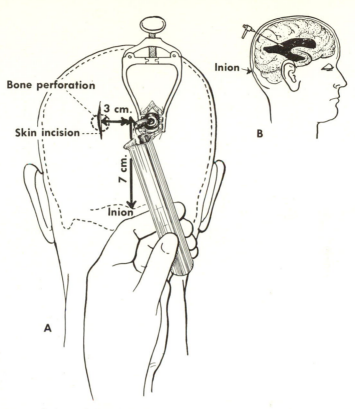

**Fig. 11-22.** Occipital burr holes for ventriculography. (From Richards, V.: Surgery for general practice, St. Louis, 1956, The C. V. Mosby Co.)

is closed with a no. 4-0 silk suture on milliners' or small cutting needles.

10. The wound is dressed and the patient taken to the x-ray department for completion of the examination. X-ray films must be taken immediately, since patients with a space-occupying lesion often cannot tolerate the air for long periods of time. The operating room must be kept available in case surgery is necessary. More recently, frontal twist drill holes performed in the radiology department under sterile conditions have largely replaced the use of parieto-occipital burr holes in cases requiring ventriculography. One hole is made anteriorly, usually just in front of the coronal suture and usually on the right side.

### Burr hole aspiration of cerebral abscess

OPERATIVE PROCEDURE. A burr hole is made as described previously, located over the lesion. The dura is incised and coagulated, and the lesion is aspirated through a coagulated incision in the brain surface utilizing a large Cone ventricular needle. Ringer's solution may be injected and removed through the needle with a plain-tipped syringe to further empty the abscess. Antibiotics and micropulverized barium sulfate are then instilled through the needle. The needle is withdrawn and the wound copiously irrigated with Ringer's solution. Closure is in the usual fashion.

Many surgeons prefer to excise brain abscesses. In this case, a craniotomy is performed. Excision of brain abscess is described subsequently in the section on craniotomy.

### Craniotomy

The instrument setup and the operative steps for an osteoplastic craniotomy for cerebral tumor will be described for illus-

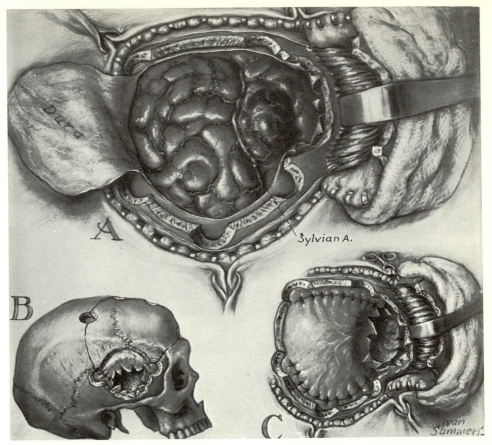

**Fig. 11-23.** Craniotomy with subtemporal decompression. (From Sachs, E.: Diagnosis and treatment of brain tumors and the care of the neurosurgical patient, ed. 2, St. Louis, The C. V. Mosby Co.)

trative purposes. Other common operations with their variations from the basic procedures will be described more briefly.

**DEFINITION.** The term *craniotomy* usually infers the fashioning of a large opening in the skull to expose and deal with intracranial disease. Depending on the location of the pathological condition, the craniotomy may be frontal, parietal, occipital, or temporal.

**SURGICAL APPROACHES.** Cerebral lesions are usually approached by removing a flap of bone from the skull. This procedure results in a minimal amount of disfigurement to the patient. To accomplish this, the skull plate, which is elevated in the exposure, is replaced at the end of the procedure so as to maintain the normal contour of the head. In performing a craniotomy, the bone plate may be left attached to the temporal muscle and turned back with the soft tissues. Alternatively, the plate may be separated from the soft tissues, including the periosteum, laid aside under sterile conditions, and replaced at the completion of the intracranial surgery.

Since subtemporal and suboccipital operations are performed in regions covered by heavy layers of muscle, it is unnecessary to replace the bone. In these locations, it is more satisfactory to rongeur bone off (craniectomy) than to fashion a bone flap (craniotomy).

When the bone is not replaced, room for cerebral decompression results (Fig.

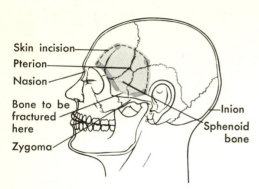

**Fig. 11-24.** Skin incision and placement of burr holes for frontal-temporal craniotomy. (From Kempe, L. G.: Operative neurosurgery, vols. 1 and 2, New York, 1968, Springer-Verlag, New York, Inc.)

11-23). If desired, skull defects left by surgery or trauma can be corrected by cranioplasty with bone grafts from a rib, tantalum plates, or one of the synthetic resins. The frontotemporal area is one of the most common operative sites (Fig. 11-24). This route is used to approach aneurysms, pituitary tumors, craniopharyngiomas, other sellar and immediate parasellar lesions, as well as lesions of the frontal and occasionally those of the temporal lobe. The scalp incision is made to ensure an adequate blood supply to the skin flap; the skin flap is usually larger than the bone flap.

SETUP AND PREPARATION OF THE PATIENT. Basic instruments for a craniotomy procedure are illustrated in Figs. 11-19 to 11-21. The instrument trays used in the basic major neurosurgical setup are shown in Figs. 11-25 and 11-26. In order to provide ease in handling, rapid setup, and efficient organization, the instruments are divided into the following three trays:

**Bone tray**

2 Hudson braces with 1 D'Errico burr
2 Mallets
1 Drill guide
1 Twist drill with drill bits
4 Gigli handles
2 Gigli guides
6 Gigli saws
1 Leksell double-action rongeur, 9¾ in.

1 Zaufal-Jansen double-action rongeur, 6¾ in.
1 Beyer double-action rongeur, 7 in.
1 Stookey single-action rongeur, ½ in. bite, 7¼ in.
1 Stookey double-action rongeur
2 Cloward rongeurs, 5 mm., 3 mm.
1 Raney rongeur
1 Kerrison rongeur, long
1 Schwartz-Kerrison rongeur
  Extra bone instruments (periosteal elevators, modified Adson elevators, staphylorrhaphy and aneurysm needles)
3 Bone curettes (sizes 1 through 2-0)
2 Vein retractors
1 Cushing subtemporal decompression retractor
2 Weitlaner self-retaining retractors, sharp, 8 in.
2 Jansen mastoid or scalp retractors, self-retaining
  Assorted brain retractors, flat ribbon spatulas
  Assorted Cushing pituitary spoons, copper malleable
  Assorted Cushing spatula spoons (brain spoons)

**Mayo tray**

1 Double-action rongeur
1 Bacon single-action rongeur
4 Lucae or Gruenwald bayonet forceps, short, 5¾ in.
4 Bayonet forceps, long, 7¼ in.
2 Tissue forceps with teeth, 6¼ in.
14 Towel clamps, small, 3½ in.
6 Bulldog towel clips with notched handles (for dural traction sutures)
18 Mosquito hemostatic forceps, 12 curved, 6 straight
36 Kolodney hemostatic forceps
18 Halsted hemostatic forceps
4 Rochester-Pean hemostatic forceps (for suction tubing)
5 Rochester-Ochsner hemostatic forceps (for tapes)
4 Towel clamps, large
6 Rochester-Pean hemostatic forceps (for fish-hook retractors)
6 Fish-hook retractors
2 Cushing periosteal elevators
1 Staphylorrhaphy (Cushing dura separator)
2 Smith-Petersen periosteal elevators
1 Sachs-Freer dural elevator, double-ended, narrow and wide, curved tips
1 Cone ventricular needle, 2 hole, 3½ in. with obturator
1 Aneurysm needle
1 Adson elevator (joker)
2 Cushing spatula spoons (small and large brain spoons)

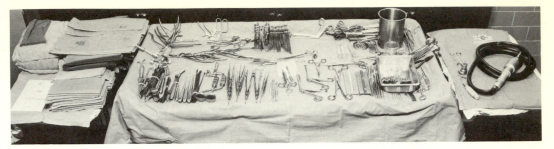

**Fig. 11-25.** Instrument table setup with the bone tray on the left and suture tray on the right.

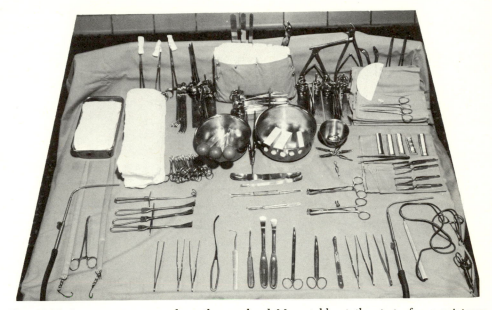

**Fig. 11-26.** Instruments arranged on the overhead Mayo table at the start of a craniotomy.

5 Sachs suction tips, 3 regular and 2 thin-tipped

3 Sachs retractors, 4-prong

1 Cushing subtemporal decompression retractor

2 Suction tubings

1 Active electrode with spatula tip

**Suture tray**

7 Sachs suction tips, 2 regular, 2 long thin-tipped, 1 large, 2 long regular

4 Potts-Smith vascular tissue forceps, 2 with and 2 without teeth

2 Tissue forceps, with and without teeth 7 in.

6 Gerald bayonet forceps, 2 fine with teeth, 2 fine without teeth, 2 heavy with teeth, 7½ in.

6 Hypophyseal bayonet cup forceps (without teeth) with assorted sizes of cups

3 Adson-Brown tissue forceps, 5 in.

3 Adson dura forceps, 5 in.

2 McKenzie silver clip applicators, 5¾ in., with clips (1 rack)

2 Penfield alligator clip applicators with clips (1 rack)

4 Weck Hemoclip applicators, 2 short 6½ in., 2 long 8 in.) with clips (1 rack)

1 Stainless steel ruler

2 Dura hooks, 6 in.

12 Needle holders, 4 fine long, 7½ in.; 4 fine short, 6 in.; 4 heavy short, 7⅛ in.

3 Schnidt gall duct forceps, half curve

3 Adson hemostatic forceps, 7¼ in.

3 Nerve hooks, 7¾ in. (small, medium, large)

1 Sachs nerve separator

3 Dural elevators, double-ended, curved tips, 1 Sachs-Freer with 1 regular, 1 fine tip, 2 with regular tips at both ends

1 Bundle of aneurysm hooks

    1 Bundle of nerve hooks
   12 Knife handles (4 each no. 3, no. 4, no. 7)
      Assorted scissors
    2 Scissors with handles angulated on flat,
      straight blade, 10 in.
    1 Needle set, neurosurgical (see basic minor
      neurosurgical set, p. 348)
    5 Disc rongeurs, pituitary, alligator
      Assorted ventricular needles
    2 Olivecrona clip applicators, with clips
    3 Asepto syringes, ½ oz.
    7 Syringes, 2 plain, 10 ml.; 3 control, 10 ml.;
      2 Luer-Lok, 10 ml.)
    1 Active electrode with spatula tip

**Supplies**

    2 Basic linen packs
    4 Packages sterile towels
    1 3-gown pack
      Gloves
      Paper craniotomy sheet
      Bone wax
      Silk no. 2-0 to 4-0
      Hemostatic material such as Gelfoam, Surgi-
        cel, etc.
      Procaine, 0.5%
    1 Polyethylene drain
    5 Wide umbilical tapes
      Raney clips
      Medicine glasses
      Culture tube
    2 Local jars, 1 for local anesthetic, 1 for
      specimen
      Fine-mesh gauze
    4 × 4 in. gauze sponges without x-ray mark-
      ers
    4 In. wide, soft gauze Kerlix roll
    3 In. wide, firm pliable gauze Kling roll
    1 In. adhesive tape

In a room adjacent to the operating room the patient's head is shaved immediately prior to the surgical procedure and after induction of anesthesia. Hair is cut before the shaving and collected in a bag, labeled with the patient's name for possible later use. The scalp is then shaved according to the surgeon's instructions.

If desired, urinary drainage is begun. For procedures requiring cerebrospinal fluid drainage, a no. 18 spinal needle is inserted into the lower lumbar spinal canal, leaving the stylet in place until drainage is desired. The patient is then positioned, and sandbags are placed to prevent him from rolling back onto the needle. The inactive electrode (stainless steel plate, coated with conductive lubricant) is placed under the patient's shoulders or flank. The patient lies more or less supine with his head turned to expose the operative area and supported with rolled towels or sandbags. Petrolatum is applied over the closed eyes to prevent corneal damage. Several towels or pillows are placed between the knees and at other possible pressure points resulting from straps and the position of the patient on the operating table. Drapes are placed under exposed portions of the body to prevent the skin from contacting metal portions of the operating table. The patient is then wheeled into the operating room.

The basic table is positioned in back of the scrub nurse. The bone and suture tray instruments are positioned on the basic instrument table with the bone instruments to the left and suture instruments to the right (Fig. 11-25). The Mayo neurosurgical table is positioned over the patient, and after the draping is completed, the Mayo tray instruments are placed on it as shown in Fig. 11-26, with the addition of knife blades and handles. It is from this table that the nurse hands instruments to the surgeon. The neurosurgical Mayo table is positioned across the patient, leaving his head and neck uncovered. A towel is placed under his head, and the shaved area of the scalp is scrubbed for 10 minutes with hexachlorophene and distilled water. The lather is removed with dry and alcohol-saturated sponges, and iodine-based solution is applied. A clean towel is placed under the head, and the line of incision is marked on the scalp with a no. 20 blade. The incision line and the areas for towel clamps may be injected with procaine or lidocaine to decrease the sensitivity of the scalp to pain.

Four or more towels are placed around the operative site, and they are secured with towel clamps or sutured with no. 2-0 silk on a cutting needle. A sterile large conductive rubber sheet is placed over the

neurosurgical Mayo table so that one edge reaches up to the line of incision. This sheet is secured to the nearest towel with Michel clips. A craniotomy sheet, with the fenestration placed over the operative site, is placed over the entire field. Disposable water-impermeable sheets are excellent for this purpose and may be secured with Michel clips. Half sheets are used for additional draping. The draping must include sufficient slack in the drapes to permit table adjustments. The contents of the Mayo tray are placed on the Mayo table. Two suction tubings with Sachs suction tips are secured to the drapes with Rochester-Pean forceps. The active electrode (Bovie pencil) with the spatula tip is secured to the operative field with towel clamps. Adequate lengths of tubing and the electrode cord must be provided for ease in handling. Two medium basins with warm Ringer's solution, one for irrigation and one for cotton strips, are placed on the table. Gauze sponges are non-Ray-Tec, 4 × 4 inches. Assorted sizes of cotton strips are used.

OPERATIVE PROCEDURE

1. With the surgeon and his assistant exerting finger pressure on gauze sponges on opposite sides of the line of incision, the scalp is incised in serial segments, each extending through the epicranial aponeurosis. At each stage, Kolodney hemostatic forceps are used on the outside skin edge for the adult. Many surgeons group these together in bundles with rubber bands or by means of opened gauze sponges or umbilical tapes passed through the rings and clamped. Bleeding from the inside skin edge at the margins of the skin flap is controlled with Michel or Raney clips (Fig. 11-27). For the infant, small Michel clips are often used on all the skin edges. Very rarely, electrocautery is necessary to control bleeding points, but this should be avoided if possible.

2. The skin-galeal flap is raised off the periosteum using a no. 20 blade on a no. 4 handle while holding the flap with a gauze sponge or tissue forceps with teeth. A Mayo scissors may be used. Hemostasis is obtained using bayonet forceps. The scalp flap is wrapped in a moist sponge and folded back over rolled sponges. The flap is retracted with fish-hook retractors that are secured to the drape with a Rochester-Pean hemostat. If a free bone flap is planned, such as may be used in cases of superficial meningioma, the skin incision

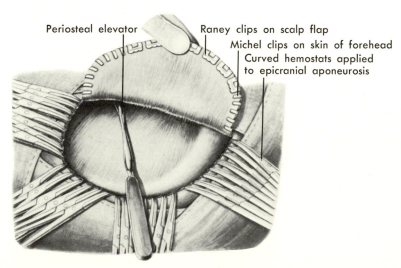

**Fig. 11-27.** Elevation of scalp flap. Hemostats on the outer rim of the incision and Raney clips and Michel clips on the scalp flap. (From Kempe, L. G.: Operative neurosurgery, vols. 1 and 2, New York, 1968, Springer-Verlag, New York, Inc.)

is carried through the periosteum down to the bone and the periosteum and muscle elevated with the skin as a single flap. In this case inappropriate portions of steps 3 and 4 are omitted.

3. The periosteum and muscle around the margins of the proposed bone flap are incised with a no. 4 scalpel and no. 20 blade or, more commonly, with the electrocautery (cutting current). The periosteum and muscle over the inferior margin of the proposed bone flap is not divided so as to maintain a bridge of muscle to provide a blood supply to the bone flap after it is elevated. The periosteum is then stripped from the line of incision with a periosteal elevator so as to expose a strip of bone corresponding to the margins of the proposed bone flap. Bone wax and coagulation are used as needed (Fig. 11-28).

4. Four-prong Sachs retractors are used to retract the muscle and periosteal edges so as to expose the bone beneath.

5. To make the bone flap, two or more burr holes are made in the skull. Either the Hall craniotome, the Smith automatic drill, or the Hudson brace with the D'Errico perforator may be used. While the skull is being drilled, warm Ringer's solution is dripped into the holes and suctioned to remove the bone dust. Alternately, the moist bone dust may be collected on an appropriately placed brain spatula spoon so that the dust may be replaced in the holes at the end of the procedure. Dust is stored in a medicine glass with a small amount of saline to keep it moist. Bleeding about the holes may be controlled with bone wax or by packing with moist cotton strips. Using a dural elevator, aneurysm needle, or small joker, the dura is freed from the bone at the margins of each hole. The dura is then stripped from the underside of the proposed bone flap and between all burr holes utilizing a staphylorrhaphy.

a. Gigli saw procedure (Fig. 11-29)
 (1) A circle of four or five burr holes is made, outlining the proposed bone flap.
 (2) With muscle and periosteal edges held apart with four-prong and subtemporal decompression retractors, a single-action rongeur is used to cut channels in the bone along the inferior edge of the proposed flap beneath its muscle bridge. A channel is cut, starting at each of the two burr holes bordering this inferior edge. A bridge of bone is left uncut to be cracked later.
 (3) The soft tissues are retracted with four-prong retractors, and a Gigli saw guide with tip previously bent upward is passed forward through one burr hole and out the next. The saw is connected to the guide, drawn through, freed from the guide, and the handles connected. The bone is sawed through. Sometimes it is necessary to use two guides for the approach. Irrigation and control of bleeding is carried out. This is repeated, using a new saw for the other holes, leaving the edge of the bone flap to be cracked intact. When muscle or periosteum is left attached to the bone flap, this edge will be beneath this attachment.

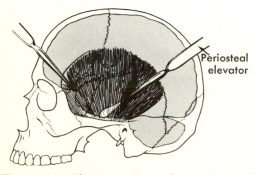

Fig. 11-28. Elevation of muscle incision with periosteal elevators. (From Kempe, L. G.: Operative neurosurgery, vols. 1 and 2, New York, 1968, Springer-Verlag, New York, Inc.)

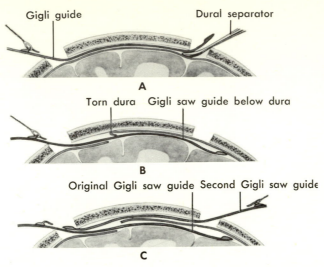

Fig. 11-29. Gigli saw insertion. **A** to **C**, Steps to be taken if Gigli saw tears dura. (From Kempe, L. G.: Operative neurosurgery, vols. 1 and 2, New York, 1968, Springer-Verlag, New York, Inc.)

b. Craniotome procedure
   (1) At least two burr holes are made.
   (2) With muscle and periosteal edges held apart with four-prong and subtemporal decompression retractors, a single-action rongeur is used to cut channels in the bone along the inferior edge of the proposed flap. A channel is cut, starting at each of the two burr holes bordering this inferior edge. A bridge of bone is left uncut to be cracked later.
   (3) The soft tissue edges are retracted with four-prong retractors, and the craniotome blade attachment with dural guard is used to cut the bone to create a flap. Cooling irrigation is carried out throughout this step.

6. The bone is cracked back, using two periosteal elevators to elevate it from the dura at a point opposite the remaining bridge of bone. A full-size moist cottonoid is placed over the dura for protection.

7. A double-action rongeur is used to remove the irregular bone along the lower edge of the bone flap (Fig. 11-30). Bleeding points in the muscle are coagulated.

8. The bone flap is wrapped and secured to the drape as described for the scalp flap.

9. Additional bone may be removed from the edges of the bony defect with the double-action rongeur after stripping off the dura with a joker. The bone edges are then waxed.

10. Cotton strips and hemostatic material may be inserted at the junction of bone edges with the dura to control bleeding.

11. Half-size cotton strips are used to cover the exposed bone and skin edges about the circumference of the operative field. This is then additionally draped with clean towels fastened with towel clamps. One of these towels is placed from the inferior edge of the exposure up to the edge of the neurosurgical Mayo table where it is also clamped into place.

12. The dura is raised with a dura hook and nicked with a no. 15 blade on a no. 3 knife handle. A cotton strip is placed beneath the dura along the line of proposed incision, and using a dura forceps and fine dissecting scissors, the incision is extended. Alternatively, the dura may be held taut by an assistant using a mosquito hemostatic forcep. A narrow

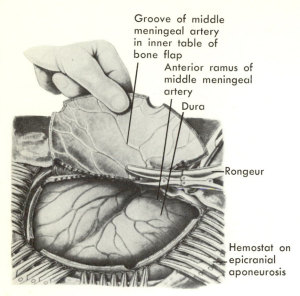

Groove of middle meningeal artery in inner table of bone flap

Anterior ramus of middle meningeal artery

Dura

Rongeur

Hemostat on epicranial aponeurosis

**Fig. 11-30.** Frontotemporal craniotomy, opening and closure. Removal of the rough bone edge from the fracture site. (From Kempe, L. G.: Operative neurosurgery, vols. 1 and 2, New York, 1968, Springer-Verlag, New York, Inc.)

brain spatula spoon may then be placed beneath the dura so as to permit its continued division with a scalpel. (Cerebrospinal fluid drainage may be instituted at this time.)

13. Stay sutures are placed in the outside edge of dura using no. 4-0 black silk tagged at the end with hemostatic forceps. For the stay sutures along the inferior edge a bulldog towel clip with notched handle is attached to the towel, placed at the inferior edge of the field up to the edge of the neurosurgical Mayo table. The end of the silk is then looped through the notched handle of the bulldog clip. Hemostatic forceps placed on sutures in other dural edges are merely hung over the adjacent side of the head. If greater tension is desired, an additional hemostat is added.

14. Moist strips of cotton, coagulation, or clips may be used to control bleeding along the dural incision.

15. Wet cotton strips are used as needed to protect the brain surface and eliminate undue exposure of the brain. Exposure

and treatment of the lesion are then carried out.

16. Instruments for exploration include suction, moistened brain retractors, bayonet cup forceps, long and short bayonet forceps, assorted nerve hooks, and various sizes of hemostatic clips. Other instruments will be selected according to procedure and the neurosurgeon's preference. Tumors may be scooped, sucked, or even cut out using pituitary rongeurs, curettes, scoops, spatula spoons, cup forceps, suction, or cautery loops (Fig. 11-31). (See following procedures for various craniotomies.)

17. When the intracranial portion of the procedure has been completed, the bleeding controlled, and the brain irrigated with warm Ringer's solution, the dura is usually closed. In those instances in which the dura is left open, gelatin film or silicone sheeting may be used to cover the defect.

18. Stay sutures of no. 2-0 or 3-0 silk tagged with straight hemostatic forceps are placed through the dura at the edges of the bony defect, as well as one central stay suture tagged with a mosquito forceps. The dura is then closed with multiple interrupted silk sutures no. 4-0 on ophthalmic needles. THE SPINAL NEEDLE IS REMOVED. Ringer's solution is used to fill the intracranial cavity just before dural closure is completed.

19. A hemostatic material is placed along the dural and bone edges. An epidural polyethylene drain may be inserted and brought out through a separate stab wound in the skin posteriorly. The point at which the bone edge is crossed by the drain is grooved with a rongeur to permit the bone flap to be replaced flush.

20. The bone flap is unwrapped. Using a craniotome with a thin drill bit, holes for anchoring sutures are drilled in the flap and at corresponding points in the edge of the bony defect. A central hole is made for the central stay suture, both ends of which are passed through this with a Keith needle. Sutures of no. 2-0 silk are passed through the peripheral holes, tied, and cut. The silk stay sutures in the dura are mounted on spring-eye needles and then

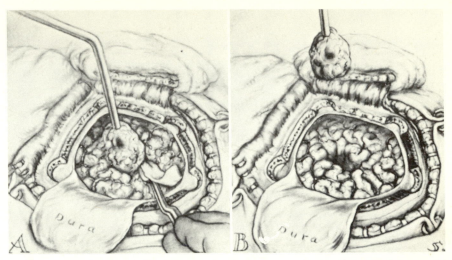

**Fig. 11-31.** Removal of brain tumor using Sachs suction tube and bayonet forceps. (From Sachs, E.: Diagnosis and treatment of brain tumors and care of the neurosurgical patient, ed. 2, St. Louis, The C. V. Mosby Co.)

sutured and tied to the underside of the periosteum. The central dural stay suture is tied to the temporal fascia or over a small piece of rolled gelatin sponge. Silk no. 3-0 on spring-eye needles is used to approximate the periosteum of the bone flap to the surrounding pericranium beneath the outer skin edges. The muscle and fascial layers are closed in similar fashion.

21. A few of the Michel or Raney clips and Kolodney clamps are removed from the skin edges, and this section is closed with buried sutures of no. 3-0 silk on spring-eye needles. This is repeated until the entire galea is closed. The ends of every six or eight of these sutures clamped several inches from the skin may be pulled taut over a rolled gauze sponge to control skin bleeding.

22. These buried sutures are then cut, one group at a time, and no. 4-0 skin sutures are placed. Skin sutures are cut and the dressing applied.

### Craniotomy for intracranial aneurysm and other intracranial vascular anomalies

**DEFINITION.** Isolation of the lesion, with or without removal of the defective intracranial vascular wall.

**CONSIDERATIONS.** An aneurysm is a vascular dilatation usually due to a local defect in the vascular wall. Within the cranial cavity the aneurysm may produce cranial nerve lesions, particularly if it impinges on the third nerve or the optic chiasm. Aneurysms usually give symptoms of stroke, since hemorrhage is generally the first evidence of the condition.

Malformations vary widely in size, area of involvement, and structure. Arteriovenous fistulas may be congenital or may result from trauma or disease. Vascular anomalies may also give rise to subarachnoid hemorrhage or may have extensive irritative effects and cause focal or generalized seizures.

Modern neurosurgical techniques of diagnosis and hemostasis have made operations on intracranial aneurysms more feasible. Overwhelming fatal hemorrhage is the greatest hazard both of the condition and of the surgery. To prevent this, control of the nerve pressure as well as the vascular supply to the region well beyond the limits of the lesion may be required. Occasionally, control of the cerebral circulation at the level of the cervical carotid artery is desired. The artery may be exposed and controlled by means

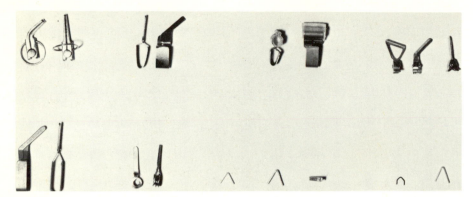

**Fig. 11-32.** Some types of vascular clips and clamps available. Top: Kerr clip, Mayfield clip, Sundt-Key clip, Heifitz clip. Bottom: Schwartz temporary clamp, Scoville clip, McKenzie silver clip, Olivecrona clip (wide), Weck Hemoclip, Olivecrona clip (narrow). (Courtesy K. Cramer Lewis, Department of Illustrations, Washington University School of Medicine, St. Louis, Mo.)

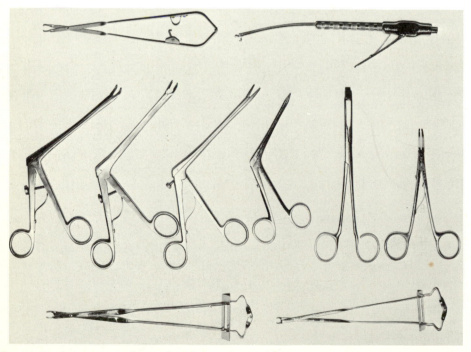

**Fig. 11-33.** Some types of vascular clip applicators. Top: Heifitz and Kerr clip applicators. Center: Right-angled Hamby, right-angled Mount-Olivecrona, Scoville-Drew, Scoville, Schwartz, and Weck Hemoclip applicators. Bottom: Mayfield and small Mayfield clip applicators. (Courtesy K. Cramer Lewis, Department of Illustrations, Washington University School of Medicine, St. Louis, Mo.)

of preplaced ligatures or clamps that may be tightened to occlude the vessel at need. This step is taken before the cranial operation is begun. A separate surgical setup is required. (See the procedure for carotid artery ligation.)

**SETUP AND PREPARATION OF THE PATIENT.** The setup is as described for craniotomy, plus Mayfield, Olivecrona, and other clips and appliers (Figs. 11-32 and 11-33) and double-suction apparatus. Supplementary strong suction must be immediately available to prevent hemorrhage from obscuring the operative field.

The aneurysm set of instruments is as follows:

  2 Scoville-Drew angular clip-applying forceps (narrow and wide Olivecrona clips)
  2 Hamby angled clip-applying forceps (left angle) (narrow Olivecrona clips)
  2 Hamby right-angled, clip-applying forceps (narrow Olivecrona clips)
  2 Mount-Olivecrona clip-applying and removing forceps, right-angled (wide Olivecrona clips)
  2 Mount-Olivecrona clip-applying and removing forceps, left-angled (wide Olivecrona clips)
  5 Schwartz temporary clamp-applying forceps, 7 ¾ in., straight and angled
 12 Schwartz temporary intracranial artery clamps, 4 straight, 4 angled (25-degree), 4 angled (45-degree)
  2 Mayfield aneurysm clip appliers (assorted angled and straight Mayfield clips)
  6 Heifitz clip appliers (straight and angled Heifitz clips of various sizes)
  2 Scoville-Lewis clip appliers (narrow and wide Scoville clips)
  2 Small Mayfield clip appliers (assorted Sundt-Key clips)
  1 Kerr clip applier (assorted Kerr clips)
  2 DeBakey vascular forceps
  2 Heavy bayonet forceps, 8 in.
    DeMartel, Edinborough, or Yasargil self-retaining retractors

**OPERATIVE PROCEDURE**

1 to 15. As described for craniotomy. If a bifrontal (coronal) skin flap is necessary, more scalp clips and hemostats will be necessary. Usually a frontal or fronto-temporal craniotomy is done. This procedure is described on p. 357.

16. The aneurysm instruments are provided.

17. A wet brain retractor is inserted over moist cotton strips and used to elevate the orbital surface of the frontal lobe of the brain in order to expose the optic nerve and the arachnoid cisterns. Another retractor may be used on the temporal lobe. The olfactory nerve may be coagulated and divided with a long scissors in order to enhance the exposure.

18. Bridging veins are coagulated; the arachnoid is dissected and torn; and a dural elevator, nerve hooks, and suction are used for further exposure. A De-Martel, Edinborough, or Yasargil self-retaining retractor is placed to maintain exposure.

19. At this time the anesthetist administers a ganglionic blocking drug (trimethaphan camphorsulfonate) to lower the blood pressure to a hypotensive level. All suctions (2 or 3) are rechecked to be sure they are in good working order.

20. Using a nerve hook, the parent artery and then the aneurysm and its neck are outlined and freed. Great care is taken not to rupture the aneurysm. If it should rupture, a large suction tip is placed over its dome, and an effort is made to place a clip so as to control the bleeding.

21. The aneurysm is then clipped across its neck. At times the surgeon will elect to ligate the neck with no. 2-0 or no. 0 silk, using an aneurysm hook and bayonet forceps. In this case, the suture is threaded down through the eye in the hook so that the short end exits below or to one side. Sometimes the aneurysm is wrapped in fine-mesh gauze and coated with methyl methacrylate (fast drying) using an eye dropper or dural elevator.

22. The blood pressure is permitted to return to normal.

23. The operative area is inspected for any unusual oozing or bleeding, and the clip, clips, or ligature is checked.

24. The wound closure and dressing are as described for craniotomy.

### Craniotomy for arteriovenous malformation

#### OPERATIVE PROCEDURE

1 to 15. As described for craniotomy.

16. The feeding arteries are exposed a distance from the malformation, then traced toward it, and occluded a short distance before they penetrate into its substance. This will spare as many of the arteries to the brain as possible. The feeding arteries may be occluded by clipping, coagulation, or ligation.

17. The malformation is then dissected out with suction and bayonet forceps. Additional vessels are clipped or coagulated along the way. Usually one or more draining veins are left to be ligated as the last step in the removal.

18. Closure and dressing is as described for craniotomy.

### Craniotomy for pituitary tumor (craniopharyngioma, optic glioma, and other suprasellar and parasellar tumors)

**PURPOSE.** The removal of the tumor to relieve pressure on surrounding structures such as the optic chiasm and optic nerve.

**SETUP AND PREPARATION OF THE PATIENT.** The setup is similar to that described for craniotomy but includes the following additional pituitary instruments (Fig. 11-34):

Ray curettes (ring, sharp)
Spinal needles no. 22 or no. 24
Luer-Lok syringe, 10 ml.
Angulated suction tips, right, left; large, small
Small curettes (sizes no. 0 through 4-0)

#### OPERATIVE PROCEDURE

1 to 15. As described for craniotomy. The incision will be either bifrontal (Souttar) or unilateral in the frontal or frontotemporal region. Most unilateral approaches are carried out from the right side.

16. Wet brain retractors over moist cotton strips are inserted for exposure of the optic chiasm and the pituitary gland. The frontal and often the temporal lobe are retracted. The olfactory nerve may be coagulated and divided with scissors.

17. A DeMartel, Edinborough, or Yasargil self-retaining retractor is placed to

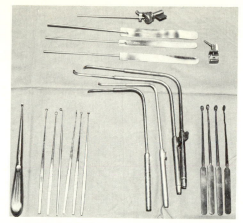

**Fig. 11-34.** Additional pituitary instruments. Top: DeMartel self-retaining retractor. Bottom: stainless steel curette, Ray curettes, Sachs angled suction tubes, Cushing pituitary spoons. (Courtesy K. Cramer Lewis, Department of Illustrations, Washington University School of Medicine, St. Louis, Mo.)

maintain exposure. Aneurysm clips and appliers of some sort should always be available to control unexpected bleeding from major vessels.

18. Using a syringe with moistened plunger and a no. 22 or 24 spinal needle, an attempt is made to aspirate the contents of the tumor in order to guard against inadvertently entering an aneurysm or vessel.

19. The tumor capsule is coagulated for hemostasis and incised with a no. 11 blade on a long handle. Using a pituitary rongeur or cup forceps, the tumor is removed.

20. Small stainless steel, copper, or Ray curettes as well as suction may be used during the tumor removal.

21. A wide Olivecrona clip may be applied to the stalk of the pituitary, which may then be cut distally. The long angulated scissors is especially helpful for this.

22. If the tumor capsule is to be removed, bayonet forceps, cup forceps, nerve hooks, and suction aid in the dissection. If the tumor capsule is not removed, Zenker's solution may be placed in the capsule of a pituitary adenoma after walling off the adjacent structures with cotton strips.

23. Closure and dressing is as described for craniotomy.

In case of a pituitary adenoma with a prefixed chiasm the surgeon will sometimes elect to remove the anterior wall of the sphenoid sinus and sella turcica with an air drill in order to gain access to the tumor. In the rare tumor with extension into the temporal fossa, a temporal approach may be utilized.

In the case of craniopharyngioma, extreme caution must be used in removing fluid from the capsule because the fluid is extremely irritating and may cause chemical leptomeningitis. Calcified pieces of tumor are dissected and removed in the same manner as the capsule of a pituitary adenoma. This is an extremely difficult procedure because of deposits on the carotid arteries, the optic nerves, and optic chiasm. Tumor capsule is often left behind on the hypothalamus in order to avoid stripping off blood vessels supplying this structure. Large amounts of moist cottonoid are used to protect the surrounding areas from the cystic contents. The technique used is similar to that for a potentially contaminated procedure.

Suprasellar meningiomas usually arise from the tuberculum sella just anterior to the optic nerves and chiasm. Tumor removal is similar to that of a pituitary adenoma except that the cutting loop of the electrocautery may be used to excavate the interior of the tumor. After the tumor has been removed, the site of its attachment to the dura is thoroughly coagulated to prevent recurrence. Other meningiomas arising at the base of the skull are treated by similar techniques.

### Craniotomy for brain abscess

The operative procedure for abscess is either excision through a craniotomy or aspiration through a burr hole.

OPERATIVE PROCEDURE

EXCISION OF ABSCESS. The abscess is approached through an osteoplastic craniotomy. The lesion is located by palpation or, more commonly, by aspiration. Care must

be taken to protect the surface of the brain with cottonoid to prevent contamination during the course of aspiration. The syringe and needle used are handled as little as possible by the nurse. They are placed in a sterile towel and handed off the field for culture and stains of the specimen. The brain abscess is then excised using suction and blunt dissection with bayonet forceps and cotton strips around the margin of the abscess capsule. The surface of the brain exposed in the course of the dissection is carefully walled off with cotton strips to prevent contamination should the contents of the abscess leak during the procedure. Cup forceps or a large brain spoon may be of aid in elevating the lesion out of the brain. After removal of the abscess copious warm Ringer's irrigation is carried out with the suction tip placed superficially inside the area of brain dissection so as to prevent the irrigation solution and any possible infected debris from washing over the surface of the brain or the more superficial levels of the wound. Antibiotics are instilled and the craniotomy closed in the usual manner.

### Craniotomy with electrocorticography for intractable epilepsy

CONSIDERATIONS. The complete cooperation of an alert patient is desired to obtain desirable results. Therefore preoperative medications are not given, and local anesthesia is used until the recordings are completed. After the recordings are completed, the anesthetist administers an intravenous neuroleptanalgesic to add to the patient's comfort while the surgery is completed. The patient is placed on a foam mattress to relieve any pressure points, and the drapes are positioned so that his face is completely visible to the anesthetist. Other precautions are taken as for craniotomy. As he operates, the neurosurgeon explains every step of the procedure to the patient.

OPERATIVE PROCEDURE

1. The skin incision site is marked using methylene blue.

2. The incision and towel clamp areas are injected with 1% lidocaine. The nurse must know the exact amount of local anesthetic used because if too much local anesthetic is given, a seizure may be produced.

3. Using a no. 4 scalpel with a no. 20 blade, one or two skin flaps are created.

4 to 15. As described for craniotomy. The bone flap usually is cut free and replaced on completion of the procedure.

16. After hemostasis is accomplished and the dura is ready to be opened, a cotton strip is saturated with 1% procaine and placed over the dura and its vessels for topical anesthesia.

17. The dura is opened as described for craniotomy, and the electrocorticography procedure is started.

18. Electrical stimulation and recording from the cortex is used to outline the motor and sensory areas and to locate the seizure focus. Small numbered or lettered squares of paper are placed at the points of stimulation in order to label them (Fig. 11-35).

19. After recordings and identification of the pathological areas are completed, the anesthetist administers the neuroleptanalgesic agent.

20. The pathological areas are removed, avoiding sensory, motor, and speech areas as much as possible. In cases of psychomotor epilepsy, it is usually the anterior temporal lobe that is resected.

21. Brain resection is carried out with suction bayonet forceps, electrocoagulation, and scissors. Ribbon retractors are used to maintain exposure.

22. Closure is as described for craniotomy. When the bone flap has been replaced, methyl methacrylate may be applied to the burr holes to further stabilize the large bone flap.

23. The patient is awake and cooperating for the application of the dressing.

### Craniotomy for cerebrospinal rhinorrhea

Cerebrospinal rhinorrhea is a rupture of the dura with evagination of the torn arachnoid through the dura into a hole or fracture in the skull communicating with one of the nasal sinuses or the nasal cavity. This results in leakage of spinal fluid from the nose. It is necessary to repair the defect to prevent air from being trapped under pressure in the brain and to prevent intracranial infection. Usually, a frontal craniotomy is carried out, and the dura is opened. The frontal lobe is elevated until the defect can be visualized. The dura is dissected from the orbital and cribriform plates. The defect in the bone is defined. If desired, the bony defect may be filled with methyl methacrylate or covered with tantalum mesh. The dural defect may be closed with sutures, but usually some type of patch should be placed over the dural defect. A piece of muscle, pericranium, fascia, gelatin foam, or silicone sheeting may be used. These may be sutured into place or glued with an adhesive such as isobutyl cyanoacrylate. Some surgeons will not fasten the patch into place. The dural incision is sutured and the wound closed. Occasionally, cerebrospinal otorrhea will occur. In this case a similar procedure is carried out in the temporal or suboccipital region.

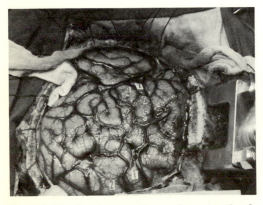

**Fig. 11-35.** Craniotomy for epilepsy with the following areas outlined: **1,** motor hand area; **2,** sensory hand area; **3,** motor face area; **6,** speech area as proven by speech arrest on electrical stimulation. (Courtesy Dr. Sidney Goldring, Department of Neurological Surgery, Washington University School of Medicine, St. Louis, Mo.)

## Supratentorial craniectomy, cranioplasty, and trephination

**DEFINITION.** Excision of a portion of the skull.

**CONSIDERATIONS.** Injury to the underlying brain frequently accompanies injury to the cranium. This procedure may be required to remove tumors, hematomas, scars, or infections of the bone. Craniectomy is also indicated as treatment for premature craniosynostosis in infants. Pressure on the brain from depressed bone or internal hemorrhage must be relieved.

**SETUP AND PREPARATION OF THE PATIENT.** Instruments are as for craniotomy. The setup may be modified according to the extent of the planned procedure. Omit tumor instruments as indicated.

## *Craniectomy with evacuation of epidural or subdural hematoma*

**DEFINITION.** The removal and drainage of blood clot and collections of liquefied blood from outside or beneath the dura caused by one or more bleeding vessels (Fig. 11-36).

**OPERATIVE PROCEDURE**

1 to 7. As described for ventriculography (p. 351). Burr holes are placed over suspected lesion site rather than the occipital area.

8. If a blood clot or collection of bloody fluid is found outside or beneath the dura, the burr hole is further enlarged using a Kerrison or double-action rongeur until adequate exposure is obtained. Bone edges are waxed and cotton strips placed along

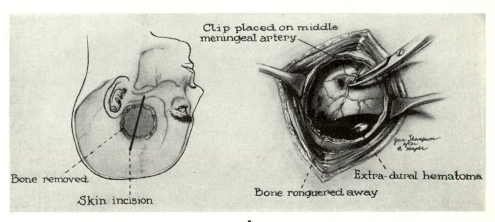

**A**

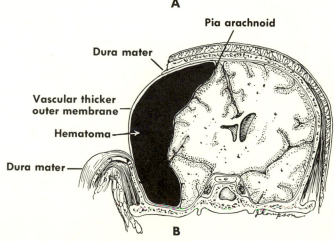

**B**

Fig. 11-36. A, Extradural hemorrhage. B, Subdural hematoma. (From Richards, V.: Surgery for general practice, St. Louis, 1956, The C. V. Mosby Co.)

edges. On occasion, craniotomy or additional craniectomy may be necessary to provide the necessary exposure for control of the bleeding (see p. 357).

9. Clot and fluid are evacuated and hemostasis accomplished with coagulation or the use of hemostatic clips.

10. In cases of chronic subdural hematoma, the inner and outer membranes are stripped with cup forceps and coagulated using bayonet forceps.

11. The brain is irrigated using French catheters or directly with an Asepto syringe. Large amounts of warm Ringer's solution are used until the return is clear.

12. For subsequent radiographical follow-up, clips may be placed. A silver or a Weck Hemoclip may be placed on the cortex at the site of a small incision created with a no. 11 blade on a no. 3 scalpel handle and electrocoagulation. Another clip is placed on the dura.

13. A small Penrose tubing or a polyethylene or red rubber (no. 12 or 14 Fr.) catheter may be inserted subdurally for additional drainage. This usually exits through a separate stab wound in the skin posterior to the incision. An anchoring suture may be placed.

14. The dura and soft tissue incision is closed and dressed in the usual manner.

15. Additional burr holes are made during the course of the procedure to be sure that clots in other areas do not remain undetected and untreated.

### Cranioplasty

**DEFINITION.** Repair of a cranial defect. The defect may be a result of accidental trauma, previous surgery, or malformation.

**PURPOSE.** To relieve subjective symptoms, headache, vertigo, fear of injury, or local tenderness or throbbing; to prevent secondary injury to the underlying brain; and for cosmetic effect.

**CONSIDERATIONS.** Many materials have been used to repair skull defects—bone and cartilage, celluloid, metals such as Vitallium and tantalum, and the synthetic resins (methyl methacrylate, silicone rub-

ber). All involve technical problems. The use of commercially prepared cranioplastic synthetics that supply the needed chemicals and mixing containers has to a large extent simplified the procedures of shaping and molding the prosthesis.

**SETUP AND PREPARATION OF THE PATIENT.** Instruments as for craniotomy, plus the materials selected for making and securing the prosthesis.

*For bone graft,* add chisels, osteotomes, and retractors suitable for exposing the donor site.

*To handle tantalum metal plates,* add molds, mallet, metal shears, files, and drills.

*For molded plastics,* add shears, files, and shaping instruments (Fig. 11-37).

**OPERATIVE PROCEDURE.** The shaped plate is fitted into the skull defect. The edges of the defect are trimmed and a ledge formed to seat the prosthesis. The plate is fastened in place with no. 2-0 black silk sutures on a taper point needle (often wire) passed through matching drill holes in the prosthesis and skull.

After the bone defect has been prepared so that it is slightly saucerized, the highly refined methyl methacrylate is mixed by adding one volume of the liquid monomer of the plastic to one volume of the powdered polymer of methyl methacrylate (Fig. 11-37, *B*). When this has formed a doughy mass, it is dropped into a sterile polyethylene bag (*C*). The soft plastic is then rolled on a flat surface into the desired shape, leaving the thickness to approximate depth of the skull edges (*D*). A sterile test tube, syringe barrel, or other round object can be used, although the stainless steel roller illustrated is preferred due to its weight and ease of operation.

The soft cranioplastic in the bag is then placed over the skull defect and, by pressing lightly with the end of the fingers, it is fitted into the missing skull area. The plastic bag is stretched by assistants as the surgeon molds the plate into the defect and forms an overlapping bevel edge (*E*). This overlapping fringe keeps the

plate from falling inside the skull. The skull saucerization helps in this regard also.

When the heat of combination begins, the plate is lifted out of the bony wound and removed from the polyethylene bag. In complicated plates, it is recommended that the surgeon supervise the latter phase of the hardening process by further molding of the hot plastic, since there is a tendency for the edges to curl and other loss of shape to take place during this period. When cool enough to handle, the excess material is trimmed away with bone rongeurs or cut with a saw and placed in the cranial defect (*F*). A sterile carborundum wheel attached to the electric bone saw or craniotome is used to smooth

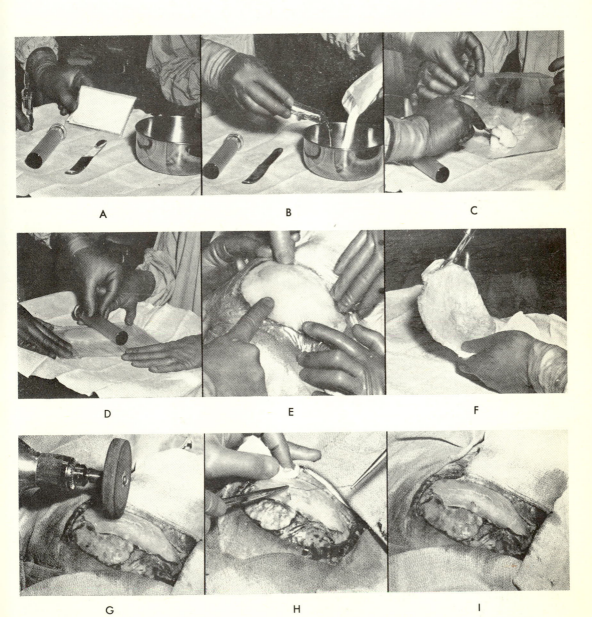

Fig. 11-37. Kit and carborundum wheel used in cranioplasty. (Courtesy Codman & Shurtleff, Inc., Randolph, Mass.)

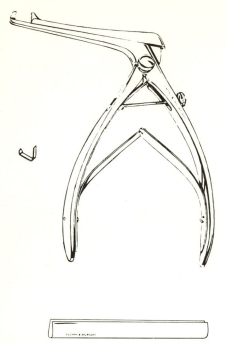

**Fig. 11-38.** Material for craniosynostosis may include Ingraham-Fowler tantalum clips, Ingraham-Fowler guillotine clip-applying forceps, and preformed silicone strip. (Courtesy Codman & Shurtleff, Inc., Randolph, Mass.)

the rough spots and bevel the edges so that the plate will blend gradually with the skull (G). Mixing and fitting the plate takes about 7 minutes and hardening about 7 minutes.

Screws or wire or no. 2-0 silk sutures may be used to hold the plate in place, generally at three or more points.

### Craniectomy for craniosynostosis

CONSIDERATIONS. This procedure is performed on infants whose suture lines have closed prematurely. In craniosynostosis a sheet of synthetic material such as silicone may be employed to keep the edges of the cranial sutures from reuniting and preventing brain growth (Fig. 11-38).

OPERATIVE PROCEDURE. These procedures are often extensive and since they are usually done on very young children, careful attention to blood replacement is mandatory. After the scalp incision is made over the appropriate skull suture, the dura is stripped off the underside of the skull with an aneurysm needle or staphylorrhapy elevator. A generous portion of the bone edges joining to form the fused suture is then removed with a heavy scissors, a craniotome, rongeur, or Kerrison punch so as to perform a strip craniectomy. The bone edges are waxed. Preformed Silastic sheeting (Fig. 11-38) is inserted over the bone edges bordering the craniectomy and is sutured or stapled in place. When sutures are used, holes must be placed in the bone edges bordering the craniectomy before the sheeting is applied to them. Closure is in the usual fashion.

### Craniectomy for trigeminal rhizotomy

CONSIDERATIONS. Trigeminal neuralgia (tic douloureux, fifth cranial nerve pain) is a condition characterized by brief, repeated attacks of excruciating pain in the face. The three divisions of the fifth cranial nerve are the ophthalmic, the maxillary, and the mandibular. Temporary relief of trigeminal neuralgia may be obtained by interruption of branches of the nerve divisions by means of alcohol injection or surgical sectioning.

SETUP AND PREPARATION OF THE PATIENT. As described for craniotomy. The patient may be placed in the supine or sitting position, depending on preference of the surgeon. (See suboccipital craniectomy, considerations and setup and preparation of the patient.)

OPERATIVE PROCEDURE
SUBTEMPORAL APPROACH

1. A vertical temporal incision extending up from the zygomatic process and through the temporal muscles and periosteum is made in the usual manner.

2. The soft tissue is freed from the bone with a periosteal elevator. The bone exposure is maintained with a Klemme self-retaining gasserian ganglion retractor to hold the soft tissues apart.

3. A burr hole is made and the dura freed from the underside of the temporal bone with an aneurysm needle.

4. The burr hole is enlarged to a diameter of about 2½ inches, utilizing a double-action rongeur.

5. Using a moist brain retractor, the dura overlying the temporal lobe is retracted upward. By means of blunt dissection with cotton strips held in bayonet forceps, the dura is elevated from the bony floor of the middle fossa.

6. The brain retractor is replaced by a heavier retractor (Cushing spatula with lip) placed deeper into the wound to hold up the temporal lobe and dura. A fiberoptic light may be attached to this retractor with rubber bands in order to provide adequate illumination.

7. As the dura is elevated, the middle meningeal artery is encountered as it leaves the foramen spinosum to join the dura. It is coagulated with bayonet forceps or a nerve hook and may be clipped prior to being divided. Occasionally a cottonoid plug or other material is packed into the foramen spinosum.

8. Additional blunt dissection will uncover the mandibular division of the trigeminal nerve and finally the trigeminal (gasserian) ganglion within its own dural sheath (dura propria). Bleeding is controlled with cotton strips and a hemostatic material.

9. Some surgeons will terminate the procedure after stripping the ganglion and its dura from that of the overlying temporal lobe. (The ganglion may be injected with saline, and the dura may be split.)

10. If a root section is to be performed, a no. 11 blade on a long scalpel handle is used to make an incision into the lateral rim of the dura propria. The sensory and motor roots of the nerve are defined using a fine nerve hook. The mandibular and maxillary sections of the root are usually then divided. These are elevated with a nerve hook and divided with a fine scissors or a fine blade. The ophthalmic portion of the root is spared as is the motor root.

11. Absolute alcohol may be injected into the affected divisions of the nerve just distal to the ganglion.

12. Saline is injected into the dura overlying the temporal lobe in order to distend it.

13. The incision is closed and dressed in the usual manner. As discussed later, some surgeons prefer to section the posterior root of the trigeminal nerve by the suboccipital route.

### Trephination for prefrontal lobotomy

**DEFINITION AND PURPOSE.** Incision into the frontal lobe of the cerebral cortex to interrupt nerve pathways (associative fibers). It is used in selected cases of psychosis and also to relieve the intractable pain in advanced stages of cancer.

**SETUP AND PREPARATION OF THE PATIENT.** The setup includes instruments and supplies as for craniotomy, as well as the following:

Bucy suction tube and cautery
Adson self-retaining cerebellum retractors with angulated arms
Trephines, 1 and 2 in. (Fig. 11-39)
1 Lobotomy needle, 8 in.
Frazier suction tubes

**OPERATIVE PROCEDURE**

1. With the patient shaved and in a supine position, the surgical approach is made through a coronal incision just back

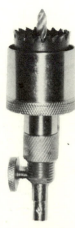

Fig. 11-39. Lobotomy trephine. (Courtesy K. Cramer Lewis, Department of Illustrations, Washington University School of Medicine, St. Louis, Mo.)

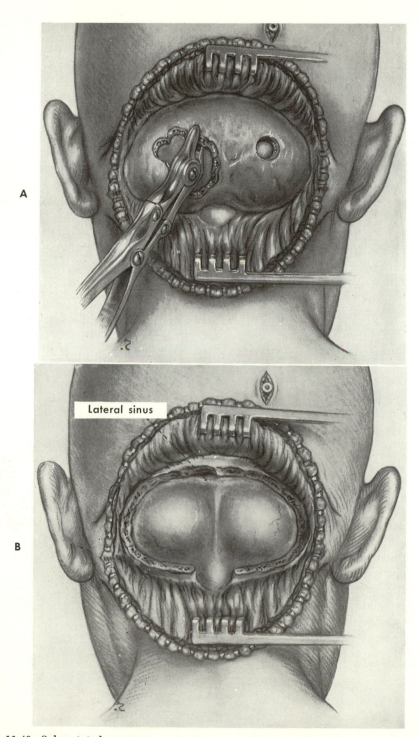

**Fig. 11-40.** Suboccipital craniotomy. **A,** Craniotomy being performed. **B,** Dura exposed. **C,** Dura incised and cerebellum exposed. (From Sachs, E.: Diagnosis and treatment of brain tumors and the care of the neurosurgical patient, ed. 2, St. Louis, The C. V. Mosby Co.)

of the hairline. This is carried down to the bone.

2. Michel clips are used for hemostasis on the skin edges. The periosteum is reflected using a periosteal elevator. Weitlaner self-retaining retractors are placed to maintain bony exposure.

3. A 1-inch trephine on a Hudson brace is used to remove a button of bone just in front of the coronal suture, just off the midline. The bone button is saved for replacement on completion of the procedure. (In the event of a future contralateral lobotomy, it is sometimes desirable to drill a hole on the other side using a D'Errico burr. A silicone button may be placed over this.)

4. Osseous bleeding is controlled in the usual manner; the dura is opened and retracted with no. 4-0 silk stay sutures.

5. The surface of the brain is coagulated and incised with a no. 11 blade at one point. A long ventricular needle is then passed vertically downward through the brain at this point until it reaches the orbital plate (floor of anterior fossa). If the tip of the ventricle is encountered, the needle is directed more anteriorly. The brain is then coagulated transversely and the surface incised, after which it is sectioned in a coronal plane following the needle tract. This is accomplished with the suction tip and exposure maintained by brain retractors placed over moist cotton strips. The brain is sectioned vertically in a transverse tract corresponding to the width of the trephine hole and extending down through the white matter until cortical gray matter overlying the orbital plate is reached.

6. Hemostasis and closure of the dura are as described previously.

7. Bone button is replaced and wedged into place with strips of gelatin, cotton, or sponge or other hemostatic material.

8. The periosteum is carefully closed.

9. The wound is closed and dressings applied in the usual manner.

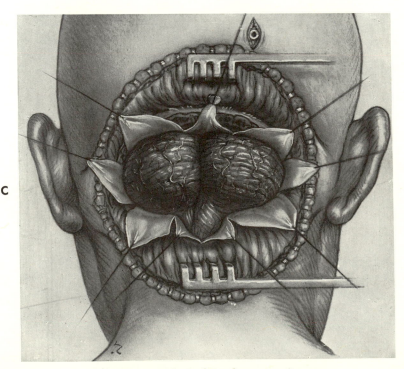

C

**Fig. 11-40, cont'd.** For legend see opposite page.

## Suboccipital craniectomy or posterior fossa exploration

**DEFINITION.** Perforation and removal of the posterior occipital bone and exposure of the foramen magnum and arch of the atlas with removal of the lesion in the posterior fossa (Fig. 11-40).

**CONSIDERATIONS.** Depending on the type and size of the lesion, the exposure may be unilateral or bilateral, and often the operation may include the removal of the arch of the atlas. The purpose is to treat lesions in the suboccipital region of the brain— in the fourth ventricle, in and about the cerebellum or about the brainstem and the cranial nerves.

**SETUP AND PREPARATION OF THE PATIENT.** The patient is anesthetized while lying flat and is subsequently positioned. The semi-sitting upright position is most often preferred for surgery of the posterior fossa. The lower extremities are wrapped with Ace bandages. In order to reduce venous bleeding and to assure a patent airway, the head must not be flexed forward too far. Correct flexion will avoid obstruction of venous drainage in the neck and kinking of the endotracheal airway. A three-prong headrest is used. If the prone position is preferred, either a padded horseshoe-shaped headrest or three-prong headrest is used. In the former case, care must be taken to avoid pressure on the eyes or malar eminences. In the prone position, pads are placed under the chest and shoulders in such a way as to assure adequate expansion of the chest during anesthesia. The supplies, instruments, equipment, and draping are as described for craniotomy. If the sitting position is used, an extra high instrument table and standing stool will be necessary for the nurse.

**OPERATIVE PROCEDURE**

1 to 7. As described for ventriculography (p. 351). Only a single burr hole is made. This is placed 3 cm. lateral to midline and 6 to 8 cm. above the external occipital protuberance, so that the lateral ventricle may be tapped during the procedure.

8. A 15 cm. silicone catheter with stylet or a Scott cannula (short, medium, or long) with stylet is inserted into the ventricle and secured to the skin with no. 2-0 silk on a large cutting needle.

9. Hemostasis is obtained, and the incision area is packed with a cotton strip and gauze sponges.

10. The site of the main incision is marked and injected in the usual manner. The incision may be made from mastoid tip to mastoid tip, in an arch curving upward 2 cm. above the external occipital protuberance.

11. Using either Michel or Raney clips, bleeding is controlled, and the skin flap is retracted with the Weitlaner retractors.

12. More commonly, steps 4 and 5 are done through a straight vertical incision made in or to one side of the midline. In this case, either clips or Halsted hemostatic forceps, held aside with umbilical tapes clamped to the drapes, are used to control skin bleeding. The skin edges are held apart with Weitlaner retractors.

13. Using a periosteal elevator to release the muscles and either 4-prong or vein retractors, the muscles are divided with the electrocautery set on cutting. As the incision is deepened, the angled Adson or the Beckman-Adson self-retaining retractor is used. The laminae of the first two or three cervical vertebrae are usually exposed in this process.

14. Several holes are drilled in the occipital bone using the preferred instrument. The Hall Neurairtome may also be used here. However, the blades break very easily in this area.

15. The dura is stripped from the bone using an aneurysm needle. Using either a double-action rongeur, Raney punch, Kerrison punch, or a Leksell rongeur, the hole is enlarged and the edges smoothed. A curette is often helpful in stripping the dura from the bone at the foramen magnum.

16. Osseous bleeding and cerebellar venous bleeding is controlled at each step by the usual methods: gelatin sponge, sponge, or, more often, bonewax and cautery. This

is essential because of the possibility of air embolism with the patient in the sitting position. (If air embolism occurs, the jugular vessels should be compressed immediately to increase venous pressure. The nurse should have large amounts of soaking wet cotton balls or sponges available to cover the exposed bone, dura, and brain. The headrest is immediately disconnected from the table, the table straightened, and the patient turned onto his left side.)

17. The bone edges are lined with moist cotton strips, and skin towels are placed. Usually the plug of the Scott cannula in the ventricle is released at this time. It must be closed before the dura of the pituitary fossa is opened.

18. The dura is opened. A small brain spoon or cotton strip is used to protect the brain as the initial nick is extended with scalpel or scissors in the same manner as during craniotomy. The dural incision is continued until the cerebellar hemispheres, the vermis, and the tonsils may be visualized. Weck Hemoclip or silver clips are used on the dura as necessary, and Olivecrona clips are used on larger vessels. Dural traction sutures are utilized as for craniotomy.

19. The cisterna magna is opened with forceps, emptied of spinal fluid, and protected with a cotton strip.

20. The cerebellar hemispheres are inspected and gently palpated. Bleeding is controlled with the electrocautery (coagulation), and a needle may be introduced through a small coagulated incision in the cerebellar hemisphere in an attempt to palpate or tap a deep lesion.

21. Brain retractors over cotton strips are placed for exposure. The handle of the retractor must be kept dry to avoid slippage in the surgeon's hand. However, the inserted edge should be wet to prevent damage or tears in the brain surface. These retractors are positioned in vital areas that may control respiration or other vital functions so that every effort must be made to avoid jarring these instruments in the operative field.

22. Using long bayonet forceps, bayonet cup forceps, nerve hooks, suction and the electrocautery loops, the lesion is removed. Olivecrona or other vascular clips may be used to aid in hemostasis. A nerve stimulator may be used to identify cranial nerves.

23. After the lesion has been removed and bleeding controlled, the posterior fossa craniectomy patient in the upright sitting position will require further checking for adequate hemostasis. This is usually accomplished by having the anesthetist press on the jugular veins in the neck.

24. The dura may be partially or completely closed in the usual manner. The muscle, fascia, and skin are closed as described for craniotomy. A check-rein dressing is applied.

25. The patient must remain anesthetized until the prongs of the headrest are removed. Particular attention must be given to the patient's head when removing these to prevent tearing the scalp or endangering the eyes. Band-aids are placed on the prong holes.

### Suboccipital craniectomy for acoustic neurinoma

CONSIDERATIONS. Usually the neurinoma arises from the vestibular portion of the eighth cranial nerve within the auditory meatus. Although it is not always possible, it is desirable to remove the complete tumor without damage to the facial nerve.

SETUP AND PREPARATION OF THE PATIENT. As described for the posterior fossa exploration operative procedure. A unilateral straight paramedian incision is used. The cerebellum is retracted gently upward with brain retractors protected with moist strips of cotton. The lower cranial nerves are defined with a nerve or aneurysm hook. A cotton strip is placed over these to protect them. Veins draining the tumor into the superior petrosal sinus are identified and either clipped or coagulated and cut. The tumor is excavated and resected, using methods similar to those utilized to remove a pituitary adenoma. A nerve stimulator

may be used to identify the facial nerve. Use of the operating microscope is advantageous because of the many nerves and vessels in this area. The high-speed drill (Hall II air drill) may be used to unroof the auditory canal and expose the remaining tumor. Constant irrigation is mandatory during drilling. More recently, very small tumors confined to the auditory canal have been approached by drilling directly through the temporal bone so as to open the auditory canal within the bone while avoiding the posterior fossa.

### Suboccipital craniectomy and trigeminal rhizotomy

**OPERATIVE PROCEDURE**

POSTERIOR FOSSA APPROACH

1. The patient lies prone or is in the sitting position. The incision is made vertically behind the mastoid process. A trephine opening or burr hole is made and enlarged with a rongeur. These steps are carried out as outlined under suboccipital craniectomy.

2. The dura is opened. The cisterna magna is pierced to empty the cerebrospinal fluid and permit backward retraction of the cerebellum. A brain spoon, brain spatula, or lighted retractor over moist strips of cotton gently lifts the cerebellar hemisphere. The eighth nerve is readily seen. The fifth is approached by opening the arachnoid of the cisterna pontis and sucking out the fluid. Veins are protected and bleeding controlled by pressure over cotton strips.

3. The nerve is elevated on a hook and carefully dissected. Some sensation in the face may be preserved by partial section or crushing rather than by complete section of the nerve. The motor root medial and anterior to the sensory root is preserved.

4. The wound is closed in the usual manner.

### Suboccipital craniectomy and glossopharyngeal nerve section

Posterior fossa exploration for glossopharyngeal neuralgia is occasionally neces-

sary. The same posterior fossa approach is used as is sometimes used for trigeminal neuralgia. The cerebellar hemisphere of the affected side is gently elevated upward and toward the midline. The ninth, tenth, and eleventh nerves are identified and defined with bayonet forceps, nerve hooks, and fine dissectors. The ninth nerve and a portion of the tenth are consecutively elevated with a nerve hook and divided with a fine-tipped scissors. Closure is accomplished in the standard fashion.

### Suboccipital craniectomy for Ménière's disease

**DEFINITION.** Complete or partial surgical section of the eighth cranial nerve.

**CONSIDERATIONS.** Ménière's disease is characterized by recurrent explosive attacks of vertigo associated with nausea, vomiting, tinnitus, and progressive deafness. It is usually unilateral. The etiology is obscure, and in intractable cases, surgical section or partial section of the eighth cranial nerve (acoustic) may be performed for relief. This operation is not commonly performed.

**SETUP AND PREPARATION OF THE PATIENT.** Same as for suboccipital craniectomy.

**OPERATIVE PROCEDURE**

1. The cerebellum is approached through a lateral vertical incision behind the ear. The cerebellum on the affected side is retracted. (See posterior fossa craniectomy.)

2. The eighth nerve is exposed with bayonet forceps and gentle manipulation. The nerve is freed from the arachnoid of the lateral cistern. It is separated from the underlying structures with a blunt nerve hook. Care is taken to avoid traction on the nearby seventh nerve (facial).

3. With a fine scissors the vestibular fibers in the anterior half of the nerve are divided over a nerve hook. If the patient has useful hearing, the posterior auditory branches are preserved. Tinnitus may be relieved by section of the anterior fibers of the auditory portion of the nerve.

4. The dura and wound are closed in the usual manner.

## Stereotaxic surgery

These procedures involve the placement of a probe capable of producing a therapeutic lesion at a precise location.

Lesions are produced in order to alleviate pain, abolish movement disorders, or change the endocrine balance of the body so as to favorably influence the course of patients with retinopathy, acromegaly, and endocrine-sensitive cancers. Since the probe must be accurately placed, the patient's head is placed in a special head holder, and the probe is introduced into the brain along one axis of the head holder. With the patient's head fixed in the holder and the path of the probe to the head chosen, x-ray films and fluoroscopy of the patient in the head holder are taken with the as yet unintroduced probe set in place, to check the axis along which the probe is to be introduced.

Stereotaxic procedures are also done in the spinal cord to achieve relief of pain (percutaneous cordotomy) and are used to place electrodes in various regions of the brain in order to determine the site of origin of seizure discharges. Such procedures are done in the radiology suite and are not discussed here.

Lesions are usually made with cold (cryosurgery) or with electrodes.

### Surgery of the globus pallidus, basal ganglia, and thalamus

DEFINITIONS. *Pallidotomy* is incision into the globus pallidus, usually made via electrocautery. *Chemopallidectomy* involves the introduction of a sclerosing solution via rigid catheter or cannula to produce a lesion. *Thalamotomy* is incision into the thalamus. *Chemothalamectomy* is the creation of a lesion in the region of the ventrolateral nucleus of the thalamus by means of a chemical solution such as alcohol with iophendylate.

PURPOSE. The surgical intervention is intended to interrupt the nerve pathways and alleviate the crippling locomotor symptoms of persistent, intractable tremor or rigidity associated with multiple sclerosis, severe brain trauma, Parkinson's disease, and various types of cerebellar degeneration. Operations of this type are also performed on the thalamus in an attempt to relieve pain.

SETUP AND PREPARATION OF THE PATIENT. Specially designed equipment is needed to facilitate precise locating of the nerve centers deep in the brain. Roentgenographic assistance is also required.

The patient must be conscious and cooperative to permit careful examination and observation of response to the procedure and the effects on the symptoms. Local anesthesia is employed. The patient may be in a supine or semisitting position.

Instruments are as for ventriculography, with electrocautery and suction, plus the following specified accessory instruments:

- 1 Basal ganglia guide or pallidotomy instrument
  Cannulae and catheters with balloons, as specified
  Radiopaque medium, as specified
- 1 Syringe, 10 ml., Luer control
- 1 Millimeter ruler
- 1 Caliper

OPERATIVE PROCEDURE

1. A short incision is made lateral and parallel to the midline at the top of the skull and crossing the coronal suture. A trephine opening or burr hole is made 14 cm. posterior to the nasion and 2.5 cm. lateral to the midline. The dura is cut and the arachnoid nicked to permit passage of the cannulae or needles. The position of the instruments is checked and regulated with x-ray assistance. It may be necessary to make ventriculograms, in addition to viewing the position of the cannulae or needles.

2. When the correct position has been achieved, tests or reversible lesions may be attempted. The patient's response is observed. Finally, the definitive lesion is created at the selected site by means of electrocautery or chemical solutions.

3. The dura and incision are closed in the routine manner.

## Cryosurgery

**DEFINITION.** Cryosurgery is the use of subfreezing temperatures to create a lesion in the treatment of disease. It is used in neurosurgery for transsphenoidal destruction of the pituitary in patients with acromegaly, diabetic retinopathy, and metastatic breast carcinoma. It can also be used for the destruction of the posterior portion of the thalamus for the treatment of Parkinson's disease or other involuntary movement disorders.

### Transsphenoidal cryosurgery of the pituitary

**CONSIDERATIONS.** This procedure is of special benefit to the patient suffering from metastatic carcinoma of the breast. These patients are more likely to respond if they have benefited from previous hormonal therapy or oophorectomy. In the patient with diabetic retinopathy, it is indicated when further laser beam coagulation of retinal lesions is considered useless. With acromegaly, if optic nerve or chiasm compression is present, a craniotomy is usually necessary.

All patients should undergo retrograde jugular venography to outline the cavernous sinuses and carotid arteries prior to surgery. The patients with tumors must also have pneumoencephalography with polytomography. The surgery is performed with fluoroscopic control with the patient under local anesthesia supplemented with neuroleptanalgesia. Transtracheal anesthesia is used prior to insertion of an endotracheal tube for maintenance of a patent airway during the procedure. The patient is instructed to answer questions with hand signals.

**ADVANTAGES**

1. Candidates in poor physical condition tolerate this procedure better than a craniotomy because it is less traumatic. Local rather than general anesthesia may be used.

2. Mortality and morbidity rates are low.

3. Complete destruction can be achieved with fair certainty in neoplastic glands and good certainty in normal glands.

**OPERATIVE PROCEDURE** (Figs. 11-41 and 11-42)

1. A local anesthetic (10% cocaine) administered with cotton applicators and 1% lidocaine injections through long needles are used to anesthetize the nasal and nasopharyngeal mucosa.

2. The head is placed in the stereotaxic head holder and fixed after injection of local anesthetic (1% lidocaine) with the skin at the points of fixation.

3. Preliminary x-ray films of the skull are taken to be sure that proper positioning has been achieved.

4. A guide is introduced, and a hole is drilled into the sphenoid sinus and the floor of the sella turcica via the nasal vault. The guide is positioned fluoroscopically.

5. A cryoprobe is introduced through the guide into the pituitary gland and its position confirmed with roentgenograms. The temperature of the probe is lowered to 180° to 190° C. for 12 to 15 minutes. The probe

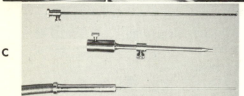

**Fig. 11-41. A,** Cryogenic unit. **B,** Stereotaxic head holder. **C,** Drill holder and cannula. (Courtesy Union Carbide Corp., Linde Division, New York, N. Y.)

can be used to feel the exact location of the dura surrounding the pituitary gland laterally and the diaphragm of the sella superiorly.

6. The probe may be introduced to several depths of penetration into the sella

and additional lesions made. Additional holes may be drilled for further lesions.

7. The probe is withdrawn, and the nasal vault is inspected for bleeding. It can be packed with nasal packing. Antibiotics can be instilled prior to packing.

FOLLOWING SURGERY. Patients are kept supine for 2 to 3 days and placed on a regimen of prophylactic antibiotics and cortisone replacement. Complications are meningitis secondary to a cerebrospinal fluid leakage, extraocular palsy, damage to the optic nerve, and injury to cranial vessels such as the carotid or cavernous sinus. These can be avoided by an accurate preoperative evaluation and precise probe placement during surgery.

### Cryothalamomectomy

DEFINITION. Destruction of the posterior aspect of the thalamus for treatment of pain or movement disorder.

CONSIDERATIONS. The following steps are necessary to obtain a good result: (1) placement of a probe with x-ray control; (2) localization of the lesion by clinical findings; and (3) gradual production of the lesion in a conscious, cooperative patient (so that the neurosurgeon can detect the point at which involuntary movements or pain perceptions are abolished, and avoid the undesirable neurological and psychological results of too large a lesion).

OPERATIVE PROCEDURE

1. The patient is placed on the operating table and the special head holder applied as in the cryohypophysectomy procedure. This is attached to the operating table.

2. After injection of local anesthetic, an incision is made with a no. 15 blade on a no. 3 handle at the level of the coronal suture.

3. Michel clips are placed on the skin edges and a Weitlaner or mastoid retractor placed for exposure.

4. A trephine opening in the skull is made with a special large burr.

5. The dura is opened, and stay sutures of no. 4-0 silk are placed for retraction. Hemostasis is obtained.

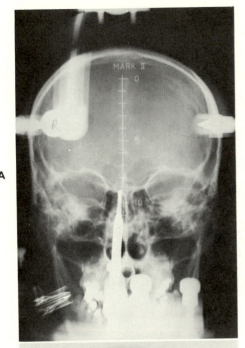

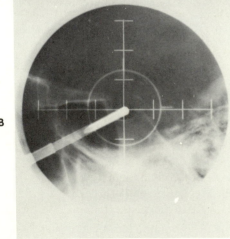

**Fig. 11-42.** Cryosurgery. Anterior, posterior, and lateral views of **A,** placement of drill, and **B,** insertion of cannula. (Courtesy William Coxe, Department of Neurological Surgery, Washington University School of Medicine, St. Louis, Mo.)

6. The cortex is coagulated with a bayonet forceps or dural elevator. It is incised with a no. 11 blade.

7. A Scott cannula is inserted into the frontal horn of the ipsilateral ventricle and air exchanged for cerebrospinal fluid. Radiopaque oil may be injected.

8. X-ray films are taken and compared with previous ones for positioning.

9. The basal ganglia guide is attached to the head holder. This guide permits adjustments of cannula position so as to direct it to the target area as well as to hold it firmly during the production of the lesion.

10. The cryosurgical cannula is fixed in the guide, and the tip is brought to the surface of the cerebral cortex. It is directed at the thalamus but is not inserted until its correct aim has been verified by x-ray film, with anterior-posterior and lateral projections (Fig. 11-42).

11. The cannula is advanced gently until its tip resides in the thalamus. Verification of placement by roentgenography is obtained. The flow of refrigerant is started, and the patient is checked regularly as the lesion is being produced.

12. Motor and sensory functions of the limbs, as well as tremor, rigidity, or ability to perceive painful stimuli, are evaluated by the neurosurgeon. Speech and consciousness are also checked.

13. After a satisfactory lesion is created, the flow of the refrigerant to the cannula is stopped. Cannula position is verified by final x-ray films.

14. The cannula is removed, and the incision is closed in the usual manner.

## Microsurgery as applied to neurosurgery

The use of the operating microscope in neurosurgery has helped to permit new procedures as well as to enhance old ones. Precise observation and manipulation of tissues are made possible by bright illumination and stereoscopic magnification. Specially constructed microscopes, microsurgical instruments, and microcoagulation units, as well as new techniques, are necessary. These new techniques have made

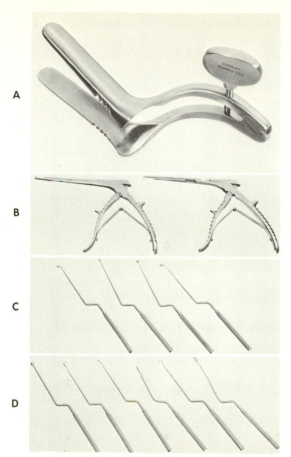

Fig. 11-43. Special instruments for transsphenoidal hypophysectomy. A, Hardy's modified Cushing bivalve speculum. B, Angell James punch forceps, extra small, upbiting and Angell James punch forceps, extra small, downbiting. C, Hardy modifications of Bronson-Ray curette. D, Left to right: Hardy's fork with bayonet handle, Hardy's enucleator (right), Hardy's dissector, angled knife handle, Hardy's enucleator (left), Hardy's modification of Cushing's malleable pituitary spoon. (Courtesy Down Bros. and Mayer & Phelps, Ltd., Toronto, Ontario, and Codman & Shurtleff, Inc., Randolph, Mass.)

possible procedures in previously inaccessible areas and permitted better accuracy in executing common procedures. The development of procedures for reconstruction and repair of small vessels and nerves without damage to the surrounding structures has been particularly enhanced by the use of the operating microscope.

Some of the equipment and instruments used in microsurgery are as follows (Fig. 11-43):

1. Electrically driven binocular surgical microscopes such as the Zeiss or the Twinscope are commonly employed. They must be draped with some type of sterile covering. A prepackaged sterile stockinette or plastic covering with side openings for observer arms or a large plastic bag secured with rubber bands can be used. Air inlet and outlet tubing with suction to provide constant fresh air under the drape is necessary so that the plastic bag will not be destroyed by the heat of the bulb.

2. Existing microsurgical instruments have been modified and adapted to the requirements of neurosurgery. These instruments often possess the following characteristics: bayonet shape so that the hand of the surgeon remains outside the line of vision and the beam of the microscope light, finely sprung and fluted grip, long length for access to deep basic structures, slender and delicate tips that take up as little space as possible (Fig. 11-43).

3. The vacuum rotary dissector may be used for tumor removal (Fig. 11-18).

4. A bipolar coagulator is essential for correct application of microsurgical techniques.

5. Very fine microsutures are available. The neurosurgeon should open the suture pack himself and ready the suture for use.

6. Fine drills such as the standard dental drill or the Kerr drill are used in conjunction with a House sucker-irrigator.

Some procedures in which microsurgery is of value are posterior fossa explorations (especially for tumors of the fourth ventricle or cerebellopontine angle), translabyrinthine and transpetrosal removal of small acoustic neurinomas with resulting preservation of the facial nerve, and transsphenoidal hypophysectomy and transsphenoidal operations for small intracranial tumors such as pituitary adenomas or even craniopharyngiomas. Transclival operations are also performed. Vascular surgery such as small vessel endarterectomy, cerebral arterial bypass graft, cerebral aneurysm surgery, and excision of A-V malformations may be carried out under the microscope. There are also advantages to microsurgery in the treatment of tumors and A-V malformations of the spinal cord.

### Transsphenoidal hypophysectomy

#### INDICATIONS

1. Endocrine pituitary disorders such as Cushing's syndrome, acromegaly, malignant exophthalmus, and hypopituitarism due to intrasellar tumors

2. Nonpituitary disorders such as advanced metastatic carcinoma of the breast and prostate, diabetic retinopathy, and uncontrollable severe diabetes

#### ADVANTAGES

1. Rapid access to the sella turcica

2. Complete extracapsular enucleation of the pituitary in cases of hypophysectomy and possible complete removal of small pituitary tumors, with the remaining normal portion of the gland left intact

3. Patient relatively pain free postoperatively

4. No visible postoperative scar

SETUP AND PREPARATION OF THE PATIENT. This procedure is performed with the patient under light general endotracheal anesthesia, with a local anesthetic injected for further anesthesia. The position used is semisitting, with the patient's head attached to the headrest and positioned in a portable image intensifier. The horizontal beam is centered on the sella turcica. A subnasal midline rhinoseptal approach is used.

#### OPERATIVE PROCEDURE

1. The face, mouth, and nasal cavity are prepped with an aqueous antiseptic solution (Zephiran). Infiltration of the nasal mucosa and the gingiva with 0.5% procaine containing 1:2000 epinephrine is helpful in initiating submucosal elevation, as well as diminishing oozing from the mucosa.

2. A sterile adhesive plastic drape is applied to the entire face with additional sterile drapes to assure a relatively sterile

operative field. Sterile sponges or cotton are placed in the patient's mouth so that only the upper gum margin is exposed.

3. Using a biopsy setup on a separate small Mayo table, a small piece of muscle is taken from the previously prepared thigh to be used later in the procedure. This is kept in a moist sponge.

4. The operating microscope is used for the cranial portion of the procedure.

5. Incision is made in the midupper gum margin. The soft tissues of the upper lip and nose are elevated from the bone with an elevator, and the nasal septum is exposed. The nasal mucosa is elevated from either side of the nasal septum, which is flanked by the blades of a Cushing bivalved speculum. The inferior third of the anterior cartilaginous septum and osseous vomer are resected, as is the floor of the sphenoid sinus. This exposes the sinus cavity. The floor of the sella turcica can be identified at this time.

6. The floor is opened with a sphenoid punch, and the dura is incised. (The hypophyseal cavity should not be opened.)

7. The extracapsular cleavage plane is identified, and the superior surface of the pituitary is dissected until the stalk and the diaphragmatic orifice are found. Cotton pledgets are applied for exposure, hemostasis, and protection of the structures.

8. The stalk is sectioned low with a "sickle" knife, and the lateral posterior and inferior surface of the pituitary is dissected with an enucleator.

9. The gland is removed in toto, and the sellar cavity is packed with muscle obtained previously. The floor is reconstructed using cartilage from the nasal septum.

10. Antibiotic powder may be used and a nasal packing introduced for 2 days. The gingiva incision is closed with catgut. In patients operated on for pituitary adenoma, the pituitary capsule is entered (step 3) and the gland searched for tumor. The latter is then defined and removed.

Some surgeons prefer to do this opera-

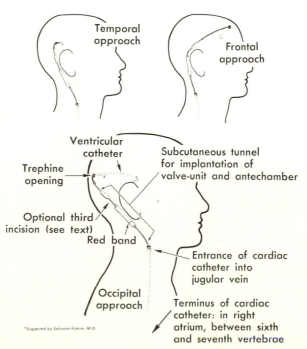

Fig. 11-44. Diagram of placement of a Hakim ventriculoatrial shunt. (Courtesy Cordis Corp., Miami, Fla.)

tion by means of a lateral rhinotomy with a transantral-transsphenoidal approach.

## Shunt operations (Figs. 11-44 to 11-47)

DEFINITION AND PURPOSE. These operations are designed to remedy obstruction of the noncommunicating type at the ventricular level in the circulation of the cerebrospinal fluid. They may also be used in cases of communicating hydrocephalus. Accumulation of fluid in the ventricles (hydrocephalus) causes dilatation and brain damage due to increased intracranial pressure. Bypass drainage via a catheter passed from the ventricles into the spinal canal or another body cavity or vessel is provided. Some of the available shunt devices include the Pudenz, Mischler-Pudenz, Ames, Holter, Hakim, and Denver valves. These devices are made of implantable materials for the continuous controlled drainage of cerebrospinal fluid from the ventricles to another body cavity or organ in cases of hydrocephalus. They are also occasionally used to obtain satisfactory drainage of chronic subdural hematomas in children. They are available in a variety of operating pressures.

Lumbar subarachnoid (thecal) shunts are also performed. These are usually subarachnoid-peritoneal shunts, but occasionally subarachnoid-ureteral shunts are done. Such shunting procedures are sometimes performed in cases of communicating hydrocephalus or pseudotumor cerebri. They are discussed in the section on laminectomy. Ventricular shunts are described here.

SETUP AND PREPARATION OF THE PATIENT. The position of the patient will vary, depending on the location of the shunt. For ventriculocisternostomy, the patient lies prone with his head in the cerebellar rest. For the ventriculoatrial shunt, the patient lies supine with his neck extended and padding under the shoulders. His head is rotated to one side, usually the left. An x-ray cassette holder is placed under the neck and chest so that roentgenograms can

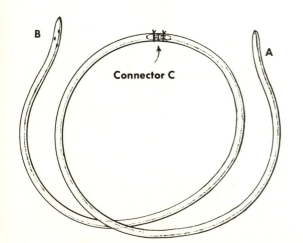
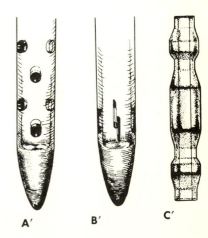

Fig. 11-45. Shunt is made from silicone tubing of special formula and consists of three component parts: A, cardiac tube with slit valve in side wall near the tip, B, ventricular tube with side perforations, and C, nylon connector. Materials used in shunt can be sterilized in autoclave. Slit valve is designed to allow cerebrospinal fluid to flow freely when pressure in tube exceeds 4 to 8 cm. of water. When intraventricular pressure falls below this level, valve slits remain closed and prevent escape of fluid. Prior to implanting it in patient, operation of valve should be checked by filling tube with sterile physiological saline solution and holding it in vertical position. If valve is functioning satisfactorily, top of fluid column should reach point 4 to 8 cm. above valve in 30 to 60 seconds. Although valve slits are coated with compound to prevent sticking, heat sterilization may increase adhesion. If this occurs, film may be broken by rolling valve end *gently* between thumb and index finger. (Courtesy Codman & Shurtleff, Inc., Randolph, Mass.)

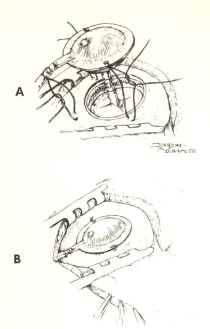

**Fig. 11-46.** Final step in attachment of ventricular and cardiac tube to flushing device is illustrated in **A** and **B.** Care should be taken not to puncture capsule while placing securing ligatures through holes in flange. These ligatures may be used to fasten flange to either skull or pericranium. Operation of flushing device should be checked before closing wounds. (From Neurosurgical News, 1963.)

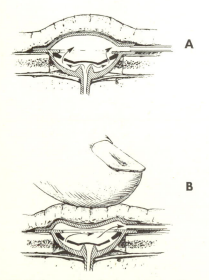

**Fig. 11-47.** Pudenz valve flushing device for ventricular shunts. **A,** Flanged silicone capsule and diaphragm valve shaped to fit into burr hole in skull. Pressure on capsule, **B,** closes ventricular inlet and flushes shunt tube. (Courtesy Codman & Shurtleff, Inc., Randolph, Mass.)

be obtained during the procedure. Preoperative films of the chest are used to determine the distance from the suprasternal notch to the middle of the right atrium. This is done to estimate the length of shunt tube that must be introduced into the jugular vein. Positioning for ventriculoperitoneal shunting is the same as for ventriculoatrial shunting, but no x-ray cassette is necessary. A much larger field, extending to the abdomen, must be prepared and draped. Instruments needed are the basic minor neurosurgical set. Rubbershod mosquito hemostatic forceps are also provided.

NURSING CONSIDERATIONS. Some precautions that must be taken during the valve implant procedures include the following:

1. Avoid the trapping of air in the valve assembly unit.

2. Remove storage fluid from about the valve, pump it out of the valve, and then replace with Ringer's solution.

3. Be extremely careful in handling the unit. Never place on gauze or linen so as to avoid lint or other foreign body. ALWAYS PLACE THE UNIT IN A BASIN.

4. Never use lubricants on the unit. The patient's body fluid adequately lubricates the device.

5. Be certain the valve is properly oriented. It permits only one-way passage of fluid.

6. The valve system must not be pumped too much immediately after surgery. This can cause too rapid a fluid loss, leading to a rapid decrease in ventricular size. This is poorly tolerated and may lead to subdural hemorrhage.

7. Check labeling of contrast medium to be sure it is appropriate for intravenous administration.

### Ventriculocisternostomy (Torkildsen procedure)

1. A burr hole is made on one side of the midline in the parieto-occipital region as discussed in the section on ventriculography.

2. A catheter is inserted into the lateral

ventricle through the burr hole, and some of the fluid under pressure is released. A specimen may be collected.

3. A midline suboccipital craniectomy is performed to expose the cisterna magna as discussed in the section on suboccipital craniectomy. The cistern is opened.

4. The end of the catheter is passed subcutaneously from the burr hole down to the craniectomy and down into the subarachnoid space of the cisterna magna. It is anchored to the dura with a no. 3-0 silk suture.

5. The incisions are closed in the usual fashion.

Alternatively, steps 3 and 4 may be replaced by a laminectomy of $L_2$ and $L_3$ with insertion of the distal catheter into the spinal subarachnoid space (see laminectomy discussion).

*Ventriculoperitoneal shunt*

1. A small, curved parieto-occipital incision is made down to the bone well behind and above the ear. Michel clips or mosquito forceps are used for hemostasis of the skin edges.

2. The periosteum is reflected with the skin flap, and either a D'Errico or Rickham burr is used for trephination.

3. A Kerrison cervical punch or narrow rongeur may be used to remove more bone inferiorly to make a channel for the correct seating of the valve if a Holter or Hakim valve is to be used.

4. Using a small hand drill with a very small point, holes are drilled on the bone edges for placement of the valve. A brain spatula is placed beneath the bone edge to protect the dura and brain as the hole is drilled. A large towel clamp is used to make the holes in the newborn.

5. No. 3-0 silk is passed through the holes for future anchoring of the valve assembly.

6. Using a bayonet forceps, the dura is coagulated and perforated. The underlying brain is also coagulated and then incised with a no. 11 blade.

7. A ventricular catheter with stylet is inserted into the ventricle until fluid returns. If a Holter or Hakim valve is to be used, a Rickham reservoir may be attached to the catheter and secured in place using no. 3-0 or 2-0 silk. If a Pudenz or Mischler-Pudenz valve is to be used, these are attached to the catheter.

8. Using a rubber-shod mosquito forceps, the ventricular catheter and whatever reservoir or valve has been attached at this stage is occluded to prevent air from entering the ventricle and cerebrospinal fluid from escaping too rapidly.

9. A small horizontal or vertical abdominal incision is made just below the liver edge (about 2 fingerbreadths below the lower costal margin). Exposure is maintained with a Weitlaner retractor.

10. The divided muscles are retracted with vein retractors. Individual fascial and muscle layers on each side of the incision may be marked with silk tagged with a different type of clamp for each layer.

11. The peritoneum is grasped with fine Adson forceps without teeth. With a no. 15 blade on a no. 3 handle, a very small opening is made into the peritoneum. No. 5-0 silk on an ophthalmic needle is used to place a purse-string suture about this. The catheter is inserted into the peritoneum and the purse-string suture drawn up snugly and tied.

12. A small incision is made in the neck (occasionally an intermediate incision over the chest wall is also necessary). A Rochester-Pean or a uterine dressing forceps is used to create a subcutaneous tunnel from the neck to the abdomen. The forceps is used to grasp the free end of the peritoneal catheter, which is then passed upward to the neck.

13. If a Holter or Hakim valve is to be used, the distal end of the valve is now tied to the free end of the peritoneal catheter with no. 3-0 or 2-0 silk. Be sure the valve is oriented in the proper direction, that it pumps fluid well (pressure characteristics may be checked utilizing a manometer filled with saline attached to the proximal end of the valve by a blunt needle and a

short length of shunt tubing), and that it is full of saline without air bubbles.

14. A subcutaneous tunnel is then created from the head incision down to the neck. An appropriate valve passer may be screwed into or onto the proximal end of the valve and grasped in the forceps used to create the tunnel. Alternatively, the proximal end of the valve or, in the case of the Pudenz and Mischler-Pudenz valve shunts, the free end of the catheter may be grasped with the forceps and brought up into the head incision.

15. The two ends of the system are then joined and tied together with no. 2-0 or 3-0 silk. If a Hakim or Holter valve is used, the valve is seated in the bony channel previously created and fixed into position with the silk tie running through the drill holes alongside the channel. If a Pudenz-type valve is used, the silk ties running through the drill holes about the burr hole are passed through the rim of the valve and tied.

16. All wounds are closed in layers.

### Ventriculoatrial shunt

CONSIDERATIONS. The neck incision and the insertion of the atrial catheter are performed first so as to utilize the time involved for the x-ray procedures.

OPERATIVE PROCEDURE

1. A small neck incision is made over the jugular vein, and mosquito forceps or Michel clips are used for hemostasis.

2. The neck tissues are incised down to the vessel and bleeding controlled by ligatures or coagulation.

3. Using a small Schnidt right-angled clamp, the selected vein (external jugular, facial, or internal jugular) is bluntly dissected, and no. 3-0 silk ties are looped about the proximal and distal ends. The proximal silk is tied.

4. Using a bayonet forceps or dural forceps without teeth, the vessel is incised with a no. 15 blade or a strabismus scissors.

5. The atrial catheter is threaded into the vein and clamped. The distal end should lie in the right atrium (at the level

of the sixth or seventh vertebra on the x-ray films). Contrast medium may be injected into the catheter to aid in the x-ray identification of the catheter and its placement. This may also be checked by electrocardiogram after the catheter has been filled with 3% saline and properly connected.

6. If necessary, the catheter is repositioned. After the catheter is properly positioned, it is tied into place in the vein with the distal suture and again occluded with a rubber-shod mosquito forceps to prevent air embolus.

7. The wound is covered, and the skull procedure is as described for ventriculoperitoneal shunt, steps 1 to 8 and 13 to 16. This portion of the procedure is begun while the x-ray films of the chest are being developed.

### Shunt revisions

If a valve procedure requires revision for nonfunctioning due to disengagement of tubing or obstruction, extra tubing is attached to various points in the assembly with a blunt no. 15 needle, and each part of the system is tested for patency and functioning. When the problem has been located, the appropriate portion of the assembly is replaced.

## Application of Crutchfield (skull traction) tongs

PURPOSE. To provide skeletal traction in the treatment of fractures or dislocations of the cervical spine.

SETUP AND PREPARATION OF THE PATIENT. Positioning the patient in slight cervical extension is of primary importance. The surgeon supervises the handling of the patient. The procedure can be carried out with the patient under local anesthesia. Instruments include a minor dissecting set, plus one scalpel handle no. 3 with blade no. 11, one Stille bone drill, one pair of Crutchfield skull traction tongs, and two Crutchfield drill points (Fig. 11-48).

OPERATIVE PROCEDURE

1. A wide strip of hair is shaved across the head from ear to ear and the skin dis-

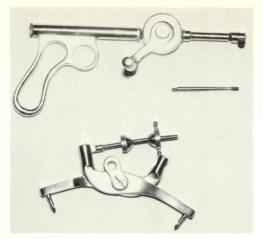

**Fig. 11-48.** Crutchfield hand drill, Crutchfield drill point, Crutchfield skull tongs, Raney-Crutchfield skull tongs. (Courtesy Codman & Shurtleff, Inc., Randolph, Mass.)

infected with antiseptic and draped with towels.

2. The placement sites are lightly marked on the scalp by pressing the tips of the almost completely open tongs on the skin. These points are infiltrated with procaine, and the scalp is nicked.

3. The outer table of the skull is perforated, using the Crutchfield drill points and the bone drill. The tongs are inserted and tightened. The skin wounds are dressed.

## Operations on the spine and its contents

DEFINITIONS. *Laminectomy* is the removal of one or more of the vertebral laminae to expose the spinal cord. Laminectomy, hemilaminectomy, and interlaminar approach are performed in order to reach the spinal cord and its adjacent structures for the purpose of treating lesions such as compression fracture, dislocation, herniated intervertebral disc (nucleus pulposus), and cord tumor. Section of the spinal nerves, cordotomy, and rhizotomy require similar surgical exposure. Laminectomy is also done when performing subarachnoid (thecal) shunts for hydrocephalus or pseudotumor cerebri.

*Cordotomy* is surgical division of the anterolateral tracts of the spinal cord for intractable pain.

*Rhizotomy* is interruption of the roots of the spinal nerves within the spinal canal. *Anterior rhizotomy* is division of the anterior or motor spinal nerve roots for the relief of spasm. *Posterior rhizotomy* is division of the posterior or sensory spinal nerve roots for the relief of intractable pain.

*Meningocele* is a hernial protrusion of the meninges through a defect in the skull or vertebral column.

### Laminectomy

SETUP AND PREPARATION OF THE PATIENT. The patient lies prone for spinal surgery. The face may be turned to the side or placed in the cerebellar headrest on the cerebellar extension (necessary for cervical laminectomy). Appropriate pads are placed under the shoulders and sides of the chest to ensure adequate chest expansion during anesthesia. These or additional pads are placed so as to avoid abdominal compression. For lumbar cases the table is flexed at the hips, and the patient's arms may be placed out in a relaxed position on padded arm boards. For thoracic and cervical procedures, the arms are kept straight down alongside the body. Alternatively, this procedure may be performed in the cervical region with the patient in the sitting position as for suboccipital craniectomy. Whatever the position, cervical patients with large discs, tumors, or spondylosis are usually positioned with the head in the neutral position, and extremes of flexion and extension are avoided during endotracheal intubation as well as positioning so as to avoid additional pressure on the spinal cord.

Laminectomy instruments (Fig. 11-49) include the basic major neurosurgical set and the following:

3 Scoville hemilaminectomy retractors
2 Basins with assorted blades and hooks (Scoville and Hibbs blades)
4 Beckman-Adson self-retaining laminectomy retractors, 12 in., 2 regular sharp, 2 large sharp

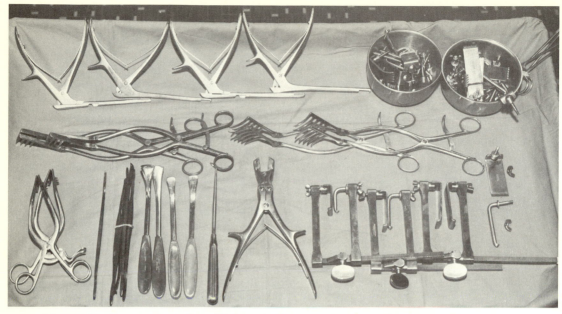

**Fig. 11-49.** Instruments to be added to the basic major neurosurgical set for laminectomy. Top: Spurling-Kerrison laminectomy rongeurs, Schlesinger cervical punches, basins with assorted retractor blades and hooks. Center: Beckman-Adson retractors, 2 regular and 2 large. Bottom: Adson self-retaining cerebellum retractors, copper nerve root retractors, Campbell angled periosteal elevators, angled curette, Horsley bone cutter, Scoville hemilaminectomy retractors with blades. (Courtesy K. Cramer Lewis, Department of Illustrations, Washington University School of Medicine, St. Louis, Mo.)

2 Adson self-retaining cerebellum retractors, angled
1 Large Horsley bone cutter, 10 ½ in.
2 Spurling-Kerrison laminectomy rongeurs, downbiting, 3 mm., 5 mm.
2 Schlesinger cervical punches, thin-lipped rongeur, 3 mm., 5 mm.
1 Bundle of assorted copper nerve root retractors
4 Campbell angled periosteal elevators, 2 wide, 2 narrow
1 Angled curette (size 1)
2 Diamond-jawed needle holders, 8 in.
1 Love nerve root retractor, angled 90-degree
Assorted bone curettes (sizes 3 through 4-0)
Additional Halsted hemostatic forceps

### Hemilaminectomy for herniated disc
(Fig. 11-50)

**OPERATIVE PROCEDURE**

1. The incision is marked and local anesthetic agent injected.

2. Draping is completed.

3. A midline vertical incision is made with a no. 20 blade on a no. 4 handle.

4. Straight Halsted hemostatic forceps are applied on the underside of the skin edge and everted for hemostasis. Deeper vessels are either ligated or coagulated.

5. Two Weitlaner retractors are inserted for exposure.

6. The fascia is incised next to the midline with either a heavy Mayo scissors or electrocautery current.

7. One side of the spinous processes is dissected out using the cutting cautery. Retraction is obtained with angled periosteal elevators.

8. The paraspinous muscles are then stripped off the laminae utilizing sharp subperiosteal dissection with periosteal elevators and cutting current dissection with the electrocautery.

9. As each area is cleaned off, a gauze sponge is packed around the bony structures with a periosteal elevator to aid in the bony exposure and to tamponade bleeding. The paraspinous muscles are dis-

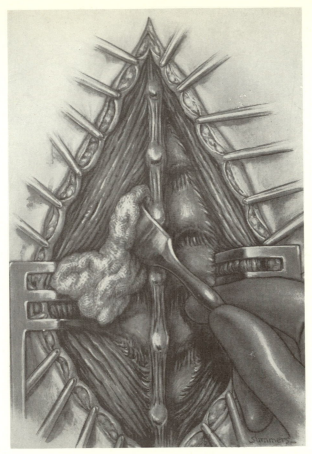

**Fig. 11-50.** Laminectomy. Exposing vertebrae by dissecting muscles away from spine. (From Sachs, E.: Diagnosis and treatment of brain tumors and the care of the neurosurgical patient, ed. 2, St. Louis, The C. V. Mosby Co.)

sected from all the laminae. In disc surgery this is only done on one side, the side of the lesion.

10. A laminectomy retractor is then placed in position. Either a Scoville (1 blade on tissue side and a slightly shorter hook on bone side) or Beckman-Adson retractor can be used.

11. Cotton strips are placed in the extremes of the field for hemostasis.

12. The edges of the laminae overlying the interspace with the herniated disc are defined with a curette. A partial hemilaminectomy of these laminal edges extending out into the lateral gutter of the spinal canal is performed with a Schwartz-Kerrison rongeur. The bone edges are waxed.

13. The flaval ligament is grasped with a vascular or a bayonet forceps with teeth, and a no. 15 blade on a no. 7 handle is used to incise it as close to midline as possible. Cotton strips are passed through this incision to protect the underlying dura, and a window is cut in the flaval ligament with a no. 15 blade on a no. 3 handle.

14. Additional ligament out in the lateral gutter of the spinal canal may be removed with a large curette or a Cloward punch after first protecting the dural sac and nerve root with a cotton strip (Fig. 11-51).

15. A dural elevator and a Love or copper nerve root retractor are used to retract the nerve root and dural sac so as to expose the disc space.

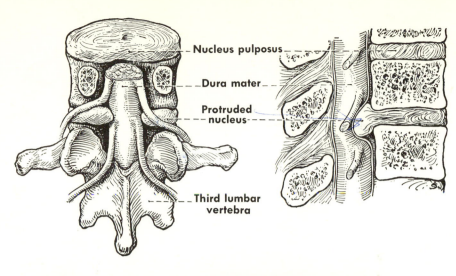

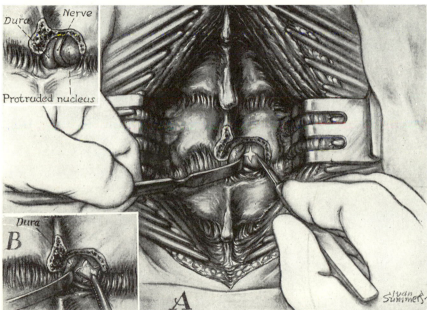

**Fig. 11-51.** Herniation of lumbar intervertebral disc. (From Sachs, E.: Diagnosis and treatment of brain tumors and the care of the neurosurgical patient, St. Louis, The C. V. Mosby Co.)

16. Troublesome epidural veins are controlled by packing with narrow cotton strips and if necessary by careful coagulation.

17. Any herniated fragment of disc is removed with a pituitary rongeur.

18. After coagulation of its surface, an opening is cut into the posterior aspect of the interspace with a no. 11 blade on a no. 7 handle.

19. Pituitary rongeurs, straight and angled, narrow and wide, are used to remove the disc material from the interspace. (The specimen is saved and weighed.)

20. Straight and angled curettes help to further clean out the interspace. Disc material so loosened is removed with the pituitary rongeurs.

21. The area is irrigated with warm

Ringer's solution and the interspace explored with a suction tip.

22. The nerve roots and extradural space are explored with a nerve hook.

23. If no further specimen is obtained, hemostasis is secured with cotton strips. Gelatin sponge or gauze or other hemostatic material is avoided if possible.

24. The cotton strips are removed from the epidural space, the table is unflexed, and the area is further irrigated. A change of position sometimes will cause more disc material to protrude, and the interspace is reexposed with a root retractor to rule out this possibility.

25. All cotton strips and retractors are removed and the wound closed with no. 2-0 silk on a Kelly no. 4 spring-eye needle for fascia, then no. 3-0 silk on Kelly no. 4 spring-eye needle for the subcutaneous tissue. Milliner or cutting needles with no. 4-0 silk are used to close the skin.

For cervical or thoracic discs, only the protruding fragment is removed and limited if any exploration of the interspace is performed. This is because attempts at adequate interspace exploration require retraction of the dural sac, which contains the spinal cord at these levels. Such retraction would result in cord injury and paralysis.

### Laminectomy for spinal cord tumors, spondylosis, etc.

1 to 9. As described for hemilaminectomy for herniated disc (p. 388), except that the fascial incision is made in the midline, both sides of the spinous processes are dissected out, and the paraspinous muscles taken down bilaterally, one side at a time.

10. One or more double-bladed Scoville or Beckman-Adson self-retaining retractors are placed to maintain the bony exposure.

11. A midline laminectomy is performed, with the spinous processes excised with a Horsley bone cutter. Various rongeurs ( Leksell, double-action, Cloward, etc.) are used to remove the laminae after defining their edges with a curette. The bone edges are waxed.

12. The remaining flaval ligament is removed with scissors, scalpel, and Kerrison or Cloward rongeurs. Epidural fat is coagulated and, if necessary, removed with dissecting scissors so that the dura is exposed fully.

13. Wide moist cotton strips are placed over the superficial soft tissues and muscle down to the bone bordering the exposed dura. This provides additional hemostasis.

14. The dura is elevated with a small hook and nicked with a no. 15 scalpel blade. A grooved director is inserted beneath the dura and the dural incision extended over it, using long forceps and fine scissors. Alternatively, the incision may be lengthened by pulling apart the two edges of the dural incision with bayonet forceps or by pushing at the ends of this incision with the edge of a dural elevator. Traction sutures of no. 4-0 silk on dura needles are placed in the dural edges, and the cord is exposed ( Fig. 11-52).

15. The cord is explored for the pathological area. Aspiration through a no. 22 needle on a plain-tipped syringe may be carried out. The tumor may be encountered extradurally or intradurally. Whenever possible, the tumor mass is dissected free and removed, using suction, dissecting scissors, the cutting electrocautery, forceps, cotton strips, small (pituitary) scoops, curettes, and pituitary rongeurs. Bleeding is controlled with moist cotton strips, silver clips, gelatin gauze, and gelatin sponge. Cautery is used very cautiously around the nerves and spinal cord. If desired, the spinal subarachnoid space is explored with a small rubber catheter to detect any blockage.

16. The wound is irrigated, using Ringer's solution, Asepto syringes, and suction.

17. Hemostasis is obtained; the dura is closed with no. 4-0 or 5-0 silk on an Ethicon TF or TF-4 needle.

18. The incision is checked for further bleeding and the paraspinous muscles approximated with no. 2-0 silk. The remainder of the wound is closed as in the previous

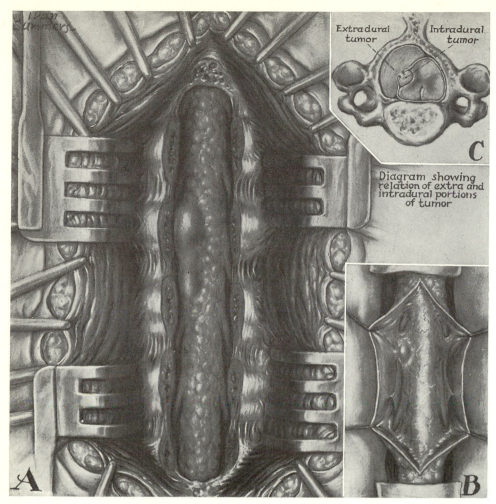

Fig. 11-52. A, Laminectomy completed showing dura and a tumor exposed. B, Dura has been incised and retracted showing spinal cord covered by pia arachnoid and portion of tumor area. C, Cross section of tumor area. (From Sachs, E.: Diagnosis and treatment of brain tumors and the care of the neurosurgical patient, ed. 2, St. Louis, The C. V. Mosby Co.)

procedure. In the case of extradural tumors, intradural exploration (step 14) is omitted.

### Laminectomy for meningocele

CONSIDERATIONS. Malformations such as meningoceles are usually congenital. They are a threat to the life of the newborn infant, since the defect may predispose to infection (meningitis) or to spinal cord damage. Defects of the cord and spinal nerves are often associated with the condition. There may also be spina bifida, a congenital defect resulting from incomplete closure of the vertebral canal.

Operation for repair of meningocele is directed at preserving intact the neural elements involved and at closing the cutaneous, muscular, and dural defects.

For surgery on infants, small hemostats, retractors, and other instruments are provided. Large bone-cutting instruments may be omitted. The small basic neurosurgical instrument set is needed, and the nerve stimulator may be needed.

### Cervical cordotomy (Schwartz technique, thoracic cordotomy, rhizotomy)

DEFINITION AND PURPOSE. Cervical cordotomy is the division of the spinothalamic tract for the treatment of intractable pain.

High cervical cordotomy is a most effective and frequently used procedure.

**SETUP AND PREPARATION OF THE PATIENT.** This procedure may be performed with the patient under general anesthesia, but in order to permit intraoperative testing of the level of analgesia achieved, local anesthesia (procaine or lidocaine) is preferred. An anesthetist should always be available. The nurse should keep an accurate account of the amount of local anesthetic agent used. In a very ill or apprehensive patient a drop in blood pressure or cardiac symptoms may develop if too much local anesthetic is injected.

The patient is placed in a prone position with his head slightly flexed to a level below the horizontal level of the cervical spine. It is essential to reassure the patient frequently and keep him as comfortable as possible.

**OPERATIVE PROCEDURE**

1. Using a 10 ml. control syringe with a 24-gauge 1-inch needle, the skin is infiltrated with the local anesthetic agent, the incision line is marked, and longer needles are used to block the second and third cervical nerves at their point of emergence from the spinal canal.

2. A midline incision is used, hemostatic forceps placed to control bleeding, and the Weitlaner retractor inserted for exposure.

3. Using the electrocautery (cutting current) with the spatula blade, the muscles are separated from one side of the arches and laminae of the first and second cervical vertebrae. An angled periosteal elevator may be used for further dissection. A gauze sponge may be packed into the wound to enhance the dissection as well as to aid hemostasis.

4. A Scoville hemilaminectomy retractor with short hook and longer blade is inserted between the midline structures and the reflected paraspinous muscles. The flexion of the head is increased when the retractor is inserted.

5. The Schwartz self-retaining retractor (modified Gelpi) is placed, with the multitoothed end in the occipital bone and the sharp point penetrating the spinous process of $C_2$ to widen the interlaminar space between $C_1$ and $C_2$ vertebrae. (For additional exposure it may be necessary to remove some of the laminae using a Kerrison rongeur.)

6. Large moist cotton strips are placed over the superficial tissues and muscle down to the bone bordering the exposed dura.

7. With the use of a dural hook, the dural incision is made with a no. 7 scalpel with a no. 15 blade. A vascular or Metzenbaum scissors is used to lengthen the incision.

8. Using no. 4-0 silk stay sutures on an ophthalmic needle, the dural edges are retracted and secured with curved mosquito or straight hemostatic forceps.

9. Using suction on cotton strips to remove spinal fluid, the dentate ligament is identified at its dural attachment with bayonet forceps and followed to the cord and left attached to prevent distortion of the cord.

10. A fine bayonet forceps (Gerald) is used to elevate the dentate attachment to provide visualization of the anterolateral quadrant of the cord and the anterior nerve rootlets.

11. The cord is incised with a slightly curved cordotomy knife (Fig. 11-53), 4.5 to 5 mm. in length.

12. After the incision is made, the patient is checked for adequacy of the level of analgesia. If the level is not satisfactory, the cord incision is deepened.

13. Hemostasis is obtained, the dural incision is closed, retractors are removed, and the wound is checked for bleeding and closed in the usual manner.

For *bilateral cordotomy,* the muscles are separated from both sides of the arches and laminae of the vertebrae. A double-bladed Scoville retractor is used, and the Schwartz retractor (modified Gelpi) is placed according to the side of the cord being approached. The cordotomy is performed on one side and then on the other. With bilateral high cervical cordotomy, falls in blood pressure and respiratory difficulty may occur.

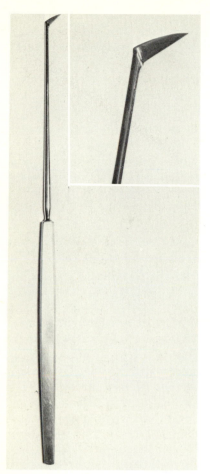

Fig. 11-53. Schwartz cordotomy knife. (Courtesy K. Cramer Lewis, Department of Illustrations, Washington University School of Medicine, St. Louis, Mo.)

*High thoracic cordotomy* is performed unilaterally or bilaterally in a similar manner, but a hemilaminectomy or total laminectomy at two levels must usually be performed in order to gain adequate exposure.

*Rhizotomy* is performed through a similar exposure with the appropriate nerve roots dissected free of any large radicular vessels, held up with a nerve hook, crushed with a hemostatic forceps, and divided with fine-tipped scissors. The roots may have a silver clip placed on their distal ends prior to division. This aids in hemostasis and permits subsequent radiological visualization of the extent and precise level of the root section.

### Subarachnoid peritoneal or ureteral shunt

**DEFINITION.** This operation provides a shunt for the cerebrospinal fluid from the lumbar subarachnoid space to the peritoneal cavity (or ureter) in cases of communicating hydrocephalus and pseudotumor cerebri. If ureteral anastomosis is done via polyethylene catheter or valve apparatus, the kidney is removed on the selected side (pp. 387 and 423) and a high lumbar laminectomy performed. Almost always, lumbar subarachnoid shunts are drained into the peritoneum, since the operation is simpler and does not require sacrifice of a kidney.

### Removal of anterior cervical disc with fusion (Cloward technique) (Fig. 11-54)

**PURPOSE.** To relieve pain in the neck, shoulder, and arm due to cervical spondylosis or herniated disc by removal of the disc with fusion of the vertebral bodies.

**SETUP AND PREPARATION OF THE PATIENT.** The patient is placed in the supine position, with his head turned very slightly to the left and his right hip well elevated for better exposure of the ilium. The skin preparation, draping, linens, and supplies are similar to those for laminectomy. The basic minor neurosurgical set with the following instruments added is used:

Cloward anterior fusion instruments (Fig. 11-54)
4 Cloward self-retaining retractors, 2 large and 2 small, with assorted blades (with and without teeth)
4 Sizes of drill guards, cervical drills, and dowel cutters
1 Cloward bone graft holder and impactor
1 Cloward bone graft impactor, double-ended
6 Cloward hand retractors
4 Cloward vertebral spreaders, 2 regular, 2 self-retaining
2 Deaver retractors, narrow
1 Rasp
1 Mallet
2 Adson cerebellum retractors, angled

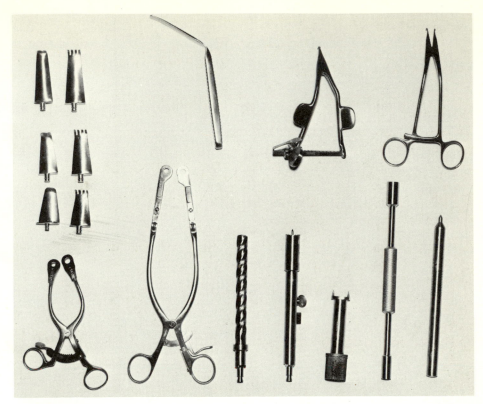

**Fig. 11-54.** Instruments for anterior cervical disc with fusion. Left to right: Cloward blade retractors, Cloward small cervical self-retaining retractor, Cloward large cervical self-retaining retractor, small Cloward hand retractor, Cloward cervical vertebral self-retaining spreader, Cloward cervical vertebral spreader, Cloward cervical drill, Cloward dowel cutter, Cloward guard guide, Cloward impactor, Cloward drill guard. (Courtesy Codman & Shurtleff, Inc., Randolph, Mass.)

Assorted spinal fusion curettes, straight and angulated, sizes 0 to 4-0
Meyerding finger retractors

**OPERATIVE PROCEDURE**

1. Drapes are sutured to the skin of the neck. Towel clamps are used over the hip.

2. A transverse skin incision is made on one side of the neck (usually the right) directly over the involved disc space; curved mosquito forceps or preferably Michel clips are placed on the skin edges for hemostasis.

3. A Weitlaner retractor is placed, and the platysma muscle is divided transvertically with Metzenbaum scissors and tissue forceps with teeth or with the cutting electrocautery.

4. The medial edge of the sternocleido-mastoid muscle is defined with the scissors by blunt and sharp dissection.

5. A vertical plane of dissection between the carotid sheath laterally and the trachea and esophagus medially is created by blunt finger dissection. This plane is held open with Cloward hand retractors, Meyerding finger retractors, or U. S. Army retractors.

6. The anterior surface of the spine is identified and the long muscles of the neck peeled off the anterior surface of the spine with periosteal elevators. Bleeders are coagulated with a dural elevator or bayonet forceps.

7. A short needle is inserted a short distance into the disc space and a lateral x-ray film taken to determine the level of the exposure.

8. While x-ray films are being developed, the neck incision is covered, an incision is made over the iliac crest, and straight hemostats are applied and retracted.

9. Soft tissue is dissected until the crest is reached, using Mayo scissors, tissue forceps, cutting electrocautery, and Richardson retractors for exposure.

10. A Hudson brace with the Cloward dowel cutter is used to remove the bone graft (care must be exercised to use dowel cutter, Cloward guide, and cervical drill guards matched for size). The dowel obtained should have cortex at both ends. The dowel hole is inspected and waxed if needed. The incision is packed with gauze sponge and covered.

11. The Cloward self-retaining retractors (2 long and 2 short) are inserted. The right blade should generally be slightly longer than the left. Care is used to protect the carotid artery and the esophagus. A combination of short and dull blades is used to acquire the best retraction. If a toothed blade is used, the teeth are carefully hooked beneath the long muscle of the neck.

12. A long knife no. 15 or 11 blade on no. 7 handle is used to cut into the disc space, and a fine pituitary rongeur is used to remove the disc material. (This is saved and weighed as a specimen.) A vertebral spreader is inserted in the vertebral space to widen the area, and further disc material is removed with the rongeur or small curettes (angled or straight, sizes no. 0 to 4-0) until the entire surfaces of both vertebrae are clean. A Hall II air drill with a small burr may also be used.

13. The Cloward bone guide is inserted into disc space to measure its depth.

14. After the drill guard is adjusted so that the drill can protrude no farther than the measured depth of the interspace, the cervical drill guard is inserted about the disc space. This is done with the aid of a mallet until the points catch the vertebral bodies above and below the interspace.

15. After the guard is in place, the vertebral spreader is removed or spread to a more limited degree.

16. The Cloward drill on a Hudson brace is inserted into the guard and the hole drilled. (The bone dust on the drill point is inspected and saved in a medicine glass.) Cotton strips or gelatin sponge is used for active bleeders. Bone wax should not be used on the walls of the disc hole. Thrombin-soaked cotton pledgets may help control troublesome bleeding.

17. The bottom of the hole is checked for further disc or cartilaginous material, which is removed. The guide may be removed and replaced, and drilling may be done several times until the desired depth is reached. The drill and guide are then removed.

18. Further bone is removed by use of the Cloward cervical punch or curettes until complete anterior decompression of the nerve root or dural sac is obtained. Nerve hooks may be used here for demonstration of adequate dissection. The Hall II air drill may also be of help.

19. The depth of the hole is measured and compared to the dowel. The dowel may be trimmed using a drill, rongeur, or rasp. The shaped dowel attached to the impactor is inserted into the hole and tapped into place. The double-edged impactor is used to drive the dowel in deeper if necessary. The spreader is removed, and bone dust may be applied.

20. Hemostasis is obtained and the wound irrigated; the vertebral spreader and retractors are removed and both incisions closed.

Alternatively, no dowel hole is made, and steps 13 to 16 are omitted. In this case, a wedge of bone rather than a dowel is removed from the iliac crest and inserted into the disc space after all disc material and bony spurs have been removed (Smith-Robinson approach). It is also possible to perform this latter procedure without placement of a bone graft.

## Carotid surgery of the neck
### *Carotid endarterectomy*

DEFINITION. Removal of occlusion of the internal carotid artery (in its extracranial part).

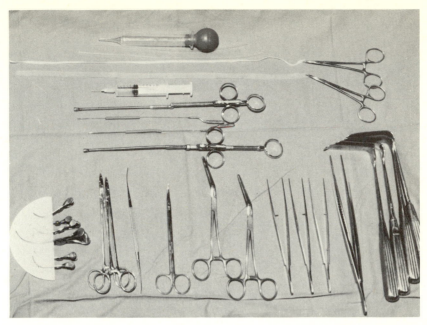

**Fig. 11-55.** Carotid endarterectomy instruments. Top: Asepto syringe, shunt material, umbilical tape on a curved mosquito hemostat, piece of rubber drain on a curved mosquito hemostat, 10 ml. syringe, Roper-Rumel tourniquets, and stylets. Bottom: Potts bulldog clamps, burlishers, dural elevator, DeBakey clamps, DeBakey forceps (very small tips), DeBakey forceps (regular), Meyerding finger retractors.

**SETUP AND PREPARATION OF THE PATIENT.** Instruments used are the basic minor neurosurgical set. Additional instruments needed are as follows (Fig. 11-55):

DeBakey arterial clamps
DeBakey arterial forceps, 10 in.
Potts bulldog clamps
Roper-Rumel tourniquet with stylet guide
Fogarty catheters (4-5-6)

**OPERATIVE PROCEDURE**

1. Using a no. 15 blade on a no. 3 scalpel, a 6 to 7 cm. skin incision is made along the anterior margin of the sternocleidomastoid muscle at the level of the thyroid cartilage.

2. Mosquito hemostatic forceps or Michel clips are used for hemostasis on the skin edges, and the Weitlaner self-retaining retractor is inserted for exposure.

3. Using the Metzenbaum scissors, the soft tissue is dissected for exposure of the carotid artery and its bifurcation.

4. Blunt dissection, using vascular tissue forceps and a small, right-angled Schnidt tonsil clamp, is used to dissect and free the carotid artery, including the bifurcated portion. A small Penrose tubing or a small moistened umbilical tape is passed around the vessel for ease of handling. A no. 2-0 silk suture is doubly looped around the superior thyroid artery and clamped at its end.

5. The internal and external carotid artery are dissected 3 to 4 cm. farther in the cranial direction.

6. The external carotid artery is clamped with a DeBakey clamp or looped with the Roper-Rumel tourniquet using small Penrose tubing or a small red rubber catheter. The common carotid artery is occluded below the bifurcation with a DeBakey clamp, and the internal carotid artery is either clamped or occluded with the use of the Roper-Rumel tourniquet.

7. Heparin solution is injected proximal and distal to the occluding clamps on the common, internal, and external carotid arteries.

8. With DeBakey tissue forceps and a no. 15 blade on a no. 3 scalpel, the arteriotomy is made over the stenotic area. The incision is lengthened with Potts angulated

scissors in order to expose the full extent of the occluding plaque.

9. Using the dural elevator, the plaque or plaques are dissected free from the arterial wall. Heparin solution is used as an irrigant to clean the intima, thereby preventing thrombosis formation. A Fogarty catheter may be used for further exploration of the artery.

10. Arteriotomy is closed with no. 5-0 or 6-0 cardiovascular suture. Before complete closure, the blood flow is restored through the artery to wash away any free plaques, air, or thrombus. To do this, the occluding clamps are opened and tightened individually: first the external, then the internal, and last the common carotid clamps. The closure of the arteriotomy is completed.

11. The occluding clamps are removed from the external and common carotid arteries, permitting blood flow through the carotid tree, and then the internal carotid clamp is removed. The suture on the superior thyroid is cut and removed.

12. Gentle pressure is applied to the suture line and the area inspected for leakage. Additional interrupted sutures may be needed to control the leakage.

13. The wound closure is accomplished in the usual manner, using no. 3-0 or 4-0 silk sutures, and dressings are applied.

### Carotid endarterectomy with temporary bypass

**OPERATIVE PROCEDURE**

1 to 8. As described for endarterectomy.

9. A piece of tubing (polyethylene, Silastic, or rubber) with a suture tied about its center is passed from the common carotid artery upward into the internal carotid artery and held in place inside the vessel with a Roper-Rumel tourniquet or Javid ring clamps at points beyond the arteriotomy. The occluding clamps are then removed from the common and internal carotid arteries.

10. The plaque is removed as described for endarterectomy.

11. After all sutures for arteriotomy clos-

ure have been placed but before the last sutures have been tied, the ring clamp or tourniquet on the internal carotid artery is released and retightened. The clamp occluding the external carotid is released. The ring clamp or tourniquet holding the shunt in place in the common carotid artery is then released, followed by the clamp or tourniquet on the internal carotid artery. At each step, blood flow through the arteriotomy is permitted to wash out any small pieces of clot or plaque remaining.

12. The shunt tubing is then quickly removed by pulling on the suture tied about its midportion. During this maneuver, gentle tension is exerted on the untied arteriotomy sutures to prevent excessive blood loss. After shunt removal, the sutures are tied individually.

13. The wound is closed as described for arteriotomy.

### Carotid endarterectomy with graft

In some cases a graft (synthetic or venous) is sutured in place to widen the artery and prevent stenosis caused by scarring. It is sutured in the usual manner for vascular surgery (Chapter 15).

### Carotid artery ligation

**DEFINITION.** Occlusion of the internal carotid artery.

**CONSIDERATIONS.** This procedure may be done to control anticipated hemorrhage during intracranial surgery for vascular anomalies. A permanent occlusion may be necessary for the control of intracranial hemorrhage or small, repeated strokes from an intracranial lesion that is not amenable to direct attack. Special clamps such as the Selverstone (Fig. 11-56) and the Crutchfield carotid artery clamps are available for gradual occlusion of the artery (Fig. 11-57). Occlusion may protect the patient from debilitating or fatal intracranial hemorrhage from aneurysm and may be used to treat carotid-cavernous fistula.

**SETUP AND PREPARATION OF THE PATIENT.**

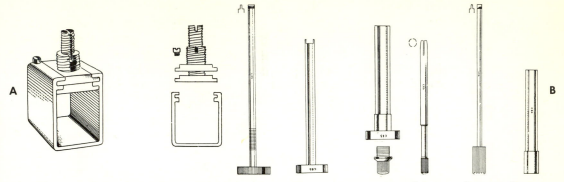

Fig. 11-56. **A,** Selverstone carotid artery clamp. **B,** Selverstone carotid artery clamp tools. (Courtesy Codman & Shurtleff, Inc., Randolph, Mass.)

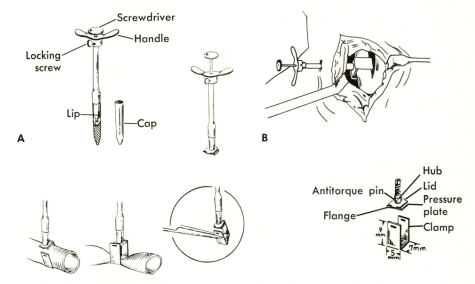

Fig. 11-57. Crutchfield clamp. **A,** Control assembly. **B,** Clamp assembly. (Courtesy Codman & Shurtleff, Inc., Randolph, Mass.)

Only the basic minor neurological instrument set is used.

**OPERATIVE PROCEDURE**

1. The skin is incised with a scalpel.

2. Mosquito forceps are used for hemostasis, and a mastoid or Weitlaner retractor is inserted for exposure.

3. The carotid artery is freed by blunt dissection using Metzenbaum scissors and a small right-angled Schnidt tonsil forceps. A small Penrose tubing or umbilical tape is passed around the vessel for retraction.

   a. For temporary control of the carotid artery (during procedures for very large aneurysms or A-V anom-

alies): the vessel is looped about with an umbilical tape and fixed, using the Roper-Rumel tourniquet in such a manner that occlusion can be accomplished immediately if necessary.

   b. For permanent occlusion: two heavy silk ligatures are used, and the artery may be divided between ligatures. Transfixing suture ligatures may be used as well if the artery is divided.

   c. For gradual occlusion:

     (1) A Crutchfield or other clamp is placed in position around

the artery (Figs. 11-56 and 11-57).

(2) Using a no. 3 scalpel with a no. 11 blade, a small stab wound is made adjacent to the incision (Fig. 11-57).

(3) The control assembly with cap is passed through the stab wound. By loosening the locking screw and pressing down on the screwdriver, the cap is removed (Fig. 11-57).

(4) The control assembly is snapped on the lid of the clamp, and with a Rochester-Pean hemostatic forceps holding the clamp, each flange is gently forced into position (Fig. 11-57).

(5) Using the dot on the screwdriver as an indicator, the number of turns for complete occlusion is noted. The clamp is then unscrewed a measured number of turns, and the screwdriver is locked.

4. The incision is closed in the usual manner, and a dressing is applied.

### Carotid surgery for carotid-cavernous fistula

In cases of carotid-cavernous fistula, ligation of the common (or internal) carotid artery may be performed. However, many surgeons will attempt to embolize the fistula with muscle or other material. When this is done, the segment of external carotid artery just distal to the carotid bifurcation may be isolated with clamps, incised, and used as a point of entry for the muscle embolus. This piece of muscle is labeled with a metal clip and attached to a length of silk so that it can be visualized by roentgenograms and withdrawn if necessary. It is introduced into the internal carotid artery through the arteriotomy in the external carotid artery after clamps have been placed on the internal and common carotid arteries and after the proximal external carotid artery clamp is removed. The internal and then common

carotid artery clamps are released as the clamp is removed. The proximal external carotid artery clamp is reapplied, leaving a small proximal opening in the arteriotomy unclamped for the suture on the embolus. The blood flow in the common internal carotid artery system then pushes the embolus up to the fistula. Alternatively, an appropriately controlled internal carotid artery may be embolized by forcing the muscle plug up into the area of the fistula with saline injected through polyethylene tubing. In either case, internal carotid ligation is usually done after satisfactory placement of the embolus. In some cases a frontotemporal craniotomy is also performed and the internal carotid artery clipped intracranially as well.

### Sympathectomy

DEFINITION. The excision of a portion of the sympathetic division of the autonomic nervous system. Most sympathectomies are performed on the paravertebral chain and are named for the region resected; for example, cervical, thoracolumbar, and lumbar. The periarterial sympathectomy, vagotomy, and presacral neurectomy are other procedures that are occasionally applied to the autonomic system.

PURPOSES. The diseases for which sympathectomy is beneficial have been suggested previously in the section on the autonomic nervous system and its function. The principal diseases requiring surgery are vascular disorders of the extremities and intractable pain from certain nerve injuries or chronic abdominal conditions.

SETUP AND PREPARATION OF THE PATIENT. The selected position of the patient on the operating table will depend on the type of procedure to be performed (Chapter 7). Skin preparation for various procedures is described in Chapter 4, and draping procedure is discussed in Chapter 5. The basic neurosurgical and laminectomy instruments will be used, plus the following:

*For retropleural and transthoracic approaches,* add Doyen rib raspatories, rib cutters, and rongeurs (Fig. 11-58).

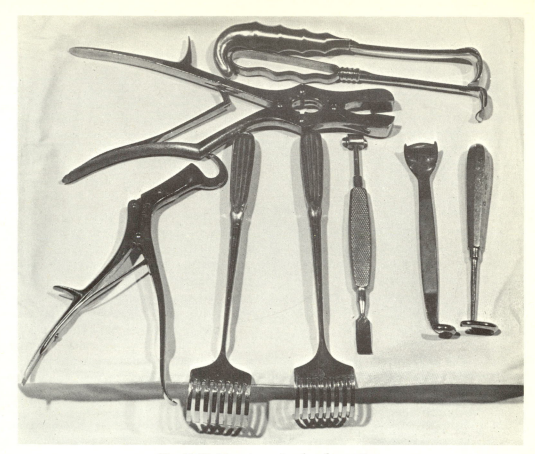

**Fig. 11-58.** Mayo tray setup for rib resection.

*Top*
Richardson retractors
Sauerbruch rib rongeur

*Bottom* (left to right)
Stille rib shears
Broad, blunt rake retractors
Lempert-Berry rib raspatory
Doyen rib raspatories

*For thoracic and lumbar approaches,* add the following:

2 Volkmann rakes, large, 8-pronged, blunt
3 Malleable copper retractors
2 Richardson retractors, large
2 Retractors, elephant-deep, right-angled
2 Deaver retractors
Retractors, self-retaining, if desired
 Thoracic approach: Beckman or Scoville laminectomy
 Lumbar approach: Beckman for posterior approach
 Abdominal approach: Balfour

### Cervicothoracic sympathectomy (dorsal)

**DEFINITION.** Removal of the cervicothoracic chain, often from the middle cervical to the third thoracic ganglion.

**PURPOSE.** Sympathetic denervation of the upper extremities and heart may be accomplished by this procedure. The vasospastic phenomenon of Raynaud's disease is relieved by this procedure, and, in addition, it may be beneficial in relieving intractable angina pectoris.

**SETUP AND PREPARATION OF THE PATIENT.** For the anterior approach, use basic neurosurgical instrument set, laminectomy set, and rib instruments (Fig. 11-58), adding deep retractors and stimulator. The setup for the posterior approach is as for anterior approach, adding rib-cutting instruments, periosteal elevators, small rib retractors, firm rubber pad, and operating table attachments for posterolateral position.

**OPERATIVE PROCEDURE**

**ANTERIOR APPROACH**

1. The patient is placed in a supine position and his head rotated to the opposite side as in mastoidectomy (Chapter 7). General endotracheal anesthesia is necessary, since there is always a possibility of puncturing the pleura.

2. A transverse incision is made one fingerbreadth above the clavicle; the clavicular head of the sternocleidomastoid muscle is severed; the deep cervical fascia is divided.

3. The phrenic nerve and the jugular vein are protected, and the anterior scalene muscle is divided to expose the underlying subclavian artery. This vessel is isolated, and the thyroid axis, which is one of its branches, is ligated and divided.

4. The stellate ganglion lying deep against the vertebral body is then brought into view, and it is lifted on a nerve hook. The sympathetic chain is traced upward to the middle cervical ganglion and divided. Deep dissection behind the pleura allows exposure of the upper thoracic ganglia, which are removed to below the third thoracic. Silver or other clips may be placed on the sympathetic nerves prior to their division.

5. The wound is closed with silk sutures and without drainage.

**POSTERIOR APPROACH (DORSAL SYMPATHECTOMY)**

1. The paravertebral incision is centered over the third rib. The trapezius muscle is divided and the rhomboid split in line with its fibers. The third and fourth ribs are isolated extrapleurally, and the posterior 4 or 5 cm. are resected. The transverse processes may be removed, using a rongeur to provide for better exposure.

2. The sympathetic trunk, which lies on the anterolateral aspect of the vertebral body, is reached by carefully reflecting the pleura. The trunk is picked up on a nerve hook, traced up and down, and removed, usually from the stellate ganglion to the fourth thoracic. Clips may be used.

3. A firm rubber tube may be left in the wound during closure. Suctioning apparatus is applied to this tube as the last deep fascial suture is drawn tight; all air is aspirated and the tube quickly withdrawn.

4. The subcutaneous tissue and skin edges are closed.

### Thoracolumbar sympathectomy and splanchnicectomy

**DEFINITION.** Through a paravertebral incision the greater splanchnic nerve is dissected, and lower sympathetics from the diaphragm down to the third lumbar are removed.

**PURPOSES.** This extensive procedure, which denervates the majority of the viscera, reduces vascular tone over such a large area that the blood pressure is markedly reduced. It has proved successful in the treatment of essential hypertension; however, medical treatment is almost invariably used to treat this disease today. A more limited resection is used occasionally to interrupt the visceral pain pathways from the upper abdomen and to relieve the intractable pain involving the biliary tract.

**CONSIDERATIONS.** The patient may be placed in a prone position, with his face resting in the cerebellum headrest and his shoulders slightly elevated, or he may be placed in a lateral decubitus position.

**SETUP AND PREPARATION OF THE PATIENT.** Instruments as described previously for the selected approach. The operation is carried out bilaterally, usually in two stages, 10 days apart. A retropleural or retroperitoneal approach is generally employed, although a transpleural or transdiaphragmatic exposure is preferred by some surgeons. The classic Smithwick procedure will be described.

**OPERATIVE PROCEDURE**

1. A paravertebral incision is made downward from the ninth rib and curved anteriorly toward the iliac crest.

2. The latissimus dorsi muscle is divided in line with the skin incision, and the sacrospinal muscle is retracted medially to ex-

pose the eleventh and twelfth ribs. These two ribs are resected subperiosteally, leaving the intercostal neurovascular bundle intact.

3. The pleura is gently stripped off both the inner chest wall and the diaphragm by blunt dissection. The renal fascia is incised, and the retroperitoneal space is opened and enlarged to expose the undersurface of the diaphragm. The latter structure is divided down to its attachment to the vertebral bodies.

4. The greater splanchnic nerve is dissected out with a staphylorrhaphy elevator at the level where it pierces the diaphragm. The nerve is divided as it enters the celiac plexus. It is then traced upward to the ninth rib and avulsed.

5. The sympathetic chain is similarly dissected out and traced upward, clipping each ramus in turn with silver clips; then the communicating rami are divided. Attention is directed to removing the lower sympathetics from the diaphragm down to the third lumbar.

6. When all bleeding has been controlled, a large, firm rubber tube is placed in the retropleural space, and the wound is closed. A purse-string suture, which is placed around the exit of the tube, is tightened. Suction apparatus is applied to the tube to remove any remaining air in the retropleural space, and the tube is rapidly removed as the purse-string suture is tied down.

7. If the pleura has been opened during the operation, an indwelling chest tube may be inserted into the chest cavity and connected to an underwater-seal drainage set.

### Lumbar sympathectomy

**DEFINITION.** The denervation of the lower extremities.

**PURPOSE.** Lumbar sympathectomy is useful in treating such vasospastic disorders as Buerger's disease and some selected cases of vascular insufficiency secondary to peripheral arteriosclerosis. It may also be of benefit in combating excessive sweating of the feet.

**SETUP AND PREPARATION OF THE PATIENT.** Same as in thoracolumbar sympathectomy, except that rib-cutting instruments are not required. The patient may be placed in a supine position if an anterior approach is to be used or in a lateral position for a posterolateral incision.

**OPERATIVE PROCEDURE** (Fig. 11-59)

1. Lumbar sympathectomy may be done transperitoneally or retroperitoneally, but the latter is more commonly used. A long McBurney-type incision or a straight or curved paramedian incision is employed.

2. The muscles are split in line with their fibers, or portions are divided to expose the retroperitoneal space.

3. The sympathetic chain is picked up on a long nerve hook and resected from above the second to below the third lumbar ganglion, clipping the rami as in a thoracolumbar sympathectomy. Deep retractors usually are necessary for adequate exposure; care is taken not to tear the lumbar veins that lie over the nerves.

4. The wound is closed in layers and dressed as for hernial repair.

### Surgery of peripheral nerves

**DEFINITION.** Suturing the divided nerve in precise approximation without tension.

**CONSIDERATIONS.** Peripheral nerve injuries are the commonest indication for surgery of these structures. Nerve tumors are rare in comparison. During wartime, injuries of nerves assume particular importance because of their frequency and disabling results.

When the continuity of a nerve is destroyed, function distal to the site of injury is lost. Recovery will occur only if regeneration of nerve axons takes place from the healthy proximal segments. These axons must grow down the axis cylinders of the nerve beyond the injury if they are to reinnervate their end organs and allow function to return (Fig. 11-60).

When a nerve is divided, the cut ends retract, become scarred, and form neuromas. Regenerating axons from the proximal segment cannot bridge such a gap or

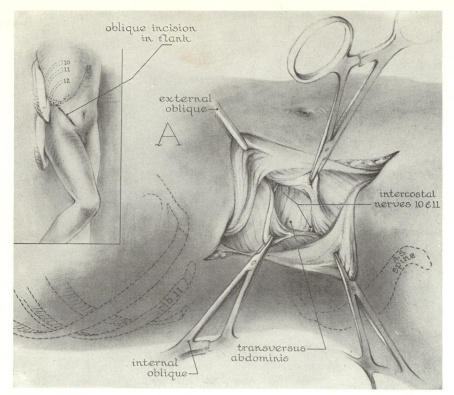

**Fig. 11-59.** Lumbar sympathectomy. (From Moseley, H. F., editor: Textbook of surgery, ed. 3, St. Louis, 1959, The C. V. Mosby Co.)

penetrate the scar tissue. An unobstructed path down the axis cylinder must be made available to them if they are ever again to move muscles or transmit sensation. All procedures are directed toward obtaining the best possible conditions for regeneration to occur.

**SETUP AND PREPARATION OF THE PATIENT.** Basic minor neurosurgical set, including the following:

Nerve stimulator
Nerve forceps (jewelers')
Special nerve sutures (no. 5-0 to 8-0 silk or polyester swaged on)
Tongue blades
Sterile razor blades

For lesser procedures such as spinofacial anastomosis in the neck, division of the volar carpal ligament for median nerve compression at the wrist, or repair of a small digital nerve, suitable modification may be made.

The positioning, skin preparation, and draping of the patient depend on the site of the injury. A large area is prepared.

General anesthesia is usually preferred, with the patient positioned for maximum accessibility to the injured nerve. Exposure must be adequate, since considerable mobilization of the nerve is often necessary. A dry field may be achieved by using a tourniquet on the extremities. This is usually unnecessary.

### Nerve anastomosis

**OPERATIVE PROCEDURE**

1. The site of injury is explored with careful attention to hemostasis. Nerve ends are dissected out from surrounding scar tissue, and neuromas are excised. Moist umbilical tapes or Penrose tubing may be passed about the nerve in order to handle it more easily and with less trauma.

2. The nerve repair (anastomosis) is made with multiple fine sutures placed only through the nerve sheath or epi-

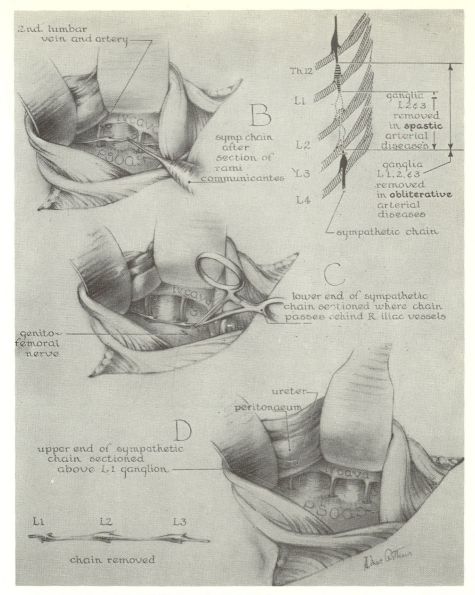

**Fig. 11-59, cont'd.** For legend see opposite page.

neurium (Fig. 11-60). Tension at the suture line is eliminated by such maneuvers as freeing up a long length of nerve on either side of the point of injury, transposition of the nerve in order to shorten its course, appropriate positioning of the extremity with plaster splinting during the postoperative period and, rarely, use of a nerve graft. Some surgeons apply a cuff of inert material such as silicone about the anastomosis.

### Hypoglossal facial nerve anastomosis

PURPOSE. With certain lesions in the posterior fossa and during some procedures on the posterior fossa the facial nerve may be damaged. In order to restore some

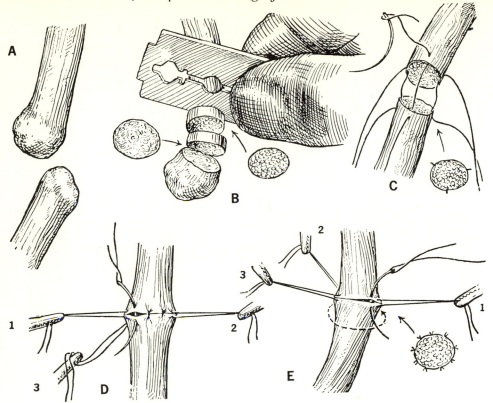

**Fig. 11-60.** Nerve repair. **A,** Divided nerve with neuroma. **B,** Serial resection of neuroma to healthy nerve fibers. **C,** Placement of sutures in perineurium. **D** and **E,** Approximation and tying of sutures. (From Sachs, E.: Diagnosis and treatment of brain tumors and care of the neurosurgical patient, ed. 2, St. Louis, The C. V. Mosby Co.)

function to the facial muscles a hypoglossal facial anastomosis may be performed.

**OPERATIVE PROCEDURE.** This is accomplished by an incision made over the anterior edge of the sternocleidomastoid muscle extending from the mastoid process downward for a distance of approximately 11 to 12 cm. The fascia and muscles are divided, and further dissection is carried out until the hypoglossal nerve is exposed and divided distally. Dissection continues until the facial nerve is exposed and divided close to its exit from the stylomastoid foramen deep to the front of the mastoid process. The proximal end of the hypoglossal nerve is anastomosed with the distal end of the facial nerve with fine arterial or nerve sutures and the wound closed.

Occasionally the surgeon may elect to use the accessory nerve or even the phrenic nerve instead of the hypoglossal nerve.

### Carpal tunnel syndrome

**SETUP AND PREPARATION OF THE PATIENT.** Basic minor neurosurgical set.

**OPERATIVE PROCEDURE**

1. A longitudinal skin incision is made in the thenar palm crease. This runs perpendicular to and stops at the most distal transverse skin crease in the wrist. This incision generally suffices but may be extended into an ʟ or a ⊤.

2. Michel clips or mosquito hemostats are used for hemostasis. A Weitlaner or mastoid retractor is placed.

3. With a curved mosquito hemostat, the fibers of the carpal tunnel ligament are divided transversely in blunt fashion at the

most proximal point of exposure. The hemostat is then introduced through this opening in the ligament, pointed distally, and spread. This protects the underlying median nerve. The ligament is then divided between the jaws of the hemostat with a Mayo scissors.

4. After this incision has been carried well into the palm, the remaining proximal fibers of the ligament are divided in the same fashion. A small vein retractor is placed on the proximal skin edges to facilitate this step.

5. A biopsy of the ligament may be obtained.

6. The skin is closed with silk or nylon suture and a bulky dressing applied, leaving the fingers visible.

### Ulnar nerve transposition at the elbow

OPERATIVE PROCEDURE. A long incision is made, and the nerve is dissected free from the surrounding soft tissues with Metzenbaum scissors and hemostatic forceps. Moist umbilical tapes or Penrose tubing is passed around the freed segments of the nerve to aid in handling for further dissection until a satisfactory length of nerve has been freed from above to below the elbow. The muscle and fascia entered by the nerve at each end of the field may be slit with a scissors to prevent tethering and kinking at these points after the nerve has been transposed. A flap of fascia overlying the medial epicondyle of the humerus is cut and elevated and the nerve transposed beneath it. The fascia is then loosely reapproximated to the fascial edge remaining on the epicondyle with no. 3-0 silk. The wound is closed in layers.

An alternative procedure, medial epicondylectomy, is sometimes performed. In this case the nerve is not dissected out, but the medial epicondyle of the humerus is removed with a rongeur and the residual bone waxed. The fascia and muscle tending to tether or kink the nerve, particularly distally, may be slit with a scissors as in the transposition procedure.

### REFERENCES

1. Berman, J. K.: Principles and practice of surgery, St. Louis, 1950, The C. V. Mosby Co.
2. Carini, E., and Owens, G.: Neurological and neurosurgical nursing, ed. 5, St. Louis, 1970, The C. V. Mosby Co.
3. Chusid, J., and McDonald, J.: Correlative anatomy and functional neurology, Los Altos, Calif., 1970, Lange Medical Publications.
4. Cloward, R. V.: Anterior surgical approach for removal of ruptured cervical intervertebral discs and vertebral body fusions. In Neurosurgical instrument catalog, Randolph, 1967, Codman & Shurtleff, Inc.
5. Hakim valve system for ventriculo-atriostomy, ed. 2, Miami, Cordis Corporation.
6. Hardy, J.: Transsphenoidal hypophysectomy, J. Neurosurg. 34:582, 1971.
7. Kempe, L. G.: Operative neurosurgery, vols. 1 and 2, ed. 2, New York, 1968, Springer-Verlag, New York, Inc.
8. Mettler, F. A.: Neuroanatomy, ed. 2, St. Louis, 1948, The C. V. Mosby Co.
9. Neurosurgical instrument catalog, Randolph, Mass., 1967, Codman & Shurtleff, Inc.
10. Poppen, J. L.: An atlas of neurosurgical techniques, Philadelphia, 1960, W. B. Saunders Co.
11. Rand, R., Renfut, A., and von Leden, H.: Cryosurgery, Springfield, Ill., 1968, Charles C Thomas, Publisher.
12. Richards, V.: Surgery for general practice, St. Louis, 1956, The C. V. Mosby Co.
13. Sachs, E.: Diagnosis and treatment of brain tumors and the care of the neurosurgical patient, ed. 2, St. Louis, 1949, The C. V. Mosby Co.
14. Schwartz, H. G.: High cervical cordotomy, J. Neurosurg. 26:452, 1967.
15. Yasargil, M. G.: Microsurgery applied to neurosurgery, Stuttgart, 1970, Georg Thieme Verlag.

# CHAPTER 12

# Operations on
# the genitourinary organs

BETTY J. DAVIES TAGUE

## ANATOMY AND PHYSIOLOGY
## OF THE GENITOURINARY TRACT

The urinary organs in the male or female comprise two kidneys that excrete the urine, two ureters that convey urine from the kidneys to the bladder, which in turn serves as a reservoir for the reception of urine, and a urethra through which the urine is discharged from the body (Fig. 12-1). In the male, the reproductive system consists of the testes, seminal vesicles, penis, urethra, prostate, and bulbourethral glands. These organs have a direct or indirect function in the process

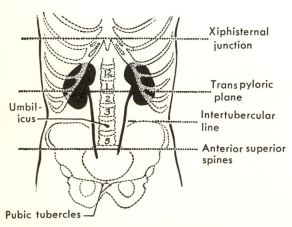

**Fig. 12-1.** Surface anatomy of kidneys, ureters, and bladder. (From Moseley, H. F., editor: Textbook of surgery, ed. 3, St. Louis, 1959, The C. V. Mosby Co.)

of procreation. The reproductive system in the female is described in Chapter 24.

**KIDNEYS.** The kidneys are situated in the retroperitoneal space on the muscles of the posterior abdominal wall, one on each side of the vertebral column at the level of the twelfth thoracic to third lumbar vertebrae. Their position may vary slightly, but usually the right kidney lies lower than the left because of the space occupied by the liver (Fig. 12-1).

Each kidney is surrounded by a mass of fatty and loose areolar tissue, known as *perirenal fat*. Each kidney and fat capsule are surrounded by a sheath of fibrous tissue called *Gerota's capsule*, or renal fascia, which is connected to the fibrous tunic of the kidney by trabeculae. The kidneys are held in place by the renal fascia, which connects with the fascia of the quadrate muscle of the loins, the psoas major muscles, and the diaphragm and also by pressure of the associated organs. The anterior and posterior relationships of the kidney are shown in Fig. 12-2.

On the medial side of each kidney there is a concave notch, called the *hilum*, through which the ureter, arteries, and veins enter and leave and at which site the renal pelvis is found (Fig. 12-3).

The substance of the kidney consists of an outer portion, called the *cortex*, and an inner portion, called the *medulla*. The cortex contains the glomeruli and the func-

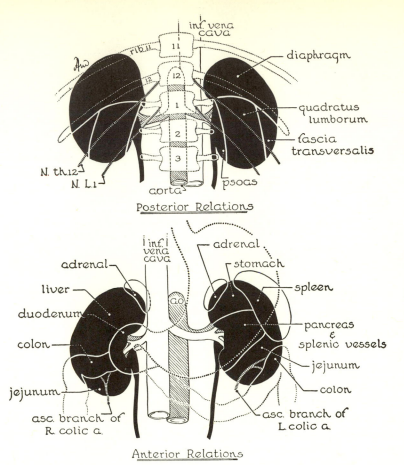

Posterior Relations

Anterior Relations

**Fig. 12-2.** Anterior and posterior relations of kidneys and ureters to organs in peritoneal cavity, to ureteral column posteriorly, and to the main arteries and veins. (From Moseley, H. F., editor: Textbook of surgery, ed. 3, St. Louis, 1959, The C. V. Mosby Co.)

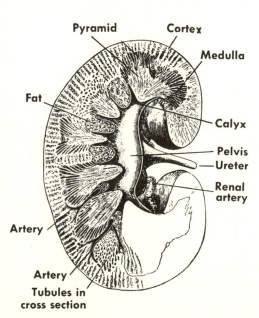

**Fig. 12-3.** Cross section of kidney. (After Tyson; from Tuttle, W. W., and Schottelius, B. A.: Textbook of physiology, ed. 15, St. Louis, 1965, The C. V. Mosby Co.)

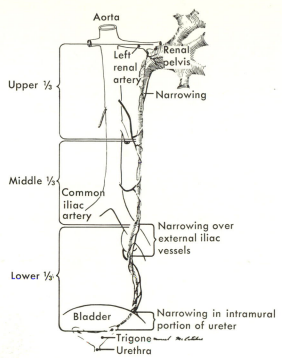

**Fig. 12-4.** Anatomy of the ureter. (From Colby, F. H.: Essential urology, ed. 4, Baltimore, copyright 1961, The Williams & Wilkins Co.)

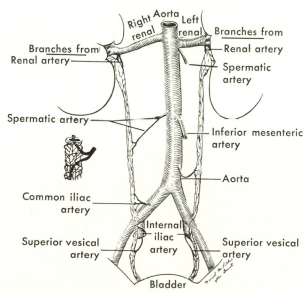

**Fig. 12-5.** Most kidney substance, in both cortex and medulla, is composed of minute tubules, closely packed together with sufficient connective tissue to carry a large supply of blood vessels and a number of lymphatic vessels and nerve fibers. Arrangement of these tubules is called *nephrons*. Flow of blood is from afferent arteriole → glomerulus → efferent arteriole → peritubular capillaries → venules → vein. (From Colby, F. H.: Essential urology, ed. 4, Baltimore, copyright 1961, The Williams & Wilkins Co.)

tioning tubules. The medulla contains many collecting tubules and papillary ducts. Each of the latter empties on a papilla within a minor calyx. Several of these join to form a major calyx. These unite to form—and therefore in turn empty into—the renal pelvis, consisting of smooth muscle lined with epithelium (Fig. 12-3). The funnel-shaped renal pelvis of each kidney is continuous with the ureter below (Fig. 12-4).

The kidneys are very vascular because one fourth of the entire volume of blood passes through them at any one time (Fig. 12-5). They receive their blood supply through the renal arteries, which originate from the aorta. Each renal artery divides into several branches, called *afferent vessels* (Fig. 12-5).

The lymphatic supply, for the most part, drains into the lymph nodes that are located between the renal vessels and the aorta, and it accompanies the venous drainage.

The nerves of the autonomic (involuntary nervous) system carry pain sensations from the urinary organs. The nerve supply to the kidney comes from the lumbar sympathetic trunk and from the vagus and vesical nerves. Removal of the nervous pathways disrupts the ability to feel pain,

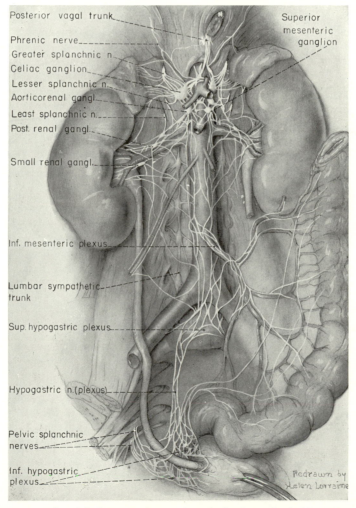

**Fig. 12-6.** Nerve supply of kidneys, ureters, adrenal glands, and bladder. (From Campbell, M. F., editor: Urology, ed. 2, Philadelphia, 1963, W. B. Saunders Co.)

without impairing kidney function (Fig. 12-6).

**URETERS.** Each ureter is a continuation of the cuplike calyces and renal pelvis. The ureter extends from the renal pelvis to the base of the bladder as a cylindrical tube (Fig. 12-4). Each tube is about 25 to 30 cm. long (10 to 12 inches) and 4 to 5 mm. (⅕ inch) in diameter. Each consists of three layers: an outer adventitial layer, a muscular layer, and an inner epithelial lining (Fig. 12-8).

**URINARY BLADDER.** The urinary bladder is a musculomembranous sac situated in the pelvic cavity behind and below the symphysis pubis, in front of the rectum, and above the prostate gland in the male. The bladder lies in front of the neck of the uterus and the anterior wall of the vagina in the female. When the bladder becomes distended, it begins to ascend above the symphysis pubis, pushes its peritoneal covering ahead of it, and partially becomes an abdominal structure.

The bladder is connected to the pelvic wall by fascial attachments that extend from the back of the pubic bones to the front of the bladder. Other muscular fibers also pass from the base of the bladder to the sides of the rectum.

The bladder consists of a thick muscular wall with outer adventitial and inner mucosal layers. In addition, a peritoneal layer partially covers and is attached to the bladder dome (Figs. 12-7 and 12-8). The blood supply of the bladder is derived from branches of the anterior trunk of the hypogastric artery.

As a result of the peristaltic muscular contraction of the renal pelvis and ureter, the urine is actively propelled from the kidney to the bladder and expressed from the ureteral orifice (Figs. 12-8 and 18-9).

The size, position, and relation of the bladder to the intestines, rectum, and reproductive organs vary according to the

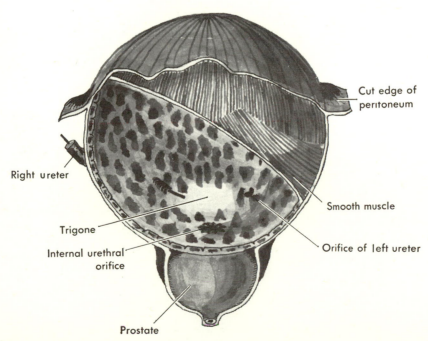

**Fig. 12-7.** Male bladder. Part of wall cut away to show muscle coat and interior. (From Anthony, C. P.: Textbook of anatomy and physiology, ed. 6, St. Louis, 1963, The C. V. Mosby Co.)

amount of fluid it contains. The process of emptying the bladder appears to be initiated by nerve cells from the sacral divisions of the autonomic nervous system. These sacral reflex centers are controlled by higher voluntary centers in the brain. Stimulation from the sacral centers results in contraction of the bladder muscle and relaxation of the bladder outlet sphincters. Muscle tone maintains closure of the sphincters when the bladder is at rest.

MALE URETHRA. The male urethra is a tube about 20 cm. (8 inches) in length that forms an S curve. It is the terminal portion of both the urinary and reproductive tracts. In the posterior portion of the urethra, there are two divisions: the prostatic urethra (Figs. 12-8 and 12-10), which passes through the prostate gland, and the membranous portion, which contains the external sphincter of the bladder. The anterior urethra has two distinct divisions: the bulbous urethra and the pendulous portion. The male urethra is composed of mucous membrane that is continuous with that of the bladder and merges with the submucous tissue, which in turn connects the urethra with other structures that it traverses.

FEMALE URETHRA. The female urethra is a narrow membranous hollow tube about 4 cm. in length (1½ inches) and 6 mm. (¼ inch) in diameter. When it is not in use, however, its walls collapse. This structure lies behind and beneath the symphysis pubis and anterior to the vagina. The external urethral orifice (urinary meatus) lies anterior to the vaginal opening

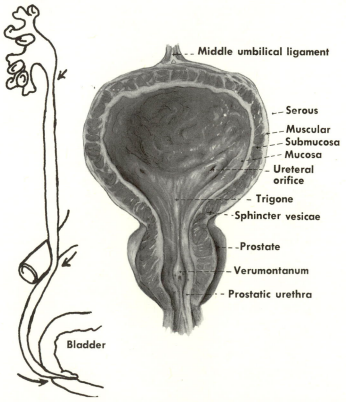

Fig. 12-8. Bladder and prostate, sectioned to show structure of bladder wall and points of interest in base of bladder and posterior urethra. Diagram showing normal areas of urethral constriction. (Modified from Campbell, M. F., editor: Urology, ed. 2, Philadelphia, 1963, W. B. Saunders Co.)

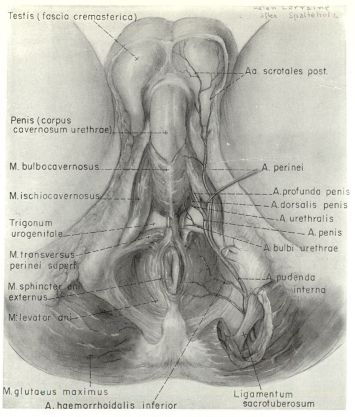

**Fig. 12-9.** Anatomy of male perineum. (After Spalteholz; from Campbell, M. F., editor: Urology, ed. 2, Philadelphia, 1963, W. B. Saunders Co.)

and posterior to the clitoris (Chapter 24).

REPRODUCTIVE MALE ORGANS. These organs include the two testes, epididymides, seminal ducts (vas deferens), seminal vesicles, and ejaculatory ducts, as well as the single reproductive organs of the prostate, penis, and urethra. The *scrotum* (Figs. 12-9 and 12-10) is located behind the base of the penis and in front of the anus. This loose sac contains and supports the testes, the epididymides, and some of the spermatic cord. The two sides of the scrotum are separated from each other by a median raphe. Within the scrotum there are two cavities or sacs that are lined with smooth and glistening tissue, known as the *tunica vaginalis*. Normally, a small amount of clear fluid is contained in the tunica vaginalis. The condition known as *hydrocele* denotes an abnormal accumulation of this fluid.

The *testes* manufacture the spermatozoa and also contain a specialized cell (Leydig) that produces the male hormone. Each testis consists of many tubules in which the sperm are formed, surrounded by a dense capsule of connective tissue. The tubules coalesce and continue into the adjacent epididymis, where the sperm mature and are stored.

The *epididymis* is a long narrow organ that lies along the top and side of each testis. It connects the testis with the seminal duct (Fig. 12-11). The *vas deferens* (ductus deferens, or seminal duct) is a distal continuation of the epididymis. Each is the excretory duct of the testis (Fig. 12-10) and conveys the sperm from the epididymis to the seminal vesicle.

The vas deferens lies within the *spermatic cord* in the inguinal region. The spermatic

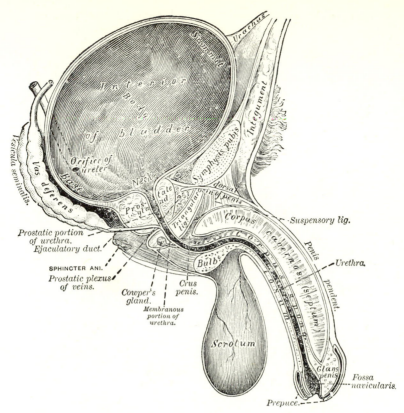

Fig. 12-10. Vertical section of bladder, penis, and urethra. (From Lewis: In Gray's anatomy, Philadelphia, Lea & Febiger.)

cord also contains the veins, arteries, lymphatics, nerves, and surrounding connective tissue (cremaster muscle) that give support to the testes.

The seminal vesicles are structures that unite with the vas deferens on either side. The terminal portion of each vas deferens is called the *ejaculatory duct,* which passes between the lobes of the prostate gland and opens into the posterior urethra (Fig. 12-11).

The *prostate gland* is an accessory sex organ. It lies just below the bladder in front of the rectum and surrounds the prostatic portion of the urethra (Figs. 12-10 and 12-11). The entire prostate gland, which consists of five lobes, is surrounded by a fibrous capsule, through which the ejaculatory ducts enter to pass through the gland (Fig. 12-11). Behind the prostatic

capsule, there is a fibrous sheath that separates the prostate gland and the seminal vesicles from the rectum. The lobes of the gland secrete a highly alkaline fluid that dilutes the testicular secretion as it comes from the ejaculatory ducts. The prostate gland receives its blood supply from the internal pudendal, inferior vesical, and hemorrhoidal arteries.

*Cowper's glands* (bulbourethral glands) (Fig. 12-11) are two small bodies situated on either side of the membranous portion of the urethra. Each gland via its duct empties mucous secretions into the urethra.

The *penis* is a pendulous organ suspended by the fascial attachments of the pubic arch and supported by the suspensory ligaments (Fig. 12-10). The penis contains three distinct vascular sponge-like bodies: the two upper bodies are

called the *right and left corpus caver-*
*nosum* and the lower body, the *corpus*
*spongiosum urethrae.* The tissue contains
a network of vascular channels that fill
with blood on erection. At the distal end
of the penis, the skin is doubly folded
to form the so-called prepuce, or foreskin,
which serves as a covering for the glans
penis (Fig. 12-10). The glans penis contains the urethral orifice.

ADRENAL GLANDS. The adrenal glands lie
retroperitoneally beneath the diaphragm at
the medial aspect of the superior pole of
each kidney. On the right side, the gland
is adjacent to the inferior vena cava; on
the left side, the gland is posterior to

the stomach and pancreas. Each adrenal
gland has a medulla, which secretes adrenaline, and a cortex, which secretes steroids
and other hormones. The glands are freely
supplied with arterial branches from the
phrenic and renal arteries and from the
aorta. The venous drainage is accomplished
on the right by the inferior vena cava;
on the left, by the left renal vein (Fig.
12-2).

## NURSING CONSIDERATIONS
## IN GENITOURINARY SURGERY

Operating room personnel must have a
good understanding of the procedure that
is planned in order to properly prepare

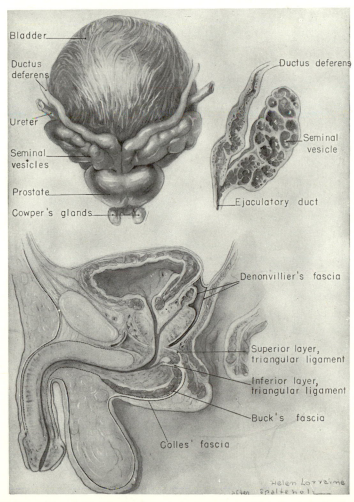

**Fig. 12-11.** Relationship of bladder and genital structures. (After Spalteholz; from Campbell,
M. F., editor: Urology, ed. 2, Philadelphia, 1963, W. B. Saunders Co.)

the patient, room, equipment, and supplies. Safety is the prime consideration, since the patient is positioned in lateral, prone, or lithotomy position (Chapter 7). These positions are frequently exaggerated to give better access to the organs involved, as for a radical operation on the prostate and bladder. Care must be taken to avoid displacement of the joints in lithotomy as the anesthetized patient is positioned. This is especially true in aged or debilitated patients.

In positioning a patient laterally for kidney surgery, the spine is extended to give more access to the retroperitoneal space. This patient should have padding and stabilizing support from rubber-covered pillows, sandbags, and straps. If the electrocautery unit is to be used, care must also be taken to see that no part of the patient touches metal equipment other than the indifferent electrode plate attached to the cautery unit.

In some procedures involving stones of the kidneys or ureters, it may be necessary to make x-ray examinations during the procedure. A cassette holder must be placed under the patient who is in the

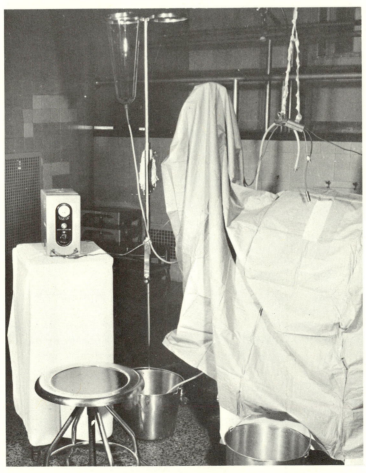

**Fig. 12-12.** Arrangement for bladder irrigation during surgery showing Valentine irrigating flasks, battery box with cords, and suspenders. Flexible rubber cords with clips provide convenient way of presenting needed attachments to surgeon and keeping them out of working field. Suspenders, cords, and flask with its tubing are sterilized. Note metal lid for Valentine flask.

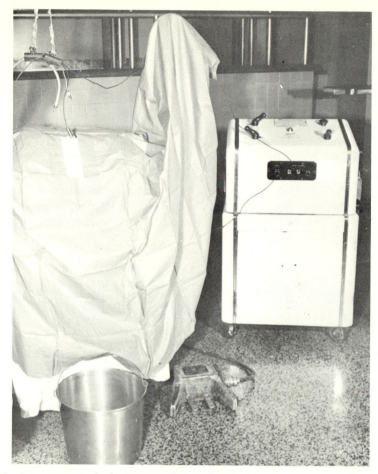

Fig. 12-13. Arrangement of electrosurgical unit for use during surgery. Note placement of foot pedal controls. Active cord is suspended with other working attachments. Indifferent cord leads to plate under patient.

supine, prone, or lithotomy position. The patient positioned laterally will be x-rayed by a cassette held in a sterile wrap.

ASEPTIC TECHNIQUES AND SAFETY MEASURES. Aseptic techniques in skin preparation and draping must be carefully maintained (Chapters 4 and 5). Difficulty may be encountered in cleansing and preparing the perineal area. Spray apparatus may be preferred to gauze sponges on forceps to apply antiseptic in perineal skin preparations.

Draping procedures for laparotomy are described and illustrated in Chapter 5. Arrangement of irrigating items and electrosurgical equipment for surgery via the

perineal route is shown in Figs. 12-12 and 12-13.

The disposable O'Connor perineal drape with finger cot may be used.

Transurethral passage of instruments and catheters requires meticulous technique to prevent retrograde infections of the urinary system (Chapter 5). The use of transurethral instruments is facilitated by darkening the room. There should be provision for proper adjustments in lighting (Chapters 1 and 5).

Electrosurgical units and battery cords are frequent adjuncts in urological surgery (Fig. 12-13). The staff must be familiar with their use and with the precautions

necessary to prevent fire, explosion, or burns (Chapter 5).

**DISTENTION OF BLADDER.** When the bladder is to be opened or manipulated, it is frequently distended with irrigating fluid prior to surgery. Provision must be made in positioning and draping of the patient and in instrument selection for filling and draining the bladder prior to or during the course of the operation.

**CYSTOSCOPY INSTRUMENTS AND CATHETERIZING TELESCOPES.** Ureteral catheterization may also precede radical operations. Preoperative preparations of the patient and cystoscopy instruments with catheterizing telescopes are needed (Figs. 12-49 and 12-59).

**DRAINAGE TUBES AND CATHETERS.** Whenever the urinary tract is opened, there is the danger of leakage of urine. All such wounds require careful drainage. Drainage tubes in the urinary tract must be kept open at all times and the surgeon immediately notified if there is no drainage. The tube or catheter used to drain the bladder suprapubically must be stiff enough to prevent collapse. An angulated tube or catheter may be useful in preventing kinking if bulky dressings are used. The catheters or tubes should be tested for patency, flushed, and suctioned prior to use. Modern vacuum drainage collectors (of the Hemovac type) have been successful in maintaining drainage and keeping wounds dry.

Ureterostomy and nephrostomy tubes must be carefully identified, fixed in position, and guarded to prevent dislodgment or obstruction (Fig. 12-27). There are various types of catheters available for specific situations. Catheters are used for diagnostic purposes and to explore the urethra for stenosis, discover residual urine in the bladder, and introduce contrast medium into the bladder.

Filiform tips and followers are used to dilate narrow strictures. Graduated woven ureteral catheters are used to introduce radiopaque material or obtain a sterile urine specimen from the renal pelvis and to help determine renal function (Fig. 12-14).

The olive-tipped bougies are used to calibrate the urethra. The silk woven catheter may be used to manipulate past enlarged prostatic lobes (Fig. 12-14). In some cases, a catheter stylet is used to insert a catheter (Fig 12-30). The catheter should be lubricated before the stylet is inserted. The catheter is drawn taut over the stylet so that its tip cannot become dislodged. Catheters with inflatable balloons are used for drainage and for pressure to help control bleeding.

## OPERATIONS ON THE KIDNEY AND THE URETER

**GENERAL CONSIDERATIONS.** Stones, infections, and tumors are the most common causes of urinary tract obstruction necessitating operation to prevent renal destruction or failure. Obstruction may also be due to malformations or the consequence of previous operations on the urinary tract (Fig. 12-15).

Although the causes of kidney stones are obscure, certain conditions such as obstruction, stasis, or body chemistry predispose to their formation. Stones may form from various elements: calcium oxalate, calcium phosphate, magnesium ammonium phosphate, uric acid, and calcium carbonate, or combinations of these substances may be found. All stones removed at operation are usually subjected to chemical analysis. Stones obtained as surgical specimens are best submitted in a dry jar. Fixative agents such as Formalin can obscure the results of the analysis.

Stones in the renal pelvis may drop down into the opening of the ureter (the ureteropelvic junction) and occlude it, or they may pass into the ureter and lodge at the ureterovesical junction or where the ureter passes into the bony pelvis at the level of the iliac crest (Fig. 12-15). A stone may lodge in a renal calyx and continue to enlarge, eventually filling the entire calyx or renal pelvis (staghorn stone).

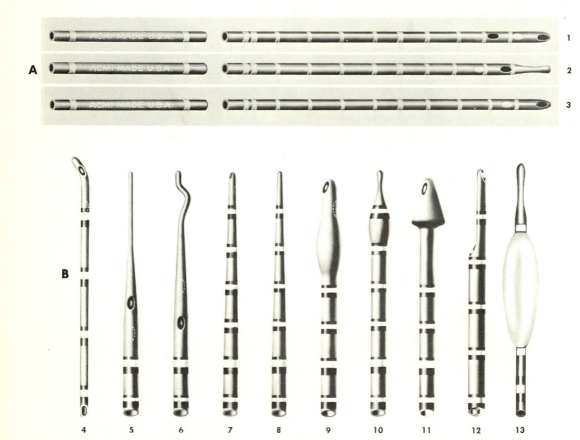

**Fig. 12-14. A,** X-ray graduate woven ureteral catheters are made of nylon or plastic material and have outer surfacing to provide for flexibility, for easy entry without kinking. Eyes provide for adequate high flow rate. Catheter's tip is constructed for specific procedures as shown. **1,** Whistle tip; **2,** olive tip; **3,** round tip. **B,** X-ray graduated woven ureteral catheters and bougies. **4,** Wishard catheter, flat, coude tip; **5,** Blasucci catheter, flexible filiform tip; **6,** Blasucci catheter, flexible spiral filiform tip; **7,** Garceau catheter, tapered for dilatation, whistle tip; **8,** Garceau bougie, tapered for dilatation, conical tip; **9,** Braasch bulb catheter, whistle tip; **10,** Braasch bougie, bulb tip; **11,** Foley catheter, cone tip (for ureteropyelography); **12,** Hyams double-lumen catheter; **13,** Dourmashkin dilator with inflation balloon, olive tip. (Courtesy American Cystoscope Makers, Inc., New York, N. Y. )

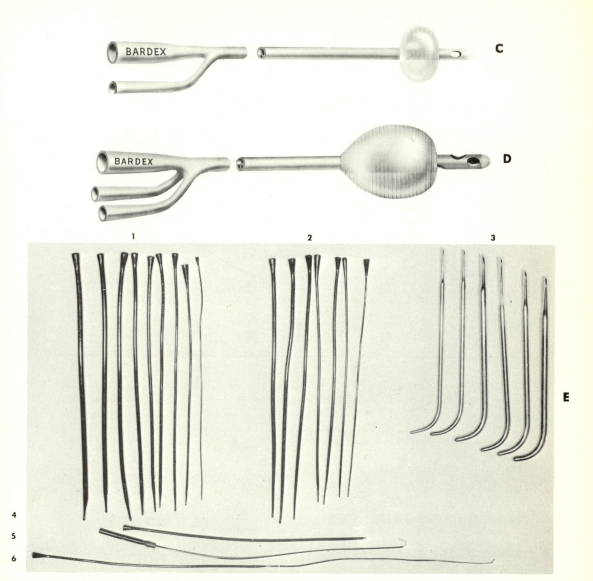

Fig. 12-14, cont'd. **C,** Foley retention catheters. **D,** Bard hemostatic catheter, 75 ml. nonfluted ovoid balloon. **E,** Urethral sounding appliances. **1,** Nylon woven catheters; **2,** nylon woven sounds; **3,** metal sounds; **4,** Philips follower; **5,** Bugbee electrode; **6,** Philips filiform with follower attached. Threaded filiform fits either urethral bougie or catheter. (**C** and **D** courtesy C. R. Bard, Inc., Murray Hill, N. J.)

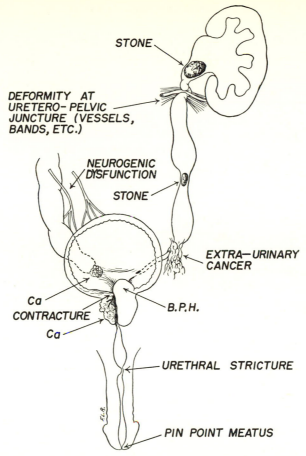

STONE

DEFORMITY AT
URETERO-PELVIC
JUNCTURE (VESSELS,
BANDS, ETC.)

NEUROGENIC
DYSFUNCTION

STONE

EXTRA—URINARY
CANCER

Ca
CONTRACTURE

Ca

B.P.H.

URETHRAL STRICTURE

PIN POINT MEATUS

Fig. 12-15. Some common causes of obstruction vary in location and nature, but all can destroy renal function, usually in the presence of infection. **B.P.H.**, Benign prostatic hypertrophy. (From Marshall, V. F.: Textbook of urology, ed. 2, New York, 1964, Harper & Row, Publishers.)

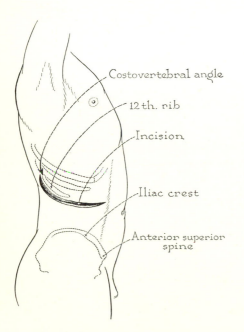

Costovertebral angle

12th. rib

Incision

Iliac crest

Anterior superior
spine

Fig. 12-16. Incision for lumbar approach to kidney. It is made parallel to twelfth rib and 1 cm. below it, extends from costovertebral angle to a point 3 cm. above anterosuperior iliac spine. (From Barnes, R. W., and Hadley, H. L.: Urological practice, St. Louis, 1954, The C. V. Mosby Co.)

Hydroureter, hydronephrosis, and fibrosis and destruction of the renal parenchyma can result from unrelieved obstruction (Figs. 12-8 and 12-15).

## Nephrectomy

**DEFINITION.** Removal of a kidney.

**CONSIDERATIONS.** Nephrectomy is performed to treat some congenital unilateral abnormalities causing renal obstruction or severe hydronephrosis, tumor of the kidney, a severely injured kidney, renal tuberculosis, calculous pyelonephrosis, and sometimes cortical abscess.

**SETUP AND PREPARATION OF THE PATIENT.** The position of the patient on the operating table will depend on the type of lesion, the position of the kidney, and the surgical approach selected (Fig. 12-16). The most common position for kidney operations is the lateral when a lumbar, transpleural, or extrapleural transthoracic approach is to be used. A supine or a modified Trendelenburg position is employed when an abdominal approach is to be used (Chapter 7).

Routine skin preparation and draping procedures are carefully carried out (Chapters 4 and 5).

The instrument setup includes the routine major laparotomy setup, as listed in Chapter 17, plus kidney instruments.

These should include the following (Fig. 12-17):

2 Satinsky, Herrick, or Mayo pedicle clamps
5 Randall stone forceps, varied sizes
1 Lewkowitz lithotomy forceps
1 Silver probe (Bakes dilators may be used)
Rubber catheter, size 8 or 10 Fr.
Asepto syringe
Penrose-type drain
Mushroom, Pezzer, or Malecot catheter

In certain operations, the chest or the gastrointestinal tract may be opened. If the chest is opened, appropriate instruments, drainage, and suction will be needed (Chapter 14). When the gastrointestinal tract is opened, precautions must be taken in the anastomosis and closure techniques. (Chapter 21). *For rib resection* (Chapter 14), add the following to the basic setup:

1 Finochietto rib retractor, large
1 Matson costal periosteotome
1 Alexander costal periosteotome
2 Doyen rib raspatories, right and left
1 Giertz rib shears
1 Double-action duckbill rongeur
1 Bailey rib approximator

### APPROACHES TO THE KIDNEY

**LUMBAR OR SIMPLE FLANK INCISION.** This incision begins at the costovertebral angle and parallels the twelfth rib. It extends forward and downward between the iliac crest and the thorax (Fig. 12-18).

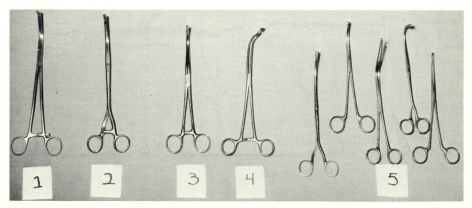

**Fig. 12-17.** Kidney instruments. **1,** Satinsky pedicle clamp; **2,** Herrick pedicle clamp; **3,** Mayo pedicle clamp; **4,** Lewkowitz lithotomy forceps; **5,** set of Randall stone forceps.

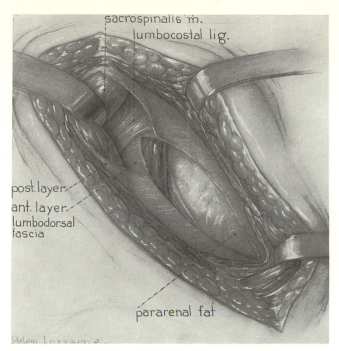

**Fig. 12-18.** Through lumbar incision, superficial fascia, and division of latissimus dorsi muscle, posterior fibers of internal oblique muscle and lumbar fascia have been divided, thereby exposing fat and fascia that surround kidney. Lumbocostal ligament is exposed and divided to provide for better exposure of upper angle of wound. (From Dodson, A. I.: Urological surgery, ed. 3, St. Louis, 1956, The C. V. Mosby Co.)

NAGAMATSU INCISION. This is a modification of the simple flank incision and is made over the eleventh and twelfth ribs, removing a section of each.

THORACOABDOMINAL INCISION. The tenth and eleventh ribs are removed, and the chest cavity is opened, collapsing the lung. Rib spreaders and approximators and chest drainage are required. When the lumbar, Nagamatsu, or thoracoabdominal approach is used, the patient is placed in a lateral position (Fig. 7-16).

TRANSPERITONEAL AND RETROPERITONEAL INCISIONS. The patient is placed in a supine position. A vertical incision is made in the epigastric and umbilical region on the affected side. This approach is used for a large kidney tumor or when the kidney and ureter are extensively involved in the surgery.

OPERATIVE PROCEDURE (LUMBAR APPROACH)

1. The incision is carried through the skin, fat, and fascia. Bleeding vessels are clamped with hemostats and ligated (Fig. 12-18).

2. The external oblique, the latissimus dorsi, and the internal oblique muscles are exposed. The required portions of the dorsi, external oblique, posterior inferior serratus, and internal oblique muscles are split or divided and retracted with dull rake or Richardson right-angled retractors. Bleeding is controlled. The transversalis fascia is cut with scissors. Then the iliohypogastric and ilioinguinal nerves are identified and retracted (Fig. 12-6). The sacrospinal muscle is retracted. The deep lumbar fascia is separated. The quadrate muscle of the loins may be divided.

3. The pleura, peritoneum, and twelfth thoracic artery and nerve are identified and retracted. Laparotomy pads and Deaver retractors are placed to protect the adjacent structure and afford exposure.

4. If necessary, a rib or ribs (twelfth, eleventh, or tenth) may be resected to

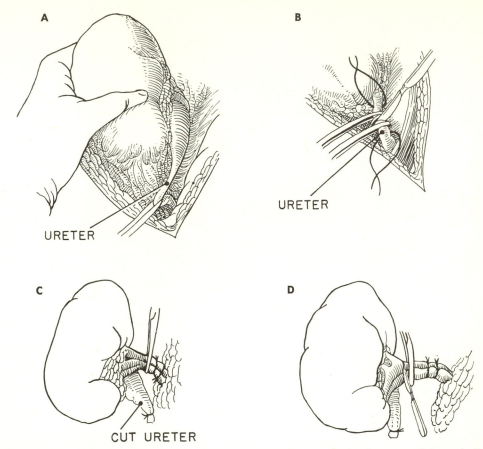

**Fig. 12-19.** Nephrectomy. **A** and **B**, Upper portion of ureter is freed, cut, and ligated. **C**, Chromic gut ligatures are placed; kidney clamps are applied between proximal ligature and kidney itself. **D**, Renal vascular pedicle is doubly ligated with suture ligatures, and kidney is removed. (From Flocks, R. H., and Culp, D.: Surgical urology, Chicago, 1954, Year Book Medical Publishers, Inc.; drawings by Paul Ver Vais.)

give access to the kidney (Chapter 14). The periosteum is stripped with an Alexander costal periosteotome and Doyen rib raspatory.

5. A scalpel and heavy scissors may be used to cut through the lumbocostal ligaments. The rib is grasped with an Ochsner clamp and cut with rib shears, removing the portion necessary to expose the kidney.

6. Retractors and pads are placed. Gerota's fascia, the perirenal capsule, is grasped with long tissue forceps and incised with a scalpel. The incision is extended, using dissecting scissors, and the kidney and perirenal fat are exposed. The kidney is dissected free, using sharp and

blunt dissection with long tissue forceps, scissors, and sponges on forceps. Crile hemostats are used on bleeding vessels.

7. The ureter is identified, separated from its adjacent structures, and retracted. Holding forceps such as long Babcock or long Allis clamps may be used, or a length of Penrose tubing may be passed around the ureter to retain and retract it. The ureter is occluded by double clamping and then divided and ligated (Fig. 12-19).

8. The kidney pedicle containing the major blood vessels is isolated, doubly clamped by using long kidney clamps of a size suitable to the structures. The vessels are securely ligated with heavy chro-

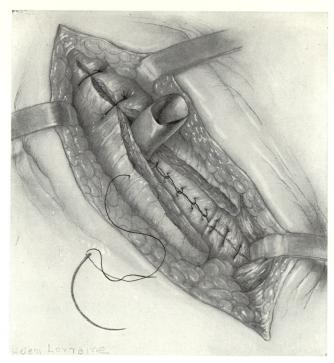

Fig. 12-20. In closing lumbar incision, each muscle layer is accurately approximated with chromic gut no. 2-0 sutures before superficial fascia is approximated with chromic gut no. 4-0 sutures; skin edges are approximated with silk nylon or stainless steel no. 4-0 or 5-0. (From Dodson, A. I.: Urological surgery, ed. 3, St. Louis, 1956, The C. V. Mosby Co.)

mic gut or transfixed with heavy sutures on Atraumatic needles. The pedicle is severed and the kidney removed (Fig. 12-19).

9. The wound is explored for bleeding, hemostasis secured, and the cavity cleansed by irrigating, sponging, and suctioning as necessary. A drain of Penrose tubing, which may be wicked with gauze, or a drain made of heavy rubber or plastic tubing is placed whenever leakage of urine may occur.

10. The fascia and muscles are closed in layers with interrupted chromic sutures. If necessary, tension sutures may be used. The skin edges are approximated with interrupted sutures of silk or wire or with skin clips (Fig. 12-20).

11. The drain is secured and the wound dressed with gauze sponges, abdominal pads, and adhesive strips.

### Heminephrectomy

**DEFINITION.** Partial excision of the kidney.

**SETUP AND PREPARATION OF THE PATIENT.** As described for nephrectomy.

**OPERATIVE PROCEDURE.** This procedure is usually indicated when one pole of the kidney has been destroyed by localized disease, such as an obstructed calculus. The rest of the kidney is healthy. This condition may be the result of a kidney being formed with two collecting systems. The capsule is pushed back, and a wedge of kidney tissue is resected, which includes the diseased or damaged cortex, pelvis, and vessels. The healthy kidney tissue is sutured with gut; the capsule is replaced; then a pad of fat is sutured over the line of closure. A nephropexy will probably be done also to ensure good position and drainage (Fig. 12-21).

### Procedures for opening the kidney

**DEFINITIONS.** *Nephrotomy* is incision into the kidney. Simple incision and drainage

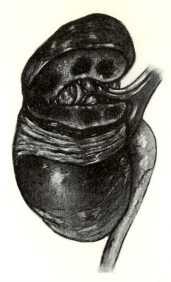

**Fig. 12-21.** Heminephrectomy (partial nephrectomy). Capsule incised and peeled back. Anterior parenchymal incision exposes vessels to upper pole, which are tied and divided. Resection then completed. (From Smith, D. R., Schulte, J. W., and Smart, W. R.: In Campbell, M. F., editor: Urology, ed. 2, Philadelphia, 1963, W. B. Saunders Co.)

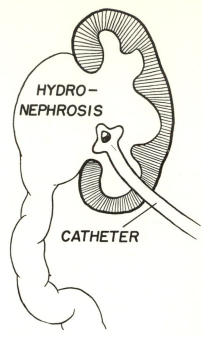

**Fig. 12-22.** Catheter used in nephrostomy crosses renal parenchyma to reach usually dilated vessels. If opening is to be maintained temporarily or permanently, the suffix *-ostomy* is used, indicating formation of an ostium; thus the term nephrostomy. (From Marshall, V. F.: Textbook of urology, ed. 2, New York, 1964, Harper & Row, Publishers.)

may be required for hydronephrosis, cyst, or perinephritic abscess (Fig. 12-15).

*Pyelotomy* is an incision into the renal pelvis.

*Pyelostomy* is an incision into the renal pelvis to establish drainage or to permit irrigation of the renal pelvis.

*Pyelolithotomy* is the removal of a stone or stones through the opening made in the renal pelvis.

*Nephrostomy* is an opening into the kidney to maintain temporary or permanent drainage. A nephrostomy is used to correct an obstruction of the urinary tract, conserve and permit physiological restoration of renal tissue that has been impaired by disease, provide permanent drainage when a ureter is unable to function, treat anuria as an emergency measure, or drain a kidney during the postoperative period following a plastic repair on the kidney or renal pelvis (Fig. 12-22).

*Nephrolithotomy* and *pyelonephrolithot-*

*omy* are essentially the same, since one is simply an extension of the incision. This is done in order to remove a large stone intact or to explore a calyx where a small stone or fragment has slipped. The presence of a staghorn calculus is an indication for this procedure.

SETUP AND PREPARATION OF THE PATIENT. As described for nephrectomy, adding the following:

  2 Kimball nephrostomy hooks
  2 Mayo duct scoops
  5 Randall kidney stone forceps

The kidney pedicle clamps should be added to the setup for these procedures, since the surgeon may find a condition that necessitates a nephrectomy.

OPERATIVE PROCEDURES

FOR OPENING. The kidney is approached as described for nephrectomy, using the

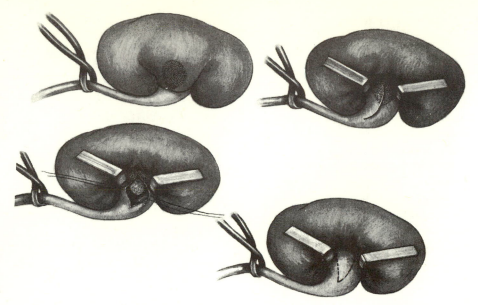

**Fig. 12-23.** Pyelotomy and pyelolithotomy. Linear incision is made in pelvis between stay sutures (pyelotomy). If pelvis is small and stone large, V-shaped incision may be used (pyelolithotomy). (From Smith, D. R., Schulte, J. W., and Smart, W. R.: In Campbell, M. F., editor: Urology, ed. 2, Philadelphia, 1963, W. B. Saunders Co.)

desired incision. The renal pedicle is identified; the ureter is identified and retracted as necessary. The kidney is mobilized to permit approach to the aspect desired.

FOR PYELOTOMY OR PYELOSTOMY. The pelvis of the kidney is incised with a small blade. Traction sutures of no. 3-0 black silk on French eye or swaged-on needles may be placed at the edges of the incision to hold it open while the pelvis and calyces are explored. In pyelostomy the catheter is placed through the incision directly into the renal pelvis. (Fig. 12-23).

FOR NEPHROSTOMY. A curved clamp or stone forceps is passed through a pyelotomy incision into the renal pelvis and then out through the substance of the renal parenchyma via a lower pole minor calyx. The tip of a Malecot or Pezzer catheter is then drawn into the renal pelvis, and the pyelotomy incision is closed (Fig. 12-22). The distal end of the tube is brought out through the flank incision. Penrose drains are placed, and the incision is closed in the regular manner (Fig. 12-20).

FOR PYELOLITHOTOMY. The renal pelvis is opened, and the ureter may be probed for stones or strictures by passing a ureteral catheter and irrigating. Stones are removed. A multieyed catheter—Pezzer, Malecot, or Foley type—is placed. The catheter is secured with sutures. A pursestring suture may be placed around the nephrostomy tube.

After removal of a staghorn calculus, mattress sutures are usually tied over a pad of renal fat to support the long parenchymal incision.

FOR CLOSURE. An incision in the renal pelvis may be closed with fine chromic gut swaged-on needles or left alone. The wound is drained and closed, as for nephrectomy. Reinforced absorbent dressings or special wound decompression apparatus is required for draining wounds.

### Nephroureterectomy

DEFINITION. Removal of a kidney and the entire ureter that drains it.

CONSIDERATIONS. Nephroureterectomy is indicated for the presence of hydrone-

phrosis, a hydroureter too damaged to repair, or carcinoma of the renal pelvis or ureter. This procedure usually requires two separate incisions, the first one in the flank and the second in the abdomen. Two separate instrument sets are not required, but a second skin preparation setup and set of sterile drapes are required.

**OPERATIVE PROCEDURE**

1. The patient is placed in a lateral position. The kidney and upper ureter are exposed, as described for nephrectomy, freed from their supporting structures, and brought out of the wound, taking as much ureter as possible. The ureter is not cut at this time. The wound is drained and closed in layers, leaving the kidney and ureter outside the wound, and lightly dressed.

2. Care must be taken not to contaminate the kidney, exposed ureter, and incision as the patient is repositioned in a supine manner.

3. The abdomen is prepped, sterile drapes are applied, and an abdominal incision is made to expose the lower ureter and bladder. These structures are freed. The ureter and a small cuff from the bladder are removed.

4. At this time the kidney and entire ureter are gently pulled free through the flank incision.

5. A Penrose-type drain or catheter is placed in the bladder, and it is closed with chromic suture no. 2-0. The abdomen is closed in layers as described in Chapter 17, and both wounds are dressed with gauze sponges and abdominal pads.

## Reconstruction operations on the kidney

**DEFINITION AND PURPOSE.** *Pyeloplasty* is a revision or reconstruction of the renal pelvis.

**CONSIDERATIONS.** This operation is done to create a better anatomical relationship between the pelvis of the kidney and the ureter and to relieve pain and obstruction to the flow of urine from the kidney (Fig. 12-15). It may be necessary to ligate aberrant vessels, divide fibrous bands, resect stenotic areas, or reconstruct a redundant kidney pelvis to accomplish this and prevent or relieve hydronephrosis and hydroureter.

*Ureteroplasty* is a reconstruction of the ureter, usually at the ureteropelvic junction (Fig. 12-15).

A *Foley-Y pyeloureteroplasty* may combine correction of a redundant kidney pelvis with resection of a stenotic area of the ureter (Fig. 12-24).

**SETUP AND PREPARATION OF THE PATIENT.** As described for nephrectomy, adding the following (Fig. 12-25):

  1 Small Schnidt gall duct forceps
  1 Metzenbaum dissecting scissors, small, straight, and fine
  1 Metzenbaum dissecting scissors, small, curved, and fine
  1 Iris scissors, curved
  2 Vascular tissue forceps, plain, 7 in.
  2 Vascular tissue forceps, with teeth, 7 in.
  2 Vascular needle holders, 7 in.
12 Mosquito hemostats, 5 in., straight and curved
    Ureteral catheter for splinting
    Red rubber catheters, 8 and 10 Fr.
  5 Randall stone forceps
    Fine chromic gut sutures on Atraumatic needles

**OPERATIVE PROCEDURE**

1. The kidney and upper ureter are exposed, as described for nephrectomy, using the desired approach.

2. The kidney pelvis and ureter are incised, trimmed, and shaped to the desired contour, using fine forceps and scissors. A caliper and a ruler may be used for establishing more precise relationships to improve urinary drainage. Anchoring sutures or soft rubber drains may be used for traction during handling and repair. The repair is completed using fine sutures and needles, as specified by the surgeon.

The technique followed is designed to provide a direct funnel-shaped, enlarged outlet.

The Foley Y-V-plasty technique may be followed as shown in Fig. 12-24. It converts a Y-shaped incision into a V-shaped one by suturing point *A* to point *B* and resecting the redundant tissue between the

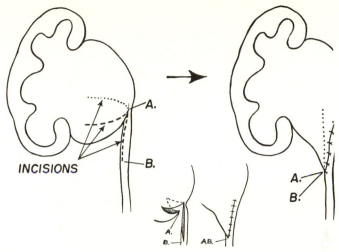

**Fig. 12-24.** Plastic Y-V repair (Foley type) for ureteropelvic obstruction at outlet of renal pelvis. This is actually conversion of a Y incision in three dimensions into two-dimensional V incision. Nephrostomy and splinting catheter through anastomosis are usually employed. (From Marshall, V. F.: Textbook of urology, ed. 2, New York, 1964, Harper & Row, Publishers.)

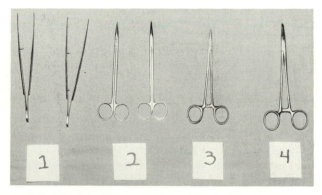

**Fig. 12-25.** Fine instruments for surgery of the ureter. **1,** Fine vascular tissue forceps with and without teeth, 7 in.; **2,** fine Metzenbaum scissors, straight and curved; **3,** fine vascular needle holder, 7 in.; **4,** small Schnidt cell duct forceps.

arm and the stem of the Y. Fine, interrupted stitches are placed to make the repair. Stenotic areas of the ureter are excised as necessary and the ureter anastomosed with fine, everting stitches (ureteroureterostomy).

3. A nephrostomy tube may be placed through a stab wound in the renal parenchyma. A splinting latex catheter 8 or 10 Fr. may be placed to extend along the nephrostomy drain through the kidney pelvis and into the ureter beyond the site of the plastic repair.

4. The incision is closed in layers and the wound dressed.

**Kidney transplant**

DEFINITION. Removal of a donor kidney by means of a nephrectomy and ureterectomy with transplant of the donor's kidney in the recipient's iliac fossa (Fig. 12-26).

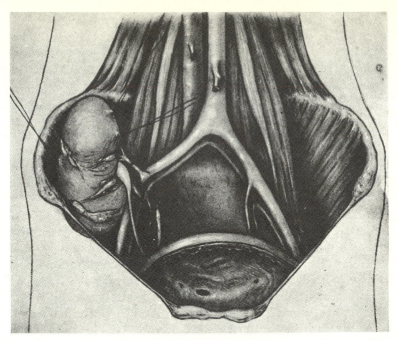

**Fig. 12-26.** Kidney transplant. Donor's left kidney is placed in recipient's right iliac fossa. End-to-end anastomosis of hypogastric and renal arteries; end-to-side anastomosis of renal and iliac vein and oblique ureterocystostomy are accomplished. (From Smith, D. R., Schulte, J. W., and Smart, W. R.: In Campbell, M. F., editor: Urology, ed. 2, Philadelphia, 1963, W. B. Saunders Co.)

CONSIDERATIONS. Kidney transplant is performed in an effort to restore kidney function and thus maintain life in a patient who is succumbing to renal failure.

PATIENT. The patient selected for kidney transplant is usually young, well advanced in irreversible uremia, free of other significant disease or infection, free of obstruction in the lower urinary tract.

DONOR. A kidney for replacement may be chosen from a living donor or from a cadaver that is without disease and of the same blood group as the recipient. The ideal living donor is an identical twin, although family members—mothers, for example—or other volunteers may be selected.

It is important that the time lapse between donor nephrectomy and transplantation of the organ to the recipient be kept to a minimum. In living donors, hypothermia may be used to reduce the oxygen requirements of the kidney.

FACILITIES; SETUP AND PREPARATION OF THE PATIENT. Two adjacent operating rooms are prepared for the surgery, and the operations on donor and recipient proceed simultaneously. On a cadaver donor the supine position is used, and a laparotomy sheet with a large fenestration is used to provide adequate exposure for bilateral nephrectomies. For a living donor, either the lateral or supine position may be used.

The recipient lies in supine position.

The instrument setup for the donor procedure requires a nephrectomy set. The nurse should also provide a sterile basin to receive the donor kidney and provide light and sterile equipment for kidney perfusion. For the recipient procedure, a nephrectomy setup, plus bladder retractor, fine vascular instruments (Chapter 15), Atraumatic vascular suture of nonabsorbable material, nos. 4-0 and 5-0 and absorbable material, nos. 4-0 and 5-0, and one size 8 to 10 Fr. red rubber catheter to ir-

rigate the ureter and to splint the ureter if necessary are required.

DONOR OPERATION. In living donors, angiography assists in selection of the preferred donor kidney.

The donor nephrectomy is done much as the procedure already described, but the surgeon will do a delicate dissection to prevent trauma to the renal vessels and ureter.

The patient may be given intravenous mannitol before the kidney is excised, and the surgeon may inject 1% lidocaine (Xylocaine) about the renal pedicle before its dissection to prevent vasoconstriction. The scrubbed nursing team member should have sterile iced normal saline available to cool the kidney immediately after it is removed.

If the donor kidney is cooled by intra-arterial perfusion, cold (15° C.), sterile, lactated Ringer's solution to which heparin and procaine have been added will be introduced into the vessels by means of small polyethylene catheters under strict aseptic conditions. The sterile basins and donor kidney should be covered with a sterile drape and taken to the recipient operation by the surgeon.

RECIPIENT OPERATION

1. The incisional approach is carried out.
2. The donor kidney is placed in the contralateral iliac fossa of the patient and rotated 180 degrees so that the posterior surface is anterior in the patient (Fig. 12-26). Placing the organ extraperitoneally may prevent peritonitis if an infection develops.
3. The renal artery is anastomosed to a branch of the hypogastric artery and the renal vein to the external iliac vein.
4. The ureter, depending on its length, may be implanted into the bladder directly, by a tunneling technique, or it may be anastomosed to the recipient ureter. A cystostomy tube may be inserted into the bladder.

(*Note:* Bilateral nephrectomies and splenectomy may be performed on the recipient at the time of transplant or at another time, depending on the patient's general condition and the surgeon's program of management. This is done to prevent hypertension or urinary tract infection.)

### Reconstructive operations on the ureter

DEFINITIONS AND PURPOSE. *Ureterostomy* (ureterotomy) is opening of the ureter for continued drainage from it into another part.

*Cutaneous ureterostomy* (anastomosis or transplant) is diversion of the flow of urine from the kidney via the ureter away from the bladder onto the skin, usually on the abdomen.

*Ureterectomy* is complete removal of the ureter. This procedure includes nephrectomy, as well as the excision of a cuff of the bladder.

*Ureterolithotomy* is an incision into the ureter and removal of a stone.

*Ureteroureterostomy* is the division of the ureter and reconstruction in continuity with another ureteral segment (Fig. 12-27).

*Ureteroileostomy (ileal conduit)* or *ureterosigmoidostomy* (anastomosis) is the diversion of the ureter into a segment of the ileum (Fig. 12-28) or into the sigmoid colon.

*Ureteroneocystostomy (ureterovesical anastomosis)* is the division of the ureter from the urinary bladder and reimplantation of the ureter into the bladder at another site.

CONSIDERATIONS. Reconstructive operations may be indicated because of a pathological condition of the urinary bladder or lower ureter that interferes with normal drainage. Conditions requiring urinary diversion or reconstruction of the urinary tract include malignancy, cystitis, stricture, trauma, or congenital malformations such as ureteral reflux. Pelvic malignancy or an anomaly requiring removal of the bladder necessitates urinary diversion.

SETUP AND PREPARATION OF THE PATIENT. The site of incision and position of the patient will depend on the indications for surgery and the nature of the proposed reconstruction or anastomosis. The patient may

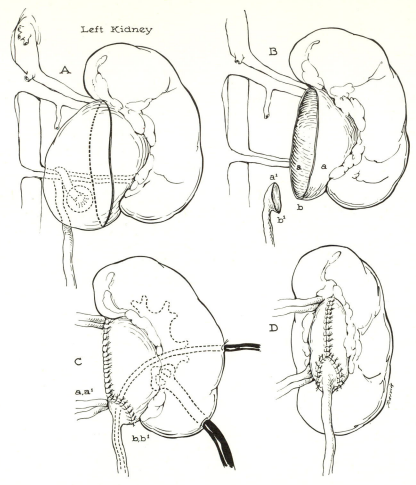

**Fig. 12-27.** Technique of reimplantation of ureter at kidney pelvis. Correction of ureteral obstruction by aberrant vessels that cannot be divided without producing muscular renal damage. **A,** Outline of proposed pelvic (ureteral) cuff and extent of redundant pelvic wall resection. **B,** Ureter, with its funneled end, is brought approximated to dependent part of resected pelvic wall ($a^1$ to **aa** and $b^1$ to **b**). **C** and **D,** Anastomosis completed. Nephrostomy drainage and ureteral splint may be inserted. (From Smith, D. R., Schulte, J. W., and Smart, W. R.: In Campbell, M. F., editor: Urology, ed. 2, Philadelphia, 1963, W. B. Saunders Co.)

be placed in a supine position for an abdominal approach or in a modified Trendelenburg position for a low abdominal or pelvic incision. The patient may also be placed in a lateral position for high ureteral stones.

Instruments include the nephrectomy setup with the instrumentation for pyeloplasty and the Mason-Judd bladder retractor added. Other items may be required, depending on the type of operation and the surgical approach used.

**OPERATIVE PROCEDURE**

FOR URETERAL ANASTOMOSIS

1. The ureter is exposed through the desired incision. A ureteral catheter, passed retrograde, may be used to facilitate identification and isolation of the ureter. The ureter is identified and dissected free, using long forceps and scissors.

2. The ureter is picked up with fine traction sutures, freed from the surrounding tissues, and severed at the desired level.

*Text continued on p. 438.*

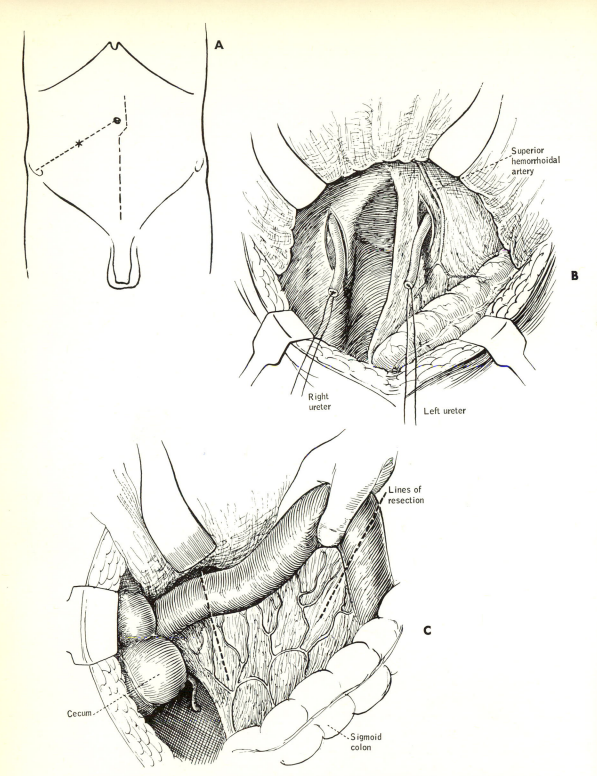

Fig. 12-28. Major steps of operation for ileal conduit, urinary diversion. **A**, Location of ileal stoma. **B**, Ureters freed. Left ureter brought under base of mesosigmoid. **C**, Location of ileal segment. **D**, Closure of proximal end of segment. **E**, Anastomosis of severed ends of ileum. **F**, Closure of opening at base of mesentery of segment showing transverse approximation. **G**, Preparation of stoma. **H**, Ureteroileal anastomosis. **I**, Fixation of segment, obliteration of mesenteric openings. **J**, Completed segment. (From Cordonnier, J. J.: In Campbell, M. F., editor: Urology, ed. 2, Philadelphia, 1963, W. B. Saunders Co.)

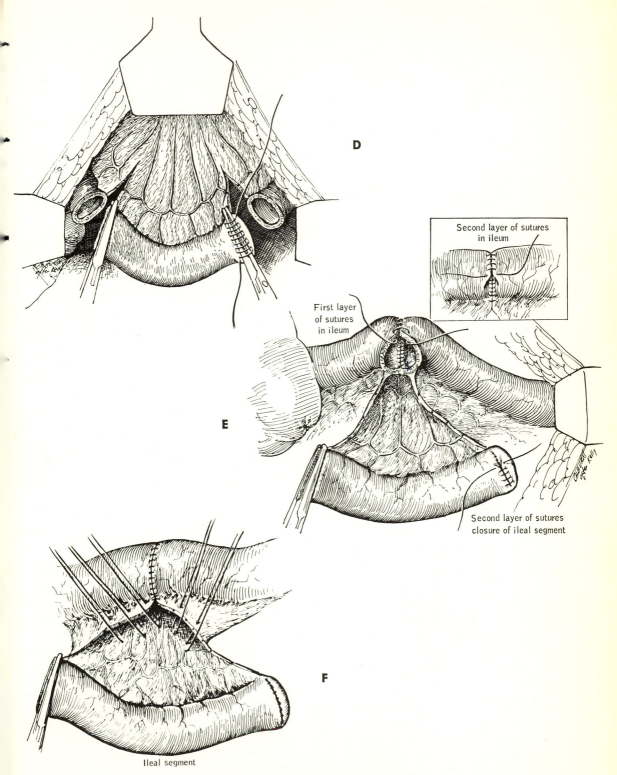

**D**

Second layer of sutures in ileum

First layer of sutures in ileum

**E**

Second layer of sutures closure of ileal segment

**F**

Ileal segment

**Fig. 12-28, cont'd.** For legend see opposite page.

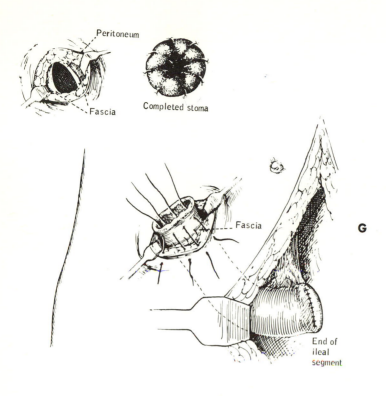

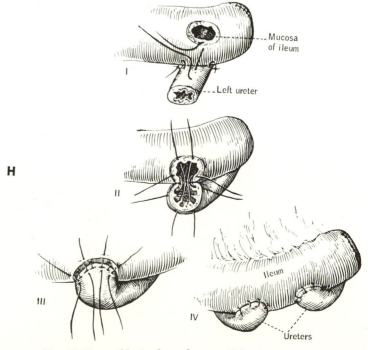

**Fig. 12-28, cont'd.** For legend see p. 434.

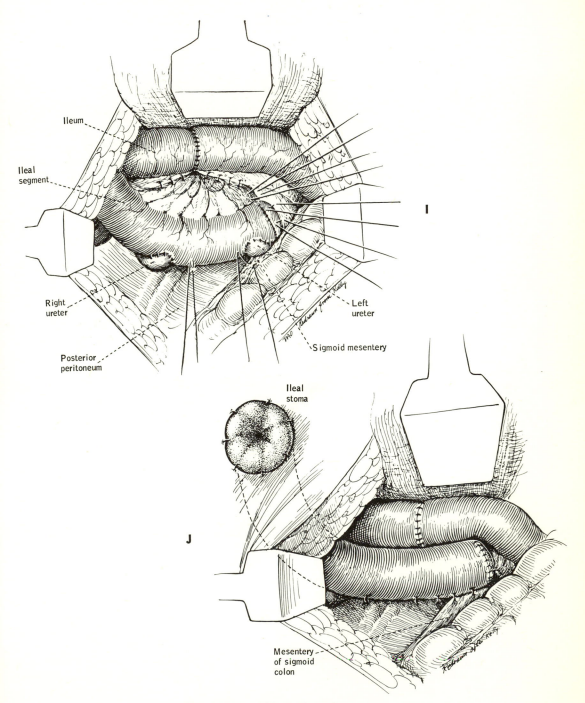

**Fig. 12-28, cont'd.** For legend see p. 434.

3. The distal end of the ureter is ligated, and the proximal stoma is transferred to the site of anastomosis. The anastomosis is accomplished with fine dissection instruments and fine swaged-on sutures.

4. A soft splinting catheter is usually left in place until healing has taken place and free drainage is assured.

5. The wound is closed in layers and dressed in the routine manner.

FOR URETEROLITHOTOMY. The patient usually has a kidney, ureter, and bladder x-ray examination immediately before surgery to determine the exact location of the stone. The surgeon may also schedule a cystoscopic examination preoperatively and may attempt to manipulate the stone through the ureter.

The position of the stone determines the surgical approach. A stone high in the ureter will require a flank incision, whereas one closer to the bladder will require an abdominal incision. Both of these have been described previously. The incision into the ureter is made with a small surgical blade above the stone. The Randall stone forceps will be used to locate and remove the stone. The ureter may be closed with fine chromic gut sutures no. 4-0, or it may be left open and the site drained well. Either of the approaches requires minimal routine closure, as already described.

Ureterocutaneous transplant, ureterosigmoid anastomosis, and ileal segment are all urinary diversion procedures performed when the bladder no longer serves as a proper urine reservoir. The cause may be a congenital disorder, as in the neurogenic bladder, exstrophy, trauma, or tumor.

FOR URETEROCUTANEOUS TRANSPLANT (ANASTOMOSIS). The surgical approach is the same as for a low ureterolithotomy, and the ureter is severed from the bladder. The severed ureter is passed through a stab wound in the flank and sewn to the skin with an everting suture of no. 4-0 chromic gut on an Atraumatic needle to form a stoma. The structures are handled with plastic instruments, fixation forceps, and iris scissors. A small catheter is passed into the ureter and irrigated for patency. The patient must have a urine collecting bag postoperatively.

FOR URETEROSIGMOID ANASTOMOSIS

1. The abdomen and peritoneal cavity are entered in the routine manner through a left rectus incision. A portion of the large bowel is protected with pads. Deep retractors are placed, and with long forceps and scissors the posterior peritoneum is incised.

2. The ureters are severed close to the bladder. The ureter is brought through the posterior peritoneal incision to the sigmoid. Traction sutures and smooth tissue forceps are used to retain and handle the severed ureters.

3. The sigmoid colon is immobilized to prevent traction and tension on the ureter by securing the former to the pelvic peritoneum at a point where the ureter falls easily on the bowel, and a silk no. 3-0 traction stitch is taken. Using a scalpel with blade no. 15, an incision is made through the taenia of the sigmoid muscle layer, separating it from the mucosal layer. A tunnel is created by blunt dissection.

4. The ureter is laid on top of the mucosa, and a small slit is made in the mucosa, using a scalpel with a no. 11 blade.

5. With fixation forceps and iris scissors, the ureter is slit to match the bowel incision. The ureter is anchored to the bowel with no. 4-0 chromic ureteral sutures on Atraumatic needles. The other ureter is anastomosed in the same manner in a position slightly above the first.

6. The posterior peritoneum is closed with fine silk sutures. Drainage is established. The abdominal wound is closed in layers.

FOR ILEAL CONDUIT

1. A urethral catheter is inserted to decompress the bladder, and a rectal tube is placed in the rectum. Before the incision is made, the stoma site is marked on the skin. Through a midline abdominal inci-

sion, the abdomen is entered and the peritoneum incised in the routine manner; abdominal retractors are placed.

2. The ureters are mobilized and brought through the retroperitoneum.

3. The distal ileum and mesentery are inspected to identify the blood supply. A Penrose drain is passed through the mesentery midway between the two main arterial arcades adjacent to the ileum at the proximal and distal ends of the selected segment. This segment usually comprises 6 to 10 inches of the terminal ileum, a few inches from the ileocecal valve (Fig. 12-28).

4. The vessels of the mesentery are ligated. Care is exercised to preserve the ileocecal artery and adequate circulation to the isolated ileal segment. The peritoneum is incised over the proposed line of division of the mesentery. Allen or other intestinal clamps are placed across the ileum, and the bowel is divided flush with the clamps (Fig. 12-28, *D*). Using gastrointestinal technique (Chapter 21), the proximal end of the conduit is closed with a chromic layer of sutures. The remaining ileum is reanastomosed end-to-end (Fig. 12-28, *E*).

5. The mesentery is closed with interrupted silk sutures.

6. The closed proximal end of the conduit segment is fixed to the posterior peritoneum. The ureters are implanted in the ileal segment using plastic technique, with fine instruments and ureteral sutures of chromic no. 4-0 catgut on Atraumatic needles (Fig. 12-28, *G* to *I*). The peritoneum and muscle of the abdominal wall lateral to the original incision is separated by blunt dissection. The distal opening of the ileal conduit is drawn through and sewn to the skin with fine chromic or silk sutures (Fig. 12-28, *J*). The wound is drained, closed, and dressed. An ileostomy bag is placed over the stoma.

The surgeon may do a cystectomy either before or after this procedure. In some cases he may choose to leave the bladder rather than subject a debilitated patient to further surgery. This procedure is discussed later in this chapter.

## ADRENALECTOMY

**DEFINITION.** Partial or total excision of one or both adrenal glands.

**CONSIDERATIONS.** Adrenalectomy may be done to treat hyperfunction of the adrenals, remove tumors of the glands themselves, or treat tumors elsewhere in the body that are affected by adrenal hormonal secretions, such as carcinoma of the prostate and breast.

**SETUP AND PREPARATION OF THE PATIENT.** For unilateral adrenalectomy, the patient may be placed in the lateral kidney or supine position (Chapter 7). More often, however, both glands are explored, and the supine position is selected.

**FOR LATERAL APPROACH.** As described for nephrectomy, with omission of urethral instruments and including rib resection instruments, vascular instruments, and silver clips, magazine, and appliers.

**FOR ABDOMINAL APPROACH.** As described for laparotomy, including vascular instruments, extra long scissors, tissue forceps, Rochester-Pean forceps, Mixter forceps, and needle holders. A Penrose-type tubing is needed for retraction. Silver clips, magazine, and appliers may also be needed. Supply various sizes of silk sutures.

**OPERATIVE PROCEDURE**

**LATERAL APPROACH**

1. An incision curving from the midline and extending from the rib cage to the iliac crest is made with the scalpel through the skin fat and muscle. The lumbodorsal fascia is cut to reveal the sacrospinal muscle. This muscle is detached from the ribs, using forceps and dissecting scissors.

2. The rib is resected (Chapter 14).

3. An opening is made through the transverse fascia with scissors. The pleura and diaphragm are protected with wet pads, and *Gerota's capsule* is incised to expose the kidney and adrenal gland.

4. The gland is dissected free, using scissors and Babcock forceps. The blood supply of the gland is identified, clamped or

clipped, and divided. Bleeding vessels are ligated. To release the glands, the left adrenal vein, a branch of the left renal vein, is separated by clamping and cutting. The right adrenal vein, a tributary of the vena cava, is also divided. Fine vascular sutures may be required to repair inadvertent injury to the vena cava.

5. When hemostasis has been assured, the wound is closed in layers—muscle, fascia, subcutaneous tissue, and skin.

ABDOMINAL APPROACH

1. The abdominal wall is incised, and the peritoneal cavity is opened and explored. Bleeding vessels are clamped and ligated.

2. The abdominal wound is retracted and the surrounding organs protected with laparotomy pads, using instruments and sutures as described for routine laparotomy (Chapter 17).

3. The retroperitoneal area near the diaphragm is opened on the left side, exposing the renal fascia.

4. The renal fascia is opened to reveal the left kidney and adrenal gland.

5. The adrenal gland is freed from the kidney by sharp and blunt dissection, clamping and ligating all bleeding vessels with silk sutures no. 3-0.

6. After all bleeding is controlled, the kidney is gently replaced in the renal fascia, which is closed with interrupted chromic sutures no. 0.

7. The peritoneum is closed over the left kidney and renal fascia.

8. The abdominal retractors are rearranged to give access to the peritoneum over the right kidney and adrenal gland. Care must be taken here to avoid trauma to the liver.

9. The right retroperitoneal space is opened to reveal the renal fascia.

10. The renal fascia is opened, exposing the right kidney and adrenal gland.

11. The adrenal gland is freed in the same manner as the left one and excised.

12. The right kidney is replaced in the renal fascia, which is sutured closed.

13. The right retroperitoneal area is closed with chromic sutures no. 0.

14. The abdomen is inspected for bleeding vessels, which are ligated.

15. The wound is closed in the routine laparotomy fashion.

## OPEN OPERATIONS ON THE BLADDER

DEFINITIONS AND PURPOSE. *Cystotomy* is a procedure in which the bladder is cut open.

*Cystolithotomy* is a procedure in which the bladder is opened to remove stones.

*Cystostomy* is a procedure in which an opening is made into the bladder for continuous drainage.

*Cystectomy (total)* is a procedure in which the bladder and adjacent structures are excised.

CONSIDERATIONS. The urinary bladder may be opened to remedy acute retention; relieve obstruction and distention; control hemorrhage; remove stones, tumors, or foreign bodies; or repair congenital or traumatic defects.

Radical procedures are done to treat cancer. Total cystectomy requires permanent urinary diversion.

SETUP AND PREPARATION OF THE PATIENT. To facilitate identification and dissection, the bladder is usually drained of urine and filled with a sterile irrigating or antiseptic solution as a part of the preoperative preparation. Equipment and instruments for catheterization and irrigation should be prepared, in addition to the surgical setup. Irrigating solutions should be sterile, isotonic, and at body temperature.

An electrosurgical unit with a cutting and coagulating current may be desired in selected open operations. The surgeon should be consulted regarding preference for cords and electrodes (Fig. 12-13).

The patient lies in the supine position for most open operations on the bladder (Chapter 7). The Trendelenburg position may be desired, since it tilts the pelvis high and offers good visualization of the pelvic organs, including the bladder (Chap-

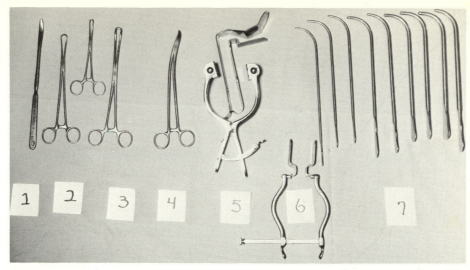

Fig. 12-29. Bladder instruments. 1, Prostatic enucleator; 2, prostatic lobe forceps; 3, Lahey thyroid traction forceps; 4, retropubic (Stratte) needle holder; 5, Millin retropubic bladder retractor; 6, Mason-Judd bladder retractor; 7, Van Buren urethral sounds, sizes 14 to 30 Fr.

ter 7). The patient may be draped with a nonabsorbent disposable skin drape (Chapter 5) and a fenestrated laparotomy sheet.

The basic setup for open bladder operations is a laparotomy set, adding to it the following (Figs. 12-29 and 12-30):

2 Mason-Judd bladder retractors
9 Van Buren urethral sounds, sizes 14 to 30 Fr.
3 Thyroid traction forceps, long
3 Thyroid traction forceps, short
2 Prostatic enucleators
2 Retropubic needle holders or other long needle holders as desired
1 Trocar (optional)
   Penrose-type drain
   Assorted Foley, Mushroom, and Malecot catheters in available sizes
   Catheter stylet
   Electrocautery unit and sterile cord

**Suturing items**

1 Basic needle set
   Plain gut ligatures no. 3-0
   Chromic gut sutures nos. 1, 0, and 2-0 swaged to Atraumatic needles
   Chromic gut ligatures no. 2-0

FOR CYSTOLITHOTOMY ON THE BLADDER. The basic setup for operations on the bladder, plus the following:

2 Millin T-shaped stone forceps
2 Millin capsule forceps
1 Lewkowitz lithotomy forceps

FOR PARTIAL CYSTECTOMY AND REPAIR OF VESICAL FISTULAS. The basic set for open bladder operation is used. When vesicointestinal fistula is present, an intestinal resection setup is necessary (Chapter 21). For vesicovaginal fistula, vaginal preparation and colporrhaphy set (Chapter 18), with colostomy or ileostomy items, is used.

FOR RADICAL CYSTECTOMY AND LYMPHADENECTOMY. Two setups may be required, including a laparotomy setup (Chapter 17) and a perineal prostatectomy setup for the male or a major vaginal plastic repair setup for the female (Chapter 18). For abdominal procedure, 3 Mayo kidney pedicle clamps are added to the open bladder setup.

STERILE SYSTEM FOR BLADDER IRRIGATION. Each hospital has its own system for bladder irrigation. Solutions suitable for this purpose should be specified by the surgeon. The system may consist of prepackaged irrigating solutions and sterile sets of connecting tubing, or it may be a flask, rubber tubing, and connector set such as

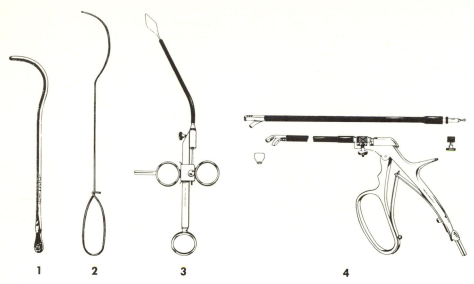

**Fig. 12-30.** Special bladder and urethral instruments. **1,** Guyon urethral sound; **2,** Guyon catheter guide (stylet); **3,** snare; **4,** punch. (Courtesy Codman & Shurtleff, Inc., Randolph, Mass.)

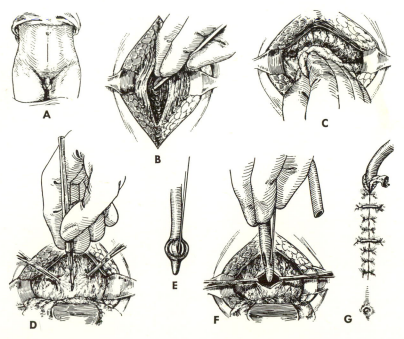

**Fig. 12-31.** Suprapubic cystostomy. **A,** Incision. **B,** Separation of rectus muscle. **C,** Prevesical fascia has been stripped upward on bladder. **D,** Bladder is grasped with two Allis forceps; stab wound is made in bladder, into which catheter is introduced. **E,** Catheter introduced with director. **F,** Straightened catheter. **G,** Wound closed and drained with Penrose tubing. (From Campbell, M. F.: In Campbell, M. F., editor: Urology, ed. 2, Philadelphia, 1963, W. B. Saunders Co.)

the Valentine irrigator (Fig. 12-12), which is prepared and sterilized by the operating room personnel as part of the instrument setup. With the Cotter system, the irrigating fluids are usually mixed and poured by the operating room personnel also. Sterile pitchers or other containers for mixing and pouring will then be needed (Fig. 12-12).

OPERATIVE PROCEDURE (SUPRAPUBIC CYSTOTOMY AND CYSTOSTOMY)

1. The bladder is distended preoperatively, with the prescribed irrigating solution instilled via catheter. A vertical or transverse suprapubic incision is made through the skin and subcutaneous layers to the muscle, using a scalpel, thumb forceps, and scissors. Bleeding vessels are controlled with hemostats and ligated. Wound towels and retractors are placed. The rectus muscle is incised or split by blunt dissection and retracted (Fig. 12-31). The prevesical fat and peritoneum are retracted upward with Deaver retractors.

2. The top of the bladder is dissected free, using thumb forceps and Metzenbaum scissors. The wall of the bladder is grasped on either side of the midline with Allis forceps. Two traction sutures of no. 0 chromic gut may be placed through the bladder wall and held with straight Halsted hemostats. The muscle of the bladder is spread by blunt dissection with the tip of a clamp or scissors until the mucosa is seen. Two Allis clamps are placed, and the bladder is incised with a sharp blade (Fig. 12-31, *A* to *D*). At this point the distended bladder may be emptied via the urethral catheter, which is unclamped under the drapes by the circulating member of the team, or a suction tube may be introduced through the stab wound to remove the fluid as the bladder mucosa is incised.

3. The bladder opening is extended with scissors. Bladder retractors are placed, and the bladder is explored for diverticula, calculi, or tumor. Removal of the pathological area or other corrective procedure is carried out and wound closure begun. A Malecot catheter may be used to drain the bladder suprapubically and a Foley retention catheter to drain through the urethra. The prevesical space may be drained with Penrose tubing (Fig. 12-31, *G*).

4. The bladder is sutured in two layers. A continuous suture of catgut is used on the mucosa and interrupted stitches of chromic catgut on the muscle layer. The abdominal muscle fascia and subcutaneous tissue are closed with catgut. Tension sutures of nylon or silver wire may be needed for some patients. A suture is placed around the cystostomy tube and affixed to the skin. The skin may be closed with silk or stainless steel wire.

5. The wound is dressed with bulky dressings. The wound and cystostomy tube are held in place by adhesive tape strips.

## Trocar cystostomy

DEFINITION. Opening the bladder, drainage by blind puncture with needles or trocar, and insertion of a catheter.

SETUP AND PREPARATION OF THE PATIENT. The minor set of instruments, which includes the following:

**Cutting instruments**
   1 Knife handle no. 4 with blade no. 20
   2 Knife handles no. 3 with blades nos. 11 and 15
   2 Mayo scissors, 6¼ in., straight and curved
   1 Metzenbaum scissors, 7½ in., curved

**Holding instruments**
   4 Towel clamps, 5¼ in.
   4 Towel clamps, 3 in.
   2 Babcock forceps, 6 in.
   2 Tissue forceps with teeth, 5½ in.
   2 Tissue forceps without teeth, 5½ in.
   2 Adson forceps with teeth
   2 Adson forceps without teeth

**Clamping instruments**
   16 Mosquito hemostats, 5½ in., straight and curved
   8 Crile hemostats, 6½ in., straight and curved
   4 Allis forceps, 6½ in.
   4 Ochsner forceps, 6½ in.

**Exposing instruments**
   2 Cushing vein retractors
   2 Green fenestrated retractors, blunt

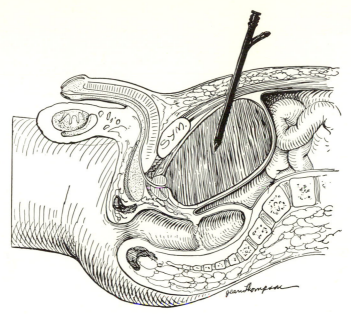

**Fig. 12-32.** Trocar cystostomy. (From Richards, V.: Surgery for general practice, St. Louis, 1956, The C. V. Mosby Co.)

4 Richardson retractors, 2 pair small and medium
2 Army-Navy retractors

**Suturing items**

2 Crile needle holders
Sutures and needles as needed

**Accessory items**

1 Silver probe
1 Grooved director
1 Anthony suction tube and tubing
1 Trocar
Catheters as required

A local anesthesia setup may be used.

**OPERATIVE PROCEDURE.** The skin at the site of the puncture is nicked with the scalpel, and the trocar is inserted into the bladder (Fig. 12-32). The trocar obturator is withdrawn, and a catheter is passed into the bladder over a catheter guide. The cannula is withdrawn, and the catheter is sutured to the wound edges. The wound is dressed.

## Partial cystectomy

**DEFINITION.** Resection of a portion of the bladder with the lesion.

**SETUP AND PREPARATION OF THE PATIENT.** As described for partial cystectomy and repair of vesical fistulas, suprapubic approach, with the patient in a supine position. Or a perineal approach, with the patient in a lithotomy position, may be carried out. Setup will be dependent on the approach selected.

**OPERATIVE PROCEDURE**

1. The bladder and lesion are exposed via suprapubic abdominal, perineal, or vaginal approach. Usually the bladder is opened suprapubically, as described for suprapubic cystostomy.

2. The ureteral orifices are identified and ureteral catheters passed.

3A. The diseased portion of the bladder is excised, using clamps and ligatures of the type required for the organs and tissues involved. Vessels are tied with no. 2-0 plain gut.

3B. *For vesicointestinal fistula,* bowel resection with colostomy or ileostomy may be indicated. *For vesicovaginal fistula,* a vaginal plastic repair is done.

3C. *For diverticulum,* excision of the de-

fect is done intravesically or extravesically.

4. The bladder is drained suprapubically, as well as by an indwelling urethral catheter. Penrose drains may also be placed in the wounds.

## Cystectomy

DEFINITION. Total and radical excision of the urinary bladder.

CONSIDERATIONS. The extent and nature of the excision of the bladder depends on the extent and nature of the pathological area. Total excision is usually carried out if the malignancy has not infiltrated the entire bladder or shown evidence of extension or distant metastasis and if the patient is in condition to withstand the procedure with hope of an appreciable period of relief. More conservative measures may be taken when the tumor is hopelessly advanced or when the pathological area is limited. If a radical procedure is to be done, combined abdominal and perineal approaches may be made.

SETUP AND PREPARATION OF THE PATIENT. As described previously for radical cystectomy and lymphadenectomy. For the male, if the prostate and seminal vesicles are to be removed, add the instruments for prostatectomy to the setup. For the female, add the instruments for major vaginal plastic repair (Chapter 18).

OPERATIVE PROCEDURE (SUPRAPUBIC APPROACH)

1. The bladder is approached as for cystostomy.

2. Deep retractors and laparotomy pads are used to retract the peritoneum. Long tissue forceps, stick sponges, and long scissors are used for dissection. Long hemostats or right-angled clamps are placed across the major vessels and ureters. Suture ligatures of no. 2-0 chromic gut are placed and the structures divided. Large pedicle or intestinal clamps are placed across the urachus and its vessels anterior to the bladder. The structures are ligated and divided by sharp dissection.

3. In the male the bladder is lifted up, using long Allis forceps. The peritoneum is dissected free from the bladder. The bladder is retracted to expose the vesicle neck. The bladder is dissected from the prostate and the vas deferens ligated. A large pedicle or intestinal clamp is placed across the urethra and ligated with no. 2-0 chromic sutures. The urethra is divided and the specimen removed.

4. The seminal vesicles are removed with the bladder. Ureteral transplant is performed if not done previously.

5. Penrose drains are placed in the suprapubic wound, which is closed in layers with no. 0 chromic interrupted sutures. Silver wire or nylon tension sutures may be placed. The skin is sutured with silk no. 3-0 or steel wire gauge 35. The abdominal and perineal wounds are dressed.

(*Note:* In the female, cystectomy will depend on the extent and nature of the pathological lesion. A vaginal approach may be used and then, via the abdominal approach, lymphadenectomy and pelvic exenteration completed [see Chapters 17 and 18].)

## Bladder neck operation (Y-V-plasty)

DEFINITION. Plastic repair of the bladder neck.

CONSIDERATIONS. A Y-V-plasty is done to overcome contracture of the bladder neck due to primary or secondary stricture.

SETUP AND PREPARATION OF THE PATIENT. The patient lies in the modified Trendelenburg position.

The instrument setup is as listed previously for operations on the ureters.

OPERATIVE PROCEDURE

1. The bladder is approached as for cystostomy. The prevesical fat is removed, using long forceps and dissecting scissors. With a right-angled clamp the vessels over the bladder neck are occluded, ligated with no. 2-0 plain gut, and divided. The self-retaining bladder retractor is placed.

2. Traction sutures of fine silk on small, fine, cutting-edge needles (cleft palate–type) are placed at the base and on either side of the urethra to start the pattern for the plastic dissection.

3. With the aid of the traction sutures and an Allis forceps, the Y is incised through all layers as evenly as possible, using sharp-pointed scissors. Bleeding vessels in the wall of the bladder and bladder neck are ligated with plain no. 2-0 gut on small Ferguson needles. The V flap is folded free, and the length of the Y arm is determined with a caliper and ruler.

4. The apex of the V is brought to the neck of the bladder to overcome the stricture and broaden the outlet. A catheter is placed in the urethra to guide the needle and prevent the suture from penetrating the urethral mucosa. A stitch of chromic no. 2-0 suture is taken through the apex of the V under the urethra to the base of the Y and tied. The closure of the plastic repair is completed with mattress suture of no. 2-0 chromic on Atraumatic needles.

5. A cystostomy tube is placed in the bladder, and the bladder and abdominal wall are closed in the usual manner for cystostomy.

### Vesical-urethral suspension (Marshall-Marchetti operation)

DEFINITION. Suspension of the bladder neck to the posterior surface of the pubis in the female patient for treatment of stress incontinence.

SETUP AND PREPARATION OF THE PATIENT. The patient is usually placed in a supine position with Trendelenburg modification, but the surgeon may prefer a frog-leg modification and vaginal preparation with the insertion of a Foley catheter. The basic laparotomy set is used, and the following instruments are added:

Mason-Judd bladder retractor
Extra-long needle holders, retropubic needle holders, or Heaney needle holders
Chromic gut sutures nos. 0 or 1 swaged to ⅝-circle needles

OPERATIVE PROCEDURE

1. A suprapubic incision is made to expose the prevesical space of Retzius. The bladder and urethra are separated from the posterior surface of the rectus muscles and pubis by gentle, blunt dissection.

2. Heavy chromic sutures are placed on each side of the urethra and then also sewn to the periosteum and cartilage on the posterior side of the pubis.

3. The outside of the bladder wall is then sutured with chromic gut suture to the rectus muscle to further suspend the urethra and bladder.

4. The area is drained, and the wound is closed in layers.

## OPEN OPERATIONS ON THE PROSTATE
### Suprapubic prostatectomy with cystostomy

DEFINITION. Enucleation of the prostatic adenomas or hypertrophied masses via a suprapubic approach.

CONSIDERATIONS. As the male ages, the prostate gland enlarges and gradually obstructs the urethra, giving rise to symptoms of urinary obstruction. The enlargement may be benign or malignant. In benign hypertrophy only the periurethral portion of the gland is removed (Figs. 12-8 and 12-10).

Total or radical prostatectomy involving excision of the entire gland and its capsule, together with associated structures, a portion of the trigone of the bladder, and the seminal vesicles, may be required in the case of malignancy (Fig. 12-11).

SETUP AND PREPARATION OF THE PATIENT. The patient is placed in the supine or modified Trendelenburg position, with the legs apart and the weight of the torso supported by shoulder braces (Chapter 7). Routine skin preparation is carried out (Chapter 4).

An O'Connor drape may be fanfolded at the pubis, with the penis exposed through the fenestration and the finger cot in the rectum. A towel folded lengthwise is placed over the fanfolded drape at the pubic level, and a fenestrated laparotomy sheet is used at the site of the suprapubic incision (Chapter 5).

The instrument setup is as listed in the basic set for operation on the bladder. For *suprapubic and retropubic prosta-*

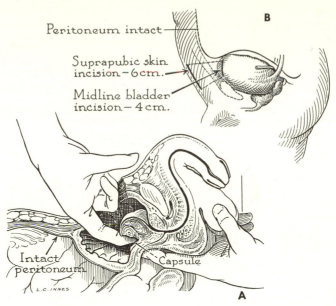

Fig. 12-33. Enucleation of prostate by suprapubic approach. (From Barnes, R. W., and Hadley, H. L.: Urological practice, St. Louis, 1954, The C. V. Mosby Co.)

*tectomy* the basic instrument setup for bladder operations is also used.

### OPERATIVE PROCEDURE

1. The bladder is distended via catheter irrigation, as for cystotomy. Vasectomy is frequently done as a preliminary procedure to prevent postoperative epididymitis.

2. The bladder is approached through the routine cystotomy incision, and the top of the bladder is dissected free, using long thumb forceps and Metzenbaum scissors (Fig. 12-31, *A* to *C* ).

3. The wall of the bladder is grasped on each side of the midline with Allis forceps (Fig. 12-31, *D* ). Two traction sutures of chromic gut no. 0 on Ferguson no. 12 needles may be placed through the wall of the bladder at this point and retained on straight hemostats.

4. The muscle layers of the bladder are spread by blunt dissection with a hemostat until the mucosa is exposed. Allis forceps are placed on either side, and the bladder is incised, using a scalpel with a no. 10 blade. The opening is extended with scissors. Bladder retractors—either

long-bladed loops or self-retaining type— are placed, and the bladder is explored.

5. The surgeon places the forefinger of one hand into the rectum via the finger cot in the O'Connor drape and pushes the prostate gland forward. With the forefinger of the operating hand, the lobes of the gland are enucleated from the capsule (Fig. 12-33). Bleeding is controlled with hemostats and ligatures, sutures, or electrocoagulation. Long forceps, half-length sutures, and long needle holders are required for placing sutures.

6. Following removal of the prostate and control of bleeding, a hemostatic catheter with an inflatable bag—Foley 24 Fr. with a 30 ml. bag—may be placed in the fossa (Fig. 12-34); the balloon is adjusted under direct vision and inflated, using sterile water in a 30 ml. syringe with an adapter. A hemostatic cone of Gelfoam may be used if preferred.

7. The bladder is closed as for suprapubic cystostomy with a Malecot catheter in place. One or two wide Penrose drains may be placed in the prevesical space of

Retzius. The wound is closed in layers and dressed.

## Retropubic prostatectomy

**DEFINITION.** Enucleation of the prostatic hypertrophied lobes directly through a cap-sular incision in the upper surface of the prostate rather than through the bladder.

**SETUP AND PREPARATION OF THE PATIENT.** As described for suprapubic prostatectomy, plus a Millin bladder retractor.

**OPERATIVE PROCEDURE**

1. Through a vertical or transverse su-prapubic incision, the abdominal wall is opened to expose the space of Retzius. The bladder is not directly opened. The precystic fat is extracted, using long, smooth tissue forceps. Large vessels are ligated, using 18-inch transfixion sutures of chromic gut no. 0 threaded on small Mayo needles.

2. The prostatic capsule is incised trans-versely, using a no. 7 scalpel with a no. 10 blade. The prostate is freed and enucleated, employing scissors and Allis forceps (Fig. 12-35). Deep bleeding ves-sels are clamped with long hemostats and ligated with long plain gut no. 2-0 or 3-0 sutures with medium curved taper point Atraumatic needles.

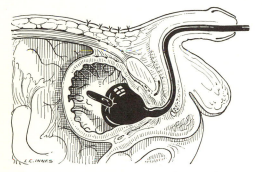

**Fig. 12-34.** Hemostatic bag (Foley), which can be deflated and removed through urethra. It is used following most prostatectomies by any ap-proach. (From Barnes, R. W., and Hadley, H. L.: Urological practice, St. Louis, 1954, The C. V. Mosby Co.)

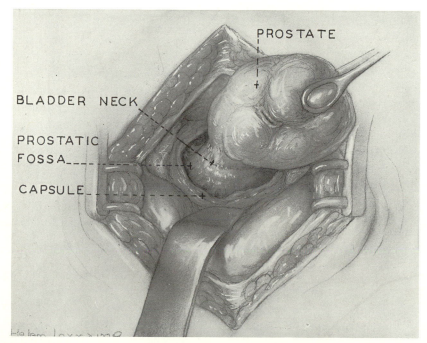

**Fig. 12-35.** Retropubic prostatectomy. Prostate ready to be liberated from prostatic fossa, which is exposed through incision made just below umbilicus and extending downward over symphysis pubis or through Pfannenstiel incision. (From Dodson, A. I.: Urological surgery, ed. 3, St. Louis, 1956, The C. V. Mosby Co.)

3. A wedge excision of the posterior bladder neck is made, using long Allis forceps, a long scalpel, and scissors. A wedge of tissue may be sutured over the defect in the bladder neck after removal of the prostate. In radical prostatectomy a V-shaped portion of the bladder mucosa may be sutured over the defect in the bladder neck.

4. A multieyed Robinson or Foley retention catheter is placed via the urethra. A Malecot cystostomy tube may be placed in the bladder if the surgeon desires.

5. The incision in the prostatic capsule is closed with a continuous suture of chromic gut no. 0. Penrose drains are placed in the retropubic space, the abdominal incision is closed in layers (Chapter 17), and the wound is dressed.

### Perineal prostatectomy

**DEFINITION.** Through perineal exposure the two types of prostatectomy may be carried out: the enucleation of adenomas or radical prostatectomy.

**CONSIDERATIONS.** Radical perineal excision for carcinoma involves removal of the entire gland, its capsule, a portion of the bladder, and the seminal vesicles.

**SETUP AND PREPARATION OF THE PATIENT.** The patient is placed on the operating table in an extreme lithotomy position (Fig. 7-13). The buttocks are elevated on pads sufficient to tilt the pelvis and flatten the perineum on the vertical plane. The thighs are fully flexed with the knees to the chest, and the feet are supported in stirrups (Chapter 7). The arms are extended on armboards and shoulder braces applied with the usual precautions. Measures must be taken to reduce strain on the muscles and nerves of the back and legs and also prevent respiratory embarrassment from compression of the abdomen and chest.

The perineal structures are cleansed, and the patient may be draped with an O'Connor drape folded and secured in place below the line of incision. The patient is also draped with a perineal sheet (Fig. 12-12).

The instrument setup is as described previously for suprapubic prostatectomy, omitting abdominal self-retaining retractors and adding the following (Fig. 12-36):

1 Prostatic enucleator
2 Prostatic lateral retractors
2 Prostatic anterior retractors
1 Prostatic bifurcated retractor (optional)
1 Electrosurgical unit and suitable electrodes (Fig. 12-13)
1 Lowsley tractor, curved
1 Lowsley tractor, straight

**OPERATIVE PROCEDURE** (Fig. 12-37)

1. Through a curved incision made just above the anal margin, the skin, fat, and

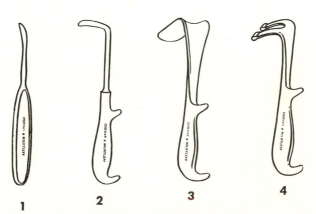

Fig. 12-36. Young perineal prostatic instruments. 1, Prostatic enucleator; 2, prostatic lateral retractor; 3, prostatic anterior retractor; 4, prostatic bifurcated retractor. Instruments shown are one third actual size. (Courtesy Codman & Shurtleff, Inc., Randolph, Mass.)

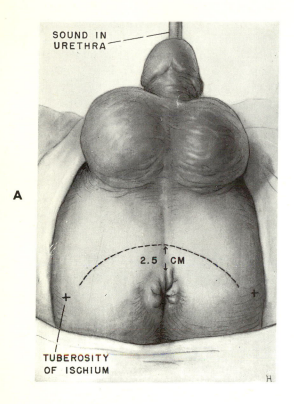

A

SOUND IN
URETHRA

2.5 CM

TUBEROSITY
OF ISCHIUM

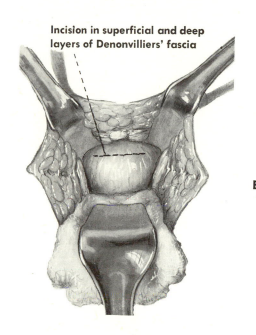

B

Incision in superficial and deep
layers of Denonvilliers' fascia

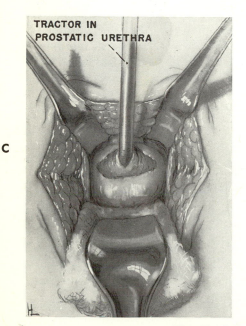

C

TRACTOR IN
PROSTATIC URETHRA

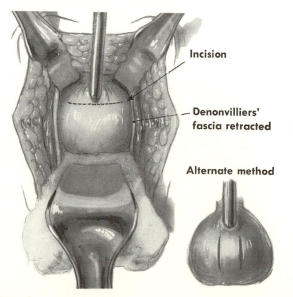

D

Incision

Denonvilliers'
fascia retracted

Alternate method

Fig. 12-37. For legend see opposite page.

E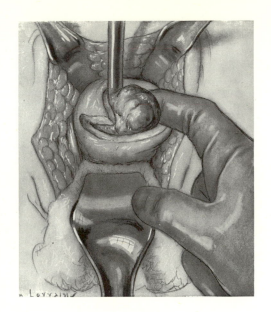

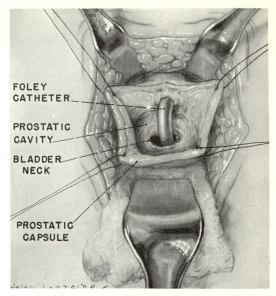 F

FOLEY
CATHETER

PROSTATIC
CAVITY

BLADDER
NECK

PROSTATIC
CAPSULE

G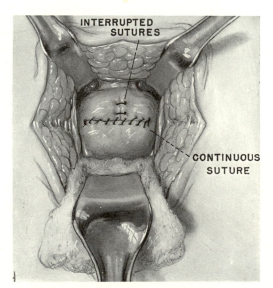

INTERRUPTED
SUTURES

CONTINUOUS
SUTURE

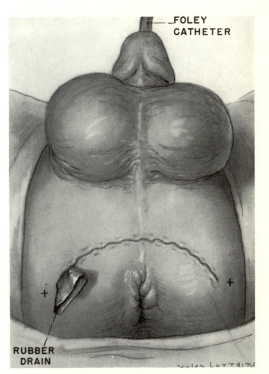 H

FOLEY
CATHETER

RUBBER
DRAIN

**Fig. 12-37.** Perineal prostatectomy. **A,** Proposed incisional site. **B,** Rectourethral muscle has been incised and pushed downward from central tendon, and levator ani muscles on each side have been divided; incision in superficial and deep layers of Denonvilliers' fascia is shown. **C,** Urethrotomy in prostatic urethra. **D,** Incision in prostatic capsule. **E,** Enucleating entire prostate with aid of finger. **F,** Catheter in urethra and bladder, exposure of prostatic bed. **G,** Closure of inverted-т incisions. **H,** Closure of perineal wounds. (From Dodson, A. I.: Urological surgery, ed. 3, St. Louis, 1956, The C. V. Mosby Co.)

subcutaneous fascia are divided (Fig. 12-37, *A*). Straight hemostats are used for bleeding vessels in the superficial tissues and curved hemostats for deeper tissues (Fig. 12-37, *B*). The tissue on either side of the central tendon is dissected, using Metzenbaum scissors and forceps. McBurney retractors followed by Young bifurcated prostatectomy retractors are placed as dissection progresses. The levator ani muscles are exposed and retracted.

2. The gland is exposed and enucleated, as shown in Fig. 12-37, *E*. The surgeon manipulates the gland with a finger in the rectum via the O'Connor drape finger cot or with the hand protected by a second glove.

3. Bleeding is controlled with sutures and electrocautery. A multieyed Robinson or Foley retention catheter is inserted into the urethra. In radical prostatectomy, the bladder neck is approximated to the urethra to cover the defect of the excision.

4. A Penrose drain is placed in the wound. The wound is closed in layers with chromic no. 0 gut sutures with swaged-on medium Ferguson no. 14 needles. The skin edges are approximated with interrupted sutures on straight needles.

(*Note:* Transurethral resection of prostatic tumor is described later in this chapter [Figs. 12-57 and 12-58].)

## OPERATIONS ON THE SCROTUM
### Hydrocelectomy

DEFINITION. Excision of the tunica vaginalis of the testis to remove the fluid-filled sac.

CONSIDERATIONS. A hydrocele is an abnormal accumulation of fluid within the scrotum around the capsule of the testis and the tunica vaginalis. Excessive secretion or accumulation may be due to infection or trauma.

SETUP AND PREPARATION OF THE PATIENT. The patient is placed in supine position (Chapter 7). Preparation and draping of the patient include routine cleansing of the external genitalia and draping of the patient with a fenestrated sheet. The minor basic instrument setup is needed, including a small Penrose drain, 30 ml. syringe, 20-gauge, 2-inch aspirating needle, and suspensory dressing.

OPERATIVE PROCEDURE

1. An anterolateral incision is made in the skin of the scrotum over the hydrocele mass, using a scalpel with a no. 2-0 blade. Bleeding is controlled with Crile hemostats and vessels ligated with no. 3-0 plain gut ligatures (Fig. 12-38).

2. Small retractors may be placed, and then the fascial layers are incised to expose the testis and tunica vaginalis. With fine scissors and forceps, the sac is delivered and dissected free (Fig. 12-38, *B* and *C*). The hydrocele may be aspirated. The adherent tunica vaginalis is separated from the internal fascia layers and the sac opened. When the tunica vaginalis has been trimmed as desired, the testis is returned to the scrotal sac.

3. A Penrose drain is placed, and the wound is closed in layers with Atraumatic sutures of plain gut no. 3-0 on curved cutting needles. The wound is dressed, and a supportive sling dressing or suspensory is usually applied.

### Vasectomy

DEFINITION. Excision of a section of the vas deferens.

CONSIDERATIONS. Vas ligation or vasectomy involves interruption of the vas deferens (Fig. 12-10). The operation is performed electively as a permanent method of sterilization or birth control and also prior to prostatectomy to prevent spread of infection from the urethra to the epididymis.

SETUP AND PREPARATION OF THE PATIENT. The patient usually lies in the dorsal supine position, although the operation can be done in the lithotomy position prior to transurethral surgery. This procedure may be done under local or general anesthesia. A minor instrument setup and collodion dressing or a suspensory is needed.

OPERATIVE PROCEDURE

1. The vas is located by palpation in the upper part of the scrotum. A small

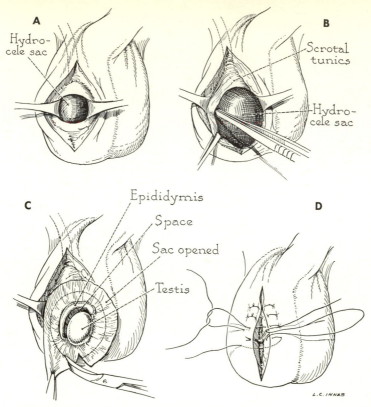

**Fig. 12-38. Hydrocelectomy. A,** Incision through anterior scrotum, exposing hydrocele sac. Characteristic dark blue shiny appearance of tunica vaginalis, which is sac wall, is due to deep shadow within sac. **B,** Hydrocele sac enucleated and removed from scrotum. It is left attached to groin by spermatic cord. **C,** Sac opened and excised from testis. **D,** Skin edges and subcuticular tissues approximated with single mattress sutures of no. 3-0 plain catgut. (From Barnes, R. W., and Hadley, H. L.: Urological practice, St. Louis, 1954, The C. V. Mosby Co.)

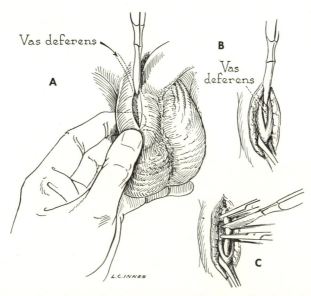

**Fig. 12-39. Vasectomy (vas ligation). A,** Vas grasped between thumb in front and first and second fingers behind. Incision 2 cm. long is made over vas. **B,** Vas grasped with Allis clamp and incision deepened into it. **C,** Vas clamped with two hemostats and incised between them. (From Barnes, R. W., and Hadley, H. L.: Urological practice, St. Louis, 1964, The C. V. Mosby Co.)

incision is made in the skin over the vas (Fig. 12-39).

2. An Allis forceps is inserted to grasp the vas and bring it to the surface of the wound. The vas is denuded of surrounding tissues of the cord, and straight clamps are placed on either side of the Allis to crush the vas.

3. The vas is cut between the clamps and a section removed. The cut ends are ligated with silk or cotton no. 3-0.

4. The clamps are removed, and the skin incision is closed with plain gut no. 3-0 on a needle. A collodion dressing and scrotal suspensory may be applied.

## Epididymectomy

**DEFINITION.** Excision of the epididymis from the testis.

**CONSIDERATIONS.** This operation is rarely done but may be indicated to treat persistent infection.

**SETUP AND PREPARATION OF THE PATIENT.** As described for hydrocelectomy, plus an electrosurgical unit with cutting and coagulation electrodes, if desired.

**OPERATIVE PROCEDURE.** Incision is made over the testis in the scrotum to expose the tunica vaginalis. This is incised to expose the testis and overlying epididymis. An incision is made between the upper pole of the epididymis, which is then carefully freed from the testis. Bleeding is controlled and the wound closed with fine sutures and small drain.

## Spermatocelectomy

**DEFINITION AND PURPOSE.** Removal of a spermatocele, which usually appears as a lobulated cystic mass within the scrotum attached to the upper pole of the epididymis.

**CONSIDERATIONS.** This condition is usually caused by an obstruction of the tubular system that conveys the sperm. An epididymovasostomy may be attempted after excision of the mass to maintain the system.

**SETUP AND PREPARATION OF THE PATIENT.** As described for hydrocelectomy as listed

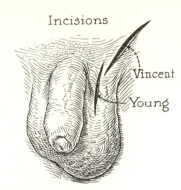

**Fig. 12-40.** Types and location of optional incisions commonly used for varicocelectomy. (From Manual of operative procedure, Somerville, N. J., 1950, Ethicon, Inc.)

previously, plus items for testing patency of anastomosis, if performed.

1 Syringe, 10 ml.
1 Needle, blunt, no. 20
Methylene blue solution
Hydrogen peroxide
Polyethylene tubing, 20 Fr., or other size as desired
Silkworm gut or fine wire
Chromic gut sutures, no. 4-0 or 5-0, on fine plastic curved needles
Lead shot
Isotonic saline solution
Microscope and slides, if desired

**OPERATIVE PROCEDURE**

1. The mass is approached through a scrotal incision as for hydrocelectomy (Fig. 12-38), or varicocelectomy (Fig. 12-40).

2. The structures of the testis and spermatic cord are identified (Fig. 12-10), and the cyst is dissected free. Bleeding is controlled with clamps and ligatures in routine fashion.

3. The wound is closed and dressed as described for hydrocelectomy.

## Varicocelectomy

**DEFINITION.** Ligation and partial excision of dilated veins in the scrotum.

**CONSIDERATIONS.** This operation is done to reduce congestion of the testes and to improve spermatogenic function. Previous-

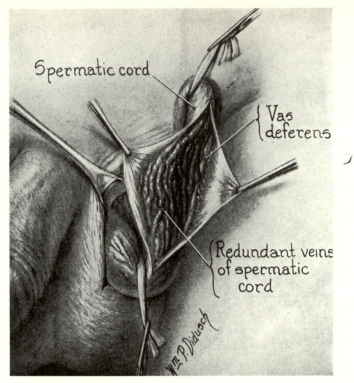

Fig. 12-41. Varicocele. Redundant veins of spermatic cord can be seen in relation to vas deferens through inguinal incision in elevation of external oblique flaps and freeing of spermatic cord. (From Aberhart, C.: In Campbell, M. F., editor: Urology, ed. 2, Philadelphia, 1963, W. B. Saunders Co.)

ly, the veins of the pampiniform plexuses were ligated and divided individually.

This condition occurs more frequently on the left, since the vein of the left testis connecting with the renal vein is under greater pressure. The veins of the pampiniform plexuses of the spermatic cord become tortuous and engorged, resembling a bag of redundant veins.

**SETUP AND PREPARATION OF THE PATIENT.** As described for hydrocelectomy.

**OPERATIVE PROCEDURE**

1. The incision may be made low in the inguinal canal or in the upper portion of the scrotum (Fig. 12-40). The structures of the spermatic cord are identified and the vessels dissected free from the vas deferens.

2. The abnormal vessels in the inguinal canal are clamped and ligated (Fig. 12-41). The redundant portions are excised. The remaining structures are sutured to the external oblique fascia above the external inguinal ring to support the testicle.

3. A Penrose drain may be placed. The incision is closed in layers.

## Orchiectomy

**DEFINITION.** Removal of the testis or testes.

**CONSIDERATIONS.** Removal of both testes is castration and renders the patient both sterile and deficient in male hormones. Because of the social implications, this operation, like vasectomy, requires particular attention to legal permission. Bilateral orchiectomy is usually performed to control carcinoma of the prostate. A unilateral orchiectomy may be indicated because of cancer, trauma, or infection. In benign conditions, a prosthesis may be implanted for cosmetic or psychological reasons. Prostheses are usually made of silicone rubber.

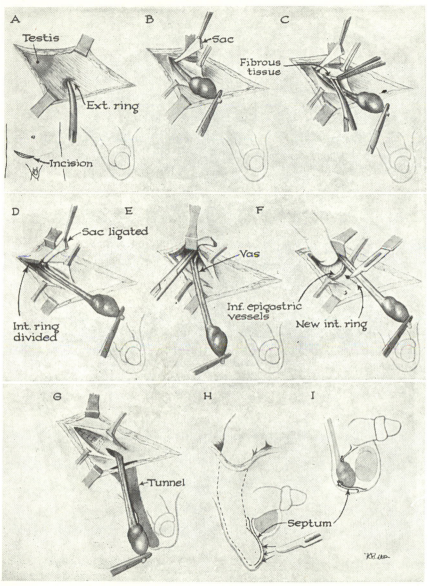

**Fig. 12-42.** Orchiopexy (operative repair for management of undescended testicle). **A,** Transverse incision at level of internal inguinal ring. **B,** Inguinal canal opened and hernial sac, if present, dissected from cord structures. **C,** Fibrous tissue on cord structures carefully removed. **D,** Hernial sac is suture-ligated. Muscles are divided laterally to the internal ring. **E,** Peritoneum is held forward with a retractor as vessels are carefully dissected from back side of posterior peritoneum as far as can be reached with long forceps and dissecting scissors. **F,** Space behind posterior wall of inguinal canal is bluntly dissected with finger. Incision is made through this at level of external inguinal ring. **G,** Testis is brought through this incision. Structures lateral to internal ring are closed. **H,** Scrotum is bluntly dissected, and incision made through skin of opposite side of scrotum and then through septum. **I,** Testis is brought through septum to its opposite side and secured with sutures to remaining divided septum. Skin wound of scrotum is closed with interrupted plain gut no. 3-0 or 4-0 sutures. (From Bill, A. H., Jr., and Shanahan, D. A.: Surg. Clin. North Am. 44:1571, 1964.)

SETUP AND PREPARATION OF THE PATIENT. The patient is placed in the supine position. A minor instrument setup is used, prosthesis if specified, and a fenestrated sheet.

OPERATIVE PROCEDURE

1. The upper anterior surface of the scrotum is incised over the testicle. The incision is carried through the skin and fascial layers to expose the tunica vaginalis. Retractors are placed and bleeding vessels clamped and tied.

2. The tunica vaginalis is grasped and mobilized. The spermatic cord is dissected free up to the external abdominal ring, clamped, and ligated. The testis is removed. Bleeding is controlled. A small Penrose drain may be placed in the wound. Fine sutures of plain gut no. 3-0 or nylon no. 4-0 are used to close the wound.

## Orchiopexy

DEFINITION. Suspension of the testis within the scrotum.

CONSIDERATIONS. An undescended or cryptorchid testis is located elsewhere than the normal intrascrotal position. A retractile testis is one that has descended through the inguinal canal but lies either within or superficial to the external ring. An ectopic testis is one that has descended through the canal and rests in an abnormal position (the perineal femoral area or lateral to the canal).

The primary goal of orchiopexy in young boys is to obtain adequate length of the spermatic vessels and the vas to allow the testis to lie in the scrotum.

SETUP AND PREPARATION OF THE PATIENT. As described for hydrocelectomy. Preparation and draping include the lower abdomen, genitalia, and thighs. Since this operation is usually performed on children, a pediatric setup consisting of *small delicate* instruments and sutures suitable to structures involved is required.

OPERATIVE PROCEDURE (TRANSVERSE INGUINAL APPROACH)

1. The major steps of Bill's technique for orchiopexy are illustrated in Fig. 12-42.

2. The reconstruction of the muscle closure of both the internal ring and the external oblique is accomplished, using fine interrupted silk or chromic sutures.

3. The subcutaneous tissue and skin are closed with fine sutures, as desired.

(*Note:* These operations may be done in two or more stages.)

# OPERATIONS ON THE PENIS AND URETHRA
## Hypospadias repair

DEFINITION. Penile straightening and urethral reconstruction (urethroplasty), usually done in two or more stages (Figs. 12-43 and 12-44 and Chapter 10).

CONSIDERATIONS. *Hypospadias* is a deformity of the penis and malformation of the urethral wall in which the urinary meatus is located on the underside of the penis, either short of its normal position at the tip of the glans or on the perineum or scrotum. This condition is often associated with chordee.

*Chordee* is a downward bowing of the penis due to the congenital malformation of hypospadias with fibrous bands.

*Epispadias* is the condition in which the urethral meatus is situated in an abnormal position on the upper side of the penis.

Because of the multiple deformities, correction of the conditions is usually accomplished in several stages, allowing several months to elapse between each operation.

The purpose of the various techniques followed is to provide a straight penis and to establish an effective urethral orifice. Many different techniques are employed.

SETUP AND PREPARATION OF THE PATIENT. The patient lies in the supine lithotomy position. Children are maintained in the frog-leg position by strapping the thighs apart and flexing the knees (Chapter 7).

The instrument setup includes a minor dissecting set with plastic instruments, as well as sutures, catheters, drains as desired, and the following.

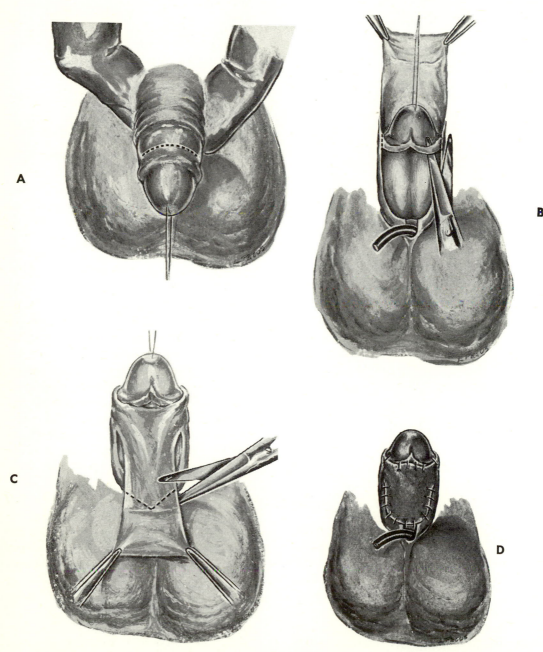

**Fig. 12-43.** Chordee repair. **A,** Transverse dorsal incision line through reflected layer of prepuce behind corona. **B,** Dorsal quadrilateral flap, with narrow bands of skin about to be divided. **C,** Penis threaded through buttonhole and ventral flap about to be trimmed to required size. **D,** Preputial flap now sutured into position to cover extensive raw area on ventral surface of penis. (From Fraser, Sir K.: Br. J. Surg. **51**:167, 1964.)

Urethral sounds, 14 and 16 Fr.
Retention sutures, nonabsorbable
Paraffin gauze dressing strips
Occlusive dressing
Nonallergenic adhesive tape

### OPERATIVE PROCEDURES

#### CHORDEE REPAIR (FRASER OR NESBIT TECHNIQUE)

1. A transverse incision is made across the penis. Restricted fibrous tissue is dissected off the undersurface of the penis. Fine plastic scissors, a scalpel with blade no. 10, and fine plastic tissue forceps are needed.

2. With the penis held forward and the prepuce retracted, the skin is incised (Fig. 12-43, *A*), and the dorsal quadrilateral flap is freed from the body of the penis (Fig. 12-43, *B*).

3. On each side, a narrow penile band of skin is divided (Fig. 12-43, *B*).

4. A transverse buttonhole is made to accommodate the head of the penis, which is threaded through it (Fig. 12-43, *C*).

5. The proximal edge of the buttonhole is sutured to the mucosa behind the corona. The preputial flap is trimmed and sutured to the raw area on the undersurface of the penis (Fig. 12-43, *D*).

6. An indwelling catheter is placed, and the wound is dressed.

#### URETHRAL RECONSTRUCTION

1. The urethra is dilated, and a Malecot catheter 14 or 16 Fr. over a sound 8 Fr. is used to accomplish a perineal urethrostomy.

2. On the ventral side of the penis the Duplay flap is made to create the new urethra. The edges of the flap are inverted and united over a catheter 8 or 10 Fr. with interrupted chromic gut sutures no. 5-0 or 6-0 on Atraumatic needles (Fig. 12-44).

#### PENILE REFORMATION

1. The scrotal flaps are made prior to lifting the penis from the scrotum (Fig. 12-45, *A*). A catheter is placed in the penile urethra. By dissection the penis with its established new urethra is lifted off the scrotum.

2. The flaps are sutured, providing the ventral and proper penoscrotal angle.

3. The scrotal fascia of the flap may be sutured (Fig. 12-45, *B*).

4. A catheter may be placed. The wound is dressed.

(*Note:* The Michalowski-Modelski urethral reconstruction technique is shown in Fig. 12-46.)

### Circumcision

**DEFINITION.** Excision of the foreskin (prepuce) of the glans penis.

**CONSIDERATIONS.** This operation is done prophylactically in infancy and is commonly performed in the newborn period. For Jewish patients, this may be a religious rite performed by a rabbi. Provision should be made in a hospital to observe the religious needs and preferences of parents in this regard.

Circumcision is done for the relief of phimosis, a condition in which the orifice of the prepuce is too small to permit easy retraction behind the glans. Circumcision may be done to relieve paraphimosis, a condition in which the prepuce cannot be reduced from a retracted position.

**SETUP AND PREPARATION OF THE PATIENT.** Newborn infants are generally positioned on specially constructed boards that facilitate restraint by immobilizing the limbs and exposing the genitalia. No anesthesia is used for newborn infants. Older patients may be given a general or local anesthetic.

For infants, the setup includes plastic cutting and clamping instruments, circumcision clamp, or bell, if desired (Fig. 12-47). The Hollister disposable circumcision device and sutures are sealed in a sterile packet ready for use. For older patients, a minor dissecting tray is used, including Allis forceps, fine hemostats, and probe and grooved director.

**OPERATIVE PROCEDURE**

1. If the foreskin is adherent, a probe or hemostat may be used to break up adhesions. The foreskin is grasped with an Allis forceps and stretched taut over the glans. A superficial, circumferential incision

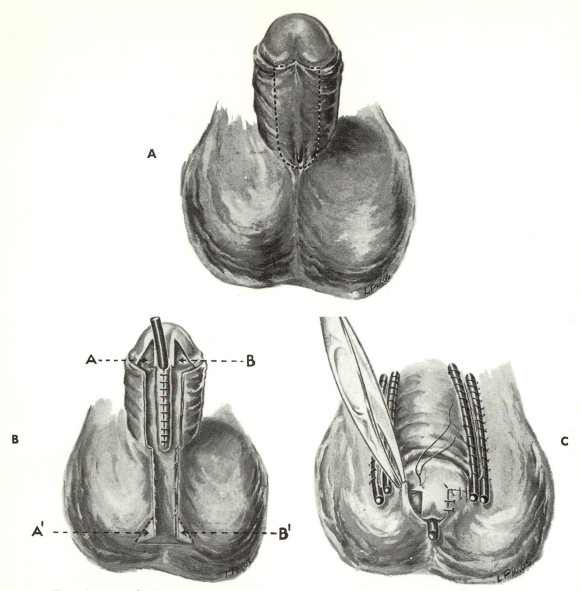

**Fig. 12-44.** Urethral reconstruction in hypospadias. **A,** Duplay flap outlined prior to commencement of urethral reconstruction. **B,** New urethra, rawed areas on glans (*A* and *B*), and midline incision in scrotum, with important triangular scrotal flaps (*A'* and *B'*). **C,** Penis is shown held firmly down on scrotal flaps, which are being sutured snugly down onto the glans to give added security. (From Fraser, Sir K.: Br. J. Surg. **51:**167, 1964.)

is made in the skin at the level of the coronal sulcus at the base of the glans with a scalpel. A straight hemostat may be placed at the medial dorsal aspect and the foreskin cut from the meatus to the sulcus with a straight scissors or scalpel. The foreskin is then completely excised

at the level of the sulcus. Bleeding vessels are clamped with mosquito hemostats and tied with fine no. 4-0 plain gut ligatures.

2. The raw edges of the skin incision are approximated along the corona with fine no. 4-0 chromic sutures on Atraumatic needles. The wound may be dressed

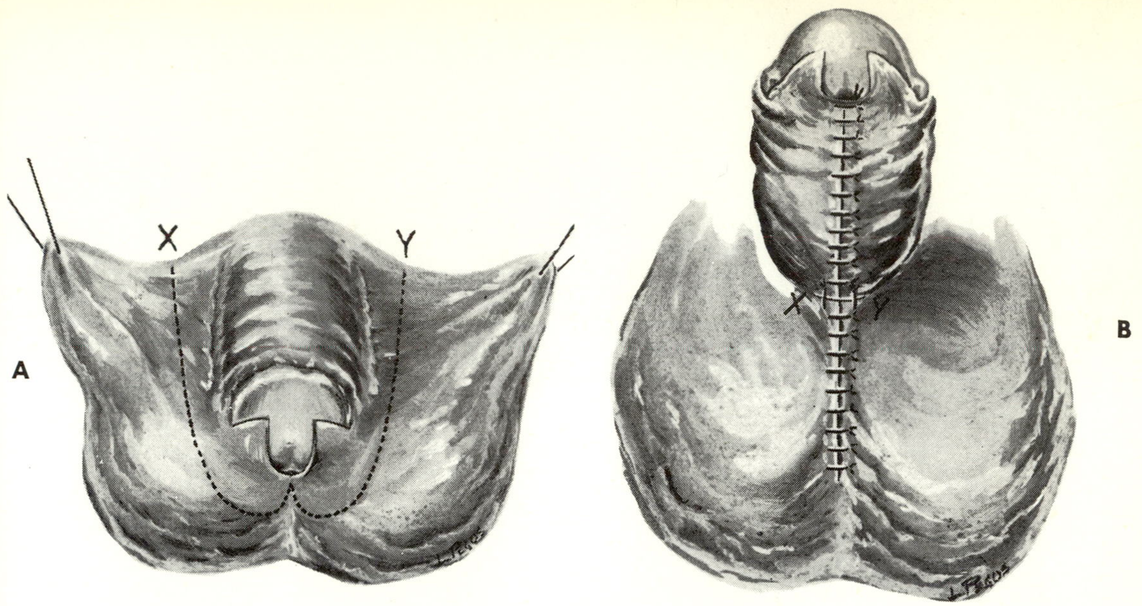

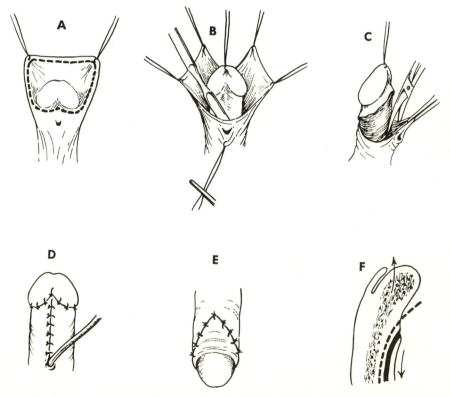

**Fig. 12-45.** Penile reformation. **A,** Scrotal flaps outlined prior to reformation of penis. Acute angle at which flaps meet near tip of penis shown and liberal length of flaps terminating at X and Y indicated. **B,** Suturing completed with X approximated to Y. Adequate ventral length and well-defined penoscrotal angle clearly shown. (From Fraser, Sir K.: Br. J. Surg. **51:**167, 1964.)

**Fig. 12-46.** Urethroplasty. Straightening and lengthening of curved penis. Circular incision of penile skin. Penis is partially denuded with dissection of the chordee and urethra from corpora cavernosa penis. Preputial skin flaps are transposed onto ventral surface of penis. Suture line at end of operation. (From Michalowski, E., and Modelski, W.: J. Urol. **89:**698, 1963.)

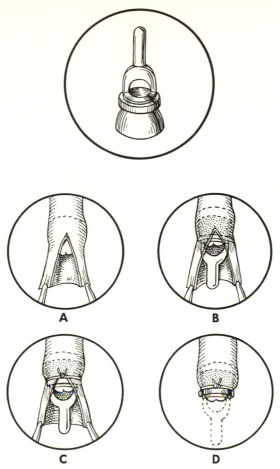

**Fig. 12-47.** Circumcision of newborn infant with Plastibell. (From Kariher, D. H., and Smith, T. W.: Obstet. Gynecol. 7:50, 1956.)

with petrolatum or hemostatic gauze, if desired.

FOR INFANT, USING PLASTIBELL. A dorsal slit is made, adhesions freed, and the bell placed over the glans inside the foreskin; a suture is tied lightly about the bell, compressing the foreskin into the groove. The free skin is trimmed, and the bell handle is broken off (Fig. 12-47).

## Urethral meatotomy

DEFINITION. Incisional enlargement of the external urethral meatus.

CONSIDERATIONS. Meatotomy is done to relieve stenosis or stricture.

SETUP AND PREPARATION OF THE PATIENT. For the male, a supine position is generally used, and the penis is elevated on a small folded sheet. For the female, the lithotomy position is used. General anesthesia or topical anesthesia of the lower urethra may be used. Cocaine, 5%, is used for the meatus and 2% procaine with a bulb syringe for instillation into the urethra. A minor perineal setup is needed, including fine instruments and petrolatum gauze dressings.

OPERATIVE PROCEDURE. A straight hemostat is applied to the ventral surface of the meatus. An incision is made along the frenum to enlarge the opening and overcome the stricture. Bleeding vessels are clamped and ligated with fine plain surgical gut sutures. The mucosal layer is su-

tured up to the skin with fine plain gut sutures. A dressing of petrolatum gauze may be applied.

## Excision of urethral caruncle

DEFINITION. Removal of papillary or sessile tumors of the urethra.

CONSIDERATIONS. Urethral caruncle is an inflammatory prolapse from the lower lip of the female urinary meatus.

SETUP AND PREPARATION OF THE PATIENT. The patient is placed in the lithotomy position. A minor or plastic dissecting setup is used, plus an electrosurgical unit and an indwelling urethral catheter of appropriate size.

OPERATIVE PROCEDURE

FOR REMOVAL OF PAPILLARY GROWTH. The growth is exposed, clamped at its base with curved hemostats, and excised. A urethral indwelling catheter is inserted into the bladder. The wound is closed.

FOR REMOVAL OF SESSILE GROWTH. A circular skin incision is made around the meatus and carried through the submucosal layer. The urethra is freed from the caruncle, the meatus is dissected back to the healthy tissue, and the diseased portion of the urethra is excised. The mucocutaneous junction is approximated with fine chromic gut sutures. An indwelling urethral catheter is introduced and is kept in the bladder for at least 5 days.

## Urethral dilatation and internal urethrotomy

DEFINITION. Gradual dilatation and removal of a urethral stricture to provide for adequate urinary drainage of the kidney.

SETUP AND PREPARATION OF THE PATIENT. The setup includes the following:

Cystoscopy pack
Electrosurgical unit
Urethral sound set (Fig. 12-14)
Valentine irrigation set (Fig. 12-12)
Retention catheters, as desired
Ellik evacuator (Fig. 12-52)
Filiform bougies, various sizes (Fig. 12-48)
Urethrotome, Maisonneuve or Otis type

A cystoscopy examination setup may be requested (Figs. 12-49 to 12-57).

The male patient may be placed in a supine position for the dilatation procedure. For other procedures the patient is placed in a lithotomy position.

OPERATIVE PROCEDURE

FOR GRADUAL DILATATION. The urethra is lubricated and anesthetized. In the male patient the penis is clamped and the urethra anesthetized. A filiform bougie is

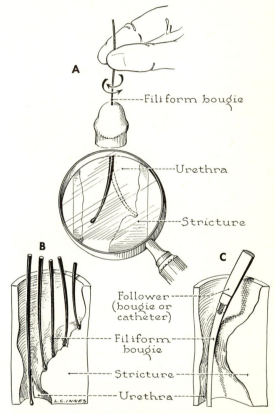

**Fig. 12-48.** Method of using coude-tipped bougie for passing stricture. **A,** Bougie is withdrawn 1 to 2 cm. each time obstruction is met, is rotated, and then is passed inward again. **B,** Method of using multiple bougies to pass through urethral stricture. Pocket is filled with bougie tips; this displaces one to opening through stricture. **C,** Philips filiform and follower. Follower is screwed onto end of filiform. Filiform passed through stricture guides follower through. (From Barnes, R. W., and Hadley, H. L.: Urological practice, St. Louis, 1954, The C. V. Mosby Co.)

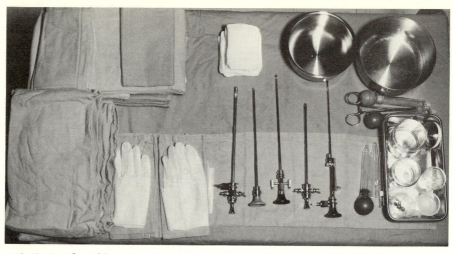

**Fig. 12-49.** Sterile table setup for cystoscopic examination includes drapes, gowns, gloves, specimen containers, lubricating jelly, and cystoscopes. Also to be added are light cord and tubing for irrigating fluid.

passed through the urethral stricture into the bladder (Fig. 12-48). Sounds or followers of desired type attached to filiform bougies are then passed into the bladder.

FOR INTERNAL URETHROTOMY. The filiform bougie is passed into the bladder; the urethrotome is connected and inserted. The Otis urethrotome consists of a curved sound with a groove on its upper side, along which is a triangular knife. Its sides are sharp and its apex blunt. The urethrotome is inserted, and then the blade is released to cut the stricture. Electrosurgical cutting and coagulating electrodes may be used.

## Cystoscopy

DEFINITION. Visual inspection of the interior of the bladder and examination of adjacent structures by means of an instrument (cystoscope) introduced via the urethra into the bladder.

CONSIDERATIONS. The urethra, the bladder neck, the interior of the bladder, and the ureteral orifices may be examined in the course of simple cystoscopy, or it may be done as the first step in a series of examinations or treatments that may be accomplished transurethrally.

SETUP AND PREPARATION OF THE PATIENT. The patient is placed in the lithotomy position (Chapter 7), perineal preparation is carried out, and the patient is draped with a lithotomy fenestrated sheet and leggings (Chapter 4 and 5). Surgical jelly is required to lubricate instruments passed into the urethra. A local or general anesthetic may be administered.

Instruments include a cystoscope, battery, irrigating fluid system, test tubes and materials for labeling and identifying specimens from right and left kidney, appropriate laboratory slips, and urethral and ureteral catheters as specified (Figs. 12-12, 12-13, 12-48, and 12-54).

For *x-ray examination* a radiopaque contrast medium of choice and syringes and needles are needed for the injection. Retrograde x-ray examination may be performed by injecting the medium into ureteral catheters.

Many cystoscopic and transurethral procedures are done under x-ray control. Special x-ray tables are available for urological use. These do not have mattresses since mattresses interfere with radiography. Measures for the patient's comfort and safety mut be provided.

Nursing service is responsible for prep-

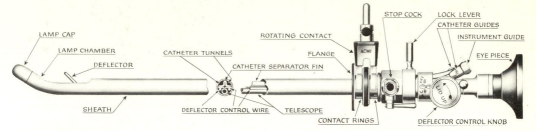

Fig. 12-50. Cystoscope assembled. Telescope in concave sheath showing essential parts. Cystoscope incorporates lens system for magnification and to permit visualization from angle. Cystoscopic view in general is at right angles to shaft of instrument, whereas panendoscope has smaller field of vision, but its view is almost in line with shaft of instrument. Cystoscope with its wide-angle lens provides for inspection of bladder, with limited visualization of the prostatic urethra. (Courtesy American Cystoscope Makers, Inc., New York, N. Y.)

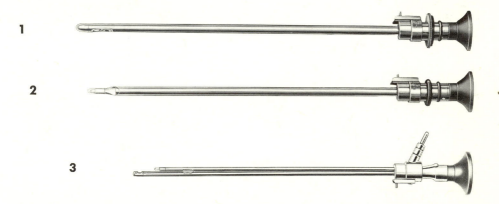

Fig. 12-51. 1, Right-angle examining telescope; 2, Foroblique examining telescope; 3, retrospective examining telescope. Retrograde lens permits viewer to look back toward himself as if he were inside the bladder viewing vesical outlet. (Courtesy American Cystoscope Makers, Inc., New York, N. Y.)

aration and arrangement of equipment and instruments as requested by the surgeon (Fig. 12-57); preparation, positioning, and draping of the patient; and the comfort and safety of the patient. The surgeon usually does not require a scrubbed assistant once the setup and draping has been completed. The surgeon sits at the foot of the table between the patient's legs. A receptacle for drainage is placed at the surgeon's feet, and the instruments are arranged on a small table at his side.

Care and handling of lensed instruments and catheters have been described in Chapter 5. In using an electrosurgical unit, the electrodes, the active cords, and the irrigating set must be sterile (Figs. 12-12 and 12-13).

The cystoscope or resectoscope must be connected to its respective power source and the irrigating system arranged. The surgeon hands out the appropriate connecting parts to the circulating team member. There are three attachments to the operating instrument. The cords and irrigating tubing are usually suspended over the patient's abdomen or legs in a set pattern. The level of the irrigation container is set about 4 to 6 inches above the level of the patient's bladder.

*Urological endoscopy instruments* include a cystoscope such as the Brown-

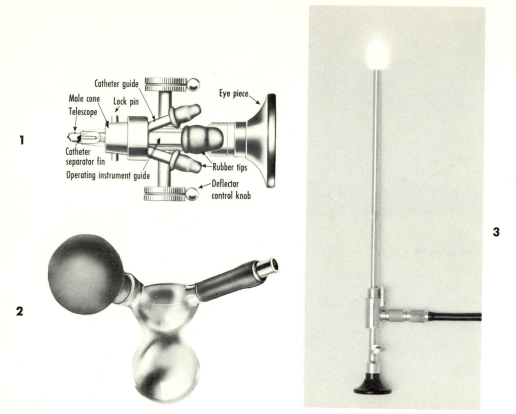

Fig. 12-52. 1, Convertible telescope showing eyepiece with catheter guides; 2, Ellik bladder evacuator—rubber bulb and connector tip with glass trap; 3, urethroscope. (Courtesy American Cystoscope Makers, Inc., New York, N. Y.)

Buerger on McCarthy with the following parts (Figs. 12-50 to 12-56):

1 Sheath (concave and convex), obturator, and telescopes as required for examining, operating, or catheterizing
Battery box and cords (Fig. 12-12)
Irrigating system (Fig. 12-13)
1 Set urethral sounds (Fig. 12-29)
1 Catheter stylet (Fig. 12-30)
2 Ellik evacuators (Fig. 12-52)
1 Asepto syringe, 2 oz.
1 Syringe, 30 ml.
Catheters as required:
Urethral type—Robinson, 12 to 20 Fr. and Foley, retention, 20 Fr. with 30 ml. bag (Fig. 12-14)
Ureteral type, 4 to 6 Fr.
*For fulguration*—add McCarthy, foroblique panendoscope with sheath obturator, telescope, and bridge assembly (Figs. 12-51 and 12-54)

*For lithopexy*—add lithotrite (Alcock model has a telescope and Bigelow-type blind) and Lowsley grasping forceps
*For ureteral catheterization*—add catheterizing telescope and ureteral catheters (Figs. 12-14, 12-52, and 12-53)
*For electrodissection of bladder tumor, prostate gland, or urethral lesions*—Electrotomes or resectoscopes: Stern-McCarthy, Nesbit, or Iglesias; complete resectoscope consisting of Bakelite sheath 24, 26, and 28 Fr., Timberlake obturator, working element, cutting loops, telescope, rotating contact, rubber tips (Figs. 12-54 to 12-56), and electrosurgical set, with electrodes as desired

The cystoscope incorporates a lens system through which the anatomy is viewed, a light to illuminate the interior structures, and a channel for irrigating fluid with which to distend the bladder so that it may

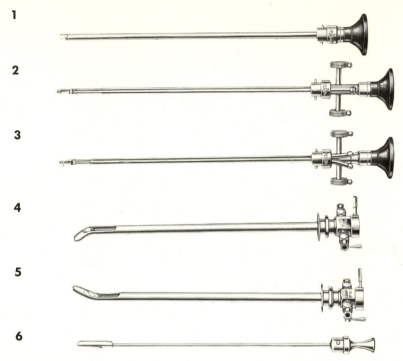

Fig. 12-53. Instruments for cystoscopy and transurethral surgery. Brown-Buerger Universal cystoscope: **1**, operating telescope; **2**, single catheterizing telescope; **3**, double catheterizing telescope; **4**, convex sheath; **5**, concave sheath; **6**, obturator. (Courtesy American Cystoscope Makers, Inc., New York, N. Y.)

be seen (Figs. 12-50 and 12-56). Fiberoptic lens systems are now commonly being used, supplanting the incandescent lamp and battery box method of illumination.

OPERATIVE PROCEDURE

1. The surgeon assembles the cystoscope, fitting the obturator into the sheath. The light is tested, and the circulating team member adjusts the current to the proper brightness.

2. The instrument is lubricated and inserted into the patient's urethra. The obturator is removed and the telescope inserted into the sheath. The surgeon puts his eye to the eyepiece and makes his examination. The bladder is distended with irrigating fluid. The surgeon adjusts the flow and volume with the stopcock. When the obturator or telescope is removed, the irrigating fluid flows out.

3. Other procedures such as ureteral catheterization, biopsy, or stone removal are carried out by exchanging or supplementing the cystoscope lens with the appropriate accessory instrument.

4. Kidney function studies, cystometry, and x-ray examinations may be performed and various specimens of urine collected. When the examination is concluded, the instrument is removed. A urethral catheter may be inserted as required.

## Transurethral surgery

DEFINITION. By means of a resectoscope passed into the bladder via the urethra, piecemeal resection of the prostate gland and of tumors of the bladder and bladder neck may be carried out, and bleeding vessels and tumors may be fulgurated.

SETUP AND PREPARATION OF THE PATIENT. As described for cystoscopy with selection of necessary instruments. Transurethral resection setup is shown in Fig. 12-57. Instruments may be supplemented for ad-

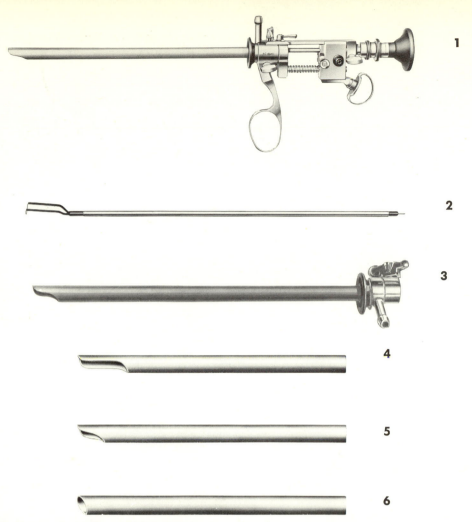

Fig. 12-54. 1, Nesbit modification of Stern-McCarthy electrotome; 2, resectoscope cutting loop; 3, Bakelite sheath for resectoscope; 4 to 6, beak models (long, short, and slanted) for resectoscope sheaths. Fiberoptic instruments permit better illumination, and viewer can continually see around changing angulations in all directions. Resectoscope is visual instrument used to accomplish transurethral resection of prostate or vesical lesions. (Courtesy American Cystoscope Makers, Inc., New York, N. Y.)

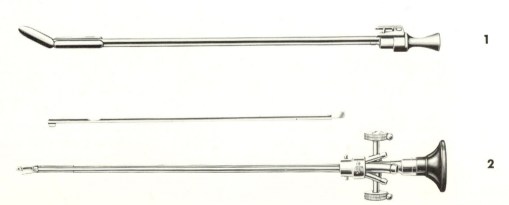

Fig. 12-55. Resectoscope components. 1, Timberlake obturator with "knee-joint" action; 2, cystoscope with convertible telescope and fin. (Courtesy American Cystoscope Makers, Inc., New York, N. Y.)

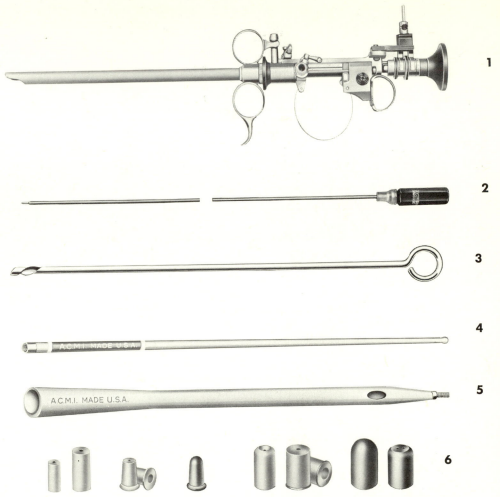

Fig. 12-56. **1,** Iglesias modification of Nesbit resectoscope assembled; **2,** Bugbee fulgurating or coagulatory urological electrode; **3,** cleaning rod for endoscopic sheaths (a spill of cotton is twisted onto lumen of instrument—supplied in fitted lengths); **4,** olive-tipped urethral filiform; **5,** Philips urethral catheter threaded for filiform; **6,** cystoscopic rubber tips for endoscopes—left to right: perforated rubber tips (small and large), blind tip, large perforated tips (recessed and blunt), large blind tip, and large double perforated tip. (Courtesy American Cystoscope Makers, Inc., New York, N. Y.)

ditional procedures such as vasectomy, urethral dilatation, or meatotomy. Consideration must be given to the presence of any inflammable or explosive gases when an electrosurgical unit is used.

The electric current that powers the electrode attached to the working element of the resectoscope is supplied from a source such as the Bovie machine. Current is varied for cutting and coagulating. It is regulated at the machine according to the surgeon's instructions, and the surgeon presses the foot pedal to select the current he desires during the course of the procedure.

Proper positioning of the indifferent plate under the patient and careful inspection of all electrical apparatus and connections must be carried out prior to each procedure.

The fluid used for distending and irrigating the bladder during the course of the operation increases the hazards of contamination and shock or short circuits

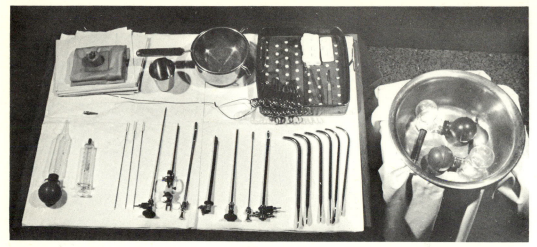

**Fig. 12-57.** Setup for transurethral resection. Square table. Top, left to right: drape sheets; O'Connor drape; Monel cup; specimen basin with strainer; instrument tray with minor dissecting set. Middle: tapered syringe adapter; catheter stylet. Bottom, left to right: Asepto 30 ml. syringe with Luer hub; 3 loop electrode for oblique telescope, working element, Timberlake obturator, resectoscope sheath, cystoscope telescope, cystoscope, obturator, cystoscope sheath; 5 sounds. Right: basin in ring stand containing 2 Ellik evacuators.

from the electrical apparatus. The operative field and environment must be kept as dry as possible to ensure safety and sterility of instruments. Properly positioned drainage and collecting items are helpful.

RESECTOSCOPE AND ITS PARTS. The resectoscope consists of five major parts. The sheath, obturator, working element, telescope, and loop electrode (Figs. 12-54 and 12-56). The *sheath* of metal or Bakelite composition forms a passage for the working element. The sheath with the obturator in place is passed into the bladder via the urethra. The *obturator* fills the cavity in the sheath and provides a smooth tapered point that acts as a sound to ease the entrance and passage of the instrument (Figs. 12-53 and 12-55). The Timberlake type of obturator has a flexible end.

The *working element* has two grooves running lengthwise to accommodate the loop electrode and the telescope. It is equipped with a level that is used to manipulate the loop electrode during cutting and coagulating (Fig. 12-54). At the top of the proximal end of the working element is the terminal part. It is attached to the active cord connected to the electrosurgical unit.

The *telescope* affords the view inside the bladder. The telescope is equipped with a lens system and a light at the distal end. The lenses of various telescopes are arranged to magnify and give various angles of view—either a forward oblique, right angle, or retrospective (Figs. 12-51 and 12-55).

The *loop electrode* has a long metal stem that conducts the current and a delicate wire loop on the end for cutting or coagulating. The wire is activated by pressing the pedal for the current desired.

*To use the resectoscope,* three accessory items are needed: an irrigation system for fluid to distend and wash out the bladder and urethra, the battery box, which supplies current for the illuminating lamp of the telescope or the fiberoptic light source, and the electrosurgical unit that transforms the electric current for cutting or coagulating (Figs. 12-12 and 12-13).

The *electrosurgical machine* is con-

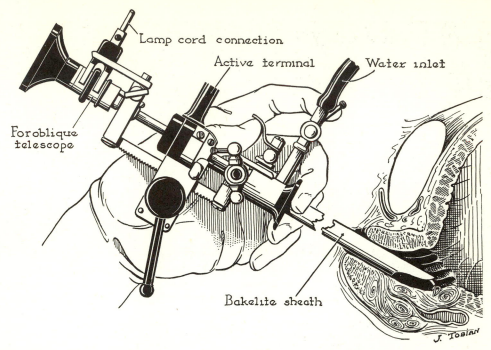

**Fig. 12-58.** Endoscopic prostatectomy with Stern-McCarthy electrotome (resectoscope). (From Barnes, R. W., and Hadley, H. L.: Urological practice, St. Louis, 1954, The C. V. Mosby Co.)

nected to the resectoscope working element by the active cord. The current flows through the electrode to the patient and is returned through the indifferent plate and cord. The indifferent plate is a piece of metal used to ground the patient. An area of patient's skin must make effective contact with the plate. A substantial surface in contact with the clean, hair-free skin will spread the current and reduce the hazard of burn from a concentration of the electrical energy in one small spot. Special electrode jellies are available and are sometimes used between the patient's skin and the indifferent plate. Lubricants in general tend to insulate, however, and it is usually better to take care that a clean contact is made.

There are two pedals on the electrosurgical unit: one for cutting current, the other for coagulating. The current intensity is controlled by dials on the machine. The settings must be specified by the surgeon.

**OPERATIVE PROCEDURE**

1. The resectoscope is assembled. The sheath is fitted with its obturator. The electrode and telescope are attached to the working element. The irrigating system is connected to the sheath. The lamp cord or fiberoptic bundle is fitted to the telescope. The electrode is attached to the electrosurgical unit. The currents are adjusted as the surgeon directs (Fig. 12-58).

2. The surgeon lubricates the sheath containing the obturator and inserts it into the urethra and bladder. The obturator is removed, and the operating element is introduced through the sheath.

3. Viewing the anatomy through the telescope, the surgeon begins the electrodissection, alternately cutting and coagulating. The bladder is permitted to drain—washing out blood tissue and clots—and refill at intervals. The operating element may be removed and evacuating devices such as the Ellik applied, to flush out the bladder (Fig. 12-59).

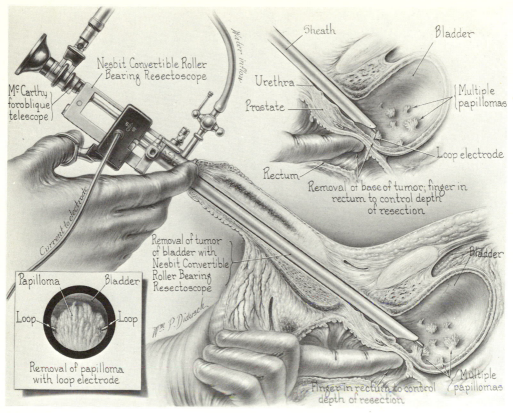

**Fig. 12-59.** Transurethral resection of bladder tumor. (Courtesy American Cystoscope Makers, Inc., New York, N. Y.)

4. When the stones are present, they are trapped or crushed with dislodgers or lithotrites, and copious irrigations are done.

5. When resection of the lesion is completed and bleeding controlled, the operating instrument is removed. A Foley catheter is introduced. A catheter stylet may be employed. The bag of the catheter is filled, using a 30 ml. syringe and adapter. The catheter may be a self-inflating type or have a valve that requires no clamp to retain the fluid in the hemostatic bag. The catheter is flushed for patency, irrigating with an Asepto syringe. When the surgeon is satisfied that the patient's condition is good, the patient is transferred from the operating table.

**REFERENCES**

1. Barnes, R. W., and Hadley, H. L.: Urological practice, St. Louis, 1954, The C. V. Mosby Co.

2. Bill, A. H., Jr., and Shanahan, D. A.: The management of undescended testicle, Surg. Clin. North Am. 44:1571, 1964.

3. Campbell, M. F., editor: Urology, vols. 1 to 3, ed. 2, Philadelphia, 1963, W. B. Saunders Co.

4. Colby, F. H.: Essential urology, ed. 4, Baltimore, 1961, The Williams & Wilkins Co.

5. Creevey, C. D.: Outline of urology, New York, 1964, Blakiston Division, McGraw-Hill Book Co.

6. Dodson, A. I.: Urological surgery, ed. 4, St. Louis, 1970, The C. V. Mosby Co.

7. Dowd, J. B., and Velasco, C.: Urologic uses of the small and large intestine, Surg. Clin. North Am. 44:849, 1964.

8. Flocks, R. H., and Culp, D.: Surgical urology, Chicago, 1954, Year Book Medical Publishers, Inc.

9. Fraser, Sir K.: Hypospadias, Surg. Clin. North Am. 44:1551, 1964.

10. Hutch, J. A.: Ureteric advancement operation: anatomy, technique, and early results, J. Urol. 89:180, 1963.

11. Kariher, D. H., and Smith, T. W.: Imme-

diate circumcision of the newborn, Obstet. Gynecol. **7:**50, 1956.

12. Leavell, L. C., Stackpole, C. E., Miller, M. A., and Chapin, F. M., editors: Kimber and Gray's anatomy and physiology, ed. 15, New York, 1966, The Macmillan Co.

13. Lowsley, O. S., and Kerwin, J.: Clinical urology, ed. 3, Baltimore, 1956, The Williams & Wilkins Co.

14. Marshall, V. F.: Textbook of urology, ed. 2, New York, 1964, Harper & Row, Publishers.

15. Michalowski, E., and Modelski, W.: Operative treatment of hypospadias, J. Urol. **89:** 698, 1963.

16. Politano, V. A., and Leadbetter, W. F.: An operative technique for the correction of vesicoureteral reflux, J. Urol. **79:**932, 1958.

17. Smith, D.: General urology, ed. 5, Los Altos, Calif., 1966, Lange Medical Publications.

18. Spratt, J. S., Shieber, W., and Dillard, B. M.: Anatomy and surgical technique of groin dissection, St. Louis, 1965, The C. V. Mosby Co.

19. Swinney, J., and Hammersley, D. P.: A handbook of operative urological surgery, Edinburgh, 1963, E. & S. Livingstone, Ltd.

# CHAPTER 13

# Orthopedic surgery

ELIZABETH COLTER

The derivation of orthopedics is from the Greek, *orthos* meaning straight and *paid-, pais* meaning child, the literal translation being to straighten the child. Nicholas Andry coined the term orthopaedic in 1741. The American Academy of Orthopaedic Surgeons stated in 1960, "Orthopaedics is the medical specialty that includes the investigation, preservation, restoration and development of the form and function of the extremities, spine, and associated structures by medical, surgical and physical method."

## ANATOMY

Knowledge of the normal anatomical structures involved in an orthopedic operation helps the nurse to become an efficient member of the operating team. The anatomy will be summarized briefly.

The bones of the body form a framework that supports the soft tissue and provides stability for the body as a whole. The framework or skeleton supports the weight of the body and forms several levers that, when acted on by the muscles, bring about body movements.

Bones are divided into four types according to their shape: long, short, flat, and irregular (Fig. 13-1). *Long* bones are present in the limbs and consist of a shaft and two ends; the ends provide a surface for articulation and muscle attachment. *Short* bones are present where strength but limited movement is required. *Flat* bones are found in the shoulder and in locations where protection of the underlying organs or space for muscle attachment is essentially needed (Figs. 13-1 and 13-2). *Irregular* bones are found in the skull and vertebral column.

## Shoulder and upper extremity

The *clavicle*, which is a long doubly curved bone attached to the spinal vertebrae by muscles, serves as a prop for the shoulder and holds it away from the chest wall. The clavicle rests almost horizontally at the upper and anterior part of the thorax above the first rib. It articulates medially with the manubrium of the sternum and laterally with the acromion of the scapula.

The *scapula* (shoulder blade) is a flat triangular bone that forms the posterior part of the shoulder girdle. Lying over the upper chest, its head or outer portion provides a socket, the glenoid cavity, for the humerus, and its acromion process articulates with the clavicle (Figs. 13-2 and 13-3). The scapula is attached to the trunk by muscles.

The *sternoclavicular joint* is the articulating structure (joint) between the outer end of the clavicle and a flattened articular facet situated on the inner border of the acromion (Figs. 13-2 and 13-3). The convex head of the humerus articulates with the shallow glenoid cavity of the scapula.

The *shoulder joint*, a ball-and-socket joint, is formed by the head of the humerus and the glenoid cavity. This joint is sur-

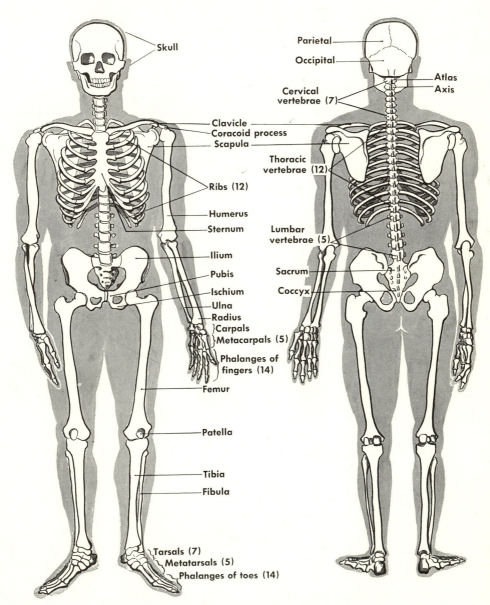

**Fig. 13-1.** Human skeleton, ventral and dorsal views. Numbers in parentheses indicate number of bones in that unit. In comparison with other mammals, man's skeleton is type of patchwork of primitive and specialized parts. Erect posture brought about by specialized changes in legs and pelvis enabled primitive arrangement of arms and hands (arboreal adaptation of man's ancestors) to be used for manipulation of tools. Development of skull and brain followed as consequence of premium natural selection put on dexterity, better senses, and ability to appraise environment. (From Hickman, C. P.: Integrated principles of zoology, ed. 4, St. Louis, 1970, The C. V. Mosby Co.)

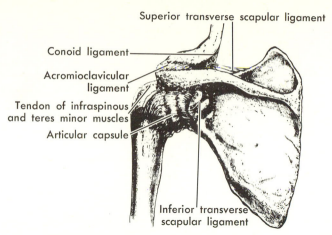

**Fig. 13-2.** Shoulder joint and related parts: anterior view. Position of clavicle in schematic. (From Anson, B. J., editor: Morris' human anatomy, ed. 12, New York, 1966, McGraw-Hill Book Co. Used with permission of the publisher.)

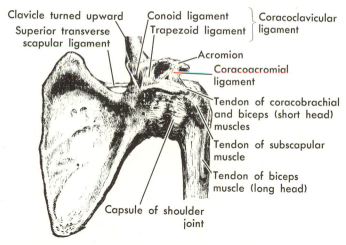

**Fig. 13-3.** Shoulder joint and related parts: posterior view. Position of clavicle in schematic. (From Anson, B. J., editor: Morris' human anatomy, ed. 12, New York, 1966, McGraw-Hill Book Co. Used with permission of the publisher.)

rounded by a loose capsular ligament that is strengthened by the coracohumeral ligament. The coracohumeral ligament extends from the coracoid across the top of the joint to the greater tuberosity of the humerus (Figs. 13-4 and 13-5).

The muscles surrounding the shoulder joint are the supraspinous and infraspinous, the teres minor and teres major, and the subscapular muscles. These muscles steady the glenohumeral joint in movements of the entire arm.

The *humerus,* the longest and largest bone of the upper extremity, is composed of a shaft and two ends.

The upper end or head has two projections, the greater and lesser tuberosities (Figs. 13-1 and 13-6).

The head articulates with the glenoid cavity of the scapula. The circumference

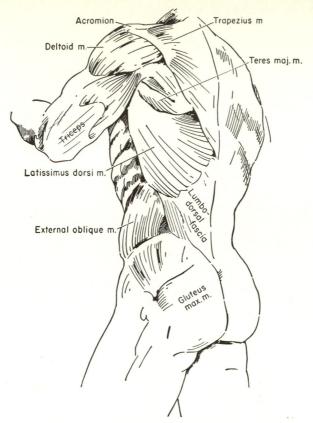

**Fig. 13-4.** Superficial muscles of trunk, shoulder, and hip. Posterior view. (From Howorth, M. B., et al.: A textbook of orthopedics, Philadelphia, 1952, W. B. Saunders Co.)

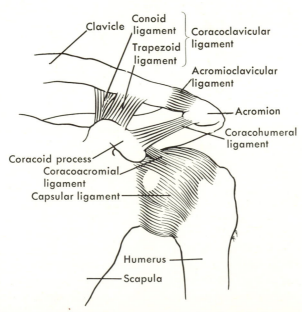

**Fig. 13-5.** Ligaments of the acromion and of the clavicle and the anterior aspect of the shoulder joint. (From Hollinshead, W. H.: Anatomy for surgeons, vol. 3, ed. 2, The back and limb, New York, 1969, Harper & Row, Publishers.)

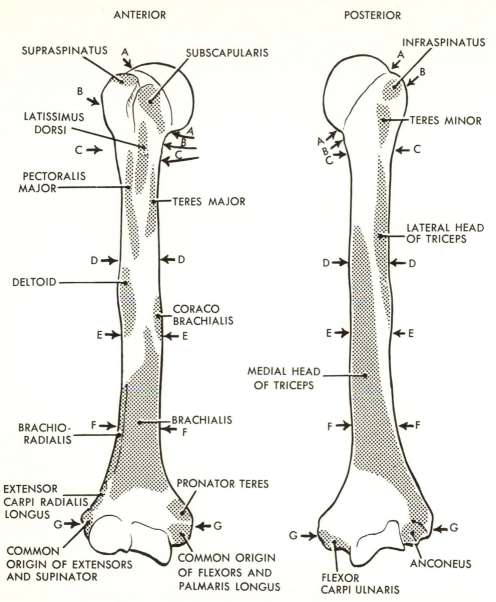

**Fig. 13-6.** Anterior and posterior views of humerus showing muscle attachments. Arrows lettered **A** to **G** indicate typical locations of fractures. These various fracture sites have different muscle groups asserting pull on fracture fragments; thus fragments assume different characterisic position in each. (From Brantigan, O. C.: Clinical anatomy, New York, 1963, Blakiston Division, McGraw-Hill Book Co.)

of the articular surface of the humerus is constricted and is termed the *anatomical neck*. The constriction below the tuberosoties is called the *surgical neck* and is the site of most fractures. The anatomical neck marks the attachment to the capsule of the shoulder joint.

The greater tuberosity is situated at the lateral side of the head. Its upper surface has three impressions; these give insertion to the supraspinous, the infraspinous, and the teres minor muscles. The lesser tuberosity is situated in front of the neck and has an impression for the insertion of the

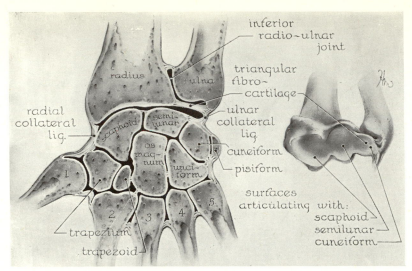

Fig. 13-7. Anatomy of wrist and carpus. (From Moseley, H. F., editor: Textbook of surgery, ed. 3, St. Louis, 1959, The C. V. Mosby Co.)

tendon of the subscapular muscle. The tuberosities are separated from each other by a deep groove (bicipital groove), in which lies the tendon of the biceps muscle of the arm. The tendon of the latissimus dorsi inserts at the bicipital groove's medial margin (Fig. 13-6).

The body of the shaft has three borders and three surfaces. The anterior border serves above for the insertion of the tendon of the greater pectoral muscle and below for the tendon of the brachial muscle. The lateral border serves for the insertion of the tendon of the teres minor, and the medial border serves for the attachment of the tendon of the teres major.

The lower portion of the humerus is flattened and ends below in a broad articular surface, which is divided into two parts by a slight ridge. On either side of the ridge are projections, the lateral and medial condyles. On the lateral condyle the rounded articular surface is called the *capitellum;* it articulates with the head of the radius. On the medial condyle the articular surface is termed the *trochlea;* it articulates with the ulna.

The *ulna* is placed at the medial side of the radius. The upper portion of the ulna presents two curved processes—the olecra-

non posteriorly and the coronoid process anteriorly—as well as two cavities, the articular cavities. The curved semilunar notch that connects them articulates with the trochlea. On the lateral side is the radial notch, which articulates with the circular border of the radial head (Figs. 13-1 and 13-7).

The *radius* rotates around the ulna. At the proximal end is the head, which articulates with the capitellum of the humerus and also with the radial notch of the ulna. The tendon of the biceps muscle is attached to the tuberosity below the proximal end. The distal end of the radius is divided into two articular surfaces. The distal surface articulates with the carpal bones of the wrist, while the other on the medial side articulates with the distal end of the ulna (Fig. 13-7).

### Wrist and hand

The skeletal bones of the wrist and hand consist of three distinct parts: (1) the carpus, or wrist bones, (2) the metacarpus, or bones of the palm, and (3) the phalanges, or bones of the digits (Fig. 13-7).

The carpal bones consist of eight bones arranged in two rows. The proximal row,

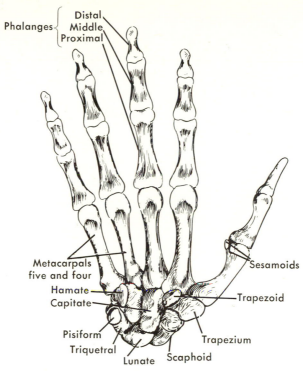

**Fig. 13-8.** Skeleton of the wrist and hand, palmar view. (From Hollinshead, W. H.: Anatomy for surgeons, vol. 3, ed. 2, The back and limb, New York, 1964, Harper & Row, Publishers.)

proceeding from the radial to the ulnar side, includes the scaphoid, semilunar, cuneiform, and pisiform, and the distal row includes the trapezium, trapezoid, os magnum, and unciform (Fig. 13-7).

Each bone, except the pisiform bone, presents six surfaces. Their surfaces consist of rough areas for the attachment of muscles and tendons and smooth articular surfaces for contact with the adjacent bones. The pisiform bone forms a projection at the front of the wrist on the ulnar side and has a single articular facet.

The five metacarpal bones are situated in the palm. Each bone has a shaft and two extremities. Proximally they articulate with the distal row of carpal bones, and distally the head of each metacarpal articulates with its proper phalanx. The heads of the metacarpals form the knuckles. (See Figs. 13-1, 13-7, and 13-8.)

The phalanges, called *finger bones*, consist of fourteen bones, two in the thumb and three in each of the fingers. Each phalanx consists of a shaft and two ends.

### Hip and femur

The *hip joint*, a ball-and-socket joint, is formed by the acetabular portion of the innominate (pelvic) bone and the proximal end of the femur (Fig. 13-1). The hip joint is surrounded by a capsule, ligaments, and muscles (Figs. 13-4 and 13-10).

The acetabulum is a deep round cavity that receives the head of the femur. The proximal end of the femur consists of the femoral head and neck, the upper portion of the shaft, and the greater and lesser trochanters (Fig. 13-9).

The greater trochanter is a broad process of cancellous bone, which protrudes from the outer upper portion of the shaft and projects upward from the junction of the superior border of the neck with the outer surface of the shaft. It serves as a point of insertion for the abductor and

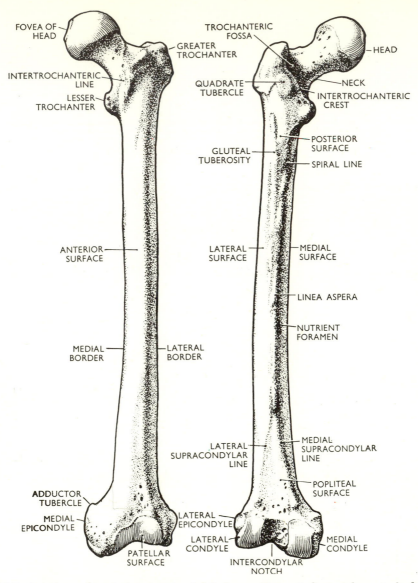

**Fig. 13-9.** Anterior and posterior aspects of left femur. Femur is longest bone in body, consisting of upper end with prominent rounded head, shaft, and expanded lower end. Head articulates with pelvis at hip joint, and lower end articulates with tibia and patella to form knee joint. (From Johnson, W. H., and Kennedy, J. A.: Radiographic anatomy of the human skeleton, Edinburgh, 1961, E. & S. Livingstone, Ltd.)

short rotator muscles of the hip. (See Fig. 13-10.)

The lesser trochanter is a conical process, which projects from the posterior and inferior portion of the base of the neck of the femur at its junction with the shaft and serves as a point of insertion for the iliopsoas muscle (Fig. 13-10). The lower end of the femur terminates in the two condyles. In front, the condyles are separated from one another by a smooth depression, called the *intercondylar groove,* forming an articulating surface for the patella. Behind, they project slightly, and the space between them forms a deep fossa, the *intercondylar fossa* (Fig. 13-9).

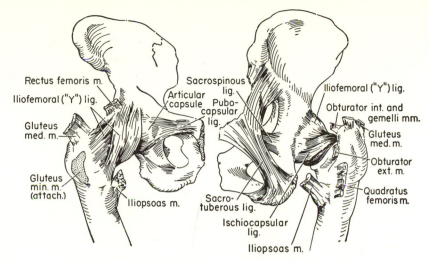

**Fig. 13-10.** Ligaments and muscles of the hip. Anterior and posterior views. (From Howorth, M. B., et al.: A textbook of orthopedics, Philadelphia, 1952, W. B. Saunders Co.)

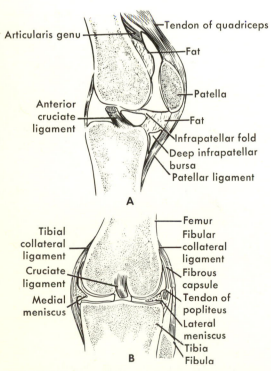

**Fig. 13-11.** Sagittal, **A**, and frontal, **B**, sections through the knee joint. (From Hollinshead, W. H.: Anatomy for surgeons, vol. 3, ed. 2, The back and limb, New York, 1964, Harper & Row, Publishers.)

The upper or condylar end of the tibia presents an articular surface corresponding with those of the femoral condyles. The articular surface of the two tibial condyles forms two facets, which are deepened by the semilunar cartilages into fossae for the femoral condyles.

**Knee and knee joint**

The patella or so-called kneecap is situated in front of the knee joint in the anterior intercondylar groove of the lower end of the femur (Fig. 13-11). It is developed within the quadriceps tendon and is composed mainly of cancellous bone. The anterior and inferior surfaces of the patella are united with the patellar tendon (Fig. 13-11). The posterior surface of the patella is intra-articular and is related closely to the fat pad of the knee. The knee joint is formed by three articulations in one. They are two condyle joints, one between each condyle of the femur and the corresponding meniscus and condyle of the tibia, and a third articulation between the patella and femur.

The bones of the knee joint are connected by sets of ligaments classified as

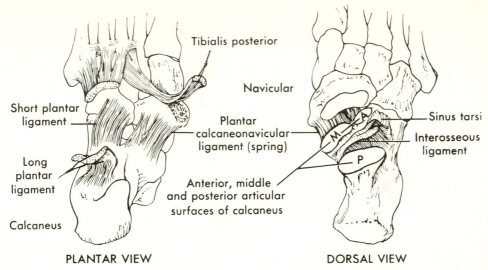

Tibialis posterior

Navicular

Short plantar ligament

Plantar calcaneonavicular ligament (spring)

Sinus tarsi

Interosseous ligament

Long plantar ligament

Anterior, middle and posterior articular surfaces of calcaneus

Calcaneus

**PLANTAR VIEW**     **DORSAL VIEW**

**Fig. 13-12.** Ligaments of the foot. (From DuVries, H. L.: Surgery of the foot, ed. 2, St. Louis, 1965, The C. V. Mosby Co.)

extra-articular and intra-articular structures (Fig. 13-11). The extra-articular attachments include the capsule, the quadriceps muscle, two collateral ligaments, and the oblique popliteal ligament. The intra-articular ligaments include the cruciate ligaments and the attachments of the menisci (so-called semilunar cartilages).

The capsule of the knee joint is attached above to the lateral surfaces of the condyles and to the posterior surface of the shaft of the femur, and it is attached below to the condyles of the tibia and to the upper end of the fibula. The capsule is reinforced—in front by the patellar and quadriceps tendon, on the sides by the internal and external lateral ligaments, and posteriorly by the popliteus and gastrocnemius muscles.

The cruciate ligaments, consisting of two fibrous bands, extend from the intercondylar fossa of the femur to attachments in front of and behind the intercondylar surface of the tibia (Fig. 13-11).

The semilunar cartilages, known as the *menisci*, are interposed between the condyles of the femur and those of the tibia. Each cartilage is attached to the joint capsule. The ends of the cartilages are at-

tached to the tibia in the midarea of its upper articular table.

Synovial membrane lines the capsule of the joint and covers the infrapatellar fat pad, parts of the crucial ligaments, and portions of the bone.

The portion of the knee joint cavity that extends upward in front of the femur is called the *suprapatellar* or *quadriceps bursa.* The infrapatellar bursa lies between the patellar tendon and the upper margin of the tibia (Fig. 13-11).

**Ankle and foot**

The ankle joint, a hinge joint, is formed by the lower end of the tibia and its malleolus, the malleolus of the fibula, and the inferior transverse ligaments. These structures form a mortise for the reception of the upper surface of the talus and its facets (Figs. 13-11 to 13-13).

The bones are connected by ligaments, which spread out from the malleoli to be attached to the os calcis, astragalus, and navicular bones. The joint is surrounded by a thin capsule (Figs. 13-11 to 13-13).

The astragalus, known as the *talus,* consists of a body, neck, and head. It is an irregular bone that fits into a mortise

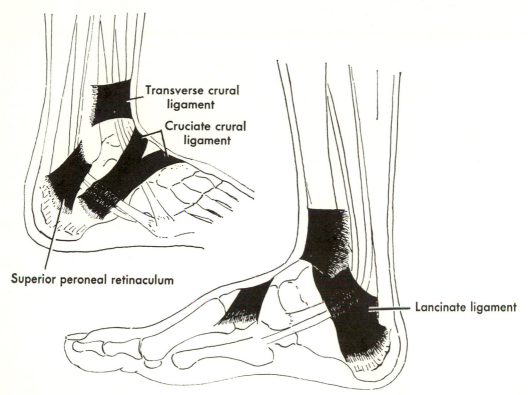

**Fig. 13-13.** Superficial ligaments of the ankle-binding tendons of the leg as they course into the foot. (From DuVries, H. L.: Surgery of the foot, ed. 2, St. Louis, 1965, The C. V. Mosby Co.)

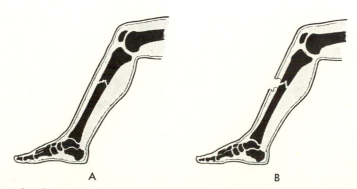

**Fig. 13-14. A,** Closed, or simple, fracture. No communication between fractured bone and body surface. **B,** Open, or compound, fracture. Wound leading down to site of fracture. Organisms may gain access through wound and infect bone. (From Adams, J. C.: Outline of fractures, ed. 4, Edinburgh, 1964, E. & S. Livingstone, Ltd.)

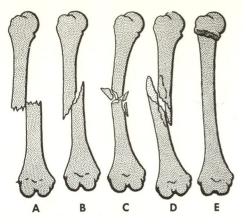

Fig. 13-15. Types of fractures, right humerus in the anteroposterior projection. **A,** Transverse fracture of midshaft with medial displacement of the distal fragment. (The fragments are in poor apposition but good alignment.) **B,** Oblique fracture with overriding. (The fragments are in partial apposition but good alignment.) **C,** Comminuted fracture with lateral angulation. (Apposition is not unsatisfactory.) **D,** Spiral fracture with lateral angulation. (Both apposition and alignment are poor.) **E,** Impacted fracture of the neck in good apposition and alignment. (From Rhoads, J., et al.: Surgery: principles and practice, ed. 4, Philadelphia, 1970, J. B. Lippincott Co.)

formed by the malleoli. It articulates with the calcaneus and navicular bones (Fig. 13-1).

The bony framework of the foot comprises seven tarsal bones, five metatarsals, and fourteen phalanges.

The os calcis, a large bone, forms the heel and gives support to the astragalus. The cuboid bone articulates posteriorly with the os calcis and anteriorly with the fourth and fifth metatarsals and the external cuneiform bones.

The navicular bone articulates with the cuneiform bones, which lie side by side in front of the scaphoid. The metatarsal bones articulate proximally with the tarsal bones and distally with the bases of the first phalanges of the corresponding toes. The phalanges of the toes consist of two for the great toe and three for each of the other toes.

# FRACTURES AND DISLOCATIONS

A fracture is a break in the continuity of a bone. If it involves the entire cross section of the bone, it is a complete fracture; if it involves only a portion of the cross section, it is an incomplete fracture. Every fracture, therefore, is either complete or incomplete. The care of fractured bones or dislocation of a joint is always complicated because of trauma to the soft parts of the body, including the muscles, nerves, and blood vessels.

## Types of fractures

Fractures are classified into two main groups: the nonpenetrating (closed) fractures and penetrating (compounded or open) fractures.

*Closed,* or nonpenetrating, fractures are those in which no wound of the skin communicates with the break in the bone (Figs. 13-14 to 13-16). *Incomplete* fractures are those in which the whole thickness of the bone is not broken but is bent or buckled, as in the so-called greenstick fractures that occur in children before puberty.

*Open,* or penetrating, fractures exist when the break in the bone communicates with a wound in the skin. Since these fractures are contaminated, measures are carried out to control potential infection. There are two types of open fractures, direct and indirect. (See Figs. 13-14, *B,* and 13-17 to 13-19.) The *direct* types are those in which violence opens the fracture from without. *Indirect* types are those in which the fractured fragments come through the soft tissue from within.

There are many varieties of fracture architectures, including (1) the *transverse* fracture, in which the fracture line runs at a right angle to the longitudinal axis of the bone; (2) the *longitudinal* fracture, which runs along the length of the bone; (3) the *oblique* fracture and the *spiral* fracture, which are similar except for the length; (4) the *comminuted* fracture, in which the bone fragments splinter into many pieces; (5) the *impacted* fracture,

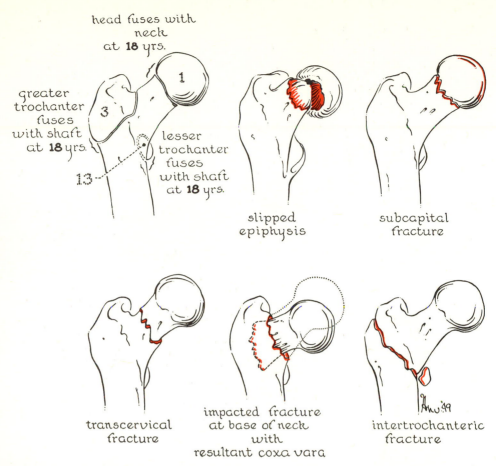

**Fig. 13-16.** Ossification, slipped epiphysis, and fractures of upper end of femur. (From Moseley, H. F., editor: Textbook of surgery, ed. 3, St. Louis, 1959, The C. V. Mosby Co.)

in which one fragment is driven into the other end and is relatively fixed in that position; and (6) the *pathological* fracture, which may occur when a bone is weakened by disease, thereby permitting a bone to break under trivial violence (Figs. 13-16, 13-17, and 13-20).

An *epiphyseal separation* occurs when a fracture passes through or lies within the growing area of a bone (Fig. 13-17).

An *avulsion fracture* may result from a joint displacement where the ligament or tendon avulses its bony attachment instead of rupturing its fibers. A *dislocation* is a complete displacement of one articular surface of a joint from the other. A *subluxation* is a partial dislocation (Figs. 13-18 and 13-19).

## Locations of fractures

A fracture in the shaft of a long bone is usually described as being in the proximal, middle, or lower third or at the junction of two of these divisions.

A fracture of one of the bony prominences of the end of a long bone is described as a fracture of that prominence by name; for example, a fracture of the olecranon, a fracture of the medial malleolus, or a fracture of the lateral condyle of the femur.

## PRINCIPLES OF FRACTURE TREATMENT

The purpose of fracture treatment is to reestablish the length, the shape, and the alignment of the fractured bones or joints

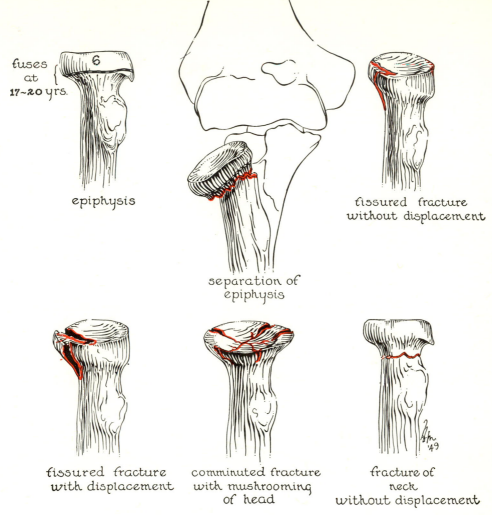

fuses
at
17~20 yrs.

6

epiphysis

separation of
epiphysis

fissured fracture
without displacement

fissured fracture
with displacement

comminuted fracture
with mushrooming
of head

fracture of
neck
without displacement

**Fig. 13-17.** Types of fractures of head and neck of radius. (From Moseley, H. F., editor: Textbook of surgery, ed. 3, St. Louis, 1959, The C. V. Mosby Co.)

and restore their physiological function to normal or to as near normal as possible.

Fractures of a bone involve two parts: the proximal and the distal fragments (Fig. 13-20). The position of the proximal fragment (the one closer to the body) is controlled by pulling the attached muscles. For this reason, the distal fragment is manipulated into the position that is assumed by the proximal fragment. The surgeon selects the method whereby this can be accomplished.

In fractures involving the treatment of the upper extremity, the surgeon endeav-

ors to preserve mobility because the individual needs a wide range of motion to perform skilled and delicate work. In fractures of the lower extremity, the objectives of surgery are to restore alignment and length and provide stability of the extremity for weight bearing.

In the presence of open fractures involving soft tissues, several conditions may arise. These include (1) secondary hemorrhage, (2) infection, (3) severe debilitation of tissues, (4) puncture of blood vessels by motion of short bone fragments, (5) invasion of spore-forming, gas-produc-

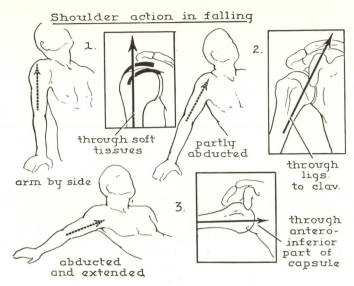

**Fig. 13-18.** Injury to shoulder: force of transmission to shoulder in falling. **1,** Results in arm at side; **2,** results with arm partly abducted; **3,** results with arm abducted and extended. (From Bateman, L. E.: The shoulder and environs, St. Louis, 1955, The C. V. Mosby Co.)

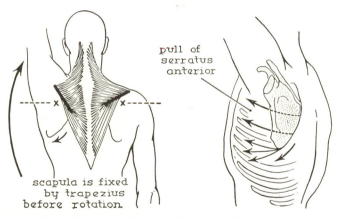

**Fig. 13-19.** Action of two important fixators of scapula. Trapezius prevents rotating swing; serratus anterior prevents posterior swinging. (From Bateman, L. E.: The shoulder and environs, St. Louis, 1955, The C. V. Mosby Co.)

ing organisms due to infection, (6) traumatic arterial spasm due to contusion of the main artery of the limb, and (7) Volkmann's contracture resulting from ischemia.

To accomplish the objectives of surgery, the operating team keeps in mind the following principles: (1) the extremity must be handled gently, (2) the body must have adequate support, (3) proper equipment and personnel must be readily available to treat impending or existing shock and control hemorrhage, (4) aseptic surgical techniques and chemotherapy must be maintained to control infection, (5) the patient must be positioned properly to provide for adequate circulatory and respiratory functioning, and (6) the comfort of the patient must be considered.

## Bone-healing process of fractures

The healing process involves several stages. When a bone is fractured, hemor-

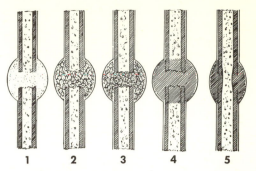

Fig. 13-21. Schematic drawing of the five stages of regeneration of bone. 1, Hematoma; 2, granulation; 3, callus; 4, consolidation; 5, remodeling. (From Adams, J. C.: Outline of fractures, including joint injuries, ed. 5, Edinburgh, 1964, Churchill Livingstone, Medical Division of Longman Group, Ltd.)

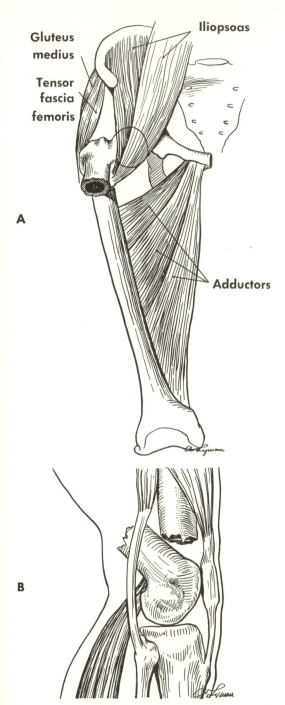

Fig. 13-20. **A,** Muscle action in subtrochanteric fractures of femur. **B,** Supracondylar fracture of femur (transverse). Note pull exerted by gastrocnemius muscle. (From Larson, C. B., and Gould, M.: Orthopedic nursing, ed. 7, St. Louis, 1970, The C. V. Mosby Co.)

rhage occurs. The amount of extravasated blood depends on the size and number of ruptured vessels and the vascularity of the fracture site. The blood exudate infiltrates the surrounding area, where it forms clots. The vascular granulation tissue coming from the ends of the bone fragments invades the clots (Fig. 13-21).

After several days, calcium deposits may form in the granulation tissue. These deposits eventually form new bone, known as *callus*. Within the callus, cartilage cells develop a temporary semirigid tissue that helps to stabilize the bone fragments (Fig. 13-21). The callus is immature bone that is remodeled by new connective tissue cells (osteoblasts of the periosteum and the intramembrane of the bone cavity). Through this process, mature bone is formed, and the excess callus is reabsorbed. (See Fig. 13-21.)

After several or many months, depending on the age and physical condition of the individual, the fractured bone becomes firmly united, although the ossification process is not yet completed. Complete union of the fractured bone or joint is determined by means of clinical and radiological examination.

*Nonunion* of a fracture signifies that the process of healing has ended without producing bony union.

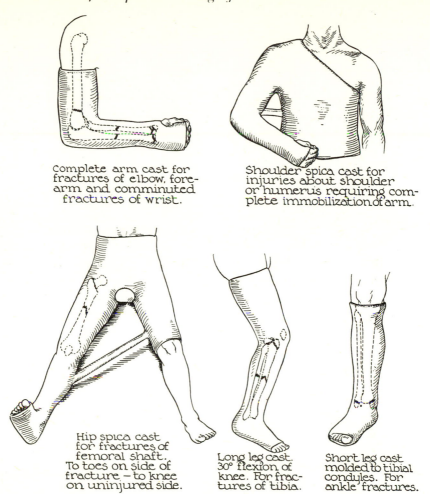

Complete arm cast for fractures of elbow, forearm and comminuted fractures of wrist.

Shoulder spica cast for injuries about shoulder or humerus requiring complete immobilization of arm.

Hip spica cast for fractures of femoral shaft. To toes on side of fracture — to knee on uninjured side.

Long leg cast. 30° flexion of knee. For fractures of tibia.

Short leg cast molded to tibial condyles. For ankle fractures.

**Fig. 13-22.** Several types of plaster casts and some of the fractures for which they may be indicated. (From Compere, E. L., Banks, S. W., and Compere, C. L.: Pictorial handbook of fracture treatment, ed. 5, Chicago, 1963, Year Book Medical Publishers, Inc.)

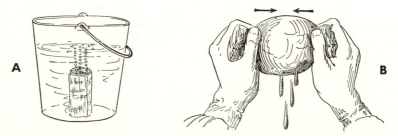

**Fig. 13-23.** Correct handling of plaster roll. **A,** Roll of plaster placed on end in pail of water. Roll saturated when bubbles cease to appear. **B,** Excess water squeezed from plaster roll by pushing both ends toward middle. Do not twist. (From Compere, E. L., Banks, S. W., and Compere, C. L.: Pictorial handbook of fracture treatment, ed. 5, Chicago, 1963, Year Book Medical Publishers, Inc.)

*Delayed union* signifies that a specific fracture has not healed in the time considered as average for this fracture. The average time for healing of a fracture depends on many variables, and delayed unions must never be considered nonunions until the healing process has ceased without bony union.

*Malunion* signifies that the fracture has united with deformity sufficient to cause impairment of function or a significant cosmetic defect.

### Closed reduction for fractured bones

Reduction of fractured bones by the closed method is usually performed in the fracture (plaster) room, not in the general surgical suite.

#### Immobilization by plaster-of-Paris cast

DEFINITION. A form of external mold that places the fractured extremity or joint at rest by immobilizing the joint and both ends of the fractured bone in a plaster or similar type of casing (Fig. 13-22).

SETUP. The essential items needed include the following:

Plaster-of-Paris bandages, appropriate sizes
Sheet wadding
Lining and padding materials
Braces and supports
Fracture table with proper fixtures (when necessary)
Sink with running water and pail (Fig. 13-23)
Table work area
Buckets
Plaster knives and scissors
Tape
Ruler
Marker

TYPES OF CASTS. A plaster boot or short leg cast may be used for fractures of the foot or sometimes for the ankle. A *complete long leg cast* may be applied to treat fractures of the tibia and fibula. A *cylinder leg cast* (Fig. 13-22) may be applied to treat a fracture of the patella.

Spica casts are designed for different parts of the body. For example, a *single spica cast* involving the trunk, the affected leg, and foot may be applied to treat a

fracture of the femur. A *body jacket cast* encircling the body but not the extremities may be used to treat a dorsal and lumbar fracture.

#### External fixation of fractured bones

DEFINITION. Fixation of bone fragments by means of metal pins or wires that are passed through the skin and soft tissue into the bone at two points and incorporated in a casing if necessary (Fig. 13-24).

CONSIDERATIONS. An external fixation method may be used in the presence of a mechanically unstable fracture such as a complicated fracture of the wrist. This method may be selected to treat a fracture when the powerful muscles involved prevent reduction of the fragments.

SETUP. The following items are sterilized and prepared on a sterile table:

Scalpel
Drill
Wires or pins, desired type and size
Gauze dressings

**Nonsterile items**

Plaster-of-Paris bandages of appropriate size
Traction equipment, desired type (Fig. 13-24)

Local or general anesthetic may be administered.

PROCEDURE. This procedure may be performed in the plaster room or in the patient's room, depending on the condition of the patient. Aseptic techniques are followed to prevent wound infection that may result in permanent stiffness of a joint or chronic osteomyelitis.

### PREPARATION OF THE PATIENT FOR ORTHOPEDIC SURGERY

The skin preparation of the operative site, the positioning of the patient on the operating table, and draping the patient with sterile sheets and towels are essential steps for a successful operation. An understanding of tourniquets is also essential to the nursing service staff.

INITIAL SKIN PREPARATION. The principles of skin cleaning have been described in Chapter 4. Improper skin preparation may

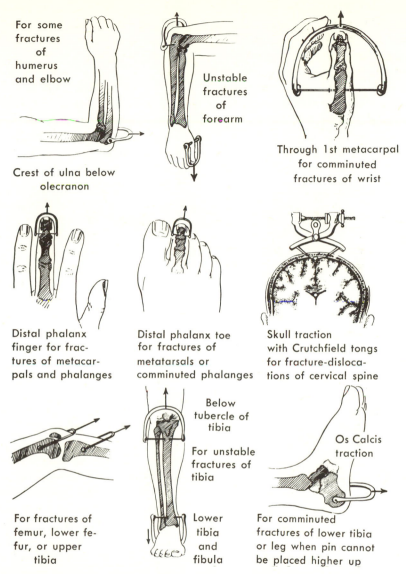

For some fractures of humerus and elbow

Crest of ulna below olecranon

Unstable fractures of forearm

Through 1st metacarpal for comminuted fractures of wrist

Distal phalanx finger for fractures of metacarpals and phalanges

Distal phalanx toe for fractures of metatarsals or comminuted phalanges

Skull traction with Crutchfield tongs for fracture-dislocations of cervical spine

For fractures of femur, lower fefur, or upper tibia

Below tubercle of tibia

For unstable fractures of tibia

Lower tibia and fibula

Os Calcis traction

For comminuted fractures of lower tibia or leg when pin cannot be placed higher up

Fig. 13-24. Skeletal traction. (From Compere, E. L., Banks, S. W., and Compere, C. L.: Pictorial handbook of fracture treatment, ed. 5, Chicago, 1963, Year Book Medical Publishers, Inc.)

result in dysfunction of an extremity or joint or in disfigurement. When the extremity has been exposed to contaminants or encased in a cast for a long time, or the thick horny epidermis has become embedded with debris, scrupulous cleansing of the operative area is a most important preventive measure against wound infection.

PREPARATION OF VARIOUS REGIONS FOR SURGERY. The proposed operative site and the immediate region above and below it should be prepared. The extent of skin preparation on the different extremities and joints is described in Chapter 4.

POSITIONING OF THE PATIENT. Proper positioning of the patient on the operating table provides for good body alignment

without undue strain or pressure on nerves and muscles, adequate exposure of the operative area, freedom of respiratory and circulatory functions, and adequate stabilization of the body.

The surgeon is primarily responsible for instructing the nursing service team members as they position the patient on the table. The nursing service staff should know the meaning of terms such as flexion, abduction, and adduction, which are used in positioning a patient. The nursing service assistants should know how to manipulate the operating table and apply the attachments and other supports.

The principles of positioning and the different types of positions used in orthopedic surgery are described and illustrated in Chapter 7.

The selection of the position depends on several factors: (1) the type of operation to be performed, (2) the location of the injury or lesion, and (3) the age and physical condition of the patient.

DRAPING. Application of sterile sheets and towels is the third important step in preparing the patient for the operation. The sterile packs containing sheets, towels, and other textiles should be standardized (Chapter 5). The sterile sheets, towels, and stockinette for operations on the ankle and foot, the knee and midthigh, the hip, the spine, and the upper extremity are described in Chapter 5.

TOURNIQUETS. A pneumatic tourniquet may be applied to an extremity to provide for a bloodless field during surgery on a joint, nerve, or tendon. Even though the surgeon often applies the tourniquet, the nursing staff should know its proper application. It is a dangerous instrument when it is not used properly or is not in good working order.

Before a tourniquet is applied to the upper region of an arm or thigh, the region should be well padded. After the pneumatic tourniquet is evenly applied, smooth out the underlying skin so that wrinkles are not allowed to form. The limb may then be wrapped tightly with an Esmarch rubber bandage or elevated prior to inflating the tourniquet.

The pneumatic tourniquet is inflated quickly to prevent filling of the superficial veins before the arterial blood flow is occluded. The degree of pressure to be applied depends on several factors. These include the patient's age, the blood pressure rate, and the size of the extremity. To control bleeding, usually the average adult arm requires a pressure of 250 mm. Hg (almost 6 pounds) and the average thigh, about 500 mm. Hg (almost 10 pounds). The period of time a tourniquet can be safely inflated on an extremity also depends on the patient's age and the vascular supply of the extremity. In many clinics, the tourniquet is inflated on an arm for about 1 hour and then released for 10-minute periods before reinflation.

After use, pneumatic tourniquets must be checked for leaking valves and gauges. The casing of the inner tube must be completely intact so that the tube will not protrude through an opening, allowing the pressure to fall. So-called tourniquet paralysis may result from insufficient or excessive pressure, too long an application, or improper application.

Germicides applied to the operative area must not be allowed to run beneath the tourniquet because a chemical burn may result.

## INSTRUMENTS, SUTURES, AND SUPPLIES

The instruments and sutures of the basic orthopedic setup should be suitable for most procedures. A special set should be selected for orthopedic pediatric surgery. Instruments required for specific operations should be added to the basic setup. The sterile items of a basic setup (Chapter 17) may include the following:

Cutting instruments (Figs. 13-25 and 13-26)
  2 Scalpel handles nos. 3 and 4 with blades nos. 20, 10, and 15
  2 Mayo scissors, 6½ in., 1 curved and 1 straight
  1 Suture scissors, straight

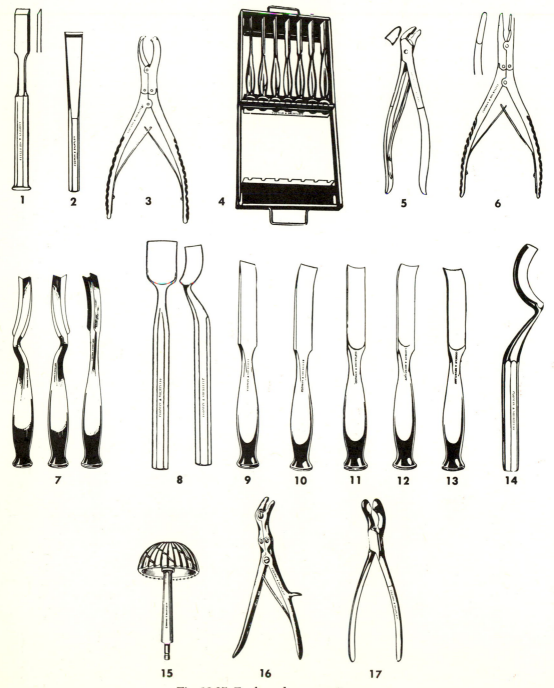

Fig. 13-25. For legend see opposite page.

1 Metzenbaum dissecting scissors, curved
1 Wire-cutting scissors, serrated blades
2 Volkmann bone curettes (Fig. 13-26)
2 Liston bone-cutting forceps (Fig. 13-26)
1 Kerrison rongeur
1 Bacon rongeur, double-action (Fig. 13-25)
3 Osteotomes, ¼, ½, and ¾ in. wide (Fig. 13-25)
2 Chisels, ¼ and ½ in. wide (Fig. 13-25)
2 Gouges
1 Bone drill and drill points, if desired
1 Kermission periosteal raspatory (Fig. 13-28)
1 Langenbeck periosteal elevator (Fig. 13-24)

### Holding instruments

6 Foerster sponge forceps, 10 in. (Chapter 17)
16 Backhaus towel clamps, 5 in.
2 Tissue forceps with 2 and 3 teeth, 5½ in. (Chapter 17)
2 Tissue forceps without teeth, 5½ in.
1 Tissue forceps without teeth, 7 in.
2 Adson tissue forceps
4 Allis forceps
2 Lowman bone-holding clamps (Fig. 13-27)
1 Bone-holding forceps (Fig. 13-27)
2 Bone hooks, 1 blunt and 1 sharp
2 Skin clip holders and clips on rack

### Clamping instruments (Chapter 5)

16 Halsted mosquito forceps, 10 curved and 6 straight
16 Crile or Kelly forceps, 5½ in., 10 curved and 6 straight
2 Ochsner forceps, straight, 6¼ in.
4 Mixter forceps, right-angled, 7½ in. (optional)
2 Mayo-Pean forceps, curved, 6¼ in.
2 Adson forceps, slightly curved jaws

### Exposing instruments

1 Set Scofield or 4 Hibbs retractors, various sizes (Fig. 13-28)
2 Bennett retractors (optional) (Fig. 13-28)
2 Roux or U.S. Army retractors (Chapter 17)

2 Volkmann retractors, 4-pronged, 1 dull and 1 sharp (Chapter 17)
1 Staphylorrhaphy narrow retractor
2 Langenbeck retractors, suitable size (Fig. 13-28)

### Suturing items

2 Needle holders, medium, 6 in.
1 Needle holder, heavy, 7½ in.
Needles:
*For bone fragments and ligaments*—2 Martin type, ½-circle, cutting edge, no. 5; 3 Mayo, ½-circle, trocar point, no. 2, free or swaged-on to sutures
*For fascia*—2 Mayo, ½-circle, taper point, no. 4 or 3; 2 Murphy, ½-circle, taper point, no. 1, free or swaged-on to suture
*For skin*—Keith abdominal, straight, 2¼ in.; 2 regular Surgeon's, ⅜-circle, cutting edge, no. 10 or 12
Suture material (preferably swaged-on to needle):
*For bones*—chromic gut no. 1
*For tendons and ligaments*—silk nos. 6-0 to 2-0 or heavier; or Dacron or nylon
*For nerves*—surgical gut or silk nos. 6-0 to 9-0, cardiovascular silk, or Dacron
*For tension sutures*—silk nos. 2-0 to 3, wire, or nylon
*For fascia and muscle*—chromic gut nos. 3-0, 2-0, or 0; silk nos. 4-0 to 2-0
*For control of bleeding*—bone wax, cautery, or no. 3-0 gut ligatures

### Accessory items

1 Mallet (Fig. 13-29)
1 Disposable Asepto syringe, 30 ml.
1 Suction set, tube, tubing, and connector
1 Metal ruler
2 Specimen containers
Bovie pencil and tip
1 Culture set
1 Orthopedic draping pack and supplies

---

**Fig. 13-25.** Various kinds of bone-cutting instruments used in orthopedic surgery. **1,** Hibbs bone chisel, various sizes; **2,** Meyerding bone chisel; **3,** double-action bone-cutting forceps; **4,** Smith-Petersen osteotomes in case; **5,** Bacon angular rongeur; **6,** Smith-Petersen double-action bone rongeur, available sizes 7½ and 9½ in., straight and slightly curved or full curved jaw; **7,** Smith-Petersen gouges for hip surgery; **8,** Smith-Petersen arthroplasty gouges, large or small sizes; **9,** Smith-Petersen osteotome, straight, 8 in., various sizes; **10,** Smith-Petersen osteotome, curved, 8 in., various sizes; **11,** Smith-Petersen gouge, straight, 8 in., various sizes; **12,** Smith-Petersen gouge, curved, various sizes; **13,** Smith-Petersen gouge, reverse curve; **14,** Smith-Petersen arthroplasty gouge, short, for starting cut, ⅞ in. wide; **15,** Smith-Petersen hip reamer; **16,** Stille bone rongeur; **17,** Horsley bone rongeur. (Courtesy Codman & Shurtleff, Inc., Randolph, Mass.)

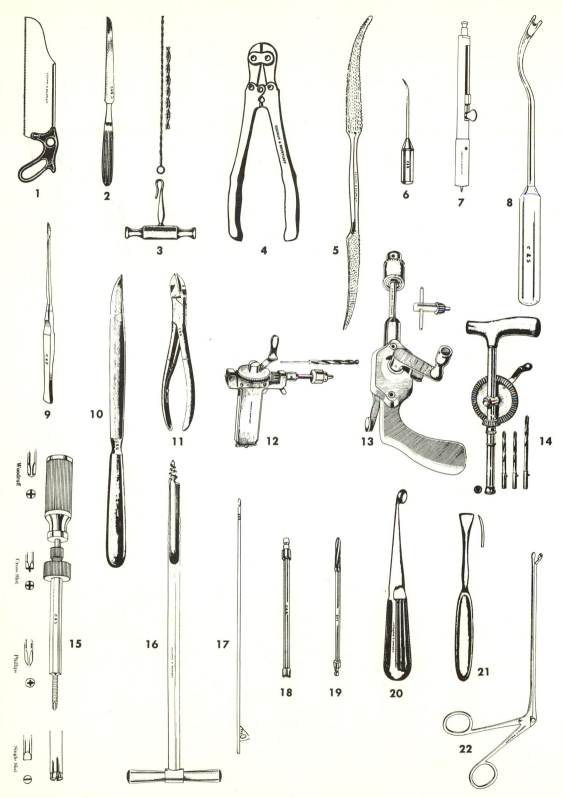

**Fig. 13-26.** For legend see opposite page.

*Unsterile equipment*

   1 Pneumatic tourniquet, desired type
   1 Fracture table with appropriate attachements (Chapter 7)
   2 Sandbags and sponge rubber pads for supports
   1 Immobilization cast setup
     X-ray machine
     Electrocautery unit

## Air-powered surgery instruments

The introduction of air-powered surgery instruments into the operating room has proved to be a most advantageous development. They eliminate the need for many hand tools, thereby reducing operating time. Fingertip control is available and allows the surgeon to control speed and power instantly. This is especially important in arthroplastic surgery. The source of power is a tank of compressed nitrogen. This is a nonflammable, inert, dependable dry gas and, most important of all considerations, is explosion free. Fig. 13-30 demonstrates some of the uses of air-powered tools.

## BASIC TECHNIQUE FOR OPEN REDUCTION OF FRACTURED BONES
### Internal fixation

DEFINITION. Through an open wound the fractured site is exposed, and the fragments are fixed by means of pins, nails, and

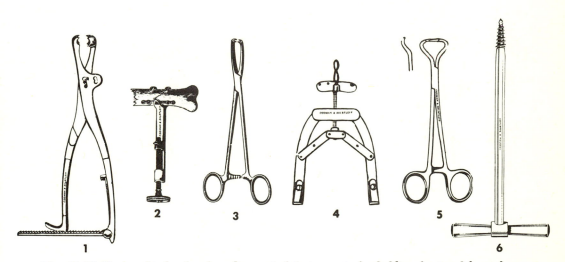

Fig. 13-27. Various kinds of orthopedic surgical instruments for holding fractured bone fragments. **1**, Lambotte bone holder; **2**, Lowman bone clamp; **3**, Jacobs vulsellum forceps; **4**, Kirschner wire tractor; **5**, Joplin bone-holding forceps; **6**, corkscrew auger. (Courtesy Codman & Shurtleff, Inc., Randolph, Mass.)

Fig. 13-26. Various kinds of orthopedic surgical instruments for cutting or dissecting ligaments and bony structures. **1**, Satterlee bone saw for amputation of long bones; **2**, Langenbeck metacarpal saw; **3**, Gigli saws, various lengths and holders; **4**, multiple-action bone pin cutters; **5**, Putti bone rasp; **6**, bone awl; **7**, Cloward dowel cutter; **8**, Downing knee cartilage knife; **9**, semilunar cartilage knife; **10**, Liston amputation knife; **11**, Liston bone-cutting forceps; **12**, Bunnell hand drill; **13**, Smedberg drill; **14**, Stille-Sherman drill; **15**, screwdriver handle and bits; **16**, shaft reamer; **17**, femur guide pin for intramedullary nails; **18**, trochanteric counter bore; **19**, medullary canal reamer; **20**, curette; **21**, Langenbeck periosteal elevator; **22**, Smith-Petersen intervertebral disc rongeur. (Courtesy Codman & Shurtleff, Inc., Randolph, Mass.)

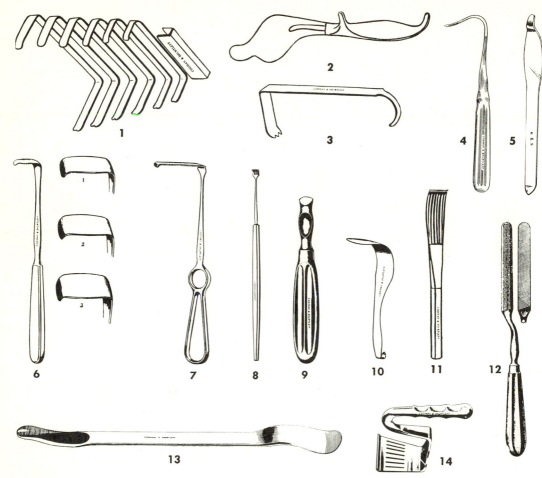

Fig. 13-28. Various kinds of orthopedic surgical instruments for exposure of structures. 1, Scofield retractors (set of six); 2, Bennett tibia retractor; 3, Hibbs retractor, various sizes; 4, Cave knee retractor; 5, Blount single-pronged blade retractor; 6, Langenbeck retractors, 4 sizes; 7, Kocher retractor; 8, 4-pronged retractor; 9, Kermission periosteal raspatory; 10, Deaver retractors, small and medium sizes; 11, Meyerding bone skid; 12, bone rasp; 13, bone skid; 14, Davidson scapula retractor. (Courtesy Codman & Shurtleff, Inc., Randolph, Mass.)

screws or with plates and screws. A blind method of fixation may be used by applying a short nail (Smith-Petersen) or a long nail (Kuntscher or Lottes) through the bone without opening the fracture site.

**CONSIDERATIONS.** Internal fixation is used when a satisfactory closed reduction cannot be obtained or maintained or when soft parts are situated betweeen the fractured fragments (Figs. 13-20 and 13-36).

Whenever possible, this operation is done before swelling has occurred or after swelling has subsided. It is not routinely done in the presence of an infection.

**SETUP AND PREPARATION OF THE PATIENT.** The basic orthopedic setup, plus intramedullary nailing or plating instruments as requested (Figs. 13-27 to 13-32). The patient is placed on the operating or fracture table in a supine position and the affected extremity supported (Chapter 7).

*Text continued on p. 503.*

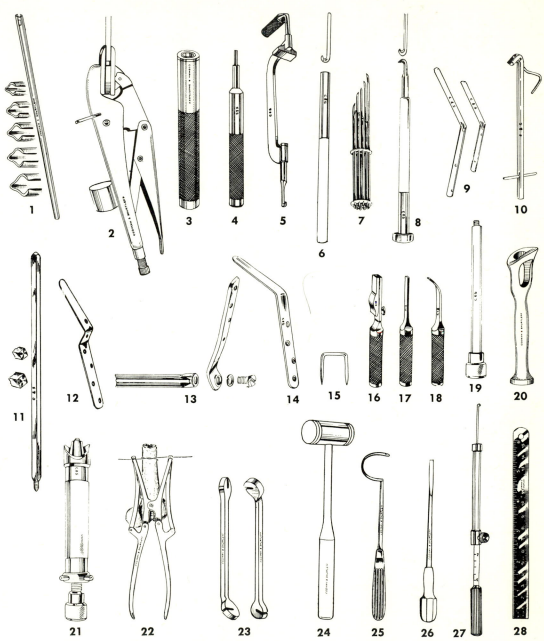

**Fig. 13-29.** Various kinds of appliances and instruments for internal fixation of fractured bones. **1,** Kuntscher intramedullary fixation; **2,** extractor pliers for intramedullary pins; **3,** Kuntscher nail driver; **4,** Kuntscher pin set; **5,** Kuntscher nail extractor; **6,** driver for Rush nails; **7,** Rush intramedullary nails; **8,** extractor for Rush nail; **9,** Neufeld plate; **10,** Neufeld plate driver; **11,** Hansen intramedullary nail; **12,** Blount blade plate; **13,** Thornton intertrochanteric bone plate for Smith-Petersen; **14,** Moore blade plate; **15,** staples; **16,** holder for staples; **17,** driver for staples; **18,** extractor for staples; **19,** Smith-Petersen nail driver handle; **20,** Smith-Petersen nail impactor; **21,** Smith-Petersen impactor extractor; **22,** Harris bone-wiring instrument; **23,** plate benders; **24,** Neufeld hammer mallet; **25,** Borchard wire threader; **26,** Lane screwdriver; **27,** depth gauge; **28,** ruler. (Courtesy Codman & Shurtleff, Inc., Randolph, Mass.)

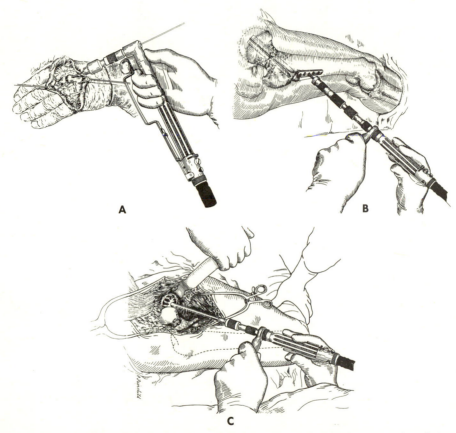

**Fig. 13-30.** Some uses of air-powered tools. **A,** Insertion of threaded or unthreaded wires (using a right-angle attachment). **B,** Insertion of screws using fingertip controlled torque in both forward and reverse rotation. **C,** Reaming of the acetabulum using the cutting power. (From Hall, R. M.: Orthairtome, Warsaw, Ind., 1966, Zimmer of Canada, Ltd., The Fred Schad Co., Inc., Columbus, Ohio.)

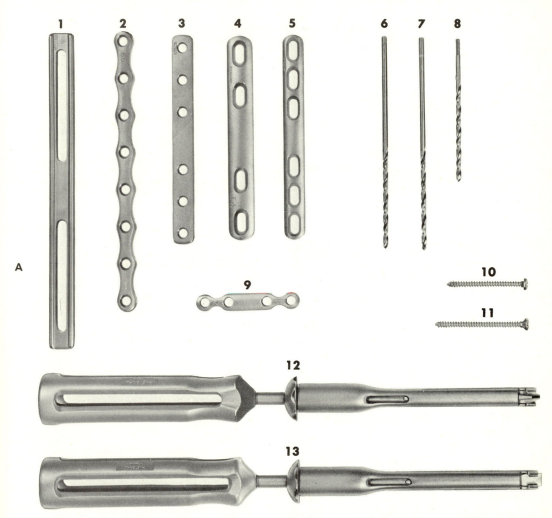

**Fig. 13-31A.** Vitallium surgical appliances, which are available in various sizes, for internal fixation of bone fragments. 1, Eggers contact splint; 2, Sherman plate; 3, Venable plate; 4, heavy-type slotted plate; 5, light-type slotted plate; 6, bone drill with perforated tip; 7, bone drill; 8, bone drill for Trinkle or Stryker drill; 9, modified Sherman bone plate; 10, Eggers screw; 11, Sherman screw; 12, Phillips screw-holding screwdriver; 13, Sherman screw-holding screwdriver. (Courtesy Austenal Co., Division of Vitallium Surgical Appliances, Howe Sound Co., New York, N. Y.)

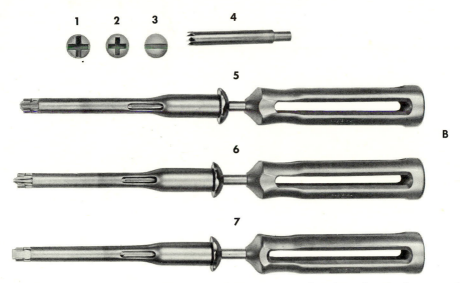

**Fig. 13-31B.** Vitallium surgical appliances, available in various lengths and sizes, for internal fixation of bone fragments—cont'd. **1,** Cruciform screw-type head and Woodruff-type screw head; **2,** Phillips-type screw head; **3,** Sherman screw-type head; **4,** Crown drill-screw; **5,** Cruciform screw-holding driver; **6,** Phillips screw-holding driver; **7,** Sherman screw-holding driver. (Courtesy Austenal Co., Division of Vitallium Surgical Appliances, Howe Sound Co., New York, N. Y.)

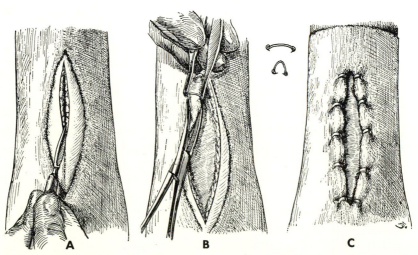

**Fig. 13-32.** Draping of edges of skin incision. **A,** Sterile stockinette incised in line of skin incision. **B** and **C,** Stockinette overlaps edges of incision and is held in place by skin clips. (From Speed, J. S., and Knight, R. A., editors: Campbell's operative orthopaedics, ed. 3, St. Louis, 1956, The C. V. Mosby Co.)

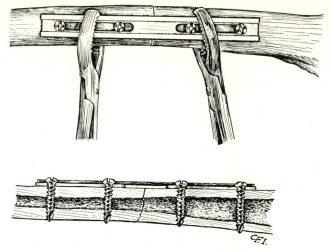

**Fig. 13-33.** Internal fixation of fracture with Eggers plate and screws. Screws must be snugly sealed in bone and must engage both cortices. (From Crenshaw, A. H., editor: Campbell's operative orthopaedics, ed. 4, St. Louis, 1963, The C. V. Mosby Co.)

Routine skin cleansing and draping procedure are carried out, as described in Chapters 4 and 5.

**OPERATIVE PROCEDURE**

1. The stockinette, if used, is cut with heavy suture scissors to expose the proposed incisional site (Fig. 13-32). The skin and subcutaneous tissue are incised with a scalpel. The skin edges are protected with towels or gauze pads that are secured in place with sutures or metal skin clips. A synthetic surgical skin drape may be used, eliminating the need for towel clips (Chapter 5).

2. The muscles are separated and retracted (with retractors). With a periosteal elevator, the periosteum is divided and elevated. Scar and granulation tissue is removed. Bleeding is controlled with hemostats and fine gut ligatures or cautery. The fractured bone ends are grasped and approximated by means of bone-holding forceps or with clamps (Figs. 13-27 and 13-33).

3. The fractured fragments are fixed by means of desired plates and screws (Figs. 13-31A and 13-34). The drill used should be approximately the same diameter as the screws. This is accomplished with the screw measure and guide. Holes are drilled in the bone in this fashion. An Asepto syringe filled with normal saline solution is used to prevent the spread of bone dust and eliminate unnecessary heat from the drilling process. The screws are inserted when the desired holes are obtained (Figs. 13-34 to 13-36).

4. The periosteum, muscle, and fascia are closed with chromic gut or silk sutures. The skin drape or towels or pads are removed. The wound edges are protected with clean towels. The subcutaneous tissue is approximated, skin edges are sutured together, and dressings are applied to the wound.

5. When applicable, the extremity is immobilized in a cast.

**Bone-grafting of fractured bone**

**DEFINITION.** Exposure of the fractured fragments, attachment of healthy bone onto the bone fragments, and insertion of screws through holes made in the graft and into the cortex of the fragments.

**INDICATIONS.** Bone grafts may be used in the following circumstances:

1. To fill cavities or defects from cysts, tumors, or other causes
2. To bridge joints and thereby provide arthrodesis

*Text continued on p. 508.*

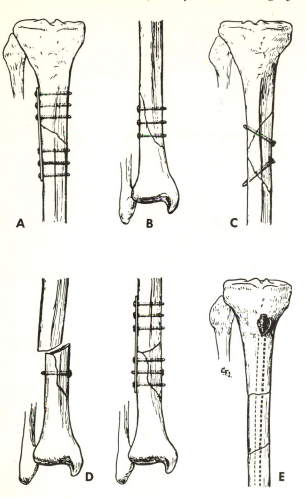

Fig. 13-34. Techniques of internal fixation. **A,** Plate and six screws for transverse or short oblique fracture. **B,** Transfixion screws for long oblique or spiral fractures. **C,** Transfixion screws for long butterfly fragment. **D,** Fixation of fracture with short butterfly fragment. **E,** Medullary fixation. (From Crenshaw, A. H., editor: Campbell's operative orthopaedics, ed. 4, St. Louis, 1963, The C. V. Mosby Co.)

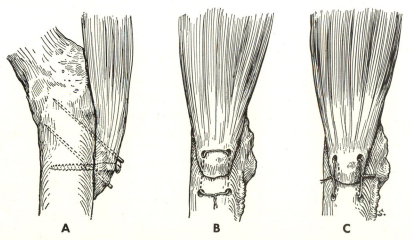

Fig. 13-35. Fixation of osseous attachment of tendon to bone. **A,** Fixation by vitallium screw or nail. **B,** Fixation by mattress suture of stainless steel wire through holes drilled in bone. **C,** Fixation by wire loops. (From Crenshaw, A. H., editor: Campbell's operative orthopaedics, ed. 4, St. Louis, 1963, The C. V. Mosby Co.)

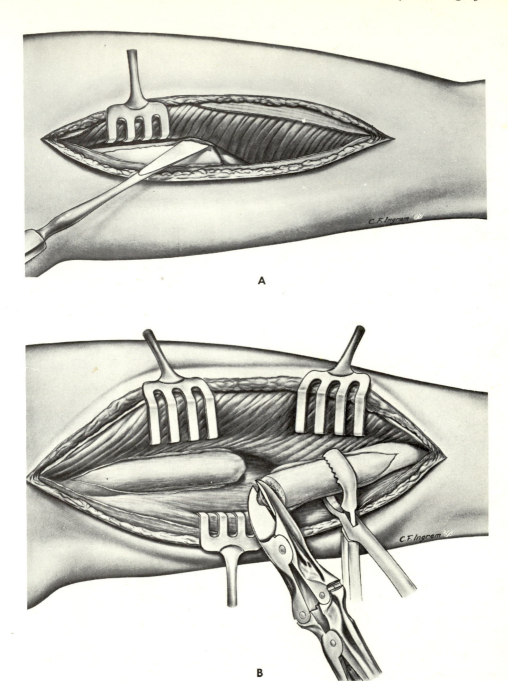

A

B

*Continued.*

**Fig. 13-36. A,** Exposure of nonunion of middle third of femur. **B,** Excision of eburnated bone from ends of fragments. Soft tissue attachments to bone are preserved as far as possible. **C,** Shavings removed from small portion of circumference of shaft, forming flat surface 3 to 4 inches long on each fragment. **D,** Each medulla is reamed out. Graft of endosteum is placed in medullary canal as fracture is reduced. **E,** Fragments and cortical graft are held in position by bone clamp; fixation is secured by screws that traverse graft and both cortices. **F,** Onlay bone graft completed by insertion of cancellous bone about fracture from medullary surface of graft and from tibial condyle. (From Crenshaw, A. H., editor: Campbell's operative orthopaedics, ed. 5, St. Louis, 1971, The C. V. Mosby Co.)

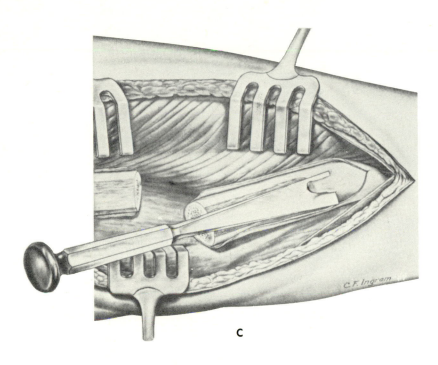

C

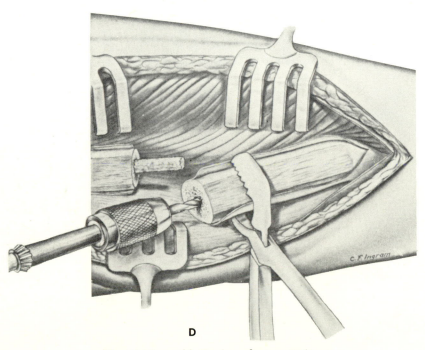

D

Fig. 13-36, cont'd. For legend see p. 505.

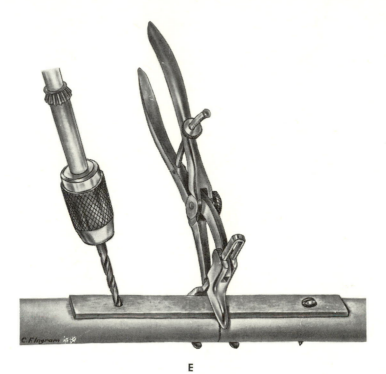

E

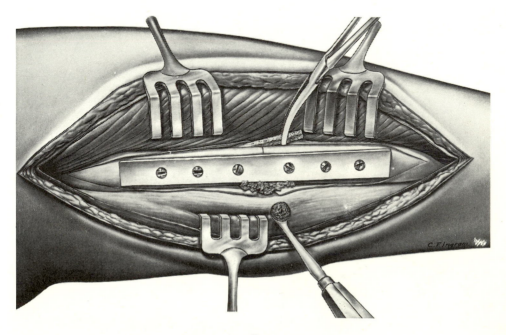

F

Fig. 13-36, cont'd. For legend see p. 505.

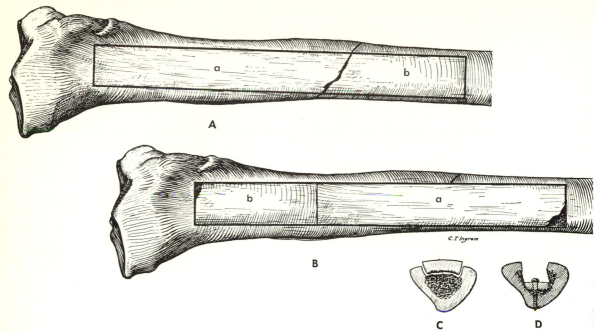

**Fig. 13-37.** Albee sliding inlay graft. **A,** Grafts cut on each fragment, **B,** Grafts reversed, longer segment placed across fracture. **C,** Cross section of inlay graft. **D,** Massive sliding graft (Buchanan-Wagner), similar to sliding inlay method, although graft is placed in medullary canal and fixed with metal screws. (From Crenshaw, A. H., editor: Campbell's operative orthopaedics, ed. 5, St. Louis, 1971, The C. V. Mosby Co.)

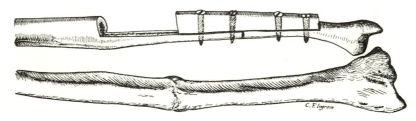

**Fig. 13-38.** Gill massive sliding graft. (From Crenshaw, A. H., editor: Campbell's operative orthopaedics, ed. 5, St. Louis, 1971, The C. V. Mosby Co.)

3. To bridge major defects or establish the continuity of a long bone
4. To promote union or fill defects in delayed union, malunion, fresh fractures, or osteotomies

CONSIDERATIONS. The type of graft to be done generally depends on the location of the nonunited bone, the condition of the ends of the fragments, and the preference of the surgeon. An autogenous graft may be taken from the tibia, ilium, or fibula; or a homologous graft may be obtained from the bone bank or a donor. The donor and patient need not have the same Rh or blood type. (See Chapter 5.)

A massive onlay graft may be taken from the tibia, including the periosteum and the full thickness of the cortex (Figs. 13-37 to 13-39). However, this extensive borrowing from the tibia is a hazardous procedure that may be followed by infection or may cause immediate or late fatigue-type fracture at the donor site. A cancellous graft comprising the spongy

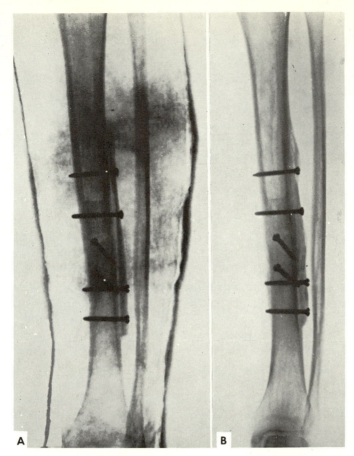

Fig. 13-39. Roentgenograms of onlay bone graft for ununited fracture of the tibial shaft. **A,** Massive cortical graft from the proximal half of the tibia has been fixed across the fracture site with two transverse screws in each fragment. The two middle screws transfix the oblique ends of the fracture fragments. Note cast, which is essential for further immobilization during the healing period. **B,** Six months after operation. Note consolidation of the onlay graft with the tibial shaft. (From Raney, R. B., and Brashear, H. R.: Shand's handbook of orthopaedic surgery, ed. 8, St. Louis, 1971, The C. V. Mosby Co.)

bone of the ilium may be used as a non-rigid graft. When there is sclerosis of the bone ends with nonunion, a bone graft may be used to stimulate osteogenesis in each fragment.

SETUP AND PREPARATION OF THE PATIENT. The setup includes the basic orthopedic setup. Electric or air-driven drills and saws are extremely helpful if available. One hand drill, drill points nos. 8 to 10, and three bone curettes of various sizes are included (Fig. 13-26).

Two sterile instrument setups and other unsterile equipment, such as two instru-ment tables and two Mayo stands, are needed. One setup is used to obtain the graft, and the other is used to fix the graft to the bone fragments.

The patient is prepared as described for internal fixation. The graft site and the fractured extremity are usually draped separately (Chapters 4 and 5).

OPERATIVE PROCEDURE

1. The skin overlying the fractured bone is incised, and the scar tissue is excised, as in open reduction. To encourage heal-ing, the sclerosed bone may be drilled

or removed to stimulate granulation tissue foundation.

2. The graft is obtained, and the affected fragments are prepared to suit the graft. To form a bed for an onlay graft, the periosteum and a portion of the outer cortex are removed from the fragmented ends of the bone. To perform an inlay or sliding grafts, a special slot is made in the bone fragments for the reception of the graft. (See Fig. 13-36.) Occasionally a sliding graft is used for tibial fractures. The graft is cut from the proximal fragment of the fractured bone and is slid into the prepared bed over the distal fragment of the bone.

3. To obtain an inlay graft (Figs. 13-37 to 13-39) from the tibia, a curved incision is made along the anteromedial surface of the tibia, with its convexity to the medial side. The periosteum is incised and reflected with an osteotome. The size and shape of the graft are outlined with drill holes, and the graft is removed with an electric oscillating bone saw that has a double blade. A fracture of the entire thickness of the donor bone may occur if the osteotomy is not outlined by drill holes.

4. In an onlay grafting operation (Figs. 13-37 to 13-39), bone-holding forceps are used on the operative site as the drill holes are placed through both the graft and fragments. Screws are then inserted through the holes of the graft and into the cortex of the bone's fragments. In some cases, bone chips are laid over the fragments to be united (Fig. 13-36).

5. A cancellous graft consists of spongy bone, usually taken from the crest or wing of the ilium. Depending on the position of the patient, the anterior or posterior third of the ilium is used. Exposure of the ilium is relatively easy, but considerable bleeding may occur. An incision is made along the subcutaneous border of the iliac crest. The muscles on the outer table of the ilium are elevated. If chip grafts are required, they are removed with an osteotome parallel to the crest of

the ilium. After removal of the crest, the cancellous bone may be obtained by curetting the cancellous space between the two intact cortices.

6. The wounds are closed in layers and dressings applied. A plaster casing may be applied to the fractured extremity.

## OPERATIONS ON THE HIP
### Treatment of fractured hips

DEFINITION OF TERMS. Fractures of the hip are in reality fractures of the upper end of the femur and are classified under three main groups: (1) the intracapsular types, which include the capital, subcapital, and transcervical fractures (Fig. 13-16); (2) the extracapsular types, which include the intertrochanteric fractures; and (3) the upper femoral epiphyseal separation, usually occurring in young obese boys (Fig. 13-17). The term *intracapsular* refers to the *inside* of the hip joint, and *extracapsular*, to the *outside* of the hip joint (Figs. 13-9 and 13-10).

GENERAL CONSIDERATIONS. A *subcapital* fracture is one that occurs in the upper end of the femur, that is, within the hip joint, just beneath the femoral head. Older persons usually are the sufferers because they may fall more often. A subcapital fracture, which may be impacted or grossly displaced, may be caused by indirect violence, such as slipping on a rug or polished floor. The bone gives way, and the patient falls to the floor. After the injury, the leg becomes externally rotated if the fracture is not impacted.

The patient with a displaced subcapital fracture is treated by the insertion of a suitable appliance at the earliest time his general condition permits. If the fracture is close to the femoral head, internal fixation may be supplemented by means of a bone-grafting operation. Delay or nonunion may occur in subcapital fractures, especially in those where the fracture line is unstable. The strong pull of the hip muscles often tends to produce a loss of normal angulation between the shaft and femoral neck, resulting in shortening, ex-

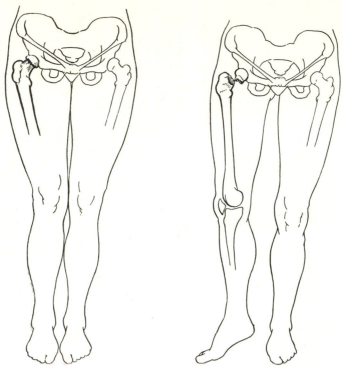

**Fig. 13-40.** Position of leg following intracapsular fracture of hip. (From Compere, E. L., Banks, S. W., and Compere, C. L.: Pictorial handbook of fracture treatment, ed. 5, Chicago, 1963, Year Book Medical Publishers, Inc.)

ternal rotation, and adduction deformities. Subcapital fractures are sometimes impacted. These are frequently managed without surgery if they are inherently stable.

A *transcervical (intracapsular)* fracture occurs in the midportion of the femoral neck. These fractures almost always require surgery. If possible, internal fixation of the fracture is carried out. Otherwise, a femoral head prosthesis may be used.

An *intertrochanteric* fracture is located farther from the region of the trochanter and may occur when the person falls directly on the trochanteric region or when his leg is twisted. After the injury, the limb generally shows a full external rotation deformity. The fracture lines of intertrochanteric fractures usually run in different directions, but they generally heal (Fig. 13-42).

Reduction of intertrochanteric fractures

may be maintained by plaster hip spica cast, external fixation and traction, or open operation. The latter includes the insertion of a pin or nail into the neck of the femur and the attachment of a plate and screws, such as a Jewett nail and plate, a Smith-Petersen nail with a McLaughlin plate, or a Neufeld angled nail and plate, to the other side of the femur (Figs. 13-29 and 13-36).

A *separation or slipping of the upper femoral epiphysis* (adolescent coxa vara) may occur quickly or gradually. This condition causes a decrease of the angle between the femoral neck and shaft. When this occurs, the femoral head rotates posteriorly and inferiorly, and the femoral shaft and neck move forward. This lesion usually is seen in obese children between the ages of 10 and 16 or following a

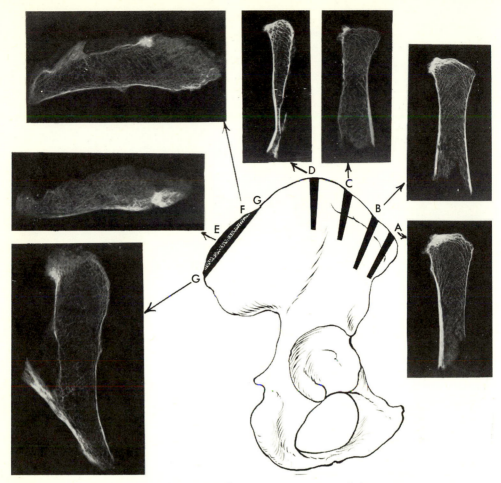

**Fig. 13-41.** Coronal sections (**A** to **D**) from anterior portion of ilium. Accompanying cross sections show width of bone and its cancellous structure. Iliac grafts for fusion of spine are ordinarily removed from posterior third of crest (**E** to **G**). (From Crenshaw, A. H., editor: Campbell's operative orthopaedics, ed. 5, St. Louis, 1971, The C. V. Mosby Co.)

traumatic injury. Acute displacement or a chronic disability in the hip is usually accompanied by a limp (Figs. 13-16 and 13-17).

An acute displacement of the upper femoral epiphysis is treated by manipulative reduction and introduction of multiple pins across the epiphysis or by manipulative reduction and immobilization with a plaster spica cast. When a chronic condition exists and is accompanied by gross displacement, more elaborate procedures are required.

### Intertrochanteric fracture

**DEFINITION.** Through an open wound the fragments are fixed by a metal appliance such as a Jewett angled nail, a Smith-Petersen nail with a McLaughlin- or Thornton plate, a Neufeld nail, a Blount-Moore blade plate and screws, or a Lorenz screw nail and plate (Figs. 13-31A to 13-45).

**CONSIDERATIONS.** If fixation of intertrochanteric fractures is done with a nail alone, angulation and coxa vara may occur because the upper portion of the nail as it lies in the thin lateral cortex of the

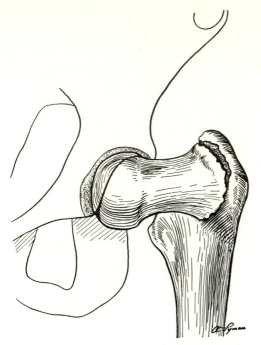

Fig. 13-42. Fracture at base of neck of femur (intertrochanteric type). Note decrease in angle of neck and eversion. Lesser trochanter shows up prominently, denoting outward rotation. (From Larson, C. B., and Gould, M.: Calderwood's orthopedic nursing, ed. 6, St. Louis, 1965, The C. V. Mosby Co.)

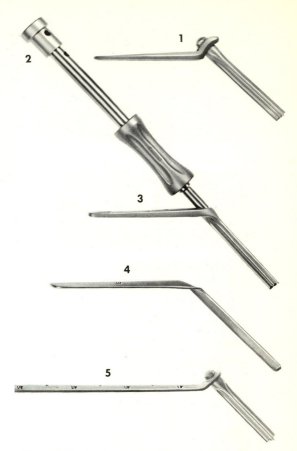

Fig. 13-43. Appliances used in treatment of intertrochanteric fractures. **1,** McLaughlin model VI plate and nail; **2,** driver extractor for removal of nail; **3,** Jewett plate-nail; **4,** Neufeld nail plate; **5,** Thornton plate and nail. (Courtesy Austenal Co., Division of Vitallium Surgical Appliances, Howe Sound Co., New York, N. Y.)

femur may cut through this inadequate support. Hence a nail-plate combination to give fixation to the shaft of the femur is needed.

**SETUP AND PREPARATION OF THE PATIENT.** The setup includes a basic orthopedic setup, plus the preferred metal appliances, screws, and screwdrivers (Figs. 13-43 to 13-46). The patient is placed in a supine position on the fracture table. The hip region is cleansed, as described previously. In some cases, the entire affected extremity, the abdomen, and the anterolateral portion of the chest are cleansed. The patient is draped, using a fenestrated sheet and regular sheets. (See Chapters 4 and 5.)

**OPERATIVE PROCEDURE**

1. With a scalpel, a skin incision is made in the thigh, beginning at the level of the superior aspect of the greater tro-

chanter and extending along the shaft of the femur. Bleeding is controlled. Wound edges are protected with skin towels or pads.

2. The deep fascia is incised and retracted with retractors, and the lateral great muscle is split and retracted to expose the shaft and trochanter of the femur.

3. With a Kirschner or Smedberg bone drill, a hole is drilled at a point midway between the anterior and posterior cortex of the femur, using at the same time an Asepto syringe filled with normal saline solution.

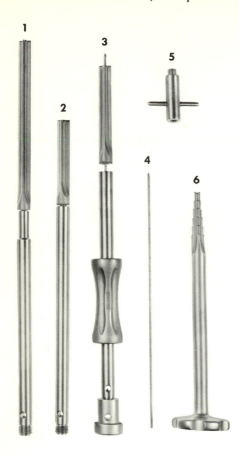

Fig. 13-44. Intertrochanteric appliances for fractures of hip—cont'd. 1, Driver shaft, ¼ in. × 20 thread and Smith-Petersen nail; 2, Thornton driver shaft, ⁵⁄₁₆ in. × 24 thread and Thornton nail; 3, driving head, extractor hammer, and Thornton nail; 4, calibrated guide wire; 5, adapter, 1¼ in. × 20 to ⁵⁄₁₆ in. × 24 threads; 6, Ritchie nail starter. (Courtesy Austenal Co., Division of Vitallium Surgical Appliances, Howe Sound Co., New York, N. Y.)

4. The desired guide wire is inserted at a 45-degree angle to the shaft and may be changed by starting the insertion of the wire at a lower point on the shaft of the femur. The guide pin is driven up the neck of the femur. This is checked by x-ray films. The guide pin may be removed before, during, or after insertion of the nail appliance.

5. A desired nail appliance of the appropriate size is driven into the bone so that its plate will be flush with the shaft (Figs. 13-46 to 13-48). The plate attachment is fixed to the shaft with appropriate size screws. X-ray films are taken before closure to determine the proper location and fixation of the nail.

6. If the fracture is subcapital or intracervical, multiple Knowles pins or a Smith-Petersen nail may be used. The exposure need not be as extensive as for the nail and plate combination, since no side plate is attached to the femoral shaft. If multiple pins are used, they are placed in much the same manner as a guide pin. Usually four are inserted parallel to each other in a boxlike pattern.

7. If the fracture is subcapital or intracervical, the surgeon may decide to use a primary prosthesis rather than attempt fixation of the fracture.

8. The wound is closed in layers. Skin towels or pads are removed. Dressings are applied, and in some cases plaster-of-Paris is applied.

### Intramedullary femoral fracture

**DEFINITION.** The insertion of a nail through the intramedullary canal of the proximal and distal fragments of the femur, usually through a posterolateral incision (Figs. 13-49 to 13-52).

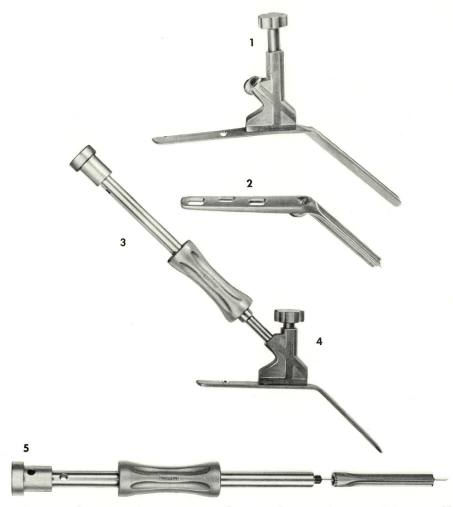

**Fig. 13-45.** Appliances used in treatment of intertrochanteric fractures of hip—cont'd. **1,** Neufeld nail driver and Neufeld appliance; **2,** modified Jewett (cannulated) appliance; **3,** driver retractor interchangeable with most appliances such as Neufeld, Jewett, and Moore; **4,** Moore blade plate driver; **5,** Austenal hip nail driver—extractor—driving head, extractor hammer, driver shaft, and Thornton nail. (Courtesy Austenal Co., Division of Vitallium Surgical Appliances, Howe Sound Co., New York, N. Y.)

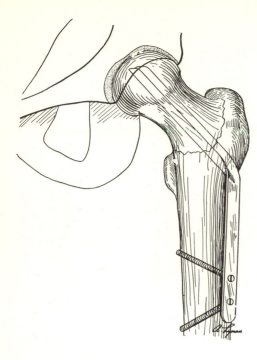

**Fig. 13-46.** Open reduction of intertrochanteric fracture, with Neufeld nail inserted into neck and head and down shaft of femur, using divergent screws. Nail is one-piece stainless steel with V-shaped flanges into neck and head. (From Larson, C. B., and Gould, M.: Orthopedic nursing, ed. 7, St. Louis, 1970, The C. V. Mosby Co.)

**CONSIDERATIONS.** Most fractures of the femoral shaft are caused by direct violence, which results in short, oblique, or transverse fractures; few result from indirect violence, which produces a torsion force. The latter situation usually causes a spiral fracture. Others are considered pathological fractures due to the presence of metastatic carcinoma, Paget's disease of the bone, and dysplasia. Patients with a fractured femur suffer severe pain and shock not only due to the injury itself but also as a result of associated injuries as well.

**SETUP AND PREPARATION OF THE PATIENT.** The basic orthopedic setup, plus desired plates and screws and intramedullary nails such as the Kuntscher, cloverleaf-shaped, or Hansen-Street diamond-shaped nail (Fig. 13-50). The patient is positioned on his side. Proper supports to stabilize the patient and x-ray equipment are required.

**OPERATIVE PROCEDURE**

1. Through a posterolateral incision made with a scalpel, the fracture site is exposed and retracted, and wound edges are protected. Bleeding vessels are clamped and ligated or cauterized.

2. A nail is selected (Fig. 13-50) and tested to fit the distal portion of the fractured bones according to their width and size and then the proximal fractured fragments. The fragments are reamed with a reamer that is the same size as the nail.

3. The proximal fragment usually is reamed out up through the isthmus. This is the narrowest portion of the intramedullary canal, where the nail might get caught during its insertion.

4. A guide wire is driven in retrograde fashion up through the proximal fragment and out through the greater trochanter until it emerges through the skin at the level of the posterior lateral buttocks. Before this step is carried out the thigh must be adducted and flexed so that the guide pin will not be driven up into the chest or abdomen (Fig. 13-52).

5. A skin incision is made around the guide pin; then a reamer is inserted over the guide wire. A hole is reamed into the top of the femur at the greater tro-

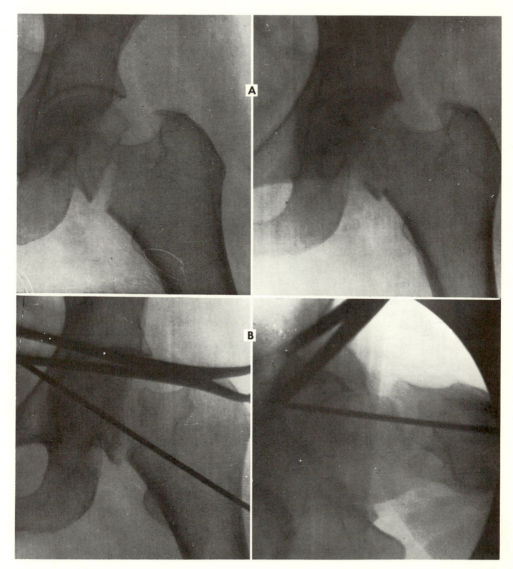

*Continued.*

**Fig. 13-47.** If reduction is unstable, multiple pins are used in preference to Smith-Petersen nail, their removal incident to poor position of pins or tilting or displacement of head is easier than removal and reinsertion of the Smith-Petersen nail. **A,** Unsatisfactory reduction after first attempt corrected by second maneuvers. Reduction in lateral view (not shown) satisfactory after both attempts. **B,** Guide pin purposely inserted through head into ilium to increase stability. Satisfactory position of pin in anteroposterior view but distraction at fracture. In lateral view, pin is in satisfactory position in neck fragment but engages head in anterior quadrant, tilting it posteriorly. **C,** Fracture has been fixed with four Knowles pins. Usually three pins are preferred. **D,** Fracture has united at 1 year. (From Crenshaw, A. H., editor: Campbell's operative orthopaedics, ed. 5, St. Louis, 1971, The C. V. Mosby Co.)

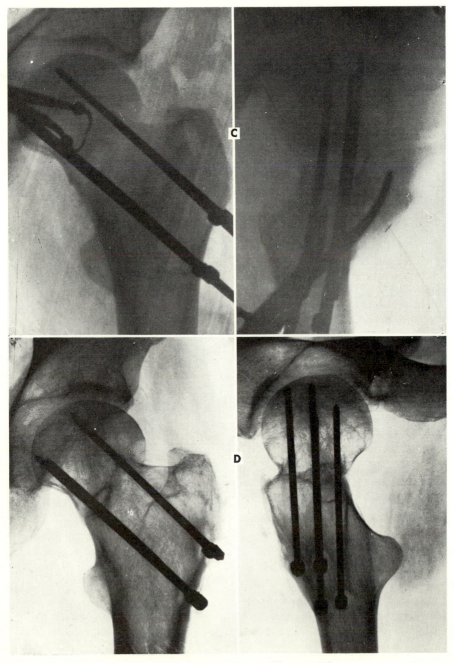

**Fig. 13-47, cont'd.** For legend see p. 517.

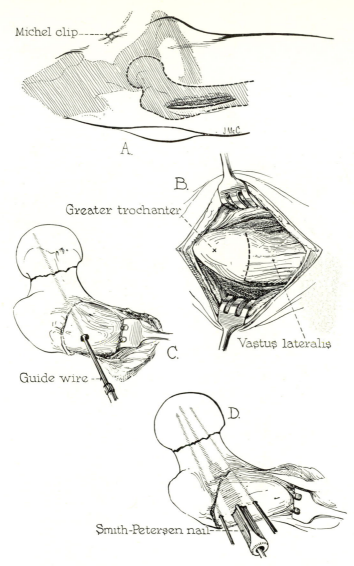

**Fig. 13-48.** Introduction of Smith-Petersen nail for internal fixation of intracapsular fractures of neck of femur. (From Compere, E. L., Banks, S. W., and Compere, C. L.: Pictorial handbook of fracture treatment, ed. 5, Chicago, 1963, Year Book Medical Publishers, Inc.)

chanter; then the nail is driven down over the guide wire until it emerges at the fracture site. The guide wire should be withdrawn as soon as the nail is firmly seated in the proximal fragment. Otherwise, the nail may bind on the guide pin.

6. The fracture is reduced and aligned correctly in regard to rotation. The nail is then driven into the distal fragment, and its position is checked with x-ray films.

7. The wound is closed, and dressings are applied. The affected leg usually is placed in balanced suspension (Thomas splint), and, on occasion, traction is applied, or the leg may merely be placed on a pillow.

### Dislocation of the hip

GENERAL CONSIDERATIONS. Although dislocation of the hip does not commonly occur, it may be caused by a severe blow that displaces the head of the femur out

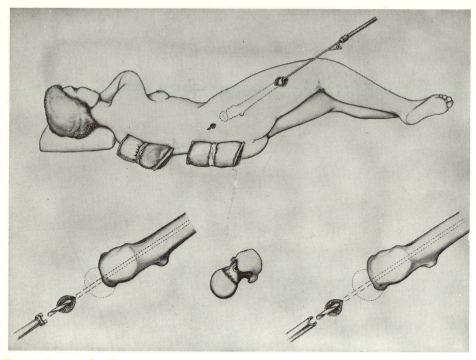

**Fig. 13-49.** Details of insertion of medullary nail. Guide pins emerge through small incision in upper outer quadrant and buttock. Trochanteric reamer placed over guide pin and holes drilled in correct alignment with medullary canal. Kuntscher nail inserted into proximal femoral fragment over guide pin. When nail has been driven down to level of fracture site, guide pin is removed and fracture reduced. Nail is then driven correct distance in distal fragment. (From Smith, H.: Radiology **61:**194, 1953.)

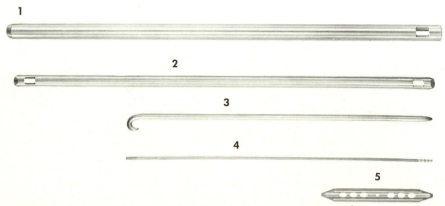

**Fig. 13-50.** Intramedullary vitallium appliances. **1,** Cloverleaf intramedullary nail, available in 6 to 15 mm. diameters and lengths ranging from 26 to 52 cm.; **2,** Kuntscher-type cloverleaf intramedullary nail; **3,** Rush hooked intramedullary pin; **4,** Street forearm pin; **5,** Livingston intramedullary bar used with vitallium Sherman, Phillips, or cruciform-type screws, $\frac{9}{64}$ in. (Courtesy Austenal Co., Division of Vitallium Surgical Appliances, Howe Sound Co., New York, N. Y.)

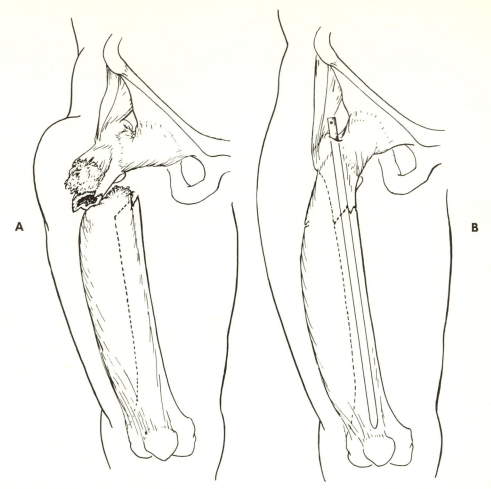

Fig. 13-51. **A,** Fracture of upper end of shaft of femur. Displacement fracture at sub-trochanteric site with interposition of torn vastus muscle. This is most common type of fracture in upper end of shaft causing nonunion. **B,** Treatment by Kuntscher rod. (From Miller, D. S.: Surg. Clin. North Am. **45:**38, 1965.)

of the acetabulum. In some injuries the head of the femur is pushed centrally, carrying with it the floor of the acetabulum. In such conditions the lower extremity on the affected side appears to be shortened, and occasionally the rim of the acetabulum or head of the femur may be fractured.

A pathological dislocation of the hip may be caused by (1) a severe infectious disease such as scarlet fever, typhoid fever, or tuberculosis; (2) infantile paralysis; or (3) a chronic arthritis resulting in destruction of the femoral head or the acetabulum.

The term *congenital dislocation* includes various degrees of displacement of the femoral head from its normal position, as well as subluxations. In some advanced cases a shelf reconstruction operation is done; however, open reduction sometimes is necessary in the early stages of the disease.

The *choice of operation* depends on the degree of injury and the condition of the patient. The types of operations that may be done to treat a dislocation of the hips include (1) closed reduction with immobilization by plaster spica cast, (2) open

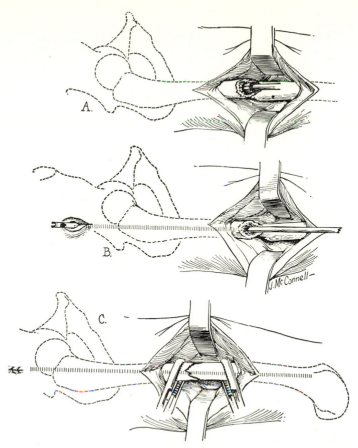

Fig. 13-52. Introduction of intramedullary rod into femur by retrograde method. Fracture is exposed through lateral incision. **A,** Stainless steel rod of correct size and length is driven upward through medullary canal of proximal fragment so that rod pierces cortex of neck just medial to greater trochanter. **B,** Skin incision is made over end of rod where it presents on gluteal region so that it can emerge far enough for other end of rod to be introduced into distal fragment. **C,** After fracture is reduced, rod is drawn into distal fragment at level corresponding to patella. Reamer is used to enlarge canal if it is too small to accept rod or if it is obstructed by bone. (From Compere, E. L., Banks, S. W., and Compere, C. L.: Pictorial handbook of fracture treatment, ed. 5, Chicago, 1963, Year Book Medical Publishers, Inc.)

reduction with screw fixation for the reducible fragments, (3) arthrodesis, or (4) arthroplasty.

### Arthroplasty of the hip

**DEFINITION.** Through an anterolateral, lateral, or posterolateral incision, the diseased joint is severed, the hip dislocated, and the articulating surfaces remodeled with the aid of a metallic cup or a prosthetic replacement.

**CONSIDERATIONS.** The function of the hip joint may be markedly limited by a degenerative lesion such as arthritis or by a pyogenic infection. Trauma is believed to be a most significant factor. Degenerative arthritis may follow an accident, or it may appear many years later in patients who had childhood epiphyseal disturbances. Surgery is not performed until the acute stage of infection has passed.

When a hip is reconstructed, the diseased head of the femur may be covered or replaced by a plastic or metal prosthesis.

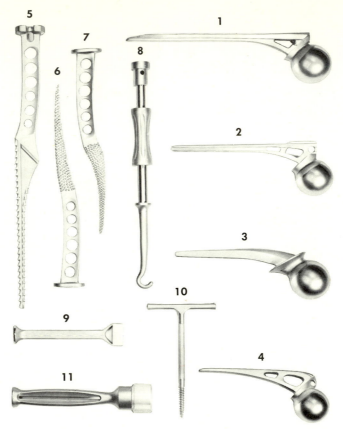

Fig. 13-53. Hip prosthesis appliances for arthroplasty procedure. **1,** Watchett-Brown hip-pinning prosthesis; **2,** Austin-Moore straight-stem hip prosthesis; **3,** Thompson modified-type intramedullary hip prosthesis; **4,** Austin-Moore-type original hip prosthesis; **5,** Moore broach; **6,** Moore rasp; **7,** Thompson rasp; **8,** Moore hooked driver-extractor; **9,** Moore hollow chisel; **10,** Moore T extractor; **11,** Universal femoral head driver. (Courtesy Austenal Co., Division of Vitallium Surgical Appliances, Howe Sound Co., New York, N. Y.)

The principle of mold arthroplasty is the interposition of a permanent inert barrier between two joint surfaces. To minimize friction, the mold must allow an adequate degree of motion between it and the adjacent reshaped surface of the femoral head or the acetabulum.

SETUP AND PREPARATION OF THE PATIENT. The basic orthopedic setup plus appropriate appliances, as well as special retractors, rasps, chisels, osteotomes, gouges, extractors, and reamers (Figs. 13-25 and 13-53). The patient is positioned on the operating table in a supine or lateral position, the operative skin area is cleansed, and the patient is draped.

OPERATIVE PROCEDURE

MOLD ARTHROPLASTY

1. The skin is incised with a scalpel, and the bleeding vessels are controlled by cautery or ligatures.

2. The necessary muscles are divided or moved with their attachments to expose the hip joint.

3. The capsule of the hip is incised or excised as necessary.

4. The hip is dislocated to expose the head of the femur and the acetabulum.

5. These are shaped and reamed to accept the mold or cup of choice (Fig. 13-54).

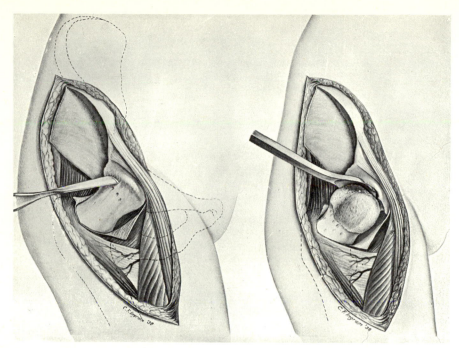

**Fig. 13-54.** Arthroplasty of hip. The articular surfaces of head of femur and acetabulum smoothed with special reamers. (From Speed, J. S., and Knight, R. A., editors: Campbell's operative orthopaedics, ed. 3, St. Louis, 1956, The C. V. Mosby Co.)

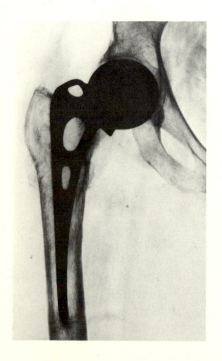

**Fig. 13-55.** Roentgenograms of the hip following replacement arthroplasty with Austin-Moore metal prosthesis in a 75-year-old woman who had had nonunion of a femoral neck fracture and a vascular necrosis of the femoral head. (From Raney, R. B., and Brashear, H. R.: Shand's handbook of orthopaedic surgery, ed. 8, St. Louis, 1971, The C. V. Mosby Co.)

6. The hip is reduced, and the position is checked.

7. The wound is closed in layers, re-attaching or transplanting as needed all muscles that were interrupted. Dressings are applied.

8. Postoperatively, abduction and neutral alignment must be maintained until the patient is capable of controlling this himself.

**PROSTHETIC ARTHROPLASTY**

1 to 4. As described in mold arthroplasty.

5. The acetabulum is examined and reamed if needed.

6. The neck of the femur is osteotomized and the medullary canal reamed at the proper angle to accept the appliance of choice ( Fig. 13-55).

7. The prothesis is seated in the femoral canal and the hip reduced.

8 and 9. As described in steps 7 and 8 under mold arthroplasty.

## Total hip replacement

**OPERATIVE PROCEDURE**

1 to 4. As described under mold arthroplasty.

5. The acetabulum is shaped and reamed to accept the acetabular portion of the appliance. The proper angle of this component is very important.

6. The acetabular component is placed and stabilized, either by the use of methyl methacrylate or by employing the proper guides and positioners for the appliance.

7. The neck of the femur is osteotomized, and the medullary canal is reamed at the proper angle for the chosen prosthesis.

8. The femoral component is seated and stabilized as required.

9. The hip is reduced, and the position is checked.

10 and 11. As described in steps 7 and 8 under mold arthroplasty.

## Arthrodesis of the hip

**DEFINITION.** The articular surfaces of the hip joint are fused together by means of

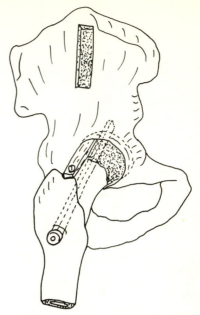

**Fig. 13-56.** Waston-Jones arthrodesis of hip joint. This arthrodesis is both intra-articular and extra-articular, combined with internal fixation with a triflanged nail. (From Mead, N. C.: Surg. Clin. North Am. **45:**171, 1965.

osteotomy, insertion of a bone graft taken from the ilium or femur, and internal fixation with a hip nail and screws (Fig. 13-56).

**CONSIDERATIONS.** Extra-articular fusion is generally performed to treat tuberculosis of the hip or relieve pain and dysfunction due to trauma or other lesions such as tumor. Some hip deformities and those produced by muscle imbalance or instability may be treated by arthrodesis.

**SETUP AND PREPARATION OF THE PATIENT.** As described for arthroplasty, plus a bone-grafting setup. In extra-articular arthrodesis with a graft to be taken from the femur, the patient may be placed on the operating table in a prone or supine position. If desired, he may be placed in the anterior half of a double hip spica cast and then positioned. If a supine position is used, the body must be adequately supported by pads and braces (Chapter 7).

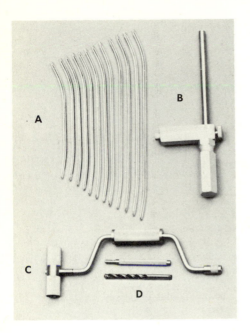

Fig. 13-57. Lottes tibial nail. A, Set Lottes tibial nails, 5/16 in. and 3/8 in. B, One driver-extractor. C, One Trinkle brace. D, One adapter, 5/16 × 3/8 in., and one twist drill, 5/16 × 6 3/8 in. (From Orthopaedic instruments and procedures, Warsaw, Ind., 1970, Zimmer of Canada, Ltd., The Fred Schad Co., Inc., Columbus, Ohio.)

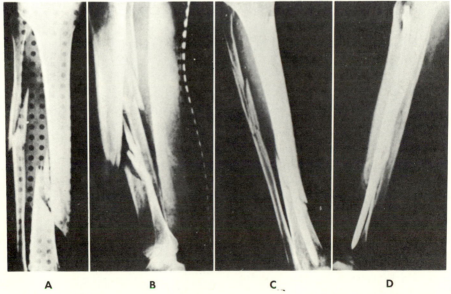

Fig. 13-58. Comminuted open fracture of both bones of leg in lower part of middle third. Treatment by debridement, internal fixation with a Lottes intramedullary nail, and primary closure of the wound. A and B, Roentgenograms in two planes with emergency splint in place. C and D, Several months after operation, showing excellent apposition and alignment and early bony union. (From Rhoads, J., et al.: Surgery: principles and practice, ed. 4, Philadelphia, 1970, J. B. Lippincott Co.)

OPERATIVE PROCEDURE. Similar to arthroplasty of the hip, as described previously.

# OPERATIONS ON THE TIBIA
## Intramedullary pinning for tibial fracture

DEFINITION. The insertion of a nail through a short incision made over the anterior aspect of the tibia and medial to the tibial tubercle.

CONSIDERATIONS. The basic requirements for intramedullary nailing are proper alignment and apposition and an accurate fit in the medullary canal. Intramedullary nailing allows the fracture to be reduced and held without plates.

SETUP AND PREPARATION OF THE PATIENT. The basic orthopedic instrument setup, plus nails such as the Kuntscher-type or Lottes nail and other instruments, as described for femoral fractures (Figs. 13-26, 13-31A, 13-50, 13-57, and 13-58). The patient is placed in the supine position, and either the leg is placed in traction to the foot or the table is bent so that the leg hangs freely, using gravity for traction. (See Chapters 4 to 7.)

OPERATIVE PROCEDURE

1. The fractured fragments are exposed in a manner similar to the procedure described for intramedullary nailing of a femoral fracture. The fracture is reduced.

2. A ⅜-inch drill hole is made through the outer cortex at the bend of the midportion of the tibial tubercle (Fig. 13-52). The nail is inserted in the drill hole with its flange facing outward. It is driven down the fracture site and its position determined. X-ray films are taken.

3. The wound is closed with chromic gut and silk sutures. The affected extremity is encased in a cast.

## Operation for tibial shaft fracture

DEFINITION. *For simple transverse fractures and many oblique fractures,* the fragments are reduced by external manipulation and the leg encased in a plaster cast. *For severe fragmented fractures,* skeletal traction or the insertion of an appropriate appliance may be used.

CONSIDERATIONS. The fractures of the tibia most commonly occur at the lower and middle thirds of the tibial shaft and at the junction of these two thirds. The fractures that result from a direct blow often are the transverse or comminuted types, whereas those that result from a twisting force are the spiral type.

SETUP AND PREPARATION OF THE PATIENT. One of the following is selected: skeletal traction and plaster cast setups, the internal reduction setup with plates and screws of desired type and size, screws alone, transfixing wires, or an intramedullary nail. In nonunion cases a bone-grafting setup is also needed.

OPERATIVE PROCEDURE. As described for open reduction of a fracture (Figs. 13-34 to 13-36).

## Compression plating of fractures

DEFINITION. The use of compression in achieving fixation and promoting union in cancellous bone is now well accepted. This plate relies on the mechanical compression prior to fixation for its function. It provides rigid fixation not only because of the compression but also because it is a very thick, heavy plate.

CONSIDERATIONS. The advantages of compression are that (1) the fixation is more rigid, (2) the gap between the fragments that must be bridged by new bone is narrowed, and (3) the external immobilization required after surgery is reduced or may even be eliminated.

Several instrument companies manufacture various types of compression instruments and implant systems (Fig. 13-59). The purpose of such a system is to approximate the bone fragments under compression during the act of applying an appliance for rigid fixation.

SETUP AND PREPARATION OF THE PATIENT. The basic orthopedic instrument setup, as previously described, with the addition of the compression plating set. Positioning and preparation of the patient depends on the fracture site.

OPERATIVE PROCEDURE. After the fracture

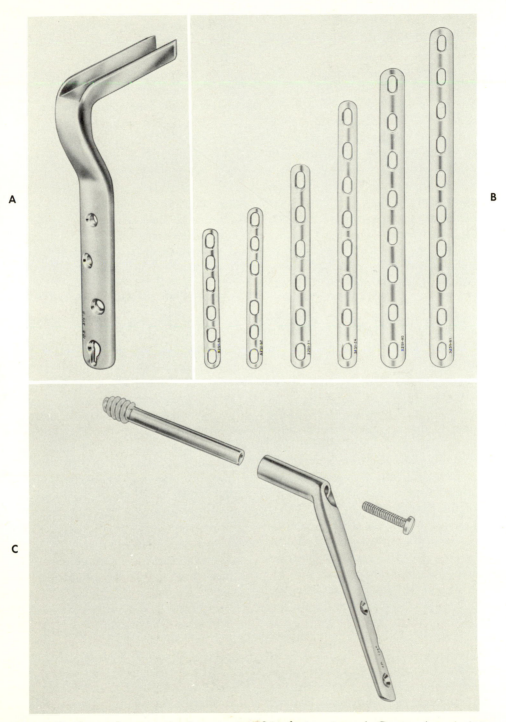

**Fig. 13-59.** Types of compression instruments and implants systems. **A,** Compression osteotomy blade-plate. **B,** Bagby compression plate. **C,** Zimmer compression hip screw. (From Orthopaedic instruments and procedures, Warsaw, Ind., 1970, Zimmer of Canada, Ltd., The Fred Schad Co., Inc., Columbus, Ohio.)

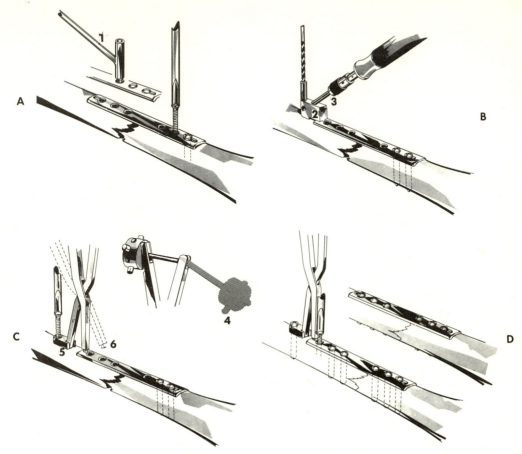

**Fig. 13-60.** Compression plating of fractures (see operative procedure below). (From Orthopaedic instruments and procedures, Warsaw, Ind., 1970, Zimmer of Canada, Ltd., The Fred Schad Co., Inc., Columbus, Ohio.)

has been reduced, the proper plate and screws are selected. The periosteum is stripped in preparation for plating (Fig. 13-60).

"1. To attach one end of the plate to bone, the plate is centered over the fracture. Holes are drilled in a proximal fragment using a hand held drill guide (1). After hole is drilled a self-tapping screw is placed. (If surgeon prefers, a separate tapping instrument is included in the set [A].)

2. The plate is affixed to the proximal end with necessary screws. A locator drill guide hook (2) is placed in the elongated slot on distal end of plate and an anchor

hole is drilled. A Trinkle handle (3) is provided which can be snapped to locator drill guide for holding in place.

3. With compression clamp capstan handle (4) in free position, the compression clamp foot (5) is placed over the anchor hole. Anchor screw is inserted. The handles are pivoted toward the anchor screw and the compression clamp hook (6) is engaged into the slot on distal end of the plate. Capstan handles are locked across compression clamp. Compression is applied by turning the capstan handle knob clockwise.

4. All remaining bone screws are then placed with full compression applied. Com-

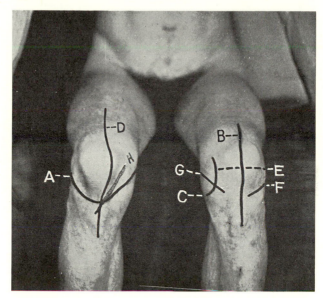

**Fig. 13-61.** Various incisions for operations on knee joint. (From Conwell, H. E., and Reynolds, F. C.: Key and Conwell's management of fractures, dislocations, and sprains, ed. 7, St. Louis, 1961, The C. V. Mosby Co.)

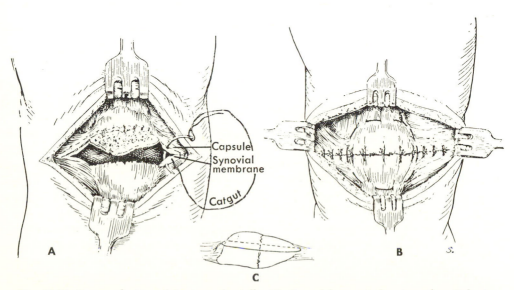

**Fig. 13-62.** Open reduction of fracture of patella. Fixation of fragments by circumferential wire loop. Lateral tears in capsule and synovial membrane repaired with catgut. (From Crenshaw, A. H., editor: Campbell's operative orthopaedics, ed. 5, St. Louis, 1971, The C. V. Mosby Co.)

pression is then released by swinging the capstan handle to a free position. The anchor screw and compression clamp are removed (D)."*

5. The wound is closed in the routine manner. The affected limb may or may not be placed in a plaster cast.

# OPERATIONS ON THE KNEE
## Patellectomy

DEFINITION. Excision of the bone portion of the patella and repair of the quadriceps expansions (Figs. 13-11, 13-61, and 13-62).

CONSIDERATIONS. Fractures of the patella are of the transverse, comminuted (stellate), or linear type. They are usually caused by direct contusion or muscular stress. The fragments of bone, especially in a transverse fracture, may separate when the torn quadriceps muscle pulls them apart. If this occurs, the quadriceps mechanism must be repaired. Linear or comminuted fractures in which the fragments do not separate are immobilized in a cast. If one pole of the patella is avulsed, it may be excised and the quadriceps repaired. A patellectomy is done to aid knee function if the patella is diseased or too severely injured to be repaired.

SETUP AND PREPARATION OF THE PATIENT. The basic orthopedic setup, including Cave knee retractors and Kocher retractor (Fig. 13-28), bone awl (Fig. 13-26), and rongeurs (Fig. 13-25).

The patient is placed on the operating table in a supine position, with the affected knee joint at a level with the break of the lower section of the table. The foot section of the table is lowered, or the knee is flexed by placing a suitable sandbag beneath its posterior aspect (Chapter 7). The extremity is cleansed, as described previously, and the patient is draped with sheets, as for draping a lower extremity. (See Chapters 4 and 5.)

---

*From *Orthopaedic instruments and procedures,* Warsaw, Ind., 1970, Zimmer of Canada, Ltd., p. 148.

OPERATIVE PROCEDURE

1. A curved, transverse, or paramedian incision is made over the knee, and the capsular tendon ligament of the joint and the quadriceps tendon are exposed (Fig. 13-62).

2. The patellar ligament is incised to expose the anterior surface of the patella.

3. The fragments of the patella are removed from the surrounding tendon by sharp dissection.

4. In some cases the quadriceps and patella tendon are sutured with chromic gut or fine stainless steel wire.

5. The defect in the patellar ligament is closed with sutures. The wound is closed and the extremity immobilized in a cast.

## Reconstruction of the patella

DEFINITION. Through an open wound, medial transplantation and fixation of the patella tendon and its bony attachments to the tibia or plication of the soft tissues on the medial side of the patella tendon.

CONSIDERATIONS. Recurrent dislocation of the patella may originate from a direct blow against its inner side when the knee is flexed. More often it is a congenital developmental phenomenon associated with a shallow groove in the femoral condyles, a ball-shaped patella, or knock-knee.

SETUP AND PREPARATION OF THE PATIENT. The basic orthopedic setup is needed, including a textile pack for the lower extremity, plus instruments for internal fixation of fractures or patellectomy. The patient is prepared as described for patellectomy (Chapters 5 and 7).

OPERATIVE PROCEDURE. One of several operations may be done, depending on the condition. The most common operations are (1) transfer of the patella tendon and its bony attachments inward on the tibia, similar to arthroplasty, (2) wedge osteotomy of the lateral femoral condyle, similar to arthrodesis, or (3) tendon or fascia lata fixation of the patella to the inner condyle of the femur, similar to patellectomy.

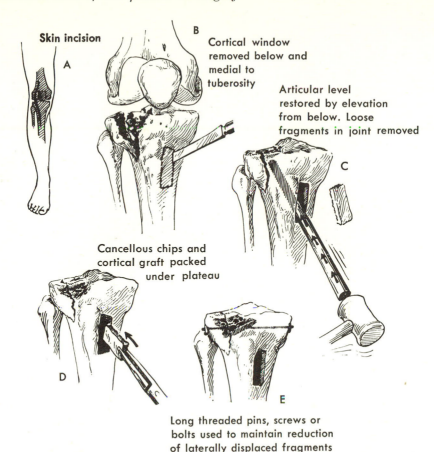

Skin incision

A

B

Cortical window removed below and medial to tuberosity

Articular level restored by elevation from below. Loose fragments in joint removed

C

Cancellous chips and cortical graft packed under plateau

D

E

Long threaded pins, screws or bolts used to maintain reduction of laterally displaced fragments

Fig. 13-63. Surgical restoration of lateral articular surface of knee. (From Compere, E. L., Banks, S. W., and Compere, C. L.: Pictorial handbook of fracture treatment, ed. 5, Chicago, 1963, Year Book Medical Publishers, Inc.)

## Arthroplasty of the knee joint

**DEFINITION.** The tibial articular surfaces are replaced by a metallic prosthesis that articulates with the femur (Figs. 13-61 and 13-63).

**CONSIDERATIONS.** Arthroplasty is done when arthritic changes in the knee are severe and when the joint appears salvageable. Otherwise, arthrodesis is done.

**SETUP AND PREPARATION OF THE PATIENT.** As described for basic orthopedic setup and patellectomy, including bone curettes, osteotomes, chisels, raspatories, and rongeurs.

The patient is placed on the operating table in a supine position, with the knees at the level of the lower break section of the table. The knee may be flexed by breaking the table. The posterior portion of the knee should be supported by a pad, and the leg should rest on the table pad.

**OPERATIVE PROCEDURE**

1. With a scalpel, a long skin incision is usually made down through the quadriceps tendon, which is dissected free from the femur by means of curved scissors, tendon strippers, and an elevator. Bleeding is controlled with hemostats and fine sutures. Skin towels are applied and secured to the wound edges if a synthetic skin drape has not been used. The patella is separated from the femur, using a tenotomy knife and bone hooks.

2. The patella is elevated and inspected.

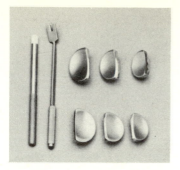

**Fig. 13-64.** Sbarbaro tibial plateau prosthesis. Left to right: impactor, driver, and six Sbarbaro tibial plateau prostheses, left or right, medial or lateral. (From Orthopaedic instruments and procedures, Warsaw, Ind., 1970, Zimmer of Canada, Ltd., The Fred Schad Co., Inc., Columbus, Ohio.)

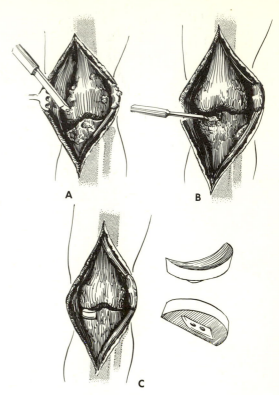

**Fig. 13-65.** Surgical reconstruction of the knee joint, utilizing the tibial plateau prosthesis. (From Sbarbaro, J. L., Jr., Warsaw, Ind., Zimmer Instrument Co., U.S.A.)

Sometimes it is removed by means of bone elevators, gouges, and rongeurs. The bony surfaces are smoothed.

3. A prosthesis (McKeever or Sbarbaro) is inserted for restoration of the anatomical contour and for elimination of friction with the opposed cartilage. The prosthesis is anatomically contoured and fits into the upper end of the tibia. It is designed to reestablish the anatomical outline of the articular surface (Figs. 13-64 and 13-65). A flat surface on the tibial condyle is first created with a saw or osteotome, and the prosthesis is inserted.

4. The wound is closed in layers. Surgical dressings are applied to the wound and secured with bandages. The leg is immobilized in a plaster splint.

## Arthrodesis of the knee

**DEFINITION.** Osteotomy and fusion of the joint with insertion of metal screws or a nail. Compression arthrodesis by means of transfixion by pins inserted through the femur and tibia and incorporated in turnbuckle clamps may be used (Figs. 13-62 and 13-66).

**SETUP AND PREPARATION OF THE PATIENT.** As described for arthroplasty of the knee, with suitable appliances such as Charnley clamps, knee plates and screws, or intramedullary rods (Fig. 13-66).

**OPERATIVE PROCEDURE.** Similar to that described for arthroplasty of the knee joint.

## Arthrotomy of knee joint for excision of torn cartilage (menisci)

**DEFINITION.** The knee joint is exposed and explored through an anteromedian, paramedian, or oblique incision, and the torn meniscus is removed (Fig. 13-67).

**CONSIDERATIONS.** Rupture of the internal and external semilunar cartilages occurs frequently because of a twisting motion. The injury may cause the anterior or posterior horn to become detached from the upper tibia. Or the cartilage may split, allowing one portion to enter the central region of the knee joint and the other portion to remain in its normal position along the outer margin of the joint (Fig. 13-68).

## INTRAMEDULLARY ROD FIXATION

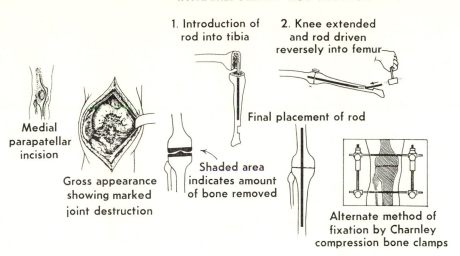

1. Introduction of rod into tibia

2. Knee extended and rod driven reversely into femur

Final placement of rod

Medial parapatellar incision

Gross appearance showing marked joint destruction

Shaded area indicates amount of bone removed

Alternate method of fixation by Charnley compression bone clamps

**Fig. 13-66.** Arthrodesis of knee for treatment of rheumatoid arthritis of knee. (From Kuhns, J. G., and Potter, T.: In Adams, J. P., editor: Current practice in orthopaedic surgery, vol. 1, St. Louis, 1963, The C. V. Mosby Co.)

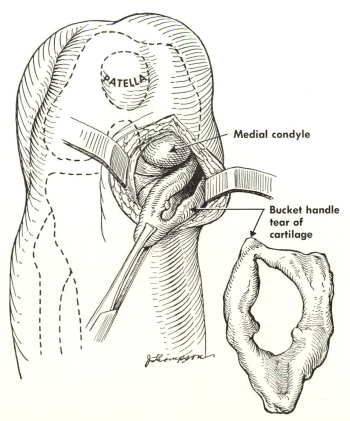

Medial condyle

Bucket handle tear of cartilage

**Fig. 13-67.** Bucket-handle tear of internal semilunar cartilage. (From Richards, V.: Surgery for general practice, St. Louis, 1956, The C. V. Mosby Co.)

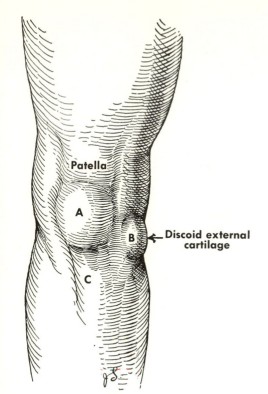

**Fig. 13-68.** Discoid external cartilage. (From Richards, V.: Surgery for general practice, St. Louis, 1956, The C. V. Mosby Co.)

**SETUP AND PREPARATION OF THE PATIENT.** As described for patellectomy, including a cartilage osteotome and tenotomy knives (Fig. 13-69).

**OPERATIVE PROCEDURE**

1. An incision is made in the knee joint and carried through the subcutaneous tissue (Fig. 13-61); wound edges are protected, as described for internal fixation.

2. The capsule of the knee is opened, and its edges are retracted; the synovial membrane is opened (Figs. 13-11 and 13-67).

3. The medial and lateral menisci are identified, and the structures of the knee joint are examined, using elevators and retractors. Broken cartilage and loose body or synovial tabs are removed, using Ochsner forceps, a long knife, tenotomes, meni-

scectomy knives, and tissue forceps. The knee joint is irrigated, using an Asepto syringe filled with normal saline solution.

4. The synovial layer is closed with plain gut no. 3-0 swaged to ½-circle, trocar point Murphy needles.

5. The wound is closed in layers and covered with dressings. The extremity is sometimes stabilized in a splint or cylinder cast.

## OPERATIONS ON THE ANKLE AND FOOT
### Treatment of fractures

**DEFINITION.** Reduction of the fracture and immobilization of the fragments by external fixation or by open reduction with fixation sutures, bolts, or screws.

**SETUP AND PREPARATION OF THE PATIENT.** The instrument setup is similar to that for patellectomy, using smaller-sized items to suit anatomical structures. Lower leg and foot preparation and draping procedure is as described in Chapters 4 and 5.

**CONSIDERATIONS.** The type of fracture or dislocation of the ankle (including Pott's fracture) is influenced by the intensity and duration of the direct or indirect force that is exerted on the ankle and foot. A fracture displacement of either the lateral or medial malleolus may involve a rupture of a main supporting ligament on the opposite side of the ankle (Figs. 13-11 and 13-24). The latter would usually require surgery to avoid interposition and malreduction.

A posterior chip fracture of the tip of the tibia, which involves more than one of the articular surfaces, is treated by internal fixation if it cannot be reduced by a closed reduction operation.

A rupture of the lower tibiofibular ligament, situated just above the ankle joint, usually is repaired by means of a transfixion bolt or screws (Fig. 13-24).

In falls from a height, the os calcis may become fractured, and the attachment of the Achilles tendon may be avulsed by muscular contraction. The avulsion of the Achilles tendon at its insertion or the dis-

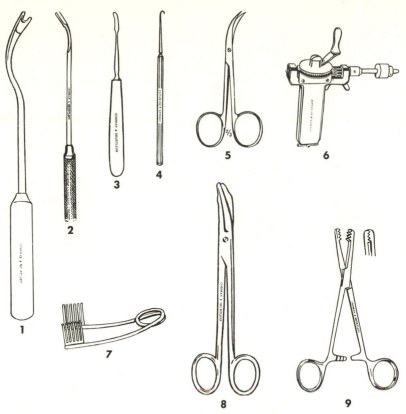

Fig. 13-69. Instruments for operations on cartilage. 1, Downing cartilage knife, 7 in.; 2, Carroll tendon stripper, curved, 8¼ in., sizes 1 and 2; 3, McKenty periosteal elevator; 4, Carroll hook; 5, side-curved scissors, 4 in., sharp points; 6, Bunnell hand drill cannulated for Kirschner wires with screw chucks; 7, Volkmann pronged retractor, 2, 3, 4, or 6 prongs, dull or sharp points, 4½ in.; 8, cartilage scissors; 9, Martin cartilage clamp. (Instruments shown here are one-third actual size.) (Courtesy Codman & Shurtleff, Inc., Randolph, Mass.)

placed fracture of the tuberosity may be treated by open reduction and insertion of sutures. If there is marked involvement of the subtalar joint, arthrodesis may be done several weeks after the original injury.

Fractures and separation of the internal malleolus are usually treated by open reduction and fixation with screws or sutures.

### Excision of exostosis

DEFINITION. Removal of the bony protuberances about the tendon or muscle insertions on a bone (Fig. 13-70).

CONSIDERATIONS. This procedure is done to restore function of the joint.

SETUP AND PREPARATION OF THE PATIENT. Basic patellectomy set, including fine chis-

els and osteotomes, curettes, and rongeurs. The position of the patient on the operating table and the draping procedure selected will depend on the location of the proposed operative site (Chapters 4, 5, and 7).

OPERATIVE PROCEDURE

1. An incision is made over the prominence of the exostosis, using a scalpel, scissors, and tissue forceps.

2. The exostosis is dissected free and cut off at its base where it connects with the cortex of the normal bone, using heavy scissors, tenaculum, Ochsner forceps, chisels, elevator, osteotome, and mallet. The remaining bony surfaces are made smooth with a rongeur and file (Fig. 13-70).

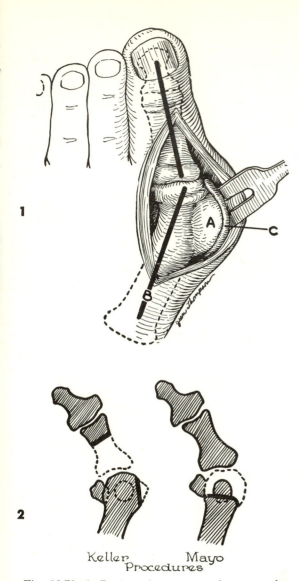

Keller Procedures    Mayo

**Fig. 13-70. 1,** Bunion: **A,** exostosis of metatarsal head; **B,** hallux valgus deformity; **C,** overlying bursa. **2,** Operations for hallux valgus. (From Richards, V.: Surgery for general practice, St. Louis, 1956, The C. V. Mosby Co.)

3. The fascial layer is closed with interrupted silk or chromic gut sutures nos. 3-0 and 2-0, and the skin edges are approximated with fine wire, nylon, or silk. Surgical dressings are applied to the wound and secured by applying a gauze bandage.

### Bunionectomy

**DEFINITIONS.** The *Mayo operation* includes a partial excision of the head of the first metatarsal. The *Keller operation* includes a resection of the proximal part of the first phalanx of the great toe. The *McBride operation* includes the attachment of the adductor muscles of the great toe to the shaft of the first metatarsal. The *Silver operation* includes the excision of the exostosis, formation of a capsular flap, and insertion of sutures in the distal flap to adduct the great toe (Fig. 13-70).

**CONSIDERATIONS.** Hallux valgus is the deviation of the great toe to the lateral side of the foot. When it is significant, surgical treatment (arthroplasty) is necessary.

**SETUP AND PREPARATION OF THE PATIENT.** The instrument setup is as for arthroplasty of a small joint and is similar to that for excision of exostosis. The patient is prepared as described for a foot operation (Chapters 4 and 5).

**OPERATIVE PROCEDURE.** A curved dorsal incision is made over the metatarsophalangeal joint on its medial side, and the bursa and exostosis are removed, as described for removal of exostosis (Fig. 13-70). The wound is sutured with fine sutures, dressings are applied, and the foot is usually immobilized in a plaster boot.

## OPERATIONS ON THE SHOULDER
### Recurrent dislocation of the shoulder joint

**DEFINITIONS.** The *Bankart operation* is the repair of a defect of the glenoid cavity through a deltopectoral incision. In some cases, this is augmented by the Putti-Platt repair, which is the bringing together of the capsule and the subscapular muscle.

**CONSIDERATIONS.** Traumatic anterior dislocation of the shoulder joint, even after treatment, may be followed by a recurrence (Figs. 13-3 to 13-5). This injury occurs when the arm is abducted and the shoulder rotated too far, thereby pushing the head of the humerus out of the

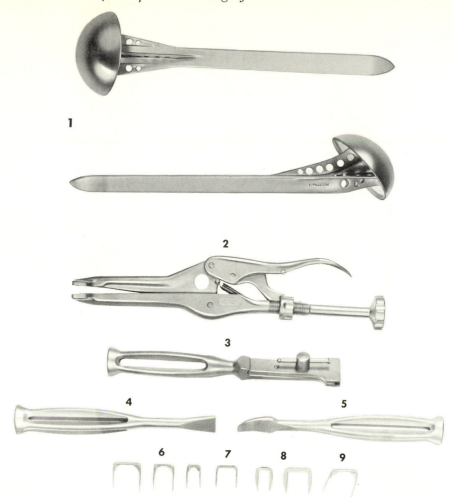

**Fig. 13-71.** Vitallium shoulder prosthesis and staple instruments. 1, Neer shoulder prosthesis; 2, Universal staple inserter set—extractor; 3, Blount staple inserter; 4, Blount staple set; 5, Blount staple extractor; 6, Blount epiphyseal staples; 7, fracture staple; 8, dePalma staples; 9, angulated epiphyseal staples. (See Fig. 13-29 for other stapler instruments.) (Courtesy Austenal Co., Division of Vitallium Surgical Appliances, Howe Sound Co., New York, N. Y.)

glenoid cavity (Figs. 13-18 and 13-19). This type of injury may cause a subglenoid, subcoracoid, or subspinous dislocation, depending on the intensity of the violence and the degree of abduction (Fig. 13-18). The muscles around the joint may be ruptured; sometimes the nerves are injured sufficiently to cause paralysis of the arm.

The Bankart, Magnuson, DePalma, Neer, and Nicola operations have been devised to treat recurrent dislocation of the shoulder (Figs. 13-72 to 13-74).

**SETUP AND PREPARATION OF THE PATIENT.** The basic orthopedic setup and internal fixation set, including narrow curved osteotomes, chisels, a bone drill and fine drill points, and a prosthesis or staples, if desired (Figs. 13-28 and 13-71). The Neer shoulder prosthesis is a Vitallium replacement for the proximal humeral articulation, thereby replacing the articulating dome (head of the humerus) (Fig. 13-76). Staples or wires are used for fixation of fragments in fractures and for arthrodesis in lesser joints (Fig. 13-75).

The patient is placed on the operating table in a supine position, with his affected side turned at a 45-degree angle

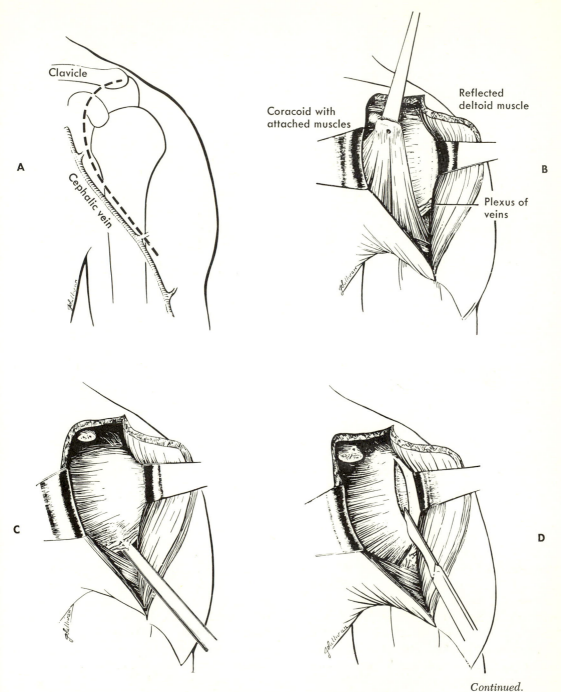

**Fig. 13-72.** Bankart operation (technique of Cave and Rowe). **A,** Skin incision. **B,** Coracoid is being divided. **C,** Inferior margin of subscapular tendon is being identified. **D,** Subscapular tendon is being divided near lesser tuberosity. **E,** Subscapular tendon has been retracted medially. **F,** Holes are being made through rim of glenoid. **G,** Free lateral margin of capsule is being sutured to the rim of the glenoid. **H,** Medial margin of capsule has been lapped over lateral part and has been sutured in place. (From Crenshaw, A. H., editor: Campbell's operative orthopaedics, ed. 5, St. Louis, 1971, The C. V. Mosby Co.)

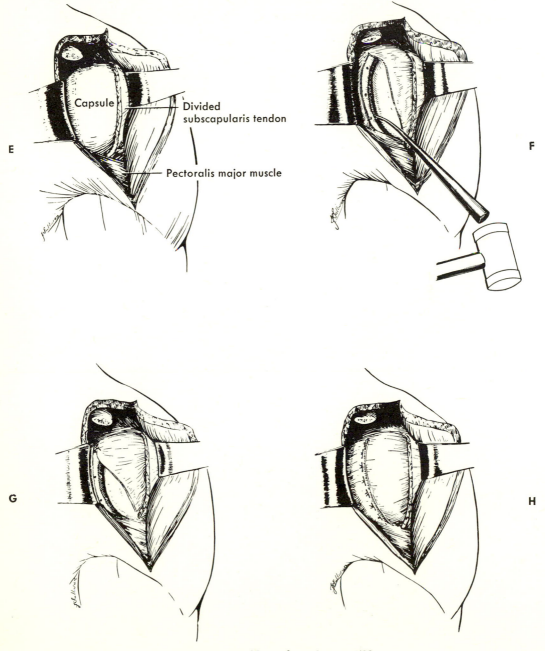

E

Capsule

Divided
subscapularis tendon

Pectoralis major muscle

F

G

H

**Fig. 13-72, cont'd.** For legend see p. 539.

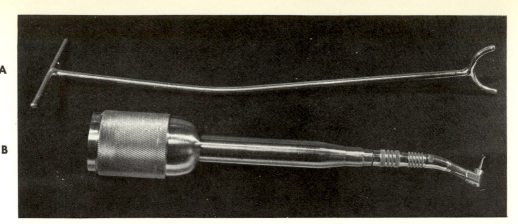

**Fig. 13-73.** Special instruments for Bankart operation. **A,** Retractor. **B,** Dental drill designed to fit Luck saw. (From Crenshaw, A. H., editor: Campbell's operative orthopaedics, ed. 5, St. Louis, 1971, The C. V. Mosby Co.)

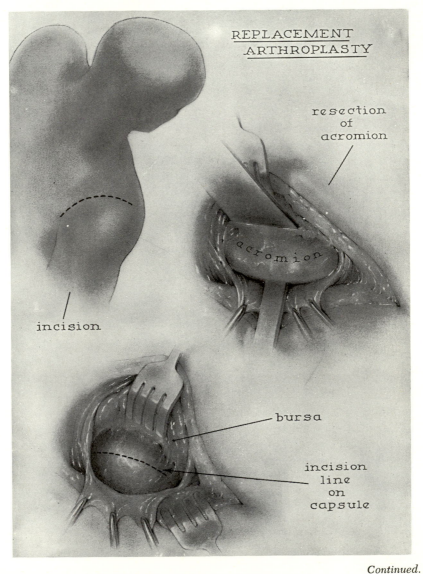

*Continued.*

**Fig. 13-74.** Technique of replacement. Arthroplasty of shoulder. (From Bateman, L. E.: The shoulder and environs, St. Louis, 1955, The C. V. Mosby Co.)

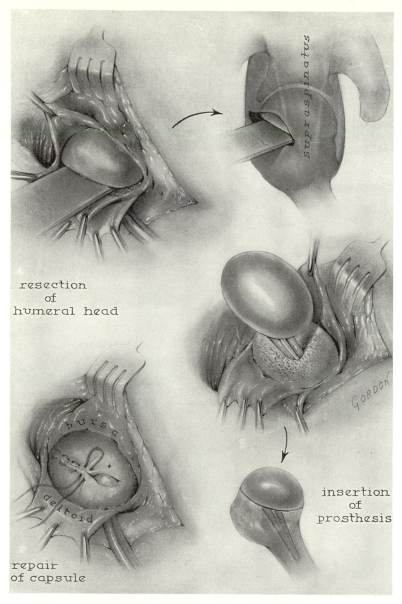

resection
of
humeral head

supraspinatus

bursa

deltoid

repair
of capsule

insertion
of
prosthesis

GORDON

**Fig. 13-74, cont'd.** For legend see p. 541.

toward the other side and supported by sandbags and padded braces. The table is tilted to provide a longitudinal operative site. Routine skin preparation and shoulder draping procedure are done. (See Chapters 4 and 7.)

**OPERATIVE PROCEDURE**

1. A curved skin incision is made over the anterior aspect of the shoulder so that the distal end of the incision is over the deltopectoral groove (Fig. 13-72).

2. The exposure is made between the deltoid and the greater pectoral muscles. The cephalic vein is ligated and retracted.

3. The coracoid process is divided by an osteotome and then pulled downward.

4. The tendon of the subscapular muscle is exposed, clamped, and divided (Figs. 13-74 and 13-75).

5. The joint capsule and the glenoid ligament are reattached to the exposed bone either by means of sutures, which

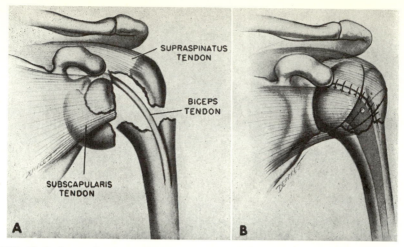

**Fig. 13-75.** Technique of repairing anterior fracture-dislocation. **A,** Biceps tendon identifies interval between greater and lesser tuberosities, and tear between subscapular and supraspinous tendons is developed. **B,** Suture is passed through hole in neck of prosthesis around greater and lesser tuberosities, and capsular defect is repaired. Biceps tendon is sutured in its groove. (From Neer, C. S.: Surg. Clin. North Am. 43:1592, 1963.)

are inserted in drill holes with staples, or by means of pullout wire sutures, as described for tendon repair. The redundant capsule is attached to the stabilized glenoid ligament and to the periosteum on the neck of the scapula (Figs. 13-74 and 13-75).

6. The subscapular muscle is reattached to the lesser tuberosity, and the coracoid process is reattached. The muscle, subcutaneous tissue, and skin are closed in layers.

7. Dressings are applied to the wound. The shoulder is supported by applying a Velpeau bandage with the arm positioned close to the chest and the elbow flexed at about a 40-degree angle.

## OPERATIONS ON ARM, FOREARM, AND WRIST
### Treatment of fractures

DEFINITION. Reduction of the fragments of the bones by means of external or internal fixation.

CONSIDERATIONS. In fractures of the humerus, there is often overriding. Injury to the radial nerve is not common. In supracondylar fractures of the humerus, the dis-

tal fragments may be displaced, resulting in tension of the nerves, tendons, and vessels. If supracondylar fractures and dislocations of the humerus cannot be reduced, they are treated by internal fixation by means of wires or plates and screws or by overhead external skeletal traction applied through the olecranon (Figs. 13-22 and 13-24).

Fractures of the olecranon process (Figs. 13-76 and 13-77) are commonly treated by open reduction with insertion of wire sutures, Rush nails, or long malleable screws (Fig. 13-31A).

Fractures of the forearm bones in children are usually treated by closed manipulation and casting. In adults, however, these fractures usually require open reduction and internal fixation in order to restore anatomical alignment. Plates, intramedullary nails, or compression devices may be used. Occasionally bone grafts are applied at the time of surgery.

Fractures of the wrist bones generally are treated by closed manipulation and casting, although some nonunions of the scaphoid may require bone grafting.

Fractures of the bones of the hand may

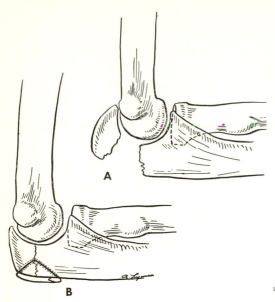

**Fig. 13-76.** Fracture of olecranon process, which always requires open reduction if fragments are separated. **A,** Fracture. **B,** Wire suture that should be fairly superficial for best results. (From Larson, C. B., and Gould, M.: Orthopedic nursing, ed. 7, St. Louis, 1970, The C. V. Mosby Co.)

require open reduction and pin fixation, although most can be treated either with traction or closed manipulation and casting.

**SETUP AND PREPARATION OF THE PATIENT.** As described for internal fixation of fractures, with instruments suitable for the involved bones, plus intramedullary appliances of proper size and similar to those used in femoral shaft fractures.

**OPERATIVE PROCEDURE.** The major steps used are similar to internal fixation of the tibia with plates of suitable size and screws or nails (Figs. 13-34, 13-35, and 13-51).

### Closed suction drainage

The use of suction drainage has become routine for most procedures involving medullary bone in which complete hemostasis cannot be obtained by the usual methods (Fig. 13-78). It is important to prevent the formation of hematomas, since there appears to be a connection between these and wound infections.

The removal of blood and fluid in arthrodesis results in closer apposition of bone chips and should facilitate revascularization. There is the possibility that by removing blood, less granulation and scar tissue is formed. This could result in better motion, particularly in arthroplastic surgery.

**OPERATIVE PROCEDURE**

1. A malleable needle comes with the closed-suction system. It is threaded onto small drainage tubes. By using the needle to make stab wounds, the tubes are brought out beyond the area of the incision.

2. These tubes are connected to a larger tubing that is part of the set.

3. The larger tubing is connected to an evacuator. This unit exerts constant negative pressure and has clear, marked walls to permit determination of the quality and quantity of drainage.

4. The evacuator may be emptied without disturbance of the system.

5. A retaining suture of silk no. 2-0 may be passed through the skin and tied around each of the drainage tubes. This minimizes the possibility of their accidental removal.

## SPINAL OPERATIONS

These procedures are performed by specialists in neurosurgery, as well as by orthopedic surgeons. Frequently new techniques such as the Cloward procedure require specially designed instruments. Basic operations on the spine, including arthrodesis and laminectomy, are described in Chapter 11.

## PLASTIC OPERATIONS

Procedures involving reconstruction of delicate structures of an extremity may be performed by specialists in plastic surgery (Chapter 10); plastic surgery may also be performed on specific structures such as the nose and ear (Chapter 8) and eye (Chapter 9).

### Repair of the tendon and nerves of the hand

**DEFINITION.** Suturing and fixation of a tendon, suturing of a nerve in the hand

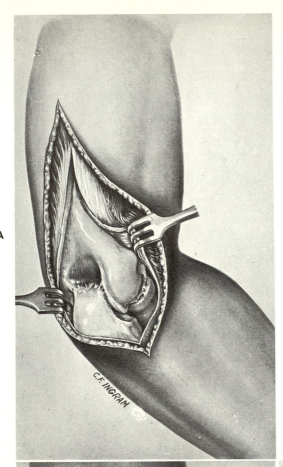

A

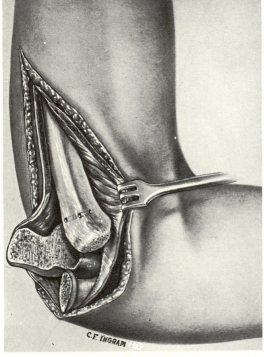

B

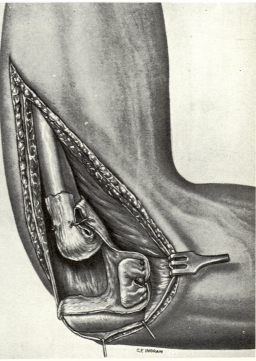

C

Fig. 13-77. Arthroplasty of elbow. **A,** Exposure of ankylosed joint; triceps aponeurosis is incised in midline and is retracted medially and laterally. **B,** Articular surfaces of elbow joint are remodeled, forming one humeral condyle. **C,** Fascia lata interposed between articular surfaces of ulna and humerus and of radius and ulna. (From Crenshaw, A. H., editor: Campbell's operative orthopaedics, ed. 5, St. Louis, 1971, The C. V. Mosby Co.)

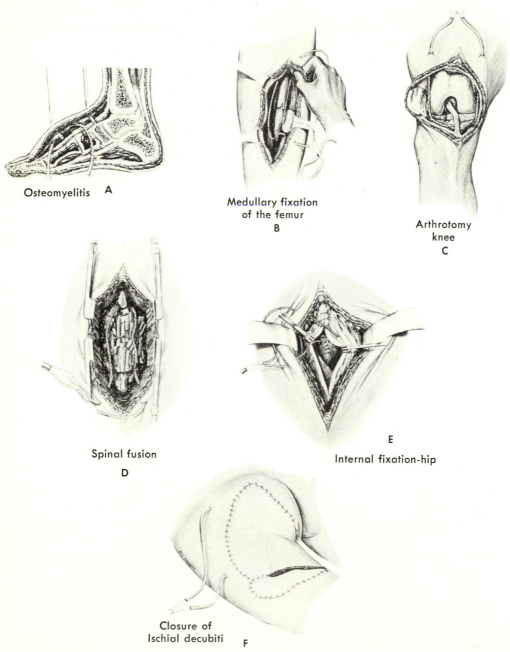

Osteomyelitis  **A**

Medullary fixation
of the femur
**B**

Arthrotomy
knee
**C**

Spinal fusion
**D**

Internal fixation-hip
**E**

Closure of
Ischial decubiti  **F**

**Fig. 13-78.** Procedures in which closed-suction drainage may be indicated. **A,** Osteomyelitis. **B,** Medullary fixation of the femur. **C,** Arthrotomy (knee). **D,** Spinal fusion. **E,** Internal fixation (hip). **F,** Closure of ischial decubiti. (From Orthopaedic instruments and procedures, Warsaw, Ind., 1970, Zimmer of Canada, Ltd., The Fred Schad Co., Inc., Columbus, Ohio.)

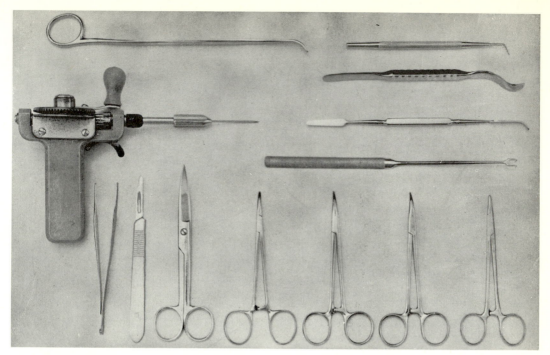

**Fig. 13-79.** Operations on small structures (tendons, nerves, and bones of hand and wrist) require fine instruments. (From Speed, J. S., and Knight, R. A., editors: Campbell's operative orthopaedics, St. Louis, 1956, The C. V. Mosby Co.)

or wrist, or reconstruction of the bones, with or without tendon repair.

**CONSIDERATIONS.** Because the hand depends for its function on the mobility of its small joints through proper balance and excursion of the tendons, the objective of surgery is to preserve the smooth gliding articular surfaces of structures in the sheath (Fig. 13-7).

**SETUP AND PREPARATION OF THE PATIENT.** The patient is placed on the operating table in a supine position, with the affected arm extended and supported (Chapter 7). Skin preparation, application of a tourniquet, and draping procedure have been described previously in Chapters 4 and 5. The basic hand setup should include the following (Fig. 13-79):

**Cutting instruments**

2 Scalpel handles nos. 3 and 7 with blades nos. 10, 11, and 15
1 Ryerson tenotomy knife
2 Mayo scissors, 5½ in., 1 curved and 1 straight
1 Cartilage scissors, lightweight
1 Metzenbaum scissors
1 Tenotomy scissors
1 Hand drill and fine drill points, assorted sizes
1 Delicate tendon dissector

**Holding instruments**

5 Foerster sponge-holding forceps, 7 in.
8 Backhaus towel clamps, 5 in.
2 Tissue forceps, 1 and 2 teeth, 5½ in.
1 Russian forceps, 6 in.
2 Adson tissue forceps
2 Plastic thumb forceps
2 Allis-Adair tissue forceps, 6 in.
2 Tendon hooks
2 Tendon passers
1 Piece nerve tape
2 Skin hooks, 1 blunt and 1 sharp

**Clamping instruments** (Chapter 5)

8 Halsted artery forceps, straight, 5 in.
6 Mosquito artery forceps, curved, 5 in.
6 Rankin artery forceps, straight, 6½ in.
4 Crile hemostats, straight, 6½ in.

**Exposing instruments**

2 Volkmann retractors, 2-pronged
2 Parker retractors, narrow blade

1 Senn retractor, double-ended
2 Greene retractors
2 Hook retractors, single-pronged
1 Cushing vein retractor
2 Little retractors
2 Crile finger retractors, appropriate sizes

**Suturing instruments**

1 Needle holder, medium
2 Needle holders, fine, light
6 Plastic sutures of wire, 34- or 35-gauge or silk and chromic gut nos. 4-0 to 6-0, with swaged-on needles (according to surgeon's preference)
6 Bone buttons, for Bunnell technique
4 Bunnell plastic needles, if desired

**Accessory items**

1 Asepto or bulb syringe
1 Pneumatic tourniquet, if desired
1 Operating pack, for arm or foot
1 Glove and gown set
1 Basin set

OPERATIVE PROCEDURE. The original incision is opened and extended parallel to the flexion crease and midlateral to the joints.

SUTURING OF A TENDON. The divided tendon ends are exposed proximally and distally and coapted with either fine monofilament stainless steel wire or silk. The severed tendon ends may be sutured by one of several methods: (1) end-to-end union with permanent silk sutures, (2) end-to-end pullout sutures (Bunnell), (3) gig pullout sutures (Bunnell), and (4) end-to-end pullout sutures at a distance (Bunnell). (See Figs. 13-80 and 13-81.)

The Bunnell traction pullout suture is most often used to ensure firm fixation at an insertion to bone or distal tendon stump. Pullout wire sutures are composed of stainless steel monofilament wires, size 34 or 35 gauge, 10 and 18 inches long. Twist closely the 10-inch length of wire, using skin hook and clamp. Thread each end of the 18-inch length of wire on straight or curved Bunnell needles, as desired, and twist the short end tightly around the strand. Secure a curved needle in a needle holder for passing pullout wire through the skin. Hand a button

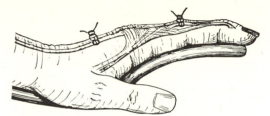

**Fig. 13-80.** Method of inserting double right-angle suture. When a tendon severed in the sheath is repaired by a pullout suture in the palm and simple approximating sutures in the finger, the sheath and any part of the pulley mechanism lying directly over the junction should be excised rather than incised. (From Boyes, J. H.: Bunnell's surgery of the hand, ed. 5, Philadelphia, 1970, J. B. Lippincott Co.)

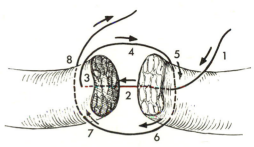

**Fig. 13-81.** For primary or secondary repair of the extensor tendons, a simple figure-of-eight stitch with 35-guage stainless steel wire is used. One loop unites the tendon ends and the other the skin edges. The stitch is without strength and is merely for approximation of tendon ends. Splinting as shown prevents ends from being pulled apart. (From Boyes, J. H.: Bunnell's surgery of the hand, ed. 5, Philadelphia, 1970, J. B. Lippincott Co.)

to the surgeon for securing the ends of the pullout wire.

After several weeks the button is clipped off, and the pullout wire is withdrawn.

FIXATION OF A TENDON TO THE BONE. The simplest method of tendon fixation consists of placing a suture in the end of the tendon by one of the techniques described previously. The bone cortex is elevated with an osteotome, and a drill hole is carried through to the opposite cortex. The

two free ends of the wire suture, which is fixed in the tendon, are threaded on a straight Keith needle and passed through the hole in the bone and out on the skin on the opposite side. The free ends of the suture may be threaded through a button. The tendon end is thus fixed in the bone tunnel.

## Skin-grafting operations
### *Free graft*

DEFINITION. A free graft of skin is one of a given thickness and area that has been completely severed from its bed and transferred to another part of the body.

CONSIDERATIONS. There are many classifications of free grafts; however, the two main types are the thin epidermal grafts and the grafts that include the dermis. The former is often called a split-thickness graft and the latter, a full-thickness graft. Skin grafting is done to fill or cover the defect from loss of skin as soon as conditions are suitable, thereby preventing infection, fibrosis, and loss of muscle and joint functions.

SETUP AND PREPARATION OF THE PATIENT. The patient is placed on the operating table in a position that will provide for exposure of the wound and the donor site. If the thigh is chosen as the donor site, it should be supported with sandbags or pads and slightly abducted to flatten the iliotibial band. The knee should be slightly flexed to reduce prominence of the hamstrings. When the back or buttock is to be the donor site, the patient is placed in a side-lying or facedown position (Chapter 7). The donor site is shaved and cleansed (Chapter 4). The patient is draped with sheets so that the wound and donor site are exposed (Chapter 5). The basic setup for skin-grafting procedures includes the following:

### Cutting instruments
2 Scalpel handles nos. 4 and 3 with blades nos. 20, 15, 11, and 10
2 Mayo scissors, 5½ in., 1 straight and 1 curved
1 Metzenbaum scissors, 7 in.
1 Suture scissors, straight

### Holding instruments
2 Tissue forceps, 1 and 2 teeth, 4½ in.
2 Dressing forceps, narrow points, 5½ in.
2 Adson tissue forceps, 2 and 3 teeth, 5½ in.
8 Towel clips
4 Sponge-holding forceps
6 Halsted mosquito hemostats, straight, 4¼ in.
6 Crile hemostats, straight, 6 in.
4 Rankin-Kelly forceps
2 Allis forceps, 3 and 4 teeth, 6¼ in.

### Exposing instruments
2 Skin hooks, sharp, 1-pronged (Fig. 13-69)
2 Delicate skin retractors, blunt, 2-pronged (Fig. 21-79)
2 Delicate blade retractors

### Suturing instruments
2 Crile needle holders, lightweight
1 Plastic needle holder
   Silk sutures nos. 4-0 and 6-0 on ⅜-circle skin needles
   Stainless steel wire or nylon sutures nos. 5-0 and 6-0 on ⅜-circle plastic needles
   Plain gut ligatures nos. 4-0 and 5-0
   Keith needles, straight, if desired

### Accessory instruments
1 Ruler
1 Grooved director
1 Metal skin-grafting board
1 Local anesthesia set with drugs, as desired
1 Drape pack, desired type
1 Plastic pack, including sponges and dressings
1 Bolus dressing set, if desired
1 Gown pack
1 Glove set, desired sizes
1 Asepto syringe, 30 oz.
1 Minor basin set
   Xeroform gauze, fine mesh, desired width
   Silver foil
   Petrolatum gauze, if desired
   Normal saline solution
   Cellophane sheets (optional)
   Paraffin gauze
   Marking pen, if desired

*For Wolfe-Krause (full-thickness) graft and Ollier-Thiersch (split-thickness) graft,* add the following:

2 Ferris-Smith or Webster knives or razor graft knives and holder
   Blair suction-box, Blair suction apparatus and rubber tubing, suction machine, and Blair retractors
   Dermatome and attachments, as desired

*For pedicle graft and flaps,* use the basic skin-grafting setup.

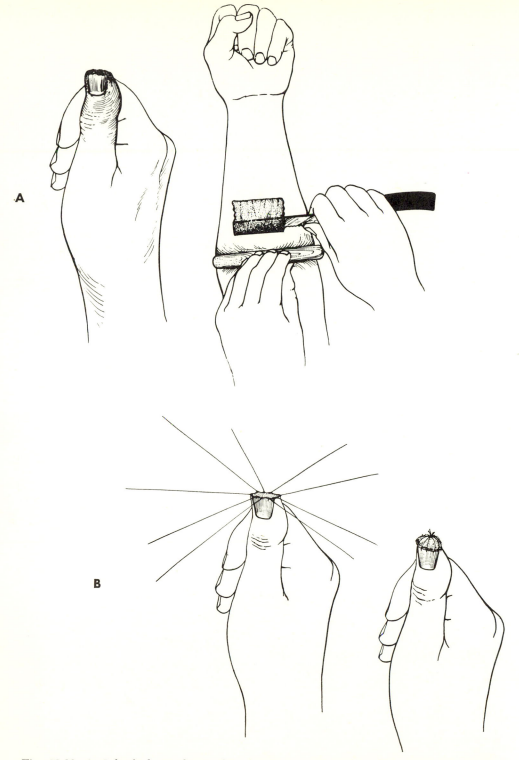

Fig. 13-82. **A,** Split-thickness skin graft technique for finger injury. Obtaining a thin, split-thickness graft from forearm. **B,** Bolus type of dressing to immobilize thin split-thickness grafts over avulsion defect. **C,** Technique of tenodesis of profundus tendon is done to stabilize distal joint in midflexion. **D,** Retrograde palmar flap of hand may be used to restore contour and length of amputated fingertip. (From Gonzalez, R. I., and Buncke, H. J., Jr.: In Adams, J. P., editor: Current practice in orthopaedic surgery, vol. 1, St. Louis, 1963, The C. V. Mosby Co.)

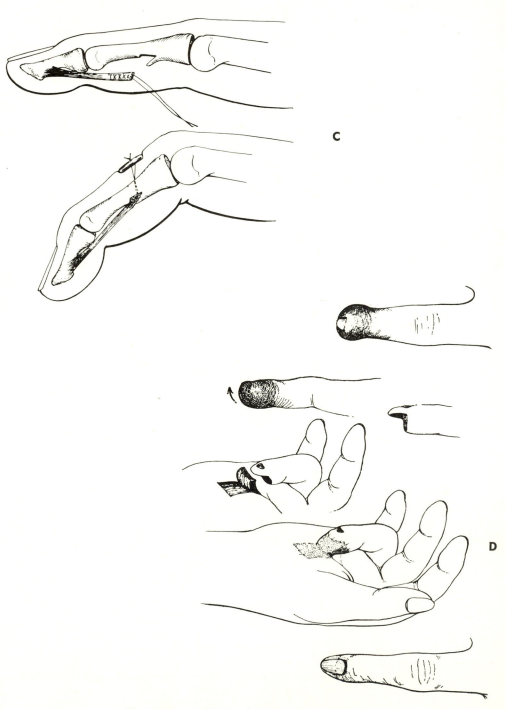

Fig. 13-82, cont'd. For legend see opposite page.

*For Reverdin-Davis pinch graft,* use the basic skin-grafting setup, and add the following:

6 Keith needles, 3 in. long
2 Razor blades and holder
1 Webster skin-grafting knife handle with two removable blades, if desired

OPERATIVE PROCEDURE

1. The recipient area is prepared by removing excessive granulation tissue to provide a smooth vascular bed for the graft.

2. The dermatome is set at the desired thickness. If a drum dermatome is used, the donor site is painted with a glue, which is allowed to dry for 4 to 5 minutes or until its glossy look has disappeared. The graft is removed from the donor site with the desired dermatome and other appliances as needed (Fig. 13-82). Skin-grafting knives may be used. The Brown dermatome does not require skin glue, but a lubricant such as mineral oil may be used on the skin.

3. The skin graft may be flattened out on a metal surface, moistened with saline solution, and transferred to the recipient area.

4. The graft is sutured in place with fine silk or nylon sutures.

5. Manual pressure is applied to the graft for several minutes, using gauze sponges.

6. A suitable dressing is applied. The type used depends on immobilization of the graft. In such a case, the individual sutures are left long and are tied diametrically over the fluffed gauze. This is a stent dressing.

7. Fine-mesh medicated gauze, fluffed gauze, and a compression bandage are applied to provide a firm dressing.

8. The donor site may be covered with fine-mesh gauze and a bandage or left free.

### Full-thickness skin graft operation (Wolfe-Krause)

DEFINITION. Transplantation of a full depth of skin, without any attached fat, from a donor site to the recipient site, to resurface freshly opened wounds in the face, neck, hands, or small areas where the skin graft will be under pressure and wear.

SETUP AND PREPARATION OF THE PATIENT. The skin-grafting setup is used, plus skin-grafting knives of desired type. The position of the patient on the operating table will depend on location of the sites to be selected. Routine skin preparation and draping procedures are carried out.

OPERATIVE PROCEDURE

1. The scar tissue on the recipient site is removed, and a pattern is made to outline the contour of the defect, using silver foil, rubber tissue, or paraffin gauze.

2. The pattern is placed over the donor site, and the skin area is outlined with a sharp knife; the desired skin is incised, and its edges are grasped; the graft is then dissected free (Fig. 13-83).

3. The graft is positioned on the recipient site, and its surrounding edges are sutured to the adjacent edges of the graft with interrupted silk or nylon sutures no. 5-0 or 6-0 swaged to cutting-edge needles.

4. The graft is held in place with a compression dressing, as described for a split-thickness graft. The donor site is dressed.

### Pedicle skin flap operations

CONSIDERATIONS. Full-thickness skin loss often requires replacement through the application of a pedicle skin flap, especially if vulnerable structures are exposed or if reconstructive surgery is required. These grafts of skin and subcutaneous fat prevent scar contracture, thereby minimizing deformity.

SETUP AND PREPARATION OF THE PATIENT. As for full-thickness graft, with a sufficient number of fine sutures and hemostats to suit the extent of the skin flap.

OPERATIVE PROCEDURE

1. The donor site is prepared as described for full-thickness graft operations. The donor site for a pedicle flap is determined by the part to be resurfaced. Full-thickness skin losses of the hand and forearm may be replaced with flaps from the

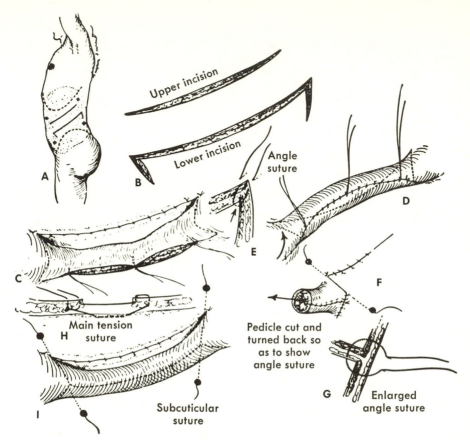

**Fig. 13-83.** Preparation of a tubular pedicle. **A** shows incisions, wide area of undermining (dotted), and four points for rubber tube drains. **B,** Incisions to have a flap of skin in each angle and to place the two main suture lines so that they will not appose each other. **C,** Three guide sutures are placed on the pedicle. The main abdominal incision is closed as in **H,** and the tips of the flaps are fastened as in **E. D,** Suture lines do not appose. **F,** A subcuticular suture is used in the angle to avoid channelways through the skin that would carry infection. By the flap method, the vulnerable x juncture is replaced by a ⊤ juncture as shown in **G** and **I.** (From Boyes, J. H.: Bunnell's surgery of the hand, ed. 5, Philadelphia, 1970, J. B. Lippincott Co.)

abdominal wall. Intact skin may be rotated from an adjacent area to cover a defect or correct a contracture, when the demand is not too great. Rotation flaps may be used as application in reconstructive surgery of the head and neck. Major soft tissue defects of the head and lower extremities can be resurfaced by tubed or "jump" pedicle flaps from the abdomen carried by way of an arm.

2. In all transfers of full-thickness skin and subcutaneous tissue, an adequate arterial and venous circuit must be maintained for survival. Extreme care must be taken in the designing and transferring of pedicle skin flaps to ensure the flap from being under too great tension and to keep its pedicle free from circulatory jeopardy.

3. Pedicle flaps require full immobilization, especially for the extremities. Approximately 3 to 4 weeks are required for the transformed portion of the pedicle flap to develop an adequate circulation from the recipient area.

4. The donor attachment may be totally or partially divided (delayed) at this

time, depending on the amount of tissue to be transferred. Pedicle flaps depend at all times on a blood supply, at first from the donor attachment and finally from that of the recipient. A free skin graft is often required to cover the area from which a flap has been taken.

### Small-thickness pinch graft operation

DEFINITION. A small free graft of skin of desired thickness is placed over the recipient site to cover a defect from loss of skin.

SETUP AND PREPARATION OF THE PATIENT. Basic skin-grafting setup, with a decrease in the number of hemostats and the addition of a razor blade and cutter, if desired. A piece of the blade may be used instead of a scalpel. The patient is prepared as described for a free skin graft.

OPERATIVE PROCEDURE

1. A cone of the skin on the donor site is elevated by piercing it with a straight needle secured to a clamp.

2. The apex of the skin's pyramid is cut off with a sharp knife or razor blade; then the skin on the needle is transferred to the raw area.

3. The donor site is covered with sponges saturated in saline solution to control bleeding vessels. The wound is covered with fine gauze saturated with an antiseptic ointment, and gauze dressings are applied. The recipient site is covered by a sterile pressure dressing.

## Amputation

DEFINITIONS. A partial or total removal of an extremity. Amputations may be classified in two main groups: the open and closed types.

The *open type* is a temporary amputation in which the surface of the wound is not covered with skin and the wound is left open to provide for adequate drainage and control of actual or potential infection. This method sometimes must be followed by a final repair but may be definitive itself.

The *closed type* of amputation is a procedure in which ample skin and muscle flaps are used to create a stump and the skin is closed.

CONSIDERATIONS. The major condition that demands amputation is a complete loss of blood supply to the extremity. An amputation also may be done in the presence of a malignant tumor, uncontrolled infection, or an extreme congenital deformity resulting in complete loss of function.

SETUP AND PREPARATION OF THE PATIENT. The type and number of instruments and other items required will depend on the extremity to be amputated. The general basic setup should include the minor dissecting setup, plus the following (Figs. 13-25, 13-26, and 13-28):

1 Amputation knife
1 Electric motor saw for large bones
1 Amputation saw
2 Gigli saws and guide (optional)
1 Rongeur
1 Bone-cutting forceps
1 Periosteal elevator
1 Bone raspatory
1 Asepto syringe, 30 ml.
  Sutures appropriate to tissues (Chapter 6)
1 Draping pack, appropriate to site
1 Linen pack and dressing
1 Pneumatic tourniquet, if desired
  Alcohol, 95% solution ½ oz.
1 Syringe, 5 ml.
1 Needle, 22-gauge, 2 in. long

The patient is placed on the operating table in a supine or lateral position. The affected joint is flexed and the extremity supported. The proposed operative site is prepared in the routine manner. The patient is draped with sterile sheets, and in some cases a tourniquet may be applied.

OPERATIVE PROCEDURE

CLOSED AMPUTATION ON A LONG BONE

1. Various types of skin flaps have been devised. Generally the anterior flap is cut longer than the posterior one in a relation of 3:2 so that the scar will fall behind the bone rather than at the end. The skin incision extends below the point of the saw line because the soft parts will retract. Bleeding vessels are clamped and ligated, using

hemostats and surgical gut sutures or cautery.

2. The muscles are divided. The major artery is dissected free from the surrounding tissue, doubly ligated, and divided.

3. The periosteum is divided by sharp dissection at the bone head.

4. The nerves are isolated and allowed to retract above the end of the bone. In some cases the nerves are infiltrated with 95% alcohol or a 10% solution of procaine hydrochloride (Novocain), if desired.

5. The skin and muscle flaps are retracted, using moist laparotomy pads and suitable retractors. The bone is divided with an electric saw or chisel, osteotome, and mallet. The sharp and projecting bony prominences are removed and the surfaces smoothed, using rongeurs, bone-cutting forceps, and bone file. The bone dust is also removed by irrigating the wound with normal saline solution.

6. The tourniquet, if used, is removed, and bleeding vessels are controlled with sutures. The fascial flaps are approximated with interrupted sutures of surgical chromic gut or silk no. 2-0 or 3-0. The skin flaps are approximated with fine nylon or stainless steel wire sutures no. 5-0 or 6-0.

7. A drain may be introduced in the wound to minimize the formation of a hematoma. The wound surface is covered with dry flat gauze sponges; then fluff gauze and sheet wadding are applied. The latter is held in place with a sterile elastic cotton or gauze compression bandage.

## REFERENCES

1. Adams, J. C.: Outline of fractures, ed. 4, Edinburgh, 1964, E & S Livingstone, Ltd.
2. Adams, J. B.: Current practice in orthopaedic surgery, St. Louis, 1963, The C. V. Mosby Co.
3. Anson, B. J., editor: Morris' human anatomy, ed. 12, New York, 1966, Blakiston Division, McGraw-Hill Book Co.
4. Bateman, J. E.: The shoulder and environs, St. Louis, 1955, The C. V. Mosby Co.
5. Boyes, J. H.: Bunnell's surgery of the hand, ed. 5, Philadelphia, 1970, J. B. Lippincott Co.
6. Brantigan, O. C.: Clinical anatomy, New York, 1963, Blakiston Division, McGraw-Hill Book Co.
7. Cole, W. H., and Zollinger, R. M.: Textbook of surgery, ed. 8, New York, 1963, Appleton-Century-Crofts.
8. Committee on Trauma: The management of fractures and soft tissue injuries, American College of Surgeons, Philadelphia, 1961, W. B. Saunders Co.
9. Compere, E. L., Banks, S. W., and Compere, C. L.: Pictorial handbook of fracture treatment, ed. 5, Chicago, 1963, Year Book Medical Publishers, Inc.
10. Crawford, A. J.: Outline of fractures, including joint injuries, ed. 4, Baltimore, 1964, The Williams & Wilkins Co.
11. Crenshaw, A. H., editor: Campbell's operative orthopaedics, ed. 4, St. Louis, 1963, The C. V. Mosby Co.
12. Crenshaw, A. H., editor: Campbell's operative orthopaedics, ed. 5, St. Louis, 1971, The C. V. Mosby Co.
13. Davis, L., editor: Christopher's textbook of surgery, ed. 8, Philadelphia, 1964, W. B. Saunders Co.
14. de Palma, A. F.: Atlas of orthopaedic surgery, Philadelphia, 1962, J. B. Lippincott Co.
15. Duvries, H. L.: Surgery of the foot, ed. 2, St. Louis, 1965, The C. V. Mosby Co.
16. Hickman, C. P.: Integrated principles of zoology, ed. 4, St. Louis, 1970, The C. V. Mosby Co.
17. Hollinshead, W. H.: Anatomy for surgeons, vol. 3, ed. 2, The back and limbs, New York, 1964, Hoeber Medical Division, Harper & Row, Publishers.
18. Howorth, M. B., and Cramer, F. J.: A textbook of orthopaedics, Philadelphia, 1952, W. B. Saunders Co.
19. Johnson, W. H., and Kennedy, J. A.: Radiographic anatomy of the human skeleton, Edinburgh, 1961, E. & S. Livingstone, Ltd.
20. Larson, C. B., and Gould, M.: Orthopedic nursing, ed. 7, St. Louis, 1970, The C. V. Mosby Co.
21. Mead, N. C.: Arthrodesis of the hip, Surg. Clin. North Am. **45:**171, 1965.
22. Mercer, W., and Duthie, R. B.: Orthopaedic surgery, ed. 6, Baltimore, 1964, The Williams & Wilkins Co.
23. Miller, D. S.: Fractures of the upper end of the shaft of the femur, Surg. Clin. North Am. **45:**38, 1965.
24. Moseley, H. F., editor: Textbook of surgery, ed. 3, St. Louis, 1959, The C. V. Mosby Co.
25. Neer, C. S.: Prosthetic replacement of the humeral head: indications and operative technique, Surg. Clin. North Am. **43:**1581, 1963.

26. Orthopaedic instruments and procedures, Warsaw, Ind., 1970, Zimmer of Canada, Ltd., The Fred Shad Co., Inc.

27. Raney, R. B., and Brashear, H. R.: Shands' handbook of orthopaedic surgery, ed. 8, St. Louis, 1971, The C. V. Mosby Co.

28. Rhoads, J., Allen, J. G., Harkins, H. N., and Moyer, C. A.: Surgery: principles and practice, ed. 4, Philadelphia, 1970, J. B. Lippincott Co.

29. Richards, V.: Surgery for general practice, St. Louis, 1956, The C. V. Mosby Co.

30. Surgery of the lower extremity, Surg. Clin. North Am. 43:1463, 1963.

31. Surgery of the shoulder region, Surg. Clin. North Am. 43:1463, 1963.

32. Taylor, S., Cotton, L. T., and Murray, J. G.: A short textbook of surgery, Philadelphia, 1967, J. B. Lippincott Co.

# CHAPTER 14

# Thoracic operations

VIRGINIA HIGGINS

## ANATOMICAL AND PHYSIOLOGICAL CONSIDERATIONS

### Anatomy of the thorax

The skeletal framework of the thorax is formed anteriorly by the sternum and costal cartilages, laterally by the twelve pairs of ribs, and posteriorly by the twelve thoracic vertebrae (Figs. 14-1 and 14-2). This airtight compartment is enclosed in the root of the neck by Sibson's fascia and is separated from the abdomen by the diaphragm.

The sternum forms the thorax wall in the anterior median line. It consists of three parts: (1) the upper part, or manubrium, (2) the body, or gladiolus, and (3) the lower cartilage, or xiphoid process. The manubrium articulates with the clavicles and the first two ribs on each side; the gladiolus articulates with the remaining true ribs by separate costal cartilages; and the xiphoid fuses with the gladiolus in early development and is attached to the diaphragm by the substernal ligament (Figs. 14-1 and 14-3).

Normally, the lateral walls of the thorax are formed by the twelve pairs of ribs. Posteriorly, each pair of ribs articulates with its corresponding thoracic vertebrae (Fig. 14-2). Anteriorly, the first seven ribs articulate with the sternum. The eighth, ninth, and tenth ribs articulate with the costal cartilages of the rib above; however, the eleventh and twelfth are not fixed to the costal arch.

The muscles of the thorax include the eleven external and eleven internal intercostal muscles, which fill the spaces between the ribs, and the twenty-four levator muscles of the ribs, which elevate the ribs to enlarge the thoracic cavity (Figs. 14-3 and 14-4).

An intercostal artery, vein, and nerve accompany each intercostal muscle. The arteries communicate with the internal thoracic anteriorly and with the aortic branches posteriorly. The intercostal veins follow the course of the arteries and communicate with the mammary veins anteriorly and with the azygos and hemiazygos veins posteriorly. (See Figs. 14-3 and 14-4.)

During surgery, great care is taken to avoid injuring the intercostal nerve, which passes forward and alongside the posterior intercostal artery and which shares with the superior branch of the artery the intercostal groove on the inferior edge of the corresponding rib. Dividing or crushing the nerve or injecting an anesthetic agent may be done to prevent postoperative pain when the nerve must be disturbed. The pericostal sutures are carefully placed in the muscles to avoid nerve injury and postoperative pain.

The chest cavity is subdivided into the right and left pleural cavities, which contain the lungs and are separated by the mediastinum, which lies medially between the two pleural membranes (Fig. 14-5). The parietal pleura, the membrane that lines the inner surface of the thorax, is

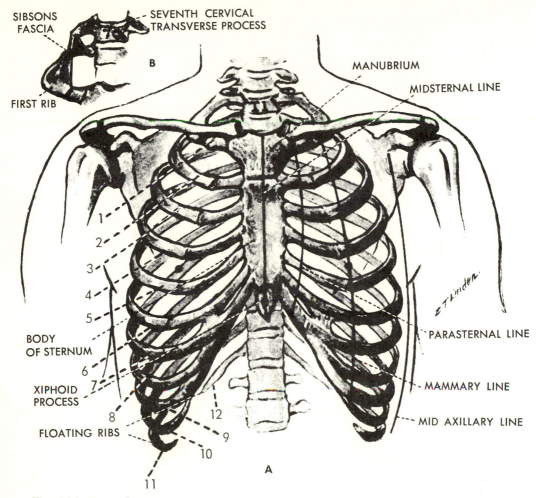

Fig. 14-1. Bony thorax. **A**, Anterior view. **B**, Sibson's fascia, which forms diaphragm for superior aperture. (From Thorek, P.: Anatomy in surgery, ed. 2, Philadelphia, 1962, J. B. Lippincott Co.)

closely associated with the inner surfaces of the ribs posteriorly and with the mediastinum medially and covers the surface of the diaphragm, except at the central portion. Part of the parietal membrane is reflected back at the root of each lung to form a sac around it. This parietal reflection is called the *visceral pleura*, and a serous secretion existing between these two membranes keeps them moist (Figs. 14-5 and 14-6).

The lungs are the essential organs of respiration. The base of each lung rests on the diaphragm, whereas its apex (upper end) projects into the base of the neck at a level above the first rib. At a point on the mediastinal surface of each lung, there is an attachment at which the bronchus, the nerves, the lymphatics, and the pulmonary and bronchial vessels enter and leave the lung. This attachment is known as the hilus, or root, of the lung. Deep fissures, comprising reflections of the visceral pleura, divide the spongy, porous lung into lobes. The primary bronchi divide, then subdivide in each lobe and eventually become bronchioles. The right lung has an upper, middle, and low-

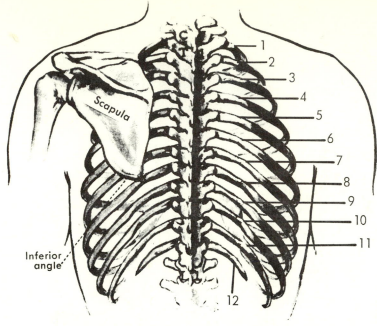

Scapula

Inferior
angle

1
2
3
4
5
6
7
8
9
10
11
12

**Fig. 14-2.** Posterior view of bony thorax. (From Thorek, P.: Anatomy in surgery, ed. 2, Philadelphia, 1962, J. B. Lippincott Co.)

er lobe, and the left lung has only an upper and lower lobe. However, the lungs are similar in that they are composed of ten major segments. Each segment extends to the pleural surface, expanding in volume from its center to its peripheral edges. Each segment also has its own bronchus and branches of the pulmonary artery and vein.

The bronchial arteries, arising from the aorta, are systemic and supply nourishment to the lungs. They vary in their number and course. The arrangement may include two branches to the left lung and one branch to the right lung, which later branches into two, or there may be one branch for each lung or two branches for each lung. The pulmonary arteries and veins (a part of the pulmonary circulation) aerate the venous blood in the lungs.

The nerves of the lungs are a part of the autonomic nervous system (Fig. 11-12). They regulate the diameter of the bronchi and that of the blood vessels within the lungs.

## Normal respiratory physiology

Although the thoracic cavity is an airtight space, the lungs communicate with the outside air by means of the bronchi, trachea, and nasal passages. The main function of the lungs is to bring venous blood into contact with the inspired air. Normally, as the thorax increases in size, the lungs expand and draw in air, and as the thorax decreases, it forces air out. Breathing normally takes place when the intrathoracic pressure is slightly below atmospheric pressure (76 cm. Hg or 760 mm. Hg, standard value, or zero) and when a partial vacuum exists between the parietal and visceral pleural (intrathoracic) surfaces. As the thoracic muscles of inspiration contract to enlarge the chest cage, the lungs passively follow the diaphragm and chest wall due to decreased intrathoracic pressure. The act of inspiration and expiration is the result of air moving in and out so that the pressure equalizes that of the atmosphere at the end of expiration.

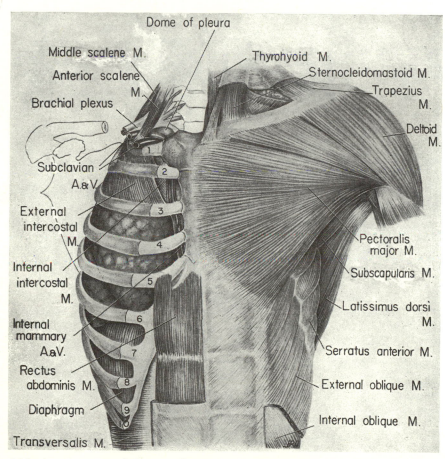

**Fig. 14-3.** Anterior view of thorax and contiguous portions of base of neck and anterior abdominal wall. Right half illustrates superficial layer of muscles and fascia. Left half illustrates relations of deep muscles of neck and abdomen to rib cage; intercostal muscles; diaphragm; internal mammary vessels; relations of muscles, nerves, and vessels with first rib; and anterior relations of lung. (From Sweet, R. H.: Thoracic surgery, ed. 2, Philadelphia, 1954, W. B. Saunders Co.)

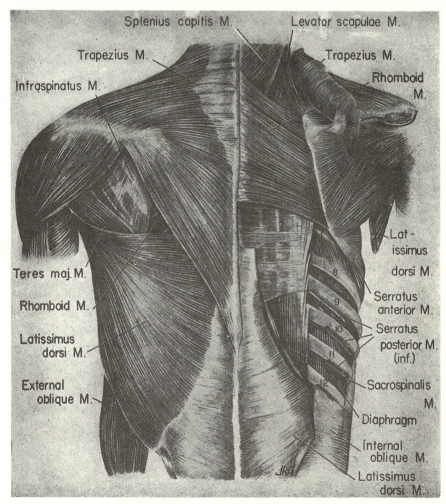

**Fig. 14-4.** Posterior view of thorax and contiguous portions of neck and abdominal wall. Left half illustrates superficial muscles. Right half illustrates deeper muscles and topographical relations of lung and diaphragm. (From Sweet, R. H.: Thoracic surgery, ed. 2, Philadelphia, 1954, W. B. Saunders Co.)

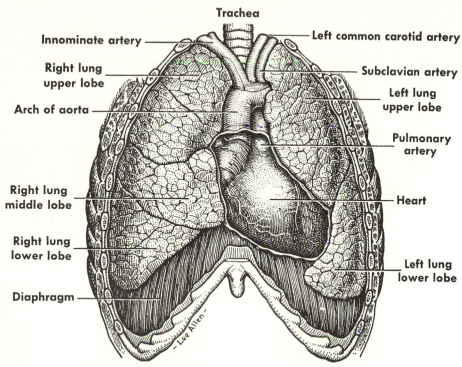

**Fig. 14-5.** Organs of thoracic cavity. Part of pericardium has been removed to expose heart. (From Tuttle, W. W., and Schottelius, B. A.: Textbook of physiology, ed. 16, St. Louis, 1969, The C. V. Mosby Co.)

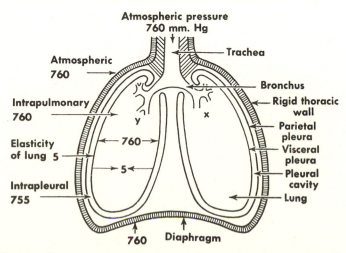

**Fig. 14-6.** Diagram illustrating intrapulmonary and intrapleural pressures with chest wall in resting position. (From Tuttle, W. W., and Schottelius, B. A.: Textbook of physiology, ed. 15, St. Louis, 1965, The C. V. Mosby Co.)

The normal intrapleural pressure varies from $-9$ to $-12$ cm. $H_2O$ on inspiration, and from about $-3$ to $-6$ cm. $H_2O$ during expiration. The greatest amount of air that can be expired after a maximum inspiration is termed the *vital capacity*. The size and vitality of the person influence the amount of expired air (Fig. 14-6). Any condition that interferes with the normally negative intrapleural pressure generally has a serious effect on respiratory function.

**RESPIRATORY COMPLICATIONS.** In the presence of pulmonary disease, the lung may not expand, causing its normal vital capacity to fall from 73% to 43%. In such cases the patient may suffer from anoxia due to diminished respiratory function and diminished cardiac output. The most common conditions that interfere with cardiorespiratory function are mucus or foreign body, pleural effusion, pulmonary edema, pneumonia, closed pneumothorax—simple and tension types, open pneumothorax, hemothorax, and multiple rib injuries that produce paradoxical motion of the thoracic cage (Fig. 14-20).

As previously mentioned, the normal function of the "pulmonary bellows" is caused by the elasticity of the lungs and by the outward traction of the negative intrapleural pressure. If the lung is not adherent to the chest wall, collapse of the normal lung will follow any condition that lowers the negative intrapleural pressure. When the pleural space is filled with air, reducing the negative pressure, the lung contracts. This action may cause a complete collapse if the pressure within the intrathoracic (pleural) space becomes positive.

Also, a diminished negative pressure or the occurrence of actual positive pressure in one pleural space may cause a shift of the mediastinum toward the opposite side. When this happens, not only will the affected lung collapse because of a positive pressure in the pleural space, but the function of the lung on the opposite side may also be impaired due to compression by the shifted mediastinum. Tension pneumothorax can produce serious effects as air continues to escape from the lung into the intrapleural space. The air is unable to return to the bronchi to be exhaled, thereby increasing the intrapleural pressure, which usually causes the lung to collapse but also diminishes the air leak on that side. However, when there is a large opening in the chest wall that allows direct communication of the pleural space with atmospheric pressure, it may cause death if the mediastinum becomes mobile. The exposure of the pleural space to atmospheric pressure collapses the affected lung; also, the positive pressure is transmitted to the mediastinum, which, in turn, shifts toward the opposite side and may cause the opposite lung to collapse.

Paradoxical motion of the chest also involves the mediastinum (Fig. 14-20). Pressure changes that are associated with respiratory movements of the unaffected lung are transmitted through the mediastinum to the affected side. Paradoxical respiration, which is the reverse of normal respiration, causes the mediastinum to shift into the unaffected side of the chest cavity, with the result that the lung on this side also is not fully inflated. Pulmonary ventilation is reduced, rebreathing of air from one lung to the other occurs, and venous return to the right side of the heart is impaired. In such a condition, the patient should be kept on his affected side in order to immobilize the affected lung and permit the unaffected one respiratory freedom. Surgical treatment is described later in this chapter.

## ENDOSCOPY

The term *endoscopy* refers to the examination of body cavities by means of instruments that permit visual inspection of the contents and the walls of certain cavities.

Proper equipment and facilities are necessary to provide for safety, comfort, and convenience of the patient, including freedom from noises and remarks that may increase his ever-present fears and apprehensions. The trend is to perform endo-

scopic examinations in a unit apart from the general operating room.

Endoscopic procedures pertinent to thoracic surgery are bronchoscopy, esophagoscopy, and mediastinoscopy. These can be used as diagnostic and therapeutic procedures.

Each endoscopist has his own preferences regarding the type of endoscope, the positioning of the patient, and the type of anesthetic to be administered.

### Preparation of the patient

A permission-consent form should be signed by the patient, and it should state the examination to be performed.

The patient's dentures must be removed, and, before examination, loose teeth are removed. The teeth are brushed just prior to sedation. The psychological preparation by the physician and assistants is as important as the drug preparation.

The patient is not permitted fluids for at least 8 hours before examination.

Drug preparation makes the examination easier for the patient. Endoscopy is not done unless the patient is sufficiently relaxed. For routine procedures, the patient is usually given a sedative orally at bedtime. One hour before examination, the patient is given a sedative such as phenobarbital (Luminal sodium), pentobarbital sodium (Nembutal), or meperidine hydrochloride (Demerol). Pentobarbital sodium (Nembutal), 50 to 150 mg., may be injected intramuscularly to allay apprehensions. Atropine or an analgesic may also be given.

### Administration of anesthetic agents

Topical or general anesthetics may be used. Infants are not given an anesthetic, but oxygen is administered.

The topical (local) anesthetic setup should include the following:

1 Head mirror
3 Laryngeal mirrors, various sizes
1 Lingual spatula

2 Sprays with straight and curved cannulae and anesthetic drugs, as ordered
1 Laryngeal syringe with straight and curved cannulae
1 Schindler pharyngeal anesthetizer, if desired
2 Medication cups
1 Emesis basin
1 Basin, small, with very warm water
1 Luer-Lok syringe, 10 ml., and needles, 20- and 22-gauge, for transtracheal injection
6 Gauze compresses, 4 × 4 in.
1 Box paper tissues
1 Reflector lamp
1 Adjustable stretcher
1 Footstool

The anesthetic drugs frequently used are a 1% solution of aqueous tetracaine (Pontocaine) to which may be added 1 ml. or a 2% solution of 1:1000 epinephrine (Adrenalin). Adrenalin reduces the rapidity of systemic absorption of the tetracaine. In some cases a mixture of 30 ml. of 2% lidocaine (Xylocaine) is used. The traditional drug has been cocaine in a 0.5% or 0.25% solution; however, because of its relatively high reaction risk, it has been replaced by less toxic agents. Cetacaine, a newer topical anesthetic, may also be used.

Pauses of 3 or 4 minutes are taken between applications of the agent to the tongue, palate, and pharynx, and then to the larynx and to the trachea. The anesthetic agent is applied by means of a spray or laryngeal syringe with a straight or curved cannula.

Some physicians prefer to have the patient sit upright and gargle with the topical anesthetic mixture, rinse it around in the mouth, and then expectorate it, thereby producing a partial anesthesia of the buccal mucosa and pharynx.

For direct bronchoscopy, a long metal cannula attached to a syringe is generally used to apply the anesthetic agent to the surface of the vocal cords; then the agent is injected through the anesthetized glottis into the trachea. This act causes the patient to produce a sharp, sudden cough.

For intrabronchial anesthesia, a portion of the anesthetic agent is introduced through the bronchoscope.

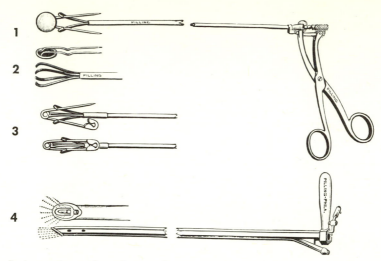

**Fig. 14-7.** Instruments used in foreign body removal. **1,** Chevalier Jackson approximation forceps; **2,** Gordon bead forceps; **3,** Clerf safety-pin closer; **4,** Jackson-Manges roller bronchoscope and esophagoscope. (From Jackson, C., and Jackson, C. L.: Bronchoesophagology, Philadelphia, 1950, W. B. Saunders Co.)

### Positioning the patient

The principles of providing comfort, safety, proper ventilation, and adequate exposure are discussed in Chapter 7.

FOR BRONCHOSCOPY EXAMINATION. The patient is placed in a dorsal recumbent position with shoulders flat on the table at a precise point to permit proper overhanging of the head and neck during the examination. The proper position of the patient is shown in Fig. 14-18.

FOR ESOPHAGOSCOPY. One of several positions may be selected. For direct esophagoscopy, the supine or the lateral position may be used. When the lateral position is used, the head holder may sit on a high stool behind the patient's head (Chapter 7).

### Draping of the patient

The eyes are draped with a towel, and long hair is encased in a disposable cap. Medical aseptic techniques are followed during endoscopy to prevent transmission of bacteria from one patient to another.

### Instruments

Instruments are designed for direct inspection and observation of the larynx, trachea, bronchi, esophagus, and mediastinum and to facilitate the removal of secretions, washings, and tissue for bacteriological and cytological studies. They are also designed to remove foreign bodies.

BRONCHOSCOPE. The standard bronchoscope is a rigid speculum for observation of the tracheobronchial tree (Fig. 14-7). Telescopic scopes such as the Broyles foroblique and the Holinger provide visualization of the upper, lower, and middle lobe bronchi (Fig. 14-8). The right-angled telescope is preferred to view the upper bronchial tree. Retrograde telescopes permit visualization of the undersurface of a tumor.

The standard bronchoscope is provided with illumination; a lamp is attached to the distal end of a metal carrier inserted into the scope. Openings are situated along the side of the lower part of the bronchoscope to permit aeration of the other lung. Oxygen may be administered through an opening in the side arm of the bronchoscope (Fig. 14-7).

The Olympus bronchofiberscope is flexible and alleviates much of the trauma associated with the insertion of the fiberscope into the bronchus. The fiberscope can be

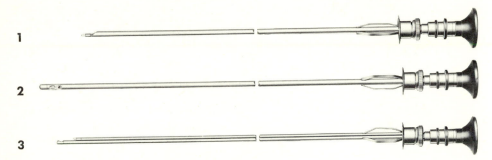

**Fig. 14-8.** Bronchoscopes: **1,** Foroblique examining telescope; **2,** right-angle examining telescope; **3,** retrospective examining telescope with shield, rotating contacts. (Courtesy American Cystoscope Makers, Inc., New York, N. Y.)

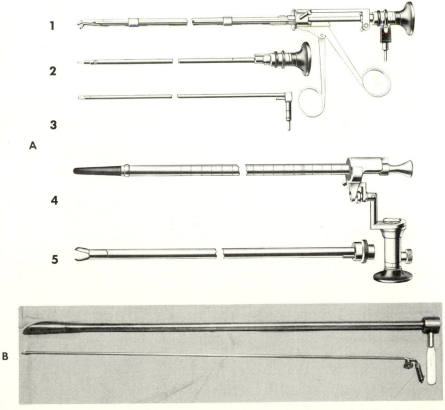

**Fig. 14-9. A,** Schindler esophagoscope: **1,** Biopsy forceps; **2,** telescope; **3,** light carrier; **4,** outer tube and obturator; **5,** inner tube. **B,** Esophagoscope and light carrier. (**A** from Palmer, E. D., and Boyce, H. W.: Manual of gastrointestinal endoscopy, Baltimore, 1964, The Williams & Wilkins Co.)

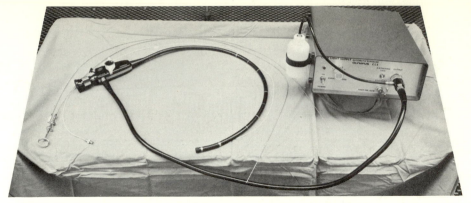

**Fig. 14-10.** Olympus Cle cold light supply; esophagofiberscope.

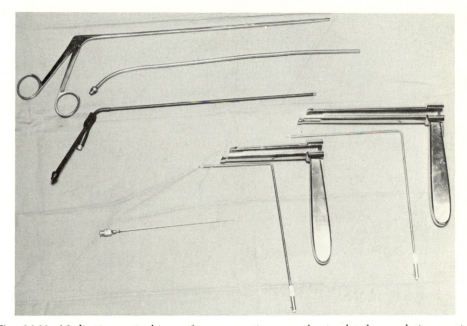

**Fig. 14-11.** Mediastinoscopic biopsy forceps, suction cannula, insulated coagulation suction cannula, endocardiac needle, and mediastinoscopes with light carriers.

inserted into the subsegmental bronchi of the upper lobe without any excess angling of the distal end, and photographs can also be taken.

**ESOPHAGOSCOPE.** One of several models —the Schindler (Fig. 14-9), Jackson, Haslinger, Broyles, Bruening, and Jesburg— is used to examine the cardiac antrum of the stomach, the cervical esophagus, and the duodenum or remove foreign bodies and tissue for microscopic study.

The Schindler esophagoscope has a rigid tube and is fitted with an obturator, the soft, flexible rubber tip of which permits safe introduction of the tube (Fig. 14-9).

The Olympus esophagofiberscope permits visual observation and simultaneous photography of the selected parts of the esophagus, with minimal patient discomfort (Fig. 14-10).

When the indirect technique is used, a flexible obturator is extended through the

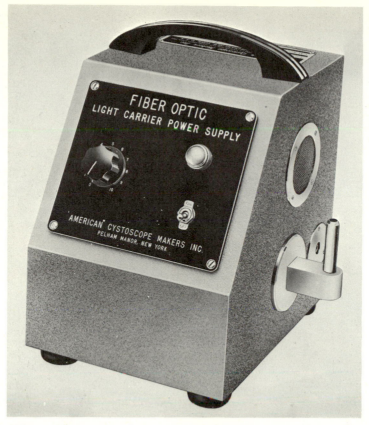

**Fig. 14-12.** Fiberoptic power supply consists of transformer that reduces voltage from 110 volts, 60-cycle A.C. to 21 volts; Variac regulates this voltage supply from 0 to 21 volts, as required. (Courtesy American Cystoscope Makers, Inc., New York, N. Y.)

hollow of the esophagoscope to assist the endoscopist in passing the scope through the pharynx and the cricopharyngeal muscle. The obturator is withdrawn after the scope has reached the esophagoscope.

When the direct technique is used, the endoscopist looks through the hollow base of the scope as he inserts the instrument.

MEDIASTINOSCOPE. The mediastinoscope is used to view lymph nodes or tumors at the tracheobronchial junction, subcarina, or upper lobe bronchi. The mediastinoscope is a hollow tube with a metal carrier and lamp attached at its distal end. (See Fig. 14-11.)

A simple battery with a rheostat switch provides for power and control of the illumination.

LAMPS, LIGHT CARRIERS, CORD, AND BATTERY BOX. Each standard scope requires a lamp, light carrier, and cord. Duplicates of each should be available for immediate use.

The battery box or power supply unit (Figs. 14-12 and 14-13) should be tested periodically and also immediately before use.

SPONGE CARRIERS AND SPONGES. The metal carrier (Fig. 14-14) consists of two parts: an inner rod, which has two jaws protruding from its distal end, and an outer band, which is screwed down on the inner rod so that the sponge is held securely within the jaws. The gauze sponges are used to keep the field dry, remove secretions, or apply a topical anesthetic agent.

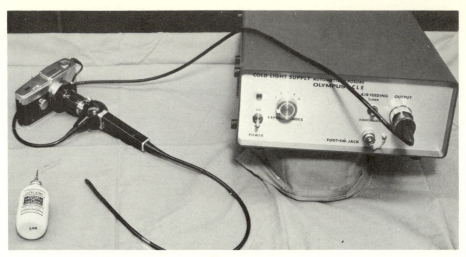

**Fig. 14-13.** Olympus Cle cold light supply.

**Fig. 14-14.** Aspirating tubes for use through bronchoscope. Tubes with curved and flexible ends are useful for obtaining cytological specimens from upper lobe bronchi, but routinely tussive squeeze forces secretions and exudates into larger bronchial stems within reach by means of straight tubes. Below is metal carrier for holding gauze sponges used for swabbing, hemostasis, or obtaining smear specimens from the bronchi. It is used similarly through esophagoscope. (From Jackson, C., and Jackson, C. L.: Bronchoesophagology, Philadelphia, 1950, W. B. Saunders Co.)

**SPECIMEN COLLECTORS.** Cytological specimen collectors such as the Clerf or Lukens are used to hold the secretions as they are obtained.

**ASPIRATORS.** Various types of aspirating tubes of different lengths and design (Fig. 14-14) are used to remove secretions and collect material for microscopic examinations. The straight aspirating tube with one or two openings at the distal end is used to remove material from the pharynx, larynx, and esophagus. The curved aspirating tube with a flexible tip is used to remove secretions from the upper and dorsal orifices of the bronchi.

**FORCEPS.** Various types of forceps are designed to remove foreign bodies or tissues for histological study. In bronchos-

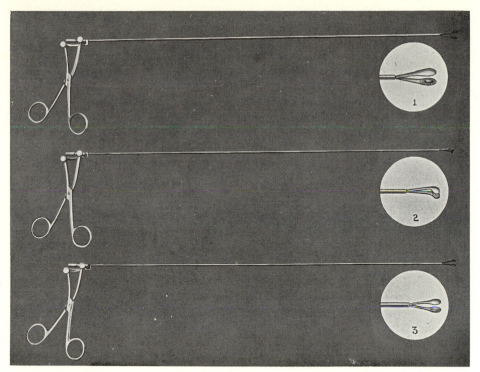

**Fig. 14-15.** Forceps for bronchoscopy: **1,** Forward-grasping forceps with serrated and slightly cupped jaws, used for all ordinary purposes; **2,** side-curved forceps, also used for general purposes—jaws are thin and flat; **3,** ball (cupped) forceps, used for taking specimens of tissue. Special forms of forceps are required for special purposes. (From Jackson, C., and Jackson, C. L.: Bronchoesophagology, Philadelphia, 1950, W. B. Saunders Co.)

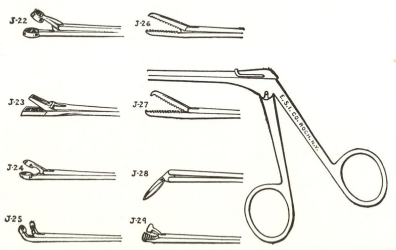

**Fig. 14-16.** Noncannulated forceps for laryngeal and bronchial regions: **J-22,** Punch forceps for tissue specimens; **J-23,** laryngeal specimen and tissue forceps; **J-24,** straight cup-bite forceps; **J-25,** angular cut-bite forceps; **J-26,** straight alligator jaw-grasping forceps; **J-27,** rotation alligator jaw-grasping forceps; **J-28,** laryngeal straight blade scissors; **J-29,** papilloma forceps for removal of recurrent laryngeal papillomas without injury to the vocal cords or delicate tissues. (Courtesy Edward Weck & Co., Inc., Long Island City, N. Y.)

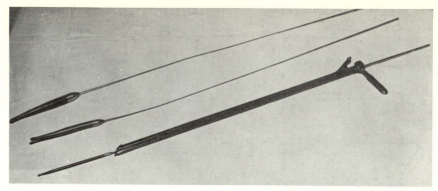

**Fig. 14-17.** Esophagoscope and Jackson dilators used for strictures. (From Saunders, W. H., Havener, W. H., Fair, C. J., and Hickey, J. T.: Nursing care in eye, ear, nose, and throat disorders, ed. 2, St. Louis, 1968, The C. V. Mosby Co.)

copy, a biting tip forceps may be used to secure tissue for study. A forceps with jaws that veer laterally at about a 45-degree angle from the instrument's axis provides for visualization during the biopsy maneuver. A bronchoesophageal forceps (Fig. 14-15) consists of a stylet, a cannula with a handle, a screw, a lock nut, and a set screw. Noncannulated forceps for laryngeal and bronchial regions are designed to remove tissue specimens (Fig. 14-16).

**BOUGIES.** Flexible, woven, silk-tipped bougies of various sizes are used either as lumen finders or to dilate an esophageal stricture. The bougie is passed through the esophagoscope (Fig. 14-17).

## Handling, terminal disinfection, and care of endoscopic instruments

**HANDLING OF INSTRUMENTS.** To ensure long life of the optical system of endoscopes, each instrument should be kept straight at all times when not in use. Flexible endoscopes such as the gastroscope should never be bent, except during introduction into or passage within the patient.

Only the instrument manufacturer should replace a part of the scope. When a telescopic scope is sent for repair, it must be properly packed in a padded instrument case and placed within a padded carton to ensure protection of the lens system during transportation. A direct blow can break the objective window of modern telescopic endoscopes. The junction of the flexible and rigid portions of the scope is the most vulnerable point.

During use the patient may bite down while the flexible portion of the scope is being passed. The sheath covering the flexible part may become perforated after contact. When new covering is needed, the instrument should be sent to the instrument manufacturer.

**CLEANING A FLEXIBLE ENDOSCOPE.** A telescopic endoscope should never be held in a horizontal position unless the objective end is supported. To clean the scope, it is held vertically by its ocular end.

**CLEANING A TELESCOPIC ENDOSCOPE.** The scope is held vertically by its ocular end and wiped downward repeatedly, using gauze sponges saturated with surgical soap and water. Special attention is given to surface joints and crevices that may retain mucus. This process is repeated, using sponges saturated with a 70% alcohol solution. The scope is then dried thoroughly, using clean gauze compresses.

Rigid endoscopes with telescopic lenses may be cleaned in ultrasonic cleaner or with soap and water and gas sterilized.

**CLEANING ASPIRATING TUBES AND SPONGE CARRIERS.** These instruments are cleaned in an ultrasonic cleaner or with soap and water and flushed and sterilized by means

of saturated steam or gas. Special care must be given to spiral-tipped aspirators. All bent or broken-tipped aspirators should be sent to the manufacturer for repair.

In caring for sponge carriers, the collar must be unscrewed before it is cleansed. After sterilization, the threads of the carrier are oiled. The carrier is assembled and stored lying straight on the shelf.

CLEANING FORCEPS. The forceps may be placed in an ultrasonic cleaner. After cleaning, each forceps is taken apart, one at a time, by unscrewing the nut and removing the stylet. All parts are examined carefully, and noncorrosive solvent oil is applied to the crotch of the forceps. Each forceps is reassembled and its action tested; then it is stored in a cabinet with jaws open. In perfect forceps (1) the jaws are close together in parallel position, (2) the handles just touch when the jaws are closed, (3) the jaws go into the cannula when the forceps is closed and protrude widely without expanding the spring when it is open, (4) the end nut, located in the stylet, is in place, (5) the side screw is tight, and (6) the distal end and jaws' edges are smooth on finger examination (Fig. 14-15).

SETTING AND TESTING THE ILLUMINATION. To test the lamp, the telescopic endoscope must be held vertically by its ocular end. The endoscope should always be tested both before and immediately prior to its passage within the patient. The rheostat should be set at the proper voltage, as specified by the instrument maker. The lamp should be switched on and off to test its function.

## Procedures
### Bronchoscopy

DEFINITION. Direct visualization of the mucosa of the trachea, the main bronchi and their openings, and most of the segmental bronchi and removal of material for microscopical study if necessary.

CONSIDERATIONS. Bronchoscopy is an integral part of the examination of patients with pulmonary symptoms such as cough,

hemoptysis, wheeze, and obstruction. Common causes of bleeding (hemoptysis) are bronchiectasis, carcinomas, and tuberculosis. Congenital anomalies and suspected presence of a foreign body, especially in infants and children, are responsible for emergency respiratory examinations.

Bronchoscopy is done to determine whether a lesion is present in the tracheobronchial passages, identify and localize that lesion accurately, and observe periodically the effects of therapy. In suspected bronchogenic carcinoma, the aspirated secretions obtained by bronchoscopy will contain the malignant cells that are not usually observed in expectorated sputum.

SETUP AND PREPARATION OF THE PATIENT. As described previously, including the following:

1 Bronchoscope, desired type, with power supply and cords (Figs. 14-7 and 14-8)
1 Suction pump and tubing
2 Aspirating tubes (Fig. 14-14)
2 Specimen collectors
2 Sponge carriers and sponges (Fig. 14-15)
2 Forceps, desired types (Figs. 14-7 and 14-15)
2 Dilators, if desired
1 Bronchial spray and cannula
1 Lubricating jelly tube
1 Topical anesthesia set, if desired
1 Emesis basin
6 Gauze compresses
1 Round basin with sterile water

The bronchoscopists are exposed to a definite risk of contamination in the presence of communicable diseases. For this reason the endoscopists and assistants should wear face masks. The endoscopist should also wear eyeglasses or an opaque disk, which is attached to a headband. Strict aseptic technique is followed to prevent any possibility of cross contamination from one patient to another.

PROCEDURE

1. The patient is positioned (Fig. 14-18), and his head is carried to the left by the head holder when the right bronchi are inspected; then it is carried to the right when the left bronchi are inspected. The head may be lowered when the right middle lobe orifices are inspected.

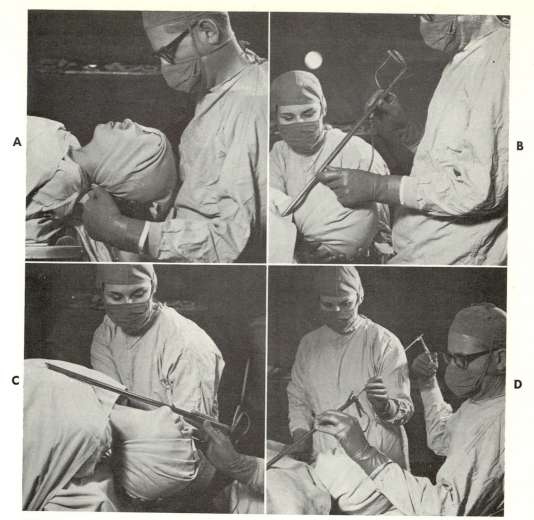

Fig. 14-18. **A,** Preparation of patient for bronchoscopy or esophagoscopy. Note relationship of shoulder to table break. **B,** Initial position for esophagoscopy. Head is held high. Shoulders must be level with or just beyond point at which table breaks. **C,** Final position that will be assumed in esophagoscopy. Head holder raises or lowers head slowly on direction of endoscopist. **D,** Demonstrating how nurse should guide forceps and sucker tips into endoscopic instruments. (From Saunders, W. H., Havener, W. H., Fair, C. J., and Hickey, J. T.: Nursing care in eye, ear, nose, and throat disorders, ed. 2, St. Louis, 1968, The C. V. Mosby Co.)

2. The bronchoscope is inserted over the surface of the tongue, usually through the right corner of the mouth. The patient's lip is retracted from the upper teeth with the finger of the endoscopist's left hand. The epiglottis is identified and elevated with the tip of the bronchoscope.

3. The distal end of the scope is passed through the glottis; the upper tracheal rings are viewed. At this time, a small amount of anesthetic solution may be sprayed through the tube on the carina and into the bronchus by means of a bronchial atomizer or spray. The patient's head is moved to the left to obtain a view of the right bronchi. A right-angled (Broyles) telescope, with its light adjusted previously, is inserted into the head of the bronchoscope. A few seconds

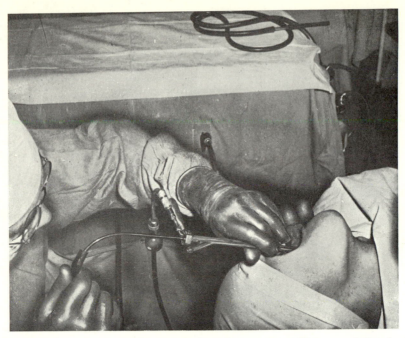

**Fig. 14-19.** Introduction of bronchoscope without laryngoscope. Fingers and thumb of endoscopist's left hand fix bronchoscope lightly against upper teeth, while right hand introduces metallic aspirating tube. Sometimes aspirating bronchoscope with integral aspirating canal is used. (From Jackson, C., and Jackson, C. L.: Bronchoesophagology, Philadelphia, 1950, W. B. Saunders Co.)

are allowed for the optical system to become free of precipitated moisture.

4. The segmental bronchial orifices of the upper right lobe bronchi are viewed. The telescope is removed. Suction and aspirating tubes are used to provide a clear dry field of vision (Fig. 14-19).

5. The scope is advanced to inspect the middle lobe branches by means of insertion of an oblique 30-degree angle telescope or right-angled telescope. The patient's head may be lowered so that the right middle lobe orifices can be viewed or head turned to the right so that the left main bronchus may be viewed.

6. Aspiration of secretions for study is done, if necessary. A biopsy may be obtained for histological diagnosis of a thoracic disorder, using suitable forceps. Or foreign bodies are removed by means of forceps.

7. The bronchoscope is removed. The patient's face is cleansed. The patient is permitted to sit up on the table for a few minutes before he is transported to the stretcher. An emesis basin and compresses must be available.

### Esophagoscopy

**DEFINITION.** Direct visualization of the esophagus and the cardia of the stomach and removal of tissue or secretions for study.

**CONSIDERATIONS.** Esophagoscopy is done to aid in the diagnosis of esophageal diverticula, hiatus hernia, stricture, benign stenosis, or varices; to obtain additional information by means of a biopsy of tissue; or to clarify the roentgenographic findings. Patients suffering with suspected obstruction, symptoms of bleeding, or regurgitation may require endoscopy. Patients with stenosis or varices may be given sclerosing treatment of varices through the esophagoscope. To perform direct therapeutic manipulations such as removal of a

foreign body or insertion of a plastic prosthesis, esophagoscopy is done.

**SETUP AND PREPARATION OF THE PATIENT.** As described previously (Fig. 14-18). The setup includes the following:

Esophagoscopes and telescopes, desired type, size, and length (Figs. 14-9 and 14-10)
Suction pump and tubing
Battery, cords, and lamps (Fig. 14-12)
Broyles dilators (Fig. 14-17)
Bougies, if desired
Forceps, desired types and length (Fig. 14-15)
Aspirating tubes
Specimen containers
Lubricating jelly
Topical anesthesia set

**PROCEDURE**

1. The indirect or direct technique may be followed. When the indirect method is used, the obturator within the scope is passed through the cricopharyngeal lumen and then removed. When the direct technique is used, the esophagoscope with the lamp is thinly lubricated. With the patient in correct position, the suction and pump are turned on. The scope is passed into the mouth. The tongue, epiglottis and laryngeal aditus, and cricopharyngeal lumen are identified, respectively. The head holder may tip the patient's head backward while extending the neck forward. If the endoscope is passed to the side of the tongue, the patient's head may be turned slightly to the opposite side.

2. When the scope is passed into the cardia of the stomach, the patient's head is moved so that all areas of the esophageal wall can be examined.

3. Specimens of secretions from the esophageal lumen may be obtained by aspirating tube and suctioning apparatus. In some cases, saline solution may be injected through the endoscope's aspirating channel and the fluid immediately withdrawn for histological study. A biopsy of tissue may be taken using forceps with jaws at a 45-degree angle.

4. The esophagoscope is removed. The patient is returned to his room.

## Treatment of esophageal varices

**DEFINITION.** Injection of a sclerosing solution into the esophageal lining.

**CONSIDERATIONS.** A varix is any submucosal vein that elevates the esophageal mucosa when the patient is horizontal and is breathing quitely and easily. Patients who are not suitable candidates for surgery may be treated by sclerosis. Only a few veins are treated at a time. Treatments are repeated at intervals.

**SETUP AND PREPARATION OF THE PATIENT.** As described for esophagoscopy, plus the following:

Sclerosing drug, such as sodium morrhuate (Morusul) in 5% solution
2 Syringes, 10 ml.
1 Piece thin rubber tubing, 15 cm. long, to connect syringe to needle
1 Straight needle suitable to dimension of scope
1 Needle, with acute bevel, to fit into other needle's shaft
1 Gastric balloon tube, such as Sengstaken type

**PROCEDURE**

1. The gastric tube is passed orally into the stomach.

2. Esophagoscopy is done as described previously.

3. The needle, tubing, and syringe with medication are then assembled. The long needle is passed through the esophagoscope, and the solution is injected into the esophagus.

4. The needle and endoscope are withdrawn. The gastric balloon of the stomach tube is inflated and pulled up lightly against the cardia. The esophageal balloon is inflated to a pressure of 600 mm. of $H_2O$ for an adult and 300 mm. for a child.

## Mediastinoscopy

**DEFINITION.** Direct visualization of lymph nodes or tumors at the tracheobronchial junction, subcarina, or upper lobe bronchi and biopsy taken.

**CONSIDERATIONS.** Mediastinoscopy usually precedes the exploratory thoracotomy in known cases of lung carcinoma. Patients with positive findings may be treated with radiation or chemotherapy as indicated.

SETUP AND PREPARATION OF THE PATIENT. As described previously, including the following:

- 2 Mediastinoscopes, desired type with power supply and cords (Fig. 14-11)
- 1 Suction pump and tubing
- 2 Aspirating tubes (Fig. 14-14)
- 1 Biopsy forceps (Fig. 14-15)
  Cautery unit
  Endocardiac needle, 20 gauge × 8 in.

The patient is placed under endotracheal anesthesia and positioned as for a tracheostomy.

### OPERATIVE PROCEDURE

1. A short transverse incision is made above the suprasternal notch and the pretracheal fascia exposed.

2. By blunt dissection the plane beneath the pretracheal fascia is developed.

3. The mediastinoscope is passed under direct vision into this fascial plane and is advanced along the ventral tracheal surface toward the mediastinum.

4. The surgeon manipulates the scope to visualize the tracheal bifurcation, bronchi, aortic arch, and associated lymph nodes.

5. Lymph nodal tissue to be biopsied is located and a needle aspiration done to positively identify a nonvascular structure.

6. A biopsy forceps is inserted through the scope and a tissue specimen excised. A bronchus sponge on a holder may be used to apply pressure to the excisional site. The mediastinum is again inspected.

7. The mediastinoscope is withdrawn.

8. The subcutaneous tissue is closed with chromic suture no. 3-0 on a taper needle; the skin is closed with silk no. 4-0 sutures on a cutting needle. A small dressing is applied.

## SPECIFIC NURSING CONSIDERATIONS FOR THORACIC SURGERY

Participation as a scrubbed or circulating nurse on the thoracic surgical team requires utilization of knowledge concerning anatomy, pathophysiology, and corrective procedures that may be performed. These nurses function as specialists skilled in the procedures encompassed in the scope of cardiothoracic nursing. In addition to the responsibilities of scrubbing and circulating, these nurses should be well versed in meeting emergency situations that may occur. Knowledge concerning the purpose, function, and utilization of defibrillators, electrocardiographs, and various monitors is imperative. The nurse is responsible for assisting the anesthesiologist and surgeon in the utilization of this equipment should an emergency arise.

ANESTHESIA. All patients undergoing thoracic surgery are given an inhalation anesthetic through a closed system, with the degree of anesthesia maintained by controlled respiration with an endotracheal tube in place.

The anesthesiologist requires efficient oral suctioning equipment to maintain a clear airway throughout the operation.

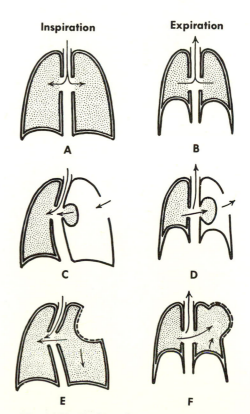

Fig. 14-20. For legend see opposite page.

Before the chest wound is closed, the lungs are reinflated after intermittent suctioning through the endotracheal tube.

POSITIONING. The principles of good positioning are followed, as outlined in Chapter 7.

The patient is placed on the operating table in a position that provides adequate exposure of the operative site, efficient ventilatory and circulatory function, and good body alignment. Since the pulmonary mechanics and venous return of blood to the right heart are influenced by the position of the patient, proper support and elimination of undue pressure areas are important to prevent circulatory difficulties. Abrupt changes of position should also be avoided to prevent serious vasomotor disturbances.

The lateral position permits a full posterolateral thoracotomy incision (Fig. 14-31), which gives the surgeon access to both the anterior and posterior surfaces of the lung and blood vessels (see Chapter 7).

The supine position is used for anterolateral thoracotomy, median sternotomy, (Fig. 14-28), and bilateral anterior transpleural incisions. The sternum may be split vertically or transected horizontally. The upper chest region is usually elevated slightly, and special attention is given to positioning the arm (or arms if bilateral) to permit access to the lateral edge of the incision.

SKIN PREPARATION AND DRAPING. Procedures are followed as described in Chapter 4.

PROVISIONS FOR BLOOD REPLACEMENT. Before the operation begins, provisions for blood replacement should be made by the physician. The circulating nurse calls the blood bank prior to the induction of anesthesia to verify the amount of blood available. She also has available facilities for estimating blood loss whenever necessary.

SUCTION AND DRAINAGE APPARATUS. An adjustable suction apparatus with a protected tube is necessary for use by the surgeon in the maintenance of a dry operative field.

One or two chest drainage tubes or catheters may be used for postoperative closed chest drainage. Drains are clamped off until each tube is connected to a separate sterile water-seal drainage bottle. When a persistent air leak cannot be controlled by drainage alone, water-seal suction may be necessary (Fig. 14-21), and the two-bottle sterile setup is needed. The first bottle provides the water seal and collects the drainage, and the second provides the suction control. All connections must be taped to provide an airtight system. A second water-seal and drainage bottle is added if two drainage tubes are used. A Y connector may be used to connect both to

---

Fig. 14-20. Pathological physiology of severe chest injuries. **A,B,** Normal physiology of inspiration and expiration. **C,D,** Open (sucking) wound of thorax. On inspiration, air at atmospheric pressure rushes in through defect, **C,** collapsing the lung. Next, positive pressure causes the mediastium to shift, compressing opposite lung. On expiration, **D,** air from lung on uninjured side reenters collapsed lung and is rebreathed in next inspiration. Impaired cardiopulmonary function in presence of sucking wound of chest is caused by (1) collapse of lung on injured side, (2) partial collapse of opposite lung, (3) increased functional dead space caused by rebreathing of unoxygenated air from collapsed lung, and (4) diminished venous return to right side of heart. **E,F,** Chief effect of paradoxical motion resulting from flail or stove-in chest is diminution of pulmonary ventilation and extensive rebreathing from one lung to the other. Venous return to right side of heart is impaired. Stabilization of chest wall, either by compression or traction, diminishes to-and-fro movement (flutter) of mediastinum, thus improving function of lung on uninjured side. (From Johnson, J., and Kirby, C. K.: Surgery of the chest, ed. 3, Chicago, 1964, Year Book Medical Publishers, Inc.)

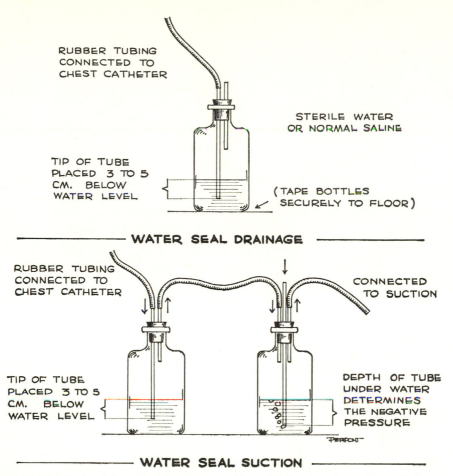

RUBBER TUBING
CONNECTED TO
CHEST CATHETER

STERILE WATER
OR NORMAL SALINE

TIP OF TUBE
PLACED 3 TO 5
CM. BELOW
WATER LEVEL

(TAPE BOTTLES
SECURELY TO FLOOR)

——— WATER SEAL DRAINAGE ———

RUBBER TUBING
CONNECTED TO
CHEST CATHETER

CONNECTED
TO SUCTION

TIP OF TUBE
PLACED 3 TO 5
CM. BELOW
WATER LEVEL

DEPTH OF TUBE
UNDER WATER
DETERMINES
THE NEGATIVE
PRESSURE

——— WATER SEAL SUCTION ———

Fig. 14-21. Methods of draining pleural space. (From Blades, B., editor: Surgical diseases of the chest, ed. 2, St. Louis, 1966, The C. V. Mosby Co.)

the suction control bottle. The surgeon is responsible for supervising the preparation and connection of the system. Regardless of the type of closed drainage system selected (there are many commercial ones available), it is imperative that it be sterile and that it *always* be maintained at a position *lower* than the patient's body to prevent reentrance of air and fluid into the chest cavity, which could cause immediate complications. Clamps for the tubing should always accompany the patient as a precautionary measure against accidental interruption of the closed system.

ISOLATION TECHNIQUE. Many thoracic operations involve patients with acute or chronic infectious conditions. For this reason, strict precautionary measures are followed whenever indicated (see Chapters 3 and 5).

In those operations involving the bronchus, the instruments and supplies used for transection are considered contaminated and must be appropriately isolated (Chapter 21).

## BASIC THORACIC INSTRUMENT SET FOR SURGERY

The thoracic setup includes the basic laparotomy instrument setup and linen pack with an appropriate fenestrated drape (see Chapter 5). The thoracic set includes the

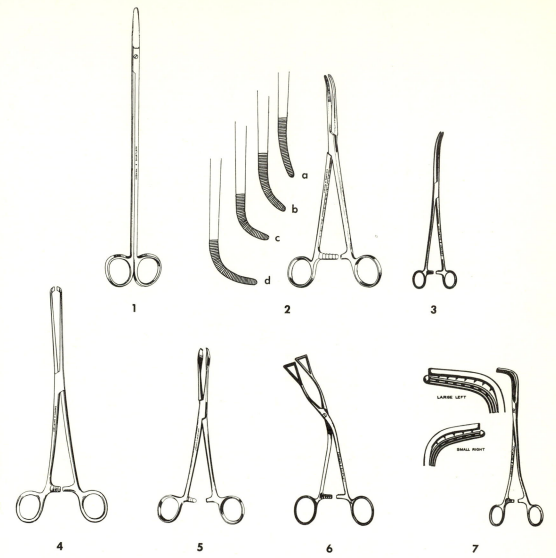

**Fig. 14-22.** Instruments for lobectomy and pneumonectomy. **1**, Willauer thoracic scissors; **2**, Rumel thoracic forceps, **a** to **d**; **3**, Harrington forceps; **4**, Willauer-Allis thoracic tissue forceps, 10 in.; **5**, Overholt segmental forceps; **6**, Lovelace lung-grasping forceps; **7**, Sarot bronchus clamps, right and left, small or large. (Courtesy Codman & Shurtleff, Inc., Randolph, Mass.)

following instruments (Figs. 14-22 to 14-24):

**Cutting instruments**

4 No. 4 knife handles with no. 20 blade
4 No. 3 knife handles with nos. 10, 11, 12, 15 blades
4 No. 3 knife handles, long, with nos. 11 and 15 blades
4 Metzenbaum scissors, 2 7 in. and 2 12 in.
2 Willauer or Nelson scissors, curved, 10 in. (Fig. 14-22)

4 Mayo scissors, straight, curved, 9 in.
1 Potts tenotomy scissors, 7½ in.
1 Potts dissecting scissors, angulated 60-degree, 7½ in.
1 Wire cutter

**Holding instruments**

36 Backhaus towel clamps, 5 in.
12 Backhaus towel clamps, 3 in.
 2 Tissue forceps, 10 in., with teeth
 1 Roberts ring forceps
 1 Ferguson forceps, smooth

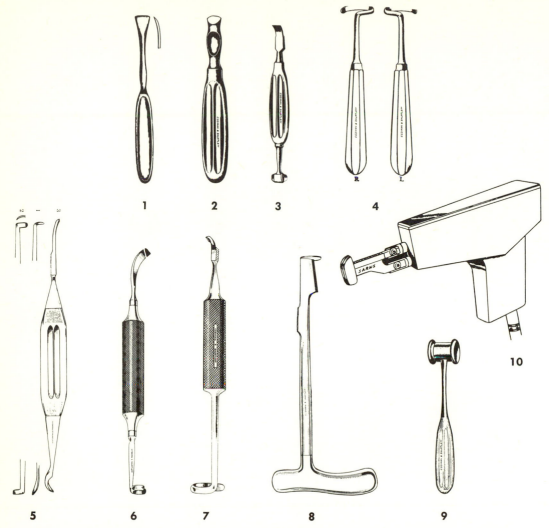

**Fig. 14-23.** Instruments for thoracotomy. **1,** Langenbeck periosteal elevator, 7½ in.; **2,** Kermission periosteal raspatory; **3,** Alexander costal periosteotome; **4,** Doyen rib raspatories, right and left, 6 in.; **5,** Overholt elevators, nos. 1, 2, and 3; **6,** Wilson rib stripper; **7,** Lambert-Berry raspatory, double-ended; **8,** Lebsche sternum knife, 10 in.; **9,** Hibbs bone mallet; **10,** Sarns sternal electric saw. (Courtesy Codman & Shurtleff, Inc., Randolph, Mass.)

2 Stille-Adson forceps, fine-toothed, 4¾ in.
4 Potts-Smith vascular forceps, smooth, 7 in.
4 Potts-Smith vascular forceps, fine-toothed, 7 in.
2 DeBakey vascular clamps, 10 in.
6 Rochester-Pean clamps, 10 in. (for small, dry dissectors)
6 Rumel thoracic clamps, 10 in. (for tapes and suture passes)
4 Lovelace lung-grasping forceps (Fig. 14-22)
1 Overholt segmental forceps
1 Semb forceps, 9¼ in. (ligature carrier)

**Clamping instruments**

36 Halsted mosquito clamps, straight, curved, 5 in.
60 Crile forceps, straight, 5½ in.
24 Rochester-Pean clamps, curved, 6¼ in.
8 Carmalt clamps (optional for clamping pump lines)
12 Rumel thoracic clamps, 10 in. (Fig. 14-22)
6 Harrington forceps, 12 in.
6 Right-angle clamps, assorted lengths and angulations
4 Sarot or Lees bronchus clamps, right and left for resection (Fig. 14-22)

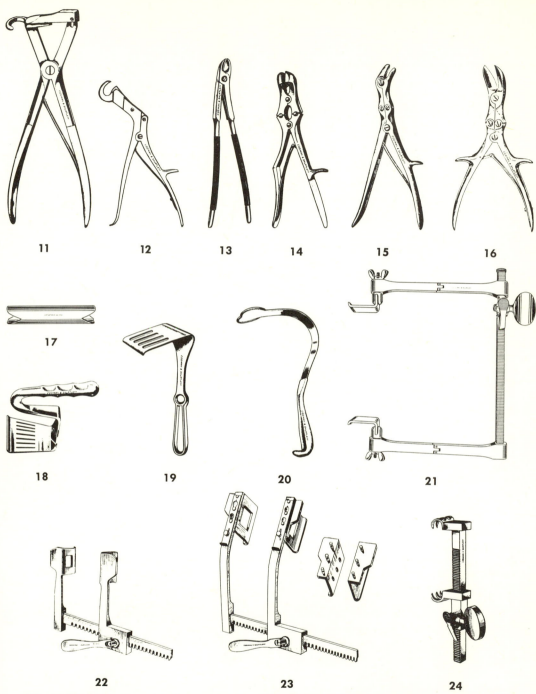

**Fig. 14-24.** Instruments for thoracotomy—cont'd. **11,** Shoemaker rib shears; **12,** Stille-Giertz rib shears; **13,** Bethune rib shears; **14,** Sauerbruch rib rongeur; **15,** Stille-Luer bone rongeur; **16,** Stille-Liston bone-cutting forceps, straight; **17,** New York Hospital emergency rib spreader; **18,** Davidson scapula retractor; **19,** Coryllos retractor, large size; **20,** Harrington splanchnic retractor; **21,** Himmelstein sternal retractor with hinged arms; **22,** Finochietto rib retractor; **23,** Burford-Finochietto rib retractor with two sets detachable blades; **24,** Bailey rib contractor. (Courtesy Codman & Shurtleff, Inc., Randolph, Mass.)

**Vascular instruments** (Chapter 15)

2 Crafoord coarctation clamps
4 Patent ductus clamps, 2 angulated, 2 straight
4 Bulldog clamps
2 Satinsky clamps
  Cooley clamps, 2 of each size and curvature

**Bone instruments**

1 Alexander periosteotome
1 Overholt elevator
2 Doyen rib raspatorys and elevators, right and left
1 Stille-Liston bone-cutting forceps
1 Bethune rib shears
1 Sauerbruch rib rongeur, double-action, square jaw
1 Stille-Luer bone rongeur, multiple action

**For median sternotomy**

1 Electric saw (Stryker, Sagital, or Sarns sternal)
1 Lebsche sternum knife (Fig. 14-23)
1 Mallet
1 Sternum spreader
1 Nunez sternum approximator
2 Gigli saws with handles
2 Bone tenacula, single hook
1 Bone punch or awl with fenestrated tip
  Stainless steel wire suture no. 22

**Exposing instruments**

4 Volkmann rake retractors, dull, 2 4-prong and 2 6- or 8-prong
2 Cushing vein retractors
2 Parker, Roux, or McBurney retractors
1 Set Richardson retractors
2 Kelly retractors, large
2 Deaver retractors, wide and narrow
1 Set malleable retractors
2 Doyen abdominal retractors
1 Burford rib retractor with 2 sets blades (Fig. 14-24)

3 Finochietto retractors, assorted sizes (or similar)
2 Bailey rib contractors
2 Weitlaner retractors, blunt

**Suturing items**

8 Vascular needle holders, various lengths
6 Sarot needle holders, 10 in. and 12 in.
1 Needle set, including assorted taper and cutting needles
  Assorted sizes silk sutures and chromic sutures; *for intrathoracic use,* intestinal, general closure, or vascular needles should be swaged on the suture strand
3 Nylon or silk sutures, fine, for skin closure

**Accessory items**

1 Local anesthesia set, if desired (see Chapter 5)
2 Electrocautery cords and tips (optional)
2 Rubber or plastic chest catheters, selected sizes (with appropriate connectors)
2 Robinson catheters, size 14 and 16 Fr.
1 Bone wax
1 Culture tube
1 Basin set
1 Pitcher, 1000 ml.
4 Medicine glasses
1 Luer-Lok syringe, 50 ml.
3 Asepto syringes, 2 oz.
1 Closed drainage set (Fig. 14-21)
1 Bronchoscopy set, if indicated
  Assorted sponges (laparotomy packs, 4 × 4 in., and dissecting sponges)
  Assorted aspirating needles, desired sizes
2 Suction tubings, 6-foot lengths
6 Pieces umbilical tape, 18 in.
  Dacron tape, silk suture no. 4 for occlusion, compression, or traction for blood vessels
2 Penrose tubings, narrow, 12 in., for traction
1 Gelfoam, size 100 (optional)
1 Surgicel absorbable hemostat (optional)
1 Dural elevator

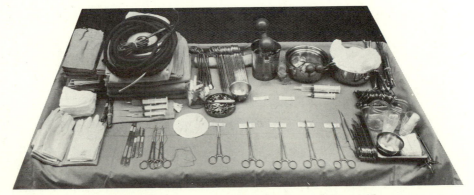

**Fig. 14-25.** Thoracic setup arrangement of nurse's front table.

2 Nerve hooks, dull
1 Ruler

Preparation of other sterile items has already been described in Chapter 5.

Thoracic surgery setup arrangment of items on table (Figs. 14-25 and 14-26) and Mayo table (Fig. 14-27) should be determined by the nursing staff, depending on an effective standard method that applies principles of work simplification and body mechanics.

Sutures are supplied according to the surgeon's preference. Ordinarily, chromic gut no. 0 is used for the muscles and fascia. The subcutaneous tissue is closed with chromic gut no. 2-0; running nylon suture no. 4-0 is used for the skin (Chapter 6).

## OPERATIONS
### Types of incisions

The incision selected provides access to the involved structures. Frequently both the anterior and posterior surfaces of the lung and the associated blood vessels and tissues are involved. The position of the patient, as previously discussed, must permit adequate surgical exposure of the involved lesion (Figs. 14-28 and 14-31).

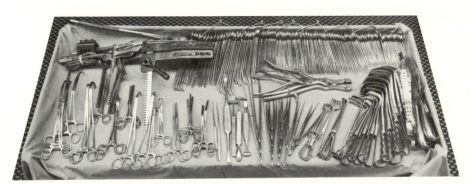

**Fig. 14-26.** Thoracic setup arrangement of instrument table.

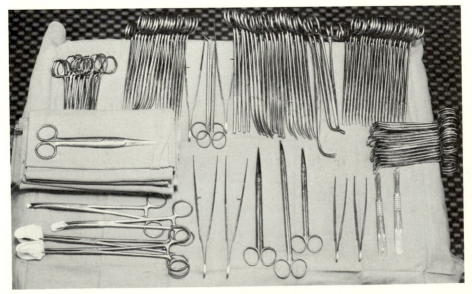

**Fig. 14-27.** Thoracic Mayo table setup arrangement of instruments.

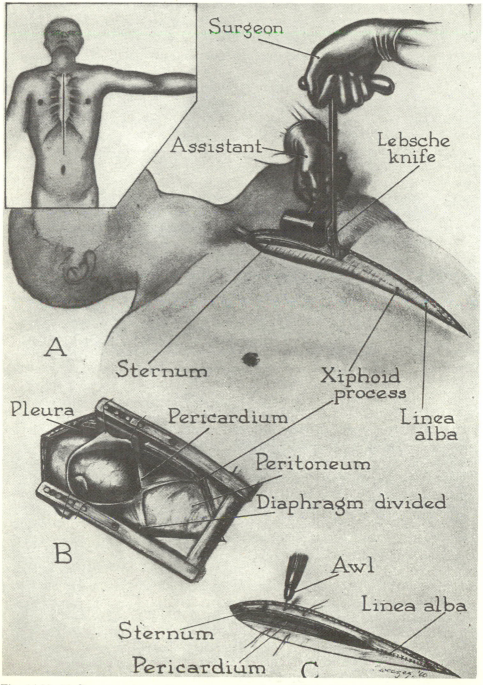

Surgeon

Assistant

Lebsche knife

A

Sternum

Xiphoid process

Linea alba

Pleura

Pericardium

Peritoneum

Diaphragm divided

B

Awl

Linea alba

Sternum

Pericardium

C

**Fig. 14-28.** Median sternotomy. Sternum may also be split from below upward, or it may be divided with oscillating saw. (From Dobell, A. R. C.: In Gibbon, J. H., Jr., editor: Surgery of the chest, Philadelphia, 1962, W. B. Saunders Co.)

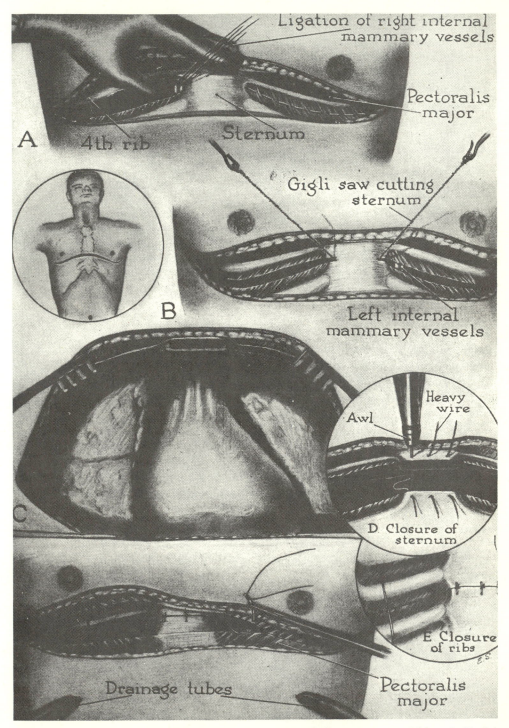

**Fig. 14-29.** Transsternal bilateral thoracotomy. (From Dobell, A. R. C.: In Gibbon, J. H., Jr., editor: Surgery of the chest, Philadelphia, 1962, W. B. Saunders Co.)

## Funnel chest operation
### (correction of pectus excavatum)

DEFINITION. Resection of the lowest costal cartilages, division of the xiphoid from the gladiolus, and severance of the substernal ligament and the diaphragmatic attachments from the resected portion of the costal cartilages; then, formation of a wedged transverse osteotomy of the sternum, excision of malformed articulations, and repositioning of the ends of the cartilages.

PURPOSE. This operation is performed for cosmesis and to establish normal respiratory and circulatory functions of the organs in the chest by eliminating the abnormal inward inclination of the sternum and by straightening the attachments of the cartilages to the sides of the sternum.

CONSIDERATIONS. A deformity of the chest wall, which is also known as trichterbrust or chonechondrosternon, is a structural depression of the anterior thoracic wall. Many theories have been proposed regarding cause—fetal position in utero, upper respiratory tract obstruction, inherited tendency, and obstruction in breathing that necessitates an increased amount of pull by the diaphragm, thereby increasing the negative pressure.

This protruding deformity is characterized by a posterior depression of the sternum, which has its deepest depression at the junction of the xiphoid with the gladiolus. The sternal ends become elongated and depressed in a posterior direction, forming a narrow inverted cone- or funnel-shaped configuration. This causes a mild compression of the thoracic viscera. The lower end of the sternum may push the mediastinum back against the anterior surface of the vertebral bodies, thus occasionally causing cardiac symptoms. Surgery is done primarily for cosmetic reasons and occasionally for symptoms of the respiratory and circulatory systems.

An anterior midline incision may be made through the level of the second rib to a point halfway between the xiphoid and umbilicus (Figs. 14-28 and 14-30), or a bilateral inframammary incision may be preferred, since it results in less keloid formation than does the midline approach.

SETUP AND PREPARATION OF THE PATIENT. The patient is placed on the operating table in a supine position, the upper half of the chest slightly elevated with a rolled sheet (see Chapter 7). The setup is as described for basic thoracic set and median sternotomy, minus lung resection instruments and long hemostatic clamps; the following are added:

1 Periosteal elevator (small)
1 Gigli saw set (optional)
  Circular blade for Stryker saw
1 Osteotome
1 Bone-holding forceps
6 Stainless steel wire sutures, various sizes
  Other traction and immobilization apparatus, if desired: Jacob sternal ladders, metal bridge ladders, light plaque or plaster with heavy wire loops attached, or wooden spreaders with wire loops
2 Skin hooks

OPERATIVE PROCEDURE

1. The selected incision is carried through the skin to the fascia. Bleeding points are controlled with electrocautery and silk ligatures. The wound edges are protected with towels; moist packs and retractors are placed. (See Fig. 14-30.)

2. The fascial insertions of the greater pectoral muscles into the sternum are cut and retracted. Dissecting scissors, Pean hemostats, and suture ligatures of silk no. 2-0 are used. Rib cartilages are freed from the sternum with an elevator and knife.

3. A transverse incision is made, separating the xiphoid from the sternum and dividing the substernal ligament and extension of abdominal muscles. A knife, periosteal elevator, sternal knife (Gigli saw or chisel may be preferred), and heavy scissors are used.

4. The xiphoid is grasped with bone forceps as the anterior mediastinum is entered. Using sharp and blunt dissection, the pericardium is freed from the sternum.

5. The posterior cartilages are cut with heavy scissors to free the depressed bone. (This allows the pleura and pericardium

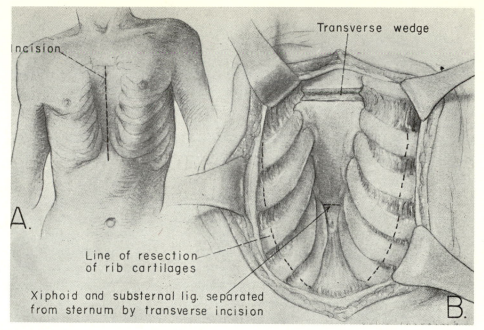

Incision

Transverse wedge

Line of resection of rib cartilages

Xiphoid and substernal lig. separated from sternum by transverse incision

A.

B.

Fig. 14-30. Operation for correction of funnel chest. **A,** Deformity and line of incision. **B,** Sternum has been divided. Dotted lines show division of costal cartilage. (From Horsley, G. W., and Bigger, I. A.: Operative surgery, ed. 6, St. Louis, 1953, The C. V. Mosby Co.)

to drop back posteriorly and the heart to shift to a normal position.)

6. A wedge-shaped transverse osteotomy is made with a circular saw in the outer table of the sternum at a point where the deformity begins (Fig. 14-30).

7. The sternum is trimmed, using rongeur and shears; cartilages are shortened or resected so that new surfaces fit flat against each other. The depressed sternum is bent forward so that it may assume a normal position.

8. The sternum is maintained in the corrected position by mattress sutures of heavy silk or steel wire that are placed across the osteotomy. (The special sternal osteotomy sutures with swaged-on needles are best suited for this purpose.) The pectoral muscles are sutured back to the sternum; the intercostal muscles are sutured to the undersurface of the sternum; and the xiphoid is left free.

9. The wound is closed with interrupted silk or synthetic sutures after pleural drainage has been established.

10. Dressings are applied.

## Repair of penetrating thoracic wounds

**DEFINITION.** Closure of the wound and decompression of the pleural cavity by closed thoracotomy.

**CONSIDERATIONS.** The physiological respiratory complications in the presence of thoracic injuries or in disease of the lung have been discussed previously.

An open penetrating wound, which is known as an open pneumothorax, permits air to reach the pleural cavity with each inspiration, but with each expiration the air is partially removed. This condition builds up a positive pressure in the pleural cavity. The dangers of open pneumothorax depend on the individual's preinjury or pulmonary status and the size of the external wound. A large penetrating wound causes the lung on the affected side to collapse.

**SETUP AND PREPARATION OF THE PATIENT.** Thoracotomy or thoracostomy setup and chest tubes, as for closed thoracotomy with a water-seal drainage set. The lateral or

supine position is used, depending on the site of injury.

OPERATIVE PROCEDURE

1. Cleaning of wound, debridement, control of hemorrhage, closure of wound, removal of air, application of pressure bandage, and administration of oxygen are done.

2. For tension pneumothorax, the chest tubes are inserted and the chest closed. Tubes are connected to a water-seal drainage set (Fig. 14-21).

## Injury of blood vessels of chest or lungs (hemothorax)

DEFINITION. Control of hemorrhage and establishment of drainage of pleural cavity.

CONSIDERATIONS. Hemothorax may be produced by an injury to the intercostal vessels, the vessels within the lung, or the major vessels in the mediastinum. When blood accumulates in the thoracic cavity, the increased pressure will displace the mediastinum and cause circulatory and respiratory problems, as in tension pneumothorax.

SETUP AND PREPARATION OF THE PATIENT. For hemorrhage of major vessels of the lung, thoracotomy setup.

OPERATIVE PROCEDURES

1. Aspiration (thoracentesis), which is the procedure of choice.

2. Cessation of progressive hemorrhage (thoracotomy).

3. Expansion of a compressed and constricted lung (decortication).

## Repair of fractured ribs and chest injuries

Injury of the chest wall may be so severe, with fracture of numerous ribs, that the integrity of the chest wall is destroyed. Segments reveal paradoxical respiration and require stabilization.

CONSIDERATIONS. Operative fixation of multiple fractures is neither feasible nor necessary. Tracheostomy is beneficial because it (1) removes tracheal secretions and (2) provides a mode of positive pressure ventilation. This is the single best mode of effective therapy for a flail chest.

## Operations for empyema

GENERAL CONSIDERATIONS. Before the existence of chemotherapeutic agents and antibiotics, *acute* empyema usually developed as a secondary complication of lobar pneumonia, streptococcal infections, or tuberculosis. Today *Staphylococcus aureus* is found to be the most frequent offender (see Chapter 3). Infection is usually associated with a lung abscess and pneumonia. Since organisms are usually virulent when drainage is established, special precautions must be taken in handling articles used during surgery and in decontaminating soiled equipment after surgery.

In *chronic* empyema, the pleural membranes become thick and rigid as a result of a prolonged infection. The chest wall becomes rigid and smaller, thus distorting the lungs. The fibrous pleural covering may extend over a part or all of the lung and chest wall. Chronic empyema is the failure of the chest cavity to become obliterated. This condition, in turn, prevents the unexpanded lung from returning to normal function (Figs. 14-6 and 14-20). Chronic empyema creates additional complications such as mediastinal shift, difficulties in swallowing, deformity of the chest, and respiratory limitations.

One of several operations is carried out to treat empyema. They include (1) thoracoplasty to obliterate the cavity and collapse the overlying portion of the chest and (2) decortication of the lung to eliminate the cavity so that the expanded lung can fill it.

### Closed thoracostomy (intercostal drainage)

DEFINITION. Insertion of a catheter through the intercostal space and the establishment of closed drainage.

CONSIDERATIONS. This procedure is done to restore a negative pressure in the cavity, which is essential to the normal function-

ing of the respiratory and circulatory system, to provide continuous aspiration of an infectious fluid from the pleural cavity and avoid an ingress of air at a time when the lung may collapse.

SETUP AND PREPARATION OF THE PATIENT. As described for routine skin preparation (Chapter 4), positioning (Chapter 7), and draping (Chapter 5), using the basic instruments (Chapter 17), plus the following:

1 Local anesthesia set, including syringes, needles, and 1% procaine solution
2 Hemostatic clamps, straight
2 Patterson or Davidson trocars and cannulae to fit catheters
2 Catheters, desired size
2 Catheter clamps, screw-type
1 Luer-Lok syringe, 30 ml.
2 Aspirating needles, 16-gauge, 3½ in.
2 Culture tubes
1 Water-seal drainage set (Fig. 14-21)

The patient is placed in a lateral or sitting position.

During the operation, air is prevented from entering the cavity by having the catheter fit snugly, clamping it on insertion into the cavity, and then attaching the catheter to the drainage set.

OPERATIVE PROCEDURE

1. The prepared operative site is anesthetized. An aspirating needle, attached to a syringe, is introduced into the chest cavity to verify presence of pus.

2. The trocar and cannula are introduced through the puncture wound, intercostal space, and then into the pleural cavity.

3. A catheter, desired size, which has been marked for its correct length, is introduced into the cavity immediately after withdrawal of the trocar obturator. The free end of the catheter is clamped to prevent the ingress of air.

4. When the cannula is withdrawn and a second forceps is placed between the end of the cannula and the patient, the terminal forceps is removed so that the cannula can be slipped off the distal end of the catheter.

5. The skin edges are sutured, and the free ends of the suture are tied around the catheter to prevent its accidental withdrawal.

6. A dressing is then applied to the wound.

7. For continuous drainage without the entrance of air into the pleural cavity, the free end of the catheter is attached to a long rubber tube that is placed beneath the water within the sterile drainage bottle; then the forceps is removed. For continuous aspiration of fluid and the creation of a negative pressure, a water-seal drainage set is used (Fig. 14-21).

### Open thoracotomy (rib resection)

DEFINITION. Partial resection of a selected rib or ribs, usually the ninth in the posterior axillary line, to treat empyemic lesions by the establishment of continuous drainage, with the eventual healing and reexpansion of the lung.

SETUP AND PREPARATION OF THE PATIENT. Basic thoracic setup, as listed previously.

The patient is usually placed in the lateral position, with the affected side uppermost (see Chapter 7). The sitting position and local anesthesia may be used. Skin cleansing and draping are described in Chapters 4 and 5.

Rigid precautions are carried out during and following the procedure to prevent cross contamination of both the patient and surgical team.

OPERATIVE PROCEDURE

1. If local anesthesia is used, the local anesthetic is injected. The incision is made over the selected rib and carried through all tissue layers (Figs. 14-31 and 14-32). The wound edges are protected by towels and laparotomy packs. Bleeding vessels are controlled by hemostats, fine silk or gut ligatures, and electrocautery.

2. The periosteum is incised with a scalpel, and the intercostal muscles (Figs. 14-31 and 14-32) are freed from the superior and inferior borders of the rib with a periosteal elevator, Doyen raspatory, and scissors (Figs. 14-22 and 14-23).

3. The segment of rib or ribs is resected with bone shears and rongeur (Fig. 14-31).

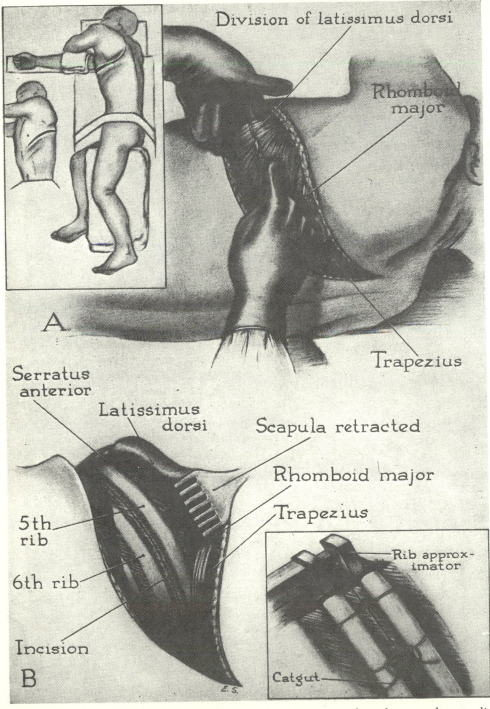

**Fig. 14-31.** Posterolateral thoracotomy incision. Wide exposure is dependent on adequate division of trapezius. (From Dobell, A. R. C.: In Gibbon, J. H., Jr., editor: Surgery of the chest, Philadelphia, 1962, W. B. Saunders Co.)

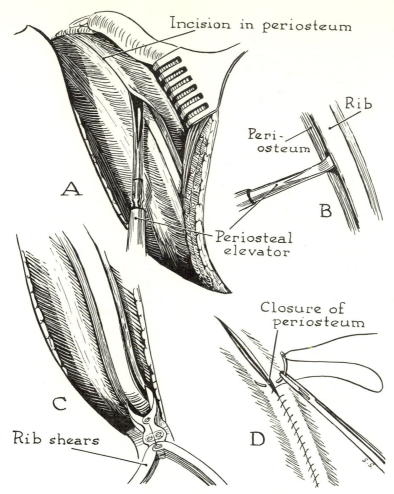

Incision in periosteum

Rib

Peri-
osteum

A

B

Periosteal
elevator

C

Closure of
periosteum

Rib shears

D

**Fig. 14-32.** Technique of rib resection in posterolateral thoracotomy. Posteriorly, rib is divided close to transverse process. (From Dobell, A. R. C.: In Gibbon, J. H., Jr., editor: Surgery of the chest, Philadelphia, 1962, W. B. Saunders Co.)

Bone wax may be applied to the ends of the ribs to help prevent infection and control bleeding.

4. The pleura is incised at the site of aspiration; suction is available as cultures are obtained, and the cavity is evacuated.

5. Drainage tubes are inserted through the pleural opening, and the margins of the wound are fitted snugly to prevent leakage at this point.

6. A suture of no. 2-0 silk on a cutting needle is passed through both sides of the tube, then it is tied around the tube.

7. Tubes are clamped with tubing clamps until connected with drainage bottles.

8. The intercostal muscles, fascia, and skin are approximated in layers, using chromic gut no. 2-0 or 0 interrupted sutures for muscle and fascia and nylon for skin closure.

9. Dressings are applied over the wound. An adhesive strip around each tube may be used for fixation.

### Thoracoplasty

**DEFINITION.** Resection of several ribs.

**CONSIDERATIONS.** Thoracoplasty is done to induce a permanent collapse of the underlying lung, which is maintained by the regeneration of bone from the periosteum of the resected ribs. This operation

is selected for those patients with a pro-ductive · unilateral fibrocavernous type of pulmonary tuberculosis when therapeutic pneumothorax, phrenic nerve paralysis, and drug therapy have failed to control the disease. This procedure is not used when the patient's general condition is poor, when inadequate respiratory or circulatory reserve is present, or when the tubercle bacilli are in an active stage.

An extrapleural thoracoplasty is per-formed in one or two stages. The initial stage includes the complete resection of the first through the fifth ribs; the second stage may include the resection of portions of the next four to five ribs.

SETUP AND PREPARATION OF THE PATIENT. Basic thoracic setup, as described pre-viously, minus drainage tubes and lung resection instruments. The lateral position is used for a posterolateral approach.

OPERATIVE PROCEDURE

1. The skin incision is carried down to the muscles and bleeding vessels are clamped and ligated.

2. The serratus anterior, trapezius, rhom-boid, and latissimus dorsi muscles (Fig. 14-31) are divided in order to expose the neck of each rib. Bleeding is controlled with electrocautery and suture ligatures. The scapula and muscles are retracted.

3. The periosteum of the third rib is incised and the third rib removed to facili-tate removal of the second and first ribs. Intercostal insertions are cut, and the pos-terior end of the rib is freed (Fig. 14-31). Tendinous and ligamentous attachments to the rib process are divided, exposing the transverse process of the corresponding vertebrae. The rib is resected, and re-maining portions of the transverse process and short segment of the rib are smoothed off. Bleeding is controlled.

4. The second rib, the first rib, the transverse processes of the vertebrae, and the neck of the second rib are resected.

5. All bleeding vessels are controlled by ligation and electrocautery.

6. The scapula is pushed back into place. The divided muscles are approximated with two rows of sutures placed in the deep fascial portion of each muscle. The second row is placed in the superficial muscle layer.

7. Skin towels are removed, and super-ficial fascial and subcutaneous tissue layers are closed. The skin is closed without drainage. Dressings are applied.

### Anterior thoracoplasty

DEFINITION. The excision of the ribs and their costal cartilages, which prevents col-lapse of the remaining residual cavities following extensive posterolateral thoraco-plasty.

SETUP AND PREPARATION OF THE PATIENT. As described for posterior thoracoplasty procedure. The patient is placed on the operating table in a supine position, with the affected side slightly elevated. The arm is positioned to permit access to the lateral edge of the incision. Skin prepara-tion and draping are completed.

OPERATIVE PROCEDURE

1. A semicircular incision is made along the anterior axillary fold or along the outer margin of the breast. The superficial muscles overlying the thorax are divided and retracted.

2. The anterior stump of the ribs and the first costal cartilage are resected.

3. The wound is closed, as described for extrapleural posterior thoracoplasty.

### Poudrage

DEFINITION. Liberal application of sterile talcum powder to the visceral and parietal pleural surfaces in order to stimulate the growth of adhesions between the pleurae.

CONSIDERATIONS. The creation of pleural adhesions is indicated in the presence of recurrent idiopathic spontaneous pneumo-thorax or as a palliative measure in the presence of excessive pleural effusions re-lated to inoperable malignancies.

SETUP AND PREPARATION OF THE PATIENT. Basic thoracic setup plus talcum powder.

The patient is usually placed in the lateral position, with the affected side uppermost.

**OPERATIVE PROCEDURE.** Same as for open thoracotomy, plus talc is sprinkled on a wet sponge held by a forceps and then wiped on all surfaces of the pleurae.

## Operations on the lung
### Decortication of the lung

**DEFINITION.** Removal of the fibrinous deposit or restrictive membrane on the pleural lining that interferes with pulmonary ventilatory function.

**CONSIDERATIONS.** Since one of the major objectives is to return the chest wall to as near normal function as possible, an intercostal incision is preferred; however, rib resection may be necessary to permit adequate exposure.

**SETUP AND PREPARATION OF THE PATIENT.** As described for lobectomy procedure.

**OPERATIVE PROCEDURE**

1. The incision is carried through skin, superficial fascia, deep fascia, and muscles; wound edges are protected, as described for lobectomy.

2. One rib, usually the fifth or sixth, is resected (Fig. 14-32).

3. A Finochietto rib retractor is placed, with ribs protected by moist gauze. It is opened slowly to achieve exposure.

4. The parietal adhesions to margins of the lung, mediastinal surface, and pericardium are divided if necessary. Long curved thoracic scissors, forceps and hemostats, moist sponges on holders, and long ligatures no. 3-0 are needed.

5. The fibrous membrane of the chest wall is incised and peeled away from visceral pleura, using blunt and sharp dissection. Gentle handling is imperative to prevent damage to the lung as thickened outside layers are removed.

6. During its liberation, the lung is expanded by positive pressure via the closed anesthesia system. The lung assumes its normal relation to the chest, and the negative pressure in the pleural cavity is stabilized by an airtight wound closure.

7. Bronchiolar openings are repaired with sutures on taper point needles as necessary.

8. The drainage of serous material in the pleural space and removal of air are accomplished by insertion of two or three chest catheters.

9. The wound is closed in layers as described for lobectomy. Drainage apparatus is connected, and dressings are applied.

### Segmental resection of the lung

**DEFINITION.** Removal of individual bronchovascular segments of the pulmonary lobe, the ligation of segmental branches of the pulmonary vein and artery, and division of the segmental bronchus, followed by closure of the wound and establishment of closed drainage.

**CONSIDERATIONS.** Segmental resection of the lung is done to treat pulmonary tuberculosis or bronchiectasis in order to save the nondiseased portion or, in some cases, to remove a chronic, localized, pyogenic lung abscess, excise congenital cysts or blebs, or remove a benign tumor.

**SETUP AND PREPARATION OF THE PATIENT.** Basic thoracic setup. The patient is placed on the operating table in a right or left full lateral position, with the affected side uppermost.

**OPERATIVE PROCEDURE**

1. A posterolateral incision is made; the wound edges are protected; the rib or ribs are resected as indicated; moist packs are applied to wound edges, and a Finochietto retractor is inserted and opened (Fig. 14-31) as described for lobectomy.

2. The parietal pleura is incised with a scalpel and long curved scissors, and adhesions are divided. Moist sponges on holders are used.

3. The bronchus of the diseased segment is identified, using Rumel or fine right-angled cystic duct forceps. Suture nos. 0 and 2-0 is used to ligate the segmental pulmonary vein and segmental branches of the pulmonary artery.

4A. The bronchus is clamped with a Sarot or Lees bronchus clamp (Fig. 14-33), and the lung is inflated. The line of demarcation quickly confirms the proper

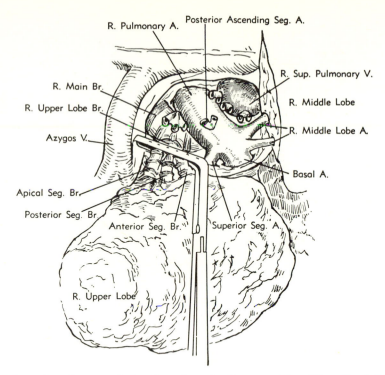

**Fig. 14-33.** Bronchus clamp applied to bronchus of right upper lobe. (From Reed, W. A., and Allbritten, F. F., Jr.: In Gibbon, J. H., Jr., editor: Surgery of the chest, Philadelphia, 1962, W. B. Saunders Co.)

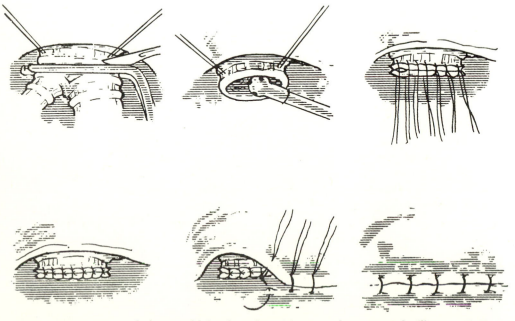

**Fig. 14-34.** Division and closure of lobar bronchus. (From Reed, W. A., and Allbritten, F. F., Jr.: In Gibbon, J. H., Jr., editor: Surgery of the chest, Philadelphia, 1962, W. B. Saunders Co.)

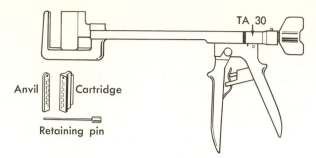

**Fig. 14-35.** Auto Suture instrument model TA 30 is used to close the bronchus or pulmonary artery and veins. A blue or green cartridge is used for bronchi, depending on the tissue thickness. A white cartridge is used for the vessels.

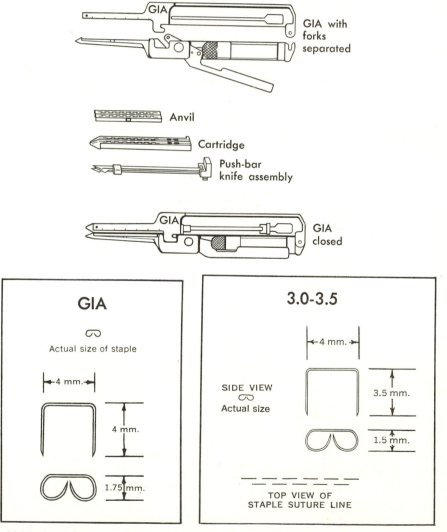

**Fig. 14-36.** Auto Suture instrument model GIA is used to create wedge resections or interlobar fissures. A gray cartridge is used.

placement of the clamp; the bronchus is divided, using a scalpel or angled scissors (Fig. 14-34).

4B. Or the thoracic Auto-Suture instrument (Figs. 14-35 and 14-36) may be used as described in the lobectomy operative procedure, step 8B.

5. The visceral pleura is completely incised around the diseased segment, beginning at the hilum and progressing toward the periphery. Narrow malleable retractors facilitate exposure. The intersegmental vessels are clamped with thoracic hemostats and ligated with nos. 2-0, 3-0, or 4-0 sutures.

6A. The segmental bronchus is transected, using a knife or scissors, and the wound closed with interrupted mattress sutures of silk no. 3-0 or 4-0 on swaged-on needles.

6B. See 8B, lobectomy procedure. Contaminated items are discarded.

7. The raw surfaces of the remaining segments are not closed. The parietal pleural flap may be placed over the bronchial stump with silk sutures no. 4-0 on swaged-on needles (Fig. 14-34).

8. The lung is reinflated; bleeding vessels are controlled. The operative field is prepared for closure, and the thoracic wall is examined for ragged bone edges.

9. A catheter is inserted in the pleural space through a stab wound for closed drainage (Fig. 14-21).

10. The thoracotomy incision is closed, as described for lobectomy. Dressings are applied and closed drainage established.

### Wedge resection

**DEFINITION.** Excision of a small, wedge-shaped section from the peripheral portion of a lobe.

**CONSIDERATIONS.** A wedge resection is preferred in certain cases of peripherally located benign primary tumors of the lung. No effort is made to isolate and ligate separately the pulmonary vessels or to secure the bronchi individually.

**SETUP AND PREPARATION OF THE PATIENT.** As described for segmental resection procedure.

**OPERATIVE PROCEDURE**

1. The incision is carried through skin, superficial fascia, deep fascia, and muscles. Wound edges are protected, as described for lobectomy (Fig. 14-31).

2. One rib, usually the sixth, is resected (Fig. 14-32).

3. A Finochietto rib retractor is placed, with ribs protected by moist gauze.

4. The lobe containing the lesion is grasped with a lung clamp, and the thoracic Auto-Suture instrument is applied to the parenchymal portion of the lung along the limits of the wedge that is being excised. The Auto-Sutures are released, and a scalpel is used to cut between the staples and the Auto-Suture instrument. The instrument is removed and reloaded. It is then reapplied to the other side of the lesion adjoining the already applied staples, and another line of staples is applied (Fig. 14-36).

5. The specimen is removed.

6. Hemostasis is maintained by ligatures and electrocautery.

7. The chest tube is inserted and connected to closed drainage bottles.

8. The thoracotomy incision is closed as described for lobectomy.

9. Dressings are applied. The chest tube is anchored to the chest wall with sutures and adhesive strips.

### Lobectomy

**DEFINITION.** Excision of one or more lobes of the lung—right upper, middle, or lower lobe or left upper or lower lobe.

**CONSIDERATIONS.** This operation is performed through a right or left posterolateral thoracotomy incision to treat a wide variety of pulmonary disease.

**SETUP AND PREPARATION OF THE PATIENT.** As previously described for basic thoracic surgery. The lateral position is used for a posterolateral thoracotomy incision.

**OPERATIVE PROCEDURE**

1. The skin incision is begun halfway between the medial edge of the scapula and the third or fourth thoracic spinous process and is continued downward medially below the angle of the scapula and

anteriorly beyond the end of the fifth, sixth, or seventh ribs, depending on the location of the lesion (Fig. 14-4). Hemostasis is obtained by clamping, ligatures, and electrocautery.

2. The subcutaneous tissue is divided in line with the skin incision, and skin towels are applied with small towel clamps. As the latissimus dorsi, trapezius, and rhomboid muscles are divided with a scalpel or electrocautery (Fig. 14-31), clamps are applied in pairs by the first assistant. Fixation sutures of silk no. 2-0 are inserted and tied, or electrocautery is used.

3. The scapula is retracted, and the rib is selected for resection.

4. The periosteum over the center of the rib is divided longitudinally with a scalpel, and exposure is completed, using elevators and rib raspatories (Fig. 14-32).

5A. Resection is accomplished, using rib shears to cut each end. Rough edges may be trimmed with a broad, blunt, box-type rongeur. A Finochietto-type retractor is placed and opened. If exposure is not adequate, adjustments may be necessary (wedge section of the rib or complete resection of a second rib).

5B. The surgeon may prefer to enter the chest through the intercostal space rather than resect the rib (Fig. 14-31).

6. The pleura is entered, and adhesions are freed. Suction is available as exploration is carried out and location of the pathological area is determined.

7. The visceral pleura is incised and dissected free from the hilum of the involved lobe. The branches of the pulmonary artery and vein of the involved lobe are isolated, clamped, ligated, and divided. Fine right-angled and vascular forceps are used. Ligatures may be silk no. 0, 2-0, or 3-0. The lung is deflated.

8A. The bronchus is doubly clamped with selected bronchus clamps and the lung inflated to identify the line of demarcation (Fig. 14-34). Division of the bronchus is completed with a scalpel or heavy-angled scissors. Bronchial secretions are aspirated. Closure of the bronchus is

completed, using mattress sutures of silk no. 3-0 or 4-0 with swaged-on needles (Fig. 14-35). Contaminated items are discarded.

8B. Or the thoracic Auto-Suture (Figs. 14-35 and 14-36) loaded with bronchus staples may be applied to the bronchus. The Auto-Suture is released, and a scalpel is used to complete the division of the bronchus. The jaws of the Auto-Suture device are then loosened after transection.

9. Incomplete fissures are divided between hemostats, using fine Metzenbaum scissors. Raw edges are closed with a continuous intestinal type suture of fine chromic gut.

10. The specimen is removed, and the bronchus suture line is covered with a pleural flap (Fig. 14-34).

11. A large pleural drainage catheter (28 to 30 Fr.) is brought out through the eighth or ninth interspace near the anterior axillary line. If indicated, an upper tube is also inserted to evacuate leaking air. Tubes are connected to separate closed drainage set (Fig. 14-21).

12. Interrupted sutures of chromic no. 0 or 1 are used to reapproximate the ribs. A Bailey rib contractor (Fig. 14-23) is inserted, and sutures are tied in place. The periosteum may be closed with a continuous chromic gut no. 0 suture (Fig. 14-32).

13. The muscles and superficial fascia are closed in layers with chromic gut no. 0, and the subcutaneous tissue is closed with chromic gut no. 2-0. Skin sutures may be interrupted or continuous silk or nylon no. 4-0.

14. Dressings are applied. Drains are anchored to the chest wall with sutures and adhesive strips.

### Pneumonectomy

**DEFINITION.** Removal of the entire lung.

**CONSIDERATIONS.** This procedure is done to treat malignant neoplasms of the lung or an extensive unilateral bronchiectasis involving the greater part of one lung, drain an extensive chronic pulmonary abscess involving portions of both or all lobes, re-

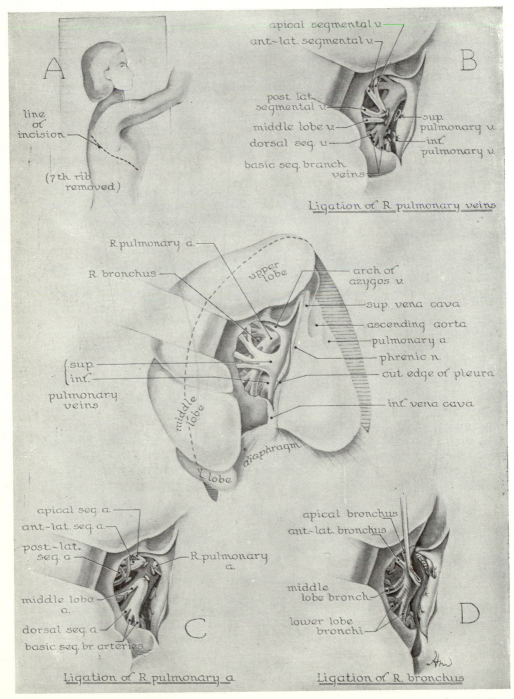

**Fig. 14-37.** Hilar anatomy and technique of right pneumonectomy. (From Moseley, H. F., editor: Textbook of surgery, ed. 3, St. Louis, 1959, The C. V. Mosby Co.)

move selected benign tumors, or treat extensive tuberculosis, mainstem endobronchial tuberculosis, or any extensive unilateral lesion (Fig. 14-37).

**SETUP AND PREPARATION OF THE PATIENT.** The basic thoracic setup is used, as described previously. A posterolateral approach is used, and the patient is placed on the operating table in a lateral position (Chapter 7). The proposed operative site is cleansed (Chapter 4). The patient is draped (Chapter 5). Isolation technique is followed to control infection.

**OPERATIVE PROCEDURE**

**OPENING OF THE CHEST CAVITY.** The chest wall is opened. The pleura is incised, the lung immobilized, and the hilum exposed. The mediastinal pleura is opened.

**RESECTION OF THE LEFT LUNG**

1. The pulmonary artery is freed from the aorta, the pulmonary vein, and a portion of the pericardial sac; then the artery is doubly clamped, ligated, and divided.

2. The pulmonary veins within the pleural cavity are ligated and divided.

3A. The bronchus is doubly clamped, ligated, and divided near the tracheal bifurcation. This step may be done before ligation of the pulmonary artery if a posterolateral approach has been used.

3B. Same as 8B under lobectomy procedure.

4. The bronchial stump is closed with several layers of mattress sutures and covered with mediastinal pleura, as for lobectomy.

5. The mediastinal pleura is closed with interrupted silk sutures no. 2-0 or 3-0, swaged to ¼-circle taper point needles; then the chest wall is closed in layers.

**RESECTION OF THE RIGHT LUNG**

1. The superior vena cava and the superior pulmonary vein are identified.

2. The pulmonary veins and artery are doubly clamped, ligated, and divided (Fig. 14-37).

3A. The bronchus is clamped, ligated, and divided near the tracheal bifurcation; then the bronchial stump is sutured with several layers of silk mattress sutures swaged to curved, taper point needles.

3B. Same as 8B under lobectomy procedure.

4. The azygos vein is ligated with silk no. 2-0; then it is divided between the Mayo-Pean clamp.

5. The chest wall is closed, with or without drainage, according to the surgeon's preference. Dressings are applied.

## Operations on the mediastinum
### Excision of tumors in upper anterior mediastinum

**DEFINITION.** The cysts most frequently found in the mediastinum are the "clear water" cysts, the dermoid, and the bronchogenic. The solid tumors of the mediastinum may be benign or malignant.

**SETUP AND PREPARATION OF THE PATIENT.** A thyroidectomy setup (Chapter 18), plus the basic thoracic setup and the sternal cutting instruments, is used.

The patient is prepared on the operating table as described for thyroidectomy (Chapter 18) and also as described for median sternotomy (Fig. 14-28).

**OPERATIVE PROCEDURE**

1. Median sternotomy is carried out.

2. The tumor is dissected free.

3. Bleeding is controlled with ligatures and electrocautery.

4. Chest catheter may or may not be inserted, depending on the entry into the pleural space and the surgeon's preference.

5. The sternum is then reapproximated and closed with no. 22-gauge wire.

6. The subcutaneous tissue is closed with chromic gut sutures no. 3-0 and the skin with interrupted or running silk or nylon suture no. 4-0.

7. If a chest catheter is used, it is anchored to the chest wall with sutures and adhesive tape. Dressings are applied.

### Thymectomy

**DEFINITION.** Removal of the thymus gland.

**CONSIDERATIONS.** An attempt to alleviate the severity of symptoms in a patient with myasthenia gravis is a frequent indication for the removal of the thymus gland, as well as thymic tumors.

SETUP AND PREPARATION OF THE PATIENT. Basic thoracic setup and sternum cutting instruments.

OPERATIVE PROCEDURE. Median sternotomy gives the best exposure for excision of the thymus gland. Dissection of the gland is carried out, and blood vessels are clamped and ligated. If either pleural space has been inadvertently opened during dissection, one need only have the anesthetist maintain full expansion of the lung during the closure of the incision with chromic gut to avoid any subsequent respiratory embarrassment. Refer to the procedure for excision of anterior mediastinal tumors for closure technique.

## Operations on the posterior mediastinum

DEFINITION. Removal of segments of rib or ribs, removal of a tumor, drainage of an abscess, or exposure of the esophagus through an incision made in the mediastinum.

SETUP AND PREPARATION OF THE PATIENT. Major thoracic setup, as described previously. The lateral position and a posterolateral incision are used.

OPERATIVE PROCEDURE

1. The thoracic wall is opened as for posterolateral thoracoplasty. The pleura is freed from the posterior mediastinum, and retractors are placed.

2. The great blood vessels and intercostal arteries are identified and isolated. Bleeding vessels are ligated.

3. If the pleura is opened inadvertently, it is closed before an abscess is drained. The abscess, if present, is aspirated and drained. Contaminated instruments are discarded. If a tumor is present, it is resected, and bleeding is controlled.

4. The intercostal muscles, rib periosteum, overlying muscles, fascia, and skin are closed in layers, as for thoracoplasty. Dressings are applied.

## REFERENCES

1. Artusio, J. F., Jr., and Mazzia, V. D. B.: Practical anesthesiology, St. Louis, 1962, The C. V. Mosby Co.
2. Banyai, A. L.: Pneumoperitoneum treatment, St. Louis, 1946, The C. V. Mosby Co.
3. Beecher, H. K.: Chest surgery, Springfield, Ill., 1952, Charles C Thomas, Publisher.
4. Benedict, E. B., and Nardi, G. L.: The esophagus; medical and surgical management, Boston, 1958, Little, Brown & Co.
5. Davis, L., editor: Christopher's textbook of surgery, ed. 8, Philadelphia, 1964, W. B. Saunders Co.
6. DeWeese, D. D., and Saunders, W. H.: Textbook of otolaryngology, ed. 3, St. Louis, 1968, The C. V. Mosby Co.
7. Gibbon, J. H., Jr., editor: Surgery of the chest, Philadelphia, 1962, W. B. Saunders Co.
8. Grant, A. R., and Melick, D. W.: Bone chip plastic repair of congenital chest deformities, Arch. Surg. 86:940, 1963.
9. Hardy, J. D., et al.: Lung homotransplantation in man, J.A.M.A. 186:1065, 1963.
10. Hinshaw, H. C., and Garland, L. H.: Diseases of the chest, Philadelphia, 1963, W. B. Saunders Co.
11. Jackson, C., and Jackson, C. L.: Bronchoesophagology, Philadelphia, 1950, W. B. Saunders Co.
12. Jackson, C., and Jackson, C. L., et al.: Diseases of the nose, throat and ear, ed. 2, Philadelphia, 1959, W. B. Saunders Co.
13. Johnson, J., and Kirby, C. K.: Surgery of the chest, ed. 3, Chicago, 1964, Year Book Medical Publishers, Inc.
14. King, B. G., and Showers, M. J.: Human anatomy and physiology, ed. 5, Philadelphia, 1963, W. B. Saunders Co.
15. Laforet, E. G., and Boyd, T. F.: Balanced drainage of the pneumonectomy space, Surg. Gynecol. Obstet. 118:1051, 1964.
16. Lahey Clinic: Surgical practice of the Clinic, Philadelphia, 1962, W. B. Saunders Co.
17. Lindskog, C. E., Liebow, A. A., and Glenn, W. W.: Thoracic and cardiovascular surgery with related pathology, New York, 1962, Appleton-Century-Crofts.
18. Morris, J. D.: Surgical correction of pectus excavatum, Surg. Clin. North Am. 41:1271, 1961.
19. Nardi, G. L., and Zuidema, G. D., editors: Surgery, Boston, 1961, Little, Brown & Co.
20. Palmer, E. D., and Boyce, H. W.: Manual of gastrointestinal endoscopy, Baltimore, 1964, The Williams & Wilkins Co.
21. Selkurt, E. E., editor: Physiology, Boston, 1962, Little, Brown & Co.
22. Spain, D. M., editor: Diagnosis and treatment of tumors of the chest, New York, 1960, Grune & Stratton, Inc.
23. Thorek, P.: Anatomy in surgery, ed. 2, Philadelphia, 1962, J. B. Lippincott Co.
24. Warren, R.: Surgery, Philadelphia, 1963, W. B. Saunders Co.

# CHAPTER 15

# Cardiothoracic operations

VIRGINIA HIGGINS

Refinements in diagnostic techniques, advances in anesthesia and monitoring methods, selective uses of hypothermia, and improved cardiopulmonary bypass facilities have given the surgeon the opportunity to alter the former closed palliative surgical procedures to the more direct open corrective ones.

Many factors are involved in the selection of the procedure, including the experience and skill of the operating team, patterns of nursing care, and availability of ancillary facilities and equipment. However, the most important single factor is the patient's physiological response to the existing pathological condition, together with the possible predictable alteration in this response by surgical intervention.

## ANATOMICAL AND PHYSIOLOGICAL CONSIDERATIONS

The standard textbooks of anatomy and physiology should be consulted for detailed description and function of the circulatory structures. Certain facts are presented here as they relate to surgical procedures and operating room nursing.

The heart, a hollow muscular organ that acts as a power pump for the circulatory system, is enclosed in the pericardial sac forming the middle subdivision of the lower part of the mediastinum (Fig. 15-1). The heart lies in the region between the lungs, anterior to the esophagus and to the descending portion of the aorta. The large blood vessels enter and leave the heart at its base. Two thirds of the heart lies to the left of the midline, and the remaining third lies to the right. The right chambers of the heart are in an anterior position.

The heart wall is composed of three layers: the epicardium, consisting of the inner layer of the pericardium; the muscular layer, or myocardium, which is the important functional layer; and the endocardium, which is the inner lining.

The heart is divided into right and left halves. Within a closed system, each half contains an upper and a lower communicating chamber. The upper chambers are called the *atria,* whereas the lower chambers are called the *ventricles.* The atria receive the blood. The right atrium has three orifices through which blood enters from the superior and inferior venae cavae and from the coronary sinus. The left atrium has four orifices through which the blood enters from the four pulmonary veins, two from each lung. The ventricles discharge the blood into the arteries. The left ventricle sends the blood through the aorta and its numerous branches—to the head, upper extremities, abdominal organs, and lower extremities. This system is termed the systemic, general, or greater circulatory system. The right ventricle discharges the venous blood into the lungs by means of the pulmonary artery, which divides into a right and left pulmonary artery. These subdivide and eventually form the capillaries in the lungs. This system is called the lesser, or pulmonary, circulatory system (Fig. 15-2).

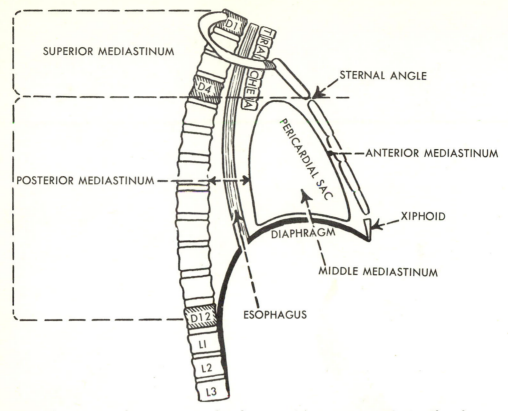

**Fig. 15-1.** Diagram showing regions of mediastinum. (From Brantigan, O. C.: Clinical anatomy, New York, 1963, Blakiston Division, McGraw-Hill Book Co.)

In both the systemic and pulmonary systems, metabolic exchange occurs only in the capillary beds. Oxygen is given off into the tissues, and carbon dioxide is taken in by the red blood cells. The capillaries empty into the veins, which bring the blood back to the right atrium. The membranous valves of the heart open and close with the cyclic fluctuations in the blood pressure within the heart chambers. Each of the four valves allows blood to flow in one direction.

The heart chambers have four valves, two atrioventricular valves, and two semilunar valves. The two atrioventricular or cuspid valves guard the openings between the atrium and ventricle of each side of the heart. The right atrioventricular valve, commonly called the *tricuspid valve,* is composed of three leaflets of endocardium,

which are attached to the right ventricle by cordlike structures, called the *chordae tendineae* (Fig. 15-2). The left atrioventricular valve, usually known as the mitral valve, has only two endocardial leaflets. Its fine chordae tendineae prevent the valve from being turned back into the atrium during the discharge phase of the heart cycle or ventricular systole. These endocardial leaflets allow the blood to flow from the atria into the ventricles and prevent the blood from flowing back into the atria. Under normal conditions, the ventricular contraction closes the valves by forcing the blood against them, thus permitting the blood to flow into the pulmonary artery and aorta. The semilunar valves are situated at the discharge openings of the left and right ventricles. These valves permit the blood to flow

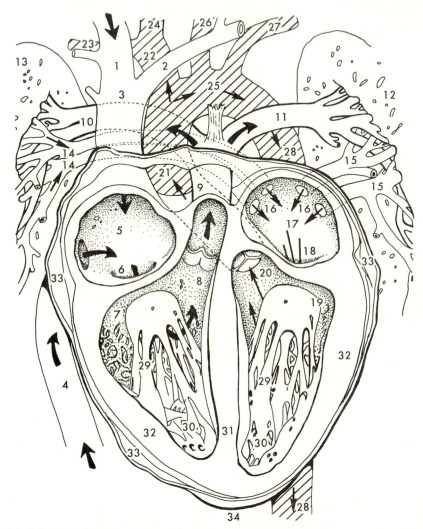

**Fig. 15-2.** Schematic diagram of heart showing related structures and direction of blood flow. **1**, Right brachiocephalic vein; **2**, left brachiocephalic vein; **3**, superior vena cava; **4**, inferior vena cava; **5**, right atrium; **6**, tricuspid valve; **7**, right ventricle; **8**, pulmonary valve; **9**, pulmonary artery; **10**, right pulmonary artery; **11**, left pulmonary artery; **12**, left lung; **13**, right lung; **14**, right pulmonary vein; **15**, left pulmonary vein; **16**, pulmonary vein orifices; **17**, left atrium; **18**, mitral valve; **19**, left ventricle; **20**, aortic valve; **21**, aorta; **22**, brachiocephalic artery; **23**, right subclavian artery; **24**, right common carotid artery; **25**, aortic arch; **26**, left common carotid artery; **27**, left subclavian artery; **28**, descending aorta; **29**, chordae tendineae; **30**, papillary muscle; **31**, interventricular septum; **32**, myocardium; **33**, pericardium; **34**, apex. (Redrawn by Maureen Jones, New York, N. Y.; from CSI Technical data sheet, Becton, Dickinson & Co., Rutherford, N. J.)

forward, and they act in the same manner as the cuspid valves in that they prevent the blood from flowing back into the ventricles from the pulmonary artery and the aorta.

When disease deforms the valves, the leaflets become fibrous and stiff and their margins swollen, uneven, and adherent to one another. Such abnormalities impair their mechanical function and alter the work load of the heart. When a valve loses its ability to close tightly, that is, when there is a valvular insufficiency, the blood flows back into the part of the heart from which it came, resulting in a condition known as regurgitation. In rheumatic heart disease, the mitral valve frequently becomes narrowed, obstructing the passage of blood from the atrium to the left ventricle and causing enlargement of the left atrium. This condition is called *mitral stenosis*. The pulmonary valve is more often affected by congenital stenosis.

The myocardium of the heart receives its blood supply from two branches arising from the aorta, the left and right coronary arteries. Their function is to carry blood to the cardiac muscle cells. Acute destruction of the blood supply may result in a loss of myocardial contractility and death.

The middle cervical nerve, composed of sympathetic fibers, and the vagus nerve, composed of parasympathetic fibers, carry nerve impulses to the heart from the medulla oblongata (Chapter 11). The sympathetic nerves promote an increase in the force and rate of the heartbeat, and the parasympathetics cause a decrease in the rate.

Certain areas of the heart muscle tissue are modified to form a conducting system. This system comprises the sinoatrial (S-A) node, which is located at the junction of the superior vena cava and the right atrium, and the atrioventricular (A-V) node with extending fibers (bundle of His), which are located medial to the entrance of the coronary sinus into the right atrium (Fig. 15-3). The extending fibers (Purkinje fibers) proceed down the posterior and inferior portion of the membranous interventricular septum to form right and left branches. The strands of these branches end in the papillary muscles and muscle wall of the right ventricle. The excitation wave passes from the sinoatrial node to

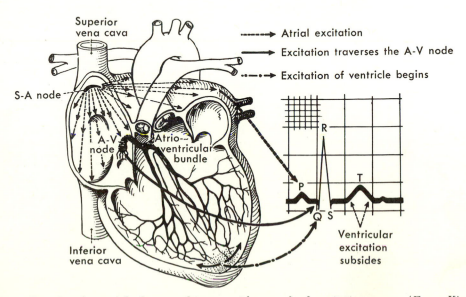

Fig. 15-3. Correlation of electrocardiogram with spread of excitation wave. (From King, B. G., and Showers, M. J.: Human anatomy and physiology, ed. 5, Philadelphia, 1963, W. B. Saunders Co.)

the atrioventricular node throughout the conducting system, which stimulates the ventricles to contract (Fig. 15-3).

## GENERAL NURSING CONSIDERATIONS FOR CARDIOTHORACIC SURGERY

All the specialized nursing considerations that are indicated for thoracic operations also apply to cardiothoracic operations (Chapter 14).

Additional general and specific information that is useful in implementing the nursing care plan for patients undergoing cardiothoracic surgery is categorized as follows.

PREINDUCTION AND ANESTHESIA. The nurse should be aware of three important considerations of the anesthesiologist in selecting the anesthetic agent for cardiac patients: (1) explosive hazards that are involved with the multiplicity of electrical equipment, (2) the level of anesthesia desired (Chapter 5), and (3) the choice of agents to minimize decrease in cardiac function.

Preoperatively, sedation is usually minimal and may be completely omitted. Operatively, a state of analgesia may be adequate. In any event, the safest possible level of anesthesia that is compatible with operating conditions is selected.

Nursing care involves duties in the preinduction preparation of an acutely alert and apprehensive patient who is subjected to the physical discomforts of positioning on the hypothermia mattress, the application of electrocardiogram (ECG) lead wires, the insertion of infusion and cutdown needles, and the skin preparation of a very large surface area. The nursing responsibilities for directing each activity toward optimum patient care are accomplished by maintaining a quiet atmosphere, reassuring the patient to relieve his emotional distress, safeguarding the dignity of the individual by preventing undue physical exposure, and giving expert technical assistance to the physicians.

DRUGS COMMONLY USED DURING SURGERY. *Heparin sodium* is used for its depressive action on the clotting mechanism of the blood. Dosage is calculated according to the weight of the patient. For open heart operations, the patient is heparinized prior to perfusion, and the fluid used to prime the pump-oxygenator is also heparinized. Heparin is added to an intravenous saline solution for irrigation of the lumen of blood vessels during anastomosis.

*Protamine sulfate* is used to neutralize the action of heparin, and dosage is calculated according to the amount of heparin previously given.

*Procaine amide (Pronestyl)* or *1% lidocaine (Xylocaine)* is used for rhythmic disorders arising in the ventricle. It abolishes ventricular premature contractions and ventricular tachycardia and may prevent the development of ventricular fibrillation.

*Epinephrine (Adrenalin)* is used as a short-acting cardiac stimulant. A dilute solution of epinephrine 1:10,000 (1 to 2 ml.) may be given in cardiac standstill; in excess, however, it may cause ventricular fibrillation.

*Calcium chloride* is used to increase the amplitude of contraction in the weakly beating heart. It increases the tone of the myocardium and opposes the effect of potassium. An excess may cause arrest; however, calcium is indispensable for coagulation of blood and for rhythmic heart activity.

*Mannitol* may be used to maintain the level of renal plasma flow during perfusion.

*Isoproterenol (Isuprel)* and *levarterenol bitartrate (Levophed)* are used to support the myocardium following total bypass.

SPECIFIC DIAGNOSTIC METHODS. Angiocardiography provides significant information in regard to the anatomical structure of the heart, and selective angiocardiography via cardiac catheterization permits preoperative determination of the abnormal physical function of the heart. This information serves as a definitive guide in selecting the operation of choice, as well

as providing a comparative basis for correction during the operative procedure.

CARDIAC CATHETERIZATION

*Definition.* A radiopaque plastic catheter is inserted into the right or left heart via a percutaneous puncture or a cut down for pressure determinations in the chambers and large vessels, determinations of oxygen saturation, dye dilution analysis, and injection of contrast media to isolate certain anatomical structural defects.

*General considerations.* This procedure is usually confined to some section of the radiology department and may or may not directly involve the operating room nursing staff.

Nursing techniques, however, include supervision of the preparation of instruments, solutions, and supplies for the sterile procedure and the maintenance of standby emergency equipment, that is, pacemaker, defibrillator, emergency drugs, and resuscitation apparatus. Nursing responsibilities consist of providing both the facilities for physical comfort and the thoughtful reassurance of the patient throughout the procedure, as well as the preparedness for capable assistance in an emergency situation.

During the fluoroscopy, the nurse may assist with observations of the patient's vital signs.

Local anesthesia is used at the site of the puncture wound or cutdown. Electrocardiographic monitoring is continued throughout the procedure.

*Procedure.* The physiological reference point is determined for pressure readings (Fig. 15-4), the skin is prepared, and sterile drapes are applied. Local infiltration is completed, and the catheter is introduced into the brachial artery and vein through puncture wounds or a cutdown. As the catheter is advanced, perfusion with heparinized saline solution prevents blood from clotting in the lumen. Fluoroscopy is used to follow the progress of the catheter as any or all tests are completed. They include the following:

1. Outline of the course of the catheter across or through a normal or abnormal pathway, such as an atrial septal defect or stenosis of a valve.

2. Injection of dye to plot an indicator dye-dilution curve. The amount of dye recovered within a specific length of time is used in determining the amount of shunted blood and cardiac output.

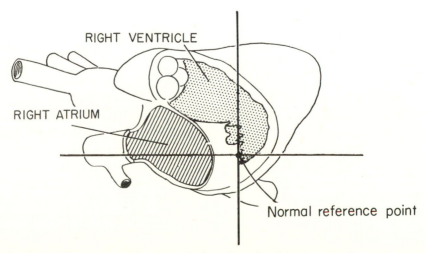

**Fig. 15-4.** Location at tricuspid valve of physiological reference point for venous pressure measurements. (Modified from Guyton and Greganti, 1956; from Guyton, A. C.: Circulatory physiology: cardiac output and its regulation, Philadelphia, 1963, W. B. Saunders Co.)

3. Intracardiac pressure measurements, variations of which from the normal may indicate valvular stenosis (Fig. 15-5).

4. Oxygen analysis, which aids in determining shunts.

5. Selective angiocardiography, rapid serial x-ray films, or cine movies of a specific area with radiopaque material, which is useful in isolating structural and functional defects.

The left heart may be approached retrograde through the aortic valve via a peripheral artery or transseptally through from the right atrium.

HYPOTHERMIA. Hypothermia may be generally defined as the deliberate reduction of body temperature for therapeutic purposes. A moderate degree of hypothermia, 37° to 28° C., as defined by Swan, will permit reduction of metabolism by 50%.

From 28° to 20° C., there is a further reduction of approximately 25%. With the lower temperature, however, ventricular fibrillation remains a constant hazard, and specific measures for treatment must be readily available.

Hypothermia is used in surgery to lengthen the period of circulatory interruption with little danger of neurological damage, thus permitting the surgeon sufficient time to repair certain cardiac lesions under direct vision. Total body hypothermia may be achieved by surface cooling, application of a cooling blanket, or ice water immersion. The cooling and rewarming process requires at least two thirds of the total anesthesia time for each patient.

Nursing activities involve maintaining the patency of intravenous infusion equip-

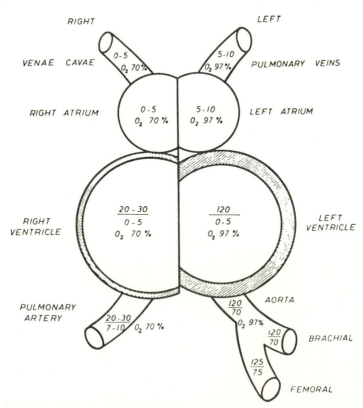

**Fig. 15-5.** Cardiac catheterization data. Schematic representation of pressures and oxygen saturation in great vessels and cardiac chambers. (From Blades, B., editor: Surgical diseases of the chest, ed. 2, St. Louis, 1966, The C. V. Mosby Co.)

ment, correctly positioning leads for accurate monitoring, preventing circulatory stasis over pressure areas, protecting fingers and toes against frostbite, and carrying out emergency procedures if the patient undergoes cardiac arrest or ventricular fibrillation.

When hypothermia is used in combination with extracorporeal circulation, it permits a reduction in rate of blood flow and provides a greater margin of safety for perfusion of other internal organs. For this method, a heat exchanger that is con-

nected within the pump-oxygenator line and supplemented by shunting devices permits total or partial body hypothermia or single organ (selective) perfusion by rapidly cooling or warming the blood. With this method, a more profound or deeper hypothermia, 10° to 8° C., may be achieved. Hypothermal cardioplegia occurs at this temperature, and circulatory arrest may be continued for periods of 30 minutes at a time to permit repair of complicated intracardiac defects.

During the rewarming process, the heart-

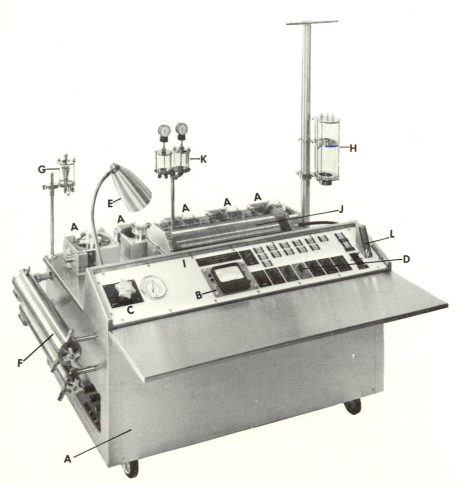

**Fig. 15-6.** Sarns console pump-oxygenator with rotating disks. **A,** Console with five pumping heads; **B,** telethermometer; **C,** water-mixing valve and thermometer; **D,** oxygenator drive unit; **E,** auxiliary light; **F,** heat exchanger; **G,** arterial bubble trap; **H,** venous collection reservoir and coronary sinus return chamber; **I,** control panel; **J,** rotating disk oxygenator; **K,** coronary perfusion pressure monitor; **L,** oxygen flowmeter. (Courtesy Sarns, Inc., Ann Arbor, Mich.)

beat may resume spontaneously when the temperature reaches 16° to 18° C. Perfusion rewarming is usually continued until the esophageal temperature has reached 33° C.

Defibrillation equipment should always be available during the entire procedure.

**EXTRACORPOREAL CIRCULATION.** Reliable equipment and established methods now exist that make the temporary substitution of a pump-oxygenator for the heart and lungs a safe clinical procedure. When this equipment is used in combination with shunting devices, heat exchangers, and varying degrees of hypothermia, the surgeon has sufficient time to complete the more complicated intracardiac repair under direct vision in a relatively dry, motionless field.

**EQUIPMENT.** Many types of pump-oxygenators are available. Generally, one of the following three methods of oxygenation is used (Figs. 15-6 and 15-7):

1. *Film method,* in which the blood is separated in a thin film over stationary plastic sheets or a series of thin, rotating, steel disks in direct contact with an oxygen atmosphere
2. *Bubble method,* in which the microscopic bubbles of oxygen are injected directly into the cylinder of blood
3. *Membrane method,* in which the oxygen is diffused through a gas-permeable plastic membrane that contains the blood

The roller pump has important basic features and is frequently used. It propels the blood through flexible plastic tubing

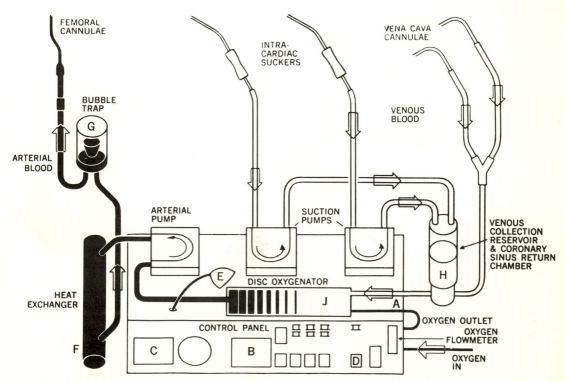

**Fig. 15-7.** Diagram of pump circuit with disk oxygenator, including three pumping heads. **A,** Pump console; **B,** telethermometer with switch; **C,** water-mixing valve and thermometer; **D,** oxygenator drive unit; **E,** auxiliary light; **F,** heat exchanger; **G,** arterial bubble trap; **H,** venous collection reservoir and coronary sinus return chamber; **J,** adult oxygenator. (Courtesy Sarns, Inc., Ann Arbor, Mich.)

by means of moving external compression. It provides for accuracy in rapid adjustment of the blood flow, with nontraumatic effect on the circulating blood components.

TECHNIQUE. To place a patient on total heart-lung bypass, the venous blood is circulated to the oxygenator by means of cannulae placed in the inferior and superior venae cavae. The catheters are inserted through small incisions in the right atrium. The oxygenated blood is returned from the machine to the arterial circulation through the arterial cannula. The ascending aorta is usually selected, although the common femoral artery was popular in the past.

The extracorporeal circulation consists of the flow of venous blood from the caval catheters by gravitation or by pumping through large-bore, flexible plastic tubing into the oxygenator reservoir. Here the process of oxygenation of the blood takes place, and carbon dioxide is released. The freshly oxygenated blood from the reservoir is pumped through the tubing into the arterial cannula to complete the return to the patient. A heat exchanger incorporated in the arterial return line facilitates accurate temperature control of the blood. Thus the heart and lungs are temporarily replaced by the artificial heart-lung machine or pump-oxygenator (Figs. 15-6, 15-7, 15-22, and 15-23).

To provide selective cooling and rewarming of individual organs or specific areas of the body, a portion of the oxygenated blood may be shunted through a second heat exchanger for direct perfusion to the heart—for example, to produce hypothermal cardioplegia.

The total body surface area serves as a guide to calculate the perfusion flow rate. Crystalloid solutions are frequently used to prime the pump-oxygenator. This is called the *hemodilution technique* and 5% dextrose alone or in a balanced salt solution is used.

MONITORING MEASURES. During modern surgery, a wide variety of electrical monitoring devices and specific laboratory techniques are utilized as adjuncts to direct observation in determining and maintaining safe physiological homeostasis of the patient.

During open heart surgery, the following physiological variables are monitored: the electrocardiogram, the arterial blood pressure, the central venous pressure, the urine output, body temperature (rectal or esophageal), blood temperature, blood flow, partial pressures of oxygen and carbon dioxide, pH, hematocrit, and a variety of electrolyte studies.

## OPEN HEART TEAM

The professional nurses, as members of the open heart team, are responsible for carrying out many varied and complicated procedures. These may include preparation and management of the pump-oxygenator. The nursing team members should have broad experience in general operating room nursing, possess technical knowledge of cardiac surgery, be capable of self-direction, and have a genuine interest in learning. Application of interpersonal relationship skills is important to maintain lines of communication and coordinate team activities. The nurses must be alert to the constant need for continual evaluation of an ever-changing situation and capable of appropriate action if the patient is to have safe, effective care (see Chapters 2 and 5).

## OPEN HEART FACILITIES

PHYSICAL FACILITIES. The unit must be of sufficient size to accept bulky, highly specialized equipment without interfering with the maintenance of aseptic technique (Chapter 1). For open heart surgery, the facilities must include multiple electrical outlets, auxiliary lighting, a water supply for the pump-oxygenator, multiple suction apparatus, equipment for handling various types of gas, proper air conditioning, sufficient space for storing equipment and sterile and unsterile supplies, and areas for preparing, cleaning, and sterilizing special equipment.

SPECIAL INSTRUMENTS. Vascular clamps,

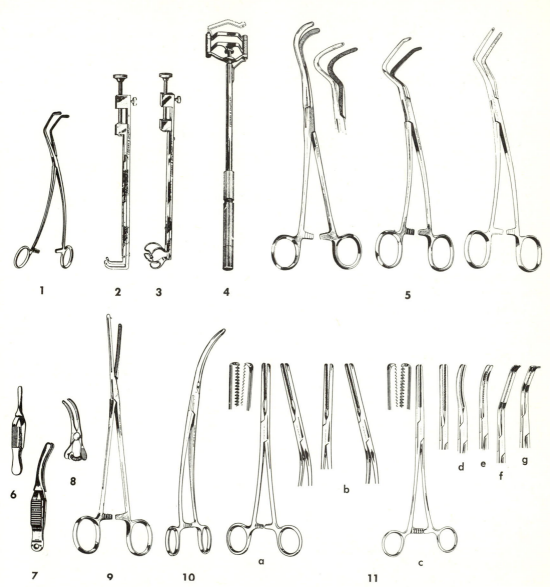

**Fig. 15-8.** Cardiothoracic instruments. **1,** Satinsky vena cava clamp; **2,** Blalock pulmonary artery clamp; **3,** Johns Hopkins modified Potts clamp; **4,** Alfred M. Large vena cava clamp; **5,** Harken auricle clamps, various sizes; **6 to 8,** bulldog clamps, straight, curved, and adjustable spring-type; **9,** Gross coarctation occlusion clamp; **10,** Crafoord coarctation clamp; **11,** vascular clamps: **a,** patent ductus, straight and curved; **b,** coarctation, straight and curved; **c,** anastomosis, straight; **d,** spoon; **e,** curved; **f,** aortic; **g,** appendage. (Courtesy Codman & Shurtleff, Inc., Randolph, Mass.)

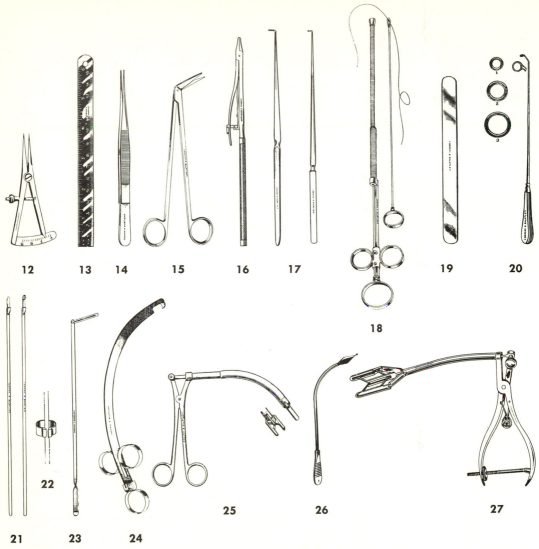

Fig. 15-9. Cardiothoracic instruments—cont'd. 12, Caliper; 13, ruler; 14, Potts thumb forceps, fine; 15, Potts 60-degree angle scissors; 16, Potts-Smith needle holder; 17, Weary nerve hooks, small and medium; 18, Rumel tourniquet; 19, silver-plated copper malleable retractor; 20, Mayo vein strippers; 21, Brock valvulotomes, unguarded and guarded; 22, Brock valvulotome ring; 23, Harken valvulotome; 24, Harken valvulotome, ring handles; 25, Brock dilator; 26, Bailey modification of Brock pulmonary valve knife; 27, Gerbode mitral valvulotome for retrograde insertion. (Courtesy Codman & Shurtleff, Inc., Randolph, Mass.)

which are designed to partially or completely occlude blood flow, must be maintained in good condition if they are to prevent fracture of the delicate intima of the blood vessel and still retain their specific holding qualities. There are many variations in construction of vascular instruments. The jaws may consist of single or double rows of fine, sharp, or blunt teeth or special cross-hatching or longitudinal serrations. All clamps are designed to hold the vessel securely without trauma.

Some basic cardiothoracic instruments and a few prostheses are shown in Figs. 15-8 to 15-19.

PROSTHETIC MATERIALS. Cardiac patches,
*Text continued on p. 619.*

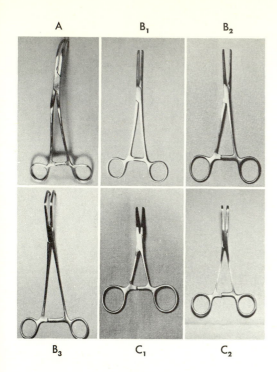

**Fig. 15-10.** Cardiothoracic instruments. **A**, Bahnson aortic clamp; **B**, Cooley clamps: **B₁**, large straight, **B₂**, small straight, **B₃**, curved; **C**, Hendrin infant clamps: **C₁**, straight, **C₂**, curved.

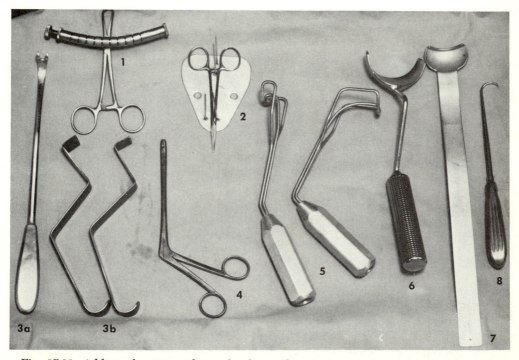

**Fig. 15-11.** Additional aortic and mitral valve replacement instruments. Top row: **1**, MacIntosh suture holder; **2**, bender suture holder. Bottom row: **3a**, Ablaza aortic retractor; **3b**, Cooley aortic retractor; **4**, Bailey aortic valve rongeur; **5**, Cooley atrial retractors; **6**, atrial retractor; **7**, Favaloro atrial retractor; **8**, hook.

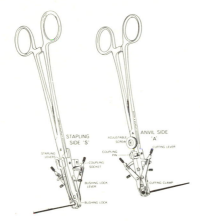

Fig. 15-12. American vascular stapler for blood vessel anastomosis. Furnished with disposable staple bushings. (Courtesy Codman & Shurtleff, Inc., Randolph, Mass.)

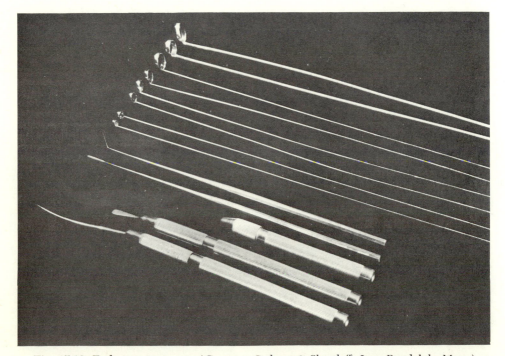

Fig. 15-13. Endarterectomy set. (Courtesy Codman & Shurtleff, Inc., Randolph, Mass.)

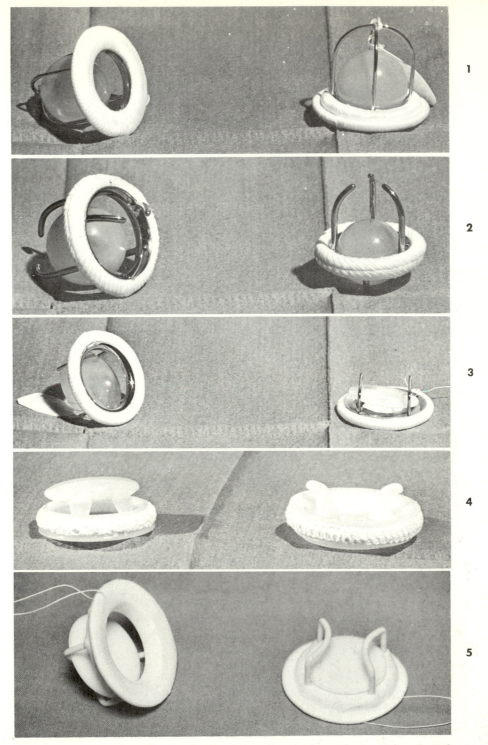

**Fig. 15-14.** Heart valve prostheses. **1,** Starr-Edwards mitral prosthesis (Edwards Laboratories, Inc., Santa Ana, Calif.); **2,** Smeloff-Cutter mitral valve prosthesis (Cutter Laboratories, Berkeley, Calif.); **3,** Kay-Shiley mitral valve prosthesis (Shiley Laboratories, Santa Ana, Calif.); **4,** Alvarez mitral valve prosthesis (Pemco Co., Cleveland, Ohio); **5,** Beall mitral valve prosthesis (Surgitool Laboratories, Division of Travenol Laboratories, Inc., Pittsburgh, Pa.).

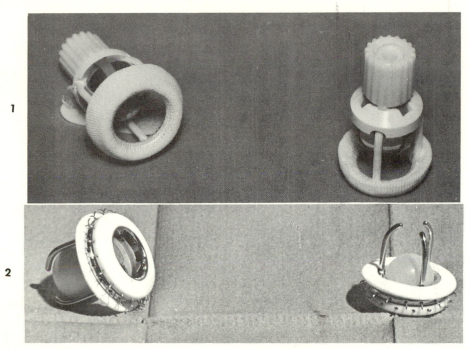

Fig. 15-15. Heart valve prostheses. 1, Starr-Edwards aortic valve prosthesis (Edwards Laboratories, Inc., Santa Ana, Calif.); 2, Magovern-Cromie sutureless aortic heart valve prosthesis (Surgitool, Inc., Pittsburgh, Pa.).

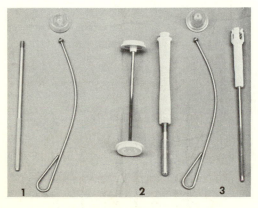

Fig. 15-16. 1, Starr-Edwards aortic valve holder and sizer; 2, Beall mitral valve sizer and holder; 3, Starr-Edwards mitral valve sizer and holder.

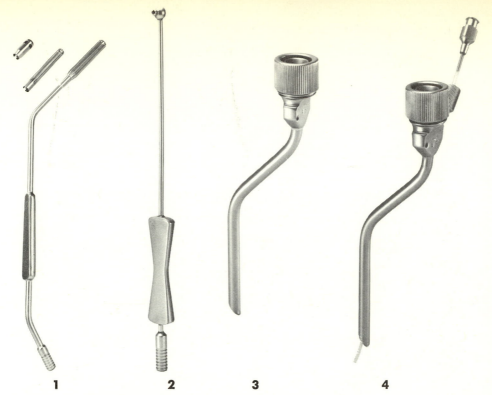

**1**  **2**  **3**  **4**

Fig. 15-17. 1, Intracardiac sucker with interchangeable tips; 2, coronary perfusion cannulae with malleable shaft, size 4, 5, or 6 mm. diameter for ¼ in. tubing; 3, femoral perfusion cannulae, sizes from 2.5 to 6.5 mm.; 4, pressure perfusion cannulae, sizes from 2.5 to 6.5 mm. with catheter. Permits simultaneous recording of central arterial pressure with separate circuit. (Courtesy Sarns, Inc., Ann Arbor, Mich.)

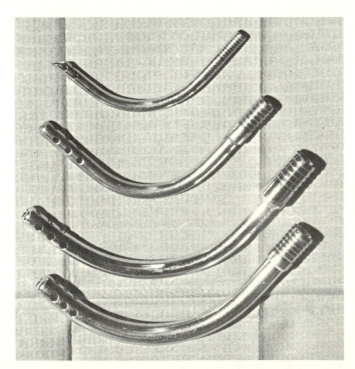

Fig. 15-18. Stainless steel cardiac sump cannulae. (Courtesy Sarns, Inc., Ann Arbor, Mich.)

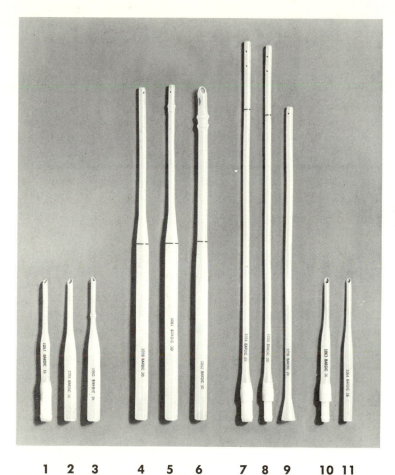

**1 2 3    4 5 6    7 8 9    10 11**

**Fig. 15-19.** Bardic translucent vinyl plastic catheters for extracorporeal systems. 1 to 3, Arterial and venous catheters; 4 to 6, venous catheters; 7 to 9, arterial and venous catheters; 10 and 11, regional and peripheral perfusion catheters. (Courtesy C. R. Bard, Inc., Murray Hill, N. J.)

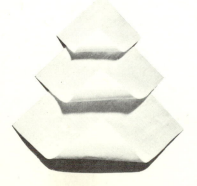

**Fig. 15-20.** Edwards Teflon intracardiac patches. For closure of intracardiac septal defects. (Courtesy C. R. Bard, Inc., Murray Hill, N. J.)

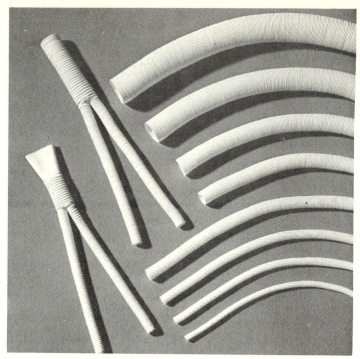

Fig. 15-21. Synthetic seamless arterial grafts with uniform crimp, as shown in Edwards Teflon, available woven or knitted. Sizes range from 4.8 to 32 mm. × 30 inches aortic bifurcation; also available in DeBakey Dacron single-crimp construction, woven or knitted. (Courtesy C. R. Bard, Inc., Muray Hill, N. J.)

heart valves, and tubular grafts made of synthetic Teflon, Dacron, and silicone rubber materials should be handled with the utmost care. Thorough cleaning and rinsing with a minimum of handling is recommended by manufacturers. Their directions for sterilization should be followed.

Edwards Teflon patches (Fig. 15-20) are made in a variety of forms for intracardiac and outflow tract use. Varying degrees of firmness, thickness, and porosity are available for specific use. Low reactivity, retention of strength, and tissue acceptance are important properties to be considered in the selection of such patches.

Teflon, a fluorocarbon fiber, and Dacron, a polyester fiber, are available in a variety of meshes, fabrics, felts, tapes, and sutures, and are also combined with other materials in the manufacture of heart valve replacements.

DeBakey Dacron seamless arterial grafts are made of polyester fiber processed specifically for use as surgical implants. They have the following qualities: high tensile and flexural strength, retention of strength with age, resistance to acids and solvents, and compatibility with the host vessels when implanted. These grafts can be clamped without harm to the fabric and can be cut at any angle. There are two types of arterial grafts, knitted and woven. The grafts are available in sizes suitable for straight arterial grafts, as well as for aortic bifurcated grafts (Fig. 15-21).

Edwards ball-valve prostheses (Figs. 15-14 and 15-15) are complete replacement prostheses for the mitral and aortic valves. A stainless steel alloy cage holds a medical grade, heat-cured Silastic or Stellite ball and a knitted Teflon cloth fixation ring.

Beall disk mitral valve prosthesis (Fig. 15-14) is a low-profile Teflon disk-type

design with a fully covered titanium base and Teflon-covered cage struts.

**SUTURE MATERIALS.** A vast array of specialized cardiovascular sutures with swaged-on needles are available from most suture manufacturers (see Chapter 6). Surgical silk is used rather extensively; however, synthetic sutures of Teflon and Dacron are usually selected for insertion of the various prostheses.

## BASIC INSTRUMENT SETUP FOR CARDIOTHORACIC SURGERY

**CLOSED HEART OPERATIONS.** The basic set-up for various closed cardiothoracic procedures consists of the basic thoracic setup, plus the following cardiothoracic instruments, sutures, and accessory items. (Additional instruments for specific procedures may be selected from the cardiothoracic instruments illustrated in Figs. 15-8 and 15-9.)

**Cardiothoracic instruments** (Fig. 15-10)

2 Bahnson aortic clamps
3 Craford coarctation clamps, various sizes
4 Blalock pulmonary artery clamps, 2 pairs
4 DeBakey multipurpose clamps
3 Beck aortic clamps, assorted sizes
2 Potts anastomosis clamps, spoon-shaped

**Sutures** (according to surgeon's preference; those listed known to be preferred by several teams)

Thoracotomy—silk nos. 4-0, 3-0, 2-0, and 0
Synthetic sutures—nos. 4-0, 3-0, 2-0, and 0
Pericostal (only)—chromic gut no. 1 or 0 for closure
Pericardium—silk or synthetic nos. 3-0 and 2-0
Atrial—purse-string, silk no. 1, or synthetic no. 2-0
Myocardiotomy—purse-string, silk or synthetic no. 2-0
Intracardiac—silk or synthetic nos. 5-0 to 0
For insertion of prosthesis—synthetic sutures of Teflon, Dacron, or polyethylene, various sizes (depending on prosthesis)
Sternotomy closure—steel wire, 22-gauge
Conductive—Flexon wire no. 0, insulated with Teflon (as indicated)

**Accessory items**

8 Syringes, 2, 5, 10, and 20 ml. (2 each)
6 Needles, 2 each nos. 25, 20, and 18, sufficient for use with emergency drugs
1 Electrocautery unit (optional)

1 Fiberoptic flexible light (optional)
1 External pacemaker unit
1 D.C. defibrillator
Drugs: Heparin, protamine sulfate, sodium bicarbonate, calcium gluconate, calcium chloride, epinephrine, isoproterenol (Isuprel), procaine amide, 50% dextrose, mannitol, levarterenol bitartrate (Levophed), and 1% lidocaine (Xylocaine)
1 Water-seal closed drainage set
1 Scale, for weighing blood
1 Gram scale, for weighing sponges
1 Body scale for weighing patient in selected cases
3 Suction aspiration units

**Prosthetic materials**

See specific operations

**OPEN HEART OPERATIONS.** As previously described for basic setup for closed cardiothoracic procedures, plus the following:

**Accessory items**

Additional suction tubing
Bard Teflon or Dacron patch material
1 Teflon felt patch, 4 × 4 in.
Heart valve prosthesis, as indicated
1 Manometer
Polyethylene catheters, 16 to 23 Fr. (available)
Pressure-recording tubing, 20 ml. syringe with threeway stopcock, and heparinized intravenous saline irrigating solution

FOR PERFUSION PROCEDURE

Perfusion cannulae or catheters (according to surgeon's preference)
Arterial, vinyl plastic, 10 to 24 Fr.
Venous, vinyl plastic, 20 to 38 Fr.
Obturators, for insertion of cannulae (optional)
Femoral, stainless steel, infant or adult, from 2 mm. to 6.5 mm. outside diameter (O.D.), for ¼ to ⅜ in. tubing.
Vena cava, stainless steel, curved 90-degree or right-angled, 3/16 in., ¼ in., 5/16 in., and ⅜ in. O.D.
Coronary perfusion cannulae with malleable shaft and stainless steel bender
Coronary suction tubes with tubing
Tubing, lengths and size determined by specific procedure, for connection of cannula to pump-oxygenator
Adapters and metal connectors (according to surgeon's preference)
Gun stapler to secure connections
Sump tubes, metal or plastic, to remove trapped air from left heart
Pressure-recording catheters and connectors

Partially frozen I.V. saline "slush" (according to surgeon's preference)

**Pump-oxygenator**

This unit, with heat exchanger, filter traps, etc., is prepared and maintained by the pump team

## BASIC OPEN HEART PROCEDURE COMBINED WITH TOTAL HEART-LUNG BYPASS

POSITIONING AND PREPARATION OF THE PATIENT. The preinduction preparation of the patient has been discussed previously and in Chapter 14. Intravenous infusions and cutdowns are completed as monitoring leads are prepared and fastened in place.

Following intubation, a venous pressure catheter may be inserted into the external jugular vein through a percutaneous needle cannula. The radial or femoral arteries may be similarly cannulated. The patient is positioned for the selected approach. A large surface electrocoagulation-indifferent plate is placed under the buttocks or back after conductive gel has been applied. An indwelling urethral catheter is connected to a receptacle. Special attention is given to pressure areas, and protective padding is utilized as indicated.

The routine skin preparation and draping of the patient is completed (see Chapters 4 and 5).

INCISIONAL APPROACHES. The heart is approached by a right or left posterolateral thoracotomy, a median sternotomy, a transsternal bilateral thoracotomy, or an anterolateral thoracotomy (Chapter 14). The selection of the incision is determined by the age of the patient, the pathological defect, the proposed correction, and the surgeon's preference.

Cannulation for the arterial return is also determined by many factors. The aorta or subclavian, iliac, or femoral arteries may be used.

The description of incisional approaches is as follows.

FOR POSTEROLATERAL THORACOTOMY, RIGHT OR LEFT INCISION. The full lateral position may be modified to permit access to both groin regions (see Chapter 14). The skin incision is made following the course of the fifth rib, which is resected. A Finochietto or Burford chest retractor is inserted. The pleura is incised, and the lung is retracted with a moist pack to expose the pericardium.

FOR MEDIAN STERNOTOMY (VERTICAL) INCISION. This incision is made over the sternum with a Y or T extension at the top and extends down over the xiphoid process. Bleeding points are clamped and electrocoagulated or tied. The incision is carried down to the periosteum, and the superior subcutaneous flap is reflected upward to expose the suprasternal notch. The sternum is split longitudinally with a Stryker or Sarns sternal electric saw or a Lebsche knife. Periosteal bleeding is controlled with bone wax and electrocoagulation.

A sternal retractor is placed in the wound. The lobes of the thymus gland may be dissected and transfixed with sutures. The pericardium is exposed.

FOR TRANSSTERNAL BILATERAL THORACOTOMY INCISION. A bilateral inframammary incision is made at the level of the fourth interspace and continued laterally on either side to the midaxillary line. The internal mammary arteries are ligated and transfixed on either side, following division of the greater pectoral muscles.

The sternum is transected horizontally with a guillotine-type rib cutter or Gigli saw. Bleeding is controlled as previously described, and two chest retractors (small Finochietto-type) are placed in the wound. The pericardium is exposed.

FOR ANTEROLATERAL THORACOTOMY INCISION. The patient is placed in a supine position with the thorax elevated about 30 degrees. The arm is flexed slightly to permit access to the lateral aspect of the incision. An inframammary incision is made from the anterior midline or the sternal border to the lateral midaxillary line. Muscles are divided, and the internal mammary vessels are doubly ligated. The fourth rib may be resected. The pleura is incised, a chest re-

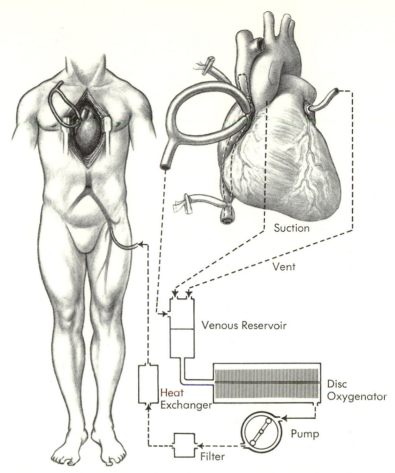

Suction

Vent

Venous Reservoir

Heat Exchanger

Disc Oxygenator

Pump

Filter

**Fig. 15-22.** Diagram of extracorporeal circulation. Using technique shown here, inferior and superior venae cavae are cannulated, and total venous return from body is led by gravity drainage into venous reservoir. Blood passes through debubbling chamber and into rotating disk oxygenator. Roller pump then passes blood through filter and bubble trap into heat exchanger, which can cool, warm, or maintain blood at normal body temperature. Oxygenated blood of desired temperature enters arterial circuit through common femoral artery, from which it perfuses patient's body in retrograde fashion. (From Advancing with surgery, Somerville, N. J., Ethicon, Inc.)

tractor is inserted, and the pericardium is exposed.

### Extracorporeal circulation

**PROCEDURE FOR PERICARDIAL INCISION AND CAVAL CANNULATION**

1. A long pericardial incision is made, and the pericardial edges are sutured to the chest wall or drapes.

2. The aorta is encircled with an umbilical tape, and a Rochester-Pean forceps is placed on each end of the tape. This maneuver will facilitate cross clamping of the aorta when indicated.

3. Each cava is encircled with a ½-inch cotton tape, the loose ends of which are threaded through a ¼- × 2-inch red rubber tubing and held taut by a hemostat (Fig. 15-22). Compression on the cava may be accomplished by tightening the tapes and resetting the hemostat. If indicated, the pulmonary artery may be similarly isolated.

4. For the return flow to the pump-oxygenator, plastic catheters are used to

cannulate the inferior and superior venae cavae (Figs. 15-19 and 15-22). An incision is usually made in the atrial appendage for the inferior caval cannula, and a transverse incision through the atrial wall is made for the superior cava. Purse-string sutures no. 2-0 are placed, and each incision is made over a Satinsky clamp. Edges may be retracted with Sarot clamps as the catheter is introduced. The purse-string suture is secured, and the catheter is permitted to partially fill with blood before the occluding clamp is applied.

PROCEDURE FOR GROIN INCISIONS AND ARTERIAL CANNULATION. To save time, a second team may be simultaneously preparing for the arterial return.

A vertical incision is made in the femoral triangle and the femoral artery exposed. Narrow umbilical compression tapes are passed around the vessel above and below the proposed arteriotomy. (Two bulldog clamps may also be applied to the vessel.) A vertical incision is made into the vessel, and the plastic catheter is inserted into the artery while the proximal bulldog clamp is released. When normal arterial blood flow has filled the catheter, it is clamped with a Carmalt forceps.

PROCEDURE FOR PUMP-OXYGENATOR PREPARATION. While the surgical team has been preparing the cannulations for connection to the pump-oxygenator, the pump team has tested and completed assemblage of the equipment (Figs. 15-6 and 15-7).

1. At the operative field, the tubing is passed off to the pump operator after the proximal ends have been secured to the drapes and the two coronary suction lines. The following will also be passed off, depending on the procedure: vent line, $CO_2$ tubing, and the fibrillation cord end if the heart is to be arrested.

2. After the venous and arterial lines are connected to the pump-oxygenator, blood is pumped through the lines to displace air in the tubing. A small basin is used to accommodate the overflow. To prevent air embolism, extreme caution is exercised as the arterial and caval connec-

tions are completed. Excess blood is returned to the oxygenator via a coronary suction catheter.

3. When all connections are properly secured and the pump-oxygenator is ready, a signal is given, and the machine is turned on. After the flow is in balance, the tapes around the cavae are tightened, and the patient is on total cardiopulmonary bypass. The perfusion rate is adjusted as the operation proceeds. (See Fig. 15-22.)

## Repair or reconstruction

The type of correction or reconstruction needed is determined first.

CONSIDERATIONS. A variety of intracardiac patches, prostheses, and sutures are prepared for specific corrections, as requested. Sterile D.C. defibrillation electrodes are kept readily available throughout the entire procedure. During the repair, elective cardiac arrest may be induced at intervals to obtain a dry, motionless field and improve visualization.

INDUCED CARDIAC ARREST. One of the following methods may be used:

1. Electrical fibrillation may be accomplished by continuous electrical stimulation of alternating current.

An alligator clip electrode is attached to the ventricular myocardium, and an indifferent electrode with a similar clip is attached to the subcutaneous tissue.

2. Anoxic arrest by cross clamping the aorta to prevent oxygenation of the myocardium for 5-minute intervals (10 minutes if hypothermal temperature is near 28° C.) usually returns to normal rhythm without complications.

3. Hypothermic arrest is achieved by selective hypothermic coronary perfusion (Figs. 15-23 and 15-24) or instillation of partially frozen isotonic saline "slush" into the pericardial sac for external bathing of the myocardium.

ELECTRICAL VENTRICULAR DEFIBRILLATION. It may be necessary to establish normal rhythm (Fig. 15-24). The D.C. defibrillator is usually requested, since it appears to be

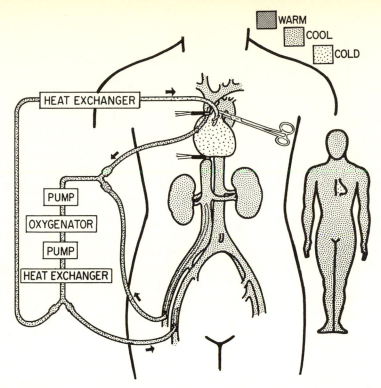

**Fig. 15-23.** Moderate general hypothermia in body core with differential deep cooling of heart. General body core temperature is reduced to 28° to 30° C., and heat exchanger supplying femoral artery inflow is maintained at this temperature. With ice water circulating through second heat exchanger, blood emerges with temperature of 2° to 4° C. and is used to perfuse coronary arteries, thereby cooling heart to low temperature. (From Brown, I. W.: In Gibbon, J. H., Jr., editor: Surgery of the chest, Philadelphia, 1962, W. B. Saunders Co.)

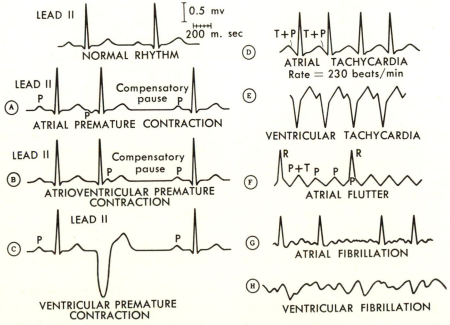

**Fig. 15-24.** Diagram showing cardiac arrhythmias. (From Bullard, R. W.: In Selkurt, E. E., editor: Physiology, Boston, 1963, Little, Brown & Co.)

more effective and less likely to injure the myocardium. The steps are as follows:

1. Connections to machine are completed with sterile electrodes.

2. Pulse duration is set—0.1 to 0.15 second.

3. Voltage is set—low 10 to high 60 watt-seconds.

4. If electrodes are covered with cloth, moisten with saline solution.

5. Electrodes are applied directly to myocardium, perpendicular to the heart's septum.

6. All other team members stand clear of the patient.

7. The surgeon squeezes the heart firmly between the electrodes and signals "fire" for the shock.

OPERATIVE PROCEDURE FOR CLOSURE OF MYOCARDIUM AND OFF BYPASS

1. After the correction has been completed, the chambers of the heart are closed with continuous synthetic cardiac sutures. Filling of the chamber is begun in order to evacuate the air before the final sutures are tied. Compression tapes around the cavae are released, and venous flow is reduced. Arterial flow is also reduced to equal the venous outflow. When heart action is sufficient and systemic arterial blood pressure is stabilized, venous suction is further reduced, and the patient is taken off bypass.

2. As the cannulation catheters are removed, the purse-string sutures are secured. Additional sutures may be required for tight closure.

3. Protamine sulfate, a heparin antagonist, is administered.

4. The pericardium may be loosely approximated with interrupted sutures. It is usually left open.

DRAINAGE. Catheters may be inserted into the pericardium, the anterior mediastinum, or either or both pleurae. They are connected by Y connectors to an underwater seal suction device.

CLOSURE OF THE CHEST

1. *For posterolateral and anterolateral thoracotomy.* Ribs are approximated by the insertion of interrupted pericostal su-

tures of chromic gut no. 2 and the application of two rib approximators. Sutures are tied in place and approximators removed. Continuous chromic sutures no. 1 swaged to general closure needles are used throughout for the muscle closure. Chromic sutures no. 2-0 are used for subcutaneous tissue, and running or interrupted nylon or silk sutures no. 4-0 may be used for skin closure.

2. *For median sternotomy.* Corresponding holes are punched or drilled on each side of the sternum to facilitate placement of no. 22 steel wire sutures. The wire sutures are twisted, cut, and buried into the sternum. A layer of interrupted synthetic sutures no. 2-0 is placed to approximate the linea alba and muscle over the sternum. The subcutaneous tissue is closed with chromic gut suture no. 3-0. Running or interrupted synthetic or silk suture no. 4-0 may be used for skin closure.

3. *For transsternal thoracotomy.* Corresponding holes are punched or drilled on each side of the transected sternum to facilitate placement of no. 22 steel wire sutures. Refer to closure for posterolateral and anterolateral thoracotomy.

CLOSURE OF THE GROIN INCISIONS

1. Femoral catheters are removed, and each arteriotomy is closed with cardiac silk suture no. 5-0 or 6-0. Compression tapes and bulldog clamps, if used, are removed.

2. Wounds are closed with interrupted silk or continuous chromic sutures no. 3-0 in the usual manner.

3. Dressings are applied to all wounds.

Final calculations of blood loss and blood replacement are determined. Any imbalance is corrected before the patient is removed to the recovery unit, where monitoring is continued for blood loss through the drainage tubes, arterial and venous blood pressure, temperature, and continuous electrocardiographic observations. A chest film is usually obtained in the recovery room.

## Operation for ventricular aneurysms

An aneurysm of the left ventricle occasionally develops after a severe myocardial infarct in which part of the myo-

cardium is replaced by scar tissue. The scar may gradually stretch due to the impact of the left ventricular pressure, thus forming an aneurysm. Surgical excision of the ventricular aneurysm using cardiopulmonary bypass has become an accepted procedure. The aneurysm is usually adherent to the pericardium, and it may not be possible to dissect it free until cardiopulmonary bypass has been established.

**OPERATIVE PROCEDURE**

1. The aorta is cross clamped to guard against systemic emboli.

2. The scar tissue of the ventricle is incised and the clot removed carefully.

3. A cuff of scar tissue is left through which to suture with cardiovascular sutures reinforced with Teflon felt pledgets. Many interrupted sutures are used.

## PERICARDIECTOMY

**DEFINITION.** Partial excision of the adhered, thickened fibrotic pericardium to relieve constriction of the compressed heart and large blood vessels.

**CONSIDERATIONS.** The heart action is constricted by the adhered portions of the scarred, thickened pericardium. As the pericardial space is obliterated and calcification of the pericardium occurs, the heart is further compressed. Ascites, elevated venous pressure, decreased arterial pressure, edema, and hepatic enlargement result. This condition is usually caused by chronic pericarditis due to tuberculosis; however, it may be of rheumatic, viral, or neoplastic origin.

**SETUP AND PREPARATION OF THE PATIENT.** The patient is placed on the operating table in a supine position. The setup is as described for closed heart surgery, utilizing a median sternotomy incision.

**OPERATIVE PROCEDURE**

1. A median sternotomy incision is completed to expose the pericardium, as previously described.

2. The lungs are displaced laterally, and the phrenic nerves are identified and carefully protected. The pericardium is incised near the left border.

3. The left atrium and then the right ventricle are freed. The outer thickened pericardium is removed, as indicated. The cartilage scissors may be used. The fibrous epicardium is carefully dissected, using dry dissectors and Metzenbaum scissors. Caution is exercised to prevent perforation of the thin wall of the right atrium. Rather than damage the wall, very small areas that are tightly adhered may be retained if the lateral edges are free.

4. Dissection is continued, and the large blood vessels are exposed and freed as indicated.

5. Adequate drainage of the pericardial wound is facilitated by catheters placed near the heart or through the pleural spaces, as indicated. Connections to closed drainage sets are established.

6. Hemostasis is carefully controlled to prevent recurrent fibrosis.

7. The chest wound is closed, as previously described. A dressing is applied.

## OPERATIONS FOR TETRALOGY OF FALLOT

**GENERAL CONSIDERATIONS.** Tetralogy of Fallot is the most common congenital cardiac anomaly in the cyanotic group. Cyanosis, as seen in the superficial vessels of the skin, is the result of an abnormally high amount of unoxygenated blood in the systemic circulation.

The essential features of this condition are pulmonary stenosis, high ventricular septal defect, overriding of the septal defect by the aorta, with resulting hypertrophy of the right ventricle—all of which may be subdivided into more complex variations (Fig. 15-25). The *infundibular* form of pulmonary stenosis is a long localized constricture in the pulmonary conus of the right ventricle. The relative position and size of this muscular band determine the condition of the chamber between the band and the pulmonary valve ring. *Valvular stenosis* and infundibular stenosis, however, may occur independently.

Physiologically, in tetralogy of Fallot blood flow into the lungs decreases as a

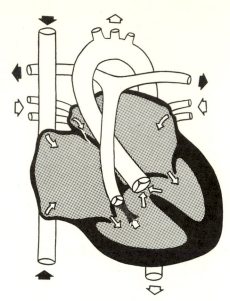

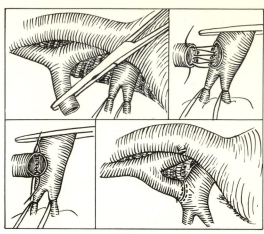

**Fig. 15-26.** Blalock-Taussig procedure. End-to-side anastomosis between right subclavian and pulmonary arteries. Posterior half of anastomosis is performed with continuous sutures and anterior half with interrupted sutures. (From Shumacker, H. B., Jr.: In Gibbon, J. H., Jr., editor: Surgery of the chest, Philadelphia, 1969, W. B. Saunders Co.)

**Fig. 15-25.** Tetralogy of Fallot is characterized by combination of four defects: pulmonary stenosis, ventricular septal defect, overriding aorta, and hypertrophy of right ventricle. (From Nursing Education Service: General signs and symptoms of congenital heart abnormalities, Columbus, Ohio, 1961, Ross Laboratories.)

result of pulmonary obstruction, and the volume of oxygenated blood into the systemic circulation decreases due to a right-to-left shunt of venous blood from the right ventricle to the left ventricle and aorta.

Symptoms of tetralogy are cyanosis, dyspnea, episodes of acute dyspnea, retarded growth, clubbing of extremities, and reduced exercise tolerance. A systolic murmur and secondary polycythemia are usually present. Cardiac catheterization and angiocardiography aid in determining the diagnosis and plan of surgical treatment.

The selection of a *closed* palliative or *open* corrective procedure will be based on the age and general condition of the patient and the severity of the pulmonary stenosis.

### Shunt operations

**DEFINITION.** These closed procedures are designed to divert poorly oxygenated blood from one of the major circulatory arteries back through one of the pulmonary arteries to the lungs for reoxygenation, thereby increasing the total blood volume of the pulmonary circulation.

The *Blalock-Taussig operation* consists of an end-to-side anastomosis between the proximal end of the subclavian and pulmonary arteries. The procedure is performed on the side opposite to the aortic arch. This shunt may be easily dismantled if a future operation for full correction is anticipated; however, the shunt has a tendency to reduce in size as the child grows (Fig. 15-26).

The *Potts-Smith operation* consists of a side-to-side anastomosis directly between the aorta and left pulmonary artery. This procedure may be selected for infants because the size of the anastomosis is not limited by the lumen of the subclavian artery as it is in the Blalock technique. The Potts technique has the advantage of enlarging as the child grows; however, it is more difficult to dismantle if future operation is anticipated (Fig. 15-27).

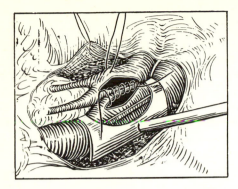

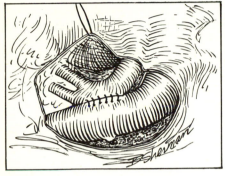

Fig. 15-27. Potts-Smith procedure. Technique of side-to-side aortopulmonary anastomosis. (From Shumacker, H. B., Jr.: In Gibbon, J. H., Jr., editor: Surgery of the chest, Philadelphia, 1969, W. B. Saunders Co.)

The *Waterston operation* consists of anastomosis of the ascending aorta and the right pulmonary artery. It is the preferred procedure when a systemic-pulmonary artery anastomosis is needed within the first several months of life.

The *Glenn operation* consists of anastomosis of the superior vena cava to the right pulmonary artery. This operation is employed infrequently in the treatment of tetralogy of Fallot.

**SETUP AND PREPARATION OF THE PATIENT.** The patient is placed in the selected position for the specific procedure. Instruments are as described for closed heart surgery, plus the following, with appropriate sizes for infants and children (Figs. 15-10 and 15-11):

2 Potts-Smith aortic occlusion clamps
2 Johns Hopkins modified Potts clamps
2 Hendrin ductus clamps
2 Cooley anastomosis clamps

## OPERATIVE PROCEDURES

### BLALOCK-TAUSSIG OPERATION

1. An anterolateral incision is made from the sternal margin to the midaxillary line. The chest cavity is opened and the lung retracted, as previously described.

2. The mediastinal pleura is incised and retracted with silk stay sutures no. 3-0 or 4-0.

3. The pulmonary artery is dissected from the surrounding tissue, using vascular right-angle forceps, dry dissector sponges, and Metzenbaum scissors. As the artery and branches are mobilized, heavy silk ligatures or moistened umbilical tapes are placed about them.

4. Branches of the vagus nerve are protected and retracted.

5. The subclavian artery is dissected completely from its origin to the place where it gives off the internal mammary and costocervical branches. Its distal end is marked with a silk suture.

6. The subclavian artery is occluded with a vascular clamp, a ligature is placed at the distal segment, and the vessel is divided.

7. The marked end of the suture is carried down to the pulmonary artery.

8. The pulmonary artery is occluded temporarily by application of a curved vascular clamp.

9. An incision of sufficient size to fit the end of the subclavian artery is made with a no. 12 knife blade and Potts scissors.

10. An end-to-side anastomosis is completed with cardiovascular suture no. 5-0 or 6-0.

11. The clamps are released, and the suture line is inspected for hemostasis (Fig. 15-26).

12. The mediastinal pleura is closed with silk no. 3-0 or 4-0.

13. Open chest drainage is established, and the chest wound is closed as previously described (Chapter 14).

**POTTS-SMITH OPERATION.** A left posterolateral incision is made in the fourth inter-

space. The pulmonary artery is dissected from its surrounding tissue, and the descending aorta is mobilized. Occluding tapes and Blalock or Potts-Smith clamps are applied. A longitudinal incision is made in each artery, and a side-to-side anastomosis is completed with cardiovascular suture no. 5-0 or 6-0. The pulmonary artery is released, and the suture line is inspected for hemostasis. The aortic clamps are then removed (Fig. 15-27).

WATERSTON OPERATION. A right anterolateral incision is made in the fourth interspace. The pericardium is opened, and the ascending aorta is exposed. The right pulmonary artery is dissected as it passes beneath the ascending aorta. A heavy suture is passed around the right pulmonary artery and used to temporarily occlude the artery. A curved Hendrin or Cooley clamp (Fig. 15-10) is placed so that one blade is behind the pulmonary artery and the other occludes a posterolateral portion of the ascending aorta. On closure of the clamp, both the right pulmonary artery and a posterior portion of the ascending aorta are occluded. Parallel incisions are made in both the aorta and the right pulmonary artery. An anastomosis with suture no. 6-0 or 7-0 is then made between the ascending aorta and right pulmonary artery.

GLENN OPERATION. A right anterolateral incision is made in the fourth intercostal space. The pericardium is opened, the right pulmonary artery is dissected, and tapes are placed around the proximal and distal ends of the right pulmonary artery. The right pulmonary artery is clamped with two straight Cooley clamps, divided medial to the vena cava, and its proximal end oversewn with cardiovascular suture no. 5-0 or 6-0. Then a curved Cooley clamp is placed on the superior vena cava. Circular section is excised from the superior vena cava, and the distal end of the pulmonary artery is anastomosed into the cava with cardiovascular suture no. 6-0.

## Open corrective operation for tetralogy

DEFINITION. Under direct vision, utilizing extracorporeal circulation, moderate hypothermia, and induced cardioplegia (surgeon's preference), corrective operation is directed toward complete repair of the infundibular stenosis or pulmonary valve stenosis and closure of the ventricular septal defect.

SETUP AND PREPARATION OF THE PATIENT. The patient is placed on the operating table in a supine position (see Chapter 7). The setup is as described for open heart surgery with the median sternotomy or transsternal approach. The selection of instruments must be suitable for the size of the patient. Additional items to be added to the basic open heart setup include the following:

1 Teflon Edwards intracardiac patch, 2 × 2 in.
1 Teflon Edwards outflow cardiac patch, 2 × 2 in.
1 Teflon felt patch, 4 × 4 in.

OPERATIVE PROCEDURE

1. A median sternotomy or transsternal incision is completed, the pericardium is incised, and the aorta and pulmonary arteries are prepared for cross clamping. All connections to the pump-oxygenator and other equipment are completed, as previously described.

2. A moderate degree of hypothermia is induced (28° C.).

3. The patient is placed on total cardiopulmonary bypass.

4. The left side of the heart is vented through a catheter inserted through the right superior pulmonary vein into the left atrium, the left atrial appendage, or the tip of the left ventricle.

5. The aorta is cross clamped at intervals to facilitate exposure of the ventricular septal defect. Considerable care must be given to the prevention of an air embolus on release of the aortic cross clamp. This is accomplished by the passage of a right-angle clamp through the aortic

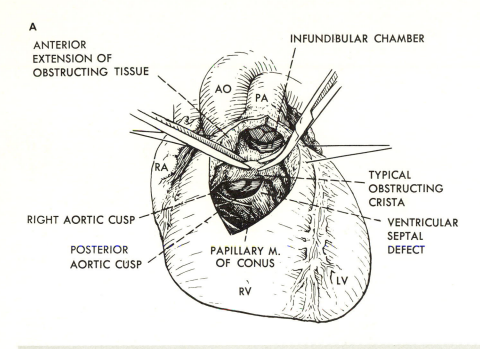

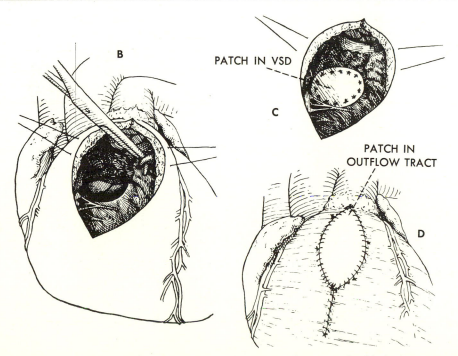

**Fig. 15-28.** Exposure of right ventricular outflow tract showing infundibular stenosis and ventricular septal defect with repair. (From Johnson, J., and Kirby, C. K.: Surgery of the chest, ed. 3, Chicago, 1964, Year Book Medical Publishers, Inc.)

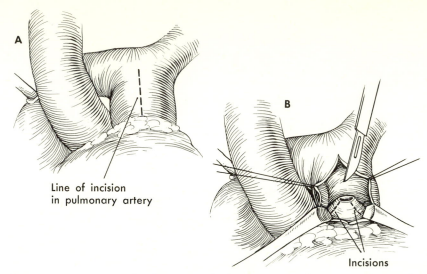

Line of incision
in pulmonary artery

Incisions

**Fig. 15-29.** Open correction of pulmonary valvular stenosis employing extracorporeal circulation. **A,** An incision is made in the main pulmonary artery, exposing the dome-shaped pulmonary valve. **B,** Radial incisions are made in each of the fused commissures with complete opening of the valve. (From Gibbon, J. H., Jr., Sabiston, D., Jr., and Spencer, F., editors: Surgery of the chest, ed. 2, Philadelphia, 1969, W. B. Saunders Co.)

valve to cause valvular insufficiency as the aortic occlusion clamp is opened.

6. Stay sutures are inserted, and a vertical oblique or transverse ventriculotomy over the infundibular area is performed (Fig. 15-28).

7. The defect is identified. Closure requires an intracardiac patch in almost all instances.

8. The hypertrophied muscle is excised as completely as possible.

9. The pulmonary valve is inspected. Fused commissures may be incised radially with a scalpel (Fig. 15-29). The pulmonary artery is closed with cardiovascular sutures no. 5-0 or 6-0.

10. Interrupted cardiovascular Teflon sutures no. 3-0 or 4-0 are placed with extreme caution into the septum, tagged with a small clamp, and placed on a bender (Fig. 15-11). It is important that the ECG and the atrial and ventricular contractions be monitored carefully while these sutures are placed. The suture should be removed and reinserted if a pattern of heart block occurs. Interrupted sutures are used in the area of the conduction system and continuous suture for the remainder.

11. After closure of the ventriculoseptal defect, an estimate is made whether the right ventricle can be closed primarily or whether a patch is necessary. If the pulmonic stenosis could not be relieved adequately by valvulotomy and infundibulectomy, an outflow patch may be needed to enlarge the outflow tract. If the pulmonary artery or valve annulus is quite small, it may be necessary to extend the patch across the valve ring to the proximal portion of the pulmonary artery. The ventriculotomy and patch are sutured with cardiovascular Teflon no. 4-0.

In recent years, a new method of total correction of the severe forms of tetralogy of Fallot has been used. An aortic allograft containing the aortic valve with the attached septal leaflet of the mitral valve and the ascending aorta has been used. The septal leaflet of the mitral valve is used as a portion of the right ventricular outflow patch. All or part of the aortic valve and ascending aorta is used either as a new conduit or an onlay patch. This technique has given good results in a group in which a high mortality rate previously existed.

## Closed valvulotomy for isolated pulmonary stenosis

**DEFINITION.** The fused leaflets of the stenotic valve are incised to increase the pulmonary flow of blood and to decrease the pressure in the right side of the heart.

**CONSIDERATIONS.** The abnormal features of isolated "pure" pulmonary stenosis are usually the result of a deformed pulmonary valve. The cusps or leaflets are fused into a domelike structure that has a very small opening, thereby permitting only a slight stream of blood to be ejected through into the lungs.

Severe stenosis in infants is characterized by right heart failure. In older patients, fatigability is an early symptom; however, as the disease progresses because of additional work load of the heart, the right ventricle hypertrophies and the pulmonary artery becomes dilated distal to the stenosis. If the stenosis is associated with other anomalies such as septal defects, cyanosis is present because of a right-to-left shunt.

*Open* technique is most frequently used for repair of this defect under direct vision; however, the *closed* Brock procedure discussed next is less traumatic and is used to treat infants and acutely ill adults.

### Brock closed procedure

**DEFINITION.** Through a left anterior thoracotomy or median sternotomy incision and right ventriculotomy, a Brock, Potts, or similar valvulotome is inserted and the stenotic leaflets are separated (Fig. 15-30).

**SETUP AND PREPARATION OF THE PATIENT.** As described for closed heart surgery, plus the following:

2 Brock valvulotomes

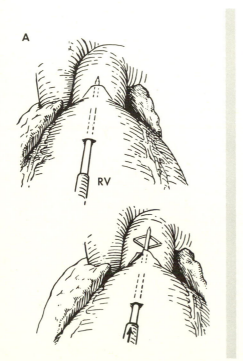
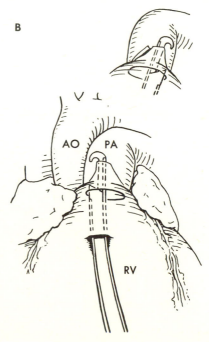

**Fig. 15-30.** Technique of closed pulmonary valvulotomy. **A,** Potts valvulotome shown in place in lumen of valve and with adjustable cutting blades open. **B,** Guillotine-type knife shown in place in lumen of valve. (From Johnson, J., and Kirby, C. K.: Surgery of the chest, ed. 4, Chicago, 1970, Year Book Medical Publishers, Inc.)

1 Set Brock valve knives
1 Set Brock or Potts-Riker dilators
1 Potts-Riker adjustable valvulotome

### OPERATIVE PROCEDURE

1. A curved submammary incision is usually made beneath the left nipple, and the chest wall is entered through the third intercostal space. The second, third, and fourth ribs may be cut at the costosternal junction to facilitate exposure. An alternate approach is a median sternotomy incision.

2. The pulmonary artery is identified and exposed, as in shunt operations for tetralogy of Fallot.

3. A mattress suture no. 4-0 or 5-0 with Teflon pledgets attached is replaced into the right ventricle. This suture is tagged with a small mosquito clamp.

4. A closed valvulotome or Brock knife is introduced into the right ventricular chamber directly into the pulmonary artery through the mattress sutures in the right ventricle. The stenotic pulmonary valve is opened (Fig. 15-30) and then dilated.

5. The ventricular wall is closed by tying down the ventricular sutures. Additional pledget sutures may be needed.

## Open valvulotomy for pulmonary stenosis

DEFINITION. This procedure involves separation of the stenosed leaflets under direct vision.

SETUP AND PREPARATION OF THE PATIENT; OPERATIVE PROCEDURE. As previously described in open heart surgery for correction of tetralogy of Fallot (Fig. 15-29).

## Closure of atrial septal defect (open technique)

DEFINITION. Under direct vision, utilizing extracorporeal circulation, a congenital defect in the atrial septum is closed by a simple suture technique or by the insertion of a synthetic prosthetic patch.

CONSIDERATIONS. Atrial septal defects are a common congenital abnormality, and their classification is based on anatomical location and associated abnormalities (Figs. 15-31 and 15-32).

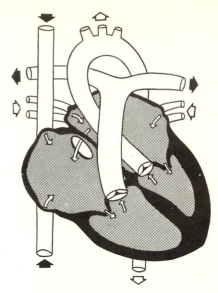

Fig. 15-31. Atrial septal defects. Abnormal opening between right and left atria. Incompetent foramen ovale, high ostium secundum defect, and ostium primum defect usually involve atrioventricular valves. (From Nursing Education Service: General signs and symptoms of congenital heart abnormalities, Columbus, Ohio, 1961, Ross Laboratories.)

The *ostium secundum defect* is located in the superior and central portion of the septum. The *ostium primum defect* is located in the lower portion of the atrial septum and associated with other defects in the atrioventricular canal, usually with a cleft of the mitral valve or occasionally of the tricuspid valve. An accompanying ventricular septal defect may also be present.

An atrial septal defect results in a left-to-right atrial shunt that may be well tolerated in early life if the opening is small. However, if the defect is large or of the ostium primum type with a marked shunting of blood, the work load of the heart is increased. The right heart and the pulmonary artery and its branches become enlarged. The vascularity of the lung field is increased, with resulting pulmonary hypertension and subsequent right heart failure.

In early life the patient may be asymp-

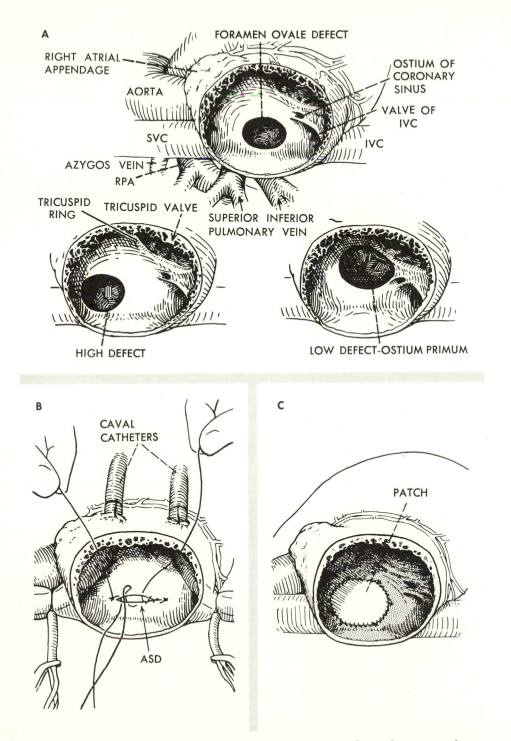

**Fig. 15-32. A,** Exposure of atrial septal defects. **B,** Open repair with simple suture technique. **C,** Open repair with synthetic patch replacement. (From Johnson, J., and Kirby, C. K.: Surgery of the chest, ed. 4, Chicago, 1970, Year Book Medical Publishers, Inc.)

tomatic. Beginning symptoms may include fatigue, retardation of normal weight gain, and increased susceptibility to respiratory infections. Later symptoms include those of right heart failure.

A systolic murmur is heard with greatest intensity over the base of the heart, and the electrocardiogram indicates a right axis deviation and incomplete right bundle branch block in the ostium secundum type. A left axis deviation and incomplete right bundle branch block are observed in the persistent ostium primum condition.

Many cardiologists and cardiac surgeons recommend that these defects be surgically repaired in early childhood, when the patient is relatively asymptomatic. The mortality for the operation is less than 1%.

SETUP AND PREPARATION OF THE PATIENT. The patient is placed in the supine position for a median sternotomy or in a right anterior oblique position for an anterolateral thoracotomy.

The instrument setup is as described for basic open heart surgery, plus 1 Teflon Edwards intracardiac patch, $2 \times 2$ inches or larger, if indicated, and 1 Teflon felt patch, $2 \times 2$ inches, $\frac{1}{16}$ inch thick.

OPERATIVE PROCEDURE

1. A right anterolateral incision is made, following the course of the fourth rib from the sternum to the midaxillary line through the pectoral and serratus anterior muscles (see Chapter 14). Blood vessels are clamped and ligated with fine silk.

2. The chest cavity is entered through the fourth intercostal space. Internal mammary vessels are exposed and ligated with silk ligatures no. 2-0, then transfixed with silk no. 2-0.

3. A median sternotomy incision is made as described in Chapter 14.

4. A small rib spreader is inserted, and the pleura is entered. The lung is retracted, using a moist pack, and the pericardium is exposed.

5. The pericardial incision is completed and cut edges sutured to drapes. Cavae

compression tapes are applied. A tape is also passed about the aorta.

6. The cannulations for perfusion are completed, and the patient is placed on total cardiopulmonary bypass, as described previously for basic open heart procedure.

7. The right atrium is incised, and the pathological defect is determined.

8. The defect is closed with a running continuous suture of no. 3-0, 4-0, or 5-0 silk, or synthetic material placed in the axis—whichever will cause less tension. Caution is exercised to prevent trapping air in the atrium by filling it with blood before the arteriotomy is completely closed with a continuous suture (Fig. 15-32). If the defect is too large for a suitable simple suture closure, a patch is fashioned to fit the opening and is sutured to the atrial wall, using four separately spaced sutures with running stitches between each one (Fig. 15-32).

For the *ostium primum* type of defect with a cleft mitral valve, repair of the *cleft* is accomplished by approximation with interrupted sutures.

9. The patient is taken off bypass, and the perfusion catheters are removed.

10. The pericardial incision is closed, leaving an opening for drainage into the right pleural cavity.

11. The pleural drainage catheters are inserted, and the chest wound is closed, as previously described. Catheters are connected to a closed drainage set. (See Chapter 14.)

12. The physiological status of the patient is determined, and any correction in blood replacement or acid-base balance is made before the patient is transferred to the recovery unit.

## Closure of ventricular septal defect (open technique)

DEFINITION. Under direct vision, utilizing extracorporeal circulation and induced intermittent cardioplegia, a congenital defect in the ventricular septum is closed by a simple suture technique or in most instances by the insertion of a synthetic

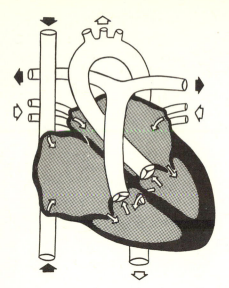

**Fig. 15-33.** Ventricular septal defects. Abnormal opening between right and left ventricles, which may vary in size and may occur in membranous or muscular portion. (From Nursing Education Service: General signs and symptoms of congenital heart abnormalities, Columbus, Ohio, 1961, Ross Laboratories.)

prosthetic patch (Figs. 15-33 and 15-34).

CONSIDERATIONS. One of the most common congenital cardiac anomalies, a ventricular septal defect, if small, is of little physiological importance (Fig. 15-33). The murmur is evident, but the patient is otherwise asymptomatic, and the heart is normal in size. At the present time, it is thought that these patients do not benefit sufficiently by surgical repair to warrant operation. Larger defects with a significant left-to-right shunt, high right ventricular pressure, increased pulmonary blood flow, and enlarged heart are selected for surgery. Patients with severe pulmonary hypertension are difficult to manage, and the operative risk is still significant.

This repair is completed through a right ventriculotomy incision. Caution is exercised in insertion of sutures to avoid damage to the conduction fibers of the bundle of His.

SETUP AND PREPARATION OF THE PATIENT; OPERATIVE PROCEDURE. As that described for repair of ventricular septal defect in the open corrective procedure for tetralogy of Fallot (Fig. 15-34).

### Pulmonary artery banding

DEFINITION. Constriction of the pulmonary artery with a tape to reduce the pulmonary artery diameter, thereby decreasing the pulmonary blood flow.

SETUP AND PREPARATION OF THE PATIENT. The patient is placed in the left lateral position (see Chapters 7 and 14). Instruments are as described for closed heart surgery, plus 8-inch pieces of various sized tapes (surgeon's preference), with appropriate sizes for children.

CONSIDERATIONS. The infant with an enlarged heart in intractable failure and a large left-to-right shunt may be treated effectively by a palliative pulmonary artery banding operation. This procedure is designed to reduce the flow of blood through the pulmonary artery to approximately one third of the existing rate. A tape is looped about the artery and secured in place by a simple suture technique. Pressures are measured by direct needle puncture before and after banding. A reduction of the distal pulmonary artery pressure by 50% to 70% is sought. Repair of the interventricular septal defect may be postponed until the child has attained sufficient growth to withstand an open heart procedure.

## OPERATIONS FOR TRICUSPID ATRESIA

GENERAL CONSIDERATIONS. Absence of communication between the right atrium and right ventricle is always accompanied by a second defect, an atrial septal defect or a patent foramen ovale, which sustains life. Other abnormalities are also present (Fig. 15-35). The infant displays cyanosis, periods of dyspnea, easy fatigability, and retardation. Congestive failure progresses rapidly. Complete corrective operations have not been developed.

Palliative operations consist of anastomotic procedures for shunting the circulation to relieve the cyanosis.

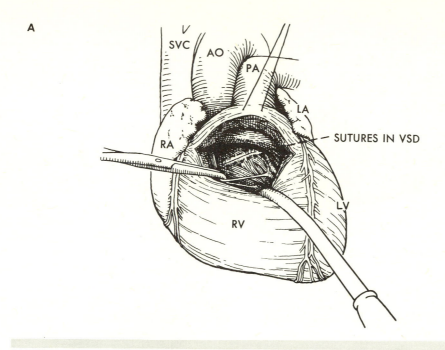

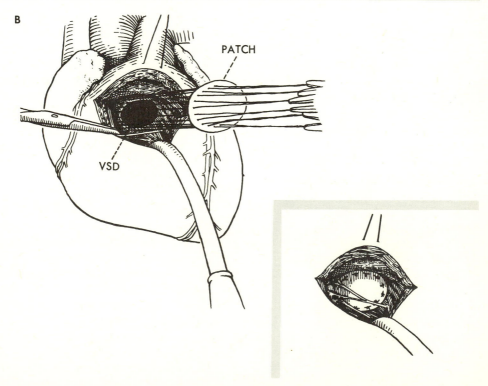

**Fig. 15-34. A,** Diagram showing closure of ventricular septal defect with interrupted sutures. **B,** Closure of defect with insertion of synthetic patch. (From Johnson, J., and Kirby, C. K.: Surgery of the chest, ed. 4, Chicago, 1970, Year Book Medical Publishers, Inc.)

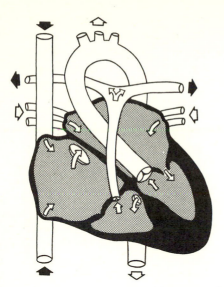

**Fig. 15-35.** Tricuspid atresia is characterized by small right ventricle, large left ventricle, and diminished pulmonary circulation. An atrial septal or other congenital defect is necessary to sustain life. (From Nursing Education Service: General signs and symptoms of congenital heart abnormalities, Columbus, Ohio, 1961, Ross Laboratories.)

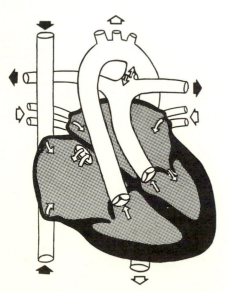

**Fig. 15-36.** Complete transposition of great vessels produces two separate circulations. Since aorta originates from right ventricle and pulmonary artery from left ventricle, abnormal communication between two chambers must be present to sustain life. (From Nursing Education Service: General signs and symptoms of congenital heart abnormalities, Columbus, Ohio, 1961, Ross Laboratories.)

## Glenn procedure

**DEFINITION.** An anastomosis is made between the superior vena cava and the right pulmonary artery to permit venous blood to bypass the right heart and go directly into the right lung.

**SETUP AND PREPARATION OF THE PATIENT.** As previously described for Blalock-Taussig anastomosis.

**OPERATIVE PROCEDURE.** As described for shunt operations.

## OPERATIONS FOR TRANSPOSITION OF THE GREAT VESSELS

**GENERAL CONSIDERATIONS.** Complete transposition of the aorta and pulmonary artery is a relatively uncommon anomaly. In this condition, the aorta arises from the right ventricle and the pulmonary artery from the left ventricle, thus producing two separate circulations (Fig. 15-36). However, to sustain life, there must be a communication between the two sides of the heart or blood vessels. This may include patent foramen ovale, patent ductus arteriosus, atrial septal defect, ventricular septal defect, or partial transposition of the pulmonary veins, which permits oxygenated blood to enter the systemic circulation.

The newborn infant with this condition is cyanotic at birth and becomes severely incapacitated with an enlarged heart, which rapidly increases and progresses to congestive failure.

*Corrective* operations for this condition are in the process of refinement and complete evaluation. The Mustard procedure is considered the most effective at present.

*Palliative* operations that tend to improve intracardiac mixing, thereby increasing the oxygen content of the systemic blood, are done to sustain life until the infant has attained sufficient growth to tolerate a long corrective procedure.

*Closed* operations that may be performed include the Blalock-Hanlon and the Baffes procedures. *Open* operation for total correction is usually performed after the first or second year of life and may be a second procedure for overcoming this

anomaly, the first having been a palliative one to sustain life.

## Blalock-Hanlon operation

DEFINITION. An opening is made between the right and left atrium at the interatrial groove.

SETUP AND PREPARATION OF THE PATIENT. Similar to shunt operations previously described.

OPERATIVE PROCEDURE

1. A right thoracotomy incision is completed, and the interatrial groove is exposed.

2. Compression tapes are placed about the right pulmonary artery and the right pulmonary veins.

3. Occlusion of these vessels is completed, and a curved Cooley clamp is applied to include a portion of both the right and left atria.

4. The segment, along with a section of the septum, is excised. The edges of the atrial walls are sutured together. Compression tapes are released.

5. Closure is completed, as previously described.

## Baffes operation

DEFINITION AND PURPOSE. This palliative procedure is designed to connect the inferior vena cava with the left atrium by means of a prosthetic tubular graft made of Teflon or Dacron and excise the right pulmonary veins from the left atrium in order to anastomose them to the right atrium. This partial correction significantly increases the oxygen content of the systemic blood.

SETUP AND PREPARATION OF THE PATIENT; OPERATIVE PROCEDURE. Similar to other shunt procedures previously described.

## Mustard operation

DEFINITION AND PURPOSE. Under direct vision and utilizing extracorporeal circulation and incisions through a median sternotomy and right atriotomy, the remaining segments of the atrial septum are excised, and a pericardial patch is sutured

in place in the atrial cavities in such a manner that the venous inflow is reversed. This permits the pulmonary venous return to be redirected into the right ventricle and the systemic venous return to be redirected into the left ventricle (Fig. 15-37).

CONSIDERATIONS. Previous creation of an atrial septal defect may serve as a first stage for this procedure. The use of the pericardial patch as a baffle permits the atrial chambers to enlarge proportionately with the growth of the child.

SETUP AND PREPARATION OF THE PATIENT. The patient is placed on the operating table in a supine position, with the chest slightly elevated (see Chapter 7). The setup is as described for open heart surgery with the median sternotomy approach. The selection of instruments must be suitable for the size of the patient and includes those listed for the closure of the atrial septal defect operation.

OPERATIVE PROCEDURE

1. A median sternotomy incision is completed.

2. A section of pericardium 2 × 3 inches is excised and placed in heparin solution.

3. Extracorporeal circulation is established after completion of cannulation of the right atrium.

4. A curved incision is made in the wall of the right atrium (Fig. 15-37, *A*).

5. The entire atrial septum is excised. The orifice of the coronary sinus is enlarged (Fig. 15-37, *B*).

6. A double-armed suture is placed three fifths of the way along the long margin of the pericardial graft (Fig. 15-37, *C*).

7. The pericardial graft or prosthetic intracardiac patch is sutured in place, excluding the coronary sinus and the left atrial appendage (Fig. 15-37, *D*).

8. An additional section of pericardium or prosthetic patch is shown in place in the wall of the right atrium that enlarges the new left atrium (Fig. 15-37, *E*).

9. Extracorporeal circulation is discontinued and closures completed in the usual manner.

## CLOSURE OF PATENT DUCTUS ARTERIOSUS

**DEFINITION.** Closure of the patent ductus arteriosus, an abnormal communication between the aorta and pulmonary artery, by ligation or by ligation and transection of the divided ends of the ductus.

**CONSIDERATIONS.** The patent ductus arteriosus is an important fetal vascular communication whereby blood is shunted in intrauterine life from the pulmonary artery into the aorta. During fetal life, the lungs are inactive and the blood is oxygenated in the placenta. Normally, the pressures

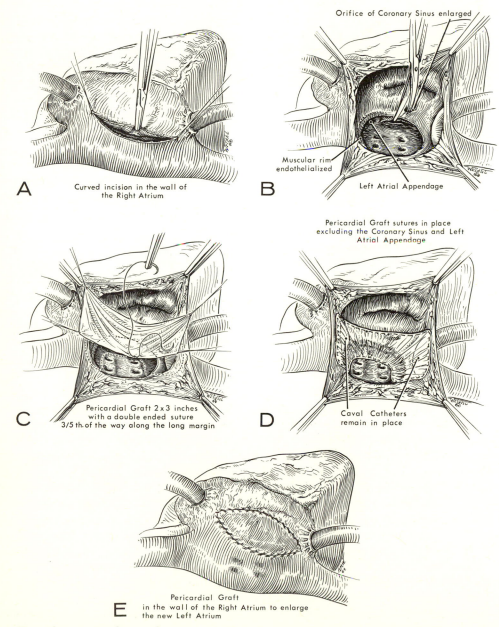

A  Curved incision in the wall of the Right Atrium

B  Orifice of Coronary Sinus enlarged
Muscular rim endothelialized
Left Atrial Appendage

C  Pericardial Graft 2 x 3 inches with a double ended suture 3/5 th. of the way along the long margin

D  Pericardial Graft sutures in place excluding the Coronary Sinus and Left Atrial Appendage
Caval Catheters remain in place

E  Pericardial Graft in the wall of the Right Atrium to enlarge the new Left Atrium

Fig. 15-37. Mustard procedure. (From Mustard, W. T., et al.: J. Thorac. Cardiovasc. Surg. 48:953, 1964.)

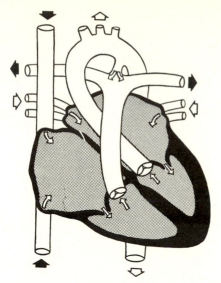

Fig. 15-38. Patent ductus arteriosus. Ductus fails to close after birth. (From Nursing Education Service: General signs and symptoms of congenital heart abnormalities, Columbus, Ohio, 1961, Ross Laboratories.)

in the systemic and pulmonary arterial circulations become equalized soon after birth, and the blood ceases to flow through the ductus. Natural changes occur, with subsequent obliteration of the lumen.

When the ductus remains patent after birth (Fig. 15-38), it creates a shunt from the aorta through the ductus into the pulmonary circulation. This increases the work of the heart and causes subsequent hypertrophy of the left atrium and ventricle. However, when persistent patency of the ductus is associated with other malformations such as tetralogy of Fallot and extreme stenosis of the pulmonary orifice, it serves as a means of maintaining life. Surgery is not performed if the patent ductus is serving in a compensatory capacity.

Many children have few symptoms because of the small size of the shunt. A frequent clinical sign associated with this disease is a harsh, continuous murmur. Since the venous blood does not escape into the systemic circulation and the blood is oxygenated, there is no cyanosis, club-

bing, or reduction in peripheral arterial oxygen saturation. However, growth is retarded in children who have a large ductus. Other symptoms may include dyspnea, palpitation, limited exercise tolerance, and cardiac failure.

SETUP AND PREPARATION OF THE PATIENT. Instruments, skin preparation, and draping procedures are as described for basic closed cardiovascular operations, with selection of appropriate equipment and supplies to suit the size of the patient, plus the following (Figs. 15-8 and 15-10):

2 Cooley curved clamps
2 Cooley straight clamps
2 Potts-Smith clamps
2 Johns Hopkins modified Potts clamps
2 Blalock clamps, small

Generally a left posterolateral approach is used; in some cases, however, a left anterolateral approach may be selected (see Chapters 7 and 14). The patient is placed in a full lateral position with the left chest uppermost.

OPERATIVE PROCEDURE

1. The incision is carried through the muscles over the fourth interspace. The chest wall is entered through the third intercostal space or bed of the fourth rib, using items as described for thoracotomy (see Chapter 14). The wound edges are protected and retracted with a Finochietto rib spreader.

2. The pleura is incised with Metzenbaum scissors, and the left lung is protected and retracted with a moist pack and a malleable retractor.

3. The mediastinal pleura is opened between the phrenic and vagus nerves over the region of the ductus. The pleura is retracted by insertion of no. 3-0 or 4-0 stay sutures. The recurrent laryngeal nerve is identified and protected. The aortic arch and pulmonary artery are dissected with fine scissors and dry dissectors. Fine arterial branches are divided and ligated, using curved Crile or mosquito hemostats and silk no. 3-0 or 4-0 ligatures and cardiac suture ligatures.

4. The pericardial membrane overlying

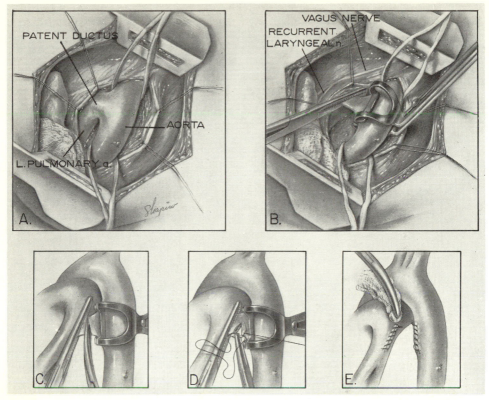

**Fig. 15-39.** Ligation and division of patent ductus arteriosus. **A,** Completed dissection and tapes in place around aorta above and below ductus arteriosus. **B,** Potts-Smith aortic clamp and ductus clamp in place. **C,** Ductus arteriosus partially divided. **D,** Closure of ductus arteriosus begun before division completed to permit better control of bleeding should one of clamps slip. **E,** Clamps removed showing completed suture lines. (From Blades, B., editor: Surgical diseases of the chest, ed. 2, St. Louis, 1966, The C. V. Mosby Co.)

the ductus is dissected free, using fine vascular forceps and scissors. Stay sutures are inserted to facilitate retraction (Fig. 15-39).

5. The adventitial layer of the ductus is dissected free. A small portion of the obscure posterior ductus is carefully freed to admit a right-angled clamp. Tapes are passed around the aorta and below the ductus.

6. Then either the suture-ligation or division method is followed.

For the *suture-ligation method,* two no. 4 silk ligatures are placed around the ductus, one near the aorta and the other near the pulmonary artery side, both of which are tied in place. Between these two liga-

tures, two transfixion sutures of no. 4-0 silk are inserted.

For the *division of the ductus method,* the patent ductus clamps are applied as close to the aorta and pulmonary artery as possible. The ductus is divided halfway through and partially sutured with mattress cardiovascular sutures no. 3-0, 4-0, or 5-0 and continued back over the free edge with an over-and-over whip suture. After both openings are sutured, a sponge is held on the area for compression while the patent ductus clamps are removed.

7. The mediastinal pleura is closed with interrupted sutures no. 3-0 or 4-0 on Atraumatic needles. The lung is reex-

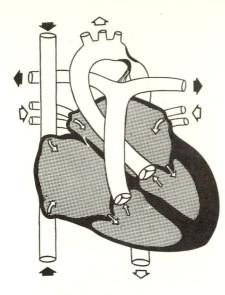

**Fig. 15-40.** Coarctation of aorta is characterized by narrow aortic lumen and exists as preductal or postductal obstruction, depending on position of obstruction in relation to ductus arteriosus. (From Nursing Education Service: General signs and symptoms of congenital heart abnormalities, Columbus, Ohio, 1961, Ross Laboratories.)

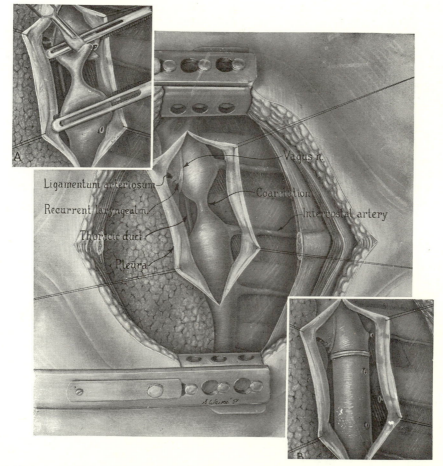

**Fig. 15-41.** Location of coarctation of aorta in mediastinal space is shown. Insets: Technique of resection. (From Moseley, H. F.: Textbook of surgery, ed. 2, St. Louis, 1955, The C. V. Mosby Co.)

panded, and a chest catheter is inserted for the establishment of closed drainage.

8. The chest wall is closed in layers as previously described, and dressings are applied.

## OPERATION FOR COARCTATION OF THE AORTA

**DEFINITION.** Through a posterolateral incision of the chest wall, the constricted segment of the aorta is excised, and an end-to-end anastomosis—with or without a graft—is performed to reestablish continuity (Fig. 15-40).

**CONSIDERATIONS.** The lesion that narrows or constricts the lumen of the aorta may be classified as *infantile* or *adult*. In the infantile type, the constriction is long and usually located in the aortic arch proximal to the junction of the aorta and ductus arteriosus. The ductus usually remains patent and may be associated with other cardiac defects (Fig. 15-41). In the adult type, the coarctation consists of a constricted area at or just distal to the junction of the aorta and the ductus, which is generally closed. This type is compatible with life for a considerable period of time.

Coarctation of the aorta (Figs. 15-40 to 15-42) is a fairly common congenital malformation, and in the adult type the patient will suffer from hypertension and complain of dyspnea, palpitation, vertigo, headache, epistaxis, and weakness. However, when the aorta is almost obstructed, hypertension will be manifested in the upper part of the body and hypotension in the lower extremities. With hypertension above the constriction the collateral blood supply, which unites the blood vessels of the shoulder, the upper extremities, and the lower extremities, increases markedly. By so doing, the intercostal vessels dilate, allowing their branches to carry blood from the subclavian arteries downward. Occasionally the vessels erode the lower margins of the ribs.

The best results of treatment are obtained when the patient is old enough to eliminate the growth factor regarding the anastomosis.

**SETUP AND PREPARATION OF THE PATIENT.** A lateral position with the left side uppermost is used (see Chapter 7). The preparation of the operative site and draping procedure are carried out as described for chest surgery (see Chapter 14). Setup is as described for basic cardiothoracic surgery, plus the following (Fig. 15-21):

> Teflon or Dacron woven or knitted vascular prosthesis, assorted sizes, to be used as necessary when primary anastomosis is not possible

**OPERATIVE PROCEDURE**

1. A left posterolateral incision is carried through the chest wall with resection of the fourth rib, as described for thoracotomy. As previously stated, the collateral blood vessels are somewhat enlarged, and bleeding may be rather profuse. Dry sponges are used throughout and weighed to determine accurate blood replacement. A Burford or Finochietto retractor is used (Fig. 15-42).

2. The pleura is incised and lung retracted, using one moist pack. The mediastinal pleura is incised over the constricted portion of the aorta. Retraction is maintained by no. 3-0 or 4-0 silk stay sutures inserted along incised edges.

3. Careful dissection with fine vascular forceps and dry dissectors is continued to mobilize the aorta and the surrounding intercostal vessels. The laryngeal nerve is identified and protected. The ductus arteriosus is ligated and divided between ductus clamps.

4. The coarctation clamps—either Potts, Glover, Gross, or straight Cooley—are applied, and the constricted segment is divided between them. A second set of clamps may be applied above and below as a safety factor in fashioning the cuffs for reapproximation (Figs. 15-41 and 15-42).

5. End-to-end anastomosis is accomplished by means of a continuous everting mattress suture of cardiovascular suture no. 5-0 for the posterior wall and interrupted everting mattress sutures for the anterior

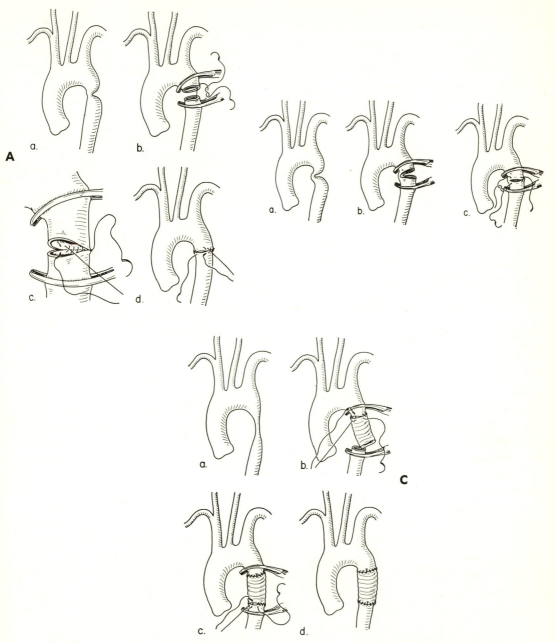

**Fig. 15-42.** Diagrams  showing coarctation of aorta—types with the methods of correction. **A,** Short narrow obstruction and steps in end-to-end anastomosis. **B,** Wedge excision with partial anastomosis completed. **C,** Segmental excision with graft replacement. (From Blades, B., editor: Surgical diseases of the chest, St. Louis, 1961, The C. V. Mosby Co.)

row. If the stricture is long, a homograft or synthetic aortic prosthesis is used to bridge the defect.

6. The clamps are released slowly, the distal one first and then the proximal. The blood pressure is noted at this time. Removal of clamps is not completed until the blood pressure is stabilized.

7. The parietal pleura is closed with no. 4-0 silk on Atraumatic needles, leaving a small opening at the lower point. Closed drainage is established, and the chest wall is closed in layers, as previously described. A dressing is applied.

## OPERATIONS ON THE MITRAL VALVE
### Commissurotomy for mitral stenosis (closed technique)

DEFINITION. Separation of the stenotic leaflets of the mitral valve.

CONSIDERATIONS. This condition, which is the most common acquired valvular lesion, is usually caused by rheumatic fever. The normal opening in the conelike valve is about 5 sq. cm. As the disease progresses, the mitral valve becomes a narrow slit in a fibrotic plaque, severely limiting blood flow into the left ventricle (Fig. 15-43). Mitral stenosis causes a rise in pressure and dilatation of the left atrium. This pressure is transmitted throughout the pulmonary vascular bed, with subsequent right ventricular hypertrophy.

The major symptoms are dyspnea, fatigue, and orthopnea. A characteristic diastolic murmur is heard, and atrial fibrillation and hemoptysis are not unusual. Embolism may result from clots in the atrial appendage. Later findings are severe pulmonary congestion and right ventricular failure.

The surgeon's selection of the open or closed method will be determined by the patient's general condition and associated pathological defect(s). For example, mitral stenosis with mitral insufficiency may be approached by the open method to accomplish complete correction.

SETUP AND PREPARATION OF THE PATIENT. As described for closed heart surgery, plus 1 set Hegar or similar dilators and 1 Gerbode or Tubbs dilator.

A supine position with the left thorax slightly elevated is used for the left anterior thoracotomy approach, or a lateral position is used for a left posterolateral thoracotomy approach. Preparation and draping is as described for cardiovascular surgery.

OPERATIVE PROCEDURE. The major steps and items used for a left lateral approach are as described in Chapter 14.

1. The pleura is opened with a knife and dissecting scissors. A small Finochietto retractor is placed, with blades over moist gauze sponges to protect the wound edges, and opened for desired exposure.

2. The phrenic nerve is protected as the pericardium is incised, using scissors and fine forceps. The pericardial silk stay sutures are placed. Free suture ends may be held with straight Halsted or mosquito clamps.

3. A thin moist gauze sponge is used, while a no. 1, 0, or 2-0 purse-string suture is placed about the base of the atrial appendage. The swaged-on needles are cut off and replaced by a Rumel rubber tourniquet.

4. A curved vascular (noncrushing) clamp is applied to the base of the appendage, and the tip of the appendage is partially amputated, using scissors and long forceps.

5. Trabeculae within the atrial appendage are divided, using a fine forceps and scissors. A second suction is connected.

6. Superficial thrombi, if present, are removed, and flushing is accomplished by momentary release of the clamp and saline solution irrigation.

Allis clamps are applied to the cut edges of the appendage.

7. The appendage traction clamps are elevated, the purse-string sutures are held taut, the surgeon introduces his finger into the atrium, and the curved vascular clamp

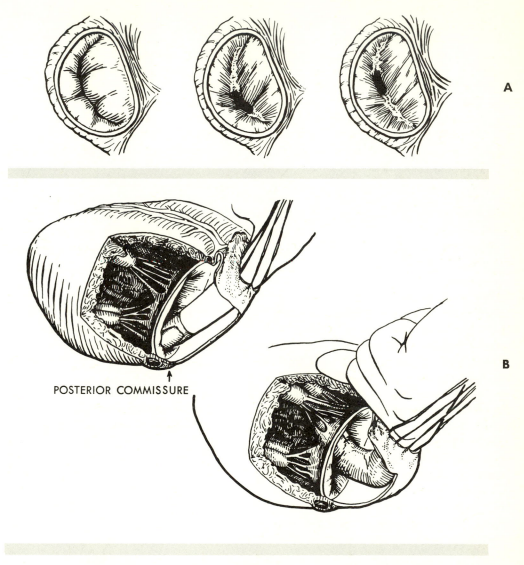

POSTERIOR COMMISSURE

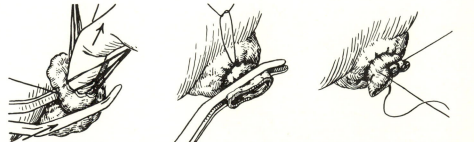

A

B

C

Fig. 15-43. A, Diagram of normal mitral valve at left; fusion and thickening of valve leaflets at center and right. B, Finger fracture of valve. C, Closure of atrial appendage. (From Johnson, J., and Kirby, C. K.: Surgery of the chest, ed. 4, Chicago, 1970, Year Book Medical Publishers, Inc.)

is slowly released. The clamp is kept on the field for reapplication if necessary.

8. The pathological condition is noted as the valve is explored. The calcified leaflets are fractured by finger pressure, first laterally, and then medially (Fig. 14-43).

9. Another method of separating the leaflets is done by a *retrograde procedure.* A purse-string suture with felt pledget attached is placed, and a ventriculotomy is made, using a no. 11 scalpel. A series of smooth metal dilators are introduced, beginning with size no. 3 and continuing through size no. 6. The Hegar type may be used. The Gerbode or Tubbs valve dilator is introduced, the tips of which are guided in place by the right index finger in the left atrium. The blades are adjusted to the desired opening, and dilation (fracture) of the valve is completed. The instrument is removed and the purse-string suture secured. Additional fine sutures with felt are used to complete hemostasis.

10. The finger is removed, and the atrial purse-string suture is tied (Fig. 15-43). The appendage is closed with cardiovascular suture no. 2-0, 3-0, or 4-0 after removal of stay sutures.

11. A pleural cavity drainage catheter is inserted through the stab wound in the lateral interspace and anchored to the skin with silk sutures.

12. The chest catheter is connected to a closed water-seal drainage system.

13. Closure of the chest is accomplished, as previously described. Dressings are applied.

### Open technique

**GENERAL CONSIDERATIONS.** Indications for open corrective procedures on the mitral valve may include previous operation, recurrent stenosis, calcification, insufficiency, atrial thrombosis, or pathological condition of other valves. The operations other than separation of stenotic leaflets may include plication of the mitral annulus for insufficiency, repair of chordae tendineae or papillary muscle, or total excision of the

valve and replacement with a ball-valve or disk-type prosthesis.

### *Mitral valve replacement with insertion of ball-valve prosthesis*

**DEFINITION.** Under direct vision and utilizing extracorporeal circulation, mild hypothermia, and incisions through a left atriotomy, the damaged leaflets of the mitral valve are excised and replaced with a ball-valve or disk-type mitral prosthesis.

**CONSIDERATIONS.** This procedure is usually performed when the pathological condition is complicated by combined stenosis and insufficiency and the valve is calcified, rigid, and deficient.

**SETUP AND PREPARATION OF THE PATIENT.** The patient may be placed in a right anterolateral position and rolled back somewhat to expose the groin, or a supine position for median sternotomy may also be used. The setup is as described for open heart procedures, plus the following:

1 Wire coil
6 Benders
2 Cooley atrial retractors
3 Favaloro atrial retractors (various sizes)
1 Complete set of Starr-Edwards mitral ball-valve prostheses, sizers, and holders (Figs. 15-14 and 15-16)
1 Complete set of Beall mitral valves, sizers, and holders (Figs. 15-14 and 15-16)
3 Masson-type needle holders, heavy, 14 in.
1 Special valve scissors (surgeon's preference)
1 Plain gauze packing, ½ × 1 in.
1 Foley catheter

**OPERATIVE PROCEDURE**

1. The thoracotomy incision is made starting below the vertebral border of the scapula following the course of the fifth rib and continuing downward and anteriorly almost to the midline; muscle layers are divided; and the fifth rib is resected, followed by hemostasis with electrocoagulation and silk ligatures (see Chapter 14).

2. The groin incision is completed for cannulation of the femoral artery by a second surgical team, as described for general open heart procedures.

3. The pump-oxygenator team is com-

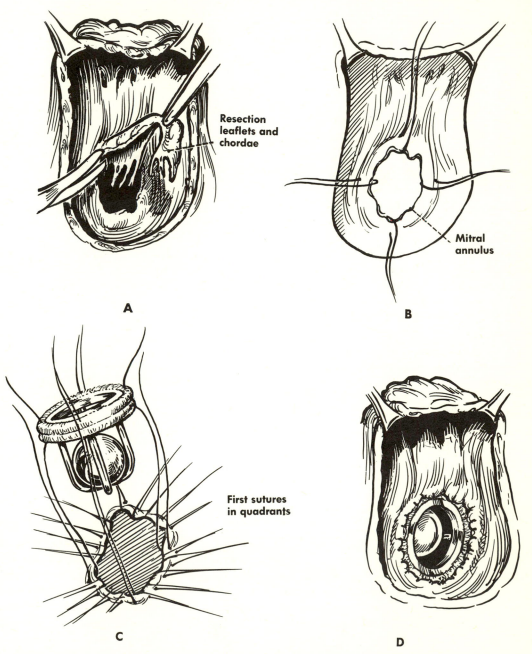

**Fig. 15-44.** Mitral valve replacement. **A,** Diagram showing resection of leaflets and chordae. **B,** Mitral annulus with quadrant sutures in place. **C,** Suturing Starr-Edwards prosthesis in place. **D,** Appearance of valve after sutures have been tied and cut. (From Julian, O. C., Dye, W. S., Hushang, D., and Hunter, J. A.: Cardiovascular surgery, Chicago, 1962, Year Book Medical Publishers, Inc.)

pleting the preparation for bypass as the pleural cavity is opened.

4. The ribs are retracted with a Finochietto or Burford-type retractor. The cavity is inspected, and adhesions are freed as indicated. A suction set is connected.

5. The pericardium is opened anterior and parallel to the phrenic nerve. Adhesions are freed, and pericardial stay sutures are inserted and attached to the drapes in the usual manner.

6. The caval and femoral cannulations are completed. The patient is heparinized, and all connections are made. The patient is placed on total bypass as the perfusion rate is adjusted. Mild hypothermia (32° C.) is produced.

7. The left atrium is incised, blood is suctioned away, and the incision is enlarged to expose the mitral valve, as shown in Fig. 15-44.

8. The pathological condition is determined, and the excision of the valve leaflets is completed with division of papillary muscles and chordae tendineae (Fig. 15-44, A and B). Selection of the cutting instrument will depend on the degree of calcification present and the method of excision. A small margin of the valve is retained in place for insertion of fixation sutures to the valve. The ventricle is inspected, and all loose debris is removed.

9. The valve sizer is temporarily placed to determine the correct size of the prosthesis.

10. Synthetic sutures no. 0 (about twenty) are first placed in the retained margin of the valve with the ends held by a wire coil to prevent tangling or tagged with mosquito clamps, which are placed on Beuller holders, and then inserted into the Teflon ring of the prosthesis.

11. The sutures are held taut as the prosthesis is guided into position and secured. Tying is completed, additional sutures are added as needed, and loose ends are cut off. The valve is kept incompetent with a Foley catheter to avoid air embolism.

12. Additional continuous sutures are used to close the atriotomy. The catheter

is retained in place as the atrium is permitted to fill with blood. The patient is placed in a reverse Trendelenburg position. Air aspiration of the left ventricle is completed through a no. 9 needle, the catheter is removed, and the atrial closure is completed.

13. Proper functioning of the valve is noted. The patient is rewarmed and taken off bypass. Cannulae are removed in the usual manner. Pressures are recorded and hemodynamic changes noted.

14. Protamine sulfate, a heparin antagonist, is given.

15. Hemostasis is controlled, and the pericardium is closed loosely to provide small openings for drainage.

16. Pleural drainage catheters are brought out through stab wounds in the lower intercostal spaces. Chest catheters are connected to a closed drainage system.

17. Chest and groin incisions are closed as previously described. Dressings are applied.

18. The patient's general condition is evaluated; corrections in blood loss, acidosis, and so forth are made before transfer to the recovery room.

## OPERATION ON THE AORTIC VALVE (OPEN TECHNIQUE)

GENERAL CONSIDERATIONS. Restriction of left ventricular outflow is usually caused by valvular stenosis in which the valve leaflets are fused together, resulting in a restriction in the valve opening that reduces the blood flow through the orifice. Restriction caused by subvalvular and supravalvular stenosis is very rare.

Aortic valvular stenosis may be of congenital origin, but it is more frequently an acquired lesion due to complications of rheumatic fever. Extensive fibrosis and heavily calcified deposits make it difficult to release the fused leaflets and restore normal function (Fig. 15-45).

In most patients, symptoms are not evident in early life. Fatigue and dyspnea on exertion are prominent symptoms that may not appear until the late teens. Late find-

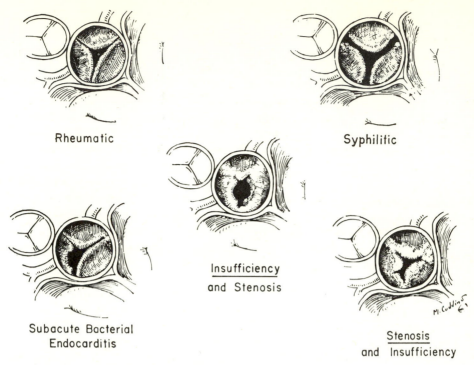

**Fig. 15-45.** Diagram showing pathological patterns of aortic insufficiency. (From Blades, B., editor: Surgical diseases of the chest, ed. 2, St. Louis, 1966, The C. V. Mosby Co.)

ings of angina pectoris, syncope, and congestive failure attributable to aortic stenosis present a grave prognosis. Sudden death is not uncommon.

A systolic aortic murmur is present, and electrocardiograms and catheterization studies reveal left ventricular hypertrophy and varying pressure gradients across the aortic valve. Surgical procedures are designed to improve valvular function, which may be accomplished by meticulous separation of the commissures, repair of individual leaflets, or total excision of the valve and replacement with a prosthesis (Figs. 15-45 and 15-46).

The open technique is the most satisfactory approach to these corrections, and the open procedure for aortic valvulotomy will be described.

## Aortic valvulotomy; aortic valve replacement (open technique)

**DEFINITION.** Under direct vision and utilizing extracorporeal circulation and moder-

ate hypothermia, the fused commissures of the aortic valve are meticulously separated in an effort to restore normal valvular function, or the valve may be excised and replaced by a prosthetic valve.

**SETUP AND PREPARATION OF THE PATIENT.** The patient is placed on the operating table in a supine position. Skin preparation of the anterior thorax for a median sternotomy incision and of the lower abdomen and upper thighs for groin incisions is completed, and the patient is properly draped. The instrument setup is as described for open heart surgery, with a median sternotomy incision, plus the following:

1 Wire coil
6 Benders
1 Ablaza aortic retractor
2 Cooley aortic retractors
1 Special valve scissors (surgeon's preference)
4 Bailey aortic valve rongeurs, assorted sizes
   Complete set of aortic valves, sizers, and holders (Figs. 15-15 and 15-16)
1 Plain gauze packing, ½ × 1 in.
1 Foley catheter

2 complete sets coronary artery perfusion cannulae, surgeon's preference
1 Fibrillator cord

**OPERATIVE PROCEDURE** ( Fig. 15-47 )

1. The pericardium is exposed through a median sternotomy incision while femoral arteries are being cannulated, as described for basic open heart procedure.

2. The pericardium is incised and edges sutured to wound margins. The cavae are prepared for cannulation, pulmonary artery and aorta are prepared for compression and cross clamping. A venting catheter is placed in the left atrium through the right pulmonary vein or through a stab wound in the left ventricle.

3. Pump-oxygenator preparations are completed, and the patient is placed on total bypass.

4. Selective cooling of the heart is begun. The left atrium is vented as the aorta is cross clamped.

5. A transverse aortotomy is completed, and coronary ostia are identified and cannulated for perfusion and selective cooling of the heart.

6A. The valve is inspected, and the extent of the pathological defect is confirmed. Separation of the commissures is completed by sharp dissection, as indicated. Calcium deposits are removed as carefully as pos-

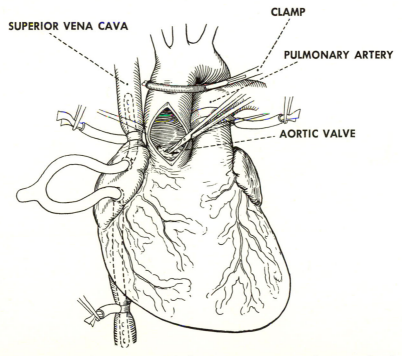

**Fig. 15-46.** Technique of open aortic valvulotomy. Scissors are used to open fused commissures. Compression tapes are shown around both cavae and pulmonary artery. Aorta is cross clamped. (From Holswade, G. R., and Arditi, L. I.: Surg. Clin. North Am. **41:**463, 1961.)

**Fig. 15-47.** Technique of aortic valve replacement. **A,** Incision. **B,** Cannulation and aortotomy. **C,** Total excision of valve. **D** and **E,** Valve being sutured in position. **F,** Ivalon collar inserted to cover suture line. **G,** Closure of aortotomy after ball replaced. Coronary perfusion cannulae removed just prior to final closure. (From Blades, B., editor: Surgical diseases of the chest, ed. 2, St. Louis, 1966, The C. V. Mosby Co.)

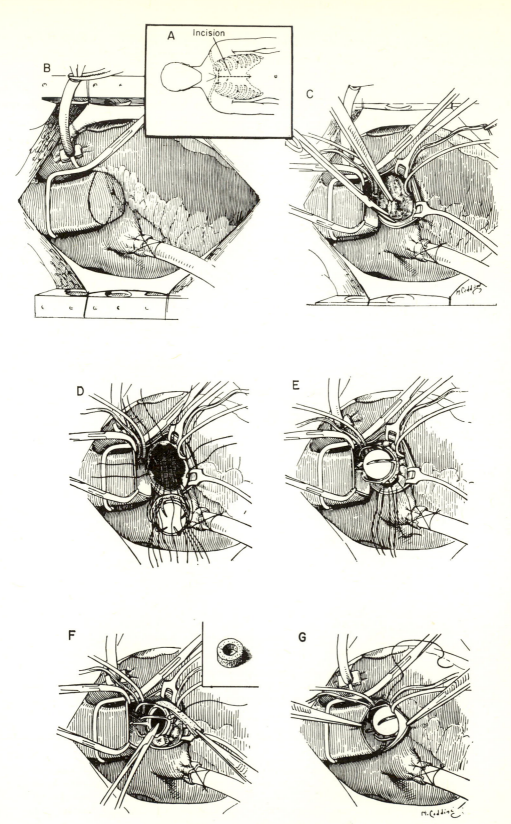

**Fig. 15-47.** For legend see opposite page.

sible to prevent damage to underlying structures and permit mobilization of the leaflets. Narrow packing may be used to confine small, loose, calcified fragments.

6B. The valve is inspected; the pathological condition is confirmed. Total excision of the valve is completed. (Total replacement is usually the method of choice.) The correct prosthesis is selected. Insertion is completed, using technique similar to that previously described for mitral valve replacement.

7. The left heart is flushed to remove air, and the aortotomy is closed with cardiovascular suture no. 4-0. The aortic clamp is removed, and rewarming of the heart is begun.

8. Defibrillation is accomplished, as indicated.

9. The venting catheter is removed from the left atrium or ventricle. Cavae compression tapes are released.

10. When the heart is rewarmed, action is competent, and the perfusion rate is adjusted, the patient is taken off bypass.

11. Cavae cannulae are removed and incisions closed, as previously described.

12. Pressures in the left ventricle and aorta may be recorded to determine valve competency.

13. The femoral cannula is removed and the incision closed, as previously described.

14. The pericardium is closed, leaving a small opening for drainage into the right pleural cavity.

15. Two drainage catheters are placed in the right pleural cavity and one in the mediastinum, as previously described. All are exteriorized through stab wounds and secured. Connections are completed to a closed drainage system.

16. The sternal incision is closed, as described in the basic procedure. Dressings are applied.

17. The physiological status of the patient is determined, with any correction in blood replacement and acid-base balance completed before transfer to the recovery unit.

## OPERATIONS FOR OCCLUSIVE DISEASE OF THE THORACIC AORTA

GENERAL CONSIDERATIONS. Obliterative arterial disease is highly significant as a common cause of death for the patient in the middle or older age group. Two important acquired pathological conditions may be found, together or separately. The term *atherosclerosis* refers to the deposition of lipid material confined to local areas of the intima. *Arteriosclerosis* is defined as a thickening of the arterial wall, with fibrosis and calcification of the medial coat. Further degeneration and destruction may lead to aneurysm formation. Any artery may become involved. Surgical intervention becomes necessary when the presenting symptoms indicate a compromise in circulation or danger of perforation of an aneurysm.

Aneurysms may be caused by atherosclerosis and arteriosclerosis, trauma, or infection. The congenital type is relatively uncommon and usually associated with other anomalies. Pathologically, aneurysms may be classified as true or false. The true type usually results from a weakness in the arterial wall, and the sac includes one or all the layers of the artery. The false type usually results from trauma with development of a hematoma, which increases in size and eventually becomes a well-organized, pulsating blood clot within the arterial wall.

Aneurysms are also categorized morphologically as follows: (1) saccular—a sac-type formation with a narrowed neck projecting from the side of the artery, (2) fusiform—a spindle-shaped formation with complete circumferential involvement of the artery, and (3) dissecting—a splitting of the intima of the aorta, permitting blood to pass in between the layers of the wall to form a false channel; as the channel extends and enlarges, the blood flow is obstructed, with a consequent perforation.

Surgical treatment is directed toward restoration or reconstruction of the affected artery to maintain its proper function. This may be accomplished by end-

arterectomy to remove fibrotic materials, with resulting restoration of normal function; excision of constricting lesions; and excision of aneurysms that may or may not require additional materials for reconstruction.

Continuity may be reestablished by a primary closure, an end-to-end or end-to-side anastomosis, or insertion of a vascular graft or synthetic prosthesis. In some patients for whom total excision of the obstructive lesion might endanger other vital organs, the surgeon may elect to substitute a bypass graft to maintain functional continuity.

The location of the lesion will determine the necessary adjuncts to the operative procedure. For example, extracorporeal circulation, temporary shunt, or hypothermia may be employed.

The external shunt may be a permanent prosthesis sutured to the aorta proximal and distal to the aneurysm, or the shunt may be removed after a second permanent prosthesis has been sutured in place in the normal aortic bed. With the use of cardiopulmonary bypass, it is now possible to excise aneurysms in any portion of the aorta.

SETUP AND PREPARATION OF THE PATIENT. The type of incision is dependent on the operative approach. The setup is as described for closed heart or open heart surgery, depending on the surgeon's operative approach, plus available assorted sizes of grafts and shunt devices.

OPERATIVE PROCEDURE. Several methods of surgical treatment are available, including thromboendarterectomy, excision with replacement and bypass.

Thromboendarterectomy is used for any well-localized, short obstruction that can be removed easily.

Graft replacement is used for a localized obstruction of a vessel when the continuity of the vessel is altered.

Bypass replacement may be used in a variety of procedures. It is helpful when there is widespread occlusion or long areas of stenosis.

# OPERATIONS FOR REVASCULARIZATION OF THE CORONARY ARTERIES

CONSIDERATIONS. The surgical treatment of coronary heart disease up to the present time has had limited popularity. However, moderate success has been reported by various surgical teams in performing myocardial implantation of the internal mammary artery and saphenous vein graft and the coronary endarterectomy. These operations are designed to improve the blood supply to the myocardium.

SETUP AND PREPARATION OF THE PATIENT. The patient is placed in a supine position. Skin preparation of the thorax, lower abdomen, upper thighs, and circumference of both legs is completed, depending on chosen operative procedure. The patient is properly draped. The instrument setup is as described for open heart surgery, plus the following fine microsurgical instruments (Fig. 15-48):

2 Microscissors, curved and straight
6 Microneedle holders
4 Microvascular forceps
4 Vascular dilators, varied sizes
6 Bulldog clamps, smooth and very small
2 Edwards spring clips

OPERATIVE PROCEDURES

MYOCARDIAL IMPLANTATION OF SAPHENOUS VEIN GRAFTS. The saphenous vein is used as a bypass graft connecting the aortic root with the distal coronary artery. The surgical approach is through a median sternotomy incision, and the usual preparations for extracorporeal circulation are undertaken. A segment of the saphenous vein is also taken prior to cannulation and placed in heparinized normal saline. A bulldog clamp is placed on the distal end of the graft for identification so that the graft will not be placed in reverse position, in which case its valves might obstruct coronary flow. The saphenous vein is measured for appropriate length, and the proximal end of the graft is sutured into the aorta. The distal end of the graft is clamped with an Edwards clip after the aortic anastomosis has been completed. The heart is put on

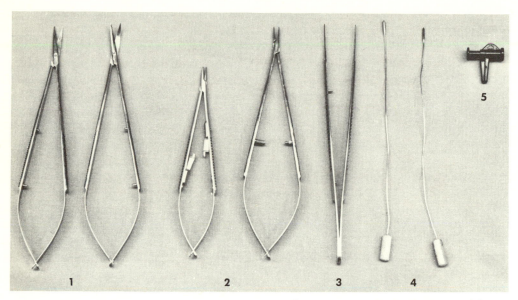

**Fig. 15-48.** Microsurgical instruments: **1,** Straight and curved microscissors; **2,** short and long microneedle holders; **3,** microforceps; **4,** vascular dilators; **5,** Edwards spring clip.

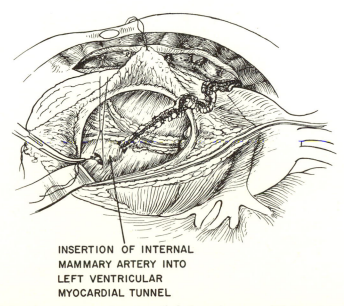

INSERTION OF INTERNAL
MAMMARY ARTERY INTO
LEFT VENTRICULAR
MYOCARDIAL TUNNEL

**Fig. 15-49.** Internal mammary artery is pulled through myocardial tunnel in left ventricle. (From Longmire, W. P., Jr.: In Gibbon, J. H., Jr., editor: Surgery of the chest, Philadelphia, 1962, W. B. Saunders Co.)

bypass circulation. The aorta is cross clamped at 10-minute intervals. The distal coronary artery is then transected distally to the occluded site; the vessel may be dissected laterally until the optimal entrance into the lumen is achieved. The distal anastomosis is made with very fine cardiovascular Teflon sutures and tagged with very small bulldog clamps. After the distal anastomosis has been completed, the Edwards clip and aortic cross clamp can be removed. The anastomoses sites are checked for hemostasis. Extracorporeal circulation is discontinued, and closure of the incision is carried out as previously described.

MYOCARDIAL IMPLANTATION OF INTERNAL MAMMARY ARTERY. Through a left thoracic incision the internal mammary artery is mobilized from the fourth to the sixth intercostal space. Ligation and division is completed at the distal end. The pericardial fat is elevated, and a section of the pericardium is excised. A small tunnel is prepared in the left ventricular myocardium to accept the free end of the mammary artery, which is sutured into place. The exposed area of the myocardium is covered with a pericardial fat pad. Pleural drainage is established, and the chest is closed in the usual manner (Fig. 15-49).

CORONARY ENDARTERECTOMY. Through a median sternotomy, the pericardium is opened, and the diseased coronary vessels are evaluated. The vessel selected for endarterectomy is isolated for operation by proximal and distal placement of silk ligatures. Incision is completed through all vessel layers. A cleavage plane is developed between the media and thickened intima, using a thin spatula-type elevator. As the

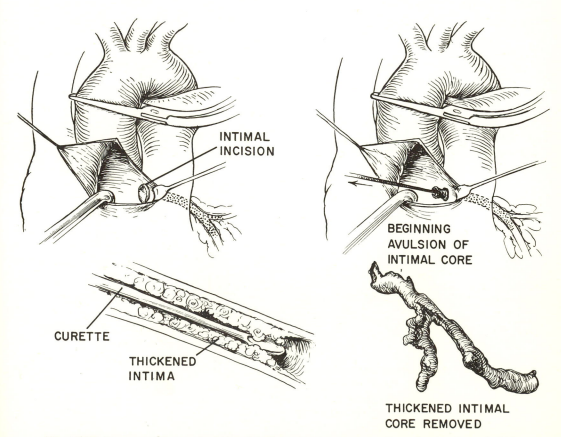

**Fig. 15-50.** Diagram showing incision of intima about coronary ostia and extraction of thickened intimal core with curette. (From Longmire, W. P., Jr.: In Gibbon, J. H., Jr., editor: Surgery of the chest, Philadelphia, 1962, W. B. Saunders Co.)

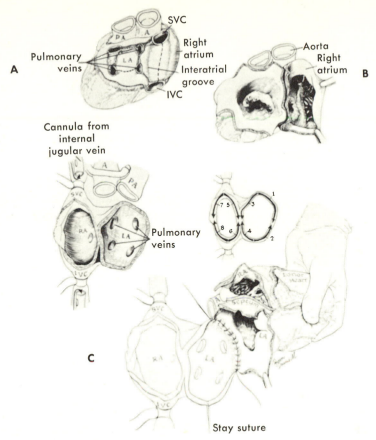

**Fig. 15-51.** Heart transplant, human-sternal incision. **A,** Donor heart. **B,** Recipient. **C,** Suturing. (From Gibbon, J. H., Jr., Sabiston, D., Jr., and Spencer, F., editors: Surgery of the chest, Philadelphia, 1969, W. B. Saunders Co.)

separation is continued, a small stripper may be introduced to aid in the removal of the thickened diseased intima (Fig. 15-50). Heparin solution may be injected for irrigation. The arteriotomy is closed with cardiovascular Teflon suture no. 6-0. When the right or left coronary artery near the aortic ostia is involved, extracorporeal circulation is utilized and the patent coronary artery perfused while the endarterectomy is performed directly through the aorta. Pleural drainage is established, and the chest wound is closed in the usual manner.

## PULMONARY EMBOLECTOMY

**DEFINITION.** The pulmonary artery is opened and the emboli removed.

**SETUP AND PREPARATION OF THE PATIENT.** The supine position is used, and the preparation of the operative site and draping are carried out as described previously. The ideal method for performance of pulmonary embolectomy is the use of cardiopulmonary bypass. Setup is as described for open heart procedures.

**OPERATIVE PROCEDURE.** The patient is placed on cardiopulmonary bypass as an emergency procedure. The aorta is cross clamped, the pulmonary artery is opened, and the emboli are removed. The artery is then closed with cardiovascular Teflon suture no. 5-0. The aortic clamp is removed. Extracorporeal bypass is discontinued, and the incisions are closed as described previously.

# HEART TRANSPLANTATION
(Fig. 15-51)

CONSIDERATIONS. Cardiac transplantation is now a clinical reality; its therapeutic value will be tested by the passage of time. Transplantation of the heart has been surgically feasible since 1960, when the essence of the surgical method was propounded. The important restrictions of the immune reaction and recipient selection remain.

SETUP AND PREPARATION OF THE PATIENT. Two individual cardiopulmonary bypass and instrument setups are necessary. The preparation of the operative site and routine draping procedures are carried out as described earlier for open heart procedures.

OPERATIVE PROCEDURE

DONOR HEART. Resuscitation of the donor heart is mandatory before proceeding with the recipient. The donor is placed on extracorporeal circulation, as soon after pronouncement of death as possible. The heart is emptied by constricting the venae cavae. The aorta and pulmonary artery are clamped with a noncrushing clamp. The venae cavae and pulmonary veins are dissected and transected individually where they enter the atrium. The atrial septum is then divided, the pulmonary artery is transected distal to the valvular commissure, and the aorta is transected distal to the coronary ostia. The donor heart is immediately placed in cold saline solution.

RECIPIENT HEART. The recipient's heart is placed on extracorporeal bypass. Peripheral venous cannulation of the venae cavae is achieved by means of the right internal jugular and left saphenous veins. This is extremely helpful because of the complete absence of tubing and catheters in the operative field. The intrapericardial venae cavae are looped by means of tapes, and occlusion is effected with rubber tourniquets. The pulmonary trunk and aorta are dissected immediately above their respective semilunar valves; the atria are incised in such a way as to leave intact portions of the right and left atrial walls and

the atrial septum of the recipient. The recipient heart is then removed.

The donor heart is removed from the vehicle of transport and placed in the pericardial well. After sutures at each end of the left atrial cavity of the recipient have been united to the extent of the left atrium of the donor, a simple over-and-over suture is utilized for joining, first, the left atria and, second, the right atria. A small catheter is placed in the left atrial appendage of the donor heart after the inflow tracts have been united, and cold saline is used to fill the left side of the heart and expel all air that has been trapped in the pulmonary veins of the host, as well as that in the combined left atrium and donor left ventricle. The aorta is sutured easily.

The aortic clamp is removed, and a bulldog clamp is placed across the donor pulmonary artery. The caval tape is removed, and vigorous ventricular fibrillation of the donor heart commences. Local cooling of the heart is discontinued at this point, and, before suturing the pulmonary artery, all atrial suture lines are carefully inspected for significant bleeding areas. The pulmonary arteries are united and the bulldog clamp removed. Defibrillation of the ventricles is usually effected by means of a single D.C. shock. A needle hole is established at the apex of the ascending aorta, so that residual air is expelled. The patient is then removed from extracorporeal bypass after some 15 to 20 minutes of partial bypass. The decannulated internal jugular vein can be either sutured or ligated. The decannulated saphenous vein is ligated at its femoral junction. The incisions are closed as described previously.

# INSERTION OF IMPLANTABLE PACEMAKER

DEFINITION. Two separate incisions, one in the left upper quadrant of the abdomen and the other in the left anterior thorax, made to expose the heart, are joined by a connecting subcutaneous tunnel. The battery portion of the pacemaker

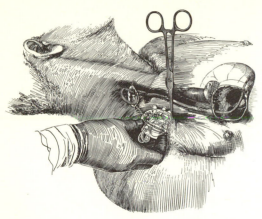

Fig. 15-52. Method of implantation of transvenous pacemaker. (Courtesy Medtronic, Inc., Minneapolis, Minn.)

is implanted in the subcutaneous "pocket" in the abdominal wound. The attached wire electrodes are channeled through the prepared tunnel into the thoracotomy wound, and the special electrode tips are sutured in place in the myocardium.

Patients who are not suitable candidates for an open thoracotomy or general anesthesia may be selected for the subcutaneous implantation of the pulse generator (pacer) and the positioning of an endocardial electrode via the right external jugular vein (Fig. 15-52). Local anesthesia and fluoroscopy are utilized. Specific directions are supplied with each pacemaker unit.

CONSIDERATIONS. An electrical pacemaker is utilized for treatment of complete heart block when the patient fails to respond to drug therapy. Coronary arteriosclerosis and rheumatic heart disease are common causes; however, during open heart surgical repair of certain septal defects, damage to the conducting bundle may produce heart block (Fig. 15-53).

Indirect stimulation may be produced by application of the electrodes to the chest wall and their connection to an external pacemaker.

Direct stimulation is possible when special electrode tips are inserted into the myocardium. The leads are exteriorized

through the chest wall and attached to the external electrical stimulus for the desired intermittent electrical response.

For long-term treatment, a small lightweight battery-type pacemaker has been developed for actual implantation (Fig. 15-54). The overall construction has been meticulously designed to resist wear, as well as the penetration of body fluids. These units have been carefully researched to ensure continuous function for several years.

SETUP AND PREPARATION OF THE PATIENT. A supine position is used. Prior to induction, all preparations are completed for the continuous electrocardiographic monitoring. The pacemaker electrodes are attached to the patient's chest, and the connections are made ready for instant pacing. The cardiologist prescribes the specific emergency medications to be administered.

The skin preparation and draping are completed for a left anterior thoracotomy and a left upper quadrant transverse incision.

The setup is as previously described for closed heart surgery, with retractors for the anterior thoracotomy approach, plus the following:

1 Sterile pacemaker with electrodes for implantation
1 Battery-operated pacemaker with 2 sterile leads, for temporary use only
1 D.C. defibrillator set, for standby
1 Hemovac drainage set, for abdominal wound (optional)

OPERATIVE PROCEDURE

1. A left anterior thoracotomy incision is made through the fourth or fifth interspace or through the bed of the resected fifth rib, as previously described.

2. A medium Finochietto retractor is placed to provide access to the left ventricular myocardium. The pericardium is incised in the usual manner.

3. If necessary, the temporary pacemaking may now be continued by direct stimulation. An external battery-driven pacemaker with two sterile lead wires is used.

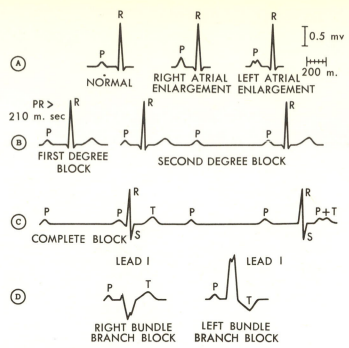

Fig. 15-53. Diagram showing conduction disturbances. (From Bullard, R. W.: In Selkurt, E. E., editor: Physiology, Boston, 1963, Little, Brown & Co.)

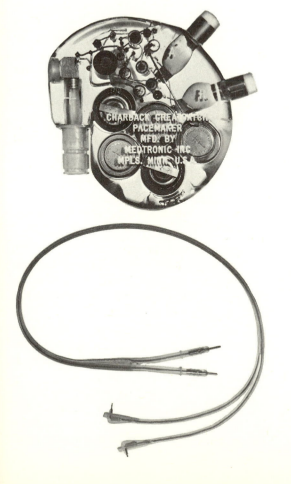

Fig. 15-54. Chardack-Greatbatch adjustable rate/current implantable pacemaker with electrodes. Chardack helical coil spring electrode consists of a platinum-iridium coil spring that moves freely within its insulating Silastic sleeve and terminates as electrode tip in myocardium. (Courtesy Medtronic, Inc., Minneapolis, Minn.)

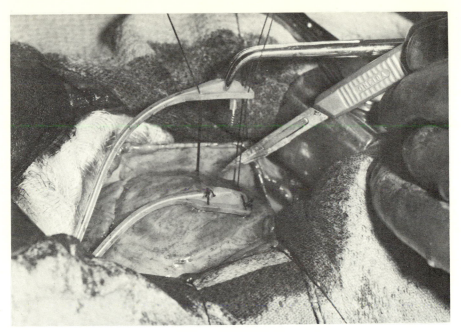

**Fig. 15-55.** Placement of sutures and method of fixation of electrodes on ventricular myocardium. (Courtesy Medtronic, Inc., Minneapolis, Minn.)

*Battery-powered* equipment must be used to eliminate hazardous circulating ground currents. One lead wire is attached to an instrument such as a rib spreader, which is in contact with the tissue. The second lead wire is attached to a hemostat, which permits the surgeon to initiate the stimulus by lightly touching the myocardium.

4. A transverse incision is now completed in the left upper quadrant. A subcutaneous pocket of sufficient size is developed to house the battery portion of the pacemaker.

5. A subcutaneous tunnel between the abdominal and thoracic incisions is made, using blunt dissection.

6. The pacemaker is implanted by placing the battery in the prepared abdominal pocket. The lead wires with special tips are carefully channeled through the tunnel to the thoracic wound.

7. The electrode tips are inserted into small stab wounds in the myocardium, utilizing cardiovascular double-armed sutures for fixation (Fig. 15-55). The procedure for the precise method of insertion

furnished by the manufacturer has been prepared by surgical research teams and provides meticulous detailed instructions for obtaining the best results. (CAUTION: If the patient is attached to a completely external pacemaker, it should be disconnected prior to the insertion of the second electrode tip.)

8. A pleural drainage tube is inserted, and the chest is closed in the usual manner. Closed drainage is established.

9. The abdominal incision may be drained with a Hemovac catheter. Closure is completed, and dressings are applied.

**REFERENCES**

1. Adams, F. H., and Hall, V. E.: Pathophysiology of congenital heart disease, Berkeley, Calif., 1970, University of California Press.
2. Advancing with surgery, vols. 1 and 2, Somerville, N. J., Ethicon, Inc.
3. Anthony, C. P.: Textbook of anatomy and physiology, ed. 8, St. Louis, 1971, The C. V. Mosby Co.
4. Artusio, J. F., and Mazzia, V. D. B.: Practical anesthesiology, St. Louis, 1962, The C. V. Mosby Co.
5. Bailey, C. P., editor: Cardiac surgery, Davis

Monograph Series, Philadelphia, 1960, F. A. Davis Co.

6. Barker, W. F., editor: Surgical treatment of peripheral vascular disease, New York, 1962, Blakiston Division, McGraw-Hill Book Co.

7. Blades, B., editor: Surgical diseases of the chest, ed. 2, St. Louis, 1966, The C. V. Mosby Co.

8. Brantigan, O. C.: Clinical anatomy, New York, 1963, Blakiston Division, McGraw-Hill Book Co.

9. Brest, A. N.: Heart substitutes, Springfield, Ill., 1966, Charles C Thomas, Publisher.

10. Brewer, L. A., III: Prosthetic heart valves, Springfield, Ill., 1968, Charles C Thomas, Publisher.

11. Burford, T., and Ferguson, T.: Cardiovascular surgery: current practice, St. Louis, 1969, The C. V. Mosby Co.

12. Clowes, G. H., Jr.: Acid-base balance during and after cardiopulmonary bypass procedures, Am. J. Cardiol. **12:**671, 1963.

13. Connolly, D. C., and Burchell, H. B.: Pericarditis: a ten year survey, Am. J. Cardiol. **7:**7, 1961.

14. Crane, C.: The choice of shunt procedure for cirrhotic patients with variceal bleeding, ascites, and hypersplenism, Surg. Gynecol. Obstet. **115:**15, 1962.

15. DeWall, R. A., and Lillehei, R. C.: Perfusions for open-heart surgery requiring only 5 per cent dextrose in water for pump priming, Surg. Clin. North Am. **44:**253, 1964.

16. Effler, D. B.: Chronic constrictive pericarditis treated with pericardiectomy, Am. J. Cardiol. **7:**62, 1961.

17. Ellis, F. H., Jr.: Surgery for acquired mitral valve disease, Philadelphia, 1967, W. B. Saunders Co.

18. Ellis, H.: Anatomy for anesthetists, Oxford, England, 1962, Blackwell Scientific Publications.

19. Erlanger, H.: Cardiac arrhythmias in relationship to anesthesia: past and present concepts, Am. J. Med. Sci. **243:**651, 1962.

20. Favaloro, R. G., and Effler, D.: Surgical treatment of coronary arteriosclerosis, Baltimore, 1970, The Williams & Wilkins Co.

21. Ferguson, D. J., and Ranniger, K.: Portography in portal hypertension, Surg. Clin. North Am. **44:**45, 1964.

22. Fonta, R. S., and Edwards, J. E.: Congenital cardiac diseases, Philadelphia, 1962, W. B. Saunders Co.

23. Galleti, P. M., and Brecher, B. A.: Heart-lung bypass; principles and techniques of extra-corporeal circulation, New York, 1962, Grune & Stratton, Inc.

24. Gibbon, J. H., Jr., Sabiston, D., Jr., and Spencer, F. C., editors: Surgery of the chest, Philadelphia, 1969, W. B. Saunders Co.

25. Glenn, F., editor: The circulatory system in surgery, Surg. Clin. North Am. **41:**265, 1961.

26. Glenn, F., and Wantz, G. E., Jr., editors: Problems in surgery, St. Louis, 1961, The C. V. Mosby Co.

27. Guyton, A. C.: Circulatory physiology: cardiac output and its regulation, Philadelphia, 1963, W. B. Saunders Co.

28. Harrison, R. W., and Moulder, P. V.: Thymectomy: indications and technique, Surg. Clin. North Am. **41:**167, 1961.

29. Holswade, G. R., and Arditi, L. I.: The diagnosis and surgical correction of aortic stenosis, Surg. Clin. North Am. **41:**462, 1961.

30. Johnson, J., and Kirby, C. K.: Surgery of the chest, ed. 4, Chicago, 1970, Year Book Medical Publishers, Inc.

31. Julian, D. G.: Cardiology, London, 1970, Bailliere, Tindall & Cassell, Ltd.

32. Julian, O. C., Dye, W. S., Hushang, J., and Hunter, J. A.: Cardiovascular surgery, 1962, Year Book Medical Publishers, Inc.

33. Lewis, F. J.: Hypothermia-physiology and clinical application, Surg. Clin. North Am. **42:**69, 1962.

34. Lindskog, G. E., Liebow, A. A., and Glenn, W. W. L.: Thoracic and cardiovascular surgery with related pathology, New York, 1962, Appleton-Century-Crofts.

35. Magovern, G. J., and Cromie, H. W.: Sutureless prosthetic heart valves, J. Thorac. Cardiovasc. Surg. **46:**726, 1963.

36. Mainardi, L. C., Bhanganada, K., Mack, J. D., and Lillehei, C. W.: Hemodilution in extracorporeal circulation: comparative study of low molecular weight dextran and 5 per cent dextrose, Surgery **56:**349, 1964.

37. McCann, F. V.: Comparative physiology of the heart: current trends, Basel, Switzerland, 1969, Birkhäuser Verlag.

38. Morse, D. P.: Indications for open-heart surgery, Springfield, Ill., 1963, Charles C Thomas, Publisher.

39. Nursing Education Service: A study guide to congenital heart abnormalities, Columbus, Ohio, 1961, Ross Laboratories.

40. Parker, B. M., Shine, L. C., Burford, T. H., and Williams, K. R.: Indwelling electronic cardiac pacemakers, J.A.M.A. **186:**754, 1963.

41. Perloff, J. K.: The clinical recognition of congenital heart disease, Philadelphia, 1970, W. B. Saunders Co.

42. Piller, L. W.: Manual of cardio-pulmonary technology, Hampshire, England, 1962, Staples Press, Ltd.

43. Redo, S. F., and Ecker, R. R.: Intrapericardial aortico-pulmonary artery shunt, Circulation **28:**520, 1963.

44. Rushmer, R. R.: Cardiovascular dynamics, ed. 3, Philadelphia, 1970, W. B. Saunders Co.

45. Selkurt, E. E., editor: Physiology, Boston, 1963, Little, Brown & Co.

46. Starr, A., and Edwards, M. L.: Mitral replacement: clinical experience with a ball-valve prosthesis, Ann. Surg. **154:**726, 1961.

47. Stewart, H. J., and Glenn, F.: Mitral valvulotomy, Springfield, Ill., 1959, Charles C Thomas, Publisher.

48. Thorek, P.: Anatomy in surgery, ed. 2, Philadelphia, 1962, J. B. Lippincott Co.

49. Warren, R.: Surgery, Philadelphia, 1963, W. B. Saunders Co.

50. Weisberg, H. F.: A better understanding of anion-cation ("acid-base") balance, Surg. Clin. North Am. **39:**93, 1959.

51. Wesolowski, S. A., and Dennis, C.: Fundamentals of vascular grafting, New York, 1963, Blakiston Division, McGraw-Hill Book Co.

52. Williams, M. H.: Clinical application of cardiopulmonary physiology, New York, 1960, Harper & Row, Publishers.

53. Wilson, J. L., and McDonald, J. J.: Handbook of surgery, ed. 2, Los Altos, Calif., 1963, Lange Medical Publications.

54. Wooler, G. H., and Aberdeen, E.: Modern trends in cardiac surgery, vol. 2, New York, 1970, Appleton-Century-Crofts.

# CHAPTER 16

# Operations on the large blood vessels

EILEEN MOEHRLE

GENERAL CONSIDERATIONS (see Chapter 15). Time is a very important factor during vascular surgery, and any delay may be hazardous to the patient. To assure a smooth-running, uninterrupted procedure, all preparations must be complete, and all equipment and supplies must be available and ready for immediate use. The heparin solution should be accurately diluted with intravenous saline solution and placed in the syringes with the desired needle attached. Arterial sutures must be placed in the proper needle holders. The bulldog clamps must be organized on a heavy paper for ease in selection and handling. The small dissecting sponges must be counted and placed on the preferred instrument. Gelfoam or Surgicel must always be on the nurse's table. Films of the preoperative arteriograms must be selected and placed on the viewing box for reference during the procedure.

During vascular surgery it is often desirable to perform an additional procedure such as sympathectomy or endarterectomy during a bypass procedure.

ARTERIOGRAMS. All parts of the vascular system can be visualized for study with arteriograms. They are usually preoperative procedures; however, an operative arteriogram may be indicated or desirable. Because preoperative arteriograms are usually performed with the patient under local anesthesia, he experiences a burning sensation during the injection of the contrast medium. It is most important to warn the patient in advance to prevent movement during the exposures. It is wise to check with the surgeon regarding the possibility of operative arteriograms so that the patient may be positioned on the cassette holder. If operative arteriograms are necessary, they can easily be done without delay, if the x-ray department is notified and the following equipment is supplied:

2 20 or 30 ml. syringes and needles
1 Ampul contrast medium (Conray, Hypaque, etc.)
2 Sterile covers for x-ray cassette
  Intravenous saline solution

VASCULAR DISSECTION. This is done initially in all vascular procedures. It is accomplished by blunt or sharp dissection using fine tissue forceps, a Potts scissors, and a small dissecting sponge. Umbilical cord tape or small Penrose tubing may be passed around the vessel to aid in handling and controlling the vessel during the dissection.

HEPARINIZATION. A 1:10 heparin solution is used at the operative site intra-arterially or topically. Intra-arterial injection is done to prevent thrombosis during the procedure, and topical application is strictly a flushing off of any clots at the proposed site for anastomosis. When it is necessary to completely occlude a vessel, the heparin solution is injected into the artery before securing the occlusion clamp. Heparin will be injected again after flushing or preclotting the prosthesis.

SUTURES. The suture material will vary between no. 3-0 and 7-0 black silk or

Dacron. Nos. 3-0 and 4-0 sutures are more frequently used in abdominal and thoracic vascular surgery, nos. 5-0 and 6-0 sutures are used for the extremities, and no. 7-0 sutures are used for very small vessels. Vascular sutures are prepared in an oil suspension to enable smooth passage through the vessel, thereby minimizing vessel trauma. If vascular sutures are not available, it may be a request of the surgeon to wax or use mineral oil on the sutures. Vascular sutures all have swaged needles in various sizes, and the suture lengths are 30 or 36 inches long. The suture may be single-armed or double-armed (for example, with one or two needles). The size and curve of the needle preferred are dependent on the vessel and its location. The diamond jaw needle holder is preferred by many surgeons to permit the placement of the needle at an angle. Sometimes the blunt angulated nerve hook is used to guide the sutures in place.

PROSTHESES. The synthetic prosthesis is a seamless, woven or knitted, Dacron, tubular, straight or bifurcated implant used for reestablishing functional continuity. The selection of the graft must be made prior to complete vascular dissection to permit adequate sterilization time. Grafts may be sterilized for 15 minutes at 250° F. or for 3 minutes in the high-speed autoclave at 270° F.

The grafts are available in various sizes. The common size used for abdominal procedures is 19 to 22 mm.; for the extremities, it is usually 8 to 10 mm.

The graft is prepared prior to insertion according to the surgeon's preference. This graft preparation is done to minimize blood loss through seepage at the graft site. Sometimes the surgeon prefers to saturate the graft with the patient's blood, or, after insertion of the graft, the occluding clamps are individually and momentarily opened to fill the graft with blood.

INSTRUMENTS. The instruments used for vascular surgery are the basic laparotomy, vascular, and, depending on the procedure and the approach, thoracic vascular instruments (see Chapter 15).

## RESECTION OF ABDOMINAL AORTIC ANEURYSM

DEFINITION. Surgical excision of the aneurysm, which may or may not include the common iliac arteries, with insertion of a vascular graft or synthetic prosthesis to reestablish functional continuity.

CONSIDERATIONS. The majority of abdominal aortic aneurysms usually begin below the renal arteries and frequently extend to involve the bifurcation and common iliac arteries, making dissection difficult. Symptoms may be vague or entirely absent until the size increases sufficiently to produce pressure on surrounding organs. The most reliable physical finding is an abnormal, pulsating, abdominal mass. Varying degrees of pain are considered an unfavorable prognostic sign, which indicates the necessity for surgery. Severe pain is usually indicative of perforation, and immediate surgery should be imminent if the patient is to be saved.

SETUP AND PREPARATION OF THE PATIENT. The nursing care is similar to that required for cardiothoracic surgery. The patient is placed on the operating table in a supine position. The skin is prepared for a midline abdominal incision and draping completed to permit access to both groin regions and exploration of femoral arteries (Fig. 16-1).

It is a good idea to mark the pedal pulses before the beginning of the procedure so that if the surgeon requests a check of the pulse, the location can be found immediately.

The setup includes the basic laparotomy set, plus the following:

**Cutting instruments**
1 Knife handle no. 7 with blade no. 11
2 Potts-Smith scissors, straight and angled

**Holding instruments**
4 Potts-Smith tissue forceps, 2 smooth, 2 with teeth

**Clamping instruments**

  8 Peripheral vascular clamps, 6 angled, 2 curved
  2 Renal artery clamps
  4 Aortic occlusion clamps
  4 Potts-Smith coarctation clamps
  3 Derra anastomosis clamps
  3 Satinsky clamps (various sizes)
10 Bulldog clamps (set of 5 pairs, nontraumatic teeth), 4 curved, 4 straight, 2 small
   Rubber-shod clamps (set of 5 pairs), curved and straight

**Suturing instruments**

  6 Needle holders (narrow diamond jaw), 8 and 10 in.

**Exposing instruments**

  2 Extra-large Kelly retractors
  2 Extra-large Deaver retractors

  2 Harrington retractors, wide and narrow
  2 Weitlaner or Beckman retractors (for extension into the legs)
   Fogarty arterial catheters (optional), 2 to 7 Fr., balloon size 4, 5, 9, 11, 13, 14 mm.; venous, 6 and 8 Fr., balloon size 12, 14, 19, 28, 45 mm.
   Endarterectomy loops (optional)

**Miscellaneous instruments**

  2 Freer elevators
  1 Right-angled blunt nerve hook
  1 Centimeter ruler
   Dural clips and applicator (optional for sympathectomy)

**OPERATIVE PROCEDURE**

1. The abdomen is opened through a generous midline incision (Fig. 17-1) from

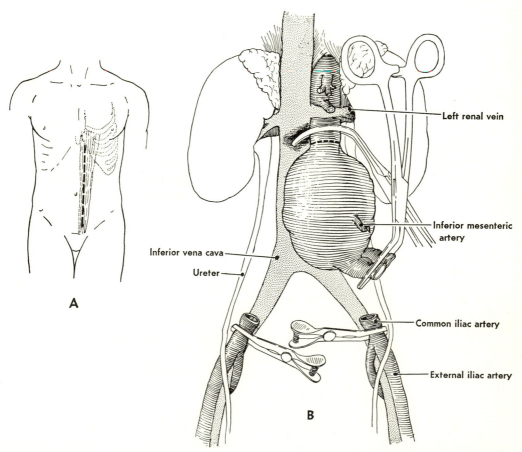

**A**

**B**

*Continued.*

**Fig. 16-1.** Resection of abdominal aneurysms. **A,** Incision. **B,** Resection of aortic aneurysm with proximal iliac arteries. (From Hershey, F. B., and Calman, C. H.: Atlas of vascular surgery, ed. 2, St. Louis, 1967, The C. V. Mosby Co.)

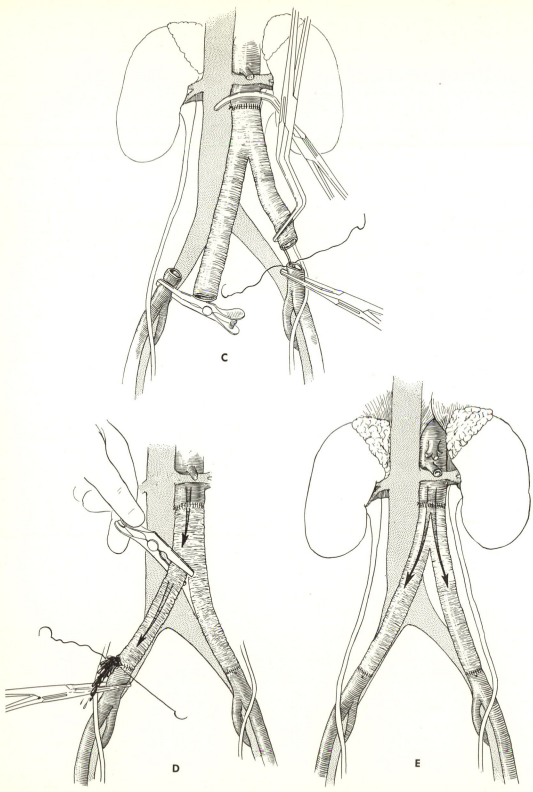

**Fig. 16-1, cont'd. C,** Showing insertion of Dacron prosthesis with bifurcation. **D,** Flushing proximal aorta. **E,** Anastomosis completed; flow restored. (From Hershey, F. B., and Calman, C. H.: Atlas of vascular surgery, ed. 2, St. Louis, 1967, The C. V. Mosby Co.)

the xiphoid to the pubis. Hemostasis is accomplished, and exploration is completed, as described for laparotomy (Chapter 17).

2. Exposure is obtained by placing a portion of the small bowel outside the abdomen and covering it with moist laparotomy packs or a Lahey bag. Kelly and Deaver retractors are inserted in the wound.

3. The parietal peritoneum is incised over the aorta and extended superiorly to expose the aneurysm and also inferiorly over the bifurcation and beyond the iliac arteries. Metzenbaum scissors, smooth forceps, and Pean hemostats are used.

4. Careful blunt and sharp dissection is continued to expose the aorta above the aneurysm to permit application of compression or occlusion tape (18-inch umbilical tape) and loose placement of an aortic clamp. The renal artery and ureters are carefully protected.

5. The iliac vessels and bifurcation are inspected for evidence of small aneurysms, thrombosis, and calcification. Moist tapes are placed about the iliac arteries, and Blalock or bulldog clamps are applied.

6. An aortic clamp such as the Satinsky, Cooley, or Swan type is applied and closed. Resection of the aneurysm is undertaken— first, by division of each iliac artery above the Blalock and, second, by dissection of the posterior surface with elevation and application of fine, right-angled forceps and Metzenbaum scissors.

7. The aneurysm is completely opened and removed in sections. The portions adherent to the vena cava wall are not excised, but all atherosclerotic deposits are removed. Bleeding is controlled.

8. A bifurcated Dacron prosthetic graft (Chapter 15) of appropriate size is prepared for insertion. Preclotting may be accomplished by immersion in a small quantity of the patient's own blood prior to the insertion.

9. The aortic cuff is prepared for anastomosis by irrigation with heparinized intravenous saline solution and by removal of all fibrotic plaques. Two no. 3-0 su-

tures are anchored to the center of the aortic cuff posteriorly. The edges of the graft are anastomosed to the aorta by through-and-through continuous stitches, with each suture being continued anteriorly to the center and tied. Additional interrupted sutures may be neeeded if the anastomosis demonstrates leakage on testing (Fig. 16-1).

10. During this time the distal vessels have been opened and inspected for back bleeding, and heparinized saline solution is injected to prevent clotting.

11. Each limb of the graft is anastomosed to the iliac artery, using a no. 4-0 suture and similar technique. After the first side of the anastomosis has been completed, blood is permitted to circulate, and the limb of the graft is clamped gently to prevent both trapping of air and leakage during the last part of the anastomosis. Pressure on the completed suture lines is exerted with moist gauze sponges. Bleeding is controlled.

12. A bilateral sympathectomy may be performed if the patient's general condition permits and in the presence of generalized arteriosclerosis with peripheral arterial disease (Fig. 16-2).

13. A nasogastric tube is inserted.

14. The parietal peritoneum is closed with silk sutures no. 3-0.

15. The abdominal wound is closed, as described for laparotomy; dressings are applied.

## AORTOILIAC ENDARTERECTOMY

**DEFINITION.** Surgical removal of the intraluminal atheromatous obstructive plaques and the restoration of arterial flow to the leg or foot. This operation is usually accomplished through a vertical arteriotomy with a primary closure. Synthetic patch material of Teflon or Dacron may be utilized if necessary to restore the normal caliber of the artery (Fig. 16-3).

**SETUP AND PREPARATION OF THE PATIENT.** The nursing care, preparation, and setup are identical with those for resection of abdominal aortic aneurysm, plus one set

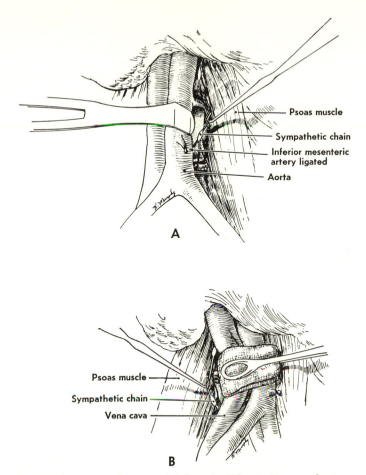

Fig. 16-2. Diagram showing technique of bilateral abdominal sympathectomy. **A,** Left. **B,** Right. (From Hershey, F. B., and Calman, C. H.: Atlas of vascular surgery, ed. 2, St. Louis, 1967, The C. V. Mosby Co.)

of endarterectomy loops or bifurcated and straight tubular synthetic prostheses if endarterectomy is not feasible.

**OPERATIVE PROCEDURE**

1 to 5. See procedure for resection of aortic aneurysm, steps 1 through 5.

6. An aortic clamp such as a Satinsky or Swan type is applied. Heparin is injected and the clamp closed immediately.

7. The arteriotomy incision is completed, and plaques are removed as shown in Fig. 16-3.

8. Arteriotomies are closed with vascular silk suture nos. 4-0 and 5-0 (Fig. 16-3).

9 to 11. The procedure is completed as in steps 12 through 15 for resection of aortic aneurysm.

## ARTERIAL EMBOLECTOMY

**DEFINITION.** A longitudinal incision is made in the affected segment, the embolus is removed, and the wound is closed.

**CONSIDERATIONS.** Emboli may be caused by a foreign body, air, fat, or a tumor that circulates through the bloodstream and becomes lodged as the vessel decreases in size. More often the direct cause is mural thrombi associated with a diseased heart. Pain is the initial symptom, followed by other signs of vascular occlusion, depending on the area affected.

**SETUP AND PREPARATION OF THE PATIENT.** The patient is positioned on the operating table, the skin area is prepared, and the

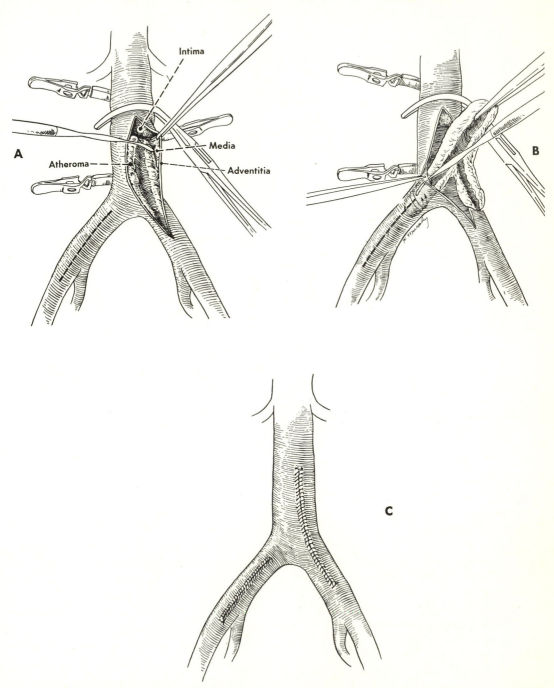

**Fig. 16-3.** Aortoiliac endarterectomy. **A,** Thin-tipped elevator is used to develop plane for dissection between plaque and media of aorta. **B,** Plaque freed from left iliac from above. **C,** Arteriotomies have been sutured. (From Hershey, F. B., and Calman, C. H.: Atlas of vascular surgery, ed. 2, St. Louis, 1967, The C. V. Mosby Co.)

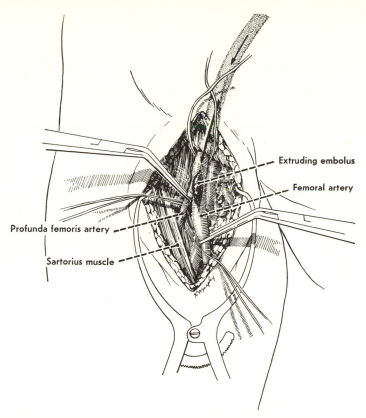

Profunda femoris artery

Sartorius muscle

Extruding embolus

Femoral artery

**Fig. 16-4.** Femoral artery embolectomy. Surgical exposure, tapes, and clamps are in place. Arteriotomy has been completed. (From Hershey, F. B., and Calman, C. H.: Atlas of vascular surgery, St. Louis, 1963, The C. V. Mosby Co.)

draping is completed to permit access to the affected area.

The instrument setup includes the basic laparotomy and vascular set, including an endarterectomy set and Fogarty arterial catheters and irrigators.

**OPERATIVE PROCEDURE**

1. The initial incision is completed, as previously described.

2. The artery is carefully exposed well above and below the site of embolus to permit application of vascular clamps (Fig. 16-4).

3. The umbilical tapes are passed about the artery above and below the proposed incision (Fig. 16-4).

4. A longitudinal incision is made with scalpel blade no. 15 or no. 11 and Potts angled scissors. The clot is grasped with suitable forceps and traction maintained as it is carefully extracted from the wound. Sometimes a Fogarty catheter is carefully inserted beyond the point of clot attachment. The balloon is inflated, and the catheter is withdrawn preceded by detached emboli.

5. As back bleeding is obtained, an artery clamp is applied above and below the wound.

6. The artery may be flushed by injection of heparin intravenous saline solution and "free" bleeding and suctioning with a small irrigating catheter or fine suction tube.

7. The arterial closure is completed with everting sutures of cardiovascular silk no. 5-0. The wound closure is accomplished in the usual manner, and dressings are applied.

## FEMORAL-POPLITEAL BYPASS

DEFINITION. The creation of a new route to restore blood flow to the leg by the insertion of a graft bypassing the occluded section of the femoral artery.

GENERAL CONSIDERATIONS. The bypass may be either a saphenous vein or straight synthetic graft. The patency of the popliteal artery must be obvious for a successful bypass procedure, and this is determined by the preoperative arteriograms. If popliteal patency is doubtful, exploration of the artery is necessary. The arteriotomy for popliteal embolectomy may be repaired with either a patch graft or preferably a vein graft.

SETUP AND PREPARATION OF THE PATIENT. The patient is placed in a supine position. The thigh is slightly rotated and abducted with the knee flexed. Preparation and draping includes the entire groin, thigh, and leg below the knee. The instrument setup includes the basic laparotomy and vascular set for extremities, including the following:

Gelpi retractors
Beckman or Weitlaner retractors
DeBakey tunneler
Supplies and equipment for operative arteriograms

OPERATIVE PROCEDURE

EXPLORATION OF POPLITEAL ARTERY

1. A vertical incision is made along the medial lateral aspect of the lower thigh extending down just past the patella.

2. The incision is lower or extended downward for the exploration of the middle or lower end of the artery.

3. The saphenous vein and nerve are retracted with small retractors.

4. A Weitlaner retractor is used to retract the muscles after blunt dissection or the exploration of the upper and lower artery. However, in exploring the midportion the gastrocnemius muscle must be divided to visualize the artery.

5. The tendons are divided if necessary, and the popliteal vein is bluntly dissected from the artery and retracted with either umbilical tape or a small blunt vein retractor.

6. The popliteal artery is dissected free, the knee is flexed, and umbilical tape is passed around it. The artery is inspected for the graft site. (It may be desirable at this time to perform arteriograms.)

EXPLORATION OF FEMORAL ARTERY

1. A vertical incision is made over the femoral artery below the inguinal area extending downward about 6 inches along the medial aspect of the thigh.

2. The femoral artery is located, the sheath of the artery is bluntly dissected in both directions, and the artery is dissected free for complete exposure.

3. Exposure of the artery is accomplished with the Weitlaner or Beckman retractor.

4. The artery is exposed and examined. (Usually the blockage occurs at the beginning of the superficial femoral artery.) The site for anastomosis is selected.

5. Umbilical tapes are passed around the common femoral, the superficial femoral, and the deep femoral artery.

6. The length and size of the graft are determined.

7. Heparinized saline solution is injected into the common femoral artery, and the vessels are occluded with DeBakey angled clamps.

8. The incision is made into the femoral artery with a no. 11 knife blade and extended with a vascular scissors.

9. The graft is anastomosed to the artery with no. 5-0 or 6-0 arterial sutures (either two single-armed or one double-armed suture).

10. The DeBakey tunneler is passed beneath the sartorius muscle from one incision to the other. Usually no bleeding occurs.

11. The knee is flexed, and a DeBakey clamp is placed on the popliteal artery at the graft site.

12. The incision is made into the popliteal artery as explained for the femoral arteriotomy.

13. The graft is pulled through the tun-

neler and adjusted to prevent kinks or twists.

14. The graft is sutured to the popliteal artery, and before completion the femoral occluding clamp will be momentarily opened to eliminate the possibility of clots.

15. All occluding clamps are removed, and a check for leaks is made before closure.

16. Incision is closed in the usual fashion.

## SHUNT OPERATIONS FOR PORTAL HYPERTENSION

GENERAL CONSIDERATIONS. Obstruction of the portal vein, which may be intrahepatic or extrahepatic, is the direct cause of portal hypertension. The intrahepatic block obstruction, which is most common, may result from cirrhosis or postinfectious hepatitis. Extrahepatic block, which represents about 15% of the total cases, may be caused by thrombosis, compression, or congenital abnormalities. One of the most important indications for surgery is to treat complications associated with potential or active hemorrhage of esophageal or gastric varices. An effective shunt between the hypertensive portal and lower caval circulation produces a fall in pressure, with subsequent disappearance of varices and protection against further hemorrhage.

Preoperatively, a portal venogram is usually performed via percutaneous splenic puncture to demonstrate the site of portal obstruction.

### Portacaval anastomosis

DEFINITION. Through an abdominal, thoracoabdominal, or thoracolumbar incision, an anastomosis is established between the portal vein and the inferior vena cava. (Fig. 16-5).

SETUP AND PREPARATION OF THE PATIENT. The patient is placed on the operating table in a supine position, with the right thorax slightly elevated to accommodate a thoracoabdominal incision (see Chapters 7 and 14). The instrument setup includes the basic laparotomy, vascular, and thoracic sets, plus the following.

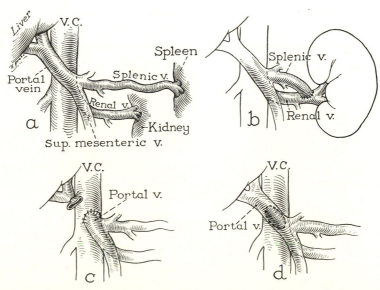

**Fig. 16-5.** Diagrammatic representation of different types of portacaval shunts. **a,** Principal structures concerned. **b,** Splenectomy with end-to-side splenorenal anastomosis. **c,** End-to-side portacaval anastomosis. **d,** Side-to-side portacaval anastomosis. (From Hallenbeck, G.: Surg. Clin. North Am. 35:1099, 1955.)

For measuring portal pressures
1 Manometer, spinal
1 Three-way stopcock
1 Polyethylene tubing
  Syringe and needles

For drainage
1 Chest tube (size according to surgeon's preference)
1 Closed chest drainage set
1 Gastrostomy tube

**OPERATIVE PROCEDURE**

1. The abdominal incision is completed, utilizing instruments and materials as previously described. The surgeon may elect to extend the thoracic incision after abdominal exploration and determination of portal pressure. Moist laparotomy packs and retractors provide exposure as exploration is carried out.

2. A jejunal mesenteric vein is isolated and cannulated with polyethylene tubing by a simple cutdown technique, using scalpel no. 11, plastic scissors, Adson forceps, two curved mosquito hemostats, and silk no. 2-0 ligatures. A spinal manometer is attached to the tubing, using a three-way stopcock, and intravenous saline solution is injected into the manometer.

3. The portal pressure is measured and determined by the height of the saline solution meniscus above the right atrium when it comes to rest. Normal limits may range from 45 to 150 mm. The abnormal range may be from 200 to 600 mm.

4. The incision is extended, the eighth or ninth rib is resected, the muscles are divided, and the pleura is incised. The diaphragm is divided from the costal cartilages. Suitable retractors and moist packs are placed to permit adequate exposure.

5. As the portal vein and inferior vena cava are dissected free, extreme caution is exercised to avoid injury to important surrounding structures, for example, gallbladder, cystic and common ducts, and the hepatic artery and its branches.

6. Compression tapes are applied to the portal vein and the vena cava both above and below the prepared sites for anastomosis.

7. Vascular clamps are placed on the portal vein—a Blalock clamp near the pancreas and a coarctation clamp near the liver. If an end-to-end anastomosis is contemplated, the vein is ligated. If a side-to-side anastomosis is to be established, the vein is incised. Small clots are carefully removed, and the lumen may be irrigated with saline solution.

8. A Satinsky or other suitable partial occluding clamp is placed on the vena cava. An elliptical section of the vessel wall that is secured within the inner aspect of the clamp is excised with Satinsky scissors (Fig. 16-6). The size of the section removed should correspond exactly to the lumen of that portion of the portal vein that has been prepared for anastomosis.

9. The anastomosis is completed by continuous mattress and interrupted sutures, using cardiovascular silk no. 5-0, fine vascular forceps, and long fine needle holders.

10. The portal pressure is taken to determine functioning of the shunt.

11. A drainage catheter is placed in the pleural cavity. The diaphragm is closed, the ribs are reapproximated, and the intercostal cartilages are closed, as previously described (Chapter 14).

12. The peritoneum is closed. Closure of the muscle, fascia, and skin is completed. Dressings are applied.

13. The chest drainage catheter is attached to an underwater-seal drainage set.

## Arteriovenous shunt

**DEFINITION.** Insertion of Silastic- and Teflon-coated vessel appliances to facilitate hemodialysis by means of an "artificial kidney."

**CONSIDERATIONS.** Arteriovenous shunts are indicated in patients with chronic renal failure. The surgeon decides on the site to insert the appliance. The left inner wrist is usually chosen for right-handed patients. Prior use of sites for this purpose may cause wide variation in the area actually used.

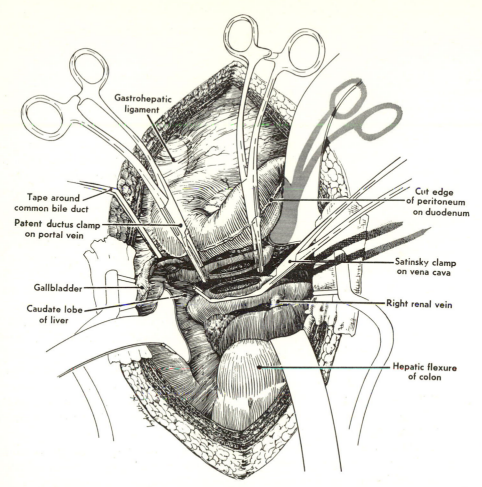

Fig. 16-6. Portacaval shunt. Clamps in place for side-to-side anastomosis. (From Hershey, F. B., and Calman, C. H.: Atlas of vascular surgery, ed. 2, St. Louis, 1967, The C. V. Mosby Co.)

**SETUP AND PREPARATION OF THE PATIENT.** The patient is placed in a supine position with the arm extended on a rather wide armboard. This procedure is usually done with local anesthesia, and care must be taken for the instruction and comfort of the patient. A basic minor instrument set is required, adding the following:

6 Bulldog vascular clamps
Penrose-type drain for use as a tourniquet
Needles and sutures as needed, vascular silk no. 4-0 or 5-0
Local setup and medication
Saline and heparin mixture (1:10) for injection into the vessels to prevent clotting

**OPERATIVE PROCEDURE**

1. After skin cleansing, sterile drapes are applied around the site. The surgeon may then apply the Penrose tourniquet. A local anesthetic is infiltrated, and a small incision is made over the venous site. Bleeding vessels are clamped and ligated. The vein is dissected free of the fascia with a small curved clamp, and two heavy silk ties are placed around the vessel and held with clamps. The tourniquet is released. A bulldog clamp is applied to the proximal end of the vein, which is then cut and ligated distally.

2. A small incision is made at the se-

lected arterial site after it is infiltrated with local anesthetic. Bleeding vessels are ligated. The artery is exposed and dissected free with a small curved clamp. Two heavy silk sutures are placed around the artery. A bulldog clamp is applied to the proximal end, and the distal end is incised and ligated.

3. Vessel tips are inserted into the open ends of the vein and artery and tied securely with the heavy silk ties. A small amount of the heparin solution is injected. The selected appliance is then connected to the vessel tips linking the vein and artery. The bulldog clamp is removed from the vein, then from the artery, and the shunt has been accomplished.

4. The fascia and the skin are closed carefully over the vessel tips and ends of the appliance to avoid twisting or occluding in any way.

5. Sterile dressings are applied and held securely in place with an elastic bandage.

### Splenorenal anastomosis

DEFINITION. Through a left thoracoabdominal incision an anastomosis is established between the splenic and the left renal vein (Fig. 16-5).

SETUP AND PREPARATION OF THE PATIENT. As for portacaval shunt, except that the patient is placed on the table with his left side uppermost.

OPERATIVE PROCEDURE

1. A transverse incision is made through the ninth rib; the recti and thoracic muscles, the costal cartilages, and the diaphragmatic pleura are incised.

2. The spleen is mobilized, and the pancreas is separated from the splenic pedicle; the phrenocolic ligament is divided.

3. The spleen is removed, using angular and curved artery forceps and silk sutures.

4. The renal vein is dissected free, and anastomosis clamps—Blalock or Potts—are applied.

5. An anastomosis of the splenic to the left renal vein is carried out.

6. The wound is closed as for portacaval shunt operation.

## VENA CAVA LIGATION

DEFINITION. The occlusion of the vena cava by ligation to prevent emboli from moving toward the heart.

GENERAL CONSIDERATIONS. Ligation of the vena cava is performed to prevent pulmonary embolism in patients when anticoagulant therapy fails or cannot be initiated. In the female patient a transabdominal incision may be used to also permit ligation of the ovarian veins.

SETUP AND PREPARATION OF THE PATIENT. The nursing care is similar to that required for lumbar sympathectomy (see Chapter 11). Gelfoam or Surgicel should be available in case of injury to the lumbar veins.

OPERATIVE PROCEDURE

1 and 2. See lumbar sympathectomy, p. 403.

3. Deep retractors are placed for adequate exposure.

4. The peritoneum and abdominal contents are bluntly dissected anteriorly with sponge holders to expose the vena cava.

5. Deep in the wound, the vena cava is dissected free with peanut sponges or a Smithwick dissector.

6. Using a Mixter forceps, two heavy silk sutures no. 2 are passed around the vena cava and tied approximately ½ inch above or below the lumbar vein. The vena cava is not cut. A Teflon clip may be used instead of silk sutures.

7. The incision is closed in layers.

## HIGH LIGATION OF THE SAPHENOUS VEINS WITH OR WITHOUT EXCISION

DEFINITION. Ligation and division of the saphenous trunk situated in the groin region of one or both sides with or without subsequent stripping and excision.

CONSIDERATIONS. A series of cup-shaped valves maintains the blood flow in the veins in a direction toward the heart. Because of disease, the normal functioning of these valves is disturbed, resulting in distention or back pressure. The veins gradually become dilated. Those in the lower extremities are most frequently af-

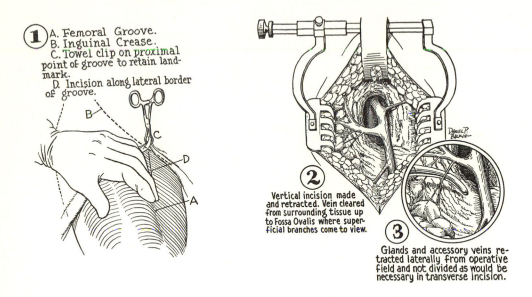

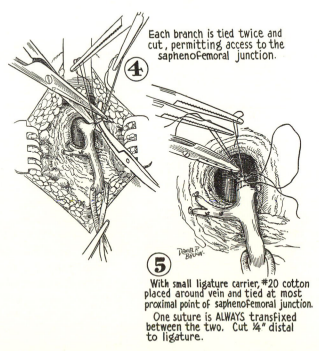

**Fig. 16-7.** Operative procedure for saphenous ligation. **1,** Palpation of femoral groove distal to inguinal crease to locate site for vertical incision and exposure of fossa ovalis and saphenofemoral junction; **2** to **5,** operation and suture. (From Theis, F. V., and Helmen, R. T.: Surg. Clin. North Am. **35**:285, 1955.)

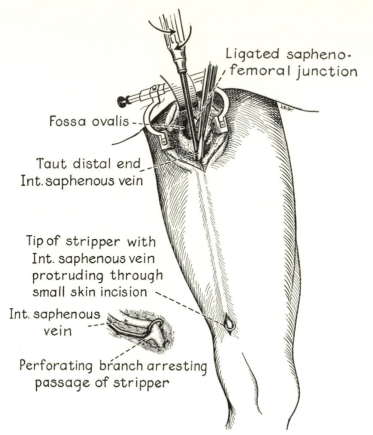

Ligated sapheno-femoral junction

Fossa ovalis

Taut distal end
Int. saphenous vein

Tip of stripper with
Int. saphenous vein
protruding through
small skin incision

Int. saphenous
vein

Perforating branch arresting
passage of stripper

**Fig. 16-8.** Extraluminal stripper showing instrument with saphenous vein arrested by large branch in midthigh. At this site, end of instrument is pushed through small incision, vein is removed from ring, and instrument is withdrawn. Segmental removal of saphenous vein is continued to ankle. (From Theis, F. V., and Helmen, R. T.: Surg. Clin. North Am. **35:**285, 1955.)

fected. Dilatation of the saphenous vein produces venous stasis, which may be followed by secondary complications.

The objective of surgical intervention is to interrupt or remove the diseased veins, thus preventing ulceration, secondary edema, pain, and fatigue in the extremity.

**SETUP AND PREPARATION OF THE PATIENT.** The patient is placed on the operating table in a supine position with the legs slightly abducted. Drapes are placed to enable flexing and lifting at the knee. Instruments include basic laparotomy instrument setup, plus the following (Chapter 17):

2 Weitlaner self-retaining retractors
6 Mosquito hemostats, 5½ in.
1 Set Mayo extraluminal vein strippers, 3 sizes

2 Intraluminal vein strippers, flexible, olive-tipped
Special sterile gauze compression dressings
Elastoplast or elastic bandages (according to surgeon's preference)

**OPERATIVE PROCEDURE**

1. The incision is made in the upper thigh, parallel to the crease in the groin. Bleeding vessels are clamped and ligated. Suture material is selected according to the surgeon's preference.

2. The saphenous vein is identified and isolated. Margins of the wound are separated, using a Weitlaner self-retaining retractor.

3. The saphenous vein and branches are doubly ligated with no. 2-0 black silk

sutures or transfixed, clamped, and divided. The proximal stump is dissected upward to the point at which it enters the femoral vein, where it is carefully religated (Fig. 16-7).

4. If the saphenous vein is to be excised, the distal end is threaded on the Mayo stripper. Traction on the vein is maintained with a hemostat or no. 2-0 suture as the stripper is pushed downward to a point near the knee (Fig. 16-8).

5. A small incision is made at this point. The vein is delivered and doubly ligated or transfixed with no. 2-0 black silk suture.

6. Stripping of other veins of the extremity may be carried out through small incisions in the same manner.

7. The groin wound is closed in layers with interrupted sutures of no. 3-0 black silk.

8. Skin incisions are closed with interrupted mattress sutures of no. 4-0 black silk.

9. Dressings and circular compression bandages are applied.

## REFERENCES

1. Barker, W. F., editor: Surgical treatment of peripheral vascular disease, New York, 1962, Blakiston Division, McGraw-Hill Book Co.
2. Crane, C.: The choice of shunt procedure for cirrhotic patients with variceal bleeding, ascites, and hypersplenism, Surg. Gynecol. Obstet. 115:12, July, 1962.
3. DeTakats, G.: Vascular surgery, Philadelphia, 1951, W. B. Saunders Co.
4. Glenn, F., and Wantz, G. E., Jr., editors: Problems in surgery, St. Louis, 1961, The C. V. Mosby Co.
5. Hershey, F. B., and Calman, C. H.: Atlas of vascular surgery, ed. 2, St. Louis, 1967, The C. V. Mosby Co.
6. Keeley, J. L., Schairer, A. E., and Pesek, I. G.: The technique of ligation and stripping in the treatment of varicose veins, Surg. Clin. North Am. 41:235, 1961.
7. Kinmonth, J. B., Rob, C. G., and Simeone, F. A.: Vascular surgery, Baltimore, 1963, The Williams & Wilkins Co.
8. McDonald, H., Jr., and Waterhouse, K.: Reprint from "Replacement of Renal Function," 1966, European Dialysis and Transplant Association.
9. Morris, G. C., Jr., and DeBakey, M. E.: Aortic aneurysms and occlusive diseases of the aorta, Am. J. Cardiol. 12:303, Sept., 1963.
10. Nardi, G. L., and Zuidema, G. D., editors: Surgery, Boston, 1961, Little, Brown & Co.
11. Warren, R.: Surgery, Philadelphia, 1963, W. B. Saunders Co.
12. Wesolowski, S. A., and Dennis, C.: Fundamentals of vascular grafting, New York, 1963, Blakiston Division, McGraw-Hill Book Co.
13. Zuidema, G. D., and Child, C. G., III: Problems in the management of portal hypertension, Surg. Clin. North Am. 41:1307, 1961.

# CHAPTER 17

# Abdominal incisions and closures; repair of hernias

EILEEN MOEHRLE

The surgeon chooses an incision that will afford maximum exposure of the structures to be operated on, ensure minimal trauma and postoperative discomfort, and provide for primary wound healing with maximum wound strength.

## TYPES, USE, LOCATION, AND CLOSURE OF INCISIONS

**PARAMEDIAN RECTUS INCISION.** When on the appropriate side, this incision can be used in any intra-abdominal surgery (Figs. 17-1 and 17-4). It is made parallel and about 4 cm. lateral to the midline. The skin and subcutaneous tissue are incised; the anterior rectus sheath is divided; and the rectus muscle is separated and retracted laterally, thus preserving the motor nerves. The posterior rectus sheath and peritoneum are opened vertically.

The advantages of a paramedian incision are as follows: the abdominal cavity can be quickly entered; the incision avoids nerve injury, limits trauma to the rectus muscle, produces less bleeding, and permits anatomical layer closure; and the original incision can be extended upward to the xiphoid process or downward to the pubis.

The peritoneum can be approximated and closed with a continuous suture of chromic gut no. 2-0 or 0 or with interrupted non-absorbable sutures of black silk no. 2-0 or 0. The posterior rectus sheath and the fas-

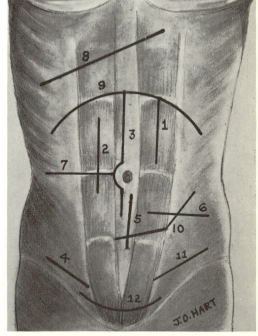

Fig. 17-1. Incisions made through abdominal wall. **1,** Left upper paramedian rectus; **2,** right midparamedian rectus; **3,** longitudinal midline; **4,** right McBurney muscle-splitting; **5,** lower midline; **6,** left lower transverse; **7,** midline transverse; **8,** right oblique (subcostal); **9,** upper inverted U; **10,** diagonal; **11,** left lower oblique; **12,** Pfannenstiel (transverse). (Drawing by Jeanne Hart, New York, N. Y.)

681

cial layers are approximated and closed with interrupted nonabsorbable sutures. Tension sutures may also be used. The superficial fascial layers are closed with finer interrupted sutures. The skin edges are approximated and closed with fine silk, cotton, or nylon.

**LONGITUDINAL MIDLINE INCISION.** This is the simplest abdominal incision. It is a good primary incision and generally preferred by many surgeons because it offers good exposure to any part of the abdominal cavity. It can be extended upward along the xiphoid, diagonally across the costal border, downward around the umbilicus (avascular, tough connective tissue), back to midline, and down to the pubis (Figs. 17-1 and 17-2). The peritoneum is incised, and the round ligament of the liver is divided.

To close the wound, the peritoneum and round ligament are approximated and sutured with surgical gut or nonabsorbable sutures. Sometimes the suture line is supported by using tension sutures, through-and-through sutures extending out through the subcutaneous tissue to the skin. Fascia,

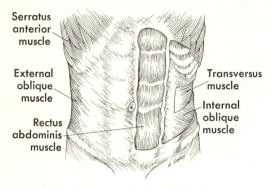

**Fig. 17-2.** Anatomy of the abdominal wall—superficial and deep. (Redrawn from Greenhill, J. P.: Surgical gynecology, ed. 2, Chicago, 1957, Year Book Medical Publishers, Inc.)

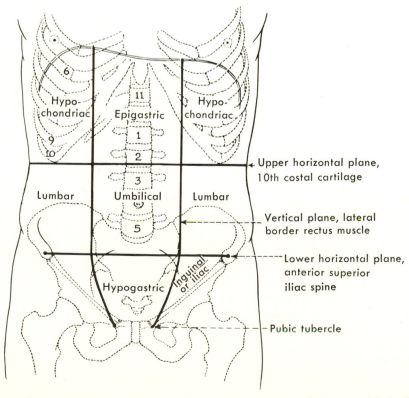

**Fig. 17-3.** Diagram of abdominal regions. (From King, B. G., and Showers, M. J.: Human anatomy and physiology, ed. 5, Philadelphia, 1963, W. B. Saunders Co.)

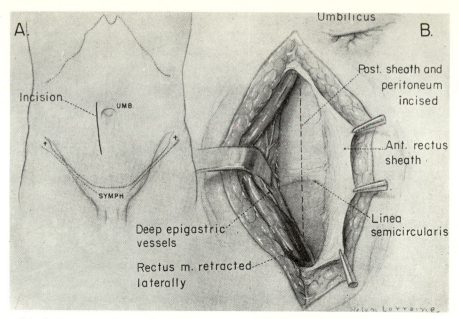

**Fig. 17-4. A,** Location of vertical paramedian rectus incision is shown on right side. **B,** Anterior rectus sheath is divided, rectus muscle retracted, and posterior sheath and peritoneum exposed. (From Horsley, G. W., and Bigger, I. A.: Operative surgery, ed. 6, St. Louis, 1953, The C. V. Mosby Co.)

subcutaneous tissue, and skin are closed as layers.

MCBURNEY MUSCLE-SPLITTING INCISION. This incision is used for the removal of the appendix. It is an 8 cm. oblique incision that begins just below the umbilicus, goes through McBurney's point, and extends upward toward the right flank (Figs. 17-1 to 17-4). The external oblique muscle and fascia are split in the direction of their fibers and retracted. The internal oblique muscle, transverse muscle, and fascia are split and retracted. The peritoneum is incised, and closure is as described in laparotomy. This incision is quick and easy to close and allows a firm wound closure. However, it does not permit good exposure and is difficult to extend. To extend the incision medially, the inferior epigastric vessels are ligated, and the rectus sheath is incised transversely.

UPPER QUADRANT OBLIQUE INCISION (SUBCOSTAL). This incision is made on the right side and preferred sometimes for operations on the gall bladder, common duct, or pancreas. When made on the left side, it may be used for splenectomy. This incision usually gives only limited exposure unless the patient is short with a wide abdomen and wide costal margins. The advantages of this type of incision are as follows: it provides good cosmetic results because it follows the skin lines; the nerve damage is limited because only one or two nerves are cut; and tension on the incisional edges is less than in a vertical incision.

The oblique incision begins in the epigastrium, extending laterally and obliquely downward to just below the lower costal margin (Fig. 17-5). Each muscle contains veins and arteries requiring ligation. If more exposure is needed, the incision is extended across the rectus muscle of the other side. The rectus muscle is either retracted or transversely divided. Vessels in the muscle must be ligated.

The closure of this incision includes approximation and closure of the falciform ligament, peritoneum, posterior rectus sheath, and anterior rectus sheath with

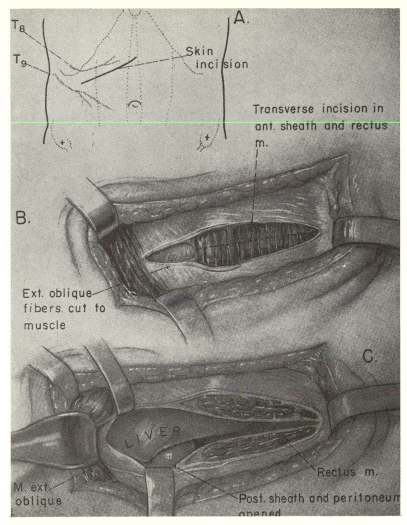

**Fig. 17-5. A,** Position of oblique (subcostal) skin incision is shown in upper right quadrant. **B,** Anterior sheath has been divided transversely, and muscle is exposed. **C,** Posterior sheath and peritoneum have been opened transversely. (From Horsley, G. W., and Bigger, I. A.: Operative surgery, ed. 6, St. Louis, 1953, The C. V. Mosby Co.)

interrupted nonabsorbable black silk sutures no. 2-0. The subcutaneous tissue and skin are closed as described for laparotomy.

**UPPER INVERTED ∪ ABDOMINAL INCISION.** This incision is not used too frequently today; however, it can be used for gastrectomy, transverse colon resection, transverse colostomy, and biliary procedures. The incision extends from a point below the costal margin on one side in the anterior axillary line to the same point on the opposite side. It is curved, with the midpoint lying mid-

way between the xiphoid process and the umbilicus. The intercostal nerves are preserved.

An upper abdominal transverse incision is closed by placing interrupted sutures in the peritoneum, anterior and posterior rectus sheaths. The muscle and fat may not be sutured. The skin edges are approximated and closed as described for laparotomy.

**MIDABDOMINAL TRANSVERSE INCISION.** This incision is used on the left or right side

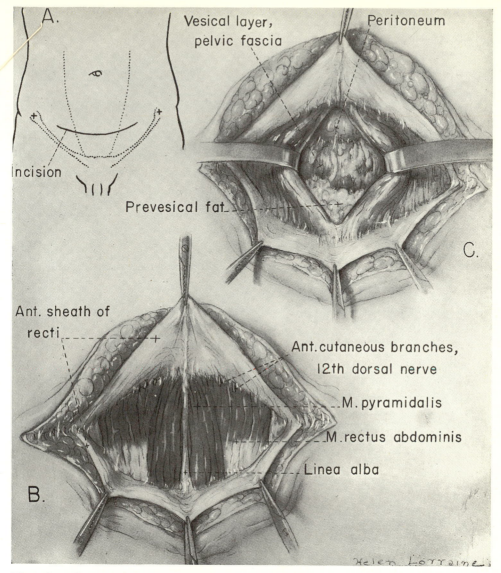

**Fig. 17-6.** Pfannenstiel incision (transverse). (From Dodson, A. I.: Urological surgery, ed. 4, St. Louis, 1970, The C. V. Mosby Co.)

or for a retroperitoneal approach. The incision begins slightly above or below the umbilicus on either side and is carried laterally to the lumbar region at an angle between the ribs and crest of the ilium (Fig. 17-1). The skin and subcutaneous tissue are incised, the anterior rectus sheath is split in the direction of its fibers (Fig. 17-2), the muscle is divided, and the vessels are clamped and ligated. The posterior rectus sheath and peritoneum are cut in the direction of the fibers, preserving the intercostal nerves. The peritoneum is incised near the midline, and the incision is extended laterally to the oblique muscle. The closure is in layers with interrupted sutures; the subcutaneous tissue and skin are closed as for laparotomy.

**PFANNENSTIEL INCISION.** This incision is used frequently for gynecological surgery.

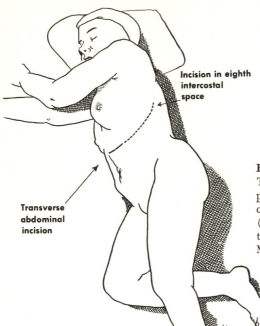

Incision in eighth intercostal space

Transverse abdominal incision

**Fig. 17-7.** Patient is placed on unaffected side. Thoracoabdominal incision is usually made from point midway between xiphoid and umbilicus to costal margin at site of eighth costal cartilage. (From Horsley, G. W., and Bigger, I. A.: Operative surgery, ed. 6, St. Louis, 1953, The C. V. Mosby Co.)

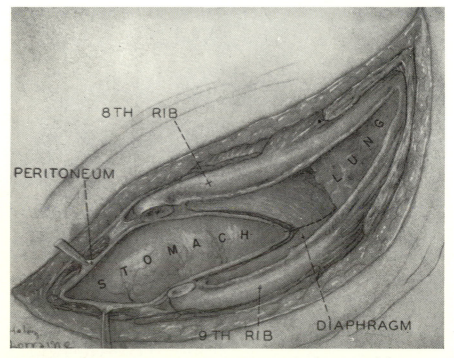

8TH RIB

PERITONEUM

S T O M A C H

LUNG

9TH RIB

DIAPHRAGM

**Fig. 17-8.** Thoracoabdominal incision (Carter). Dissection has been carried down to peritoneum and pleura. Costal cartilage and diaphragm have been divided, and stomach has been exposed. (From Horsley, G. W., and Bigger, I. A.: Operative surgery, ed. 6, St. Louis, 1953, The C. V. Mosby Co.)

It is a curved transverse incision across the lower abdomen through the skin, subcutaneous tissue, and rectus sheaths (Fig. 17-6). The rectus muscles are separated in midline, and the peritoneum is entered through a midline vertical incision (Fig. 17-2). This incision provides for a strong closure; when the rectus muscles contract, there is less strain on the fascial sutures.

**THORACOABDOMINAL INCISION.** This incision is used for operations on the upper end of the stomach and the lower end of the esophagus (Fig. 17-7). Often the abdominal part of the incision is made first for exploration and then, if necessary, extended across the costal margin into the chest.

The incision begins at a point midway between the xiphoid and the umbilicus, extending across to the seventh or eighth interspace and to the midcapsular line (Fig. 17-7). The rectus and oblique abdominal muscles and the serratus and interthoracic muscles are divided in the line of incision down to the peritoneum and pleura. Then the costal cartilage and the diaphragm are divided (Fig. 17-8).

The wound is closed in layers using interrupted sutures. Surgical gut may be used for the peritoneum and intercostal muscles. Silk, cotton, or Dacron sutures may be used for the muscle and fascial layers. Skin edges are approximated with silk.

## LAPAROTOMY

**DEFINITION.** An opening made through the abdominal wall into the peritoneal cavity. The name of the operation is usually derived from the additional procedure carried out.

**SETUP AND PREPARATION OF THE PATIENT.** After placing the patient in the desired position (Chapter 7), the routine skin preparation is done (Chapter 4), and the patient is draped (Chapter 5). The basic instruments used include the following:

**Cutting instruments** (Fig. 17-9)

  6 Knife handles—no. 3 with blade no. 10, no. 4 with blade no. 20, no. 7 with blade no. 15

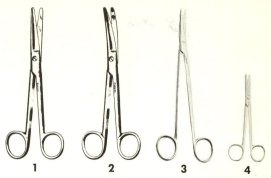

Fig. 17-9. Basic cutting instruments for laparotomy. 1, Mayo scissors, straight; 2, Mayo scissors, curved; 3, Metzenbaum scissors, curved; 4, suture scissors, straight or curved. Specific cutting instruments for various procedures are illustrated in following chapters. (Courtesy Codman & Shurtleff, Inc., Randolph, Mass.)

  1 Mayo scissors, 6¼ in., straight
  1 Mayo scissors, 6¼ in., curved
  1 Metzenbaum scissors, 7 in.
  1 Suture scissors

**Holding instruments** (Fig. 17-10)

  2 Smooth tissue forceps, 5½ in.
  2 Tissue forceps with teeth, 5½ in.
  2 Smooth tissue forceps, 7 and 10 in.
  2 Tissue forceps with teeth, 7 and 10 in.
  2 Adson-Brown forceps with teeth
  6 Sponge-holding forceps, 10 in.
 12 Towel clamps, 3½ or 5½ in.
 12 Allis forceps, 6 and 9 in.
  4 Babcock intestinal forceps, 6 in.

**Clamping instruments** (Fig. 17-11)

 24 Crile forceps, 5½ in., straight or curved
 12 Rochester-Pean forceps, 6¼ in., curved
  8 Rochester-Pean forceps, 10 in., curved
  6 Rochester-Ochsner or Kocher forceps, 6¼ in., straight
  6 Rochester-Ochsner or Kocher forceps, 9 in., straight

**Exposing instruments** (Fig. 17-12)

  2 Malleable copper retractors, 1 to 1½ in., width
  2 Small vein retractors
  2 Parker, Roux, Greene, or U. S. Army retractors
  6 Richardson or Kelly retractors, small, medium, and large pairs
  3 Deaver retractors, small, medium, and large
  4 Rake retractors, 4- and 6-pronged pairs, dull
  1 Balfour retractor with blades (optional)

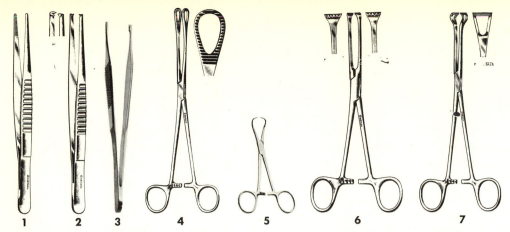

**Fig. 17-10.** Basic holding instruments for laparotomy. **1,** Dressing forceps, smooth; **2,** tissue forceps with teeth; **3,** Adson-Brown tissue forceps; **4,** sponge-holding forceps; **5,** towel clips; **6,** Allis tissue forceps; **7,** Babcock intestinal forceps. Specific holding instruments for various procedures are illustrated in the following chapters. (Courtesy Codman & Shurtleff, Inc., Randolph, Mass.)

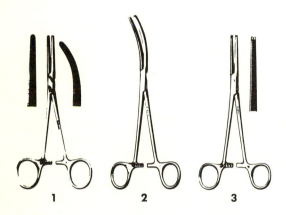

**Fig. 17-11.** Basic clamping instruments for laparotomy. **1,** Crile hemostatic forceps; **2,** Rochester-Pean hemostatic forceps; **3,** Ochsner or Kocher hemostatic forceps. Specific holding instruments for various procedures are illustrated in the following chapters. (Courtesy Codman & Shurtleff, Inc., Randolph, Mass.)

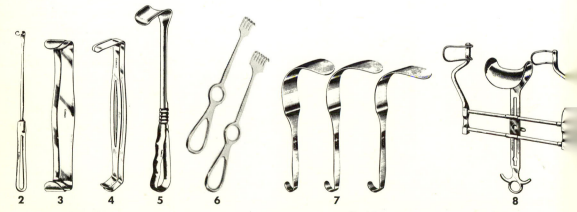

**Fig. 17-12.** Basic exposing instruments for laparotomy. **1,** Malleable copper retractor; **2,** vein retractor; **3,** Parker retractor; **4,** U. S. Army retractor; **5,** Richardson retractor; **6,** Volkmann rake retractor; **7,** Deaver retractor; **8,** Balfour self-retaining retractor with blades. Specific retractors for various procedures are illustrated in the following chapters. (Courtesy Codman & Shurtleff, Inc., Randolph, Mass.)

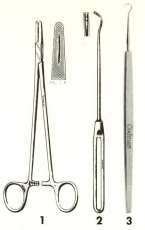

**Fig. 17-13.** Basic suturing instruments. **1,** Needle holder; **2,** ligature carrier; **3,** skin hook. Specific needle holders for various procedures are illustrated in the following chapters. (Courtesy Codman & Shurtleff, Inc., Randolph, Mass.)

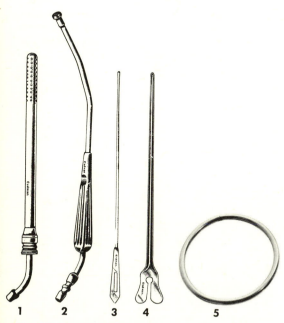

**Fig. 17-14.** Accessory items. **1,** Poole suction tube; **2,** Yankauer suction tube; **3,** silver probe; **4,** grooved director; **5,** laparotomy ring. Special accessory items for various procedures are illustrated in the following chapters. (Courtesy Codman & Shurtleff, Inc., Randolph, Mass.)

**Suturing instruments** (Fig. 17-13)

  6 Needle holders, 6 and 8 in.
  1 Needle set
  2 Ligature carriers (optional)
  2 Skin hooks (optional)

**Accessory items** (Fig. 17-14)

  1 Poole suction tube and tubing
  2 Yankauer suction tubes and tubing
  1 Silver probe
  1 Grooved director
  12 Laparotomy pack rings (optional)

### OPERATIVE PROCEDURE

#### LAPAROTOMY OPENING

1. Laparotomy packs are placed on each side of the proposed incision site to protect the surgeon's gloved hands from the skin and to provide traction for making the skin incision.

2. Suction tube and tubing are connected, tested, and secured to the field.

3. With scalpel no. 4 and blade no. 20, the skin incision is made and the scalpel discarded.

4. With scalpel no. 3 and blade no. 10, the incision is continued down to the fascia.

5. Hemostats are used to control bleeding vessels. Clamped vessels are ligated with fine surgical gut, silk, or cotton.

6. If a plastic drape is not used, skin towels are placed to evert the skin edges and exclude them from the inside of the wound. Towel clamps or silk sutures no. 2-0 may be used to secure the skin towels.

  a. Two skin towels folded in half are placed together with folded edges parallel to the incision.

  b. The folded edge of the top towel is clipped or sutured to the skin edges at various points. The operator everts the skin edges with tissue forceps.

  c. The two towels are turned onto the other side of the wound and secured as in b.

  d. The top towel is turned back, thereby exposing the wound.

  e. The ends of the towels are overlapped at each end of the incision and secured with a towel clamp.

7. The wound edges are retracted with small retractors.

8. With tissue forceps and a scalpel, the external oblique fascia is incised.

9. Using Metzenbaum scissors, the external oblique muscle is split the length of the incision. Bleeding vessels are controlled with hemostats and medium or fine ligatures.

10. The external oblique muscle is then retracted.

11. The internal oblique and transverse muscles are split, parallel to the fibers, up to the rectus sheath with a scalpel or a scissors. These muscles are then retracted. All free sponges are removed from the operative field.

12. The peritoneum is exposed, grasped with smooth tissue forceps, and nicked with scalpel no. 3 with blade no. 10.

13. Sponges and suction are used as needed. Cultures may be taken at this time.

14. The peritoneal incision is continued the length of the wound using Metzenbaum scissors.

15. The peritoneum is retracted with large Richardson retractors for exploration.

### LAPAROTOMY CLOSURE

1. Two tissue forceps are used to approximate the peritoneal edges, and the peritoneum is closed with a continuous chromic suture or interrupted nonabsorbable sutures.

2. The internal oblique transverse muscle, the small opening at the outer border of the rectus sheath, and the external oblique fascia are closed in layers using interrupted sutures. Sometimes retraction is necessary.

3. If towels and clamps were used, these are removed and discarded. Careful handling facilitates removal without contamination.

4. Place clean towels around skin edges.

5. Fine interrupted gut or silk sutures may be used to close the subcutaneous tissue. Retraction is provided with sponges or small retractors.

6. Skin edges are approximated with Adson forceps, and interrupted fine silk sutures on a cutting needle are used for skin closure.

## REPAIR OF HERNIAS

**GENERAL CONSIDERATIONS.** A hernia can be defined (although this is debatable) as the displacement of any viscus (usually bowel) or tissue through a congenital or acquired opening or defect in the wall of its natural cavity. The term *hernia* is usually applied to protrusion of abdominal viscera; however, it is actually a defect in the wall through which abdominal contents have protruded. Hernias are classified according to their anatomical site as inguinal, femoral, epigastric, umbilical, incisional, and diaphragmatic (Fig. 17-3). Hernias in general have three layers: (1) the coverings, (2) the sac, and (3) the hernial contents. In certain locations the sac or coverings may be absent.

The coverings of the hernial sac vary. In acute cases of herniation, the intestines may be pushed through the separated muscles with little covering except the peritoneum and skin.

The hernial sac is a complete peritoneal pouch, which may be acquired or congenital. In the congenital hernia, the sac, as it progresses through the abdominal wall, acquires a series of thin coverings, each one representing a layer of that wall. The neck of the sac is often thick, endurated, and adherent to the surrounding structures.

The contents of the sac may contain parts of the viscera such as the omentum, loops of small or large intestine, the appendix, or a fallopian tube. The anatomical situation of the hernia will in part determine its possible content.

A hernia is *reducible* when the hernial contents can be replaced by manipulation in their normal position and the sac remains in the abdominal wall.

A hernia is *irreducible,* or *incarcerated,* when the hernial contents cannot be replaced in their normal position. The conditions preventing the return of the hernial contents into the abdomen can be due to (1) adhesions between the contents of the sac and the inner lining of the sac, (2) adhesions between the contents of the sac,

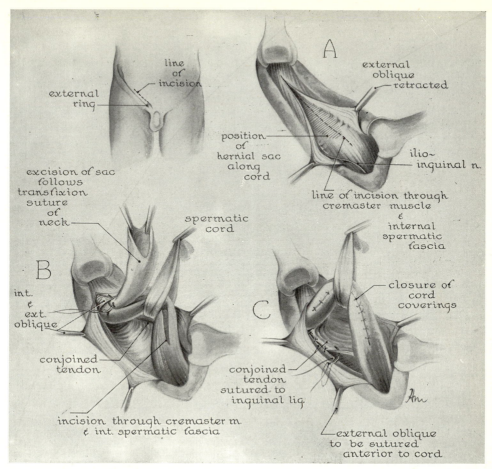

Fig. 17-15. **A** and **B**, Repair of inguinal hernia. **C**, Conjoined tendon is sutured to inguinal ligament under cord. (From Moseley, H. F.: Textbook of surgery, ed. 3, St. Louis, 1959, The C. V. Mosby Co.)

and (3) narrowing of the neck of the sac.

Strangulated hernia is a hernia in which there is a diminished or absent blood supply to the hernial contents. It is almost always irreducible.

Acquired hernia is a herniation brought on by lifting, a strain, or other injury.

SURGICAL ANATOMY. The anterolateral abdominal wall consists of an arrangement of muscles, fascial layers, and muscular aponeuroses lined interiorly by peritoneum and exteriorly by skin. The abdominal wall in the groin area seems to be composed of two groups of these structures: a superficial group, namely, Scarpa's fascia, external and internal oblique muscles, and their aponeuroses and a deep group, the

internal oblique transverse fascia and peritoneum.

## Inguinal herniorrhaphy (direct or indirect)

DEFINITION. Reconstruction of a weakened area in the abdominal wall after reduction or repair of the protruding tissue in the opening.

SURGICAL ANATOMY. The spermatic cord progresses diagonally through the muscular structures in the groin area, excluding the peritoneum (Fig. 17-15). In the female the round ligament is located in this area. This passage or groove, about 1½ inches long, is referred to as the inguinal canal, one on the right side and the other on the left.

The canal begins at the internal (deep

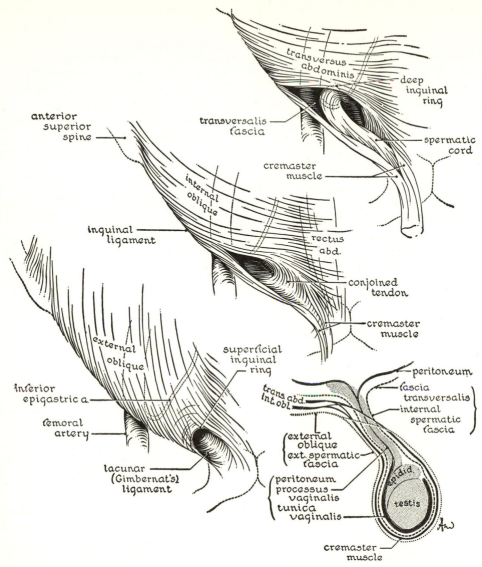

**Fig. 17-16.** Anatomy of inguinal canal is shown. (From Moseley, H. F.: Textbook of surgery, ed. 3, St. Louis, 1959, The C. V. Mosby Co.)

inguinal) ring in the transverse muscle and ends at the external (superficial inguinal) ring in the aponeurosis of the external oblique muscle. The so-called rings are actually defects or thinned-out portions of the structures (Fig. 17-16).

The following organs and tissues may be involved during the repair of an inguinal hernia: the inguinal nerves, cord structures, sac contents, femoral or epigastric vessels, and bladder. If the inguinal nerve has been

accidentally divided, the proximal end will most likely be ligated to prevent a neuroma. If the vas deferens has been accidentally divided, an end-to-end anastomosis with fine silk will be used for its repair.

An indirect inguinal hernia (weakness of the fascial margin of the internal ring) leaves the abdomen through the inguinal ring, passes through the inguinal canal, and emerges at the external ring.

A direct hernia (weakness of the fascial

floor of the inguinal canal) does not enter the canal through the internal ring, but protrudes directly through the transverse fascia below the epigastric vessels, emerging at the external ring.

**SETUP AND PREPARATION OF THE PATIENT.** The extent of the area to be shaved and the skin preparation is determined by the surgeon (Chapter 4). The patient is placed in a supine position (Chapter 7). Occasionally the surgeon requests a pillow beneath the knees of the patient to provide slight relaxation of the groin area. Draping of the patient is as described in Chapter 5.

**FOR INGUINAL HERNIA.** This is the same as for a laparotomy, excluding the longer instruments and larger retractors. The size of instruments, drapes, sponges, and sutures will depend on the age and size of the patient. For the pediatric patient, mosquito hemostats, small Kelly hemostats, and smaller retractors will be needed. Today it is desirable to use nonabsorbable sutures in the repair of hernias. Sutures may include silk or cotton nos. 0 to 4-0 and stainless steel or tantalum wire nos. 3-0 to 5-0. To repair some defects, tantalum gauze, stainless steel wire mesh, or synthetic material may be required (Chapter 6).

**FOR BILATERAL INGUINAL HERNIA.** With the addition of a plastic incisional drape, the setup is the same as described for inguinal hernia. If the plastic incisional drape is not used, a Mayo setup as described for gastrointestinal surgery is preferred (Chapter 21). Two complete setups can also be used, one for each side, that is, two separate procedures.

**OPERATIVE PROCEDURE**

1. An incision about 4 inches long is made a fingerbreadth above and parallel to Poupart's ligament, using laparotomy sponges, scalpel, and hemostats as described for laparotomy.

2. The incision is made through the skin and subcutaneous fascia down to the external oblique muscle, clamping the vessels and ligating with silk no. 3-0.

3. A pair of small retractors are used to expose the external oblique fascia.

4. With a clean scalpel, an incision is made in the external oblique fascia in line with its fibers. Metzenbaum scissors are generally used to extend the incision to the length of the wound.

5. Using four hemostats, the external oblique fascial edges are retracted, exposing the cremaster muscle and cord structures.

6. Blunt and sharp dissection of the cremasteric fibers may be necessary to free the cord structures from the inguinal floor. Smooth tissue forceps must be used to prevent injury to the nerves and spermatic artery.

7. Gentle retraction of the cord may be maintained with a Penrose-type drain secured with a Rochester-Pean forceps.

8. The nature of the hernia is determined. Bulging peritoneum beneath the cord indicates a direct hernia, whereas peritoneum protruding along the cord indicates an indirect hernia.

   a. If direct, the peritoneum bulging through the muscle is exposed, using moist gauze sponges. The sac is usually broad and shallow and if the defect is small, the bulge may be depressed and the sac reduced by imbricating the transverse fascia with no. 2-0 silk sutures.

   b. If indirect, the hernia sac is exposed, the very tip of the sac is grasped with a hemostat, and the cord is elevated as the sac is gently dissected free.

9. The hernia sac is incised, and the contents are pushed into the abdominal cavity. A moist sponge on a holder may be used.

10. Four hemostats are placed on the sac edges for traction, enabling the surgeon to insert a finger into the sac for blunt dissection. A gauze sponge is wrapped around the index finger, and the hernial sac is freed by blunt dissection.

11. The neck of the sac is twisted, trans-

fixed, and doubly ligated with silk sutures no. 2-0 or 0.

12. The sac is excised using Metzenbaum scissors. The hernial sac is saved for pathological examination and cared for according to the policy of the hospital.

There are various methods of hernia repair. However, they all have the same objectives: high ligation of the sac and an adequate reconstruction of the roof and floor of the inguinal canal. The handling of the sac is the same; the suturing may vary.

13. Interrupted silk sutures no. 2-0 or 0 are used for repair. The subcutaneous tissues are closed with interrupted silk sutures no. 3-0 or 4-0.

14. The skin edges are approximated and closed with interrupted silk sutures no. 4-0 on a cutting needle. A subcuticular closure with plain gut no. 3-0 or 4-0 is often preferred for the pediatric patient.

## Femoral herniorrhaphy

**DEFINITION.** To remove and replace peritoneum protruding through the femoral ring, which is situated just below Poupart's ligament and medial to the femoral vein, and to repair the defect in the transverse fascia at the exit of the femoral vessels.

**CONSIDERATIONS.** A femoral hernia is found more frequently in women than in men. It is seldom found in children. In the adult it may be unilateral or bilateral. Even though the femoral hernia is found predominantly in women, it is not seen as frequently as the indirect inguinal hernia.

**SURGICAL ANATOMY.** The layers in the femoral area are skin, fat, subcutaneous fascia, fascia lata, transverse fascia, and peritoneum.

**SETUP AND PREPARATION OF THE PATIENT.** Setup is the same as for laparotomy, with the inclusion of an intestinal set. The skin preparation, positioning, and draping of the patient are as previously described (Chapters 4, 5, and 7).

**OPERATIVE PROCEDURE.** There are three approaches for femoral hernia repair: (1)

the lower approach through the thigh, usually done to relieve strangulation in the critically ill patient, (2) the upper or abdominal approach (transinguinal), which is the preferred method, and (3) the preperitoneal approach, which is usually performed in addition to a pelvic or lower abdominal procedure.

**TRANSINGUINAL APPROACH**

1. The incision is made as described for inguinal hernia, and sometimes the incision is made in the groin crease.

2. The inferior epigastric vessels are divided and ligated with silk sutures no. 2-0.

3. The sac is dissected free, opened, inspected, and closed with a silk figure-of-eight or purse-string suture no. 2-0.

4. The wound is closed in layers as described earlier.

Incarcerations and strangulations are common in femoral hernias, and with this approach an intestinal resection can be performed.

**LOWER APPROACH.** A vertical incision about 3 inches long is made through the tissues overlying the sac. Sometimes the saphenous vein must be ligated. Ligation of the sac and wound closure are the same as for the transinguinal approach.

## Repair of sliding hernia

**DEFINITION.** To free and reduce the sliding viscus and to repair the abdominal tissues surrounding and overlying the inguinal canal.

**CONSIDERATIONS.** The term *sliding hernia* indicates that as the peritoneum slides into the internal ring, it carries with it mesentery and intestine. If the hernia is on the right side, mesentery carries with it a loop of cecum; however, its occurrence is more frequently on the left side. The sliding contents may be ascending, descending, or sigmoid colon, cecum, appendix, and bladder. Very rarely do the sliding contents include tubes, ovaries, and uterus. In the usual type of sliding hernia, the serosal surface of the sliding viscus forms a part of the hernial sac.

The positive diagnosis of a sliding hernia cannot always be made preoperatively.

**SETUP AND PREPARATION OF THE PATIENT.** It is the same as for laparotomy, with the inclusion of intestinal instruments (Chapter 21).

**OPERATIVE PROCEDURE**

1. An oblique incision is made in the inguinal region as described for direct and indirect inguinal hernia. If the sliding hernia is diagnosed preoperatively, the incision will be about an inch higher and more medial.

2. The sac is widely opened to permit freeing of the internal ring. The sac is usually very large and the contents bulky.

3. The adherent bowel is dissected free from the cord structures.

4. If resection is apparent, prepare field for anastomosis (Chapter 21). Supply intestinal instruments, sutures, etc.

5. The upper part of the incision is deepened, and an incision is made into the peritoneal cavity, retracting the edges with hemostats.

6. A curved hemostat is passed from the peritoneum above through the internal ring. The edges of the opened hernial sac are grasped with hemostats and brought into the peritoneal cavity.

7. The bowel is replaced within the peritoneal cavity, and the peritoneum is closed.

8. The handling of the sac, repair of the inguinal floor, and closure of the wound are as described for inguinal hernia.

## Epigastric and hypogastric herniorrhaphy

**DEFINITION.** Ligation of the preperitoneal fat or hernial sac with repair and closure of the abdominal wall.

**CONSIDERATIONS.** An epigastric hernia is usually a small hernia occurring in the linea alba several inches above the umbilicus. A hypogastric hernia occurs in the linea alba below the umbilicus. The opening is usually a small transverse slit in the linea alba and the content usually preperitoneal fat. There may be a sac containing omentum and if the omentum is adhered to the sac, the hernia is often irreducible.

**SETUP AND PREPARATION OF THE PATIENT.** Same as for laparotomy and sutures as used for inguinal hernia repair.

**OPERATIVE PROCEDURE**

1. A small transverse incision about 2 inches long is made directly over the hernial site.

2. The incision is deepened to the fibers of the linea alba.

3. Small retractors are used to expose the hernia.

4. With tissue forceps and Metzenbaum scissors, the preperitoneal fat is dissected free.

5. If a sac is found, it will be handled as described for inguinal hernia.

6. Closure is in layers; seldom is it necessary to imbricate for reinforcement.

## Umbilical herniorrhaphy

**DEFINITION.** Closure of the peritoneal opening and reconstruction of the abdominal wall surrounding the umbilicus.

**CONSIDERATIONS.** Umbilical hernia is usually found in the pediatric patient. It is a protrusion of the peritoneum through the umbilical ring, formed by the fused anterior and posterior rectus sheaths, which normally close after birth. Umbilical hernia at birth is most common in black females. There is a possibility of spontaneous healing in the small umbilical hernia during the first few years of life, but some are so large that they will not close without surgery. Incarceration or strangulation is rare in the infant.

The umbilical hernia found in the adult is usually large and more difficult to repair. The repair of larger adult umbilical hernias is as described for repair of incisional hernia.

**SETUP AND PREPARATION OF THE PATIENT.** As described for laparotomy, with the inclusion of intestinal instruments.

**OPERATIVE PROCEDURE**

1. The skin of the hernia is grasped and retracted upward with Allis forceps.

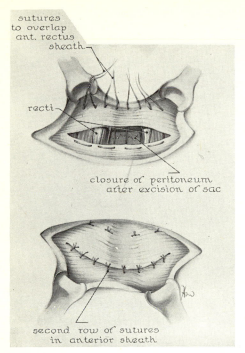

sutures to overlap ant. rectus sheath

recti

closure of peritoneum after excision of sac

second row of sutures in anterior sheath

**Fig. 17-17.** Mayo closure is shown for umbilical hernia. After peritoneum is closed transversely and ring is enlarged by incision of rectus muscles on each side, imbricating upper flap is closed over the lower flap with sutures inserted closely together. Subcutaneous tissue and skin edges are approximated. (From Moseley, H. F.: Textbook of surgery, ed. 3, St. Louis, 1959, The C. V. Mosby Co.)

2. A small curved incision is made below the hernial protrusion.

3. The Allis forceps are placed on the upper skin edges; sharp or blunt dissection is performed to free the sac from the skin.

4. The sac is handled as described for repair of inguinal hernia.

5. If intestinal resection is necessary, prepare the field as described in Chapter 21.

6. The peritoneum is closed with interrupted silk sutures no. 2-0.

7. The rectus sheath is usually overlapped by using multiple mattress sutures of silk no. 2-0. The free edge of the upper flap is secured with interrupted sutures of silk no. 2-0 (Fig. 17-17).

8. A silk suture no. 2-0 on a cutting needle is placed through the fascial layers and subcutaneous tissue at the site of the umbilicus.

9. Skin is closed as described for inguinal hernia.

### Incisional herniorrhaphy

**DEFINITION.** The reunion of the abdominal wall in layers, if at all possible.

**CONSIDERATIONS.** Incisional hernias can be of any size and found almost anywhere in the abdomen. They occur most frequently after vertical abdominal incision due to a disruption of some or all the layers of the abdomen. Some of the possible reasons for their occurrence are excessive postoperative strain, hematoma, infection, and delayed wound healing. In many cases the peritoneum has fused with the fascial layers, making dissection difficult due to the underlying intestine. After dissection, if it is impossible to pull layers of the abdominal wall together without tension, it may be necessary to make relaxing incisions. Another method of reconstruction is the use of prosthetics such as fascia lata, Teflon or Marlex mesh, or tantalum mesh.

**SETUP AND PREPARATION OF THE PATIENT.** As described for laparotomy, including heavy silk or wire sutures.

**OPERATIVE PROCEDURE**

1. An incision to excise the old scar is made.

2. One end of the scar is held with an Allis forceps; the scar is excised carefully. There may not be any peritoneum just below, only skin and intestine.

3. Abdominal contents will be explored, and adhesions will be released by blunt or sharp dissection.

4. The sides of the incision will be undermined to identify fascial layers.

5. The peritoneum may be closed with interrupted heavy sutures and the fascia closed as described for umbilical hernia. Or a figure-of-eight wire closure may be used.

6. Skin is closed as described for inguinal hernia. An abdominal binder may

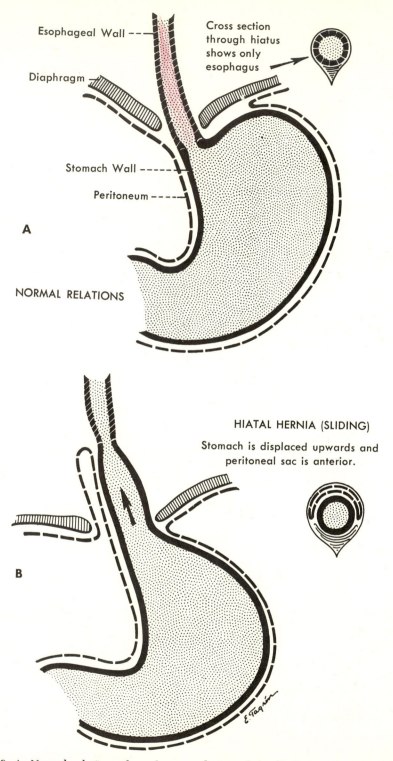

**Fig. 17-18. A,** Normal relations of esophagus and stomach to diaphragm. **B,** Hiatus (sliding) hernia. (From Nardi, G. L., and Zuidema, G. D., editors: Surgery, a concise guide to clinical practice, Boston, 1961, Little, Brown & Co.)

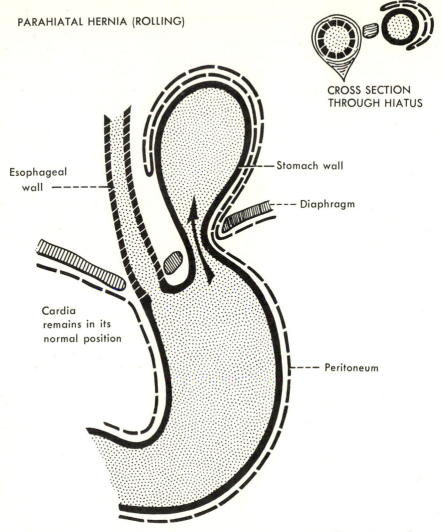

PARAHIATAL HERNIA (ROLLING)

CROSS SECTION
THROUGH HIATUS

Stomach wall

Esophageal
wall

Diaphragm

Cardia
remains in its
normal position

Peritoneum

**Fig. 17-19.** Parahiatal (rolling) hernia. (From Nardi, G. L., and Zuidema, G. D., editors: Surgery, a concise guide to clinical practice, Boston, 1961, Little, Brown & Co.)

be requested to aid in the reduction of strain from the suture line.

### Diaphragmatic herniorrhaphy

**DEFINITION.** To replace the abdominal contents that have entered the thorax and to repair the defect in the diaphragm.

**CONSIDERATIONS.** Diaphragmatic hernias may be classified in three groups. Congenital, acquired, and traumatic. With the repair of the diaphragmatic hernia, it is sometimes necessary to do an additional procedure such as gastropexy, vagectomy, pyloroplasty, subtotal gastrectomy or esophagogastrectomy, and crushing of the phrenic nerve. The esophageal (sliding) hiatus hernia (Fig. 17-18), which occurs with greatest frequency, demonstrates the upward displacement of the stomach.

The esophageal (rolling) parahiatal hernia permits the stomach wall to roll upward into it, leaving the esophagus in the normal position (Fig. 17-19). This

presents the so-called condition of upside-down stomach.

An abdominal, thoracic, or thoracoabdominal approach is selected, depending on the condition of the patient, location of the hernia, and other existing pathological conditions.

SETUP AND PREPARATION OF THE PATIENT. A laparotomy, thoracotomy, and intestinal setup is used, including extra-large retractors and long sutures.

OPERATIVE PROCEDURE (see Chapter 14)

1. A paramedian, subcostal, thoracoabdominal, or left thoracic incision is made.

2. The hiatus is exposed, and the hernial contents are reduced.

3. The sac, if present, will be carefully incised.

4. The defect in the diaphragm is repaired with mattress sutures.

5. The abdominal or chest wound is closed.

## REFERENCES

1. Allison, P. R.: The diaphragm. In Gibbon, J. H., Jr., editor: Surgery of the chest, Philadelphia, 1962, W. B. Saunders Co.
2. Altemeier, W. A., and Stevenson, J. M.: Physiology of wound healing. In Davis, L., editor: Christopher's textbook of surgery, ed. 6, Philadelphia, 1956, W. B. Saunders Co.
3. Boyd, D.: The transthoracic repair of esophageal hiatus hernia, Surg. Clin. North Am. **6:** 631, 1956.
4. Calman, C. H.: Atlas of hernia repair, St. Louis, 1966, The C. V. Mosby Co.
5. Cole, W. H., and Zollinger, R. M.: Textbook of surgery, ed. 8, New York, 1963, Appleton-Century-Crofts.
6. Cooper, P.: The craft of surgery, ed. 1, vol. II, Boston, 1964, Little, Brown & Co.
7. Goldman, L., and Wylie, E. J.: Abdominal incisions. In Allen, A. W., and Barrow, D. W., editors: Abdominal surgery, New York, 1961, Harper & Row, Publishers.
8. Gross, R. E.: The surgery of infancy and childhood, Philadelphia, 1953, W. B. Saunders Co.
9. Koontz, A., and Kimberly, R. C.: Tissue reactions to tantalum mesh and wire, Ann. Surg. **131:**666, 1950.
10. Lampe, E. W.: Surgical anatomy of the abdominal wall, Surg. Clin. North Am. **32:**545, 1952.
11. Latimer, E. O., and Werr, J. A.: Clinical experience with Dacron as a nonabsorbable suture material, Surg. Gynecol. Obstet. **112:** 373, March, 1961.
12. Leacock, A. G., and Rowley, R. K.: Results of nylon repairs in inguinal hernias, Lancet **1:**20, 1962.
13. Lichtenstein, M. D.: The abdominal wall and peritoneum. In Davis, L., editor: Christopher's textbook of surgery, ed. 6, Philadelphia, 1956, W. B. Saunders Co.
14. Mair, G. G.: Surgery of abdominal hernia, Baltimore, 1948, The Williams & Wilkins Co.
15. McVay, C. B., and Anson, B. J.: Inguinal and femoral hernioplasty, Surg. Gynecol. Obstet. **88:**473, April, 1949.
16. Moseley, H. F.: Textbook of surgery, ed. 3, St. Louis, 1959, The C. V. Mosby Co.
17. Nardi, G. L., and Zuidema, G. D., editors: Surgery: a concise guide to clinical practice, chapter 14, Boston, 1961, Little, Brown & Co.
18. Nyhus, L. M.: Hernias. In Egdahl, R. H., and Mannick, J. A.: Modern surgery, New York, 1970, Grune & Stratton, Inc.
19. Ravitch, M. M.: Repair of hernias, the handbook of operative surgery, Chicago, 1969, Year Book Medical Publishers, Inc.
20. Usher, F. C., and Ochsner, J. R.: Marlex mesh: a new polyethylene mesh for replacing tissue defects, Surg. Forum **10:**319, 1960.
21. Wilder, J. R.: Atlas of general surgery, ed. 2, St. Louis, 1964, The C. V. Mosby Co.

# CHAPTER 18

# Thyroid and parathyroid surgery

JUDITH YVONNE JACOBS

Surgery of goiter has long been a part of modern surgery. The introduction of iodine therapy in 1923 greatly reduced the incidence of endemic goiter and consequently the need for goiter surgery. Since 1941, surgery on the thyroid gland has taken on a changed role due to the use of radioactive iodine and antithyroid drugs that preoperatively decrease the size and vascularity of the gland.

## ANATOMY AND PHYSIOLOGY OF THE THYROID GLAND

The thyroid gland is a very vascular organ situated at the front of the neck. It consists of right and left lobes united by a middle portion, known as the isthmus. The isthmus is situated near the base of the neck, and the lobes lie alongside the larynx and trachea. The upper pole of the gland is hidden beneath the upper end of the

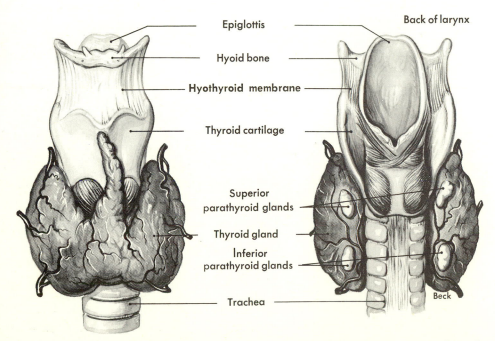

Epiglottis

Back of larynx

Hyoid bone

**Hyothyroid membrane**

Thyroid cartilage

Superior
parathyroid glands

Thyroid gland

Inferior
parathyroid glands

Trachea

Beck

**Fig. 18-1.** Thyroid and parathyroid glands. Note their relations to each other and to the larynx (voice box) and trachea. (From Anthony, C. P.: Textbook of anatomy and physiology, ed. 8, St. Louis, 1971, The C. V. Mosby Co.)

700

sternothyroid muscle. The lower pole extends to the sixth tracheal ring. The posterior surface of the isthmus is adherent to the anterior surface of the tracheal rings, and the gland is enclosed by the pretracheal fascia (Fig. 18-1).

Blood supply to the thyroid is from the external carotid arteries, via the superior thyroid arteries, and from the subclavian arteries, via the inferior thyroid arteries. The thyroid gland is drained by three pairs of veins, which are given off by a plexus formed on the surface of the gland and on the front of the trachea. The capillaries form a dense plexus in the connective tissue around the follicles.

On each side the superior laryngeal nerve lies in close proximity with the superior thyroid artery. The recurrent laryngeal nerve that supplies the vocal cord ascends from the mediastinum and is in close association with the tracheoesophageal sulcus and the inferior thyroid artery. Sympathetic and parasympathetic nerves enter the gland, probably exerting their influence primarily on blood flow.

Numerous lymphatics of the pretracheal fascia and carotid sheath drain the gland.

The thyroid gland is important in maintaining the metabolic rate at a level compatible with health and efficiency. It is not, however, essential to life. Removal of the thyroid results in reduction of the oxidative processes of the body.

The thyroid gland is primarily concerned with iodine metabolism. Ingested iodides are absorbed from the gastrointestinal tract into the circulation, from which they are sequestered by the thyroid gland. Iodides are converted into thyroid hormones, some of which are stored in the gland as thyroglobulin or secreted into the blood as thyroxin.

## THYROIDECTOMY

CONSIDERATIONS. Graves' disease (hyperthyroidism) is associated with diffuse and near symmetrical enlargement of the thyroid gland. In surgical treatment of hyperthyroidism, the objective is to resect enough

of the gland to reduce the level of circulating hormones to normal, yet leave a sufficient amount of the gland to secrete a supply of the hormone.

In Hashimoto's thyroiditis, thought to be an auto-immune disease, there is nontender enlargement of the gland. Surgery is done to relieve tracheal obstruction.

Nontoxic nodular goiter does not produce an excess of hormones and is not inflammatory in character. This condition is a proliferation of the thyroid tissue in an attempt to produce the minimal hormonal requirement despite an iodine-deficient diet. Surgery may be indicated to relieve tracheal or esophageal obstruction, forestall or rule out a malignant nodule of the thyroid gland, or relieve cosmetic disfigurement.

In the presence of papillary carcinoma and in thyroid nodules in children, a total thyroidectomy is usually done. In the presence of a primary tumor of one lobe, total thyroid lobectomy and radical neck dissection of the involved side may be performed, since the primary route of metastasis is through the regional lymph nodes.

## THYROID LOBECTOMY

DEFINITION. Removal of a lobe of the thyroid gland.

SETUP AND PREPARATION OF THE PATIENT. The patient is placed on the table in a dorsal recumbent position with the neck extended and the shoulders raised by a conductive rubberized block or rolled sheet. The table is slanted downward to elevate the upper part of the body for the convenience of the surgeon (see Chapter 7).

An endotracheal anesthetic is administered. An effective suction apparatus is most essential.

The proposed operative site, including the anterior neck region, lateral surfaces of the neck down to the outer aspects of the shoulders, and the upper anterior chest region, is cleansed in the usual manner (see Chapter 4). The patient is draped with sterile towels and a fenestrated sheet, as described in Chapter 5.

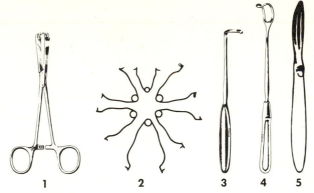

Fig. 18-2. Special instruments for thyroidectomy. 1, Lahey vulsellum forceps; 2, wire or spring retractors (set); 3, Lahey thyroid retractor; 4, Greene thyroid retractor; 5, Kocher sound. (Courtesy Codman & Shurtleff, Inc., Randolph, Mass.)

A standard instrument setup for thyroid surgery should include (1) a tracheal suction setup with a whistle-tipped type of catheter having an open end, (2) fine tissue forceps with several teeth to prevent slipping, (3) fine straight and curved hemostats to control bleeding vessels without causing trauma, (4) fine plastic scissors for isolation of facial and recurrent laryngeal nerves and for dissection of arteries and veins, and (5) tracheostomy setup ready for emergency use.

The thyroidectomy setup (Fig. 18-2) includes the following:

**Cutting instruments**

    2 Knife handles no. 3, blades nos. 10 and 15
    1 Knife handle no. 7, blade no. 12, if desired
    1 Mayo scissors, curved
    1 Suture scissors, straight
    1 Lahey goiter scissors
    1 Metzenbaum scissors
    1 Stevens scissors, if desired

**Holding instruments**

    4 Lahey gall duct forceps
    2 Martin tissue forceps with fine teeth
    1 Adson tissue forceps
    2 Tissue forceps with 1 and 2 teeth, 5½ in.
    2 Tissue forceps without teeth
    4 Lahey vulsellum forceps
    4 Allis forceps
    8 Towel forceps, small size
    5 Foerster sponge-holding forceps

**Clamping instruments** (see Chapter 5)

    48 Crile hemostats, 36 curved and 12 straight
    24 Mosquito hemostats, curved
    4 Ochsner or Kocher forceps

**Exposing instruments**

    2 Cushing loop muscle retractors
    2 U.S. Army retractors
    2 McBurney or Greene retractors
    2 Lahey retractors
    2 Volkmann retractors, 4-pronged, blunt
    2 Skin hook retractors
    1 Nerve hook

**Suturing instruments**

    3 Crile-Wood needle holders
      Suture material (see Chapter 6):
        Plain gut no. 3-0
        Chromic gut nos. 0, 2-0, and 3-0
        Silk nos. 2-0, 3-0, and 4-0
        Nylon no. 5-0
      Swaged-on needles, desirable size, or 2 Mayo or Ferguson needles, ½-circle, taper point no. 4
    2 Surgeon's regular needles, ⅜-circle, taper point no. 10
    2 Murphy needles, ½-circle, taper point, nos. 3 and 4
    8 Keith or milliner needles

**Accessory items**

    1 Suction set
    1 Tracheostomy set
    1 Penrose drain, ⅜ in. wide and 8 in. long
      Dressings

**OPERATIVE PROCEDURE**

1. A transverse incision is made through the skin and first layer of the cervical fascia and platysma muscles, approximately 2 cm. above the sternoclavicular junction or in the normal skin crease by means of a length of silk thread for marking skin, a knife with a no. 10 blade, tissue forceps, and sponges (Fig. 18-3).

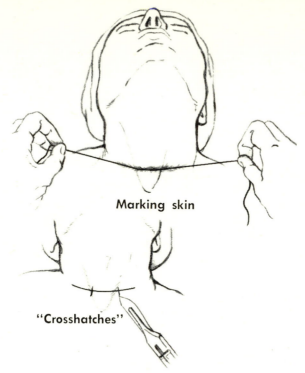

Marking skin

"Crosshatches"

**Fig. 18-3.** Thyroidectomy. Proposed area of skin incision is outlined by pressure with fine silk thread to ensure even cosmetic incision. Patient who is to undergo thyroidectomy has considerable amount of anxiety concerning incision into neck and cosmetic results, particularly women. That collar incision after surgery is barely perceptible should be explained to patient. (From Wilder, J. R.: Atlas of general surgery, ed. 2, St. Louis, 1964, The C. V. Mosby Co.)

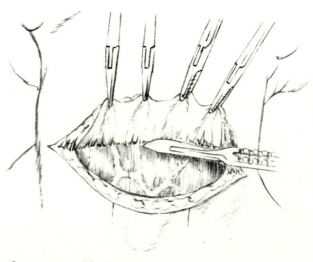

**Fig. 18-4.** Thyroidectomy—cont'd. Skin flaps are created by dissection through underlying platysma and cervical fascia. (From Wilder, J. R.: Atlas of general surgery, ed. 2, St. Louis, 1964, The C. V. Mosby Co.)

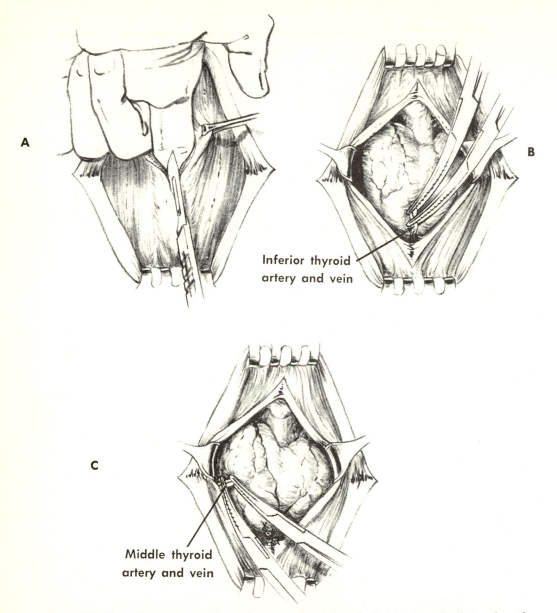

Inferior thyroid
artery and vein

Middle thyroid
artery and vein

**Fig. 18-5.** Thyroidectomy—cont'd. **A,** Strap muscles reflected. **B,** Ligation of inferior thyroid artery and vein. **C,** Ligation of middle thyroid artery and vein. (From Wilder, J. R.: Atlas of general surgery, ed. 2, St. Louis, 1964, The C. V. Mosby Co.)

2. Flaps may be held away from the wound with stay sutures inserted through the fascia and platysma, or the skin edges of flaps may be inverted and covered with skin towels by means of heavy silk sutures or small towel forceps.

3. The upper skin flap is undermined to the level of the cricoid cartilage; then the lower flap is undermined to the sternoclavicular joint, using a knife, curved scissors, tissue forceps, and moist gauze compresses (Fig. 18-4). Bleeding vessels are clamped with mosquito hemostats and ligated with white silk no. 5-0 or plain gut no. 3-0 ligatures.

4. The fascia on the midline is incised

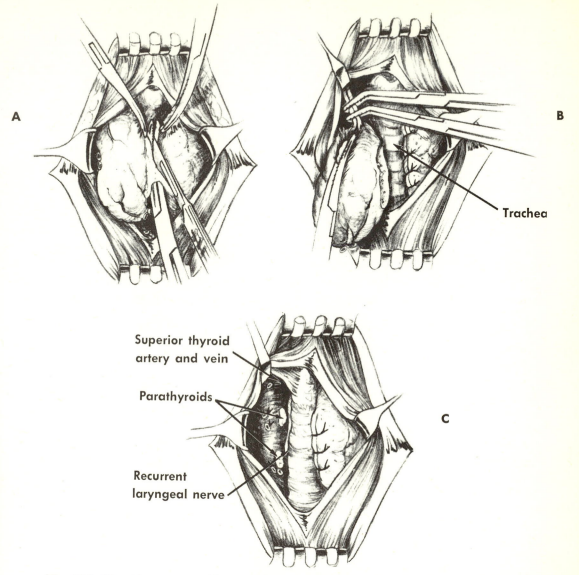

Fig. 18-6. Thyroidectomy—cont'd. **A,** Isthmus divided. **B,** Ligation of pole vessels. **C,** Anatomical structures identified and wound examined for bleeding. (From Wilder, J. R.: Atlas of general surgery, ed. 2, St. Louis, 1964, The C. V. Mosby Co.)

between the strap (sternohyoid) muscles with a knife (Fig. 18-5); the sternocleidomastoid muscle is retracted with a loop retractor; the strap muscles may be divided between clamps, using Ochsner or Crile hemostats and a knife. The divided muscles are retracted away from the operative site with Lahey vulsellum forceps, thereby exposing the diseased lobe.

5. The inferior and middle thyroid veins are doubly clamped with curved duct forceps, divided with Metzenbaum scissors, and doubly ligated with chromic gut no. 0 or silk ligatures (Fig. 18-5).

6. The lobe is rotated by means of forceps, and the loose areolar tissue is divided posteriorly and medially toward the tracheoesophageal sulcus, using hemostats and Metzenbaum scissors. Bleeding is controlled

by hemostats and ligatures. The recurrent laryngeal nerve is identified.

7. The middle thyroid artery is ligated with chromic gut no. 0 or silk no. 2-0. Fine forceps, curved hemostats, and fine scissors are needed.

8. The thyroid lobe is pulled downward, and the avascular tissue between the trachea and upper pole of the thyroid is dissected by means of Metzenbaum scissors (Fig. 18-6).

9. The superior thyroid artery is secured with two or three curved hemostats; the artery is ligated and divided and then transfixed with chromic gut or silk sutures (Fig. 18-6).

10. The inferior thyroid artery is identified and ligated by means of fine forceps, sutures, and scissors. The thyroid lobe is then dissected away from the recurrent nerve, using Metzenbaum scissors, hemostats, and retractors. Bleeding vessels are clamped with hemostats and ligated with fine chromic gut or fine silk sutures.

11. The lobe is elevated with Lahey vulsellum forceps; it is freed from the trachea with fine scissors, forceps, knife, and hemostats. The fibrous bands attached to the trachea and cricoid cartilage are divided.

12. The isthmus of the gland is elevated with fine forceps and divided between Crile hemostats with scissors. The resection of the lobe is completed and the lobe removed.

13. The strap muscles, if severed, are approximated with interrupted chromic gut or silk sutures. A Penrose drain may be inserted in the thyroid bed (Fig. 18-7) and brought out between the strap muscles and sternocleidomastoid muscle.

14. The edges of the platysma are approximated; then the skin edges are approximated with interrupted fine silk sutures (Fig. 18-7).

15. Gauze dressings are applied to the wound; a thyroid collar-type dressing is applied. This dressing consists of a strip of adhesive tape 2 inches wide and 28 inches long, with a folded gauze compress covering its center portion. The gauze prevents the hair from coming in contact with the tape. The dressing is brought from the back of the neck to the front, and the free ends of the collar are crossed and secured over the chest region. The dressing is further secured in place by additional strips of tape.

16. The vocal cords are inspected as the endotracheal tube is withdrawn to rule out possible nerve damage.

## SUBSTERNAL OR INTRATHORACIC THYROID

Extensions of enlarging goiters into the substernal and intrathoracic regions are rarely seen. They may cause tracheal and esophageal obstruction, in which case they are surgically excised.

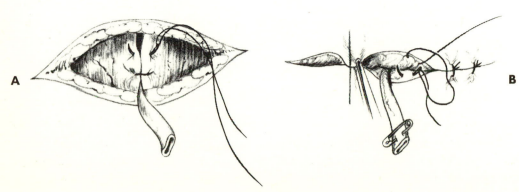

**Fig. 18-7.** Thyroidectomy—cont'd. **A,** Drain. **B,** Skin closure. (From Wilder, J. R.: Atlas of general surgery, ed. 2, St. Louis, 1964, The C. V. Mosby Co.)

## THYROGLOSSAL DUCT CYSTECTOMY

DEFINITION. Complete excision of all portions of the sac and a portion of the hyoid bone to avoid recurrent cystic formation and prevent infections.

CONSIDERATIONS. The thyroglossal duct is an embryological structure present during the descent of the thyroid gland into the anterior neck. When present in the adult, it exists as a pretracheal cystic pouch attached to the hyoid bone, with or without a sinus tract to the base of the tongue at the foramen cecum.

SETUP AND PREPARATION OF THE PATIENT. A modified thyroidectomy set, plus the following:

    1 Periosteal elevator, small
    1 Duckbill rongeur, small
    1 Bone cutter, small
      Silver probes
      Methylene blue dye for injection
      Syringe, 5 ml., and appropriate needle

OPERATIVE PROCEDURE

1. After extending the head and elevating the chin, an incision is made between the hyoid bone and the thyroid cartilage through the subcutaneous tissue.

2. The platysma muscle layers are mobilized and retracted using small muscle retractors.

3. The anterior cervical fascia is longitudinally incised and the sternohyoid muscle retracted.

4. Sharp and blunt dissection is used to mobilize the cyst down to its attachment to the hyoid bone. The hyoid is transected with bone-cutting forceps and the segment of bone and cyst freed from adjacent structures.

5. The cephalad part of the duct is identified; a transfixion suture no. 3-0 is passed through it and the duct transected. (Methylene blue dye injection will aid in visualizing the whole tract.)

6. The cyst is removed. The thyrohyoid muscles are closed with interrupted silk sutures no. 3-0. A drain may be placed. The skin is closed with interrupted nylon sutures no. 5-0.

## PARATHYROID SURGERY

Interest in the parathyroid glands began in 1880 when they were discovered by the Swedish anatomist Sandström. Through the years, continuing discoveries have been made linking disturbances of these endocrine glands with tetany, bone diseases, renal calculi, and many other systemic abnormalities. Current surgical interest is focused on definitive treatment of hyperparathyroidism.

## ANATOMY AND PHYSIOLOGY OF THE PARATHYROID GLANDS

The parathyroid glands are four small masses of tissue lying behind or within the thyroid gland, inside the pretracheal fascia. The upper pair lie behind the superior pole of the thyroid; the lower pair lie near the lower pole of the thyroid. Aberrant nodules of the parathyroid tissue may be found outside the pretracheal fascia as low as the superior mediastinum (within the thymus). The glands are a pinkish buff color and normally measure 3 to 6 mm. in diameter. Their blood supply is derived from the superior and inferior thyroid arteries (Figs. 18-5 and 18-6).

The function of these glands in body metabolism is most important. The endocrine secretion of parathormone regulates and maintains the metabolism and hemostasis of blood calcium concentration. Removal of all parathyroid tissue results in severe tetany or death. The diseases attributed to the parathyroid glands are hyperparathyroidism, which results in elevation of calcium in the blood, and hypoparathyroidism, resulting in decreased calcium in the blood.

## PARATHYROIDECTOMY

DEFINITION. Excision of one or more diseased parathyroid glands. Normal or atrophic glands are not to be damaged or resected.

CONSIDERATIONS. The presence of adenomas (hypersecreting neoplasms), hyperplasia, or carcinomas requires surgical excision. In the latter case, resection of lym-

phatics is essential, although metastasis may also occur via the bloodstream. After local excision, a metastasis may continue the hypersecretion of parathyroid hormone.

SETUP AND PREPARATION OF THE PATIENT. Same as for thyroidectomy. Presterilized specimen cups (plastic medicine cups) on the scrubbed nursing team member's table may simplify the separation and identification of the specimens.

OPERATIVE PROCEDURE

1. A transverse incision is made through the skin, first layer of cervical fascia, and platysma muscles, approximately 2 cm. above the sternoclavicular junction or in the normal skin crease by means of a knife handle no. 3 with blade no. 10, tissue forceps, and sponges (Fig. 18-4).

2. The skin edges of the flaps may be inverted and covered with skin towels using small towel forceps.

3. The upper skin flap is undermined to the level of the cricoid cartilage; then the lower flap is undermined to the sternoclavicular joint using a knife, Metzenbaum scissors, tissue forceps, and sponges. Bleeding vessels are clamped with mosquito hemostats and ligated with plain gut or silk sutures no. 3-0.

4. The midline fascia is incised between the sternohyoid muscles (Fig. 18-5); the sternocleidomastoid muscles are retracted with small muscle retractors. The sternohyoid muscles may be divided by means of Ochsner clamps and a knife for better operative exposure.

5. The thyroid gland is now visible. A thorough exploration of the "normal" locations of the parathyroids is conducted in order to find the four glands. Meticulous hemostasis by means of mosquito hemostats and fine silk ligatures is a prerequisite to location and identification of these small glands.

6. The thyroid gland is gently rotated forward by means of forceps to provide access to the posterior thyroid sulcus where the upper parathyroid is most frequently found. Identification of the parathyroid vascular pedicle as it leaves the superior thy-

roid artery is an excellent means of finding the upper gland. Metzenbaum scissors, mosquito hemostats, and Kitner sponges are used in the dissection.

7. Attention is then directed toward the posterior lateral surface of the thyroid lobe or just beneath the lower thyroid pole, where the lower parathyroid is frequently found. Again, finding the vascular pedicle from the inferior thyroid artery may aid in identification. Occasionally the lower pair may be found in the thymic capsule or tissue, in which case a portion of the thymus is resected.

8. Should one of the upper or lower pair evidence disease, it is resected by clamping the vascular pedicle with mosquito forceps, cutting with a knife and blade no. 15, and ligating with silk no. 3-0 ligatures. A portion of one gland must remain to prevent complications.

9. The neck region is explored for aberrant parathyroid tissue, which is also resected.

10. The sternohyoid muscle, if severed, is approximated with silk no. 3-0 sutures on fine taper point needles. The platysma is approximated with silk no. 4-0 sutures and the skin edges with nylon no. 5-0 sutures (Fig. 18-7).

11. A dressing is applied as decribed for thyroid surgery.

REFERENCES

1. Anthony, C. P.: Textbook of anatomy and physiology, ed. 8, St. Louis, 1971, The C. V. Mosby Co.
2. Ballinger, W. F., and Haff, R. C.: Hyperparathyroidism: increased frequency of diagnosis, South. Med. J. **63**:571, 1970.
3. Birnstingl, M.: Subtotal thyroidectomy, Nurs. Times **63**:1332, Oct. 6, 1967.
4. Cope, O.: Hyperparathyroidism, diagnosis and management, Am. J. Surg. **99**:394, 1960.
5. Davis, L., editor: Christopher's textbook of surgery, ed. 8, Philadelphia, 1964, W. B. Saunders Co.
6. Haff, R. C., Black, W. C., and Ballinger, W. F.: Primary hyperparathyroidism: changing clinical, surgical, and pathologic aspects, Ann. Surg. **171**:85, 1970.
7. Jackson, C., and Jackson, C. L.: Diseases

of the nose, throat, and ear, ed. 2, Philadelphia, 1959, W. B. Saunders Co.

8. Madden, J. L.: Atlas of technics in surgery, ed. 2, New York, 1964, Appleton-Century-Crofts.

9. Moyer, C. A., Rhoads, J. E., Allen, J. G., and Harkins, H. N.: Surgery: principles and practice, ed. 3, Philadelphia, 1965, J. B. Lippincott Co.

10. Randall, H. T., Hardy, J. D., and Moore, F. D., editors: Manual of preoperative and postoperative care, Philadelphia, 1967, W. B. Saunders Co.

11. Rawson, R. W.: The thyroid gland, Clin. Symp. **17**:35, April-June, 1965.

# CHAPTER 19

# Breast surgery

JUDITH YVONNE JACOBS

Surgery on the mammary glands is performed in the presence of disease; it is also done because of other physical and psychological determinants.

## ANATOMY AND PHYSIOLOGY OF THE BREAST

The mammary glands are bilateral organs lying in the superficial fascia of the pectoral region and extending toward the axilla. The normal global contour is secondary to this fascial support. The breasts are not encapsulated; they extend from the edge of the sternum to the anterior axillary line and from the first to the seventh rib. The deep surface of the glands rests on the connective tissue covering the greater pectoral and anterior serratus muscles.

The glands are ectodermal in origin, aris-

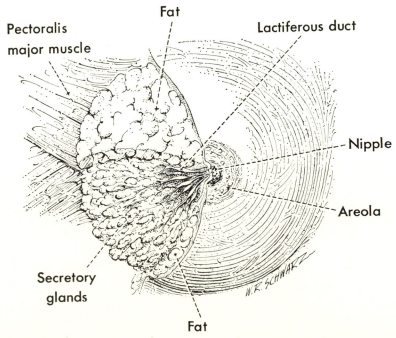

**Fig. 19-1.** Diagrammatic cross section of mammary gland showing relationship of various anatomical structures. (From Jorstad, L. H.: Surgery of the breast, St. Louis, 1964, The C. V. Mosby Co.; drawings by W. R. Schwarz.)

ing from epithelial ingrowths that divide, subdivide, and proliferate to form the lobules of the glands (Fig. 19-1). Each breast consists of fifteen to twenty lobes separated by septa of connective tissue and adipose tissue deposits. Each lobe consists of connective tissue in which are embedded the secreting cells (alveoli) arranged in grapelike clusters around minute ducts. These ducts converge to form a single duct from each lobe, which drains into the nipple. The nipple forms a conical projection in which each duct has a tiny opening to the body surface. The areola is the pigmented circular area around the nipple that contains sebaceous glands. The glandular portion of the breast is central in location, since it is surrounded and permeated by adipose tissue, the amount of which determines actual breast size.

The mammary glands are present in the male and the female; however, hormonal stimulation of the female during puberty promotes actual development. Estrogen promotes growth of the ducts, and progesterone promotes growth of the alveoli. The ultimate function of the gland is lactation, which is promoted by the lactogenic hormone after pregnancy.

The blood supply of the mammary glands is derived from branches of the internal mammary and intercostal arteries and from the external mammary branches of the lateral thoracic artery. The veins follow the courses of the arteries.

Lymphatics also follow the course of the vessels. These drain into the axillary nodes and internal mammary chain of nodes. The lymphatics act as channels for the spread of malignant disease from the breast to associated lymph glands on the chest wall or in the axilla.

The nerve supply is mainly from the anterior cutaneous branches of the upper intercostal nerves, the third and fourth branches of the cervical plexus, and the lateral cutaneous branches of the intercostal nerves.

Occasionally supernumerary nipples and aberrant breast tissue are present. These may be amenable to excision.

## OPERATIONS ON THE BREAST
### Incision and drainage of abscess

**DEFINITION.** Surgical opening of an inflamed and suppurative area of the breast.

**CONSIDERATIONS.** Abscesses are most frequently associated with infections in the lactating breast. Even after antibiotic treatment, granulation of the abscess cavity may be incomplete, and sinus tracts may exist. Surgical excision of the cavity and sinus tract is then indicated.

**SETUP AND PREPARATION OF THE PATIENT.** The patient is placed on the operating table in a supine position, and the operative area is cleansed. Instruments include the following:

1 Knife handle and blade no. 10
2 Mayo scissors, curved and straight
1 Tissue forceps with teeth
2 Crile hemostats
2 Rochester-Pean clamps, 6¼ in.
2 Allis forceps, 6 in.
1 Silver probe
  Culture tube
  Iodoform gauze packing

**OPERATIVE PROCEDURE**

1. An incision is made through the skin over the abscess using a knife handle no. 3 and blade no. 15.
2. A Rochester-Pean clamp is directed subcutaneously and the abscess cavity entered. A culture is taken.
3. Loculations are broken up by exploring the cavity with the index finger.
4. The cavity is irrigated with warm saline solution. Bleeding vessels are ligated with plain gut sutures no. 3-0; the wound is packed with iodoform gauze and allowed to heal by granulation.
5. Should a sinus tract exist, it and the old scar tissue are excised; the wound is packed and allowed to heal by granulation.

### Biopsy of the breast

**DEFINITION.** Removal of tissue to determine the exact nature of a mass in the breast.

NEEDLE BIOPSY. After cleansing the skin, a Vim-Silverman biopsy needle is introduced into the mass and a portion taken for examination.

INCISIONAL BIOPSY. The mass is incised and a portion taken for examination.

EXCISIONAL BIOPSY. Removal of the entire tumor mass from adjacent tissue for examination.

CONSIDERATIONS. Biopsy is indicated in the presence of tumor mass, nipple discharge, and skin changes. Excisional biopsy is considered most effective, since it allows examination of the whole mass and does not necessitate entering the lesion with the potential risk of seeding malignant cells.

SETUP AND PREPARATION OF THE PATIENT. Excisional biopsies are performed in the operating room, where facilities are available for frozen section, immediate diagnosis, and definitive surgery. The surgeon should prepare the patient with the knowledge that extensive surgery may be necessary. General anesthesia is preferred so that the tumor is not obscured by local infiltrate or the patient agitated by the findings.

The patient is placed on the table in a supine position, with the arm on the involved side extended on an armrest. The skin is prepped from above the clavicle to the umbilicus and from the opposite nipple to and including the upper arm. Gentle handling of the breast is encouraged to avoid dislodging tumor cells. The patient is draped in the usual manner; a cloth tray cover or Mayo felt cover may be used over the extended arm and armrest.

A Mayo setup alone is used for the biopsy. The scrubbed nursing team member may assist, or she may remain with her tables in the event that she is needed for more extensive surgery. After the biopsy, the instruments used are removed for cleaning and sterilization. Should more extensive surgery be required, the operative site is again prepped and draped; the surgical team changes gowns and gloves. The following instruments are placed on the Mayo table for the biopsy:

**Cutting instruments**

1 Knife handle no. 3 with blade no. 10
2 Mayo scissors, 1 straight and 1 curved
2 Tissue forceps with teeth
2 Tissue forceps without teeth
1 Electrosurgical unit, if desired

**Holding instruments**

2 Allis forceps
2 Rochester-Pean hemostats, 6¼ in.
6 Crile hemostats
6 Towel clamps

**Exposing instruments**

2 Small muscle retractors
2 Rake retractors, small
1 Set intraductal probes

**Suturing items**

1 Needle holder
1 Package chromic gut suture no. 3-0
1 Package silk or other skin suture

OPERATIVE PROCEDURE

1. An incision over the tumor mass is made through the skin, subcutaneous tissue, and breast tissue, using a scalpel.

2. Gentle traction is applied to the mass by Allis forceps; the tumor mass and an edge of normal tissue are removed by sharp dissection. The specimen is submitted for frozen section examination.

3A. Benign lesion—Breast tissue is approximated using chromic gut no. 3-0 interrupted sutures; fine silk sutures no. 4-0 close the skin; a firm pressure dressing is applied.

3B. Malignant lesion—The incision is tightly closed with silk sutures no. 2-0 on a cutting needle and the wound sealed with collodion to prevent the spread of tumor cells via drainage.

## Simple mastectomy

DEFINITION. Removal of breast tissue without axillary lymphatic contents.

CONSIDERATIONS. A simple mastectomy is done to remove extensive benign disease or as a palliative measure when gross malignancy is present.

SETUP AND PREPARATION OF THE PATIENT. As for excisional biopsy. Have sterile and

at hand the following supplies and instruments:

> Drapes
> Gowns and gloves

**Cutting instruments**

> 2 Knife handles no. 4 with blade no. 20
> 2 Knife handles no. 3 with blade no. 10
> 2 Mayo scissors, 1 straight and 1 curved
> 1 Metzenbaum scissors, 5½ in.
> 2 Tissue forceps with teeth
> 2 Tissue forceps without teeth
> 2 Adson forceps with teeth

**Holding instruments**

> 12 Allis forceps, 6¼ in.
> 4 Ochsner forceps, 6¼ in.
> 4 Rochester-Pean forceps, 6¼ in.

> 24 Crile hemostats, 5½ in.
> 12 Towel clamps, 5½ in.

**Exposing instruments**

> 2 U. S. Army retractors
> 4 Richardson retractors, 2 small and 2 medium
> 4 Rakes, 4-prong, 2 small and 2 medium
> 4 Skin hooks, 2-prong

**Suturing items**

> 4 Mayo-Hegar needle holders, 6 in.
> 1 Needle set
> 2 Applicators with skin clips (optional)
> Suture material

**Accessory items**

> 1 Suction tube and tubing
> 1 Tissue drain
> 1 Electrosurgical unit

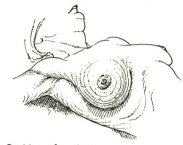

**Position of patient**

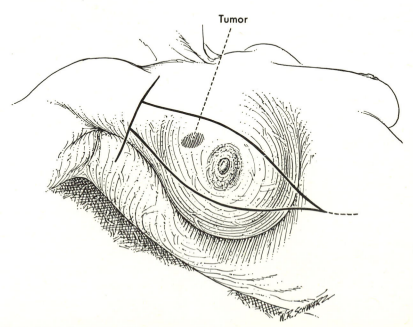

**Fig. 19-2.** Position of patient on operating table and outline of flaps, with prolongation of incision toward umbilicus for radical mastectomy. (From Jorstad, L. H.: Surgery of the breast, St. Louis, 1964, The C. V. Mosby Co.)

**OPERATIVE PROCEDURE**

1. Through a transverse elliptical incision, using a knife and curved scissors, the skin edges are freed from the fascia. Bleeding vessels are clamped with Crile hemostats and ligated with fine silk or chromic gut sutures (Fig. 19-2).

2. The skin edges of the wound are protected by warm laparotomy packs; the breast tissue is grasped with Allis forceps and dissected free from the underlying pectoral fascia with curved scissors and knife.

3. The tumor and all breast tissue are removed. Bleeding vessels are clamped and ligated.

4. A tissue drain or Hemovac may be inserted and anchored to the skin with a fine suture. The wound is closed with skin sutures, and a light pressure dressing is applied.

## Radical mastectomy

**DEFINITION.** Following tissue biopsy and frozen section, removal of the entire breast, axillary contents, and portions of the greater and smaller pectoral muscles and the rectus sheath, en bloc.

**CONSIDERATIONS.** A radical mastectomy is done to control the spread of cancerous lesions.

**SETUP AND PREPARATION OF THE PATIENT.** The biopsy Mayo setup is used. After completion of the biopsy, the draping sheets and the biopsy instruments are removed to prevent implantation of cancer cells during the operation. The operating team dons fresh gowns and gloves. The proposed operative site is repainted and redraped. The arm on the involved side may be draped in a cloth tray cover or Mayo felt cover to allow exposure of the axillary region.

When a skin-grafting procedure is to be performed, a separate setup will be needed for taking the graft from the donor site. Instruments include those described for biopsy and simple mastectomy, adding the following:

12 Crile hemostats, 5½ in.
 6 Allis forceps
 4 Babcock forceps
 1 Skin-grafting set, if desired
 2 Vein retractors
12 Mosquito hemostats, curved
   Sutures
      Plain and chromic gut nos. 3-0 and 4-0 for ligatures
      Chromic gut no. 2-0 on ½-circle, taper point needles, desired size
      Silk nos. 2-0 to 4-0, as desired for ligatures and closure
      Skin sutures on straight or ⅜-circle, cutting-edge needles, as desired

**OPERATIVE PROCEDURE (UNILATERAL)**

1. The elliptical skin incision is made down through the fat to the muscle with a knife. The bleeding points are controlled with Crile hemostats, warm moist pressure packs, and ligatures (Fig. 19-3, *A*).

2. The skin is undercut in all directions to the limits of the dissection by means of a fresh knife, curved scissors, and retractors.

3. The margins of the skin flaps are covered with warm moist packs and held away with retractors; the greater pectoral muscle at the point of insertion into the humerus is freed and divided by means of a knife, Rochester-Pean hemostats, and ligatures of chromic gut no. 0 or silk no. 2-0.

4. The vessels and nerves of the greater and smaller pectoral muscles are dissected free, clamped with Crile hemostats, and ligated with fine silk or chromic gut ligatures swaged to ½-circle, taper point needles on Crile-Wood needle holders.

5. The cut end of the greater pectoral muscle is grasped with Allis forceps and held medially by a Richardson retractor. The attachment of this muscle to the clavicle is clamped with a Rochester-Pean hemostat and cut (Fig. 19-3, *B*).

6. Then the smaller pectoral muscle is cut and ligated close to its insertion into the coracoid process of the scapula with Rochester-Pean hemostats, a knife, and ligatures.

7. The axillary dissection is completed cephalad to brachial plexus by means of Metzenbaum scissors, a knife, and tissue forceps. The axillary vein is stripped of its lymphatic tissues; preservation of the cephalic vein is imperative. Bleeding ves-

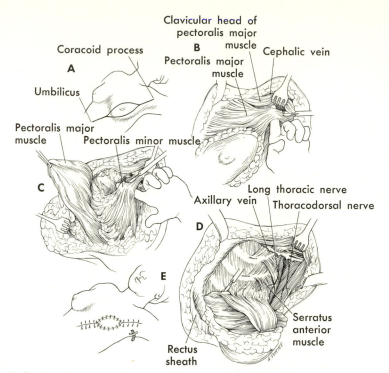

Fig. 19-3. Radical mastectomy. **A,** Lines of incision. **B,** Resection of pectoralis major muscle at clavicular attachment. **C,** Resection of pectoralis minor muscle at coracoid attachment. **D,** The axillary contents are dissected free and resected. **E,** The incision is closed (a skin graft may be necessary), and a drain is placed. (Redrawn from Moseley, H. F., editor: Textbook of surgery, ed. 3, St. Louis, 1959, The C. V. Mosby Co.)

sels are clamped and ligated with silk or fine chromic gut ligatures.

8. The fascia overlying the anterior sheath of the rectus abdominis muscle is freed from the chest wall; bleeding vessels are clamped and ligated. The sternal and costal origins of the pectoral muscles are severed by sharp dissection. The breast and tumor are removed. The wound is cleansed with laparotomy packs saturated in warm saline solution (Fig. 19-3, *C* ).

9. The skin edges are approximated with Allis forceps or towel clamps. If drainage is desired, an opening is made through the skin flap in the axillary region with a knife. A tissue drain, soft multieyed tube, or Hemovac is introduced, using tissue forceps. The free end of the drain is secured to the skin with a suture (Fig. 19-3, *D* ).

10. The wound is closed with interrupted silk sutures; a skin graft may be necessary. A light pressure dressing is applied and held in place with nonallergic tape; suction may be applied to the drainage tube.

### Radical mastectomy with internal mammary node dissection

**DEFINITION.** En bloc removal of the breast, axillary contents, portions of the greater and smaller pectoral muscles, and the internal mammary lymph nodes in the manner of Urban.

**CONSIDERATIONS.** An internal mammary node dissection may be indicated to control primary lymph node metastasis from inner quadrant or subareolar tumors.

**SETUP AND PREPARATION OF THE PATIENT.** As for radical mastectomy. In addition, periosteal elevators and rib shears are needed. Pleural drainage tubes and collection bottles should also be available.

**OPERATIVE PROCEDURE**

1. After making the skin incision and freeing the skin flaps as described for radical mastectomy, the greater pectoral muscle at the point of insertion into the humerus is freed and divided by means of a knife, hemostats, and silk ligatures no. 2-0.

2. The sternal origin of the greater pectoral muscle is divided by knife. As the first interspace is exposed, a thoracotomy is established, and through this opening into the chest the internal mammary vessels are isolated and divided lateral to the sternum.

3. Using rib shears, a segment of chest wall between 3 and 4 cm. wide is resected, including portions of the second through fifth ribs and possibly part of the sternum. The intercostal vessels are clamped and ligated with silk ligatures no. 2-0 as they are encountered.

4. The bone flap and lymphatic tissues are resected in continuity with the breast specimen. Resection is then continued on to the pectoral muscles and the axillary contents.

5. On excision of the en bloc specimen, closure of the wound is begun. The chest wall defect may be grafted with a piece of rectus sheath sewn to the intercostal muscles and sternal sheath; chest catheters are inserted into the eighth or ninth intercostal space; multieyed suction catheters are placed in the wound; the skin edges are approximated with interrupted silk sutures; and a light pressure dressing is applied.

6. A chest x-ray film may be taken while the patient is in the operating room.

## Mammoplasty

Reconstructive surgery of the breasts is increasing because of their psychological importance to the feminine image. Surgery may either reduce the amount of breast tissue or increase the size of the breasts.

### Reduction mammoplasty

**DEFINITION.** Excision of excessive breast tissue and reconstruction of symmetrical breasts.

**CONSIDERATIONS.** Reduction of the amount of breast tissue may be indicated for the patient with ptosis, disproportion of breast size and body build, or back pain related to posture and the weight of large breasts. Breast hypertrophy may be complicated by obesity, which causes lymph and venous stasis.

**SETUP AND PREPARATION OF THE PATIENT.** As for simple mastectomy, omitting the biopsy setup and adding an indelible marking pen.

**OPERATIVE PROCEDURE**

REDUCTION WITH FREE NIPPLE TRANSPLANT (Fig. 19-4)

1. The site for placement of the nipples is marked with the patient in the upright position (normal nipple position is over the fourth intercostal space, pointing inferiorly and laterally). The lines of excision are marked, and the patient is returned to the supine position. A general anesthetic is administered and the skin prepared.

2. The nipple-areolar complex is removed by sharp, nontraumatic dissection with a knife and blade no. 15. The excised nipple graft is preserved on the back table on a saline sponge.

3. The epidermis is removed from the new nipple site and the area covered with a moist sponge.

4. The redundant breast tissue is excised along inframammary incisional lines.

5. The subcutaneous tissue is closed with chromic gut sutures no. 3-0, and suction drainage catheters are inserted. The skin is closed with nylon sutures no. 5-0.

6. The nipple transplant is sutured in place with nylon sutures no. 5-0 that are left long and tied over a bolus of gauze as a stent dressing. The wound is dressed.

REDUCTION WITH NIPPLE TRANSPOSITION IN CONTINUITY WITH BREAST TISSUE (STROMBECK TECHNIQUE) (Fig. 19-5). This technique is recommended for those patients in the childbearing age who wish to preserve the potential of lactation and nipple sensation and erectability.

1. The site of nipple placement is marked as in free nipple transplant.

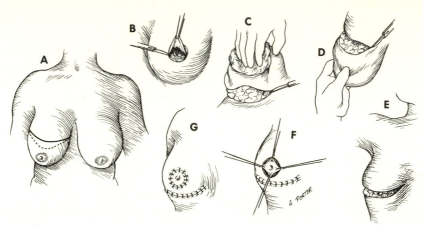

**Fig. 19-4.** Reduction mammoplasty with free nipple transplant. **A,** Pendulous breast with incisional lines marked. **B,** Nipple graft taken. **C** and **D,** Redundant tissue excised. **E,** Incisions approximated. **F,** Nipple graft transplanted. **G,** Reduced breast. (Redrawn from McGregor, I. A., and Reid, W. H.: Plastic surgery for nurses, London, 1966, E. & S. Livingstone, Ltd.)

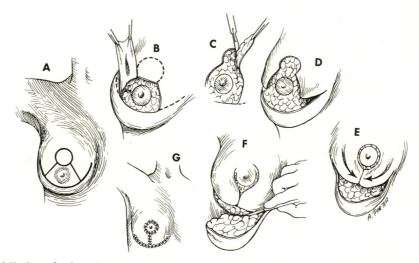

**Fig. 19-5.** Strombeck technique of nipple transposition. **A,** Skin incisions marked. **B** and **C,** Skin edges freed and 5 cm. dimension excised. **D,** Nipple prepared for transposition. **E,** Freed skin edges approximated and nipple moved upward. **F,** Redundant inferior breast tissue excised. **G,** Completed transposition and incisional closure. (Redrawn from McGregor, I. A., and Reid, W. H.: Plastic surgery for nurses, London, 1966, E. & S. Livingstone, Ltd.)

2. The skin between the new nipple site and the present nipple is incised, and a 5 cm. dimension of breast tissue is removed down to the pectoral fascia, preserving the blood supply and innervation of the nipple.

3. The medial and lateral areas of nipple are then freed of epidermis, creating new skin edges. Bleeding vessels are clamped and ligated with plain gut sutures no. 3-0.

4. The redundant segment of breast tissue inferior to the nipple is then excised through a transverse elliptical inframammary incision. The undersurface of the breast is sharply dissected from the pectoral fascia. Hemostasis is established.

5. The nipple and adjacent structures are mobilized in an upward manner to fill the 5 cm. circular defect. The nipple is secured

in the transposed position with nylon sutures no. 5-0.

6. The medial and lateral skin edges are then approximated in a vertical suture line inferior to the nipple.

7. The inframammary elliptical incision is trimmed and closed transversely with nylon sutures no. 5-0. Suction drainage catheters may be placed. The wound is dressed.

### Augmentation mammoplasty

DEFINITION. Insertion of an inert prosthesis between the breast proper and the pectoral fascia to enlarge breast size.

CONSIDERATIONS. Augmentation mammoplasty may be performed in cases of hypoplasia, postpartal involution, surgical defects, and asymmetry of the breasts. Psychological factors are important in the selection of patients; the surgeon may request a psychiatric consultation.

SETUP AND PREPARATION OF THE PATIENT. As described for simple mastectomy, omitting the biopsy setup and adding the following:

> Mammary prosthesis, assorted paired sizes
> 4 Schnidt tonsil hemostats
> 2 Malleable retractors, 1 medium and 1 wide
> 2 Deaver retractors, narrow
> 2 Brown needle holders, 5 in.
> Antibiotic solution for wound irrigation (optional)

### OPERATIVE PROCEDURE

1. A low, 3-inch, transverse incision is made below the projected site of the inframammary fold with a knife and blade no. 10.

2. The incision is deepened through the subcutaneous fat to the pectoral fascia.

3. By blunt and sharp dissection, the entire breast is elevated to the level of the clavicle superiorly, separating it from the pectoral fascia. This creates a submammary pocket.

4. Meticulous hemostasis is achieved, using Crile or the longer Schnidt tonsil forceps and ligatures of plain gut no. 3-0. The wound may be irrigated with antibiotic solution. A dry pocket is established.

5. The prosthesis is inserted, using the malleable retractor as a skid.

6. The subcutaneous fat is closed with chromic gut sutures no. 3-0 and the skin with nylon sutures no. 5-0.

7. The wound is dressed with gauze and tape to fix the incision to the chest wall. An elastic tape dressing is then applied. The nipples are left undressed for observation of viability.

### REFERENCES

1. Anthony, C. P.: Textbook of anatomy and physiology, ed. 8, St. Louis, 1971, The C. V. Mosby Co.
2. Arufe, H. N., and Juri, J.: Modification of the Strombeck technique, Plast. Reconstr. Surg. 46:604, 1970.
3. Davis, L.: Christopher's textbook of surgery, ed. 8, Philadelphia, 1964, W. B. Saunders Co.
4. Edwards, B. J., and Gatewood, J. W.: Mammary prosthesis implantation, A.O.R.N. Journal 9:54, Jan., 1969.
5. Madden, J. L.: Atlas of technics of surgery, ed. 2, New York, 1964, Appleton-Century-Crofts.
6. McGregor, I. A., and Reid, W. H.: Plastic surgery for nurses, London, 1966, E. & S. Livingstone, Ltd.
7. Moyer, C. A., Rhoads, J. E., Allen, J. G., and Harkins, H. N.: Surgery: principles and practice, ed. 3, Philadelphia, 1965, J. B. Lippincott Co.
8. Southwick, H. W., Slaughter, D. P., and Humphrey, L. J.: Surgery of the breast, Chicago, 1968, Year Book Medical Publishers, Inc.
9. Urban, J. A.: Extended radical mastectomy for breast cancer, Am. J. Surg. 106:399, Sept., 1963.

# CHAPTER 20

# Operations on the gallbladder, ducts, liver, pancreas, and spleen

PEGGY E. LILES

## ANATOMICAL AND PHYSIOLOGICAL CONSIDERATIONS

The *liver* is situated in the upper right abdominal cavity beneath the dome of the diaphragm and directly above the stomach, duodenum, and hepatic flexure of the colon (Fig. 20-1). The external covering, known as *Glisson's capsule,* is composed of dense connective tissue. The peritoneum extends over its entire surface, except at the point of posterior attachment to the diaphragm. The arterial blood supply is maintained by the hepatic artery, and blood from the stomach, intestines, spleen, and pancreas is carried to the liver by the portal vein and its branches. The hepatic venous system returns blood to the heart by way of the inferior vena cava.

The bile, manufactured by the liver cells, is secreted into the fine biliary radicals and, in turn, flows into the large ducts. It ultimately leaves the liver through the right and left hepatic ducts. These ducts join immediately after leaving the liver to form one common hepatic duct that merges with the cystic duct from the gallbladder to form the common bile duct. The common bile duct opens into the duodenum in an area called the *ampulla* or *papilla* of Vater, located slightly below the pyloric opening from the stomach.

The bile contains bile salts, which facilitate in digestion and absorption, and vari-

ous waste products. The liver is also essential in the metabolism of carbohydrates and proteins, as well as fats.

The *gallbladder,* which lies in a sulcus on the undersurface of the right lobe of the liver, terminates in the cystic duct. This ductal system provides a channel for the flow of bile to the gallbladder, where it becomes highly concentrated during the storage period. However, as food is ingested, especially fats, the musculature of the gallbladder contracts, forcing bile into the cystic duct and through the common duct. As the sphincter of Oddi in the ampulla of Vater relaxes, bile pours forth, flowing into the duodenum to aid in digestion. The gallbladder receives its blood supply from the cystic artery, a branch of the hepatic artery (Fig. 20-2).

The *pancreas* lies in a horizontal position behind the stomach, with the head firmly attached to the duodenum and the tail reaching to the spleen. The pancreatic juice, containing digestive enzymes, is collected in the pancreatic duct or duct of Wirsung, which unites with the common bile duct to enter the duodenum about 7.5 cm. below the pylorus. The ampulla of Vater is formed by the dilated junction of the two ducts at the point of entry (Fig. 20-3).

The pancreas also contains groups of cells, called *islets* or *islands of Langerhans,* which secrete hormones into the blood

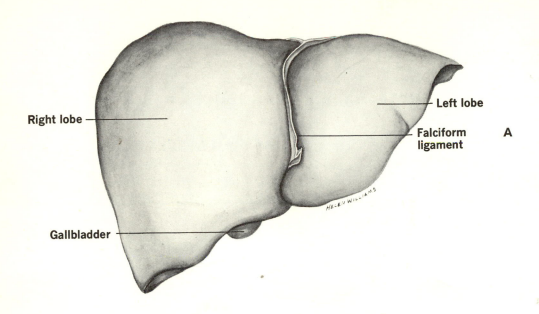

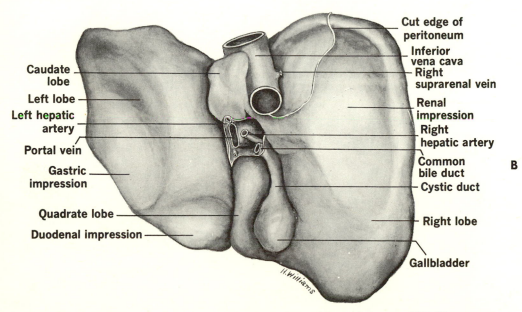

**Fig. 20-1. A,** Anterior surface of liver. **B,** Undersurface of liver. (Courtesy W.R.U. museum specimen.) (From Francis, C. C: Introduction to human anatomy, ed. 5, St. Louis, 1968, The C. V. Mosby Co.)

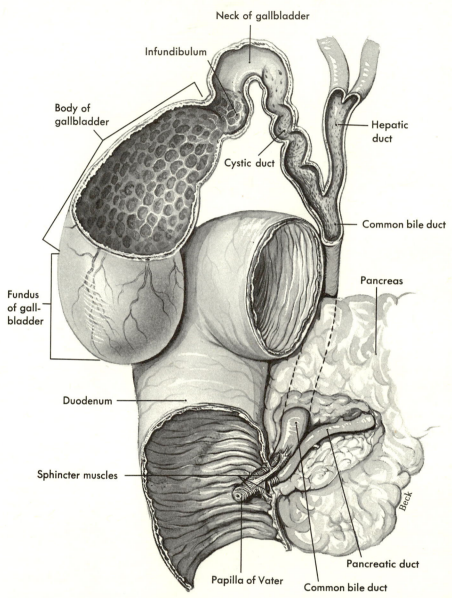

**Fig. 20-2.** The gallbladder and its divisions: fundus, body, infundibulum, and neck. Obstruction of either the hepatic or common bile duct by stone or spasm blocks the exit of bile from the liver where it is formed and prevents bile from ejecting into the duodenum. (From Anthony, C. P.: Textbook of anatomy and physiology, ed. 8, St. Louis, 1971, The C. V. Mosby Co.)

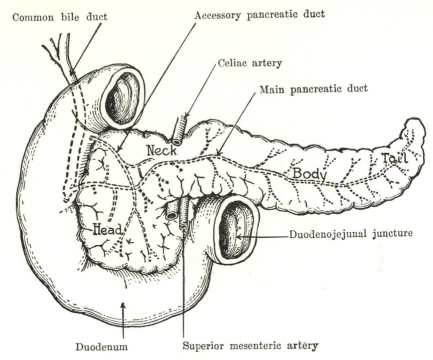

Common bile duct

Accessory pancreatic duct

Celiac artery

Main pancreatic duct

Neck

Body

Tail

Head

Duodenojejunal juncture

Duodenum

Superior mesenteric artery

Fig. 20-3. Relative positions of duodenum, pancreas, and ductile systems. (From Pitzman, M.: The fundamentals of human anatomy, St. Louis, The C. V. Mosby Co.)

capillaries instead of into the duct. These hormones are insulin and glucagon, and both are involved in carbohydrate metabolism.

The *spleen* is situated in the upper left abdominal cavity, with full protection provided by the tenth, eleventh, and twelfth ribs; the lateral surface is directly beneath the dome of the diaphragm. The anterior medial surface is in close proximity with the cardiac end of the stomach and the splenic flexure of the colon. The spleen is covered with peritoneum that forms supporting ligaments. The arterial blood supply is furnished by the splenic artery, a branch of the celiac axis. The splenic vein drains into the portal system (Fig. 20-4).

The spleen is said to have many functions. Among them are the defense of the body by phagocytosis of microorganisms, formation of nongranular leukocytes and plasma cells, and phagocytosis of damaged red blood cells. It also acts as a blood reservoir.

## SPECIFIC NURSING CONSIDERATIONS IN BILIARY SURGERY

General nursing standards of skin preparation and draping are discussed in Chapters 4 and 5. The following pertinent factors are to be considered in caring for the patient undergoing biliary surgery.

POSITIONING THE PATIENT. The patient is placed in a supine position with the patient's upper right quadrant over the gallbladder rest, which may be elevated to achieve adequate exposure. Some surgeons do not use the gallbladder rest because they do not believe that it aids in exposure and it may cause backaches postoperatively.

When an operative cholangiogram is anticipated, the operating table is prepared with an x-ray cassette holder before the patient is positioned. The holder must be directly beneath the patient's upper right quadrant, since correct positioning is im-

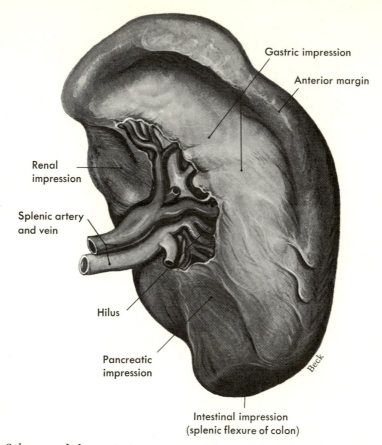

Gastric impression

Anterior margin

Renal impression

Splenic artery and vein

Hilus

Pancreatic impression

Intestinal impression
(splenic flexure of colon)

**Fig. 20-4.** Spleen, medial aspect. Arrangement of the vessels at the hilus is highly variable. (From Anthony, C. P.: Textbook of anatomy and physiology, ed. 8, St. Louis, 1971, The C. V. Mosby Co.)

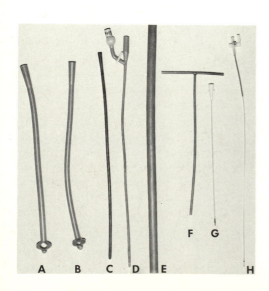

**Fig. 20-5.** Drainage tubes and catheters for biliary surgery. **A,** Malecot catheter. **B,** Mushroom or Pezzer catheter. **C,** Red Robinson catheter. **D,** Foley catheter. **E,** Penrose soft latex tubing. **F,** T-tube (latex). **G,** Biliary balloon probe. **H,** Cholangiography catheter.

perative to assure accurate visualization of the biliary tract. The cassette holder will interfere with elevating the gallbladder rest if it is not an integral part of the operative table.

DRAINAGE MATERIALS. Tubes and catheters must be in perfect condition and suitable for the areas to be drained. If a defective drain is used, a free fragment may remain in the wound on the removal of the tube (Fig. 20-5).

The scrubbed nursing team member should note the condition of all drainage materials and test them for patency before offering them to the surgeon.

Soft rubber or latex tissue drains (Penrose) are used after a cholecystectomy or a choledochotomy. The Penrose drain may be used the way it comes from the package, or it may be made into a cigarette drain. The latter can be made by passing folded gauze packing, of suitable width and length, through the lumen of the drain. The packing will serve as a wick.

A T-tube drain of latex rubber and of suitable size is prepared by the surgeon after the duct has been explored (Fig. 20-5). The center of the crossbar is notched opposite the junction of the vertical limb so that its ends will bend more readily on removal. The ends are beveled and tailored to fit the duct. In operations involving the ampulla of Vater, a Cattell-type, long T-tube may be needed to be passed through this sphincter and into the duodenum.

Drains are usually exteriorized through separate stab wounds and anchored to skin edges to prevent retraction of the drain.

ASEPTIC MEASURES. When the common duct is opened or an anastomosis is to be established between a duct and other parts of the tract, care should be exercised to isolate contaminated instruments and materials from the remainder of the operative field, as described for gastrointestinal surgery (Chapter 21).

Instruments and materials used for the exteriorization of a drain should be treated as contaminated.

## INSTRUMENTS FOR OPERATIONS ON THE BILIARY TRACT

The setup includes the basic laparotomy set (Chapter 17), plus the following:

**Cutting instruments**
1 Metzenbaum or Nelson scissors, 9¼ in.

**Clamping instruments** (Fig. 20-6)
2 Lahey gall duct forceps, 7¼ in.
2 Johns Hopkins gallbladder forceps, 8 in.
2 Mixter gallbladder forceps, 7¼ in.
6 Schnidt gall duct forceps

**Holding instruments** (Fig. 20-8)
1 Mayo common duct scoop, malleable shaft, 10½ in.
1 Mayo cystic duct scoop, malleable shaft, 10 in.
1 Set gall duct spoons, malleable copper, sizes 1 to 5
1 Moore gallstone scoop
2 Blake gallstone forceps, 1 straight and 1 curved, 8¼ in. (Fig. 20-7)
1 Desjardin gallstone forceps, 9¼ in. (Fig. 20-7)
2 Vascular thumb forceps, fine-type, 8 in.
1 Set Randall kidney stone forceps (may be used instead of the Blake and Desjardin gallstone forceps) (Fig. 20-7)

**Exposing instruments**
3 Deaver retractors, 2 with blade 2 in. wide and 1 with blade 3 in. wide

**Accessory items**
1 Ochsner gallbladder aspirating trocar, 16 Fr. (Fig. 20-8)
  Hemostatic clips and applicators
2 Penrose drains, ⅝ or ½ in. diameter, each 12 in. long
2 Safety pins
1 Yard plain gauze packing, 2 in. wide, if desired
  Drainage catheters, as desired (Fig. 20-5)
  Sutures, as listed for surgeon in card file (Chapter 6)
  Fogarty biliary catheters (Fig. 20-5)

## OPERATIONS ON THE BILIARY TRACT
### Cholecystectomy

DEFINITION. Removal of the gallbladder.
CONSIDERATIONS. This operation is performed for the treatment of diseases involving the gallbladder, such as acute or

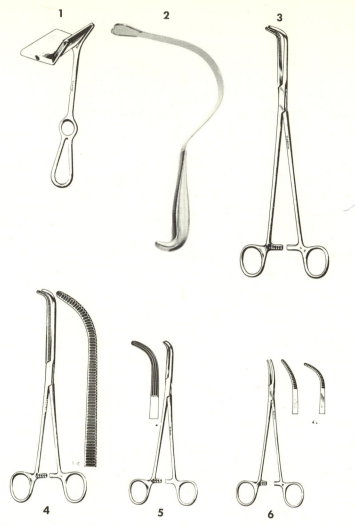

Fig. 20-6. Instruments for gallbladder surgery. Exposing: **1,** Wolfson gallbladder retractor; **2,** Harrington retractor (2 sizes). Clamping: **3,** Mixter gallbladder forceps; **4,** Johns Hopkins gallbladder forceps; **5,** Lahey gall duct forceps; **6,** Schnidt gall duct forceps. (Courtesy Codman & Shurtleff, Inc., Randolph, Mass.)

chronic inflammation with or without stones (cholelithiasis), or in the presence of polyps or carcinoma.

**SETUP AND PREPARATION OF THE PATIENT.** The setup and position are as described for laparotomy and biliary surgery.

**OPERATIVE PROCEDURE** (Fig. 20-9)

1. Through a right subcostal or right paramedian incision, the abdominal cavity is opened, as described for laparotomy (Chapter 17). Kelly retractors and lap-

arotomy packs are employed as careful examination of the abdominal cavity is carried out.

2. The common duct is palpated for evidence of stones and the pathological condition determined. Deaver retractors, moist or dry laparotomy packs, long tissue forceps, and suction are used.

3. The surrounding organs are walled off from the gallbladder region, using laparotomy packs and deep retractors.

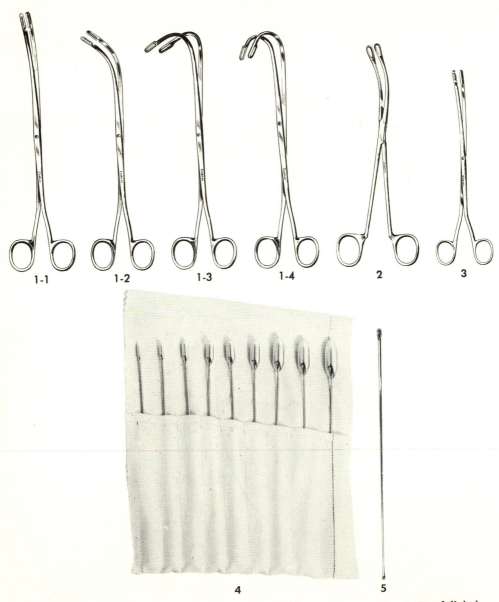

**Fig. 20-7.** Instruments for gallbladder surgery—cont'd. Duct instruments: **1,** Randall kidney stone forceps (4 sizes and shapes); **2,** Blake gallstone forceps; **3,** Desjardin gallstone forceps; **4,** Bakes common duct dilators; **5,** Moynihan gall duct probe and scoop. (Courtesy Codman & Shurtleff, Inc., Randolph, Mass.)

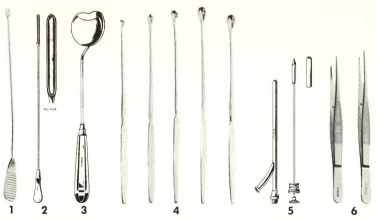

**Fig. 20-8.** Instruments for gallbladder surgery—cont'd. Duct instruments: **1,** Mayo common duct scoop; **2,** Mayo cystic duct scoop; **3,** Moore gallstone scoop; **4,** gall duct spoons; **5,** Ochsner gallbladder trocar; **6,** Potts-Smith forceps. (Courtesy Codman & Shurtleff, Inc., Randolph, Mass.)

4. To facilitate gentle traction, Rochester-Pean forceps are usually placed on the body of the gallbladder (Fig. 20-9, *A*).

5. The peritoneal fold overlying the junction of the cystic and common duct is incised, using a long no. 7 knife handle with a no. 15 blade or a no. 4 handle with a no. 20 blade, long Metzenbaum scissors, and forceps. Suction is available, and bleeding points are clamped and ligated.

6. Adhesions are separated by blunt dissection, using small, round, dry dissector sponges, sponges on holders, and blunt right-angled forceps. Dissection is continued to expose the neck of the gallbladder, the cystic artery, and the cystic duct (Fig. 20-9, *B* and *C*).

7. Blunt dissection is continued to expose the cystic artery as it enters the wall of the gallbladder. On complete exposure and visualization of the branches, the cystic artery is doubly ligated with silk or clamped with hemostatic clips and divided (Fig. 20-9, *B*). Occasionally a third ligature or clip may be used. If there is more than one branch of the cystic artery, each one of them will be ligated and divided separately.

8. The true junction of the cystic duct with the common bile duct is visualized. The cystic duct is identified and carefully dissected from the common bile duct to the gallbladder neck. It is then doubly ligated and divided (Fig. 20-9, *C*). A transfixion suture of fine chromic gut may be used on the stump of the cystic duct near the common bile duct. The gallbladder is freed from the liver, working upward to the fundus, and the specimen is removed (Fig. 20-9, *D*). In some cases it may be necessary to work from the fundus downward to the neck of the gallbladder.

9. All bleeding is controlled; reperitonealization of the liver bed, if indicated, is accomplished, using interrupted or continuous fine chromic intestinal sutures.

10. A Penrose or cigarette drain is inserted near the cystic duct stump. The free end of the drain is exteriorized through a stab wound in the lateral abdominal wall (Fig. 20-9, *E*).

11. The wound is closed in layers, as described for laparotomy (Chapter 17).

12. A safety pin is attached to the protruding drain, and a dressing is applied (Fig. 20-9, *E*).

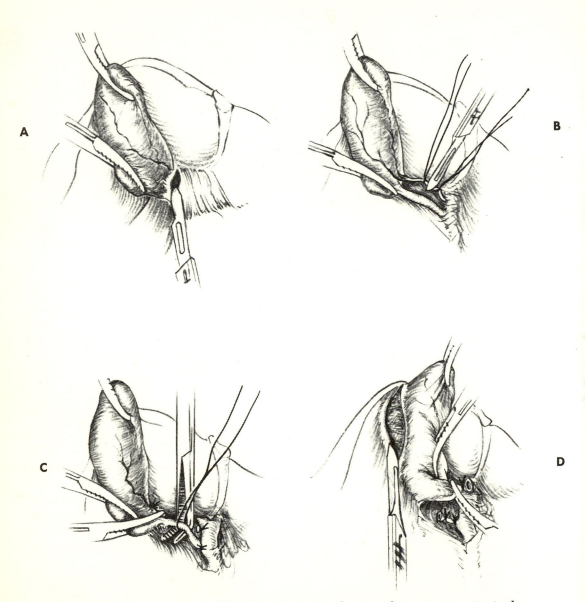

**Fig. 20-9.** Cholecystectomy. **A,** With Pean forceps in place, gentle traction is maintained as peritoneum over Calot's triangle is incised. **B,** Cystic artery is clearly visualized, doubly ligated, and divided. **C,** Cystic duct is carefully dissected and identified before clamps and ligatures are applied. **D,** Dissection of gallbladder from liver bed is completed. **E,** Liver bed is shown with reperitonealization completed. Cigarette drain has been placed in Morison's pouch and exteriorized through stab wound. (From Wilder, J. R.: Atlas of general surgery, ed. 2, St. Louis, 1964, The C. V. Mosby Co.)

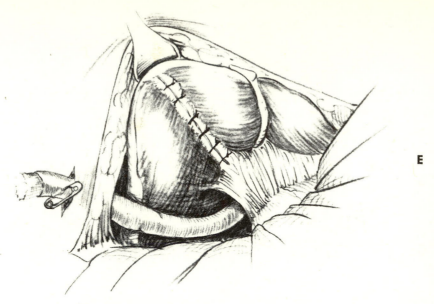

E

Fig. 20-9, cont'd. For legend see opposite page.

## Cholecystostomy

**DEFINITION.** Establishment of an opening into the gallbladder to permit drainage of the organ and the removal of stones.

**CONSIDERATIONS.** Cholecystostomy is usually selected for patients with acute gallbladder disease and a general physical condition that will not permit more extensive surgery. A local anesthetic may be administered.

Because continuous decompression of the stomach is important in the postoperative management of these patients and also because a nasogastric tube is sometimes contraindicated, a direct gastrostomy (Chapter 21) may be performed with introduction of a retention drainage tube.

**SETUP AND PREPARATION OF THE PATIENT.** As described for laparotomy and biliary surgery, plus selected drainage tubes or catheters of suitable size, such as Foley, Malecot, mushroom, or Robinson type.

A large syringe (50 ml.) or an Asepto syringe may be needed for irrigation purposes. If a local anesthetic is used, the agent and a selection of syringes and needles will be necessary.

**OPERATIVE PROCEDURE**

1. The abdomen is opened through a vertical incision, which may be somewhat shorter than that for cholecystectomy.

2. The fundus of the gallbladder is grasped with an Allis or Babcock forceps, and the proposed opening is encircled by means of a chromic purse-string suture, leaving the ends free (Fig. 20-10, *A*).

3. To protect the abdominal cavity from infection, the gallbladder is isolated by means of laparotomy packs, and suction is available.

4. At the identified site, the gallbladder is aspirated by means of a trocar with tubing and suction attached (Fig. 20-10, *A*).

5. As the contents are aspirated, cultures may be taken. The contaminated trocar is removed and discarded.

6. The opening is enlarged with Metzenbaum scissors; gallstones are removed with malleable scoops and stone forceps (Fig. 20-10, *B*). It may be necessary to irrigate the gallbladder with isotonic saline

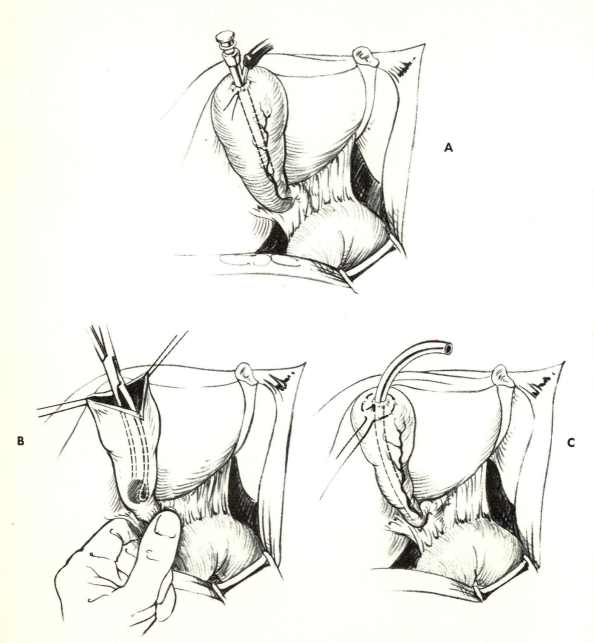

**Fig. 20-10.** Cholecystostomy. **A,** Purse-string suture and trocar are in place. **B,** Calculus is removed through opening in fundus. **C,** Drainage catheter is in place. (From Wilder, J. R.: Atlas of general surgery, ed. 2, St. Louis, 1964, The C. V. Mosby Co.)

solution to remove small stones, grit, or pastelike material. A syringe with a catheter or an Asepto syringe may be used for irrigation. Contaminated instruments are placed in a basin on the operative field.

7. A drainage tube is inserted in the gallbladder opening. The purse-string suture is tightened around the catheter. A second purse-string suture or separate mattress sutures may be used to secure the gallbladder to the peritoneum and the posterior rectus fascia (Fig. 20-10, *C*).

8. The free end of the catheter or tube is exteriorized through a stab wound and then anchored to the skin edges, as described for cholecystectomy.

9. Drainage of the abdominal cavity is established by means of a Penrose or a cigarette drain. The exterior end of each drain is secured by a safety pin.

10. The wound is closed in layers, as described for laparotomy, and dressings are applied without disturbing the drains.

## Choledochostomy and choledochotomy

**DEFINITIONS.** The establishment of an opening into the common bile duct by means of a drainage T-tube. A choledochotomy for choledocholithiasis is the actual incision into the common bile duct for removal of stones.

**CONSIDERATIONS.** This procedure is done to treat choledocholithiasis or to relieve an obstruction in the common bile duct.

Before exploration is begun, open cholangiography may be performed to locate all stones within the ductal system. X-ray films are repeated after the T-tube drain is in place to confirm the successful evacuation and patency of the ducts.

A subcostal or upper right rectus incision may be made.

**SETUP AND PREPARATION OF THE PATIENT.** As described for biliary surgery, plus the following additional instruments:

1 Set Bakes common duct dilators, malleable shafts, nine sizes—3 to 11 mm. (Fig. 20-7)
1 Ochsner flexible spiral gallstone probe, 14 in.
1 Malleable silver probe, 8 in.

1 Asepto syringe, 2 oz.
4 Syringes, 2, 20, 30, and 50 ml.
3 Aspirating needles: 24-gauge, ¾ in., 19-gauge, 3½ in., 16-gauge, 2 in.
1 Catheter adapter for saline solution irrigation
2 Ampuls contrast media
3 Robinson catheters, 8, 12, and 16 Fr.
3 T-tubes, Cattell-type, 8 to 26 Fr., as desired
  Fogarty biliary catheters (Fig. 20-5)

**OPERATIVE PROCEDURE**

1. The abdomen is opened as for cholecystectomy. If the gallbladder has not been previously removed, it is now exposed and removed or retracted by means of laparotomy packs and right-angled abdominal retractors.

2. The common duct may be identified by means of an aspirating syringe and fine-gauged needle to make certain that the suspected duct is not a blood vessel. A specimen for cultures may be obtained.

3. Two traction sutures, silk no. 3-0, are placed in the wall of the duct below the entrance of the cystic duct (Fig. 20-11, *A*).

4. The common duct region is walled off with laparotomy packs and narrow blade retractors. A discard basin for contaminated instruments is placed at the lower end of the operative field; suction apparatus is made ready for immediate use.

5. A longitudinal incision is made in the common duct, between the traction sutures, with a no. 7 handle and a no. 15 or no. 11 blade. Constant suction is initiated, using a Yankauer suction tube to keep the field free of oozing bile as the incision is enlarged with a Potts angled or Metzenbaum scissors. Additional stay sutures or Babcock forceps may be applied to the ductal opening.

6. Visible stones are removed with gallstone forceps, after which exploration of the duct is begun with small malleable scoops proximally and then distally to the opening. Probing and dilatation are continued as stones are removed from both the common and hepatic ducts. Isotonic saline solution in a bulb syringe and a small-lumen catheter or a Fogarty-type

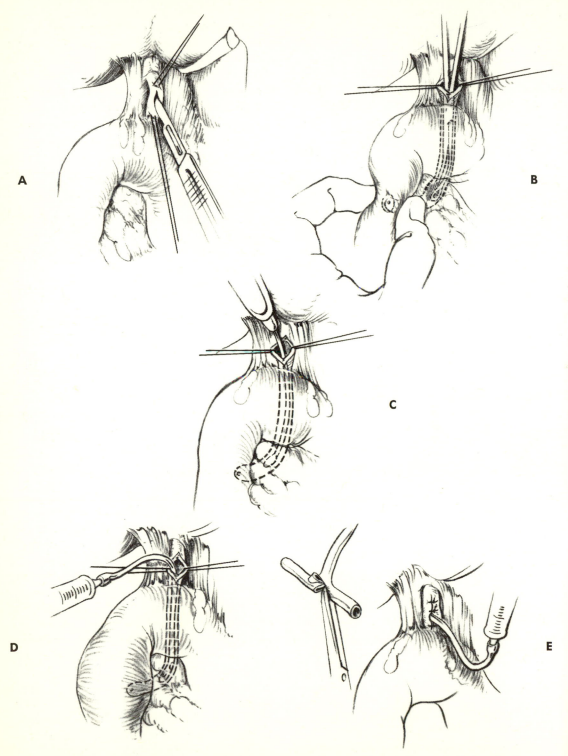

**Fig. 20-11.** Choledochotomy. **A,** Opening common duct. **B,** Stone forceps introduced. **C,** Probing common duct. **D,** Irrigating duct. **E,** T-tube in place. (From Wilder, J. R.: Atlas of general surgery, ed. 2, St. Louis, 1964, The C. V. Mosby Co.)

balloon-tipped catheter is used to facilitate the removal of small stones and debris, as well as demonstrate patency through to the duodenum (Fig. 20-11, *B* and *D*).

7. A transduodenotomy may be performed if patency of the sphincter of Oddi and ampulla of Vater cannot be demonstrated. (a) An area of the duodenum is walled off with laparotomy packs. The incision is made longitudinally with a scalpel, using blade no. 15 and Metzenbaum scissors. (b) Bleeding vessels are clamped with mosquito hemostats and ligated with fine silk or chromic sutures. (c) Fine silk traction sutures are inserted, and exploration is carried out. (d) The duodenal opening is closed transversely with fine chromic and silk intestinal sutures. (e) The T-tube is prepared by the surgeon, irrigated for patency, and introduced into the common duct with fine vascular forceps (Fig. 20-11, *E*).

8. The common duct incision is closed with chromic no. 3-0 intestinal sutures. Contaminated instruments are placed in the discard basin.

9. The T-tube is irrigated to demonstrate patency, and a cholangiogram is done (Fig. 20-11, *E*).

10. The gallbladder may be removed, as described for cholecystectomy.

11. A Penrose or a cigarette drain is introduced into the foramen of Winslow. Both drain and tube are exteriorized through a stab wound.

12. The wound is closed in layers; tube and drain are carefully anchored to the skin, and each wound is dressed individually to prevent undue tension that could result in displacement of tube and drain.

13. Sterile tubing may be used to connect the T-tube to the small drainage container.

## Cholecystoduodenostomy or cholecystojejunostomy

**DEFINITIONS.** Establishment of continuity by an anastomosis between the gallbladder and duodenum or jejunum to relieve an obstruction in the distal end of the common duct.

**CONSIDERATIONS.** An obstruction in the biliary system may be caused by a tumor of the ducts involving the head of the pancreas or the ampulla of Vater, the presence of an inflammatory lesion, or a stricture of the common duct.

**SETUP AND PREPARATION OF THE PATIENT.** As described for cholecystostomy, plus 2 Doyen intestinal forceps, curved, with rubber guards or similar nontraumatic holding forceps.

**OPERATIVE PROCEDURE**

1. The abdomen is opened, the gallbladder is exposed and aspirated, and the pathological condition is confirmed, as described for cholecystostomy.

2. The anastomosis site is prepared, posterior serosal silk sutures are placed, and open anastomosis is performed. The technique as described for gastrointestinal anastomosis is followed (Chapter 21).

3. Contaminated instruments are placed in the discard basin, and the operative field is prepared for closure.

4. A Penrose or a cigarette drain may be introduced; the wound is closed in layers, and dressings are applied.

## Choledochoduodenostomy and choledochojejunostomy

**DEFINITIONS.** Anastomosis between the common duct and the duodenum or between the common duct and the jejunum.

**CONSIDERATIONS.** These procedures are usually necessary in postcholecystectomy patients with complications to circumvent an obstructive lesion and reestablish the flow of bile into the intestinal tract.

**SETUP AND PREPARATION OF THE PATIENT.** As described for choledochostomy and cholecystojejunostomy.

**OPERATIVE PROCEDURES**

FOR CHOLEDOCHODUODENOSTOMY

1. The abdomen is opened; the common duct and duodenum are exposed.

2. The common duct is identified and dissected free.

3. The common duct and duodenum are

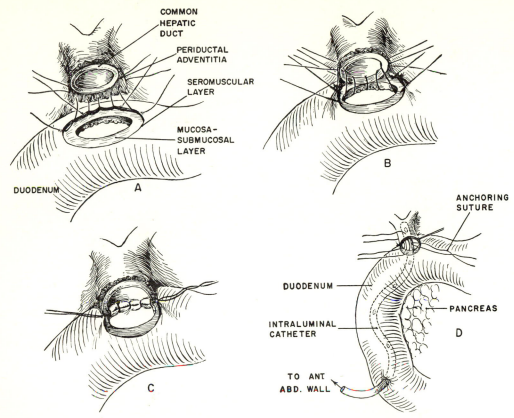

**Fig. 20-12.** Technique for choledochoduodenostomy. **A,** First posterior row of interrupted silk sutures approximates adventitia around proximal biliary segment and seromuscular layer of anterior aspect of duodenum. **B,** Second posterior row approximates full thickness of duct and mucosa-submucosal layer of bowel. Note that knots are on outside of lumen. **C,** The two posterior rows are completed. **D,** The intraluminal catheter is in place, secured by gut suture at line of anastomosis. Note extra holes in catheter providing egress of bile to bowel. (From Longmire, W. P., Jr., and Lippman, H. N.: In Allen, A. W., and Barrow, D. W., editors: Abdominal surgery, New York, 1961, Harper & Row, Publishers.)

approximated, and an anastomosis is established (Fig. 20-12).

4. The wound is closed in layers, and dressings are applied.

FOR CHOLEDOCHOJEJUNOSTOMY

1. The abdomen is opened, the jejunum is mobilized, and the common duct is identified.

2. Anastomosis is established between the common duct and the transected jejunum (Fig. 20-13, *A*). A catheter is introduced, as described for cholecystoduodenostomy.

3. Jejunal continuity is reestablished by Roux-Y anastomosis (Fig. 20-13, *B*).

4. Contaminated instruments are removed from the operative field.

5. The drain is exteriorized; the wound is closed in layers and dressings applied.

## Repair of strictures of the common and hepatic ducts

**DEFINITION.** Biliary obstruction may be relieved either by resection of a stricture of the duct and an end-to-end anastomosis over a T-tube splint (Fig. 20-14) or by means of an anastomosis between the duct or ducts and the intestinal tract.

**SETUP AND PREPARATION OF THE PATIENT.** As described for choledochostomy and

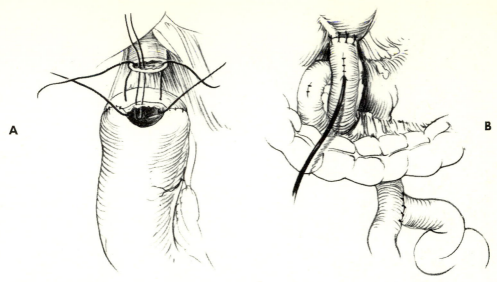

**Fig. 20-13.** Technique for choledochojejunostomy. **A,** Stay sutures are placed in lumen of prepared jejunum and common duct stump prior to anastomosis. **B,** Completed Roux-Y anastomosis is shown with intraluminal catheter in place. (From Wilder, J. R.: Atlas of general surgery, ed. 2, St. Louis, 1964, The C. V. Mosby Co.)

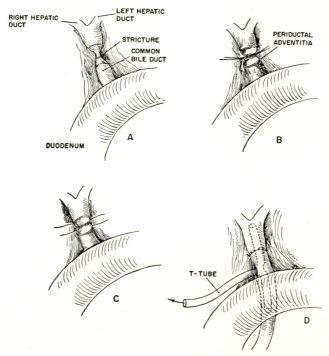

**Fig. 20-14.** Technique for duct-to-duct anastomosis with T-tube in place. **A,** Strictured area is defined. Dotted lines indicate area of duct to be excised. **B,** First posterior row of sutures has been placed in adventitia around duct. **C,** Posterior inner row of interrupted catgut sutures has been completed. **D,** Completed anastomosis with the T-tube in place, brought out below line of anastomosis. (From Longmire, W. P., Jr., and Lippman, H. N.: In Allen, A. W., and Barrow, D. W., editors: Abdominal surgery, New York, 1961, Harper & Row, Publishers.)

gastroenterostomy (Chapter 21), with a complete selection of drainage tubes and fine intestinal chromic and silk sutures with swaged-on needles.

OPERATIVE PROCEDURE

1. The abdomen is opened, and the anastomotic procedure to be performed is selected after careful exploration and evaluation of existing pathological condition (Fig. 20-14).

2. After anastomosis, the selected T-tube and drain are inserted. Extreme caution is exercised to prevent displacement of the vital drainage tubes (Fig. 20-14).

3. The wound is closed, as described in Chapter 17.

## Transduodenal sphincterotomy

DEFINITION. Partial division of the sphincter of Oddi and exploration of the common duct to treat recurrent attacks of acute pancreatitis due to the formation of calculi in the pancreatic duct or blockage of the sphincter of Oddi.

SETUP AND PREPARATION OF THE PATIENT. As described for choledochotomy, plus a ureteral knife or sphincterotome.

OPERATIVE PROCEDURE

1. The gallbladder may have been removed; the common duct is opened and explored for stones, as described for choledochotomy.

2. For the Doublet and Mulholland technique, a sphincterotome is inserted through the common duct into the duodenum and the sphincter severed; or the ampulla of Vater is exposed through an incision made in the duodenum, and a probe is passed through the common duct into the duodenum. The sphincter is incised over the probe.

3. The duodenum is closed with interrupted silk sutures. A T-tube is introduced into the common duct and held in place with sutures. The abdominal cavity is drained and the wound closed.

## OPERATIONS ON THE PANCREAS
### Drainage or excision of pancreatic cysts

DEFINITION. Surgical treatment may be excision or internal or external drainage of cysts of the pancreas.

CONSIDERATIONS. Cysts of the pancreas

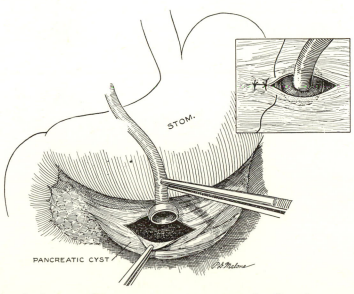

Fig. 20-15. Simple drainage of pancreatic cyst. Cyst is incised sufficiently to permit complete evacuation of contents and inspection of lining of cavity. Flanged end of Pezzer catheter is sutured into cyst, and other end is brought out through stab wound. (From Warren, K. W., and Baker, A. L., Jr.: In Lahey Clinic: Surgical practice of the Clinic, Philadelphia, 1962, W. B. Saunders Co.)

have been classified by Warren and Baker according to etiological factors as follows: developmental or congenital, inflammatory, traumatic, neoplastic, and parasitic. Their etiology and size, location, and anatomical relationships are important deciding factors in selection of the surgical procedure.

Complete excision of retention cysts is usually considered the preferred method; however, this may not be possible in the presence of an acute or secondary inflammatory reaction. In the latter, internal or external drainage of the cyst may be established.

SETUP AND PREPARATION OF THE PATIENT. As described for common duct and gastrointestinal procedures, plus appropriate drains.

OPERATIVE PROCEDURE FOR DRAINAGE OF PANCREATIC CYSTS

1. Simple external drainage is established by direct introduction of a retention-type catheter into the cyst, following decompression and inspection (Fig. 20-15).

2. Internal drainage may be accomplished by an incision into the anterior wall of the stomach directly opposite the cyst as it adheres to the posterior wall (Fig. 20-16). A fistula is established between the anterior wall of the cyst and the posterior wall of the stomach, thereby providing drainage through the gastrointestinal canal.

3. The anterior gastrotomy is closed, and the wound closure is completed in the usual manner.

## Pancreaticoduodenectomy (Whipple operation)

DEFINITION. Removal of the head of the pancreas, the entire duodenum, a portion of the jejunum, the distal third of the stomach, the lower half of the common bile duct, and a portion of the pancreatic duct, with the reestablishment of continuity of the biliary, pancreatic, and gastrointestinal tract systems.

CONSIDERATIONS. Radical excision of the head of the pancreas for carcinoma is a

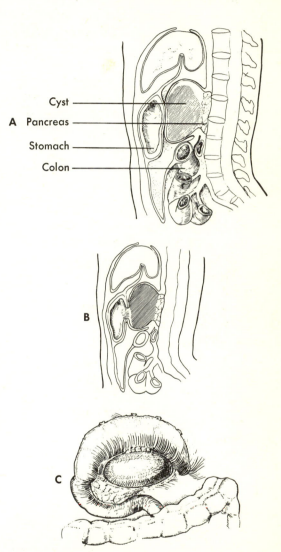

Fig. 20-16. Treatment of pancreatic pseudocyst by internal drainage by means of anastomosis of cyst to stomach. **A**, Sagittal section showing relationship of cyst of the body of the pancreas to posterior wall of stomach. **B**, Schema illustrating cystogastrostomy, sagittal view. **C**, Schema illustrating cystogastrostomy, anterior view. Stomach has been lifted cephalad to demonstrate the anastomosis between pseudocyst and the posterior wall of the stomach. (From Dreiling, D. A., Janowitz, H. D., and Perrier, C. V.: Pancreatic inflammatory disease, New York, 1964, Hoeber Medical Division, Harper & Row, Publishers.)

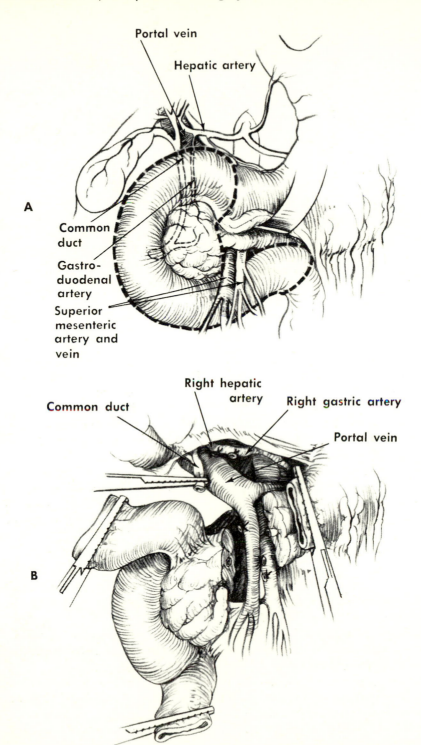

**Fig. 20-17.** Radical one-stage pancreatoduodenectomy. **A,** Anatomy. **B,** Operative field prepared for anastomosis and transection completed. **C,** Reconstruction of gastrointestinal canal completed by means of three anastomoses—establishment of continuity with pancreas and jejunum or duodenum, with gallbladder and jejunum, and with stomach and jejunum. (From Wilder, J. R.: Atlas of general surgery, ed. 2, St. Louis, 1964, The C. V. Mosby Co.)

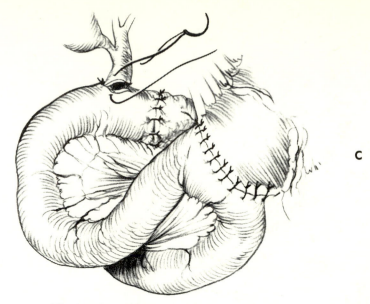

**Fig. 20-17, cont'd.** For legend see opposite page.

technically hazardous procedure because it involves many vital structures and organs. Resectability of the tumor in the presence or absence of metastasis and the general overall condition of the patient are evaluated carefully prior to resection (Fig. 20-17, *A*).

After surgery, it is important to reevaluate the insulin requirements, as well as those of supplementary pancreatin.

**SETUP AND PREPARATION OF THE PATIENT.** As described for gastrointestinal surgery, plus drainage tubes and drains, as in cholecystoduodenostomy.

**OPERATIVE PROCEDURE**

1. The abdomen is entered through an upper transverse, bilateral subcostal, or long paramedian incision. Laparotomy packs and retractors are used to expose the operative site and protect structures.

2. Mobilization of the duodenum is achieved with an adequate Kocher maneuver. Blunt dissection of loose areolar tissue is carried out, and incision of peritoneal reflection, lateral to the second portion of the duodenum, is done with Metzenbaum scissors.

3. Mobilization is continued; bleeding vessels are ligated with silk.

4. The gastrocolic ligament and the gastrohepatic omentum are divided between Pean curved forceps and transfixed, using silk suture ligatures.

5. The gastroduodenal and right gastric arteries are clamped, divided, and doubly ligated.

6. The prepyloric area of the stomach is mobilized. The operative field is prepared for open anastomosis. By placing two long Allen or Payr clamps near the midportion of the stomach, the transection is completed (Fig. 20-17, *B*).

7. The duodenum is reflected, the common duct is divided, and the distal portion is marked or tagged for later anastomosis.

8. The jejunum is clamped with two Allen forceps, and the duodenojejunal flexure is divided.

9. The pancreas is divided, and the duct is carefully identified. A temporary ligature may be used to prevent spillage into the abdominal cavity.

10. Further mobilization of the duodenum and division of the inferior pancreatoduodenal artery is done to permit complete removal of the specimen.

11. Reconstruction of the gastrointestinal

canal is completed by the following anastomoses: retrocolic end-to-end pancreato-jejunostomy, retrocolic end-to-side choledochojejunostomy, and an antecolic long-loop isoperistaltic gastrojejunostomy (Fig. 20-17, *C*).

12. Drains are introduced, as for cholecystostomy.

13. The wound is closed in layers, usually with wire sutures.

## OPERATIONS ON THE LIVER
### Drainage of liver subhepatic or subphrenic abscess

**DEFINITION.** Drainage of the liver or one or more abscesses situated in the right upper quadrant.

**CONSIDERATIONS.** Hepatic abscesses may be pyogenic and single or multiple. The pyogenic and secondary amebic types are generally treated by surgery.

Extreme care is exercised to prevent the fluid from an *Echinococcus* cyst from entering the peritoneal cavity, since it may produce an anaphylactic reaction.

Some surgeons prefer to disinfect the cyst as follows: A sufficient amount of a 10% solution of Formalin may be injected into the cyst, thus allowing the fluid to combine with Formalin. This may result in a 1.5% solution of Formalin. Instillation of Formalin for a 4-minute period usually disinfects the cavity. The solution is then completely evacuated prior to the excision of the cyst.

**SETUP AND PREPARATION OF THE PATIENT.** As described for biliary surgery, plus drainage materials such as several Penrose or cigarette drains.

**OPERATIVE PROCEDURE**

1. The incision and type of procedure selected depends on the etiology and location of the abscess. For the anterior approach, a right transperitoneal incision is made. For the posterior approach, the patient is prepared and incision selected, as described for posterior thoracotomy (Chapter 14).

2. Drainage of an abscess may be treated in one or two stages. In the one-stage procedure, the approach is through the outer third of the right twelfth rib, reaching the liver abscess retroperitoneally.

A two-stage operation may be selected to obliterate the right pleural cavity. The objective of the first stage is to seal off the pleural cavity by stimulating adhesions with the insertion of iodoform packing; then, when the second operation—which is done at a higher level—is performed, the chest cavity will not become contaminated.

### Hepatic resection

**DEFINITION.** Resection of the liver may involve a small wedge biopsy, excision of simple tumors, or a major lobectomy. Increased knowledge of liver function and circulatory physiology and improved methods of hemostasis now permit the surgeon to offer safer, more definitive treatment to the patient with liver disease or traumatic injury.

**CONSIDERATIONS.** Facilities should be available for hypothermia, electrocoagulation, portal pressure measuring apparatus, thoracotomy drainage, and accurate replacement of blood loss; special needles for suturing liver tissue are available.

**SETUP AND PREPARATION OF THE PATIENT.** The patient is placed in a supine position with the gallbladder rest elevated (Chapter 7). An incision through the midline with division of the sternum will provide access to the left lobe, whereas a combined right thoracoabdominal incision is needed to expose the right hepatic region.

Instrument setup includes those for portacaval shunt and common duct procedures, plus additional items as follows:

> Electrocoagulation cords and attachments
> Penrose or cigarette drains
> 2 Chest drainage catheters
> 12 to 18 Special liver sutures (silk or gut, according to surgeon's preference)
> Hemostatic material

**OPERATIVE PROCEDURE FOR RIGHT HEPATIC LOBECTOMY**

1. Through a right subcostal incision, the abdominal cavity is opened; examina-

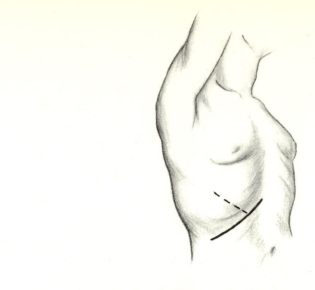

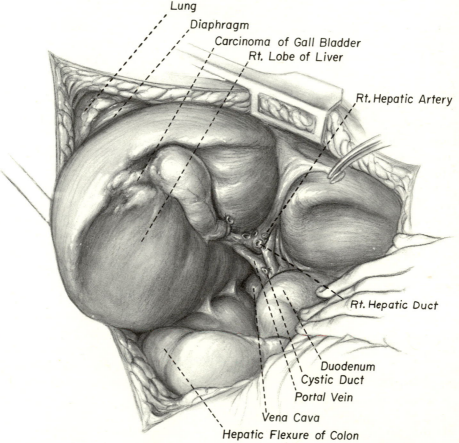

Lung
Diaphragm
Carcinoma of Gall Bladder
Rt. Lobe of Liver

Rt. Hepatic Artery

**A**

Rt. Hepatic Duct

Duodenum
Cystic Duct
Portal Vein
Vena Cava
Hepatic Flexure of Colon

*Continued.*

**Fig. 20-18.** Right hepatic lobectomy. **A,** Extension of subcostal incision through seventh or eighth interspace. **B,** Hilar structures ligated preparatory to transection of right lobe. **C,** Preparation of devascularized channel for transection by placement of interlocking sutures. **D** shows pattern of hemostatic sutures following removal of specimen. **E,** Omentum has been sutured over raw liver surface to decrease bile and serum loss. **F** shows position of drainage catheters. (From Indications and technique of right hepatic lobectomy, Somerville, N. J., 1964, Ethicon, Inc.)

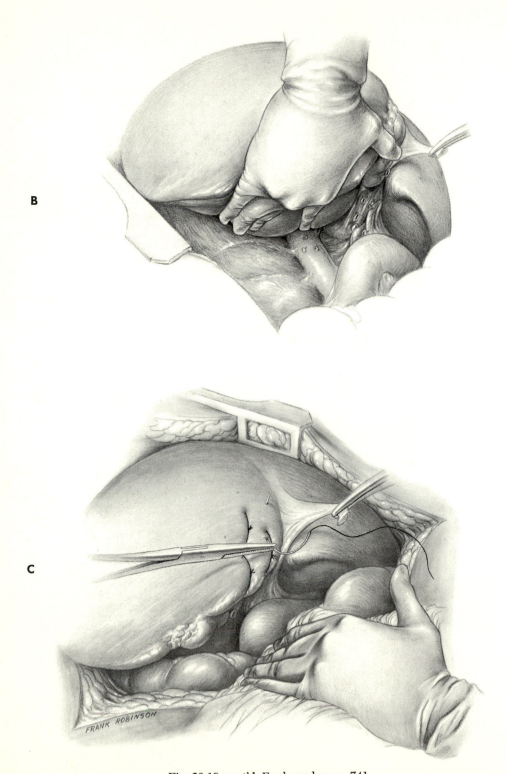

B

C

FRANK ROBINSON

**Fig. 20-18, cont'd.** For legend see p. 741.

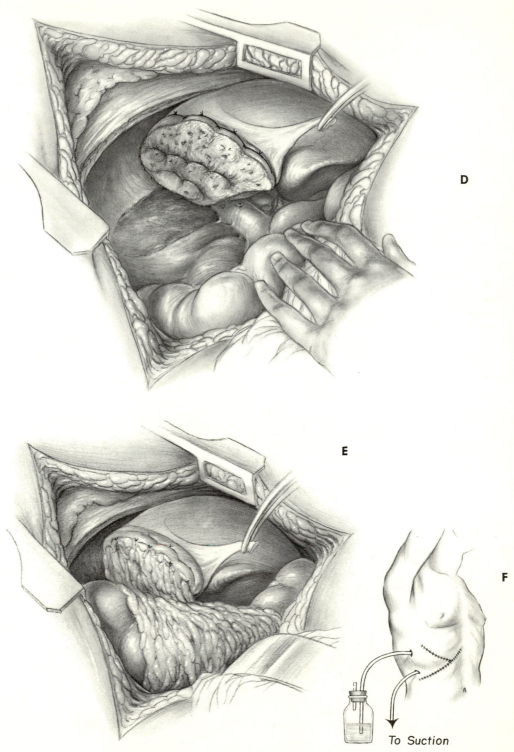

**D**

**E**

**F**

To Suction

**Fig. 20-18, cont'd.** For legend see p. 741.

tion is carried out, using items as described for biliary surgery. Pathological condition is determined and resectability evaluated.

2. Thoracoabdominal incision is completed through the seventh or eighth interspace, as illustrated in Fig. 20-18. Moist laparotomy packs are inserted, and a chest retractor is placed.

3. Exposure of the hilar structures is obtained by displacement of the right lobe into the right chest cavity, application of Pean clamp to the falciform ligament to facilitate traction, and inferior displacement of intestines with moist packs and lateral retractors.

4. The cystic duct is carefully exposed, using Metzenbaum scissors, vascular forceps, small dry dissectors on curved holders, and fine right-angled forceps. It is clamped, transected, and doubly ligated, using chromic or silk ligatures and transfixion sutures.

5. The right hepatic duct, right hepatic artery, and right branch of the portal vein are also transected and doubly ligated, using silk ligatures and transfixion sutures (Fig. 20-18, *B*).

6. The liver is rotated forward, and a double row of interlocking liver sutures are placed, as shown in Fig. 20-18, *C*. A scalpel is used to excise the specimen through the devascularized section. Fine suture ligatures of chromic gut may be needed to ligate bile ducts and small blood vessels. As additional sutures are placed, care should be exercised to avoid injury to the left hepatic veins (Fig. 20-18, *D*).

7. The omentum may be sutured to the raw liver surface to decrease bile and serum loss (Fig. 20-18, *E*).

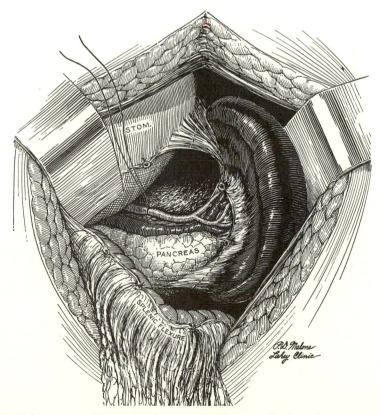

**Fig. 20-19.** Splenectomy. Upper attachments of spleen to fundus of stomach are divided. (From Sedgwick, C. F., and Parrish, C. M.: Surg. Clin. North Am. **35**:675, 1955.)

8. Chest and abdominal drainage tubes are inserted, and layer closure is completed, as previously described (Fig. 20-18, *F*).

## OPERATIONS ON THE SPLEEN
### Splenectomy

**DEFINITION.** Removal of the spleen.

**CONSIDERATIONS.** A splenectomy is usually performed to treat traumatic rupture of the spleen or specific conditions of the blood that are associated with abnormal splenic function. If accessory spleens are present, they are also removed, since they are capable of perpetuating hypersplenic function.

Splenomegaly may on occasion require a thoracoabdominal approach. Abdominal suction apparatus should be available throughout the entire procedure.

**SETUP AND PREPARATION OF THE PATIENT.** As described for biliary surgery, plus 2 large, right-angled pedicle clamps and hemostatic material.

**OPERATIVE PROCEDURE**

1. Through a long left rectus or subcostal incision, the abdomen is opened. Aspiration of the cavity is maintained by continuous suction, as indicated. Kelly retractors are placed over laparotomy packs. Gentle retraction is employed as exploration is carried out. The costal margin is retracted upward.

2. The stomach and transverse colon are exposed; the fundus of the stomach is retracted toward the midline, using a Deaver retractor and laparotomy pack (Fig. 20-19).

3. Adhesions posterior to the spleen are freed. The splenorenal, splenocolic, and gastrosplenic ligaments are clamped and divided, using long dressing forceps, long hemostats, sponges on holders, and long Metzenbaum or Nelson scissors.

4. The ligaments are ligated with silk or chromic sutures.

5. The spleen is delivered into the wound after all the attachments are freed.

6. The cavity formerly occupied by the spleen is packed with laparotomy packs if necessary.

7. The splenic artery and vein are dissected free, using long fine dissection scissors and long forceps.

8. The artery is clamped with Pean forceps and then doubly ligated with silk. The artery is ligated first and then the vein, thus permitting disengorgement of the spleen with blood and facilitating the return of the venous blood to the circulatory system.

9. The splenic vein is then clamped, divided, and ligated, as described for ligation of the artery.

10. The specimen is removed; all bleeding vessels are controlled.

11. The wound is closed in layers, as described for routine laparotomy, and dressings are applied.

**REFERENCES**

1. Anthony, C. P.: Textbook of anatomy and physiology, ed. 8, St. Louis, 1971, The C. V. Mosby Co.
2. Artz, C. P., and Hardy, J. D.: Complications in surgery and their management, Philadelphia, 1960, W. B. Saunders Co.
3. Blakemore, A.: The liver and biliary system. In Davis, L., editor: Christopher's textbook of surgery, ed. 6, Philadelphia, 1956, W. B. Saunders Co.
4. Blaustein, A., editor: The spleen, New York, 1963, Blakiston Division, McGraw-Hill Book Co.
5. Brasfield, R. D.: Right hepatic lobectomy for carcinoma of the gallbladder; a five-year cure, Ann. Surg. 153:563, 1961.
6. Child, C. G., III: Radical one-stage pancreaticoduodenectomy, Surgery 23:492, 1948.
7. Child, C. G., III: The hepatic circulation and portal hypertension, Philadelphia, 1954, W. B. Saunders Co.
8. Glenn, F.: Surgery of the gallbladder. In Allen, A. W., and Barrow, D. W., editors: Abdominal surgery, New York, 1961, Harper & Row, Publishers.
9. Glenn, F.: Atlas of biliary tract surgery, New York, 1963, The Macmillan Co.
10. Glenn, F.: Surgical treatment of biliary tract disease, Am. J. Nurs. 64:92, 1964.
11. Glenn, F., and Wantz, G. E., Jr., editors: Problems in surgery, St. Louis, 1961, The C. V. Mosby Co.
12. Gross, R. E.: Surgery of infancy and childhood, Philadelphia, 1955, W. B. Saunders Co.

13. Henderson, L. M.: Nursing care in acute cholecystitis, Am. J. Nurs. **64**:93, 1964.

14. King, B. G., and Showers, M. J.: Human anatomy and physiology, ed. 5, Philadelphia, 1963, W. B. Saunders Co.

15. Longmire, W. P., and Lippman, H. N.: Benign biliary stricture. In Allen, A. W., and Barrow, D. W., editors: Abdominal surgery, New York, 1961, Harper & Row, Publishers.

16. Maingot, R.: Abdominal operations, ed. 5, New York, 1969, Appleton-Century-Crofts.

17. Moyer, C. A., Rhoads, J. E., Allen, J. G., and Harkins, H. N.: Surgery: principles and practices, ed. 3, Philadelphia, 1965, J. B. Lippincott Co.

18. Nardi, G. L., and Zuidema, G. D., editors: Surgery, Boston, 1961, Little, Brown & Co.

19. Sedgwick, C. E.: Splenectomy: elective and emergency, Surg. Clin. North Am. **36**:725, 1956.

20. Selkurt, E. E., editor: Physiology, Boston, 1962, Little, Brown & Co.

21. Smith, R., editor: Progress in clinical surgery, series 2, London, 1961, J. & A. Churchill, Ltd.

22. Spencer, R. P.: The intestinal tract; structure, function and pathology in terms of the basic sciences, Springfield, Ill., 1960, Charles C Thomas, Pulisher.

23. Thorek, P.: Anatomy in surgery, ed. 2, Philadelphia, 1962, J. B. Lippincott Co.

24. Warren, K. W., and Baker, A. L., Jr.: In Lahey Clinic: Surgical practice of the clinic, Philadelphia, 1962, W. B. Saunders Co.

25. Warren, R., editor, with members of the Department of Surgery of the Harvard Medical School: Surgery, Philadelphia, 1963, W. B. Saunders Co.

26. Wilder, J. R.: Atlas of general surgery, ed. 2, St. Louis, 1964, The C. V. Mosby Co.

27. Zollinger, R. M., and Cutler, E. C.: Atlas of surgical operations, ed. 3, New York, 1961, The Macmillan Co.

# CHAPTER 21

# Upper gastrointestinal surgery

DORRIS JACKO

## ANATOMICAL AND PHYSIOLOGICAL CONSIDERATIONS

The alimentary canal is comprised of a series of organs joined to form a tubelike structure that extends the full length of the trunk (Fig. 21-1). The entire alimentary tract includes the mouth, pharynx, esophagus, stomach, the small intestine (duodenum, jejunum, and ileum), large intestine, colon, rectum, and anus. These organs effect the supply of nourishment to the body and the discharging of solid wastes.

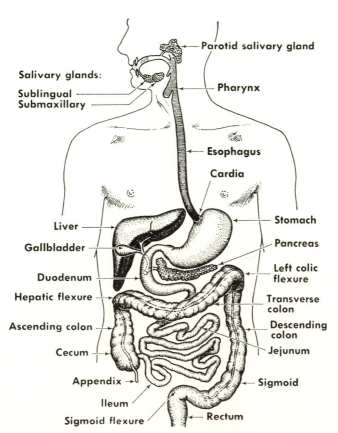

**Fig. 21-1.** Alimentary tube and its appendages. (From Tuttle, W. W., and Schottelius, B. A.: Textbook of physiology, ed. 16, St. Louis, 1969, The C. V. Mosby Co.)

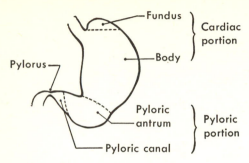

Fig. 21-2. Regional anatomy of stomach. (From Moseley, H. F., editor: Textbook of surgery, ed. 3, St. Louis, 1959, The C. V. Mosby Co.)

Gastrointestinal tract usually refers to the stomach and the small and large intestines. Colon refers to the entire large intestine exclusive of the rectum.

### Regional anatomy of the gastrointestinal organs

The *esophagus,* extending from the pharynx at the level of the sixth cervical vertebra, passes through the neck posterior to the trachea and heart and anterior to the vertebra. The lower portion of the esophagus courses in front of the aorta and passes through the diaphragm slightly to the left of the midline to join the cardia orifice of the stomach.

Blood is supplied from branches of the inferior thyroid, thoracic aorta, and celiac arteries. The nerve supply of the esophagus comes from branches of the vagi and sympathetic chain. The esophagus is a collapsible tube of musculomembranous quality about 9 inches in length.

The *stomach* is situated between the esophagus and the duodenum. It lies in the upper abdominal cavity, to the left of the midline, beneath the diaphragm. The stomach is divided into three parts: the fundus, the body, and the pyloric antrum (Fig. 21-2). The fundus lies beneath the left dome of the diaphragm behind the apex of the heart and pericardium at the level of the fifth rib posteriorly. The body and antrum lie in an oblique direction within the abdominal cavity.

The stomach is stabilized indirectly by the lower portion of the esophagus and directly by its attachment to the duodenum, which is anchored to the posterior parietal peritoneum. The stomach is associated with branches of the celiac vessel, the peritoneal ligaments, and the omenta, which provide additional support.

The convex or lower margin of the stomach is known as the *greater curvature,* and its concave margin is identified as the *lesser curvature.* Attached to the greater curvature is the greater omentum. The omentum is a double fold of peritoneum known as the "watchdog" of the belly. It covers the intestines loosely and is not to be confused with the mesentery, which connects the intestines with the posterior abdominal wall. Through the omentum runs the left gastroepiploic branch of the splenic artery and the right gastroepiploic branch of the hepatic artery. The lesser omentum, which is attached to the lesser curvature of the stomach, contains the left gastric artery, a branch of the celiac artery, and the right gastric branch of the hepatic artery. During a gastrectomy these vessels are clamped and ligated. (See Fig. 21-3.)

The *small intestine,* which begins at the pylorus and ends at the ileocecal valve, is divided into three parts: the duodenum, about 11 inches long; the jejunum, 7½ feet long; and the ileum, 11½ feet long. The length of the small intestine varies with the degree to which the muscle fibers are contracted, but it is usually about 20 feet in length and 1 inch in diameter (Fig. 21-1).

The duodenum, the proximal portion of the small intestine, begins at the pyloric opening and is continuous with the jejunum below (Fig. 21-1). It is stabilized by a fusion between the peritoneum and the head of the pancreas, which is attached to the posterior parietal peritoneum. The duodenum communicates also with the common bile duct. The duodenojejunal angle is stabilized by the ligament of Treitz that suspends the duodenum. The uppermost

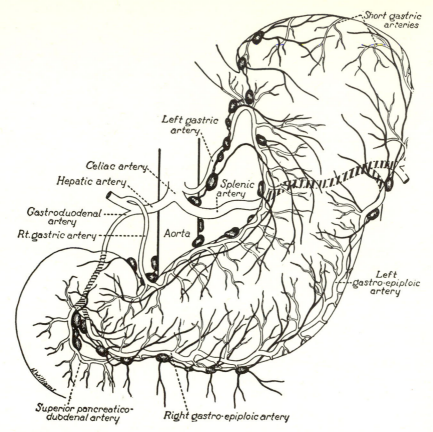

**Fig. 21-3.** Arterial supply of stomach. (After Cutler and Zollinger; from Francis, C. C, Knowlton, G. C., and Tuttle, W. W.: Textbook of anatomy and physiology, St. Louis, The C. V. Mosby Co.)

part of the duodenum forms the beginning of the C-shaped bend that encloses a portion of the pancreas, the pylorus, and the neck of the gallbladder. (See Figs. 21-1 and 21-3.)

The middle portion of the duodenum forms an acute angle in its descent. It passes along the right side; then its inferior portion transverses to the left so that it lies in front of the right ureter, the inferior vena cava, and the aorta. It then turns upward and forward to become a part of the duodenojejunal flexure that, in turn, joins the jejunum. The bile duct and pancreatic ducts enter the descending portion of the duodenum. The blood supply of the duodenum comes from arterial branches of the celiac axis (Fig. 21-4).

The jejunum, which is situated in the upper left portion of the abdominal cavity, joins the ileum, which is situated in the right lower portion of the cavity. The ileum empties into the large intestine through the ileocecal valve. The jejunum and ileum are suspended by the mesentery, which is attached to the posterior abdominal wall. The free border of the mesentery (Fig. 21-4), which is about 18 feet long, contains branches of the superior mesenteric artery, many veins, lymphatic nodes and vessels, and nerve fibers.

Distinction between the jejunum and the ileum may be made by inspection of their mesentery. The jejunal mesentery exhibits long parallels of arteries into one or two arcades with little fat distribution, whereas

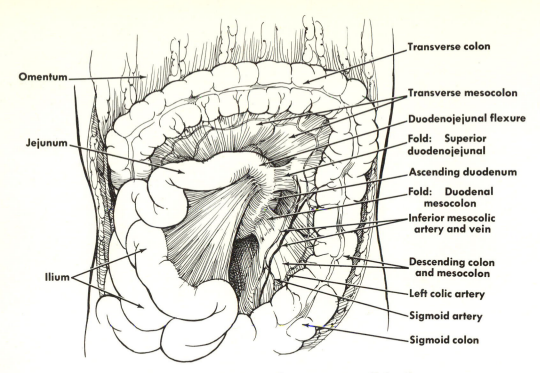

**Fig. 21-4.** Mesentery as seen when intestine is pulled aside.

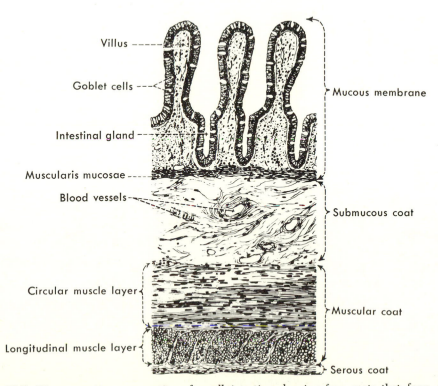

**Fig. 21-5.** Diagrammatic cross section of small intestine showing four coats that form conspicuous structural feature throughout gastrointestinal tract. (From King, B. G., and Showers, M. J.: Human anatomy and physiology, ed. 5, Philadelphia, 1963, W. B. Saunders Co.)

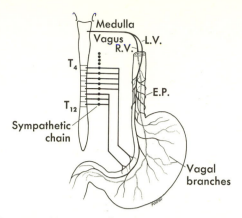

**Fig. 21-6.** Nerve supply of esophagus, stomach, and duodenum. **R.V.,** Right vagus; **L.V.,** left vagus; **E.P.,** esophageal plexus. (From Welch, C. E.: Surgery of the stomach and duodenum, ed. 4, Chicago, 1966, Year Book Medical Publishers, Inc.)

the ileal mesentery exhibits increasingly shorter arterial arcades and larger fat distribution.

### Influence of the nervous system on the gastrointestinal structures

The structural wall of the gastrointestinal tract is composed of four coats (Fig. 21-5), except in the esophagus, which does not contain a serosal layer. The four layers from within outward include a mucosal layer, containing villi, epithelial cells, and capillaries; a submucosal layer, composed of loose connective tissue containing many blood and lymph vessels; a muscular layer, composed of inner oblique, circular, and longitudinal fibers; and a serosal layer, containing fibrous tissue and visceral peritoneum.

The progress of material through the gastrointestinal tract results from muscular activity of the organs. Such activity is influenced by the sympathetic and parasympathetic nerves (Fig. 21-6). The former reach through the splanchnic nerve, whereas the latter, which are derived from the medulla oblongata in the brain, pass through the vagus nerve that acts on the muscles of the stomach, small intes-

tine, and the proximal half of the large intestine (Fig. 21-6). Other parasympathetic nerves, which are derived from the sacral portions of the spinal cord, supply the lower half of the large intestine and the rectum. The results of studies seem to indicate that the parasympathetic nerves are excitatory for all musculature except the sphincters, for which they are generally inhibitory. On the other hand, the sympathetic nerves are excitatory for the sphincters and inhibitory for the other muscles.

The effects of bilateral vagotomy include a reduction in the volume and acidity of gastric contents, a decrease in muscle tonus and motility, and an increased pyloric spasm, with resulting delayed emptying time.

Within the muscular layer of the tract the circular fibers are enlarged at points where one part of the tract joins the next. These junctions are known as sphincters because they keep the lumen of the tract closed until a stimulus causes them to relax. This action, which is controlled by the sympathetic (excitatory) nerves and by the parasympathetic (inhibitory) fibers, restrains the food units in their passage from one part of the tract to the next and also prevents regurgitation. The terms used for the sphincters correspond to those portions that are involved. They are known as (1) the cardiac sphincter between the esophagus and body of the stomach, (2) the pyloric sphincter between the stomach and small intestine, (3) the ileocecal valve between the small and large intestine, and (4) the internal anal sphincter between the rectal sigmoid colon and anal opening.

## ENDOSCOPIC PROCEDURES

Endoscopic procedures that permit direct visual inspection of the contents and walls of the esophagus and stomach may be pertinent to establishing diagnosis or to determining preferred treatment of a disease process.

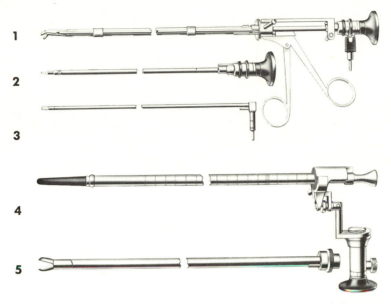

**Fig. 21-7.** Schindler esophagoscope: **1,** Biopsy forceps; **2,** telescope; **3,** light carrier; **4,** outer tube and obturator; **5,** inner tube. (From Palmer, E. D., and Boyce, H. W.: Manual of gastrointestinal endoscopy, Baltimore, 1964, The Williams & Wilkins Co.)

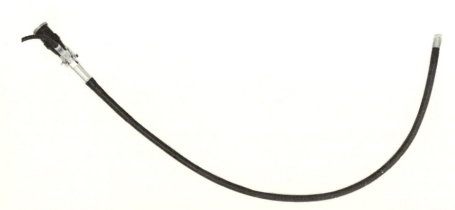

**Fig. 21-8.** LoPresti fiberoptic esophagoscope. This instrument contains flexible fiberoptic image–transmitting bundle, which transmits images by total internal reflection through multiple and spatially aligned optical fibers. Light is provided by means of separate adjacent fiberoptic carrier that has 5 cm. markings on outer corner. There are two channels: one for irrigation or suction and one for biopsy. (Courtesy American Cystoscope Makers, Inc., New York, N. Y.)

# Esophagoscopy

**DEFINITION.** Direct inspection of the esophagus and cardia of the stomach by means of a lighted instrument known as an *esophagoscope* (Figs. 21-7 and 21-8) to obtain a tissue biopsy or secretions for study.

**CONSIDERATIONS.** Esophagoscopy is done to aid in the diagnosis of esophageal diverticula, hiatus hernia, stricture, benign stenosis, and varices; to obtain additional information by means of a tissue biopsy; or to clarify roentgenographic findings. Patients suffering with suspected obstruction, symptoms of bleeding, or regurgitation may require endoscopy. Patients with stenosis or varices may be given sclerosing treatment of varices through the esophagoscope, although the results are not very satisfactory. To perform direct therapeutic manipulations such as removal of a foreign body or insertion of a plastic prosthesis, esophagoscopy is done.

**SETUP AND PREPARATION OF THE PATIENT.** Instrumentation includes the following:

Local anesthesia set (optional)
Esophagoscopes and telescopes, desired type, size, and length
Suction pump and tubing
Power source (battery or fiberoptic)
Broyles dilators
Bougies, if desired
Forceps, desired types and lengths
Aspirating tubes
Specimen containers
Lubricating jelly

An operative permit is obtained. The patient is not permitted fluids or food for at least 8 hours prior to surgery.

The patient needs to be sufficiently relaxed to make the examination easier. This is accomplished by both psychological and proper drug preparation. An oral sedative is usually given the night before and again approximately 1 hour prior to the examination. The usual preoperative medications to decrease anxiety and mucous membrane secretions are given on call to surgery.

An esophagoscopy may be done with the patient under general or local anesthesia. If a local agent is used, it is instilled into the pharynx, larynx, and trachea to prevent gagging, coughing, and discomfort.

The patient is placed in the supine or lateral position with the endoscopist at the patient's head. Dentures or bridges are removed.

The face is cleansed, and long hair is encased in a disposable cap. Medical aseptic techniques are followed during the procedure to prevent transmission of bacteria from one patient to another.

**OPERATIVE PROCEDURE**

1. The indirect or direct technique may be followed. When the indirect method is used, the obturator within the scope is passed through the cricopharyngeal lumen and then removed. When the direct technique is used, the esophagoscope with the lamp is thinly lubricated. With the patient in correct position, the suction and pump are turned on. The scope is passed into the mouth. The tongue, epiglottis, laryngeal aditus, and cricopharyngeal lumen are identified, respectively. The head holder may tip the patient's head a little backward while extending the neck forward. If the endoscope is passed to the side of the tongue, the patient's head may be turned slightly to the opposite side.

2. When the scope is passed into the cardia of the stomach, the patient's head is moved so that all areas of the esophageal wall can be examined.

3. Specimens of secretions from the esophageal lumen may be obtained by aspirating tube and suctioning apparatus. In some cases, saline solution may be injected through the endoscope's aspirating channel and the fluid immediately withdrawn for histological study. A tissue biopsy may be taken using forceps with jaws at a 45-degree angle.

4. The esophagoscope is removed and the patient returned to his room.

5. The instrument is mechanically cleansed and then terminally sterilized by ethylene oxide.

### Esophagoscopy to treat varices

Treatment of esophageal varices by injection of a sclerosing solution into the esophageal lining, although not a very satisfactory method, is still used by some.

CONSIDERATIONS. A varix is any submucosal vein that elevates the esophageal mucosa when the patient is horizontal and is breathing quitely and easily. Patients who are not suitable candidates for surgery may be treated by sclerosis. Only a few veins are treated at a time. Treatments are repeated at intervals.

SETUP AND PREPARATION OF THE PATIENT. As described for esophagoscopy, plus the following:

> Sclerosing drug such as sodium morrhuate (Morusul) in 5% solution
> 2 Syringes, 10 ml.
> 1 Piece thin rubber tubing, 15 cm. long, to connect syringe and needle
> 1 Straight needle suitable to dimension of scope
> 1 Needle with acute bevel to fit into other needle's shaft
> 1 Gastric balloon tube, such as Sengstaken type

OPERATIVE PROCEDURE

1. The gastric tube is passed orally into the stomach.

2. The patient is esophagoscoped, as described previously.

3. The needle, tubing, and syringe with medication are then assembled. The long needle is passed through the esophagoscope, and the solution is injected into the esophagus.

4. The needle and endoscope are withdrawn. The gastric balloon of the stomach tube is inflated and pulled up lightly against the cardia. The esophageal balloon is inflated to a pressure of 600 mm. of $H_2O$ for an adult and 300 mm. for a child.

## Gastroscopy

DEFINITION. Direct inspection of the stomach and removal of tissue specimen, if necessary, by means of an instrument known as a *gastroscope.*

CONSIDERATIONS. A study of the stomach by endoscopy is done to assist in the diagnosis of organic stomach disease or some systemic diseases.

SETUP AND PREPARATION OF THE PATIENT. Similar to that for esophagoscopy. The position selected depends on the areas of the stomach to be visualized. For inspection of lesions in the gastric fundus and about the cardia, an upright sitting position may be used. The instrument set includes the following:

> Local anesthesia set
> Standard flexible or fiberoptic gastroscope, as preferred by physician
> Forceps, as desired
> Suctioning set
> Emesis basin
> Tissues
> Lubricating jelly
> Gauze sponges

OPERATIVE PROCEDURE

1. The gastroscope is thinly but completely covered with water-soluble lubricating jelly.

2. During introduction of the gastroscope, the patient's head and neck must remain in the sagittal plane of his spine so that the axis of his mouth and throat is in line with that of the esophagus. As the gastroscope is passed into the mouth, the head holder slowly tips the patient's head backward and then extends the neck anteriorly.

3. The gastroscope is passed into the stomach.

4. Gastric biopsy may be done. A standard flexible gastroscope can be used, with insertion of a flexible, very thin, long biopsy forceps through its own channel. Or the vacuum biopsy device, which is built into the gastroscope, may be used.

## FACTORS RELATED TO MEDICAL ASEPSIS
### Physiological considerations

The hydrochloric acid secreted by parietal cells in the proximal two thirds of the stomach exerts an antiseptic action on ingested food in the stomach and duodenum. The digestion and absorption of foods is enhanced in the small intestine

by pancreatic juice, bile, and intestinal juice. As mucus and pancreatic secretion act to neutralize the hydrochloric acid in the duodenum and upper jejunum, the ability of the gastric juice to control pathogenic bacteria is reduced.

In the lower portion of the intestine a large number of bacteria, including certain cocci and clostridia, are usually present in the material as it moves toward the ileum and colon. These resident pathogenic organisms are rarely harmful in the intestine; however, if they enter the bloodstream or peritoneal cavity, serious infection may result.

Since the lymphatic system aids in the elimination of bacteria and their products, regional lymph nodes may be enlarged in the presence of certain infections and diseased conditions. Carcinoma in the stomach and colon may be spread by means of the lymphatics and veins that carry the cells to the liver or by direct extension through the walls to their neighboring organs.

Some protection against the spread of infection is achieved by the natural ability of the serous membranes (the peritoneum and omentum) to localize and wall off a disease process. However, the healing process of the sutured bowel is largely dependent on the accurate approximation of the serosa-to-serosa anastomosis, a minimum of tissue trauma, and the elimination of gross bacterial contamination.

Although the preoperative preventive measures of mechanically cleansing the gastrointestinal tract and administering antibacterial medications do decrease the possibility of infection, surgical methods of anastomosis and the discriminating use of aseptic technique are other means of preventing pathogenic organisms from entering the bloodstream and tissues.

### Methods of anastomosis

The technique to be followed in gastrointestinal surgery depends on the type and location of the lesion and the characteristics of the disease.

*Open anastomosis* indicates that a portion of the gastrointestinal tract is openly divided and that the two open segments are sutured together in layers while exposing the peritoneal cavity to the contents of the tract, a potentially "soiled" area (Fig. 21-26).

*Closed anastomosis* implies that specific resection instruments are placed on the involved segments prior to transection to confine the contents within the tract. Before the instruments are removed, a new passageway is established, and the incised portions are closed by sutures (Fig. 21-27).

During the anastomosis the instruments that have been placed on the involved segments form a barrier to prevent the gastrointestinal contents from coming in direct contact with the open peritoneal cavity. This closed method decreases the possibility of infection, but it does not necessarily eliminate the potential danger.

### Gastrointestinal techniques

The goal of preventing pathogenic contamination can also be met by physically separating the sterile instruments based on their anatomical utilization.

The use of *two distinct sterile* setups includes the gastrointestinal set, which is used to open the abdomen, resect the diseased organs, and reestablish bowel continuity, and the laparotomy closure set, which is used to close the abdominal wound.

1. During the preliminary preparation for the operation, the nursing team arranges the sterile laparotomy closure set on a second portable stand ready for use. It is covered with a sterile double-thickness sheet and moved to a protected area within the operating room.

2. The gastrointestinal set is prepared.

3. After the completion of the final anastomosis, all laparotomy packs are removed from the cavity, the instruments are removed from the operative field, the sponge and instrument counts are veri-

fied, and the wound is covered with a freshly moistened laparotomy pack.

4. As the surgical team changes to fresh gowns and gloves, one assistant remains at the field with the patient. The circulating nurse removes the cover from the closure set as the scrubbed nursing team member is donning fresh gown and gloves. The assistant removes the remaining laparotomy pack from the wound.

5. The second Mayo stand with instruments is moved into position, the operative field is redraped (preferably with materials impervious to furthering contamination), a fresh laparotomy pack is applied, and the abdominal wound is closed.

The use of the double setup tends to reduce marginal errors of contamination and provides a greater safety factor in long complicated operations involving many anastomotic procedures.

*The single setup,* which is commonly used and generally preferred, consists of the selected gastrointestinal set plus a small metal tray, a small sheet, and additional instruments and supplies for the abdominal closure.

1. During the initial preparation the scrubbed nursing team member drapes the portable stand in the routine manner and then places a folded sheet over the top of the tray as an extra cover. This later serves as a receptacle for contaminated instruments. The tips of an extra sponge-holding forceps are protected in a folded towel and placed on the stand conveniently near the instrument table. If it is necessary to obtain supplies from the basic set during the anastomosis, the forceps is readily available for this purpose.

2. Before the resection is started, all instruments except those actually needed for the resection and anastomosis are removed from the Mayo stand.

3. The lesion is mobilized; then the operative field surrounding the wound is draped with large towels, and the wound is draped with four laparotomy packs or other protective material. The small metal discard basin is placed on the sterile field near the lower end of the wound for the collection of soiled instruments and sponges.

4. On completion of the anastomosis the assistant surgeon removes the skin towels and clamps from the wound and discards them in the discard basin.

5. The scrubbed nursing team member and surgeons change to fresh gowns and gloves. The abdominal cavity is protected with fresh moist packs, and the wound is redraped. Instruments and sutures for closure are transferred to the Mayo stand, and the operation is completed in the usual manner.

When this method is used, fewer pieces of equipment are needed. However, the objective remains the same: mechanical elimination or reduction of a potential source of wound infection.

## SPECIFIC NURSING CONSIDERATIONS FOR GASTROINTESTINAL SURGERY

Gastrointestinal drainage or decompression may be indicated. A nasogastric tube is usually introduced before the patient arrives in the operating room. However, a variety of these and other gastrointestinal tubes should be available, together with materials for irrigation and aspiration.

Fluid and electrolyte losses should be anticipated in procedures involving obstruction and edema. Equipment for measuring and replacement should be available.

If the use of a cautery is anticipated, the unit should be operational before the surgery begins. The anesthesiologist should be informed well in advance of induction of the patient, to permit selection of an appropriate anesthetic agent for the provision of routine safety measures against explosive hazards.

If 95% phenol solution is used to cauterize tissue, 70% alcohol should be available to neutralize the action. Extreme caution should be exercised by all members of the surgical team in handling the phenol solution because inadvertent contact with tissue or instruments may cause

irreparable damage to the patient or team member. A few drops of phenol placed in a medicine cup set within a larger basin affords protection against spillage. The scrubbed nursing team member should handle *only* the outside basin, to guard against the inadvertent transfer of phenol to the patient by means of glove, sponge, or instruments. The scalpel and applicators used in the cauterization of the appendix should be carefully discarded in the designated basin. Immediately after use, the scrubbed nursing team member should pass the phenol and alcohol containers in the discard basin to the circulating nurse.

Gloves are worn by the circulating nurse for protection. The remaining alcohol is mixed with the remaining phenol and discarded immediately in the sink. Mixing is done over the sink, and complete rinsing of items is best accomplished by using a fine stream of running water.

To reduce tissue trauma, the jaws of heavy intestinal forceps may be protected by pieces of soft rubber tubing. These guards (shods) should fit the jaws firmly, but not tightly. Before sterilization, the rubber shods should be separated from forceps to facilitate steam penetration.

Stapling instruments that automatically place sutures lines in organs are often complex devices (Chapter 14). Prior to a surgical procedure the integrity and completeness of the device should be ascertained. After the procedure the device should be dismantled for thorough cleaning and terminal sterilization.

Rubber Penrose tubing for soft tissue drainage may also be used to provide effective yet gentle traction for the stomach or a loop of bowel.

Moist packs are used to exclude open and diseased portions of the stomach and bowel from the abdominal cavity. Many new disposable synthetic materials provide more effective protection.

Throughout the entire resection and anastomotic procedure, careful handling of "soiled" instruments and supplies tends to reduce the number of disseminated enteric organisms and provide a greater margin for patient safety. The gastrointestinal techniques discussed previously should be routinely followed. Instruments that have been attached to the specimen or those soiled with gastrointestinal contents are placed in the discard basin. They must not be retrieved for reuse. If these instruments are needed to complete the procedure, the circulating nurse should either arrange for their sterilization or provide replacements.

### Preparation of the patient

Positioning of the patient has been described in Chapter 7. To permit the stomach to fall below the costal margin, reduce the fundus of the stomach, or expose the cervical esophagus, a reverse Trendelenburg position may be used.

Skin preparation has been described in Chapter 4. The various incisional approaches are described in Chapter 17.

## BASIC GASTROINTESTINAL INSTRUMENT SETUP

Since there are many varieties of resection instruments available, the basic set should be standardized with the approval of the attending physicians. Frequently it is impossible for the surgeon to determine in advance the specific type of operation to be performed until he has examined the involved organs. The gastrointestinal instrument set comprises the basic major laparotomy setup (Figs. 17-9 to 17-15), plus the following (Fig. 21-9):

**Cutting instruments**

1 Metzenbaum scissors, 9 in.
2 Metzenbaum scissors, 5¾ in., 1 straight and 1 curved
2 Mayo scissors, 9 in., 1 straight and 1 curved

**Clamping instruments**

1 Von Petz stomach or DeMartel clamp or stapler clamp, if desired
4 Allen intestinal anastomosis clamps, 1 and 2 fine teeth
4 Rochester-Carmalt forceps, straight, 8 in.
4 Doyen intestinal forceps, longitudinal serrations, 9 in., 2 straight and 2 curved
2 Mayo vessel clamps, angled, 9 in.

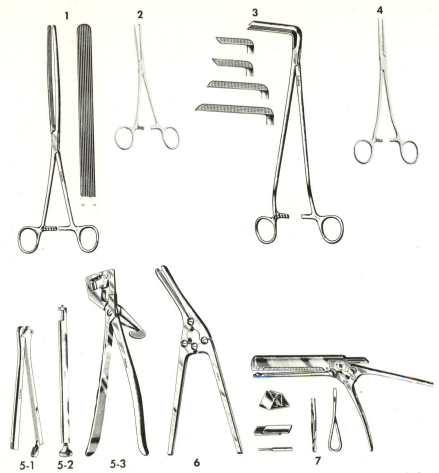

**Fig. 21-9.** Instruments for stomach and intestinal operations. **1**, Doyen intestinal forceps; **2**, Allen intestinal anastomosis clamp; **3**, Best colon clamps; **4**, Dennis intestinal forceps; **5**, DeMartel anastomosis clamp set; **6**, Payr pylorus clamp; **7**, Von Petz stomach and intestinal suturing instrument. (Courtesy Codman & Shurtleff, Inc., Randolph, Mass.)

4 Gallbladder forceps, right-angled, assorted sizes
4 Rochester-Pean forceps, curved, 8 in.
12 Rochester-Pean forceps, curved, 6¼ in.
12 Crile forceps, curved, 5½ in.
36 Halsted mosquito forceps, 5 in., 24 curved and 12 straight

**Holding instruments**

2 Thumb forceps, 6 in.
2 Fixation or Adson forceps, 5 in.
2 Potts-Smith dressing forceps, 8 in.
6 Babcock intestinal forceps, 6¼ in.

**Exposing instruments**

1 Doyen retractor, large blade 2¼ in. wide × 3½ in. deep

2 Kelly retractors, large blade 3 in. deep × 2½ in. wide

**Suturing items**

2 Fine needle holders, 6 in.
6 Intestinal needles
*Suture materials for gastrointestinal operations*
Ligatures for small blood vessels—chromic gut no. 4-0, and silk no. 5-0, 4-0, or 3-0.
Ligatures for larger blood vessels—chromic gut no. 0 or silk no. 2-0 or 0
Closure of gastrointestinal layers:
Mucosal—chromic gut no. 4-0 or 3-0 with curved Atraumatic intestinal needle; usually continuous
Seromuscular—chromic gut no. 3-0 or 2-0 and silk no. 4-0 or 3-0 with curved or

straight Atraumatic intestinal needles; interrupted silk sutures on intestinal needles may be used

Abdominal closure and retention sutures, as previously described (Chapters 6 and 17)

### Accessory items

3 Penrose drains, 12 in. long, narrow, and medium diameter
2 Malecot, Pezzer, or Foley catheters, desired size
1 Robinson catheter, desired size
1 Rectal tube (optional)
1 Baker jejunostomy tube

## OPERATIONS
## Esophageal obstruction

GENERAL CONSIDERATIONS. Esophageal obstruction may be caused by the swallowing of a caustic substance or foreign bodies, an infection, achalasia, or tumor. When an ulcer forms in the esophagus, the muscular structure is replaced by dense connective tissue, thereby narrowing the esophageal lumen. When a caustic material has been swallowed, emergency measures are first carried out; then a gastrostomy may be done. Foreign bodies are removed by means of an endoscope. Strictures may be dilated, using graduated bougies that are passed through an esophagoscope. If repeated dilatation is unsuccessful, the lesion is resected.

## Excision of esophageal diverticulum (diverticulectomy)

DEFINITION. Through an incision over the inner border of the sternocleidomastoid muscle and extending from the level of the hyoid bone to a point 2 cm. above the clavicle, the sac of the diverticulum (pouch) is freed and ligated and the pharyngeal muscles and surrounding tissues closed.

SETUP AND PREPARATION OF THE PATIENT. As described for thyroidectomy (Chapter 18). The additional instruments include the following:

2 New York Hospital lateral retractors
2 Duval lung forceps or 2 Pennington clamps
2 Rochester-Carmalt clamps
6 Halsted mosquito clamps, curved
2 Adson forceps, 5 in.

OPERATIVE PROCEDURE. The steps are described and illustrated in Fig. 21-10.

## Partial esophagectomy and intrathoracic esophagogastrostomy

DEFINITION. Through a left thoracoabdominal incision in the left chest, including a resection of the seventh, eighth, or ninth rib or separation of the two appropriate ribs, the diseased portions of the stomach and esophagus are removed, and an anastomosis is established.

CONSIDERATIONS. This procedure is performed to remove strictures of the lower esophagus that may develop following trauma, infection, or corrosion or to remove tumors that are situated in the cardia of the stomach or distal esophagus.

SETUP AND PREPARATION OF THE PATIENT. Technique is as described for gastrointestinal surgery. The instruments include a basic thoracotomy setup (Chapter 14) and the gastrointestinal setup.

OPERATIVE PROCEDURE

1. The skin incision is carried downward midway between the vertebral border of the scapula and the spinous processes to the eighth rib and then forward along that rib to the costochondral junction (Chapter 14). The extent of the vertical portion of the incision will depend on the location of the tumor. The wound is retracted. Bleeding vessels are ligated.

2. The chest cavity is opened, and the rib spreader is placed. With moist packs and a Deaver or Harrington retractor, the lung is retracted.

3. The mediastinal pleura is incised in line with the esophagus and the lesion with long plain forceps and long Metzenbaum scissors. The esophagus is dissected free from the aorta, using dry dissectors. Suture ligatures of silk nos. 2-0 and 3-0 are used for controlling bleeding vessels.

4. With a nerve hook and a right-angled clamp, the phrenic nerve is crushed. The diaphragm is opened, and a series of traction sutures are attached. The stomach is mobilized by dissection of its ligamental

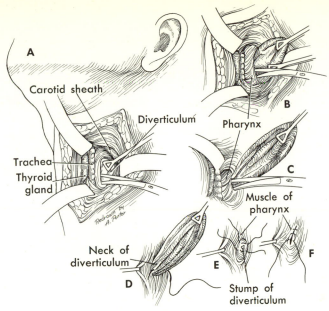

**Fig. 21-10.** Harrington technique for one-stage esophageal diverticulectomy. **A,** Wound opened, thyroid retracted medially, and carotid sheath with sternocleidomastoid retracted laterally, exposing diverticulum. **B,** Diverticulum dissected free from surrounding structures down to neck. **C,** True neck of sac dissected from surrounding muscles of posterior wall of pharynx. **D,** Neck of sac ligated with chromic gut sutures. **E,** Stump of sac invaginated into wall of pharynx. **F,** Opening in pharyngeal muscles closed. (From Harrington, S. W.: Surgery **18:**76, 1945.)

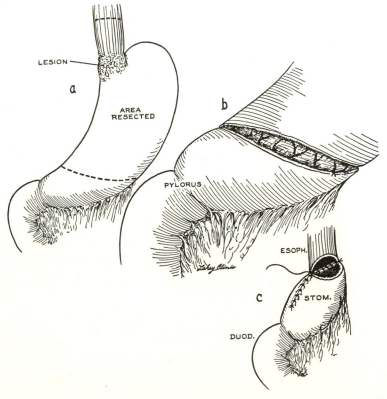

**Fig. 21-11. a** and **b,** Resection of cardia and distal esophagus for carcinoma. **c,** Tailoring of antrum for esophagogastric anastomosis. (From Adams, H. D.: In Lahey Clinic: Surgical practice of the clinic, Philadelphia, 1962, W. B. Saunders Co.)

attachment with long scissors and curved thoracic clamps.

5. A splenectomy may be done. The left gastric artery is clamped, cut, and doubly ligated with silk no. 2-0 and a suture ligature of silk no. 3-0 (Chapter 20).

6. The sterile field is prepared for the open method of anastomosis. The stomach is transected well below the lesion using the selected resection instruments. Partial closure of the stomach is completed with two rows of intestinal sutures of chromic gut no. 2-0 and sometimes also with a third row of silk sutures no. 3-0 for reinforcement (Fig. 21-11, *B*).

7. Two Allen clamps or a stapler-type clamp is applied above the stricture, and the freed esophagus is divided (Fig. 21-11).

8. Using the open method of anastomosis, the circular opening in the stomach and the severed end of the esophagus are sutured together. The mucosal layers are approximated; then the muscular layers of the esophagus and stomach are closed by two rows of interrupted sutures (Fig. 21-11, *C*).

9. The stomach is anchored to the pleura, and the edges of the diaphragm are sutured to the wall of the stomach, using interrupted sutures of silk no. 3-0 or 2-0.

10. The pleura is cleansed with normal saline solution that is suctioned off. A catheter is inserted for closed drainage. The chest wall is closed as described for thoracotomy (Chapter 14). Additional procedures are completed as necessary (pyloromyotomy).

## Heller cardiomyotomy (esophagomyotomy)

**DEFINITION.** Myotomy at the esophagogastric junction.

**CONSIDERATIONS.** This operation is done to correct esophageal obstruction due to cardiospasm. Selection of transthoracic or transabdominal incision will depend on the patient's general condition and other existing pathological conditions. The surgeon may also elect to perform a pyloro-

plasty to prevent reflux (a backward flow).

**SETUP AND PREPARATION OF THE PATIENT.** As described for gastrointestinal surgery, minus long resection clamps, and plus one set of esophageal bougie dilators and a basic thoracotomy setup, as indicated.

**OPERATIVE PROCEDURE**

1. After exposure of the esophagogastric junction as previously described, a nasogastric tube is inserted by the anesthesiologist to serve as a splint.

2. A longitudinal incision is made, using a scalpel with blade no. 15, through the muscular wall of the distal esophagus and proximal stomach, leaving the mucosa intact (Fig. 21-12).

3. Additional procedures are completed as indicated, and the wound is closed.

## Pyloromyotomy (Fredet-Ramstedt technique)

**DEFINITION.** Through a high upper right rectus abdominal incision about 3 inches long, the abdominal cavity is opened, and the thickened seromuscular layers of the pyloric ring are separated.

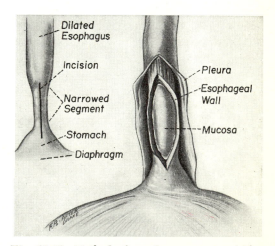

**Fig. 21-12.** Method of esophagomyotomy. (After Ellis, Olsen, Holman, and Code; from Barnes, W. A.: In Glenn, F., Moore, S. W., and Beal, J. M., editors: Surgery in the aged, New York, 1960, Blakiston Division, McGraw-Hill Book Co.)

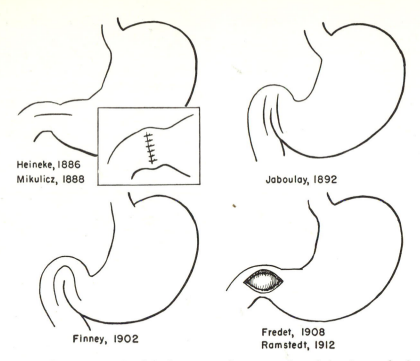

**Fig. 21-13.** Different types of pyloroplastic procedures. Heineke-Mikulicz longitudinal incision with transverse closure to enlarge lumen. Jaboulay anastomosis of two longitudinal incisions. Finney closure of inverted ∪ incision. Ramstedt longitudinal incision down to muscle layer, with mucosa pouching out to level even with adjoining serosa. (After Waugh and Hood; from Moyer, C. A., Rhoads, J. E., Allen, J. G., and Harkins, H. N.: Surgery: principles and practices, ed. 3, Philadelphia, 1965, J. B. Lippincott Co.)

CONSIDERATIONS. The cause of hypertrophied stenosis of the pyloric sphincter is unknown. It usually occurs in infants 4 to 6 weeks of age. The sphincter becomes hypertrophied; as the seromuscular coats increase in size and become thickened, the mucosal coat becomes edematous, thereby impairing the pyloric opening.

SETUP AND PREPARATION OF THE PATIENT. As described for laparotomy (Chapter 17), plus these additional instruments of appropriate size: six curved mosquito forceps, two Adson forceps, and one straight and one curved anastomosis scissors.

OPERATIVE PROCEDURE

1. The abdominal cavity is opened as previously described. The pylorus is delivered into the wound.

2. An incision is made through the serous and muscular layers of the pyloric ring, using a scalpel with a no. 15 blade.

The thickened muscle is spread apart with straight scissors, allowing the mucosal layer to bulge (Fig. 21-13).

3. The wound is closed with fine sutures, as described for abdominal closure (Chapter 17).

## Pyloroplasty

DEFINITION. Formation of a larger passageway between the prepyloric region of the stomach and the first or second portion of the duodenum and excision of the peptic ulcer, if present.

CONSIDERATIONS. A pyloroplasty may be done to treat a peptic ulcer under selected conditions but is more frequently utilized to remove cicatricial bands in the pyloric ring to relieve the spasm and permit rapid emptying of the stomach.

SETUP AND PREPARATION OF THE PATIENT. As described for gastrointestinal surgery.

Large resection clamps are not required.

**OPERATIVE PROCEDURE**

1. Through an upper right rectus incision, the abdominal cavity is opened (Chapter 17).

2. The operative field is prepared for open anastomosis.

3. An incision is made through the stomach and the duodenum. Different types of techniques are illustrated in Fig. 21-13.

4. The pyloroplasty is closed with silk or chromic gut intestinal sutures.

5. The abdominal wound layers are closed, and dressings are applied.

## Closure of perforated gastric or duodenal ulcer

**DEFINITION.** Through a high right rectus or midline abdominal incision, the perforation in the stomach or duodenum is closed.

**CONSIDERATIONS.** Perforated gastric or duodenal ulcer is treated as an "emergency," and the operation is performed promptly after the diagnosis has been made. A gastric lavage is not performed, but continuous suction is used.

A partial gastrectomy for peptic ulcer is discussed and illustrated (Fig. 21-17) under the Billroth II operation.

**SETUP AND PREPARATION OF THE PATIENT.** As described for gastrointestinal surgery.

**OPERATIVE PROCEDURE.** The abdomen is opened (Chapter 17), the involved portion of the stomach or duodenum is examined, the exudate in the peritoneal cavity is removed by suctioning, the perforation is closed, and an omental tag is sutured over the closure. The abdominal wound is closed in layers.

## Gastrostomy

**DEFINITION.** Through a high left rectus abdominal incision, a temporary or permanent channel is established from the gastric lumen to the skin to permit liquid feeding or retrograde dilatation of an esophageal stricture.

**CONSIDERATIONS.** This palliative procedure is performed to prevent starvation, which may be caused by a lesion or stricture situated in the esophagus or in the cardia of the stomach. A temporary procedure is done when the obstruction is capable of being corrected. A permanent gastrostomy, in which a stomach flap is formed around the catheter, is advised by some surgeons in cases of extensive lesion in the esophagus.

**SETUP AND PREPARATION OF THE PATIENT.** As described for gastrointestinal surgery, including suitable Pezzer, Malecot, Foley, or Robinson catheters.

**OPERATIVE PROCEDURE**

1. The abdominal cavity is opened, and the wound edges are protected.

2. The stomach is held with Allis or Babcock forceps, and a purse-string suture of intestinal chromic gut no. 2-0 is placed at the proposed site for the entrance of the catheter. The area is protected with moist packs.

3. Using a scalpel with a no. 15 blade, an incision is made within the purse-string suture, and the contents are suctioned away as mosquito clamps are applied to bleeding points. The catheter is inserted, and the purse-string suture is tied around it (Fig. 21-14).

4. Soiled instruments are discarded; the catheter is clamped and exteriorized through a stab wound made in the margin of the left rectus muscle near the costal margin.

5. The stomach may be sutured to the peritoneal layer, and the abdominal wound is closed in layers (Fig. 21-14).

## Gastrotomy

**DEFINITION.** Through a left paramedian abdominal incision, the anterior stomach wall is opened, the interior is explored, and a foreign body may be removed.

**SETUP AND PREPARATION OF THE PATIENT.** As described for gastrointestinal surgery, minus large resection clamps.

**OPERATIVE PROCEDURE**

1. The abdominal wound is protected, and a longitudinal incision usually is made through the anterior wall of the stomach,

Stamm

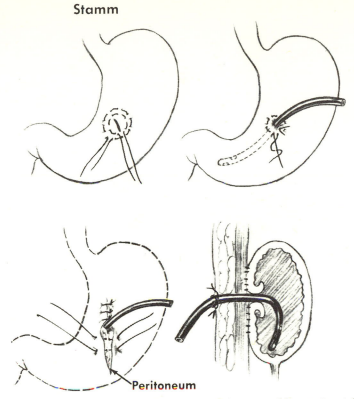

Peritoneum

Fig. 21-14. Stamm technique of simple gastrostomy. (From Wilder, J. R.: Atlas of general surgery, ed. 2, St. Louis, 1964, The C. V. Mosby Co.)

halfway between the curvatures, where fewer arteries are encountered. The stomach wall is grasped and elevated by Allis or Babcock forceps. The bleeding vessels are ligated with fine-gauged silk or chromic gut ligatures.

2. The proposed site is walled off with moist packs, and an incision is made through the mucosa; a suction tube is introduced into the stomach to withdraw the gastric contents; then the foreign body or tumor is removed, if present.

3. The layers of the stomach wall and the abdominal wound are closed.

### Gastrojejunostomy

**DEFINITION.** Through a midline or a paramedian abdominal incision a permanent communication is made, either between the proximal jejunum and the anterior wall of the stomach or between the proxi-

mal jejunum and the posterior wall of the stomach, without removing a segment of the gastrointestinal tract.

**CONSIDERATIONS.** Gastrojejunostomy may be performed to treat a benign obstruction at the pyloric end of the stomach or an inoperable lesion of the pylorus when a partial gastrectomy would not be feasible and also to provide a large opening without sphincteric obstruction.

**SETUP AND PREPARATION OF THE PATIENT.** As described for gastrointestinal surgery.

**OPERATIVE PROCEDURE**

1. Through an upper midline or paramedian abdominal incision, exploration of the peritoneal cavity is completed, as described for routine laparotomy. Pathological condition is confirmed.

2. Moist packs are placed, and a loop of proximal jejunum is grasped with Babcock forceps and freed from the mesen-

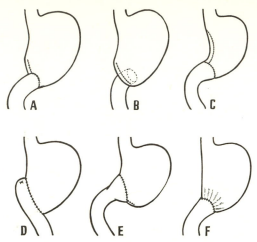

**Fig. 21-15.** Diagrams illustrating resections of stomach with anastomosis of stomach and duodenum (gastroduodenal anastomosis). All these types in which stomach brought to duodenum are modifications of Billroth I technique. **A,** Billroth I. After pylorus is removed, lesser curvature is partially closed and duodenum is sutured to open end of stomach at its lower margin. **B,** Kocher. In this case, distal end of stomach is closed and duodenum brought up to posterior margin of closed stomach. **C,** Schoemaker. In this instance, lesser curvature of stomach is sutured and brought down to same size as duodenum, and then end-to-end anastomosis is done. **D,** Von Haberer-Finney. In this operation, side of duodenum is brought up to end of stomach so that entire end of stomach is open for direct anastomosis. **E,** Horsley. Horsley type of gastroduodenal anastomosis uses lesser curvature end of stomach to suture to duodenum and closes greater curvature end. **F,** Von Haberer. Modification of operation shown in **D.** Stomach is, so to speak, narrowed or puckered so that it fits end of duodenum. Modification of this is done by some in following way: Duodenum is split longitudinally, and its ends are flared open so that opening is large enough to fit open end of stomach. (From Berman, J. K.: Principles and practice of surgery, St. Louis, 1950, The C. V. Mosby Co.)

tery. It is approximated to either the anterior or posterior stomach wall several centimeters from the greater curvature. Silk no. 2-0 traction sutures are placed through the serosal layers at each end of the selected portion of the jejunum and stomach. Rubber-shod or gastroenterostomy clamps may be placed prior to insertion of the posterior interrupted silk no. 3-0 or 2-0 serosal sutures.

3. The field is draped for open anastomosis. The jejunum and stomach are opened. Bleeding points are clamped with mosquito forceps and ligated with gut no. 3-0. The inner posterior row of sutures is placed, using continuous chromic gut no. 2-0 or 3-0 with ½-circle intestinal needle, and continued for the first anterior row. The anastomosis is completed with anterior serosal sutures of silk no. 3-0 or 2-0. Traction sutures are re-

moved. Interrupted silk no. 4-0 sutures may be used for reinforcement.

4. The contaminated instruments are discarded, and the wound is redraped. The abdominal wound is closed in layers and a dressing applied.

### Partial gastrectomy
*Billroth I technique*

**DEFINITION.** Through a right paramedian or transverse abdominal incision, the diseased portion of the stomach is resected, and an anastomosis is established between the stomach and duodenum.

**CONSIDERATIONS.** The Billroth I operation is performed to remove a benign or malignant lesion located in the pyloric half of the stomach.

One of several techniques may be followed to establish gastrointestinal continuity. These include the Schoemaker, the

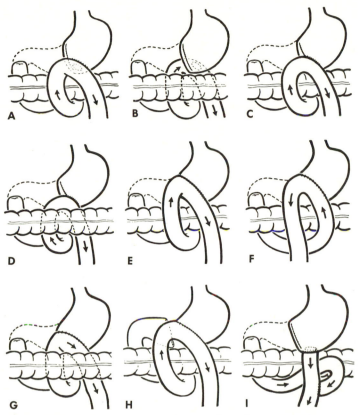

**Fig. 21-16.** Diagram illustrating resections of stomach with anastomosis to some part of jejunum. All types of gastrojejunal anastomoses are modifications of Billroth II. Modifications of this follow. (1) *End of stomach closed.* **A,** Billroth II is resected with side-to-side gastrojejunostomy anterior to transverse colon, and anastomosis is isoperistaltic. **B,** Mikulicz type is retrocolic side-to-side gastrojejunostomy with isoperistaltic alignment of jejunum. (2) *End of stomach partially closed.* **C,** Von Eiselsberg. Anastomosis is antecolic end-to-side isoperistaltic, but superior portion of stomach is closed for greater part of its surface, thereby creating small stoma. This allows resection of greater portion of lesser curvature and decreases size of stoma, thereby tending to avoid so-called dumping syndrome. **D,** Hofmeister-Finsterer. This is a *retrocolic,* end-to-side gastrojejunostomy and is isoperistaltic. (3) *End of stomach entirely open.* **E,** Kronlein-Balfour—isoperistaltic, antecolic, and end-to-side. Entire end of stomach is anastomosed to side of jejunum. **F,** Moyniham II—antiperistaltic, antecolic, end-to-side gastrojejunostomy. **G,** Reichel-Polya—isoperistaltic (that is, from lesser to greater curvature), retrocolic, end-to-side gastrojejunostomy. One of most common varieties employed today following subtotal gastrectomy. (4) *Stomach not resected.* These operations are known as exclusion operations. **H,** Stomach divided, distal portion turned in, proximal portion brought up to jejunum, usually according to Reichel-Polya or Kronlein-Balfour type of end-to-side anastomosis. **I,** Roux type—also known as Roux-en Y type of anastomosis. Jejunum severed, distal limb sutured to cut end of stoma of stomach or to side of stomach as in Billroth II, and proximal limb sutured to side of distal jejunum. Operation useful when insufficient amount of bowel is available to bring up to stomach or when technically not possible because of dense adhesions. This type of anastomosis avoids vicious circles and dumping syndromes that have been described in connection with other types of operations. (From Berman, J. K.: Principles and practice of surgery, St. Louis, 1950, The C. V. Mosby Co.)

von Haberer-Finney, and other modifications of the Billroth I operation (Fig. 21-15).

SETUP AND PREPARATION OF THE PATIENT. As described for gastrointestinal surgery.

OPERATIVE PROCEDURE

1. The abdominal wall is incised; the peritoneal cavity opened and explored. Bleeding vessels are clamped and ligated.

2. The abdominal wound is retracted and the surrounding organs protected with moist packs.

3. The gastrocolic omentum is freed from the colon mesentery to prevent injury to the middle colic artery. With Rochester-Pean hemostats and Metzenbaum scissors, the right and left gastroepiploic arteries and veins are clamped, divided, and ligated with silk no. 2-0 and suture ligatures of silk nos. 3-0 and 2-0, thereby freeing the greater curvature of the stomach. The gastrohepatic vessels are also clamped, divided, and ligated to free completely the diseased portion of the stomach (Fig. 21-16).

4. The operative field is prepared for open anastomosis. Two Payr, Allen, or other suitable clamps are placed on the upper portion of the duodenum just distal to the pylorus. Division is accomplished by scalpel or cautery, as preferred. Additional moist packs are placed for protection, and two sets of anastomosis clamps are placed across the stomach. Division is completed by a preferred method.

5. The opened stomach at the lower margin is approximated to the duodenum by a series of interrupted sutures placed in the serosal layers. Silk no. 3-0 threaded on intestinal or Atraumatic needles is used. Suture ends are held with hemostats, and the intestinal clamps are removed. Stumps of the stomach and duodenum are cleansed with moist sponges, and bleeding vessels are ligated with fine gut. During the anastomosis the involved segments may be held with rubber-shod clamps.

6. The excess of the lesser curvature in the stomach is closed on completion of the anastomosis (Fig. 21-15). Soiled instruments are discarded.

7. The wound is redraped, and routine laparotomy closure is completed.

### Billroth II technique and modifications

DEFINITION. Through an abdominal incision the distal stomach is resected and anastomosis established between the stomach and the jejunum.

CONSIDERATIONS. The Billroth II procedure is performed to remove a benign or malignant lesion in the stomach or duodenum. This technique and modifications may be selected because the volume of acidic gastric juice will be reduced and the anastomosis can be made along the greater curvature or at any point along the stump of the stomach. Modifications of the Billroth II operation include the Polya and Hofmeister operations, which also establish gastrointestinal continuity through bypassing the duodenum (Fig. 21-16). After surgery the duodenal and jejunal secretions empty into the remaining gastric pouch. The stomach empties more rapidly because of the larger opening, and a limited amount of acid gastric juice remains.

SETUP AND PREPARATION OF THE PATIENT. The items used to perform the various steps are similar to those listed for the Billroth I operation up to the point of anastomosis.

OPERATIVE PROCEDURE

1. The duodenal stump is sutured, using closed technique (Fig. 21-18).

2. The stomach is divided as shown in Fig. 21-18. The step-by-step procedure for the gastrojejunostomy is demonstrated in Figs. 21-17 to 21-21.

3. Soiled instruments are discarded.

4. The wound is redraped, and the abdominal wound is closed in layers. Retention sutures may be used.

### Total gastrectomy

DEFINITION. Complete excision of the stomach, establishment of an anastomosis

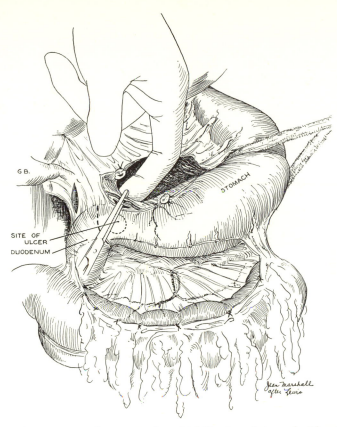

**Fig. 21-17.** Partial gastrectomy for peptic ulcer. Mobilization of stomach. Elevation of stomach by traction tape. Omentum preserved in this instance but frequently excised with stomach. Right gastroepiploic vessels ligated; right gastric artery isolated and clamped. Incision into hepatoduodenal ligament made to expose common bile duct. (Courtesy Lahey Clinic, Boston, Mass.; from Marshall, S. F.: Surg. Clin. North Am. **6:**665, 1955.)

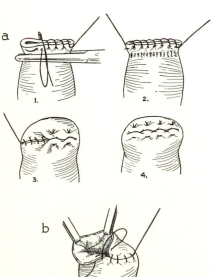

**Fig. 21-18.** Partial gastrectomy for peptic ulcer—cont'd. Closure of distal end of divided duodenum can be made with clamp on duodenum, **a,** or with open duodenal segment. **b,** If duodenal cuff remaining above ampulla of Vater is short, or if ulcer is densely adherent, duodenum is transected without clamp and inverted with Connell sutures of chromic catgut as first suture layer, **b.** (Courtesy Lahey Clinic, Boston, Mass.; from Marshall, S. F.: Surg. Clin. North Am. **6:** 665, 1955.)

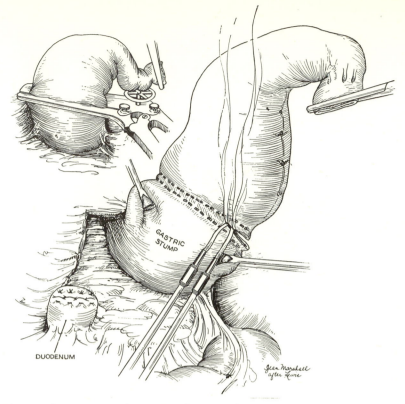

**Fig. 21-19.** Partial gastrectomy for peptic ulcer—cont'd. Application of Von Petz clamp. Note inverted duodenal stump. Stomach divided with cautery between double row of inserted metal clips. (Courtesy Lahey Clinic, Boston, Mass.; from Marshall, S. F.: Surg. Clin. North Am. 6:665, 1955.)

between the jejunum and the esophagus, and an enteroenterostomy, as indicated.

**CONSIDERATIONS.** Total gastrectomy is done as a potentially curative or a palliative procedure to remove a malignant lesion of the stomach and metastases in the adjacent lymph nodes. The incision may be bilateral subcostal, long transrectus, or thoracoabdominal (Chapters 14 and 17).

**SETUP AND PREPARATION OF THE PATIENT.** As described for partial gastrectomy. The instruments include the basic laparotomy, gastrointestinal, and thoracotomy setups, plus two blunt nerve hooks and two fine needle holders, 10 inches long.

**OPERATIVE PROCEDURE**

1. The abdomen is opened, and the wound edges are protected and retracted, as previously described.

2. Careful and complete exploration for extent of metastasis is carried out. The lesser peritoneal cavity may be examined as shown in Fig. 21-22.

3. The omentum is freed from the colon, using sharp dissection; vessels are ligated with silk no. 2-0.

4. The splenic vessels are ligated and transfixed with silk nos. 2-0 and 3-0 at the tail of the pancreas, leaving the spleen attached to the omentum.

5. The duodenum is mobilized, intestinal clamps are applied, and the operative field is protected for transection and closure of the distal duodenum.

6. The right gastric artery is ligated and transfixed, using silk nos. 2-0 and 3-0, and the gastrohepatic omentum is separated from the liver. Following ligation of the left gastric artery, the mobilized stomach, spleen, omentum, and lesser and

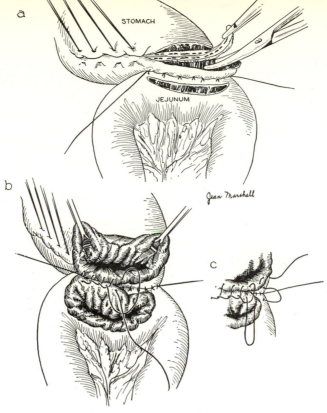

**Fig. 21-20.** Partial gastrectomy for peptic ulcer—cont'd. **a,** Upper portion of transected end of stomach inverted with running suture of chromic catgut and second layer of interrupted sutures. Gastrojejunal anastomosis placed at greater curvature end of divided stomach. Note excision of clips to open into gastric lumen. Two-layer closure used: **b,** mucosal layer of continuous catgut suture, and **c,** outer serosal layer of interrupted silk sutures. (Courtesy Lahey Clinic, Boston, Mass.; from Marshall, S. F.: Surg. Clin. North Am. **6**:665, 1955.)

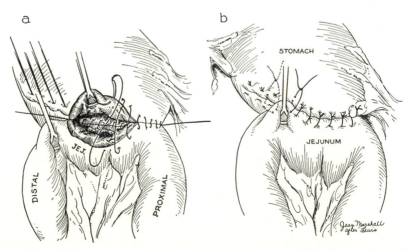

**Fig. 21-21.** Partial gastrectomy for peptic ulcer—cont'd. **a,** Completion of gastrojejunal anastomosis. Continuous catgut suture inverts gastric and jejunal mucosa; outer reinforcing serosal and muscular sutures of interrupted silk. **b,** Distal jejunal loop sutured to inverted end of stomach, thereby avoiding tension at angle of gastrojejunal anastomosis. Gastrocolic omental tag tied at corner of anastomosis at greater curvature. Gastrohepatic omentum used to reinforce corner at lesser curvature. (Courtesy Lahey Clinic, Boston, Mass.; from Marshall, S. F.: Surg. Clin. North Am. **6**:665, 1955.)

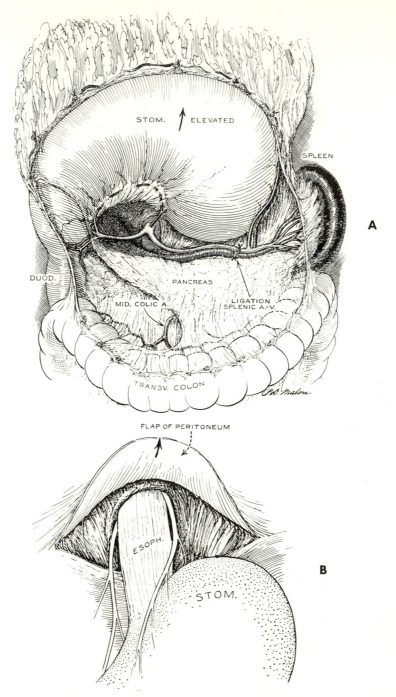

**Fig. 21-22.** Total gastrectomy. **A,** Method of detaching greater omentum from transverse colon so that entire lesser peritoneal cavity is exposed. Spleen left attached to omentum and stomach and gastrohepatic omentum are removed in one block. **B,** Flap of peritoneum cut from front surface of esophagus and reflected over diaphragm is diagrammatically shown. This flap will be used to suture to jejunum, reinforce anterior suture line, and take up weight of jejunum anastomosed to esophagus. Also shows vagi diagrammatically and how necessary it is to sever nerves before free delivery of esophagus can be obtained. (From Boyd, D. P.: In Lahey Clinic: Surgical practice of the Clinic, Philadelphia, 1962, W. B. Saunders Co.)

greater curvature ligamentous attachments are delivered into the wound.

7. Division of the coronary ligament of the left lobe of the liver permits exposure of the diaphragmatic peritoneum over the esophagogastric junction. The liver is protected by a moist pack and gentle retraction maintained with a Harrington or malleable retractor.

8. A flap of peritoneum is freed from the diaphragm, and branches of the vagus nerves are divided as seen in Fig. 21-22, B.

9. A loop of jejunum is selected and delivered antecolic to the esophagogastric junction for anastomosis. Using the specimen for traction, the posterior layer of interrupted silk no. 3-0 sutures is inserted.

10. As the jejunum and esophagus are incised, bleeding is controlled, using mosquito hemostats and ligatures of gut no. 3-0. The posterior layer is reinforced with chromic no. 2-0 intestinal interrupted sutures.

11. Division of the esophagus is completed, and the entire specimen is removed. Interrupted chromic no. 2-0 sutures are also used to approximate the mucosal anterior wall of the anastomosis. A second layer of sutures, silk no. 3-0 or chromic no. 2-0, is placed in the seromuscular and muscular coat of the intestine anteriorly. A flap of peritoneum is attached to the jejunum with interrupted silk no. 3-0 sutures to relieve traction on the anastomosis. A lateral jejunojejunal anastomosis is completed to permit irritating bile and pancreatic fluids to bypass the anastomosis line, thereby preventing esophageal regurgitation (Fig. 21-23). An alternate method of establishing continuity is a combination of a Roux-Y jejunojejunostomy and a jejunoesophagostomy, as shown in Fig. 21-24.

12. The abdominal wound is closed in layers. The absence of omentum to protect the small bowel necessitates the extraperitoneal placement of retention sutures.

### Vagectomy

**DEFINITION.** Segmental resection of the vagus nerves to the stomach as they lie

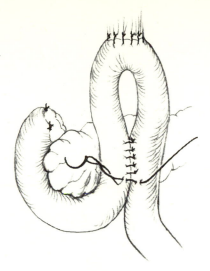

**Fig. 21-23.** Jejunojejunostomy performed to prevent regurgitation esophagitis. (From Wilder, J. R.: Atlas of general surgery, ed. 2, St. Louis, 1964, The C. V. Mosby Co.)

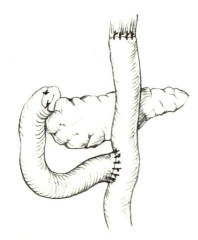

**Fig. 21-24.** Completed jejunoesophageal anastomosis with Roux-Y jejunojejunostomy. (From Wilder, J. R.: Atlas of general surgery, ed. 2, St. Louis, 1964, The C. V. Mosby Co.)

on the lower esophagus. It may be done at a level either above or below the diaphragm. This procedure should be supplemented by a gastric drainage procedure such as partial gastrectomy, pyloroplasty, or gastrojejunostomy.

**CONSIDERATIONS.** Normally, the action of the digestive chemical processes and the mucous coating dilutes and neutralizes the

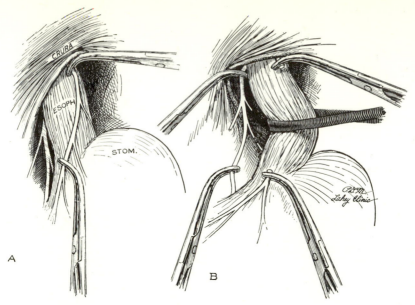

**Fig. 21-25.** Vagectomy. **A,** Lower segment of esophagus mobilized and left vagus nerve identified and clamped with right-angled ductal forceps. Small branches of nerve divided and segment of nerve between two clamps excised. Divided ends of nerve ligated. **B,** Esophagus retracted to left and ventrally by encircling Penrose drain. This maneuver stretches right vagus nerve and facilitates its identification. Segment of nerve between two clamps excised. (From Warren, K. W., and Braasch, J. W.: In Lahey Clinic: Surgical practice of the Clinic, Philadelphia, 1962, W. B. Saunders Co.)

gastric juices, thereby protecting the gastrointestinal tract from corrosive irritation. When excessive amounts of gastric secretions form in the empty stomach, ulcers may develop. This condition is influenced by the actions of the vagus nerves. When the fibers of the autonomic nervous system are overstimulated, the stomach contracts, the pyloric sphincter relaxes, and the amount of gastric secretions increases. Some patients who have had a vagectomy without a drainage procedure complain of a fullness of the stomach, which becomes atonic and empties poorly, so that food fermentation follows, accompanied by foul eructations.

**SETUP AND PREPARATION OF THE PATIENT.** As for gastrointestinal surgery, plus two 10-inch surgical hemostatic clip holders, one clip magazine, and two blunt nerve hooks.

**OPERATIVE PROCEDURE.** The peritoneal cavity is opened, and the wound edges are protected with towels and moist packs. The abdominal contents are walled off, the left lobe of the liver is retracted, and the peritoneal membrane to the esophagus is divided. The esophagus is mobilized and retracted, using Penrose tubing. The vagus nerves are clamped, resected, and ligated or clipped with the hemostatic clips (Fig. 21-25). The wound is closed without drainage and dressed.

## Procedures on the small intestine

*For ileostomy procedure,* see Chapter 22, since this operation is usually concerned with a pathological condition of the colon.

### Resection of small intestine

**DEFINITION.** Through an abdominal incision that is made over the suspected site of the lesion (generally in the right lower quadrant), the diseased intestine is excised, and a suitable anastomosis is completed.

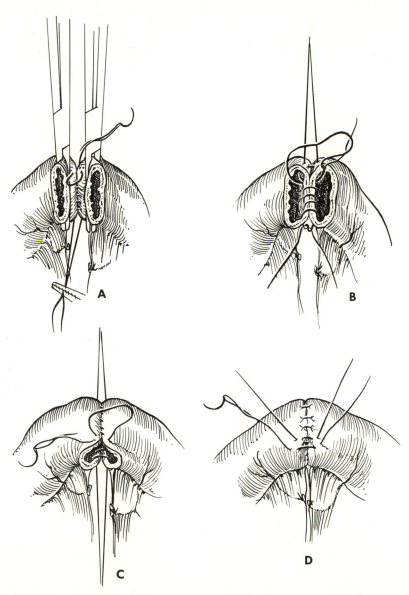

Fig. 21-26. Open anastomosis technique for gastrointestinal resection procedures. Two straight resection clamps left in place following excision of diseased portion of intestine. **A,** Posterior interrupted seromuscular sutures placed. **B,** Clamps removed and continuous chromic gut suture used to reinforce posterior layer. **C,** Gut suture may be continued anteriorly with mattress stitches, or anterior row may be completed with interrupted silk sutures. **D,** Anterior layer reinforced with silk sutures and mesentery closed. (Drawings by Shirley Baty, New York, N. Y.)

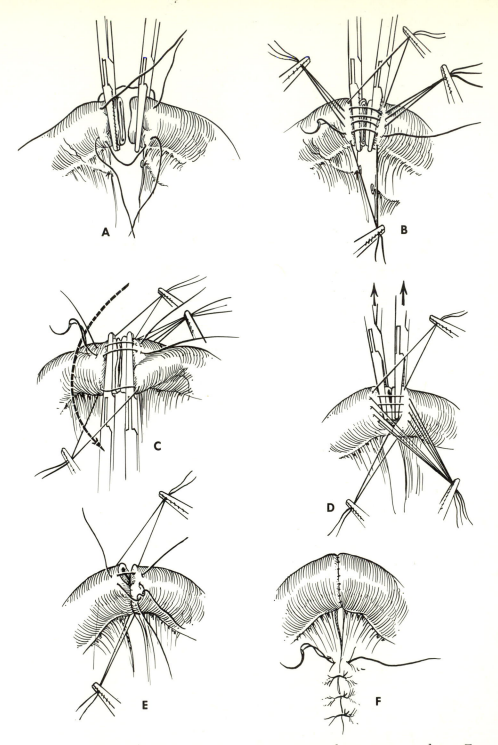

**Fig. 21-27.** Closed anastomosis technique for gastrointestinal resection procedures. Four straight resection (Allen) clamps applied following mobilization of small bowel to be resected, and diseased portion removed, leaving two clamps in place. **A,** Corner silk sutures placed. **B,** Interrupted seromuscular anterior silk sutures inserted. **C,** Clamps reversed to permit insertion of posterior sutures. **D,** Traction placed on suture ends to prevent spillage as clamps withdrawn. **E,** Sutures tied in place, and reinforcing sutures added as needed. **F,** Patency of lumen determined and mesentery closed. (Drawings by Shirley Baty, New York, N. Y.)

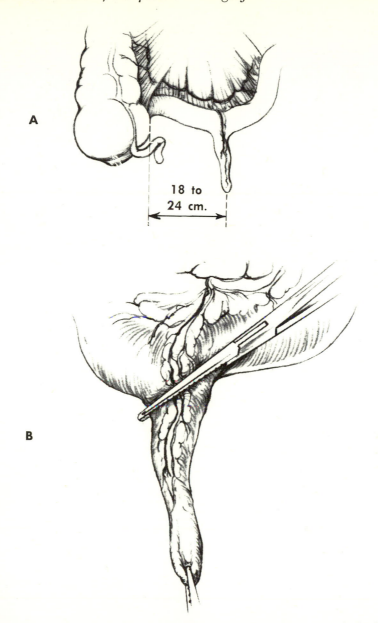

18 to
24 cm.

**Fig. 21-28. A,** Diagrammatic representation of usual location of Meckel's diverticulum. **B,** Ochsner clamp placed across base of diverticulum at its juncture with ileum. (From Wilder, J. R.: Atlas of general surgery, ed. 2, St. Louis, 1964, The C. V. Mosby Co.)

**CONSIDERATIONS.** This procedure is selected to remove certain tumors, a gangrenous portion of the intestine due to strangulation from bands of adhesions, a herniation of the intestine, or a volvulus.

**SETUP AND PREPARATION OF THE PATIENT.** As described for gastrointestinal surgery.

**OPERATIVE PROCEDURE**

1. The abdominal wall is incised and retracted; the peritoneal cavity is explored and protected with moist packs.

2. The clamps are placed above and below the diseased segment of the bowel and mesentery. The involved area is re-

moved with cautery or a scalpel (Fig. 21-26, *A*).

3. The continuity of the gastrointestinal tract is established by an end-to-end, an end-to-side, or a side-to-side anastomosis. The *open* and *closed* techniques of anastomosis are shown in Figs. 21-26 and 21-27.

4. The wound is closed and dressed.

### Operation for Meckel's diverticulum

**DEFINITION.** Removal of the diverticulum and establishment of bowel continuity.

**CONSIDERATIONS.** An unobliterated congenital duct may remain attached to the terminal ileum (Fig. 21-28, *A*). This embryonic yolk stalk may persist as an appendix-like structure arising from the lower ileum. The diverticulum may contain gastric mucosa, which may ulcerate, perforate, or bleed.

**SETUP AND PREPARATION OF THE PATIENT.** As described for gastrointestinal surgery, minus large resection clamps and twelve mosquito hemostats.

**OPERATIVE PROCEDURE.** The abdomen is opened and the peritoneal cavity explored. The procedure will depend on the size of the diverticulum. If it is long with a narrow base, the steps of the operation are similar to those for an appendectomy (Chapter 22).

When the neck of the diverticulum is broad, the loop of bowel containing the diverticulum is isolated from the mesentery, and the base of the diverticulum is doubly clamped and divided, using Allen or Ochsner clamps and a scalpel (Fig. 21-28, *B*). An anastomosis of the divided ends is completed, as described for posterojejunostomy. The wound is closed and dressed, as described for closure of laparotomy (Chapter 17).

### REFERENCES

1. Adams, H. D.: In Lahey Clinic: Surgical practice of the Clinic, Philadelphia, 1962, W. B. Saunders Co.
2. Anthony, C. P.: Textbook of anatomy and physiology, ed. 8, St. Louis, 1971, The C. V. Mosby Co.
3. Barnes, W. A.: Diaphragmatic hernia. In Glenn, F., Moore, S. W., and Beal, J. M., editors: Surgery in the aged, New York, 1960, Blakiston Division, McGraw-Hill Book Co.
4. Blades, B., editor: Surgical diseases of the chest, ed. 2, St. Louis, 1966, The C. V. Mosby Co.
5. Davis, L., editor: Christopher's textbook of surgery, ed. 7, Philadelphia, 1960, W. B. Saunders Co.
6. Dennison, W. M.: Surgery in infancy and childhood, Edinburgh, 1967, E. & S. Livingstone, Ltd.
7. Harkins, H., and Nylus, L., editor: Surgery of the stomach and duodenum, ed. 2, Boston, 1969, W. B. Saunders Co.
8. Johnson, J., and Kirby, C. K.: Surgery of the chest, ed. 3, Chicago, 1964, Year Book Medical Publishers, Inc.
9. King, B. G., and Showers, M. J.: Human anatomy and physiology, ed. 5, Philadelphia, 1963, W. B. Saunders Co.
10. Madden, J. L.: Atlas of technics in surgery, ed. 2, vol. 1, New York, 1964, Appleton-Century-Crofts.
11. Maingot, R.: Abdominal operations, ed. 5, New York, 1969, Appleton-Century-Crofts.
12. Marshall, S. F., and Adams, H. D.: Surgery of the stomach. In Allen, A. W., and Barrow, D. W., editors: Abdominal surgery, New York, 1961, Harper & Row, Publishers.
13. Mayo, C. W.: Surgery of the small and large intestine, Chicago, 1955, Year Book Medical Publishers, Inc.
14. Moyer, C. A., Rhoads, J. E., Allen, J. G., and Harkins, H. N., editors: Surgery: principles and practices, ed. 3, Philadelphia, 1965, J. B. Lippincott Co.
15. Nealon, T. F., Jr.: Management of the patient with cancer, Philadelphia, 1965, W. B. Saunders Co.
16. Thorek, P.: Anatomy in surgery, ed. 2, Philadelphia, 1962, J. B. Lippincott Co.
17. Tuttle, W. W., and Schottelius, B. A.: Textbook of physiology, ed. 16, St. Louis, 1969, The C. V. Mosby Co.
18. Warren, R., editor: Surgery, Philadelphia, 1963, W. B. Saunders Co.
19. Welch, C. E.: Surgery of the stomach and duodenum, ed. 3, Chicago, 1959, Year Book Medical Publishers, Inc.

# CHAPTER 22

# Lower gastrointestinal surgery

BARBARA ROSENBERG GRANA

## SURGICAL ANATOMICAL CONSIDERATIONS

The *cecum* is attached to the ileum and extends about 2½ inches below it (Fig. 22-1). The adult cecum is usually adherent to the posterior wall of the peritoneal cavity and has a serosal covering on its anterior wall only. The cecum forms a blind pouch from which projects the appendix. The teniae coli are concentrations of the outer longitudinal muscle coat of the cecum and colon into three narrow bands, or teniae. These are relatively shorter than the bowel itself so that the latter is puckered with typical haustrations. The teniae terminate at the appendix.

The *colon,* which within the rectum comprises the remaining portion of the large intestine, is divided into four parts: ascending, transverse, descending, and sigmoid. These portions form an inverted ∪ within the abdominal cavity (Fig. 22-2). Although the mesocolon provides some stability for the colon, its mobility varies greatly. The ascending portion of the colon, which is about 6 inches long, extends from the level of the ileocecal valve upward to the hepatic flexure. Since it is not entirely covered by peritoneum, it is rather fixed. The upper portion of the ascending colon lies behind the right lobe of the liver and in front of the anterior surface of the right kidney.

The transverse colon, about 20 inches long, begins at the hepatic flexure, lies transversely across the abdominal cavity, and ends at the splenic flexure near the spleen. It lies below the stomach and is attached to the transverse mesocolon.

The descending colon, which is about 7 inches long, extends from the left colic flexure to the region below the iliac crest. It is firmly attached to the posterior abdominal wall. The iliac portion of the sigmoid colon, which is about 6 inches long, lies on the inner surface of the left iliac muscle. The remaining portion of the colon passes over the pelvic brim into the pelvic cavity, lying partly in the abdomen and the pelvis. It forms an S curve in the pelvis, terminating in the rectum at a level with the third segment of the sacral vertebrae.

The structural wall of the colon is similar to that of the small intestine, except for the presence of teniae coli, epiploic, appendices, and haustra.

The superior mesenteric artery supplies the appendix, the cecum, and the proximal portion of the colon; the inferior mesenteric artery supplies the remainder of the colon (Fig. 22-3).

The *rectum,* which is a continuation of the sigmoid colon, terminates in the anus. The rectum, a slightly curved passage about 6 inches long, is surrounded by pelvic fascia as it lies on the anterior surface of the sacrum and coccyx (Fig. 22-4). In the male, the rectum lies behind the prostate gland and the bladder. In the female, the rectum lies behind the uterus and the vagina. The rectum dilates just before it becomes the anal canal, and this dilatation

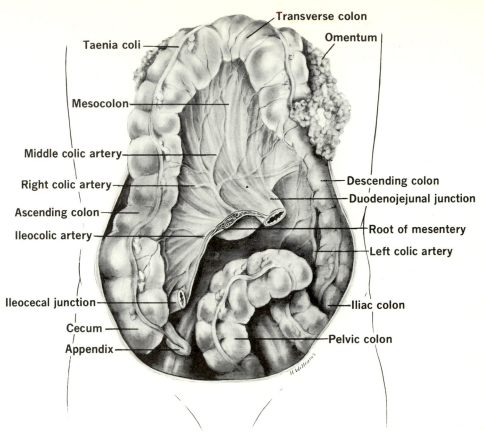

Fig. 22-1. Colon and root of mesentery. Transverse colon turned upward to show duodeno-jejunal junction. (From Francis, C. C: Introduction to human anatomy, ed. 5, St. Louis, 1968, The C. V. Mosby Co.)

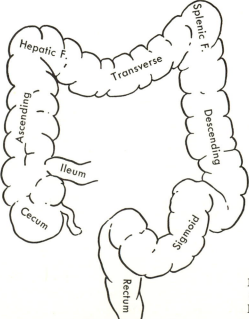

Fig. 22-2. Anatomical divisions of large intestine (colon), showing placement of ileocecal valve, hepatic flexure, and splenic flexure.

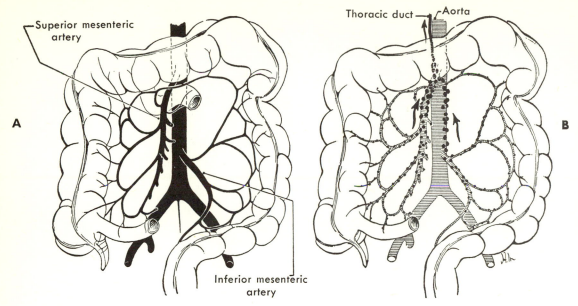

Fig. 22-3. **A,** Normal arterial supply of colon. **B,** Lymphatic drainage of colon. (From Moseley, H. F., editor: Textbook of surgery, ed 3, St. Louis, 1959, The C. V. Mosby Co.)

or ampulla, presents folds called *Houston's valves.* The wall of the rectum consists of four layers, similar to those of the small intestine.

The *anal canal* is a narrow passage about 1 inch long, which passes downward and backward. It is surrounded and controlled by two circular bands, which form the external and internal anal sphincters (Fig. 22-5). The act of defecation is accomplished by contraction of the rectal and abdominal muscles, the descent of the diaphragm, and the relaxation of the sphincter muscles.

## SPECIFIC NURSING CONSIDERATIONS

General nursing standards relating to medical and surgical asepsis (Chapters 3 to 7) and other special considerations have been discussed in Chapters 17 and 21.

The preoperative preparation is directed toward producing as complete intestinal asepsis as possible. Mechanical cleansing of the large bowel through restricted diet and soapsuds solution irriga-

tions is utilized for all elective operations. Bacteriostatic and bactericidal agents may be administered to reduce or attempt to completely eliminate the number of pathogenic organisms in the lower tract.

In some cases an indwelling urethral catheter (Foley type: female, no. 16, or male, no. 18, with a 5 ml. bag) is retained in place throughout the operative procedure. An empty bladder is necessary to allow more space for the surgeon to work in, as well as to prevent cutting of the bladder due to its large size when full.

### Preventive measures

When the team shifts a patient from a Trendelenburg or lithotomy position to a complete horizontal position, it must be done slowly. Legs must be lowered together. Slow, cautious movements prevent large shifts in blood volume away from vital organs (Chapter 7).

The skin preparation includes shaving the skin, which should be completed before the patient is brought to the operating room, and wiping the operative site with

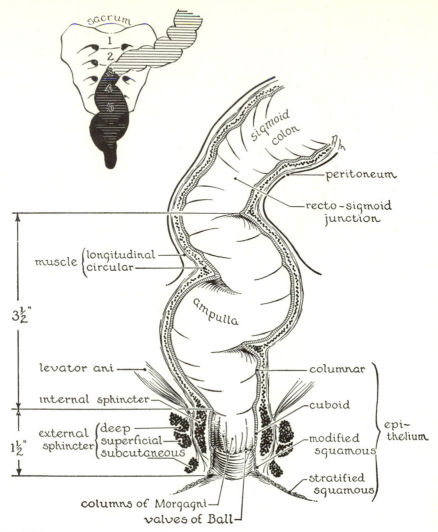

**Fig. 22-4.** Diagrammatic anatomy of rectum. (From Moseley, H. F., editor: Textbook of surgery, ed. 3, St. Louis, 1959, The C. V. Mosby Co.)

alcohol, followed by an application of povidone-iodine complex (Betadine).

## BASIC INSTRUMENT SETUPS
### Colon operations

Bowel contaminants may be effectively isolated by use of the separate anastomosis instruments. (See Chapter 21 for the basic gastrointestinal set.)

### Rectal operations

The instrument setup for major rectal procedures should include the following (Fig. 22-6):

**Cutting instruments**

  1 Knife handle no. 4 with blade no. 20
  1 Mayo scissors, 6¼ in.
  1 Suture scissors, 5½ in.

**Holding instruments**

  2 Tissue forceps, 5½ in., 1 with teeth, 1 without teeth
  6 Allis forceps, 6 in.
  6 Pratt T forceps

**Clamping instruments**

10 Crile hemostatic forceps
  3 Rochester-Pean forceps, 6¼ in., curved
    Rochester-Pean forceps, 10 in., curved
12 Ochsner forceps, 6¼ in., straight

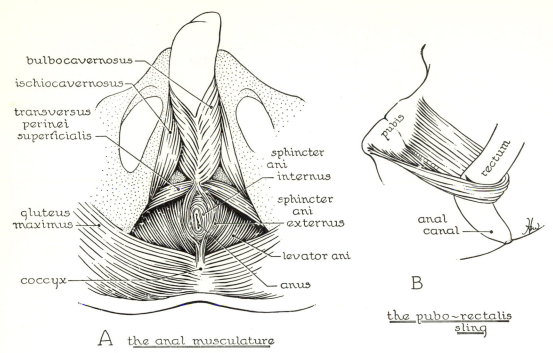

bulbocavernosus

ischiocavernosus

transversus
perinei
superficialis

sphincter
ani
internus

sphincter
ani
externus

gluteus
maximus

levator ani

coccyx

anus

A   the anal musculature

pubis

rectum

anal
canal

B

the pubo-rectalis
sling

**Fig. 22-5.** Anal musculature. (From Moseley, H. F., editor: Textbook of surgery, ed. 3, St. Louis, 1959, The C. V. Mosby Co.)

**Exposing instruments**

  2 Rectal speculums, bivalve
  2 Rake retractors
  2 Richardson retractors, small
  2 U.S. Army retractors (optional)
  1 Sponge holder, 10 in.

**Suturing items**

  2 Mayo-Hegar needle holders, 6¼ in.
  2 Large regular surgeon's ½-circle, cutting edge needles with silk sutures no. 2-0
    Chromic gut sutures No. 2-0 swaged on general closure needle

**Accessory items**

  2 Probes, silver
  1 Grooved director
  1 Suction tube and tubing, if indicated
    Packing, as indicated
    Lubricant

**Optional items**

  1 Sigmoidoscopy set
  1 Rectal biopsy forceps (Fig. 22-7)
  1 Rectal snare and coagulation unit (Fig. 22-7)

## OPERATIONS
### Appendectomy

**DEFINITION.** Through a right lower quadrant muscle-splitting incision (McBurney),

the appendix is severed from its attachment to the cecum and removed (Fig. 22-1).

**CONSIDERATIONS.** This operation is performed to remove a chronic or inflamed appendix, thereby controlling the spread of infection and reducing the danger of peritonitis. If a more extensive pathological area is suspected, the surgeon may select a right paramedian incision (Chapter 17).

**SETUP AND PREPARATION OF THE PATIENT.** A general laparotomy setup, plus a culture tube and a basin for bowel-contaminated instruments, is all that is required. Some surgeons still prefer to use 95% phenol, 70% alcohol, and cotton-tipped applicators for the stump of the appendix (Chapter 21).

**OPERATIVE PROCEDURE** (Fig. 22-8)

1. A right McBurney incision is made, utilizing items as previously described in Chapter 17.

2. Muscles are retracted with Richardson or Roux retractors to expose the peritoneum.

3. The peritoneum is grasped with tis-

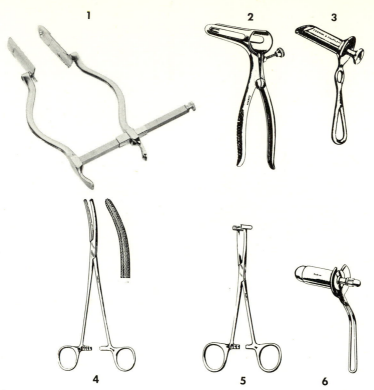

**Fig. 22-6.** Instruments for rectal and anal surgery. **1,** Smith anal retractor; **2,** Sims rectal speculum; **3,** Hirschmann anoscope; **4,** Buie pile clamp; **5,** Pratt ⊤ forceps; **6,** Fansler anal speculum. (Courtesy Codman & Shurtleff, Inc., Randolph, Mass.)

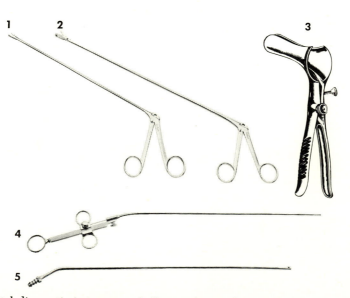

**Fig. 22-7.** Rectal diagnostic instruments. **1,** Yeoman biopsy forceps; **2,** Yeoman rotating biopsy forceps; **3,** Pratt rectal speculum; **4,** Weston rectal snare; **5,** Buie suction tube. (Courtesy Codman & Shurtleff, Inc., Randolph, Mass.)

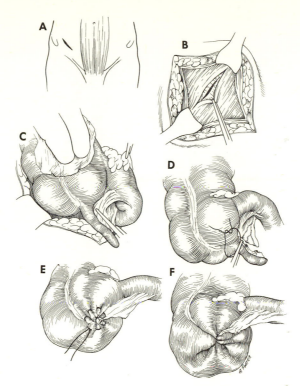

Fig. 22-8. Stages of appendectomy. **A,** McBurney incision. **B,** Approach to peritoneum. **C,** Clamp on mesoappendix. **D,** Clamp on base of appendix with suture around its base. **E,** Inversion of appendiceal stump with purse-string suture. **F,** Operation completed. (From Moseley, H. F., editor: Textbook of surgery, ed. 3, St. Louis, 1959, The C. V. Mosby Co.)

sue forceps or Allis forceps, and a small incision is made, using a scalpel with a no. 15 blade. A culture may be taken at this time with a cotton applicator. The suction set is connected. The incision is completed with Metzenbaum scissors.

4. The mesoappendix is grasped near the tip with a Babcock clamp or a hemostat for gentle traction. The mesoappendix is dissected from the appendiceal wall, using hemostats and silk ligatures no. 3-0. If a suture ligature is required, catgut suture no. 2-0 on a gastrointestinal needle is preferred.

5A. The appendix is elevated as a purse-string suture of chromic gut no. 2-0 is placed in the cecal wall at its base. (a) The appendix base is crushed with a straight hemostat, a silk no. 3-0 tie is placed over the crushed area, and a hemostat is placed above the ligature. (b) A basin for specimen

and discarded instruments is prepared. (c) Protective gauze sponges are placed over the cecum around the base of the appendix. The appendix is amputated between the clamp and catgut suture with a scalpel. (d) The appendiceal stump is inverted into the lumen of the cecum as the purse-string suture is tightened and tied by means of a fine straight hemostat and a small sponge on a holder. Soiled instruments are discarded in the basin.

5B. When the appendix has ruptured, the peritoneum is drained. A drain (Penrose) may be inserted down to the appendix bed to allow for continuous drainage. The wound may then be packed open with wet fine-mesh gauze, and healing by secondary intent is permitted. This packing method may be used in any case in which bowel contamination or an abscess

formation is present. It allows for clean healing and prevents pocketing of pus.

6. In cases in which there is no rupture, the abdomen is closed in the usual manner.

## Ileostomy

**DEFINITION.** Formation of a temporary or permanent opening into the ileum.

**CONSIDERATIONS.** An ileostomy is generally done when an extensive lesion is present to provide complete rest of the colon by means of diversion or when all of the large bowel is resected.

**SETUP AND PREPARATION OF THE PATIENT.** As described for gastrointestinal operations (Chapter 21), plus a disposable coloplast bag to place around the stoma.

**OPERATIVE PROCEDURE**

1. Through a left rectus incision the peritoneal cavity is explored and the pathological condition determined (Chapter 17).

2. The ileum is mobilized, using Metzenbaum scissors and hemostatic clamps; the mesentery is clamped, divided, and ligated with silk sutures no. 3-0 at the proposed site, usually about 15 cm. from the ileocecal junction.

3. The operative field is prepared for transection as described under gastrointestinal techniques in Chapter 21.

Two Payr intestinal clamps are then placed on the bowel, and the ileum is divided with a scalpel between the two clamps.

4. The distal end of the ileum is closed with chromic gut suture no. 2-0 on a general closure needle.

5. The proximal end is then brought out to the skin through an opening on the right side (held in place by clamps), making sure that the ileum is not overstretched or its blood supply compromised. The abdomen is then closed; wire figure-of-eight sutures may be placed through the peritoneum and fascia. The skin is closed.

6. The stoma is then sutured to the skin with chromic gut suture no. 3-0 swagged to an Atraumatic needle.

7. A disposable coloplast bag is then applied over the stroma to collect fecal material.

## Colostomy

**DEFINITION.** Through a right rectus incision to expose the transverse colon or through a left rectus incision to expose the descending sigmoid, a loop of colon is mobilized, and the layers of the wound are closed beneath or around it.

**CONSIDERATIONS.** Colostomy is done to treat an obstruction in the sigmoid colon due to a malignant lesion or an advanced inflammation or trauma that has caused a distention of the proximal portion of the colon. To decompress the bowel and give rest to the colon, a temporary colostomy (loop or double-barreled) may be performed prior to a resection of the colon (Fig. 22-9).

**SETUP AND PREPARATION OF THE PATIENT.** As described for laparotomy (Chapter 17), plus the following:

2 Babcock forceps
1 Glass or plastic rod, 6 in.
1 Length of tubing, 12 in., to fit rod
1 Penrose drain, 12 in., for traction
    Petrolatum gauze, for dressing

**OPERATIVE PROCEDURE**

**FOR FIRST-STAGE COLOSTOMY**

1. The abdomen is opened, and the wound edges are protected and retracted. The peritoneal cavity is opened and walled off with dry laparotomy packs, and appropriate retractors are inserted.

2. A small opening is made in the mesentery near the bowel, using Crile or Pean curved hemostats and Metzenbaum scissors. A piece of Penrose tubing is passed about the colon and the two ends held with a Pean hemostat to maintain gentle traction.

3. The loop of colon is brought out through an incision made on the left side of the midline.

4. The abdomen is then closed as described in Chapter 17.

5. The Penrose tubing is removed after the glass rod is in place; the length of rubber tubing is then placed over the

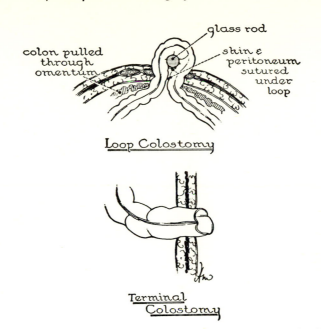

Loop Colostomy

Terminal Colostomy

**Fig. 22-9.** Types of colostomy. (From Moseley, H. F., editor: Textbook of surgery, ed. 3, St. Louis, 1959, The C. V. Mosby Co.)

loop and securely attached to either end of the rod.

6. The loop of intestine is dressed with petrolatum and 4- × 4-inch strips of gauze.

FOR SECOND-STAGE LOOP COLOSTOMY. After 48 hours, the loop of colon is completely severed with a cautery. By this time, if there is no tension, healing has advanced sufficiently to make it safe to allow feces onto the wound. This procedure is very simple and is usually performed in the patient's own room or treatment room.

FOR TRANSVERSE COLOSTOMY

1. A short incision, vertical or preferably transverse, is made to reach the transverse colon (Fig. 22-10, A).

2. A loop of transverse colon, freed of omentum, is withdrawn. A glass rod has been passed through an avascular area of the mesocolon, and this prevents the loop from returning to the peritoneal cavity (Fig. 22-10, B). A mushroom catheter, held in place with a purse-string suture, effects immediate decompression.

3. The bowel is opened 24 to 36 hours later (Fig. 22-10, C).

4. The glass rod may be removed in about 10 days (Fig. 22-10, D).

### Closure of colostomy

DEFINITION. Closure of the walls of the colon and repair of the abdominal wall to reestablish intestinal continuity.

CONSIDERATIONS. When the loop has been completely divided, a closed or open anastomosis may be performed. Preventive measures are carried out.

SETUP AND PREPARATION OF THE PATIENT. As described for colostomy operations.

OPERATIVE PROCEDURE

1. A circumferential incision is made about the colostomy to free the skin margin. Dry packs, a scalpel with a no. 20 blade, Metzenbaum scissors, and Crile hemostats are used, as the layers of the abdominal wall are identified and dissected free (Fig. 22-11, A and B).

2. An end-to-end anastomosis is completed, using silk suture no. 3-0 on an intestinal needle (Fig. 22-11, C).

3. The abdominal wound is closed in layers (Fig. 22-11, D). Soft tissue Penrose

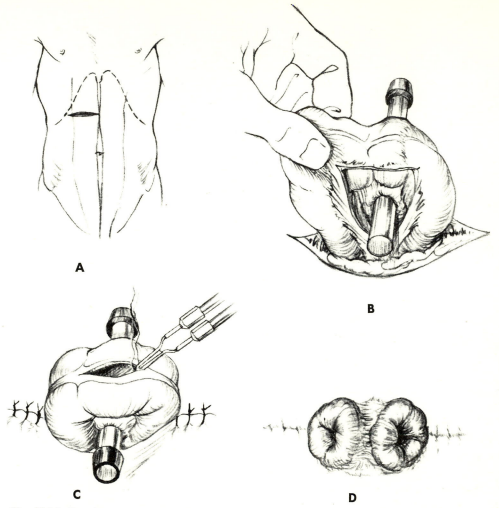

**Fig. 22-10.** Step-by-step procedure for transverse colostomy. **A,** Short incision, vertical or preferably transverse, made to reach transverse colon. **B,** Loop of transverse colon, freed of omentum, withdrawn. Glass rod passed through avascular area of mesocolon and loop prevented from returning to peritoneal cavity. **C,** Bowel opened by cautery 24 to 36 hours later. **D,** Appearance of colostomy several weeks after surgery. Glass rod usually removed in about 10 days. (From Wilder, J. R.: Atlas of general surgery, ed. 2, St. Louis, 1964, The C. V. Mosby Co.)

drain may be inserted, if indicated. A dressing is applied.

## Right hemicolectomy and ileocolostomy

**DEFINITION.** Through a right rectus abdominal incision, the right half of the colon—including a portion of the transverse colon, the ascending colon, and the cecum—and a segment of the terminal ileum and mesentery are resected, and an anastomosis between the transverse colon and the ileum is accomplished, preferably end-to-end or side-to-side or end-to-side occasionally.

**CONSIDERATIONS.** This operation is performed to remove a malignant lesion of the right colon and, in some cases, to remove an inflammatory lesion involving the ileum, cecum, or ascending colon.

When a side-to-side anastomosis is car-

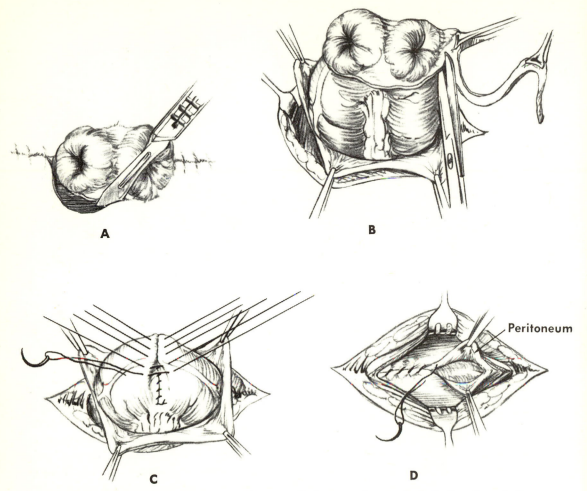

**A**    **B**

**C**    **D**

Peritoneum

Fig. 22-11. Closure of colostomy. **A,** Skin incised close to colostomy bud. **B,** Scar tissue being excised. **C,** Bowel closed transversely with interrupted Lambert sutures of fine silk and replaced in abdomen. **D,** Wound closure completed with gut or wire sutures. (From Wilder, J. R.: Atlas of general surgery, ed. 2, St. Louis, 1964, The C. V. Mosby Co.)

ried out, the severed stumps of the ileum and the transverse colon are closed before the anastomosis is done. It is completed between the side portions of the ileum and transverse colon. When an end-to-end anastomosis is performed, the layers of the severed stumps of the ileum and the transverse colon are sutured together.

SETUP AND PREPARATION OF THE PATIENT. As described for gastrointestinal operations (Chapter 21).

OPERATIVE PROCEDURE

1. The abdomen is opened and the peritoneal cavity walled off, as described for laparotomy.

2. The mesentery of the transverse colon and the terminal ileum are incised at the points where the resection is to be done. Dry packs, Metzenbaum scissors, Rochester-Pean hemostats, and silk no. 3-0 ligatures are used (Fig. 22-12).

3. The lateral peritoneal fold along the lateral side of the right colon is incised and the right colon mobilized medially. Metzenbaum scissors, Pean hemostats, and sponges on holders are used. The ureter and duodenum are carefully identified.

4. The same procedure is done concerning the terminal ileum.

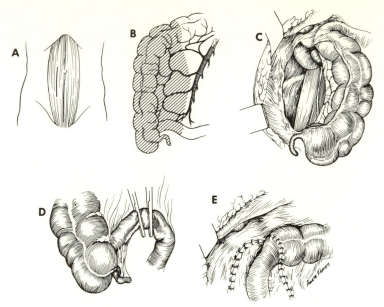

**Fig. 22-12.** Right hemicolectomy and ileocolostomy. **A,** Right paramedian incision. **B,** Specimen to be resected. **C,** Mobilization of right colon medially. **D,** Clamps on distal portion of ileum. **E,** End-to-end anastomosis of ileum and transverse colon. (Redrawn from Manual of operative procedure, Somerville, N. J., Ethicon, Inc.)

5. The mesenteric vessels are clamped and ligated with silk ligatures no. 2-0.

6. The operative field is prepared for anastomosis. Resection clamps are placed on the transverse colon and ileum (Fig. 22-12). Division is completed with a scalpel, and the specimen is removed.

7. An end-to-end anastomosis is completed between the severed ends of the terminal ileum and the transverse colon.

8. Contaminated instruments and supplies are discarded.

9. The mesentery and posterior peritoneum are closed with interrupted sutures of silk no. 3-0.

10. A separate closure set is used to complete abdominal wound closure. Retention sutures and a drain may be used. A dressing is applied.

## Transverse colectomy

**DEFINITION.** Through an upper midline or transverse incision, the transverse colon is excised and continuity reestablished by an end-to-end anastomosis.

**CONSIDERATIONS.** This operation is performed for malignant lesions of the transverse colon. A more radical procedure may be required when the lesion has perforated into the greater curvature of the stomach. If the entire lesion is resectable, a partial gastrectomy may also have to be performed.

**SETUP AND PREPARATION OF THE PATIENT.** As described for gastrointestinal operations (Chapter 21).

**OPERATIVE PROCEDURE**

1. The abdomen is opened, and the peritoneal cavity is explored to determine the extent of the pathological area, using items as described for laparotomy (Chapter 17).

2. Dry packs are used to wall off surrounding structures to expose the hepatic and splenic flexures. A Balfour retractor is inserted (this is optional).

3. The colon is mobilized by incising the lateral peritoneum on either side and transecting the transverse mesocolon. Pean

hemostats, Metzenbaum scissors, and silk no. 3-0 ligatures are used.

4. The operative field is prepared for resection. Four Allen or Payr intestinal resection clamps are applied. Transection is completed with a scalpel, and end-to-end anastomosis is completed, as previously described and illustrated (Chapter 21 and Figs. 21-26 and 21-27).

5. Contaminated articles are discarded. Approximation of mesentery and lateral peritoneum is completed with silk no. 3-0 sutures.

6. A separate closure set is used to complete the abdominal wound closure. Retention sutures may be used. The wound is dressed.

### Anterior resection and rectosigmoidostomy

**DEFINITION.** Removal of the lower sigmoid and rectosigmoid portion of the rectum, usually through a low left paramedian incision, followed by an end-to-end anastomosis.

**CONSIDERATIONS.** This operation is selected to treat lesions in the lower portion of the sigmoid and rectum that permit excision with a wide margin of safety and still retain sufficient tissues with adequate blood supply for an accurate rectosigmoid end-to-end anastomosis.

**SETUP AND PREPARATION OF THE PATIENT.** As described for gastrointestinal surgery (Chapter 21), plus the following instruments:

2 Richardson retractors, extra large
1 Harrington or Ford retractor
1 Indwelling catheter set
2 Pieces of umbilical tape, 18 in.

**OPERATIVE PROCEDURE**

1. The abdomen is entered through a left paramedian incision. The peritoneal cavity is explored for metastasis and resectability of the lesion.

2. Prior to mobilizing the colon, the tumor-bearing segment is isolated by ligatures to the lymphovenous drainage (provided these structures are accessible).

3. A loop of sigmoid is elevated as the small intestines are walled off with moist packs; retractors are placed.

4. The peritoneum on the left side of the colon is incised with a long scalpel, scissors, Pean hemostats, and sponge forceps. Traction sutures of silk no. 2-0 may be used as the peritoneum is reflected. Bleeding vessels are ligated with silk ligatures no. 2-0 or 3-0.

5. The pelvic peritoneum is exposed and dissected free to form the left side of the reconstructed pelvic floor. Long dissecting instruments are used. Vessels are ligated with 28-inch silk ligatures no. 2-0 inserted in the tip of a long Pean forceps to facilitate placement.

6. The sigmoid is turned toward the left, and the same procedure as in step 4 is carried out on the right side of the pelvis. The two incisions are then curved and joined in front of the rectum.

7. The rectum is freed anteriorly and posteriorly from the adjacent structures.

8. The sigmoid is clamped with Payr or similar resection clamps after mobilization of the proximal portion. As the sigmoid is divided distal to the clamp, the severed rectal edges are grasped with Allis or Ochsner forceps and the rectal opening exposed. The diseased portion is removed and the soiled instruments discarded.

9. Continuity is established by an end-to-end anastomosis (Fig. 21-26) of the proximal colon and the rectum.

10. The pelvic floor is reperitonealized, and drains may be placed.

11. The abdominal wound is closed in the routine manner, and a dressing is applied.

### Total colectomy

**DEFINITION.** Usually through a lower left rectus incision, the whole colon is removed, and a permanent ileostomy is made through a stab wound in the right lower quadrant.

**CONSIDERATIONS.** This operation may be selected to treat an extensive inflammatory

disease or multiple polyposis. Generally an ileostomy is performed. In some cases, continuity is reestablished by performing an ileosigmoidostomy. The retained portion of the sigmoid may be closed and left in the peritoneal cavity, or it may be exteriorized in the lower left quadrant, as described for sigmoidostomy.

**SETUP AND PREPARATION OF THE PATIENT.** As described for anterior resection and rectosigmoidostomy.

**OPERATIVE PROCEDURE.** The major steps are similar to those previously described for anterior resection and ileostomy.

## Polypectomy of the colon

**DEFINITION.** Through a low rectus incision, the involved colon, including the polyp, is resected, or the polyp is excised.

**CONSIDERATIONS.** Polyps that occur in the colon are true tumors that grow from the mucous membrane. They may be flat or pedunculated. They are usually benign, but are removed because of their tendency to become malignant.

**SETUP AND PREPARATION OF THE PATIENT.** As described for gastrointestinal surgery (Chapter 21), plus a proctoscopy set.

**OPERATIVE PROCEDURE.** The abdominal

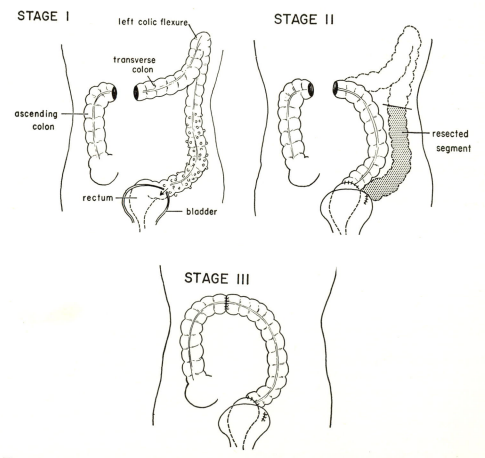

**Fig. 22-13.** Management of diverticulitis of colon. Stage I: Preliminary colostomy to put left colon at rest. Stage II: Adequate mobilization of splenic flexure, resection of diseased segment of sigmoid with anastomosis, and repair of bladder at site of fistula. Stage III: Closure of colostomy. (From Patterson, H. A.: Surg. Clin. North Am. 4:451, 1955.)

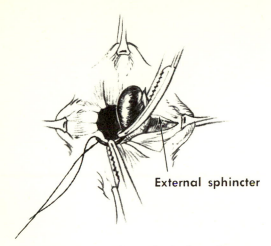

External sphincter

**Fig. 22-14.** Excising hemorrhoid above hemostat. (From Wilder, J. R.: Atlas of general surgery, ed. 2, St. Louis, 1964, The C. V. Mosby Co.)

cavity is opened, the polyp is located, and rubber-shod intestinal clamps are applied to the involved colon, which is opened. The polyp is grasped, ligated, and removed. The layers of both the colon and abdomen are closed separately.

### Diverticulitis of the colon

Diverticulitis of the colon may be treated as shown in Fig. 22-13, by the following staged operations: (1) colostomy, (2) resection of the sigmoid colon with anastomosis, and (3) closure of the colostomy.

### Hemorrhoidectomy

**DEFINITION.** Excision and ligation of dilated veins in the anal region to control bleeding and relieve discomfort (Fig. 22-14).

**CONSIDERATIONS.** Preoperative anal dilatation aids in exposing the vessels, as well as contributes to the patient's comfort in the immediate postoperative period. Many surgeons prefer to precede the operation with a sigmoidoscopy examination. Spinal anesthesia may be used.

**SETUP AND PREPARATION OF THE PATIENT.** A jackknife or lithotomy position is used (Chapter 7). The sigmoidoscopy setup is ready for immediate use. Setup is as described for rectal operations (Fig. 22-6),

with suitable drapes and operating table appliances, depending on the position selected.

**OPERATIVE PROCEDURE**

1. The anal canal is dilated and inspected through an anoscope.

2. Four Allis forceps are applied several centimeters from the anal margin for exposure.

3. The base of the hemorrhoid and tissue are grasped with Allis forceps and held.

4. An intestinal suture of chromic gut no. 2-0 is placed and tied at the proximal end of the hemorrhoid, and a Buie pile forceps is applied across the base and above the proposed incision line. Excision is completed with a scalpel (Fig. 22-14). Suturing is completed by loosely placed continuous stitches over the Buie forceps. The suture is tightened as the forceps is removed, and suture ends are tied.

5. Or traction is maintained as hemostatic forceps are applied, and dissection is completed in segmental fashion. Suture ligatures of chromic gut no. 2-0 are used as each hemostat is removed.

6. Remaining hemorrhoids are excised in a similar manner.

7. Petrolatum gauze packing is placed in the anal canal. A dressing and ⊤ binder are applied.

### Excision of anal fistulas

**DEFINITION.** Resection of the anal fistula (Fig. 22-15).

**CONSIDERATIONS.** This lesion usually originates in an anal crypt, and isolation is aided by injection of a dye solution or insertion of malleable silver probes.

**SETUP AND PREPARATION OF THE PATIENT.** As described for hemorrhoidectomy operation, plus a grooved director, a probe, a dye solution, and syringe and blunt needle.

**OPERATIVE PROCEDURE**

1. The sphincter muscle is dilated, a self-retaining retractor is inserted, and the fistulous opening is injected with dye or probed.

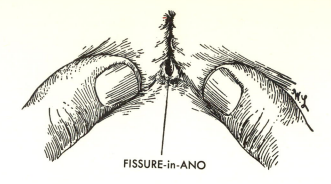

FISSURE-in-ANO

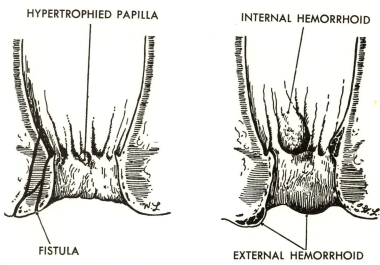

HYPERTROPHIED PAPILLA

INTERNAL HEMORRHOID

FISTULA

EXTERNAL HEMORRHOID

Fig. 22-15. Various types of anal lesions. (From Ferguson, L. K., and Sholtis, L. A., editors: Eliason's surgical nursing, ed. 11, Philadelphia, 1959, J. B. Lippincott Co.)

2. The tract is incised over a grooved director, using a scalpel with a no. 15 blade.

3. The fibrous wall of the sinus is dissected out. Allis forceps and Metzenbaum scissors are used. Bleeding points are ligated with fine gut sutures.

4. A petrolatum gauze dressing is applied.

### Excision of anal fissures

DEFINITION. Dilatation and excision of the lesion.

CONSIDERATIONS. These are benign lesions of the anal wall (Fig. 22-15).

SETUP AND PREPARATION OF THE PATIENT. As described for rectal operations.

OPERATIVE PROCEDURE

1. Dilatation of the sphincter is completed.

2. The fissure is resected. Bleeders are ligated or cauterized.

3. A drain or packing is inserted, and a dressing is applied.

### Excision of pilonidal cyst and sinus

DEFINITION. Excision of cyst with sinus tracts from the intergluteal fold on the posterior surface of the lower sacrum.

CONSIDERATIONS. This condition, which may have a congenital origin, rarely becomes symptomatic until the individual reaches adult life. Inflammatory reaction varies from a mild, irritating, draining sinus

tract to an acute abscess with secondary recurrences. Treatment consists of drainage in the acute stage and total surgical excision during remission.

The excision of a cyst, which usually contains hair, and the sinus tracts must be complete to prevent recurrence. The defect resulting from recurrences may become too large for primary closure. In such cases, the wound is left open to heal by granulation.

SETUP AND PREPARATION OF THE PATIENT. As described for rectal surgery, plus the following:

Rubber tissue drain or packing material, as indicated
Methylene blue dye with syringe and needle for injection
Table accessories for jackknife position

The patient is placed on the operating table in a jackknife position. Adhesive strapping on either side of the buttocks facilitates exposure (Chapter 7). Skin preparation and draping are completed.

OPERATIVE PROCEDURE

1. The sinus tracts are identified by insertion of silver probes.

2. An elliptical incision is made with a scalpel as digital pressure is exerted laterally for hemostasis. The incision is carried down to the fascia, and Pean hemostats are applied to bleeding points. A tissue curette may be utilized to remove gelatinous tissue. Excision is completed, and the specimen is removed.

3. Bleeding is controlled with suture ligatures of plain or chromic gut no. 2-0 or 3-0. Adhesive strappings are released to let the wound edges approximate.

4. Closing sutures will depend on the size of the defect and the surgeon's preference. Steel wire, 28-gauge, or silk no. 2-0 through-and-through stay sutures may approximate the deeper tissues; fine silk sutures are used on the skin (dead space is obliterated).

5. Packing may be indicated if complete closure is not feasible. A pressure dressing is applied.

REFERENCES

1. Amshel, A. L.: Hemorrhoidal problems, Am. J. Nurs. 63:87, Dec., 1963.
2. Brunner, L. S., Emerson, C. P., Jr., Ferguson, L. K., and Suddarth, D. S.: Textbook of medical-surgical nursing, ed. 2, New York, 1970, J. B. Lippincott Co.
3. Colcock, B. P.: Carcinoma of the colon, Surg. Clin. North Am. 47:647, 1967.
4. Culp, C.: Pilonidal disease and its treatment, Surg. Clin. North Am. 47:1007, 1967.
5. Goligher, J. C.: Surgery of the anus, rectum and colon, ed. 2, London, 1967, Bailliere, Tindall & Cassell, Ltd.
6. Lyons, A. S.: Technique of ileostomy, Surg. Clin. North Am. 45:1211, 1965.
7. Madden, J. L.: Atlas of technics of surgery, ed. 2, New York, 1964, Appleton-Century-Crofts.
8. Mayo, C. W.: Surgery of the small and large intestine, Chicago, 1962, Year Book Medical Publishers, Inc.
9. Moyer, C. A., Rhoads, J. E., Allen, J. G., and Harkins, H. N.: Surgery: principles and practice, ed. 3, Philadelphia, 1965, J. B. Lippincott Co.
10. Sheridan, B. A.: After hemorrhoidectomy, Am. J. Nurs. 63:90, Dec., 1963.
11. Swinton, N. W., and Schatman, B. H.: Colostomy, Surg. Clin. North Am. 44:821, 1964.
12. Thorek, P.: Anatomy in surgery, ed. 2, Philadelphia, 1962, J. B. Lippincott Co.
13. Turell, R., editor: Diseases of the colon and anorectum, vols. I and II, Philadelphia, 1969, W. B. Saunders Co.

# CHAPTER 23

# Deep pelvic surgery

JUDITH YVONNE JACOBS

The success of modern deep pelvic surgery for malignant abdominoperineal lesions is attributable to increased knowledge regarding aseptic technique, anesthesia, transfusions, and the pathophysiology of involved organs. Current therapeutic techniques evolved after determination of the modes of metastasis, resective possibilities, and means of reestablishing modified physiological function.

## ABDOMINOPERINEAL RESECTION

During the nineteenth century, surgeons removed rectoanal carcinomas via perineal excision. In the early twentieth century, the first abdominoperineal resections were performed. Today's surgical approach is an extension of the Miles technique to include lymphatic and areolar tissue of the pelvis and abdomen.

DEFINITION. Through a left rectus incision, extending from the pubis to several centimeters above the umbilicus, the diseased segment of the lower bowel is mobilized and divided. The proximal end is exteriorized through a separate stab wound as a single-barreled colostomy. The distal end is pushed into the hollow of the sacrum and removed through the perineal route.

CONSIDERATIONS. This operation is performed for malignant lesions of the lower sigmoid colon, rectum, and anus (Fig. 23-1). The choice of patient position depends on the surgeon. Some may prefer to start with the patient in the supine position and move him to the lithotomy or Sims position for the perineal portion of the operation. Others may originally place the patient in a modified lithotomy or "ski" position. Trendelenburg placement of the table is used in both cases. When the operation is performed by two teams, the immediate lithotomy position is necessary to provide simultaneous exposure of the abdominal and perineal wounds.

SETUP AND PREPARATION OF THE PATIENT. As described for gastrointestinal surgery (Chapter 21). The setup includes the following:

FOR THE ABDOMINAL PROCEDURE

**Cutting instruments**

   2 Knife handles no. 4L with blade no. 20
   1 Metzenbaum scissors, curved, 10 in.

**Holding instruments**

   2 Right-angled colon clamps
  12 Crile hemostats
  12 Schmidt tonsil hemostats
   8 Rochester-Pean forceps, 10 in.
   2 Tissue forceps without teeth, 10 in.

**Exposing instruments**

   1 Deep blade for self-retaining retractor
   2 Deaver retractors, large
   2 Richardson retractors, extra-large
   1 Harrington or Ford retractor

**Suturing items**

   2 Mayo-Hegar needle holders, 10 in. (all chromic sutures have Atraumatic needles; silk sutures are applied to either regular or spring-eye intestinal needles)

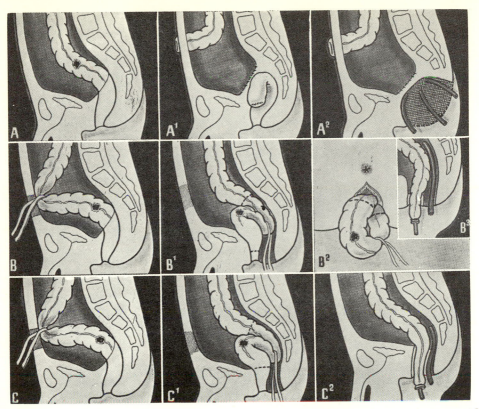

**Fig. 23-1.** Combined abdominoperineal operations for carcinoma of rectum or rectosigmoid. **A,** Miles operation. **A¹,** Abdominal portion of operation completed. Divided sigmoid placed beneath reconstructed pelvic floor and colostomy formed. **A²,** Perineal part of operation. Sigmoid, rectum, and anus removed and drains placed in perineal cavity. Operation may be performed in one or two stages. **B,** Babcock operation. Iliac and pelvic colon freed through abdominal incision. **B¹,** Perineal part of operation. Freed colon and rectum brought out through perineal incision. **B²,** Colon and rectum removed down to sphincter, which is split posteriorly. **B³,** Proximal colon brought down through sphincter. **C,** Hochenegg, or "durchzug," operation. Abdominal part shown. **C¹,** Sigmoid brought out through perineal incision and removed, leaving cuff of rectum. **C²,** Proximal colon brought down through this small portion of remaining rectum and out through sphincter. (From Berman, J. K.: Principles and practice of surgery, St. Louis, 1950, The C. V. Mosby Co.)

**Accessory items**

1 Indwelling catheterization set
2 Pieces of umbilical tape, ½ in. wide, 18 in. long
  Routine dressing for abdominal wounds

FOR THE PERINEAL PROCEDURE

**Cutting instruments**

1 No. 4L knife handle with blade no. 20
1 Mayo scissors, curved, 10 in.
1 Suture scissors

**Holding instruments**

12 Crile hemostats
6 Ochsner forceps, 6¼ in., straight

1 Tissue forceps without teeth, 5½ in.
6 Allis forceps, 10 in.

**Exposing instruments**

2 Doyen retractors
2 U.S. Army retractors
2 Richardson retractors, small
2 Rake retractors, 4-prong, medium

**Suturing items**

2 Mayo-Hegar needle holders, 6¼ in.
2 Large regular surgeon's cutting needles, large, ½-circle
  Silk sutures no. 2-0
  Chromic gut sutures no. 2-0 swaged on a general closure needle

**Accessory items**

   1 Large Penrose tissue drain with safety pin attached

     Petrolatum gauze and perineal dressings

### OPERATIVE PROCEDURE

#### FOR THE ABDOMINAL STAGE

1. The abdomen is entered through a left rectus incision, as previously described in Chapter 17. The peritoneal cavity is carefully explored for evidence of metastasis and resectability of the lesion.

2. A loop of sigmoid is elevated as the small intestines are walled off with synthetic abdominal drapes or moist packs; retractors are placed. If possible, an umbilical tie is placed proximal to the tumor in the sigmoid to prevent dissemination of malignant cells to the upper colon.

3. The peritoneum on the left side of the colon is incised with a long scalpel, scissors, Rochester-Pean forceps, and sponge forceps. Traction sutures of silk no. 2-0 may be used as the peritoneum is reflected. Bleeding vessels are ligated with silk ligatures no. 2-0 or 3-0. The inferior mesenteric vessels may be ligated to prevent metastasis from tissue handling.

4. The pelvic peritoneum is exposed and dissected free to form the left side of the new pelvic floor. The ureter is identified. Bleeding vessels are ligated with 28-inch silk ligatures no. 2-0, which are inserted in the tip of Rochester-Pean forceps to facilitate placement, or with chromic gut no. 2-0 sutures on general closure needles.

5. The sigmoid is turned toward the left, and the same procedure as in step 4 is carried out on the right side of the pelvis. The two incisions are then curved and joined in front of the rectum.

6. The superior hemorrhoidal blood vessels are doubly ligated with silk no. 2-0 and divided.

7. The rectum is freed anteriorly and posteriorly from the adjacent structures down to the sacrococcygeal junction.

8. The sigmoid is doubly clamped with DeMartel, Payr, or similar resection clamps, following mobilization of the proximal portion. The sigmoid is divided with a scalpel

or cautery, and soiled instruments are discarded.

9. The proximal end is protected with a small gauze sponge as it is drawn through a previously prepared stab wound for the colostomy. The DeMartel blade is retained in place, or the Payr clamp may be replaced by an Ochsner clamp, which is supported by gauze sponges on the abdominal wall to prevent tension on the bowel.

10. The distal end is tied off with heavy silk, or a small DeMartel blade may be left in place and the entire end covered with a rubber dam or surgical glove and then tied securely with a silk suture to prevent contamination. The closed distal end is placed deep in the pelvis in the presacral space (Fig. 23-1, *A*).

11. The pelvic peritoneum is closed over the distal divided end to make a new floor. Reperitonealization is completed, using long forceps, a long needle holder, and continuous sutures of chromic gut no. 2-0 with swaged-on needles.

12. The colostomy site is inspected. The mesentery may be anchored to the abdominal wall with carefully placed interrupted sutures.

13. The abdominal wound is closed by the Tom Jones technique, using 28-gauge stainless steel wire. Retention sutures may be used. Dressings are applied to both the abdominal wound and the colostomy.

#### FOR THE PERINEAL STAGE (Fig. 23-1, *A²*)

1. The patient is repositioned on the operating table in a Sims or lithotomy position.

2. The anus is closed with a purse-string suture of heavy silk on a cutting needle. The forceps, scissors, needle, and needle holder used for anal closure are discarded. This step may be completed prior to application of sterile sheets. Routine skin preparation and draping are completed.

3. An elliptical incision is made around the anus with a scalpel, using a blade no. 20 or 10. Tissue forceps, hemostats, gauze sponges, and chromic gut sutures no. 2-0

or 0 are used in dissection and control of bleeding vessels.

4. The levator ani muscles are divided at their point of attachment to the rectal wall. Rochester-Pean forceps, Ochsner forceps, Mayo scissors, and transfixion sutures are used.

5. The upper end of the distal bowel containing the tumor is grasped with Allis forceps, delivered into the perineal wound, and then dissected free.

6. The bleeding vessels are ligated with chromic gut no. 2-0 or 0 transfixion sutures.

7. The perineal defect is packed or drained, according to the surgeon's preference.

### Abdominoperineal resection with preservation of the external sphincter

During the abdominal operation a colostomy is not done. The specimen is excised and removed. In the perineal procedure the rectum and the internal anal sphincter are freed. The proximal end of the sigmoid is drawn through the external anal sphincter with long Allis forceps. A rectal tube may be tied inside the sigmoid to facilitate this maneuver (Fig. 23-1, *C*). The protruding sigmoid is held in place by suturing it to the anal skin. The rectal tube is left in place. A sump drain may be placed in the presacral space. The redundant sigmoid, which protrudes through the anal segment containing the external sphincter, may be trimmed by electrocautery after 10 days.

## RADICAL HYSTERECTOMY (WERTHEIM)

**DEFINITION.** Through an abdominal incision, the peritoneum is opened; the uterus, adnexa, proximal vagina, and bilateral lymph nodes are resected en bloc.

**CONSIDERATIONS.** Radical abdominal hysterectomy may be performed in the presence of cervical carcinoma with or without attendant radiation. Abdominal exploration should determine lymph node involvement.

**SETUP AND PREPARATION OF THE PATIENT.** As described for total hysterectomy (Chap-

ter 24). Add the following to the abdominal instrument set:

 8 Schnidt tonsil hemostats
 6 Lahey gallduct forceps, 9 in.
 2 Cushing vein retractors
 2 Vascular fine tissue forceps, plain, 12 in.
   Hemostatic clips and applier (optional)
   Kitner sponges

**OPERATIVE PROCEDURE**

1. The skin is incised and the abdominal layers opened as for a laparotomy.

2. The peritoneum is cut at its reflexion on the anterior surface of the uterus between the round ligaments (Fig. 23-2). By blunt dissection, the bladder surface is freed from the cervix and vagina.

3. The right round and infundibulopelvic ligaments are clamped with Rochester-Pean forceps, cut with Metzenbaum scissors, and ligated with silk no. 2-0 sutures to expose the external iliac artery. The ureter is identified and retracted with a vein retractor (Fig. 23-3).

4. The lymph and areolar tissue is dissected from the iliac artery, obturator fossa, and ureter, using Lahey forceps, Kitner sponges, and Metzenbaum scissors. The uterine artery and vein are clamped, cut, and doubly ligated with silk no. 0 suture ligatures. The block of tissue is reflected toward the uterus and the procedure repeated on the left side.

5. The uterus is then elevated; the cul-de-sac is opened (Fig. 23-4); and the uterosacral and cardinal ligaments are clamped with Heaney forceps, cut with scissors, and doubly ligated with chromic gut no. 0 suture ligatures. The pararectal and paravesical areolar tissues are dissected free to skeletonize the upper vagina.

6. The upper third of the vagina is cross clamped with Heaney forceps (Fig. 23-5) and divided with a knife handle no. 4L and blade no. 20. The uterus and surrounding tissues are removed.

7. The vagina is closed transversely with chromic gut sutures no. 0 swaged to general closure needles (Fig. 23-6). The pelvis is peritonized with chromic gut sutures no. 2-0 swaged to general closure needles.

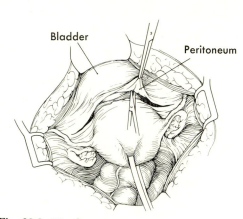

**Fig. 23-2.** Wertheim type of radical hysterectomy. Applying upward traction on the uterus, the peritoneum is incised from round ligament to round ligament at its reflexion on the anterior surface of the uterus. (Redrawn from TeLinde, R. W.: Operative gynecology, ed. 3, Philadelphia, 1962, J. B. Lippincott Co.)

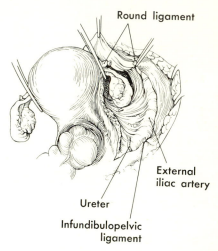

**Fig. 23-3.** Wertheim hysterectomy—cont'd. The right round ligament and the right infundibulopelvic ligaments have been ligated and cut, thus exposing the right external iliac artery. Note the ureter crossing through the areolar tissue, which is then dissected. (Redrawn from TeLinde, R. W.: Operative gynecology, ed. 3, Philadelphia, 1962, J. B. Lippincott Co.)

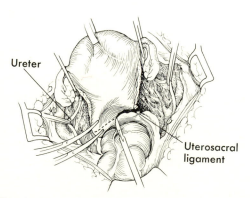

**Fig. 23-4.** Wertheim hysterectomy—cont'd. The uterus is held upward and forward, exposing the cul-de-sac, which is incised as shown by the dotted line. (Redrawn from TeLinde, R. W.: Operative gynecology, ed. 3, Philadelphia, 1962, J. B. Lippincott Co.)

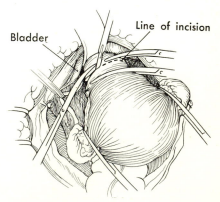

**Fig. 23-5.** Wertheim hysterectomy—cont'd. After the dissection is completed, the vagina is doubly clamped, preparatory to transection, after which the entire specimen will be lifted out en masse. (Redrawn from TeLinde, R. W.: Operative gynecology, ed. 3, Philadelphia, 1962, J. B. Lippincott Co.)

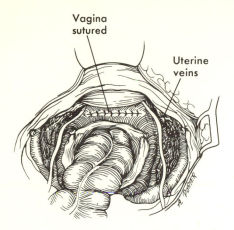

**Fig. 23-6.** Wertheim hysterectomy—cont'd. The vagina is closed. The peritoneum remains to be peritonized. (Redrawn from TeLinde, R. W.: Operative gynecology, ed. 3, Philadelphia, 1962, J. B. Lippincott Co.)

8. The abdominal wound is closed, using the Jones technique, and dressed in the usual manner.

## WIDE CUFF HYSTERECTOMY

The definition is the same as that for a Wertheim hysterectomy except that this procedure does not include removal of the lymph nodes and is done for carcinoma in situ of the cervix.

## PELVIC EXENTERATION

**DEFINITION.** An en bloc "removal of the rectum, distal sigmoid colon, the urinary bladder and the distal ureters, the internal iliac vessels and their lateral branches, all pelvic reproductive organs and lymph nodes, and the entire pelvic floor with the accompanying pelvic peritoneum, levator muscles, and perineum."* Bricker's technique will be described here. A partial exenteration, either anterior or posterior, may be performed, depending on the origin of the carcinoma and the extent of local tissue invasion.

---

*From Bricker, E. M.: Pelvic exenteration. In Welch, C. E., editor: Advances in surgery, Chicago, 1970, Year Book Medical Publishers, Inc., p. 14.

**CONSIDERATIONS.** Pelvic exenteration is the treatment of choice for recurrent or persistent carcinoma of the cervix after radiation therapy; it is also applicable to carcinomas of the endometrium or rectum. Exenteration is considered only after a thorough investigation of the patient and disease status to determine if there is a reasonable chance of cure and of return to a productive life style. Determination of the chance of resectability with cure can be made with finality at the time of abdominal exploration by the surgeon.

The need for creation of urinary and bowel diversion must also be considered, together with the patient's ability to cope with these diversions postoperatively.

**SETUP AND PREPARATION OF THE PATIENT.** Psychological preparation by the physician is a prime requisite in the care of the patient and family. Nursing care should be directed toward supporting the patient during the course of therapy and helping the patient to maintain personal dignity.

Preoperative cleansing of the bowel with antibiotics and enemas will be done. A nasogastric tube, urinary catheter, and rectal tube will be inserted in surgery. Antiembolic stockings will be placed on both legs. Constant cardiac and central venous pressure monitoring will be carried on.

A general endotracheal anesthetic is usually administered. The patient is placed in the supine position with legs elevated in a modified lithotomy or "ski" position to allow access to the perineum without disruptive position changes (Fig. 23-7). Trendelenburg placement of the table is indicated.

The circulating and scrub nurses must be alert to fluid and blood loss; irrigation solutions must be accurately measured; laparotomy packs must be weighed to assess blood volume loss; and the anesthetist and surgical team appraised of the measurement.

Two separate instrument setups are required for the abdominal and perineal approaches. Extra drapes, gowns, and gloves should be available.

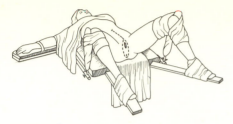

Fig. 23-7. Pelvic exenteration. Modified lithotomy position with incision shown by dotted lines. (Redrawn from Lindenauer, S. M., et al.: Arch. Surg. 96:493, April, 1968.)

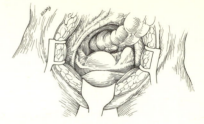

Fig. 23-8. Pelvic exenteration—cont'd. Pelvic viscera in situ as viewed from operating surgeon's vantage point after retractors are placed and the small bowel is packed off. (Redrawn from Lindenauer, S. M., et al.: Arch. Surg. 96:493, April, 1968.)

FOR THE ABDOMINAL APPROACH. As described previously for abdominoperineal resection, adding the following:

1 Metzenbaum scissors, 12 in.
8 Schnidt tonsil hemostats
6 Lahey gallduct forceps, 9 in.
6 Allis forceps, 9¼ in.
8 Pean hysterectomy forceps, 9½ in.
2 Large right-angled clamps, 12 in.
2 Stille kidney clamps, 9 in.
2 Cushing vein retractors
2 Vascular fine tissue forceps, plain, 12 in.
2 Needle holders, 12 in.
  Instruments for removal of reproductive organs of the male or female
  Electrosurgical unit (optional)
  Red rubber catheters, assorted French sizes
  Ileostomy bag
  Colostomy bag
  Sutures—various sizes of silk (long and short), chromic gut, and steel wire, 28-gauge

When the colon is transected or ureteral drainage is to be diverted into an ileosegment, the gastrointestinal technique as described in Chapter 21 should be followed.

FOR THE PERINEAL APPROACH. As described previously for the abdominoperineal resection.

Antiseptic skin preparation includes the abdomen, thighs, and perineum, including the internal vaginal vault. At this time, the bladder is catheterized and the catheter removed; the anus is tightly closed with a running silk suture no. 0 on a cutting needle.

OPERATIVE PROCEDURE

1. A long midline incision is made and the abdomen opened in the usual manner.

2. The peritoneal cavity is explored for metastasis to the liver, the nodes of the celiac axis, the superior mesenteric artery, and the para-aortic tissues.

3. The pelvis is explored and the peritoneum along the brim of the pelvis examined for lymph node involvement. Frozen sections may be indicated. The obturator fossa and the region of the uterosacral ligaments are explored. On negative findings at exploration, retractors are placed and the small bowel packed off with moist laparotomy packs (Fig. 23-8).

4. The sigmoid mesocolon is freed and sectioned by means of Payr clamps and a scalpel no. 4 with blade no. 20. The proximal end is exteriorized through an opening in the left side of the abdomen; an intestinal clamp is left across the lumen until later, when the permanent colostomy will be secured to the skin.

5. The remaining sigmoid mesentery is clamped with Rochester-Pean forceps, cut, and ligated with silk ligatures no. 2-0 down to and including the superior hemorrhoidal vessels. Long instruments and sutures are used to facilitate reaching the deep pelvic structures.

6. The distal sigmoid is closed with an inverting chromic gut suture no. 2-0. The sigmoid and rectum are freed from the sacrococcygeal area by blunt and sharp dissection.

7. The lateral pelvic peritoneum is cut along the iliac vessels; the ovarian vessels

and round ligaments on each side are clamped with Rochester-Pean forceps, cut, and doubly ligated with silk no. 2-0 ligatures.

8. The peritoneum is incised over the dome of the bladder with long knife and Metzenbaum scissors, and the bladder is separated from the symphysis pubis down to the urethra.

9. The ureters are identified and divided 2 to 3 cm. below the brim of the pelvis. The proximal end is left open to allow urinary drainage while the distal end is ligated.

10. The hypogastric artery, the internal iliac vein, and the superior and inferior gluteal vessels are exposed, clamped with hemostats, doubly ligated with silk ligatures no. 2-0, and cut. The external iliac vein is retracted to allow evacuation of the contents of the obturator fossa (leaving the obturator nerve intact). Care must be taken in dissection not to damage the sacral plexus and sciatic nerve.

11. The internal pudendal vessels are isolated, ligated with transfixion sutures of chromic gut no. 0, and cut. The remaining soft tissue attachments of the pelvis are clamped and cut. Steps 10 and 11 are then performed on the opposite side.

12. The perineum is then incised by an elliptical incision that includes the clitoris and anus. The ischiorectal fat is incised up to the area of the levator muscle.

13. The coccygeal attachment of the rectum is severed. The levator muscles are severed at their lateral attachments by means of a knife no. 4L with blade no. 20; hemostasis is maintained by pressure and traction.

14. The paravesical and paravaginal tissues are resected from the periosteum of the symphysis and pubic rami by means of a knife. The specimen is completely freed and removed from the pelvis (Fig. 23-9).

15. After residual bleeding vessels are identified and controlled by transfixing chromic gut ligatures no. 0, the subcutaneous tissue is closed by interrupted chromic gut sutures no. 0. The skin is closed with

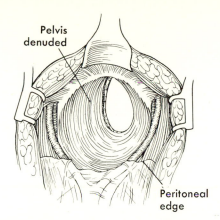

Fig. 23-9. Pelvic exenteration—cont'd. Empty pelvis after dissection of the paravesical and paravaginal tissues and removal of the specimen en bloc. (Redrawn from Lindenauer, S. M., et al.: Arch. Surg. 96:493, April, 1968.)

silk sutures no. 3-0 on cutting needles; a drain is placed in the wound.

16. On return to the abdomen, further residual bleeding vessels are controlled. Gauze pads may be left in the pelvis to be removed via the perineum after 48 hours.

17. The ileosegment is then fashioned and the ureters anastomosed to it in the manner described in Chapter 12. The external stoma of the ileal segment is placed on the right side of the abdomen.

18. A red rubber, multieyed tube size 16 Fr. is inserted into the proximal jejunum for the length of the jejunum and the ileum to aid in postoperative bowel decompression. It is sutured to the bowel with a chromic gut no. 3-0 purse-string suture and brought out to the skin, where it is sutured in place with silk no. 2-0 sutures.

19. A gastrostomy tube is placed in the stomach in the same manner.

20. Hemostasis is reappraised. The small intestines are carefully placed into the pelvis. Packs and retractors are removed (Fig. 23-10).

21. The peritoneum, rectus muscles, and fascial sheaths are closed with interrupted figure-of-eight sutures of steel 28-gauge wire. The skin is closed with interrupted silk no. 3-0 sutures.

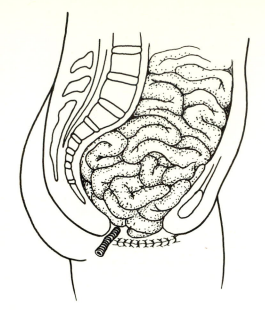

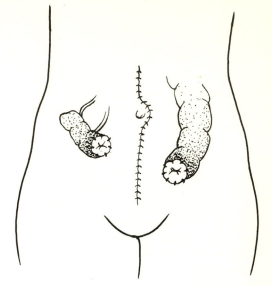

**Fig. 23-10.** Pelvic exenteration—cont'd. Sagittal view of small bowel above pelvic defect. Perineal packing and/or a drain may be used. (Redrawn from Lindenauer, S. M., et al.: Arch. Surg. **96:** 493, April, 1968.)

**Fig. 23-11.** Pelvic exenteration—cont'd. Following closure of the abdominal wall the colostomy and ileostomy stomas are sutured to the skin edges. (Redrawn from Lindenauer, S. M., et al.: Arch. Surg. **96:**493, April, 1968.)

22. The colostomy stoma is prepared by removing the intestinal clamp from the sigmoid, opening the colon, and suturing the stoma to the skin edges with chromic gut no. 3-0 sutures (Fig. 23-11).

23. The abdominal wound and tube sites are dressed in the usual manner. Drainage bags are applied to the colostomy and ileostomy stomas. A perineal dressing is secured by means of a T-binder.

### REFERENCES

1. Anson, B. J.: Morris' human anatomy, ed. 12, New York, 1966, The Blakiston Division, McGraw-Hill Book Co.
2. Black, B. M., and Walls, J. T.: Combined abdominoendorectal resection: reappraisal of a pull-through procedure, Surrg. Clin. North Am. **47:**977, 1967.
3. Bricker, E. M.: Pelvic exenteration. In Welch, C. E., editor: Advances in surgery, Chicago, 1970, Year Book Medical Publishers, Inc.
4. Brunschwig, A.: Reduction of morbidity and mortality in pelvic exenterations, Surg. Clin. North Am. **42:**1583, 1962.
5. Davis, L.: Christopher's textbook of surgery, ed. 8, Philadelphia, 1964, W. B. Saunders Co.
6. Lindenauer, S. M., Morley, G. W., and Cerny, J. C.: Multidiscipline approach to treatment of recurrent pelvic neoplasms, Arch. Surg. **96:** 493, 1968.
7. Madden, J. L.: Atlas of technics of surgery, ed. 2, New York, 1964, Appleton-Century-Crofts.
8. Moyer, C. A., Rhoads, J. E., Allen, J. G., and Harkins, H. N.: Surgery: principles and practice, ed. 3, Philadelphia, 1965, J. B. Lippincott Co.
9. Rutledge, F. N., and Burns, B. C.: Pelvic exenteration, Am. J. Obstet. Gyencol. **91:**692, 1965.
10. TeLinde, R. W.: Operative gynecology, ed. 3, Philadelphia, 1962, J. B. Lippincott Co.
11. Thorek, P.: Anatomy in surgery, Philadelphia, 1951, J. B. Lippincott Co.
12. Turell, R., editor: Diseases of the colon and anorectum, vol. 1, Philadelphia, 1969, W. B. Saunders Co.

CHAPTER 24

# Gynecological and obstetrical surgery

**DORINDA HARMON** and **JUDITH A. JONES**

A general understanding of the anatomy and physiology of the female pelvis, reproductive organs, and associated structures is necessary for the operating room nursing staff. Application of anatomy is extremely important in positioning the patient for surgery, in selecting the proper instruments and sutures for a specific type of operation, and in understanding the plan of surgery.

## REPRODUCTIVE SYSTEM

The female reproductive organs and their relationships are shown in Fig. 24-1.

The adult female structures directly and indirectly associated with the process of reproduction include the bony pelvis, the associated ligaments and muscles, the soft tissues and contents of the pelvic cavity, the external organs (vulva) (Figs. 24-2 and 24-3) and the breasts (mammary glands).

BONY PELVIS. The Latin word *pelvis* means basin. The pelvis is that part of the trunk below and behind the abdomen. The bony pelvis is made up of the ilium, pubis, ischium, sacrum, and coccyx (Fig. 24-2). The so-called pelvic brim divides the abdominal false portion from the true por-

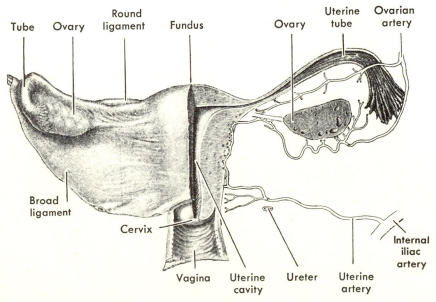

**Fig. 24-1.** Female reproductive organs. Left half, tube and ovary in their natural relationship; right half, diagrammatic section. (From Pitzman, M.: Fundamentals of human anatomy, St. Louis, The C. V. Mosby Co.)

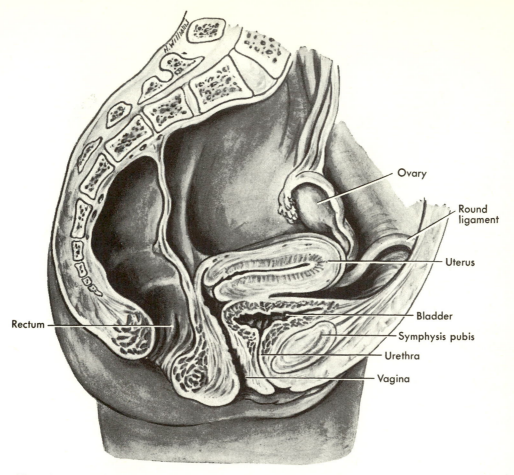

**Fig. 24-2.** Sagittal section of female pelvis. (From Anthony, C. P.: Textbook of anatomy and physiology, ed. 6, St. Louis, 1963, The C. V. Mosby Co.)

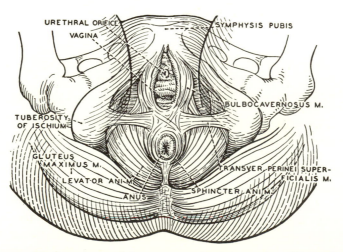

**Fig. 24-3.** Topographical anatomy of important perineal structures. (From Greenhill, J. P.: Surgical gynecology, Chicago, 1957, Year Book Medical Publishers, Inc.)

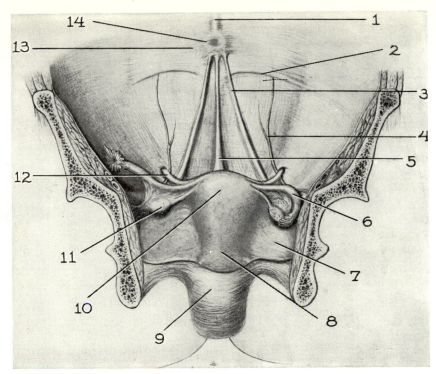

**Fig. 24-4.** Relationship of female sexual organs to anterior abdominal wall. **1,** Round ligament and liver; **2,** semicircular line of Douglas; **3,** lateral umbilical ligament; **4,** inferior epigastric artery; **5,** medial umbilical ligament; **6,** fallopian tube; **7,** broad ligament; **8,** cervix; **9,** vagina; **10,** uterine corpus; **11,** ovary; **12,** round ligament; **13,** umbilical fascia; **14,** umbilicus. (From Rubin, I. C., and Novak, J.: Integrated gynecology, New York, 1956, Blakiston Division, McGraw-Hill Book Co.)

tion of the pelvis. The abdominal (false) pelvis is the part above the arcuate line (Fig. 24-2). The true pelvis is the part below this line. It forms the passageway through which the infant passes during parturition.

The true pelvis may be considered as having three parts: the inlet, cavity, and outlet. The muscles lining the pelvis facilitate movement of the thighs, give form to the pelvic cavity, and provide firm elastic lining to the bony pelvic framework. All organs located in the pelvis are covered by pelvic fascia (Fig. 24-4). The fascia covering some muscles is dense and firm, whereas that covering other organs is thin and elastic. The nerves, blood vessels, and ureters coursing through the anatomical structures are closely associated with the muscular and fascial structures (Fig. 24-5).

The *pelvic fascia* may be divided into three general groups: parietal, diaphragmatic, and visceral. The parietal pelvic fascia covers the muscles of the true pelvic wall and the perineum. The diaphragmatic fascia covers both sides of the pelvic diaphragm, which is made up of the levator ani and coccygeal muscles (Fig. 24-6). The visceral fascia is thin flexible fascia, which covers the pelvic organs. The *floor of the pelvis,* known as the *pelvic diaphragm,* gives support to the abdominal pelvic viscera in this region. The pelvic diaphragm, consisting of the levator ani and coccygeal muscles with their respective fascial coverings, separates the pelvic cavity from the perineum. The basis of modern vaginal surgery is concerned with the function of the levator ani muscles

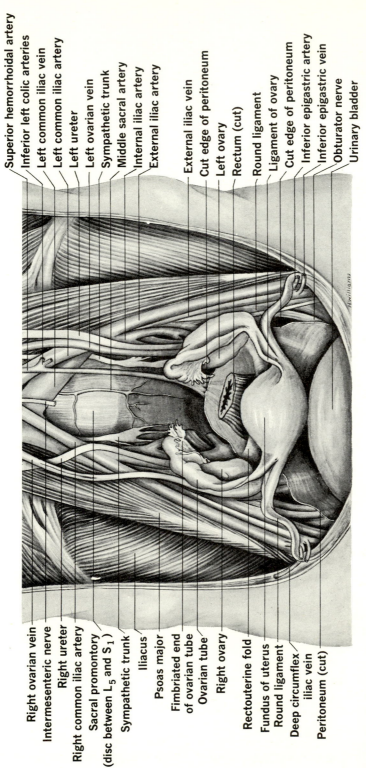

Right ovarian vein
Intermesenteric nerve
Right ureter
Right common iliac artery
Sacral promontory
(disc between $L_5$ and $S_1$)
Sympathetic trunk
Iliacus
Psoas major
Fimbriated end
of ovarian tube
Ovarian tube
Right ovary
Rectouterine fold
Fundus of uterus
Round ligament
Deep circumflex
iliac vein
Peritoneum (cut)

Superior hemorrhoidal artery
Inferior left colic arteries
Left common iliac vein
Left common iliac artery
Left ureter
Left ovarian vein
Sympathetic trunk
Middle sacral artery
Internal iliac artery
External iliac artery
External iliac vein
Cut edge of peritoneum
Left ovary
Rectum (cut)
Round ligament
Ligament of ovary
Cut edge of peritoneum
Inferior epigastric artery
Inferior epigastric vein
Obturator nerve
Urinary bladder

Rwilliams

**Fig. 24-5.** Internal female genitalia and arterial and nerve supply. Anterior view; uterus antiflexed. (W.R.U. 2975, female, 31 years of age.) (From Francis, C. C: Introduction to human anatomy, ed. 5, St. Louis, 1968, The C. V. Mosby Co.)

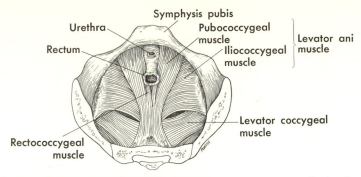

**Fig. 24-6.** Perineal musculature. (Redrawn from Anthony, C. P.: Textbook of anatomy and physiology, ed. 7, St. Louis, 1967, The C. V. Mosby Co.)

and the provision of an effective lower outlet (Fig. 24-6).

The *levator ani muscles*, varying in thickness and strength, may be divided into three parts: the iliococcygeal, the pubococcygeal, and the puborectal muscles (Figs. 24-5 and 24-6). The fibers of the levator ani blend with muscle fibers of the rectum and vagina. The fibers (pubovaginal) of the pubococcygeal part of the levator ani muscles, lying directly below the urinary bladder, are involved in the control of micturition. The pubococcygeal fibers of the levator ani control and pull the coccyx forward and assist in the closure of the pelvic outlet. The fibers pull the rectum, vagina, and bladder neck upward toward the symphysis in an effort to close the pelvic outlet and are responsible for the flexure at the anorectal junction. Relaxation of the fibers during defecation permits a straightening at this junction. During parturition, the action of the levator ani directs the fetal head into the lower part of the passageway.

The uterus gains much of its support by its direct attachment to the vagina and by indirect attachments to nearby structures such as the rectum and pelvic diaphragm (Fig. 24-7). The ligaments and muscles on each side of the uterus are the broad, round, and cardinal (Mackenrodt) uterosacral ligaments and the levator ani muscles.

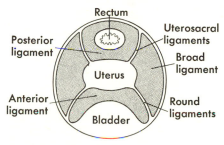

**Fig. 24-7.** Scheme to show relative positions of eight uterine ligaments formed by folds of peritoneum: two broad ligaments, double folds extending from uterus to side walls of pelvic cavity; two uterosacral ligaments, foldlike extensions of peritoneum from uterus to sacrum; posterior ligament, fold between uterus and rectum; and two round ligaments, folds from the uterus to the deep inguinal ring. (Redrawn from Anthony, C. P.: Textbook of anatomy and physiology, ed. 7, 1967, St. Louis, The C. V. Mosby Co.)

### Female pelvis

The *uterus*, which occupies a central place in the pelvis, is a pear-shaped organ directed downward and backward. At its upper lateral points the uterine cornua receive the uterine tubes (Figs. 24-1 and 24-8). The fundus of the uterus is the upper rounded portion situated above the level of the tubal openings and just below the pelvic brim. Below, the body of the uterus joins the cervix, from which it is separated by a slight constriction canal,

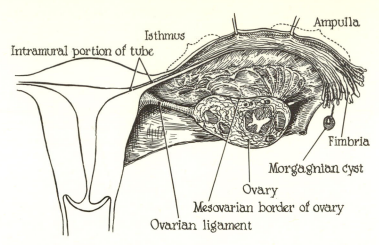

**Fig. 24-8.** Diagrammatic lateral section through uterus and tube. (From Beacham, D. W., and Beacham, W. D.: Synopsis of gynecology, ed. 8, St. Louis, 1972, The C. V. Mosby Co.)

called the *isthmus*. The cervix lies at the level of the ischial spines. The body of the uterus communicates with the cervical canal at the internal orifice, called the *internal os* (Fig. 24-1). The constriction (canal) ends at the vaginal portion of the cervix at the external orifice, called the *external os*. This is a small oval aperture situated between two lips.

STRUCTURE OF THE UTERUS. The Greek word for uterus is *hystera*. The uterus lies behind the bladder (Fig. 24-7) and in front of the rectum. The uterine body has three layers: (1) the outer peritoneal, or serous, layer, which is a reflection of the pelvic peritoneum: (2) the myometrium, or muscular layer, which houses involuntary muscles, nerves, blood vessels, and lymphatics; and (3) the endometrium, or mucosal layer, which lines the cavity of the uterus.

The *cervix* consists of a supravaginal and a vaginal portion (Fig. 24-1). The supravaginal portion is closely associated with the bladder and the ureters. The vaginal portion of the cervix projects downward and backward into the vaginal vault.

UTERINE (FALLOPIAN) TUBES. The Greek word *salpinx*, meaning trumpet or tube, is used in referring to the uterine tube (Figs. 24-1 and 24-8). Bilateral tubes, each consisting of a musculomembranous channel

about 4 to 5 inches long, form the canals through which the ova from either ovary are conveyed to the uterus (Fig. 24-8). Each uterine tube leaves the upper portion of the uterus, passes outward toward the sides of the pelvis, and ends in fringelike projections, called *fimbriae*. These are situated just below the ovaries. The fimbriae catch the ova, and the tubes convey the ova to the cavity of the uterus. This channel also transmits spermatozoa in the opposite direction. The tubes are covered on their outer surfaces by peritoneum. Each tube receives its blood supply from the branches of the uterine and ovarian arteries (Figs. 24-1 and 24-5).

How the ova are transported from the ruptured follicle into the uterus is unknown. One theory is that the transfer is accomplished through vascular changes, together with contraction of the smooth muscle fibers of the tube and that the peristaltic movements of the tube push the ova toward the uterus.

The right tube and ovary are in close relationship to the cecum and appendix, and the left tube and ovary are associated with the sigmoid flexure. Both are closely associated with the ureters.

OVARIES. Each ovary, situated at the side of the uterus, lies within a depression

(ovarian fossa) on the lateral wall of the pelvic cavity and above the broad ligament (Fig. 24-1). The ovary is attached to the posterior surface of the broad ligament by the mesovarium and is kept in place by the ovarian ligament. The ovary, a small, flattened, almond-shaped organ, is composed of an outer layer, known as the cortex, and an inner vascular layer, known as the medulla. The cortex contains ovarian (graafian) follicles in different stages of maturity. After ovulation the corpus luteum is developed within the ovary by reorganization of the graafian follicles. The medulla, lying within the cortex, consists of connective tissue containing nerves, blood, and lymph vessels. The ovary is covered by epithelium, not by peritoneum.

The ovaries are homologous with the testes of the male. They produce ova after puberty and also function as endocrine glands, producing hormones. The estrogenic hormone is secreted by the ovarian follicle. It controls the development of the secondary sexual characteristics and initiates growth of the lining of the uterus during the menstrual cycle. The progesterone hormone, which is secreted by the corpus luteum, is essential for the implantation of the fertilized ovum and for the development of the embryo.

LIGAMENTS OF THE UTERUS. The uterine ligaments are the broad, round, uterosacral, and transverse cervical ligaments (Figs. 24-4 and 24-7).

BROAD LIGAMENTS. From each side of the uterus, the pelvic peritoneum extends laterally, downward, and backward. A double fold of pelvic peritoneum forms the layers of the broad ligament, enclosing the uterus (Fig. 24-4). These layers separate to cover the floor and sides of the pelvis. The uterine tube is situated within the free border of broad ligament. The part of the broad ligament lying immediately below the uterine tube is termed the *mesosalpinx* (Fig. 24-1). The ovary lies behind the broad ligament.

ROUND LIGAMENTS. These fibromuscular bands are attached to the uterus (Figs. 24-2 and 24-4). Each round ligament passes forward and laterally between the layers of the broad ligament to enter the deep inguinal ring.

TRANSVERSE CERVICAL LIGAMENTS. These cardinal ligaments are composed of connective tissue masses with smooth muscle fibers that are strong support for the uterus in the pelvis (Fig. 24-5).

UTEROSACRAL LIGAMENTS. These are a posterior continuation of the peritoneal tissue, which forms the cardinal ligaments. The ligaments pass posteriorly to the sacrum on either side of the rectum (Fig. 24-7).

VAGINA. This is a tubelike organ for copulation and the excretory duct for the products of menstruation (Figs. 24-1 and 24-2). It is directed downward and forward, situated in front of the rectum and behind the bladder. The upper part of the vagina lies above the pelvic floor and is surrounded by visceral pelvic fascia. The lower half is surrounded by the levator ani muscles.

FORNICES. The projection of the cervix into the vaginal vault divides the vault into four regions, called *fornices*: anterior and posterior and right and left lateral.

The posterior fornix is in close contact with the peritoneum of the pouch of Douglas. The rectovaginal septum lies between the vagina and rectum. The dense connective tissue separating the anterior wall of the vagina from the distal urethra is termed the *urethrovaginal septum*.

## Female external genital organs (vulva)

The external organs are referred to collectively as the vulva. It occupies the central portion of the perineal region. The mons veneris, urethra, and Skene's glands are in close proximity to the vulva (Fig. 24-9).

The *mons pubis (veneris)* of the vulva is a rounded elevation of tissue covered by skin and, after puberty, by hair. It is situated in front of the symphysis pubis,

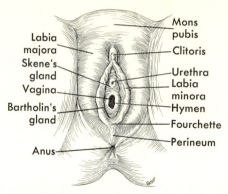

**Fig. 24-9.** External genitalia and areas most likely to harbor infection. (Redrawn from Beacham, D. W., and Beacham, W. D.: Crossen's synopsis of gynecology, ed. 6, St. Louis, 1963, The C. V. Mosby Co.)

beneath which are located the labia majora.

The *labia majora* are two folds of skin that extend downward and backward. They unite below and behind to form the posterior commissure and in front to form the anterior commissure. A Bartholin gland is situated on each side of the labia majora.

The *labia minora* comprise the two delicate folds of skin that lie within the labia majora (Fig. 24-9). Each labium minus splits into lateral and medial parts. The lateral part forms the *prepuce of clitoris,* and the medial part forms the *frenulum.* The posterior folds of the labia are united by a delicate fold extending between them. This forms the fourchette.

The *clitoris* is the homologue of the penis in the male. It hangs free and terminates in a rounded glans (small sensitive vascular body). Unlike the penis, the clitoris does not traverse the urethra.

The *vestibule* is a smooth area surrounded by the labia minora, with the clitoris at its apex and the fourchette at its base. It contains opening for the urethra and the vagina.

The *urethra,* which is about 4 cm. long, is in close relationship with the anterior vaginal wall and connects the bladder with the outside, acting as an excretory duct. At each side of the external ure-

thral orifice (meatus) lie two small ducts, termed the *paraurethral ducts,* which drain small *urethral glands (Skene's)* (Fig. 24-9).

The *vaginal opening* lies behind the urethral orifice, and in the virgin it is almost closed by the hymen, a fold of vaginal mucosa.

The *vestibular glands (Bartholin)* lie one at each side of the lower end of the vagina. They are homologues of the bulbourethral glands in the male. This narrow gland duct opens into the vaginal orifice on the inner aspects of the labium minus.

### Vascular, nerve, and lymphatic supply of the reproductive system

The *blood supply* of the female pelvis is derived from the internal iliac branches of the common iliac artery and is supplemented by the ovarian, superior rectal, and median sacral arteries—branches of the aorta (Figs. 24-4 and 24-5).

The *nerve supply* of the female pelvis comes from the autonomic nerves, which enter the pelvis in the superior hypogastric plexus (presacral nerve).

The *lymphatics* of the female pelvis either follow the course of the vessels to the iliac and preaortic nodes or empty into the inguinal glands (Fig. 24-10).

### PREPARATION OF THE PATIENT FOR GYNECOLOGICAL SURGERY

Surgery on the structures of the reproductive system in the female may be done either for diagnostic purposes or as a form of therapy in the treatment of a pelvic condition such as uterine bleeding or suspected cancer. Surgery is done to remove tumors or repair structures.

Principles and methods for positioning patients for different types of operations are described in Chapter 7. For vaginal and perineal surgery the lithotomy position is generally used. For abdominal surgery the patient is placed in a modified or extreme Trendelenburg position. Care should be taken to protect the patient from nerve injury and provide for circulatory and respiratory functioning.

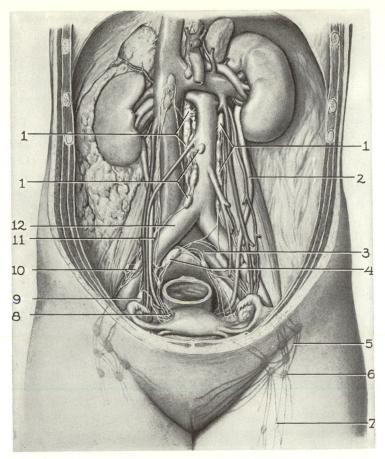

Fig. 24-10. Lymphatic system of abdomen and pelvis. 1, Lumbar or aortic nodes; 2, ureter; 3, common iliac vein; 4, sacral lymph nodes; 5, inguinal lymph nodes; 6, subinguinal or inguinofemoral lymph nodes; 7, femoral lymph nodes; 8, parametric gland of Champoniere; 9, hypogastric lymph node; 10, external iliac lymph nodes; 11, common iliac lymph nodes; 12, common iliac artery. (From Rubin, I. C., and Novak, J.: Integrated gynecology, New York, 1956, Blakiston Division, McGraw-Hill Book Co.)

Skin preparation is described in Chapter 4 and routine draping procedures in Chapter 5. A sterile lithotomy pack is needed for vaginal surgery. A laparotomy pack is needed for abdominal surgery.

Because pelvic and vaginal procedures involve manipulation of the ureters, bladder, and urethra, indwelling urinary drainage systems are frequently established during surgery. Either the urethral Foley catheter or the suprapubic Silastic cannula directly into the bladder may be used, depending on the surgeon's preference and the type of surgery.

## BASIC VAGINAL INSTRUMENT SETUP

The sterile preparation setup for the vaginal approach includes the following:

1 Graves vaginal speculum
1 Urethral catheter, 16 or 18 Fr.
1 Boseman dressing forceps
3 Sponge-holding forceps
  Gauze sponges
2 Towels
  Skin cleaning solutions, as desired

**Accessory unsterile items**

Preparation table
Kick buckets
Stools

The instrument setup includes the following (Chapter 17):

### Cutting instruments

3 Bard-Parker knife handles nos. 4 and 3, with blades nos. 20 and 10
2 Mayo uterine scissors, 6¾ in., 1 curved and 1 straight (Fig. 24-15)
1 Metzenbaum scissors, curved or flat, 7 in.
1 Suture scissors, straight

### Holding instruments

4 Foerster sponge-holding forceps, 9½ in.
6 Backhaus towel forceps, 5¼ in.
2 Tissue forceps with 2 and 3 teeth, 5½ in.
1 Tissue forceps with 2 and 3 teeth, 10 in.
2 Tissue forceps without teeth, 5½ in.
8 Allis-Adair tissue forceps, 6 in.
4 Allis forceps, 6 in.
2 Kocher forceps, 5½ in.
1 Boseman dressing forceps
1 Jacobs vulsellum forceps (Fig. 24-11)
4 Babcock forceps

### Clamping instruments

12 Crile hemostats, straight, 6¼ in.
12 Kelly hemostats, curved, 5 in. (optional)
2 Mayo-Pean hemostats, curved, 6¼ in.
4 Kocher hemostats, straight, 8 in. (optional)

### Exposing instruments

1 Jackson vaginal retractor
2 Heaney retractors
1 Uterine sound, graduated
1 Auvard speculum, weighted

### Suturing items

2 Heaney needle holders
3 Crile-Wood needle holders, 6¼ in.
Sutures:
Chromic gut, nos. 2-0, 0, and 1, swaged to ½-circle, taper point, medium-sized needle
Chromic gut, nos. 2-0 and 0, swaged to ½-circle, trocar-point, medium-sized needle
Plain gut, nos. 2-0 to 0, for free ligatures
Silk, no. 2-0, swaged to ⅜-circle, cutting-edge needle, for skin traction

### Accessory items

Indwelling urinary drainage items (Foley catheter or suprapubic cystostomy tube)
Asepto syringe, 2 oz.
Metal tray for surgeon's lap (optional)
Specimen containers
Lubricant, water-soluble
Electrosurgical unit, if desired
Suction tubing and tube
1 Lithotomy drape pack
1 Sheet, small
1 Vaginal supply pack

**MAJOR VAGINAL REPAIR SETUP.** Basic vaginal setup, plus the following:

### Cutting instruments

1 Kelly scissors, curved or flat, 6¾ in.

### Holding instruments (Fig. 24-11)

2 Allis-Adair forceps, 3 and 4 teeth, 7 in.
2 Jacobs vulsellum forceps
2 Kelly tenaculi, 9 in.

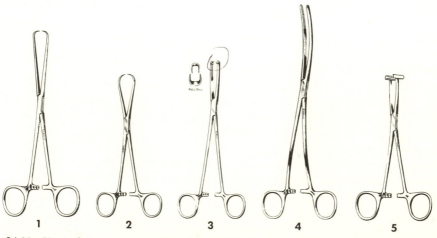

**Fig. 24-11.** Vaginal instruments: clamping and holding. **1,** Uterine tenaculum; **2,** Staude uterine tenaculum; **3,** Jacobs vulsellum forceps; **4,** Boseman dressing forceps; **5,** Pratt T-clamp. (Courtesy Codman & Shurtleff, Inc., Randolph, Mass.)

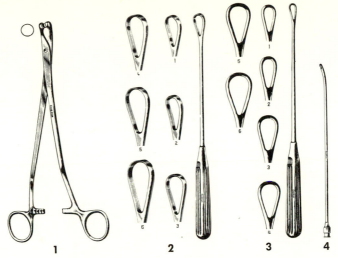

**Fig. 24-12.** Vaginal instruments: cutting. **1,** Gaylor biopsy forceps; **2,** uterine curettes (blunt); **3,** uterine curettes (sharp); **4,** endometrial biopsy suction curette. (Courtesy Codman & Shurtleff, Inc., Randolph, Mass.)

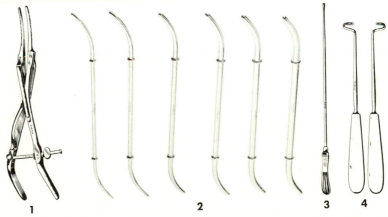

**Fig. 24-13.** Vaginal instruments: accessories. **1,** Goodell uterine dilator; **2,** Hank uterine dilators; **3,** uterine sound (graduated); **4,** Deschamp ligature carriers (right and left). (Courtesy Codman & Shurtleff, Inc., Randolph, Mass.)

3 Staude uterine tenaculum forceps, 5½ in.
1 Mayo tissue forceps with teeth, 7 in.
6 Pratt T-clamps

**Clamping instruments** (Fig. 24-16)

4 Mayo-Pean hemostats, curved, 6¾ in.
6 Crile hemostats, curved
4 Heaney hysterectomy forceps, 8 in.
8 Rochester-Ochsner hysterectomy forceps, 8 in.

**Exposing instruments**

1 Self-retaining vaginal retractor
1 Auvard speculum, weighted (optional)

2 Kelly retractors
1 Doyen vaginal retractor
2 U.S. Army retractors

**Suturing instruments**

1 Mayo-Hegar needle holder, 7 in.

## BASIC ABDOMINAL INSTRUMENT SETUP

The standard instrument setup for the abdominal approach (oophorectomy, sal-

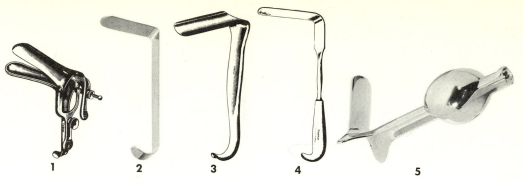

**Fig. 24-14.** Vaginal instruments: exposing. 1, Graves vaginal speculum; 2, Heaney hysterectomy retractor; 3, Doyen vaginal retractor; 4, Glenner vaginal retractor; 5, Auvard vaginal speculum (weighted). (Courtesy Codman & Shurtleff, Inc., Randolph, Mass.)

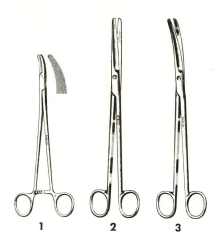

**Fig. 24-15.** Abdominal gynecological instruments: cutting and suturing. 1, Heaney needle holder; 2, Mayo uterine scissors (straight, 7¼ in.); 3, Mayo uterine scissors (curved, 7¼ in.). (Courtesy Codman & Shurtleff, Inc., Randolph, Mass.)

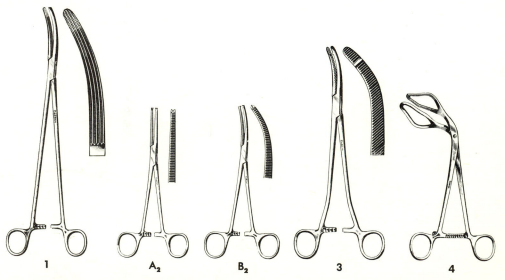

**Fig. 24-16.** Abdominal gynecological instruments: clamping. 1, Rochester-Pean forceps; A₂, Rochester-Ochsner (straight); B₂, Rochester-Ochsner (curved); 3, Heaney hysterectomy forceps; 4, Somer uterine elevating forceps. (Courtesy Codman & Shurtleff, Inc., Randolph, Mass.)

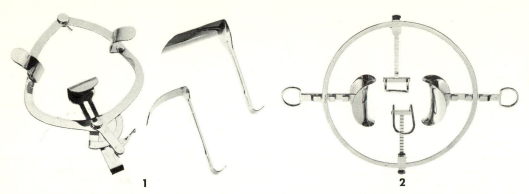

**Fig. 24-17.** Abdominal gynecological instruments: exposing. **1,** O'Sullivan-O'Connor self-retaining abdominal retractor; **2,** Martin abdominal ring retractor, self-retaining. (Courtesy Codman & Shurtleff, Inc., Randolph, Mass.)

pingectomy, hysterectomy, excision of ovarian cyst, and cesarean section) includes the basic laparotomy setup (Chapter 17) and the major vaginal repair set, plus the following:

**Holding instrument**
1 Somer uterine elevating forceps

**Exposing instrument**
1 Martin or O'Sullivan-O'Connor universal retractor with lateral and center blades (Fig. 24-17)

**Suturing items** (standard laparotomy set suturing items, plus the following)
2 Mayo-Hegar neeedle holders, long, heavy type
  Sutures:
4 Chromic gut, nos. 0 and 1, swaged to ½-circle, cutting-edge needles of desired size
4 Chromic gut, no. 0, free long ligatures
4 Chromic gut, nos. 0 and 2-0, swaged to ½-circle, taper point, medium-sized needles
1 Package silk, no. 0 or 2-0, for sutures or ligatures

*For most abdominal gynecological procedures,* a dilatation and curettage setup should be available (Figs. 24-12 to 24-14). *For cesarean section,* see setup and preparation of the patient on p. 853.

## VAGINAL SURGERY
### Simple vulvectomy

**DEFINITION.** Removal of the labia majora (Fig. 24-9), the labia minora, and possibly the clitoris and perianal area, with a Z-plasty closure.

**CONSIDERATIONS.** Simple vulvectomy may be done to treat leukoplakia vulvae because of its known association with carcinoma of the vulva, an intractable pruritus in older women, or other types of skin lesions such as kraurosis and vitiligo.

Simple vulvectomy also may be used for carcinoma in situ of the vulva, Bowen's disease of the vulva, and Paget's disease of the vulva.

**SETUP AND PREPARATION OF THE PATIENT.** The patient is anesthetized and placed in the lithotomy position, as described in Chapter 7. The operative site is cleansed, using the standard sterile vaginal set, and the patient is draped as described for lithotomy (Chapters 4 and 5). The basic vaginal setup is used, as described previously, plus an electrosurgical unit if desired.

**OPERATIVE PROCEDURE**
1. The affected skin is incised, usually starting anteriorly above the clitoris. The incision is continued laterally to the labia majora, to the midline of the perineum, and around the anus if it is involved (Fig. 24-18, *A*). A knife, holding forceps, gauze sponges on holders, tissue forceps, and Allis forceps are needed. Bleeding vessels are clamped. Bleeding is controlled by the

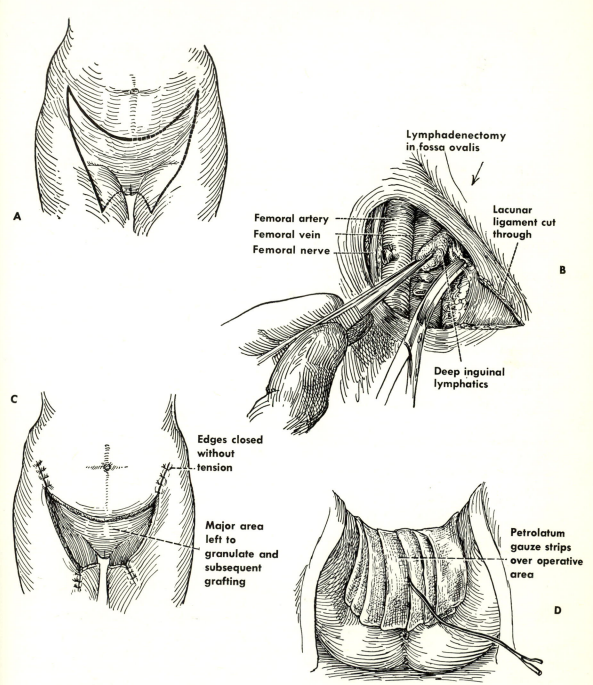

**Lymphadenectomy in fossa ovalis**

**Lacunar ligament cut through**

**Femoral artery**

**Femoral vein**

**Femoral nerve**

**Deep inguinal lymphatics**

A

B

C

**Edges closed without tension**

**Major area left to granulate and subsequent grafting**

**Petrolatum gauze strips over operative area**

D

Fig. 24-18. **A,** Outline of incisional lines for simple or radical operations for vulval cover. **B,** Dissection completed, involving nerves, saphenous veins, and muscles when dissection of distal half of femoral canal has been completed. **C,** Upper edges of abdominal incisions may be partially closed. **D,** With indwelling catheter in bladder, wound is dressed with layers of petrolatum gauze and held in place with light pressure dressing. (From Ball, T. L.: Gynecologic surgery and urology, ed. 2, St. Louis, 1963, The C. V. Mosby Co.)

electrosurgical unit or plain or chromic gut ligatures.

2. Periurethral and perivaginal incisions are made. Bleeding of this vascular area is controlled by means of Kelly or Crile hemostats, ligatures, and sponges on holders. Allis-Adair forceps are used for holding diseased tissues.

3. All skin and subcutaneous tissues are undermined and mobilized, using curved dissecting tissue forceps, scissors, Allis forceps, and sponges on holders.

4. The wound is closed, usually by simple bilateral Z-plasty closure with chromic gut no. 2-0 or 3-0. In some cases, an excision of the skin is made around the anus to accomplish a slide skin flap.

5. Drains or continuous suction sometimes is placed in the dependent areas, an indwelling system of urinary drainage is established, and gauze packing is placed in the vagina. Petrolatum gauze and dressings are applied and held in place with plastic tape and a binder.

## Radical vulvectomy and groin lymphadenectomy

**DEFINITION.** This operation involves abdominal and perineal dissection, which may be performed as a one-stage or two-stage operation.

A mass dissection comprises the following structures: a large segment of skin from the abdomen and groins, the labia majora, labia minora, clitoris, mons pubis, and terminal portions of the urethra, vagina, and other vulvular organs, as well as the superficial and/or deep inguinal nodes, portions of the round ligaments, portions of the saphenous veins, and the lesion itself. It also involves reconstruction of the vaginal walls and pelvic floor and closure of the abdominal wounds (Fig. 24-18). At a later date, placement of full-thickness pinch grafts may be done if the denuded area of the vulva appears too large for normal granulation (Chapter 10).

**SETUP AND PREPARATION OF THE PATIENT.** The patient lies supine and may be placed in the Trendelenburg and lithotomy positions, as required for the various stages. The skin preparation includes both the abdomen and vulva, and the skin of the thighs is usually prepared down to the knees. As in other radical surgery, the nursing team should be prepared to measure blood loss and anticipate procedures to combat shock.

The setups include a basic gynecological abdominal setup, plus additional incisional instruments. A minor vaginal setup is also required.

*For groin lymphadenectomy,* add the following to the basic laparotomy setup (Chapter 17):

**Clamping instruments**
  8 Schnidt gall duct forceps, full curved, right-angled (Chapter 20)
  1 Set silver clips and holders

**Accessory items**
  Drains:
    2 Latex rubber catheters, 14 Fr.
    4 Pieces Penrose tubing, 12 × ⅝ in.
    Petrolatum gauze packing, if desired

*For vulvectomy,* the basic vaginal instrument setup is used, plus the following:

**Exposing instruments**
  2 Richardson retractors, small
  2 Richardson retractors, narrow, long blades
  2 Volkmann rake retractors, 3-pronged, dull

**Accessory items**
  Drains:
    4 Pieces Penrose tubing, 12 × ⅝ in.

**OPERATIVE PROCEDURE**
**FOR GROIN DISSECTION**
**(LYMPHADENECTOMY)**

1. The first skin incision is made on the side opposite the primary lesion. The end of the incised skin is grasped with Allis forceps. The incision is carried down to the aponeuroses of the external oblique muscle.

2. The fascia over the inguinal ligament and the fascia lata of the upper thigh are exposed, separated, and freed, using retractors, knife, scissors, hemostats, and sponges.

3. Bleeding vessels are clamped and ligated, including the superficial iliac artery and vein, the epigastric artery and vein, and the superficial external pudendal artery and vein, using Crile hemostats and ligatures of chromic gut or silk no. 0 or 2-0 (Fig. 24-18, *B*).

4. The fibers of the inguinal, hypogastric, and femoral nerves are resected, using Metzenbaum or Harrington scissors, tissue forceps without teeth, and long-bladed retractors.

5. The lymphatic node beds may be identified with silk or metal clips. Fine, long, sharp dissection scissors are needed.

6. The large tissue surfaces are exposed for complete dissection by means of retractors and protected by warm, wet laparotomy packs. High saphenous vein ligation is performed, using scissors, forceps, hemostats, and chromic gut or silk suture ligatures (Chapter 16).

7. The femoral canal is cleaned of its lymphatics, and the round ligament is clamped, cut, and ligated.

8. The peritoneum is freed from the muscles, fascia is dissected free, deep lymphatic nodes and areolar tissue are removed, and vessels and their attachments are clamped, cut, and ligated, using long curved scissors, long tissue forceps, hemostats, and ligatures.

9. The lesion is removed. In deep pelvic lymphadenectomy, the ureter may be exposed and drained.

10. The inguinal canal is reconstructed, and the wound is partially closed, using chromic gut and silk sutures. An indwelling system of urinary drainage is established, and the wound is dressed (Fig. 24-18, *D*).

FOR VULVECTOMY

1. The skin incisions of the abdomen and thigh join with those for vulvectomy. The incisions in the vulva encircle the urethra.

2. In the vulval dissection, terminal portions of the urethra and vagina, the mons pubis, clitoris, frenulum, prepuce of the clitoris, and Bartholin's and Skene's glands, plus fascial coverings of the vulva, are removed with the specimen.

3. Reconstruction of the vaginal walls and the pelvic floor is completed. An indwelling system of urinary drainage is established, suction drains are placed into the denuded area, the wound is dressed with layers of petrolatum gauze, and a light pressure dressing is applied (Fig. 24-18).

### Vaginal plastic operation (anterior and posterior repair)

DEFINITION. Reconstruction of the vaginal walls, the pelvic floor, and the muscles and fascia of the rectum, urethra, bladder, and perineum.

CONSIDERATIONS. A vaginal repair is done to correct a cystocele and/or rectocele, restore the bladder to its normal position, and strengthen the vagina and the pelvic floor.

A *cystocele* is formed when the portion of the anterior vaginal wall that is between the cervix and the urethra and the base of the bladder adjacent to it herniate inferiorly (Figs. 24-2, 24-3, and 24-9). The hernia of the bladder protrudes through the torn musculofascial components of the vaginal anterior wall, with protrusion into the vaginal outlet. A defect in the anterior vaginal wall is usually caused by trauma or an inherent weakness. A large herniation may cause a sensation of pressure in the vagina or present as a mass at or through the introitus (Fig. 24-19).

A *rectocele* is formed by a herniation of the anterior rectal wall (posterior vaginal wall) into the vaginal outlet. In general, the anterior rectal wall forms a bulging mass beneath the posterior vaginal mucosa (Fig. 24-19). It is created as the mass pushes downward into the lower vaginal canal. The rectum may be torn from its dense connective tissue, the fascial and muscular attachments of the urogenital diaphragm, and the pelvic wall. The levator ani muscles become stretched or torn (Fig. 24-6). The symptomatic signs are a mass protruding from the vagina, difficulty in

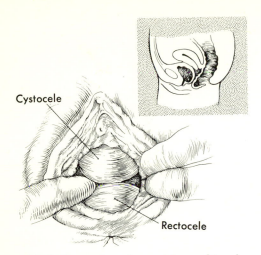

**Fig. 24-19.** Cystocele and rectocele resulting from unrepaired tears of muscles of pelvic floor and those under bladder. Usually following the birth of several infants. (From Crossen, R. J.: Diseases of women, ed. 10, St. Louis, 1953, The C. V. Mosby Co.)

evacuating the lower bowel, and a feeling of pressure.

An *enterocele* is a protrusion of the cul-de-sac of Douglas and some of the pelvic bowel within the peritoneal sac. It pierces through a weakened area between the attenuated anterior rectal and posterior vaginal walls (Fig. 24-22).

An enterocele may also be seen in multiparous women as part of a massive lesion, in which a large sac contains the bladder, lower portions of the ureters, and the prolapsed uterus. In some cases, a Kelly or Marshall-Marchetti operation may be necessary to treat urinary incontinence and uterine prolapse.

During parturition, the outer fibrous layers of the vagina may be torn, thereby permitting the adjoining viscera to herniate into the vaginal outlet. Because of unrepaired perineal lacerations, gradual pulling apart of the underlying fascia and muscles of the pelvic floor and outlet takes place. The woman has symptoms of relaxation and displacement of the pelvic organs. Accidents, gradual deterioration of the tissues, or congenital weakness may

also result in mechanical disturbances of the pelvic structures (Fig. 24-6).

SETUP AND PREPARATION OF THE PATIENT. The patient is anesthetized; positioning is as described for lithotomy (Chapter 7); vaginal preparation, including skin cleansing of the vaginal vault and vulva and draping with sterile sheets, is as described previously. Instruments are as described for major vaginal repair, plus the setup that is described later for uterine dilatation and curettage.

OPERATIVE PROCEDURE

1. Dilatation and curettage may be done.
2. The labia are sewn back, and traction sutures, silk or chromic gut on cutting needles, are placed on the anterior and posterior lips of the cervix. Adair forceps are used to retract the cervix; self-retaining or Sims retractors are used to expose the operative site.

ANTERIOR WALL REPAIR

1. Areolar tissue between the bladder and vagina at the bladder reflection is exposed with the knife handle. The full thickness of the vaginal wall is separated up to the bladder neck, using a knife, curved scissors, tissue forceps, Adair or Allis forceps, and sponges on holders. Bleeding vessels are clamped and tied with ligatures (Fig. 24-20, A).

2. The urethra and bladder neck are freely mobilized, using a knife, gauze sponges, and curved scissors (Fig. 24-20, B).

3. The urethra, bladder neck, and bladder are sutured, using chromic gut sutures no. 2-0. Sutures are placed in such a manner that after they have been tied, there results a double inverting of the tissue, a narrowing of the bladder neck, and a delineating of the posterior urethrovesical angle (Fig. 24-20, C).

4. The connective tissue on the lateral aspects of the cervix is sutured into the cervix with chromic gut no. 2-0 sutures swaged on curved needles. This is done to shorten the cardinal ligaments.

5. Allis forceps are applied to the edges of the incision, and the left flap of the vag-

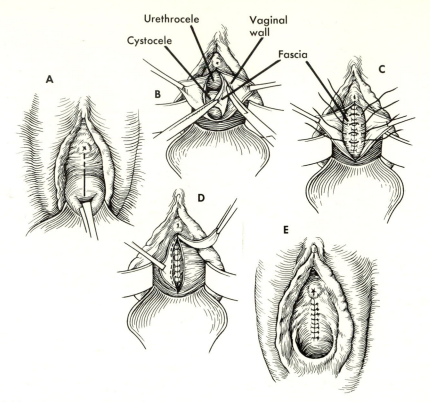

**Fig. 24-20.** Correction of cystourethrocele. **A,** Cervix pulled down as far as possible with tenaculum. Vertical incision made entirely through to vaginal wall. **B,** Vaginal flaps further dissected upward. Urethral meatus and pubocervical fascia separated from vaginal wall with Mayo scissors. **C,** Fascia brought together with continuous surgical chromic suture, beginning at lowest point and ending near external urethral meatus. A few interrupted sutures (chromic gut or silk) placed secondarily. **D,** Excess portion of vaginal wall carefully removed, leaving sufficient amount to be closed with tension. **E,** Completed operation, maintaining bladder and urethra in normal position. (From Counseller, V. S.: In Lowrie, R. J., editor: Gynecology: surgical techniques, Springfield, Ill., 1955, Charles C Thomas, Publisher.)

inal wall is drawn across the midline. Edges are trimmed according to the size of the cystocele (Fig. 24-20, *D*). This process is repeated on the right flap of the vaginal incision. Adair forceps, tissue forceps, and curved scissors are needed.

6. The anterior vaginal wall is closed with interrupted chromic gut no. 2-0 sutures in a manner resulting in reconstruction of an anterior vaginal fornix (Fig. 24-20, *E*).

POSTERIOR WALL REPAIR

1. Allis forceps are placed posteriorly at the mucocutaneous junction on each side, at the hymenal ring, and just above the anus (Fig. 24-21, *A*).

2. Skin and mucosa are incised and dissected from the musculature beneath, using a knife, tissue forceps, curved scissors, and sponges.

3. Allis-Adair forceps are placed on the posterior vaginal wall, scar tissue is removed, and dissection is continued to the posterior vaginal fornix and laterally, depending on the size of the rectocele (Fig. 24-21, *A* and *B*).

4. The perineum is denuded by sharp dissection; the trimming of the posterior vaginal wall is carried out, using Allis forceps, curved scissors, and sponges on holders.

5. The rectal wall proximal to the pu-

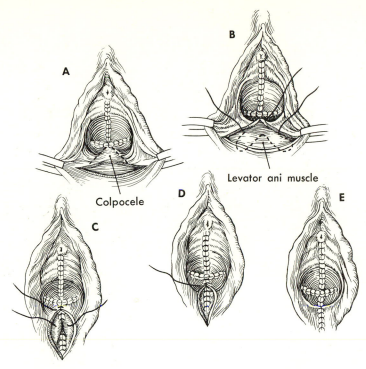

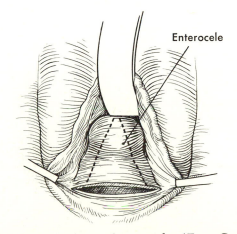

Fig. 24-21. Repair of rectocele. **A,** Exposure of perineum and portion of posterior vaginal wall excised. **B,** Excess skin and excess portion of posterior vaginal wall excised up to vaginal vault. First suture placed in vaginal vault. **C,** Levator ani muscles brought together with interrupted stitches; Colles' fascia brought together over perineum. **D,** Perineum restored and Colles' fascia repaired with interrupted sutures. **E,** Skin of perineum closed. (From Counseller, V. S.: In Lowrie, R. J., editor: Gynecology: surgical techniques, Springfield, Ill., 1955, Charles C Thomas, Publisher.)

borectal muscle is strengthened by insertion of chromic gut nos. 0 and 2-0 sutures (Fig. 24-21, *C*).

6. Bleeding is controlled, and the vaginal wall is closed from above downward to the anterior edge of the puborectal muscle, using interrupted chromic gut no. 0 sutures. The rectocele is repaired from the posterior fornix to the perineal body (Fig. 24-21, *D* and *E*). Remains of the transverse perineal and bulbocavernous muscles are used to build up the perineum. The anterior edge of the levator ani sling may be approximated.

7. The mucosa and skin are trimmed, and the remaining closure is effected by interrupted sutures. The skin is closed with subcuticular sutures, chromic gut no. 2-0.

Fig. 24-22. Exposure of enterocele. (From Counseller, V. S.: In Lowrie, R. J., editor: Gynecology: surgical techniques, Springfield, Ill., 1955, Charles C Thomas, Publisher.)

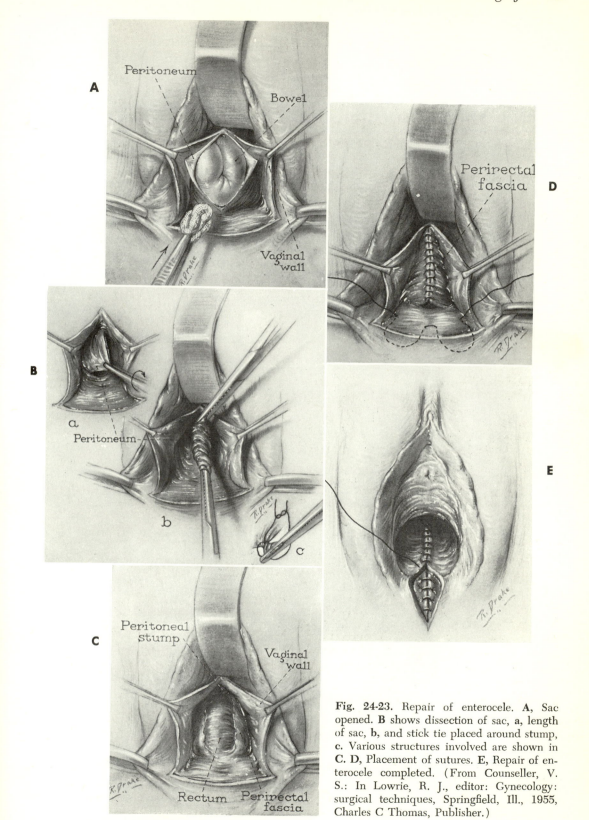

**Fig. 24-23.** Repair of enterocele. **A,** Sac opened. **B** shows dissection of sac, **a,** length of sac, **b,** and stick tie placed around stump, **c.** Various structures involved are shown in **C. D,** Placement of sutures. **E,** Repair of enterocele completed. (From Counseller, V. S.: In Lowrie, R. J., editor: Gynecology: surgical techniques, Springfield, Ill., 1955, Charles C Thomas, Publisher.)

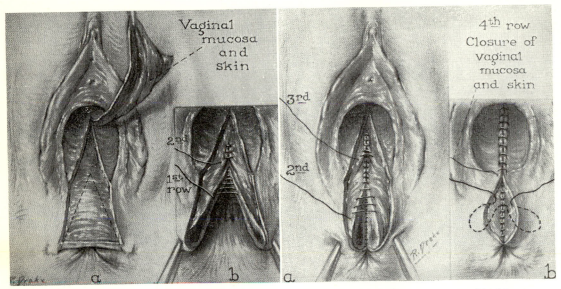

**Fig. 24-24.** Repair of complete lacerations of the perineum. **A** shows lower margins of incision, **a,** and placement of first and second rows of sutures, **b. B** shows second and third rows of sutures, **a,** and fourth row of sutures, **b.** (From Counseller, V. S.: In Lowrie, R. J., editor: Gynecology: surgical techniques, Springfield, Ill., 1955, Charles C Thomas, Publisher.)

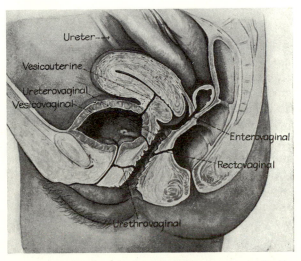

**Fig. 24-25.** Types of genital fistulas. Urogenital fistula is communication between urethra, bladder, or one of ureters and some part of genital tract. Urethrovaginal, vesicovaginal, or ureterovaginal fistulas, most common types, empty into vaginal canal. (From Huffman, J. W.: Gynecology and obstetrics, Philadelphia, 1962, W. B. Saunders Co.)

8. The vagina is packed with 2-inch vaginal packing. An indwelling urinary drainage system is established. A perineal pad may be applied to the wound and held in place by means of a perineal binder.

### Enterocele repair

Setup is as described for anterior and posterior repair; the procedure is illustrated in Figs. 24-22 and 24-23.

### Perineal repair

See basic vaginal setup; the procedure is illustrated in Fig. 24-24.

### Vesicovaginal fistula repair

**DEFINITION.** Through the vaginal outlet, the mocosal tissue of the anterior vaginal wall is dissected free, the opening from the bladder into the vagina is closed, the fascial attachments between the bladder and vagina are repaired, and temporary drainage is established (Fig. 24-25).

**CONSIDERATIONS.** The fistulas vary in size from a small opening that permits only slight leakage of urine into the vagina to a large opening that permits all urine to pass into the vagina (Fig. 24-25).

Fistulas may result from radical surgery in the management of pelvic cancer, from radium therapy without surgery, from chronic ulceration of the vaginal structures, from penetrating wounds, or from childbirth.

A *urethrovaginal fistula* usually causes constant incontinence or difficulty in retaining urine (Chapter 12). This condition occurs after damage to the anterior wall and bladder or following radiation surgery or parturition. A *ureterovaginal fistula* develops as a reult of injury to the ureter. In some cases, reimplantation of the ureter in the bladder or ureterostomy may be done (Chapter 12).

### Vaginal approach

**SETUP AND PREPARATION OF THE PATIENT.** Setup and preparation is as described for vaginal plastic repair, adding the following items:

1 Kelly fistula scissors
1 Adson dressing forceps, 7⅛ in.
2 Probes, pliable
1 Frazier suction set
2 Hooks, fine and blunt
2 Ureteral catheters
1 Robinson or Foley indwelling catheter
1 Asepto syringe, 2 oz.
1 Electrosurgical unit and attachments
2 Tubes petrolatum gauze dressings, if desired
  Distilled sterile water, if desired

**OPERATIVE PROCEDURE**

1. Traction sutures are placed about the fistulous tract; tissues are grasped with Adair forceps and plain tissue forceps.

2. The scar tissue about the fistula is excised, cleavage between bladder and vagina is located, and clean flaps are mobilized, using scissors, forceps, and sponges.

3. The bladder mucosa is inverted toward the interior of the bladder with interrupted sutures of chromic gut no. 4-0 swaged to fine curved needles held with a Mayo needle holder and tissue forceps. The suture is passed through the muscularis of the bladder down to the mucosa.

4. A second layer of inverting sutures is placed in the bladder and tied, thereby completely inverting the bladder mucosa toward the interior.

5. The vaginal wall is closed with interrupted chromic gut sutures in the direction opposite to the closure of the bladder wall.

6. The bladder is distended with distilled sterile water to determine any leaks. A catheter is left in the bladder; dressings are applied and held in place with a nonirritating plastic tape and a binder.

### Transperitoneal approach

**DEFINITION.** Through a suprapubic incision, the opening from the bladder into the vagina is closed, and the fascial attachments are repaired.

**SETUP AND PREPARATION OF THE PATIENT.** The patient is placed in slight Trendelenburg position (Chapter 7). Ureteral catheters may be introduced just prior to

surgery (Chapter 12). The vagina is cleansed and packed with moist gauze saturated with an antibiotic or antiseptic solution. The abdominal operative site is cleansed and the patient draped.

The instrument setup required, as described for laparotomy (Chapter 17).

**OPERATIVE PROCEDURE**

1. A median abdominal incision is usually made, as described for laparotomy (Chapter 17).

2. The fistulous tract is identified; the vaginal vault and the adjacent adherent bladder are separated with scissors, forceps, and sponges.

3. The vesicovaginal septum is dissected down to the healthy tissue beyond the site of the fistula.

4. The fistulous tract is mobilized. The bladder site of the fistula is inverted into the interior of the bladder with two rows of inverting sutures of chromic gut no. 4-0. The muscularis and mucosa layers of the vagina are inverted into the vaginal vault by means of two rows of sutures.

5. The flaps of peritoneum are mobilized, both from the bladder and from the adjacent vaginal vault, and are closed to form a new vesicovaginal reflection of peritoneum below the site of the old fistulous tract.

6. The wound is closed in layers, as for laparotomy. Dressings are applied and held in place with adhesive or plastic tape, and an indwelling catheter is left in the bladder.

### Rectovaginal fistula repair
#### *Vaginal approach*

**DEFINITION.** Vaginal repair of the perineum, fascia, and muscle-supporting structures between the rectum and vagina, thereby closing the fistula formed between the rectum and the vagina.

A *rectovaginal fistula* occurs between the rectum and the vagina (Fig. 24-26). In the presence of a large rectovaginal fistula in patients who suffer from incurable

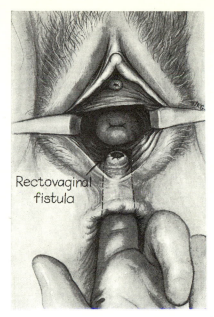

**Fig. 24-26.** Rectovaginal fistula. Examiner's finger puts tension on rectovaginal septum. (From Huffman, J. W.: Gynecology and obstetrics, Philadelphia, 1962, W. B. Saunders Co.)

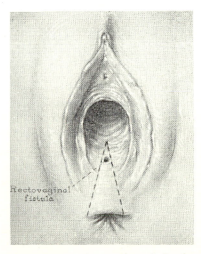

**Fig. 24-27.** Repair of rectovaginal fistulas of all types essentially same as shown here. Rectovaginal fistula; portion of scar tissue to be excised is included in dotted line; repair, as for complete lacerations of perineum (Fig. 24-24). (From Counseller, V. S.: In Lowrie, R. J., editor: Gynecology: surgical techniques, Springfield, Ill., 1955, Charles C Thomas, Publisher.)

cancer, a colostomy may be done (Chapter 22).

SETUP AND PREPARATION OF THE PATIENT. The patient is placed in the lithotomy position and prepared as described for vaginal repair. The instruments and other items needed are as for vaginal plastic repair.

OPERATIVE PROCEDURE

1. The scar tissue and tract between the rectum and vagina are excised; edges of fresh tissue are approximated with sutures of chromic gut no. 4-0 (Fig. 24-27).

2. The rectum and vaginal walls are mobilized; the rectum is closed with inversion of the mucosa into the rectal canal.

3. The vagina is closed transversely or in a sagittal plane different from that of the rectal canal; the vaginal mucosal layer is inverted into the vaginal wall; an indwelling urinary drainage system is established; and dressings are applied to the wound.

## Operations for urinary stress incontinence

DEFINITION. Through a vaginal or abdominal approach, the fascial supports and the pubococcygeal muscle surrounding the urethra and the bladder neck are repaired (Fig. 24-6).

CONSIDERATIONS. Normal micturition depends on a finely coordinated group of voluntary and involuntary movements. As a result of volitional impulses, voiding may be inhibited or stopped by contraction of the perineal and periurethral musculofascial structures (Chapter 12).

The type of operation selected depends on the severity of stress incontinence, the extent of the lesion causing it, the patient's ability to use the anatomical mechanism for voluntary inhibition of urination, and the operations that have already been performed for correcting it. Stages of stress incontinence are classified in relation to frequency and degree of incontinence, the presence of other diseases, and the function of the pubococcygeus muscle (levator ani) (Figs. 24-3 and 24-6).

The aim of any operation for urinary stress incontinence is to improve the performance of a dislodged or exhausted bladder neck. The surgeon endeavors to restore or reconstruct the supporting structures, the operation thereby resulting in the effective closure of the bladder neck.

Previous pelvic operations may have resulted in scarring and distortion, with displacement of the bladder neck to an unfavorable position for proper functioning. Conditions such as uterine prolapse, cystocele, urethrocele, cystourethrocele, or urogenital fistulas following radiation therapy may be associated with stress incontinence.

SETUP AND PREPARATION OF THE PATIENT. *For vaginal approach,* as described for vaginal plastic repair. *For partial vaginal vesicourethrolysis and plication,* as described for anterior and posterior vaginal repair. *For combined vaginal and abdominal approach,* as described for anterior vaginal plastic repair and for suprapubic cystectomy (Chapter 12).

OPERATIVE PROCEDURE

FOR VAGINAL APPROACH

1. A Foley catheter is passed into the bladder. The posterior vaginal wall is retracted, and an incision is made through the anterior vaginal wall down to the urethra and bladder.

2. The vaginal wall is dissected from the bladder and urethra; the neck of the bladder is sutured together with fine chromic gut. The wound is closed, as described for vaginal repair.

FOR VESICOURETHRAL SUSPENSION (see Marshall-Marchetti procedure, p. 446)

1. Through a suprapubic abdominal incision, the space of Retzius is entered, and the bladder and urethra are freed from the surrounding structures.

2. Mattress chromic gut sutures no. 1 or Mersilene no. 0 are inserted through the supporting fascia of the vaginal wall on either side of the urethra and bladder neck; they are then passed through the muscle associated with the symphysis pubis, there-

by providing support to the urethra and bladder neck (Figs. 24-2 and 24-3).

3. Additional sutures are introduced in the lower and lateral portions of the bladder wall and are attached to the posterior portion of the rectus muscles, thereby pulling the bladder anteriorly to obliterate the space of Retzius.

4. The wound is closed and may be drained with a Penrose drain (Chapter 17).

## Excision of fibroma of the vagina

DEFINITION. Through a transverse or longitudinal incision of the wall of the vagina, the lesion is removed.

CONSIDERATIONS. Small cysts or small benign tumors that distort the vagina or those that are ulcerated and infected are treated surgically.

SETUP AND PREPARATION OF THE PATIENT. As described for simple vaginal surgery, plus six Halsted hemostats.

OPERATIVE PROCEDURE

1. The vaginal vault is retracted, using lateral and Sims retractors. Traction sutures of chromic gut no. 0 or silk no. 2-0 are placed on each side of the tumor. The posterior lip of the cervix is grasped with a Jacobs vulsellum forceps and drawn anteriorly to expose the operative site.

2. The vaginal wall is incised, and the edges are grasped with traction sutures on curved, taper point needles or with Allis forceps.

3. The base and its capsule are excised, using a knife and curved scissors; bleeding vessels are clamped and ligated, using Halsted forceps and fine sutures.

4. The vaginal incision is closed with interrupted sutures of chromic gut no. 2-0, and dressings are applied.

## Construction of vagina

DEFINITION. This operation involves two or more stages: the taking of a skin graft and vaginal reconstruction to repair or overcome a congenital or surgical defect.

SETUP AND PREPARATION OF THE PATIENT. The patient is placed in the lithotomy position. The instrument setups include the following:

FOR SKIN GRAFTING (Chapter 10)

Cutting instruments

1 Mayo scissors, straight, 6¼ in.
1 Skin-grafting set
2 Iris scissors, 1 straight and 1 curved

Holding instruments

2 Fixation forceps

Clamping instruments

12 Halsted mosquito hemostats, 5 in., 6 curved and 6 straight

Accessory items

Metal or plastic slab for spreading and handling skin
Xeroform gauze dressing
1 Fenestrated sheet
1 Vaginal supply pack

FOR VAGINAL CONSTRUCTION. The vaginal plastic setup and dilatation and curettage setup are used, plus the following:

Cutting instruments

2 Iris scissors, 1 straight and 1 curved

Holding instruments

2 Fixation forceps
2 Skin hooks

Clamping instruments

6 Halsted mosquito hemostats, 5 in., 6 straight and 6 curved

Exposing instruments

2 Kocher appendectomy retractors, right-angled, 2 in. blade
2 Pryor-Pean retractors, right-angled, 4 in. blade

Suturing instruments

2 Crile-Wood needle holders, fine
Fine chromic, silk, or Dacron sutures, as desired

Accessory items

Metal ruler
Dental compound, approximately 18 units, or other substance, as requested

OPERATIVE PROCEDURE

1. Skin is taken from the abdomen or anterior thighs. The donor sites are dressed in the routine manner with pressure dressings over nonadhesive gauze.

2. A vaginal orifice is created by sharp dissection, and a molding is made of dental compound or plastic shaped to size. Donor skin is sutured over the mold, and the mold is secured in the vaginal opening with sutures and pressure dressings.

## Trachelorrhaphy

**DEFINITION.** Removal of torn surfaces of the anterior and posterior cervical lips and reconstruction of the cervical canal.

**CONSIDERATIONS.** Trachelorrhaphy is done to treat deep lacerations of a cervix (1) that is relatively free of infection and (2) in women past the childbearing age.

**SETUP AND PREPARATION OF THE PATIENT.** As described for plastic vaginal repair and electrosurgical unit with cone-type electrode, if desired.

**OPERATIVE PROCEDURE**

1. The labia are retracted with Allis-Adair forceps or sutures. The cervix is grasped with a Jacobs vulsellum forceps.

2. The infected tissue of the exocervix is denuded with a knife. The flaps are undermined by means of a knife and curved scissors. Bleeding vessels are clamped and ligated. The mucosa is dissected from the cervix.

3. A small distal portion of the cervical canal is coned to remove infected tissue by means of a knife. Bleeding vessels are clamped and ligated with chromic gut no. 2-0 ligatures.

4. The denuded and coned areas are covered by suturing the mucosal flaps of the exocervix transversely, using six to eight interrupted chromic gut no. 0 sutures swaged to ½-circle, trocar-point needles. Tissue forceps, hemostats, and sponges on holders are needed. The sutures are placed in such a manner that the fibromuscular tissue of the cervix is included, thereby eliminating dead space where a hematoma may form and providing a complete reconstructed cervical canal.

5. The wound is cleansed, and dressings are applied and held in place with a binder.

A retention catheter may be introduced in the bladder.

## Removal of pedunculated cervical myoma

**DEFINITION.** Removal of the tumor by the snare method or by dissection from the cervical canal with a knife or with cold-knife conization.

**CONSIDERATIONS.** Cervical polyps (small pedunculated lesions) stem from the endocervical canal and consist almost entirely of columnar epithelium with or without squamous metaplasia. They may vary in size and are soft, red, and friable. Bleeding may result from the slightest trauma. Usually, the surgeon performs an endometrial and endocervical curettage, and a cytological smear is taken.

**SETUP AND PREPARATION OF THE PATIENT.** As described for dilatation and curettage, adding a tonsil snare and medium snare wire, smear slides, and an electrosurgical unit, including pencil knife.

**OPERATIVE PROCEDURE**

1. The anterior lip of the cervix is grasped with a Jacobs vulsellum forceps. The canal is sounded and dilated to either visualize or palpate the base of the pedicle.

2. If the pedicle of the tumor is thin, a tonsil snare may be placed over the body of the tumor, permitting the snare to crush the base of the tumor and to control bleeding. If the tumor is large, its base is dissected out with a knife. Bleeding is controlled by the use of warm, moistened gauze sponges on holders.

3. Retractors are withdrawn; vaginal packing may be introduced into the cervical canal. The tenaculum is removed from the cervix, and a dressing applied and held in place with a binder.

## Amputation of the cervix

**DEFINITION.** Removal of a portion of the portio vaginalis of the cervix.

**CONSIDERATIONS.** A cervical amputation, without repair of the pelvic floor, is usually done in the presence of an intraepi-

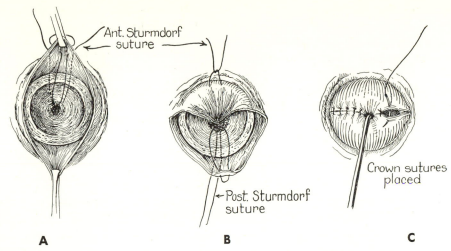

**Fig. 24-28.** Amputation of portion of cervix. **A,** Anterior Sturmdorf suture placed. **B,** Anterior suture tied and posterior suture inserted. **C,** Flaps of vaginal wall closed by interrupted sutures. (From Ball, T. L.: Gynecologic surgery and urology, ed. 2, St. Louis, 1963, The C. V. Mosby Co.)

thelial cancer, with preservation of the remainder of the female genital organs. In specific cases such as mycotic or venereal infections of the cervix, this may be done by excision of the cervix.

SETUP AND PREPARATION OF THE PATIENT. As described for anterior vaginal repair and dilatation and curettage.

OPERATIVE PROCEDURE

1. A dilatation and curettage may be performed before excision of the cervix.

2. The labia are retracted; the cervix is grasped with a Jacobs tenaculum and drawn sharply downward.

3. A circular incision is made through the full thickness of the vaginal wall by means of a knife. The distal end of each cardinal ligament is clamped, cut, and ligated, using Heaney clamps, long curved Ochsner forceps, scissors, and chromic gut no. 0 ligatures.

4. A portion of the portio vaginalis of the cervix is amputated by an oblique circular incision; the canal is coned, using a knife. Bleeding vessels are clamped and ligated with chromic gut no. 0 ligatures.

5. Anterior and posterior Sturmdorf sutures of chromic gut no. 0 and no. 2-0

on ½-circle, trocar-point needles are placed (Fig. 24-28). Bleeding vessels are clamped and ligated.

6. The vaginal wall flaps are approximated, covering the denuded cervix by means of six to eight interrupted chromic gut nos. 2-0 and 0 sutures swaged to ½-circle, taper point needles. The patency of the cervical canal is tested, using a sound; urinary drainage may or may not be established; vaginal dressings are applied and held in place with nonirritating plastic tape and a binder.

## Dilatation of the cervix and curettage

DEFINITION. Introduction of instruments through the vagina into the cervical canal and then into the uterus and, in some cases, removal of substances and blood.

CONSIDERATIONS. This operation is done either for diagnostic purposes or as a form of therapy for a variety of pelvic conditions such as incomplete abortion, abnormal uterine bleeding, or primary dysmenorrhea. Dilatation and curettage may be performed when carcinoma of the endometrium is suspected, in the study of infertility, or prior to amputation of the cer-

vix or an operation for prolapse of the uterus.

**SETUP AND PREPARATION OF THE PATIENT.** The lithotomy position, skin preparation, and draping of the patient are as described for vaginal plastic surgery. The instrument setup includes the following items:

**Exposing instruments** (Figs. 24-13 and 24-14)

1 Auvard vaginal speculum, if desired
2 Jackson and Eastman retractors
1 Uterine sound
1 Set Hegar or Hank dilators
1 Goodell uterine dilator

**Holding instruments** (Fig. 24-11)

2 Barrett tenaculi
1 Jacobs vulsellum forceps
2 Foerster sponge-holding forceps
2 Backhaus towel forceps
1 Boseman uterine forceps
2 Allis forceps
1 Tissue forceps, plain, 7¼ in.
2 Fletcher-Van Doren polyp forceps
1 Tissue forceps, 1 and 2 teeth, 5½ in.

**Cutting instruments** (Fig. 24-12)

1 Bard-Parker knife handle no. 3 with blade no. 10
2 Scissors, 1 curved and 1 straight
1 Set Sims uterine curettes, sharp
1 Set Thomas uterine curettes, blunt
1 Gaylor biopsy forceps

**Clamping instruments**

2 Crile hemostats
2 Mayo-Pean hemostats

**Suturing instruments**

1 Needle holder
1 Suture, chromic gut no. 0 or 1 on an appropriate needle

**Accessory items**

1 Specimen container
  Vaginal packing as desired
1 Ampul muscular action drug if desired
1 Urethral catheter if desired

**OPERATIVE PROCEDURE**

1. A Kelly or Auvard retractor is placed posteriorly in the vagina. A Sims or Kelly retractor is placed anteriorly to expose

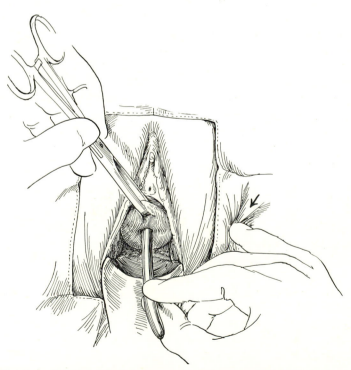

**Fig. 24-29.** Dilatation of cervix and curettage. Vaginal wall retracted; cervix held by tenaculum; cervix dilated with a dilator. Uterine cavity is curetted with sharp curettes. (From Ball, T. L.: Gynecologic surgery and urology, ed. 2, St. Louis, 1962, The C. V. Mosby Co.)

the cervix. The anterior lip of the cervix is grasped with a tenaculum (Fig. 24-29).

2. The direction of the cervical canal and the depth of the uterine cavity are determined by means of a blunt probe or graduated pliable uterine sound.

3. The cervix is gradually dilated by means of graduated Hegar or Hank dilators and a Goodell uterine dilator.

4. Exploration for pedunculated polyps or myomas may be done, using a polyp forceps.

5. The interior of the cervical canal and the cavity of the uterus are curetted to obtain either a fractional or a routine specimen. For specific identification of the site of specimens, the endocervix is scraped with the curette first, and the specimen is separated from the curettings of the uterine endometrium. In a routine curettage, all curettings are sent together for identification of tissue cells.

6. Fragments of endometrium or other dislodged tissues are removed with warm, wet gauze sponges on holders.

7. Multiple punch biopsies of the cervical circumference (at 12, 3, 6, and 9 o'clock) may be taken with the Gaylor biopsy forceps to supplement the diagnostic workup.

8. Retractors are withdrawn; packing of iodoform or plain gauze secured to dressing forceps may be inserted into the cavity. The tenaculum is removed from the cervix. A perineal pad is applied.

## Uterine aspiration

**DEFINITION.** Vacuum aspiration of the contents of the uterus.

**CONSIDERATIONS.** Aspiration has proved to be a safe and effective method for early termination of pregnancy and for use in missed and incomplete abortions. Advantages are smaller dilatation of the cervix, less damage to the uterus, less blood loss, less chance of uterine perforation, and reduced danger of infection.

**SETUP AND PREPARATION OF THE PATIENT.** The patient is placed in the lithotomy position. A general anesthetic is used. An

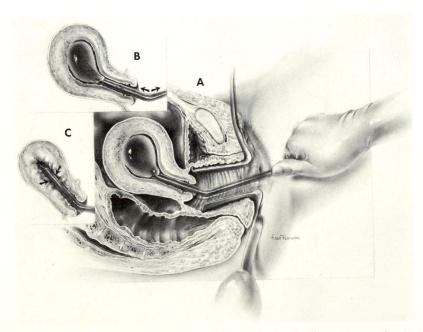

Fig. 24-30. Uterine aspiration. **A,** Insertion of the cannula. **B,** Gentle suction motion to aspirate contents. **C,** Uterus evacuated. (From Eaton, C. J.: Technic of uterine aspiration, Berkeley, Calif., 1969, Bio-Engineering, Inc.)

external and internal vaginal prep is done. The setup includes the following:

Dilatation and currettage set
Reliable controlled suction apparatus
Vacuum aspirator
Sterile cannulas and aspirating tubing
Sterile surgical gel
Oxytocic drugs available

### OPERATIVE PROCEDURE

1. The cervix is exposed using an Auvard weighted speculum and an anterior retractor; then the cervix is grasped with a sharp tenaculum and drawn toward the introitus (Fig. 24-30).

2. The cervix is dilated in the routine manner, allowing 1 mm. of cannula diameter for each week of pregnancy.

3. The appropriate sized cannula is then inserted into the uterus until the sac is encountered. The vacuum is turned on with immediate disruption and aspiration of the contents. Continued gentle motion of the cannula will remove the entire uterine content (Fig. 24-30).

4. Depending on the diagnosis, conventional curettage may then be employed.

5. Retractors and tenaculum are withdrawn; a perineal pad is applied.

6. The specimen is contained in the vacuum bottle, from which it is removed for laboratory examination.

### Shirodkar operation (postconceptional)

**DEFINITION.** Placement of a collar-type ligature or other material at the level of the internal os to close it (Fig. 24-31).

**CONSIDERATIONS.** Incompetence of the cervix is a condition characterized by habitual midtrimester spontaneous abortions. The operation is designed to prevent

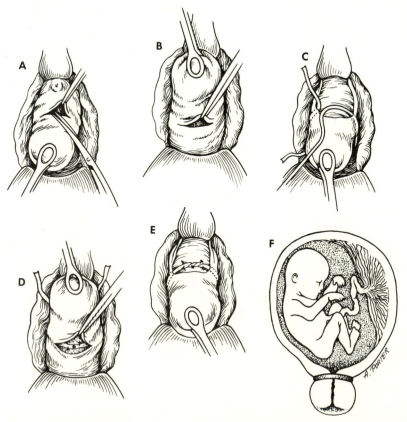

**Fig. 24-31.** Principles of Shirodkar operation for treatment of incompetent internal cervical os during pregnancy. (From Taylor, E. S.: Essentials of gynecology, ed. 2, Philadelphia, 1962, Lea & Febiger.)

the cervical dilatation that results in release of uterine contents.

**SETUP AND PREPARATION OF THE PATIENT.** The lithotomy position is used, and gentle vaginal preparation is carried out. The instrument setup includes the basic vaginal setup, using a few hemostats, and adding the following:

1 Short fine needle holder
2 Ligature carriers
1 Basic needle set
2 Trocar needles
Sutures: heavy Dacron, Mersilene, silk, or chromic (as desired)

**OPERATIVE PROCEDURE**

1. Anterior and posterior vaginal retractors are placed, and the cervix is pulled down with smooth ovum or sponge forceps. With thumb forceps and dissecting scissors, the mucosa over the anterior cervix is opened to permit the bladder to be pushed back (Fig. 24-31).

2. The cervix is lifted, and the posterior vaginal mucosa is similarly incised at the level of the peritoneal reflection. With ligature carriers, the lateral mucosa is tunneled on either side.

3. The prepared ligature is placed at the desired level and anchored posteriorly with silk suture, drawn tight in front to close the cervix. The suture is tied.

4. The collar ligature is anchored with silk sutures anteriorly. The anterior and posterior mucosal incisions are closed with chromic sutures no. 0 or 2-0 to complete the procedure.

## Conization and biopsy of the cervix

**DEFINITION.** Removal of diseased cervical tissue to treat strictures of the cervix and chronic cervicitis (Fig. 24-32). The conization may be performed either by scalpel resection and suturing or by the application of cutting electrosurgical current with an active electrode inserted into the cervical canal.

**CONSIDERATIONS.** Endometrial biopsy is done to determine the menstrual phase and carry out histological study of the endometrium. Scalpel conizations are done for diagnostic purposes, such as when a patient has a positive Papanicolaou (Pap) smear. Conization of the cervix may be done in some cases in which hysterectomy

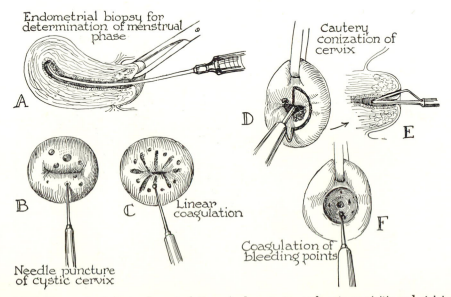

**Fig. 24-32.** Removal of diseased cervical tissue is done to treat chronic cervicitis and strictures of the cervix or to obtain an endometrial specimen for diagnostic tests. (From Ball, T. L.: Gynecologic surgery and urology, ed. 2, St. Louis, 1963, The C. V. Mosby Co.)

is indicated and in which benign disease of the cervix is present. It may also be done in those cases in which total hysterectomy is not feasible.

SETUP AND PREPARATION OF THE PATIENT. As described for vaginal surgery. The instruments include a dilatation and curettage set, minor vaginal set, 1 ml. syringe, curved metal cannula, and the appropriate scalpel and blade or an electrosurgical unit with conization and ball tip electrodes.

OPERATIVE PROCEDURE

1. The posterior vaginal wall is retracted by a speculum and the anterior vaginal wall by lateral retractors. The outer portions of the cervix are grasped with a tenaculum, and the cervix is drawn toward the introitus; then the anterior speculum is removed (Fig. 24-32). Cystic cervix may be treated with a needle electrode (Fig. 24-32, *B* and *C*). Endometrial biopsy may be done (Fig. 24-32, *A*). Bleeding points may be coagulated (Fig. 24-32, *F*).

2. For cauterization the electrode is passed into the cervical canal, and the diseased membrane is removed (Fig. 24-32, *E*).

3. The cervical canal is cleansed with an antiseptic solution. If a wide conization is performed, the cervix may be sutured.

### Radium insertion for cervical malignancy

DEFINITION. Insertion of radium into the cervix. The procedure may be accomplished with x-ray film control to ensure accurate placement of the radium. Precautions to protect personnel from undue ex-

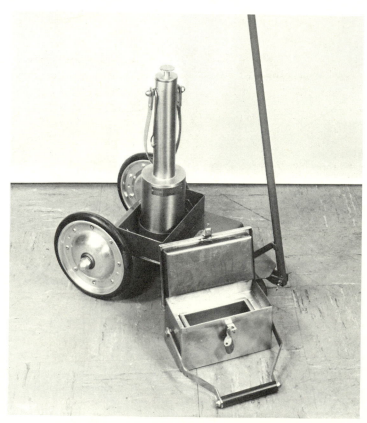

Fig. 24-33. Radium transport cart and carrying box for loaded radium applicators. Conductive rubber wheels of cart enable loaded applicators to be carried from preparation area to operating room. Short-handled case, which is Monel covered and fitted with lock, may be lifted to treatment table area. (Courtesy Radium Chemical Co., Inc., New York, N. Y.)

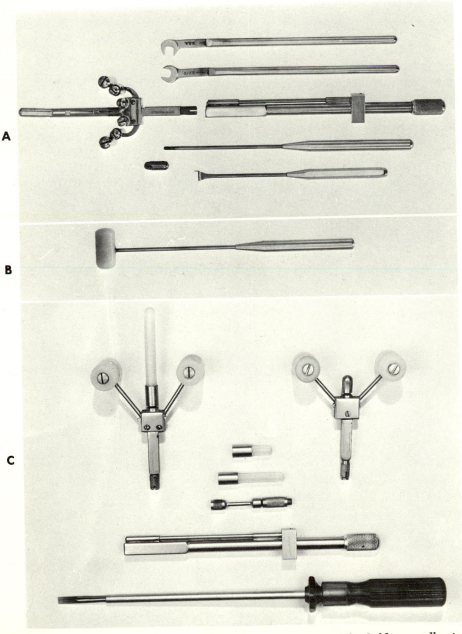

**Fig. 24-34. A,** Ernst applicator set, including standard applicator for holding needles in sections, handle for removing Ernst applicator, screwdriver for caps, and wrenches for closing tandem. **B,** London colpostat. **C,** Ter-Pogossian cervical radium applicator set. (Courtesy Radium Chemical Co., Inc., New York, N. Y.)

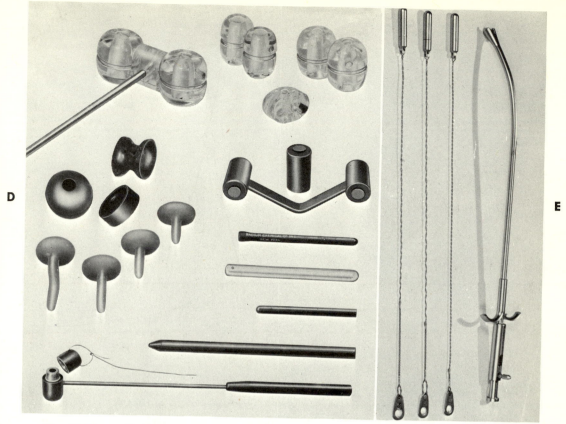

**Fig. 24-34, cont'd. D,** Various types and sizes of cervical applicators and intrauterine sounds. Top: Hankins and Hockin Lucite ovoids. Middle left: Various sizes of Manchester rubber tandems and ovoids. Middle right: Kaplan rubber colpostat, other types of rubber and flexible plastic (Raflex) tandems, and intrauterine sounds. Bottom: Applicator attached to screw handle. **E,** Campbell-type Heyman fundus applicator set, which consists of twelve numbered stainless steel capsules and inserter. (Courtesy Radium Chemical Co., Inc., New York, N. Y.)

posure are taken, and the procedure is monitored by the radiology department (Fig. 24-33).

**SETUP AND PREPARATION OF THE PATIENT.** As described for vaginal surgery. Aseptic technique must be maintained. Long-handled instruments, lead screens, and protectors are used when loading the applicators. Radium insertion instruments are shown in Figs. 24-34 and 24-35.

FOR RADIUM INSERTION FOR CERVIX. Dilatation and curettage set, plus the following:

**Holding instruments**

1 Cross-action thumb forceps
1 Needle-handling forceps, long, straight
1 Thumb forceps, long

**Exposing instruments**

2 Deaver retractors, narrow
2 Pryor-Pean retractors, right-angled (optional)

**Accessory items**

2 Ernst applicators and inserters
2 Ernst screwdrivers
1 Ernst extractor
2 Wrenches
2 Screws with wing nuts
Plastic sleeves and culpostat covers
Rubber tandems
Manchester ovoids, desired type

*Drains*

1 Foley urethral catheter, 16 Fr. with 5 ml. bag
1 Rectal tube, 24 Fr.

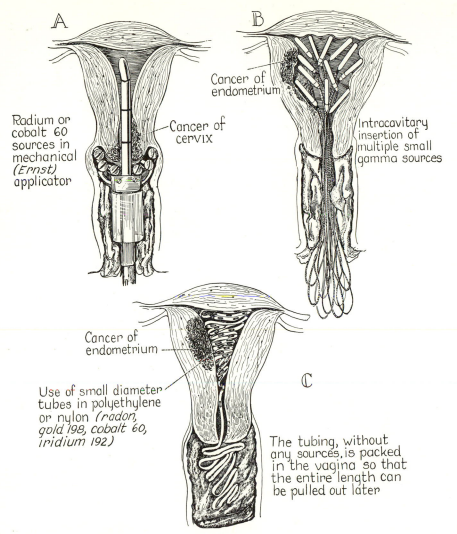

Fig. 24-35. **A,** Ernst applicator consists of central tandem divided in sections, in which gamma sources are placed. One to three can be placed in uterine cavity, depending on length of cavity. Three mechanically operated metal tubes are available on each side of central tandem. They are placed perpendicular to axis of cervical canal and mechanically spread for radiation of parametrium and pelvic side wall. **B,** Methods of intracavitary radiation of lesions of uterine fundus. **C,** Methods of intracavitary radiation for uterine lesions, utilizing polyethylene or nylon tubing as containers for small gamma sources. (From Ball, T. L.: Gynecologic surgery and urology, ed. 2, St. Louis, 1963, The C. V. Mosby Co.)

**Suturing items**

Sutures:

2 Plain gut, no. 2-0 swaged to ½-circle, trocar-point needles, medium-sized

2 Chromic, no. 2-0, swaged to ½-circle, cutting-edge needles, medium-sized

2 Chromic, no. 0, swaged to ⅜-circle, cutting-edge needles, large-sized

FOR RADIUM INSERTION FOR ENDOMETRIAL MALIGNANCY. As described for cervical malignancy, except that Ernst applicators are omitted and the following items are added:

Ernst appliances (Fig. 24-34)
Campbell-type Heyman capsules (Fig. 24-34)
Capsule holder
Intubating forceps

OPERATIVE PROCEDURE. The bladder is identified and decompressed by inserting a Foley catheter. The Foley bag is inflated with a radiopaque medium such as Conray for visualization. The patient is placed on an x-ray table or operating table with a cassette, and radium is inserted (Fig. 24-35).

FOR INTERSTITIAL THERAPY. Radium and cobalt ($Co^{60}$) needles are available in various lengths with a small diameter for insertion into the tissue surrounding the cervix. They are inserted vaginally with a needle applicator and are used as a supplement to intravaginal or intrauterine sources. To facilitate removal, the needles have wires or threads attached to their distal end.

## Culdoscopy

DEFINITION. Visualization of pelvic structures through a tubular instrument similar to a cystoscope, which is introduced through a small incision in the posterior vaginal cul-de-sac.

CONSIDERATIONS. Culdoscopy is a diagnostic procedure. Direct observation of the passage of dye from the uterus through the fimbriated ends of the tube is possible with the culdoscope to help determine infertility, tubal patency, the presence of ectopic pregnancy, unexplained abdominal or pelvic pain, and the nature of pelvic masses and to evaluate normal functioning of the genital tract (Fig. 24-8). This examination may enable the surgeon to avoid unnecessary pelvic surgery. The laparoscopy is the preferred procedure today (p. 845).

SETUP AND PREPARATION OF THE PATIENT. The patient is prepared as for vaginal operation. A local or regional anesthetic may be employed. When a general anesthetic is administered, the patient is intubated. The patient is usually placed in a knee-chest position, kneeling on the footboard with a kneestrap around the thighs, the chest supported on pillows, and the arms comfortably flexed above the head (Chapter 7). Instruments may

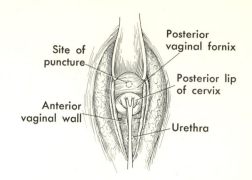

Fig. 24-36. Culdoscopy. View of vagina, with patient in knee-chest position showing site of puncture. (From TeLinde, R. W.: Operative gynecology, ed. 3, Philadelphia, 1962, J. B. Lippincott Co.)

be placed on a small accessory table; the surgeon may serve himself and require no assistance. A nurse carries out the circulating nursing duties. The instrument setup includes the following:

1 Culdoscope set
2 Syringes, 5 ml. and methylene blue
1 Piece plastic tubing
2 Barrett tenaculum forceps
1 Jacobs vulsellum forceps
2 Sponge-holding forceps
2 Retractors, 1 anterior and 1 posterior
2 Deaver or Doyen retractors, narrow blade
1 Vaginal dressing-holding forceps

The lens of the scope, if introduced when cold, may become foggy because of body heat. Thus the tip of the scope should be dipped in warm water then wiped dry before it is handed to the surgeon.

OPERATIVE PROCEDURE

1. The trocar of the culdoscope is inserted into the fornix behind the cervix; the trocar is then introduced into the pelvis between the two uterosacral ligaments (Fig. 24-36).

2. The trocar is withdrawn from the sheath; the sterile culdoscope is inserted through the sheath. The culdoscope does not touch the vaginal mucous membrane, thus reducing the possibility of infection to a minimum.

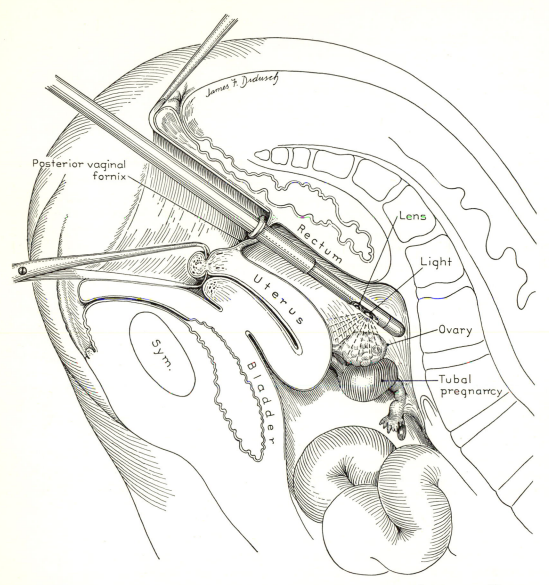

**Fig. 24-37.** Culdoscopy. Sagittal section showing culdoscope viewing pelvic viscera. (From TeLinde, R. W.: Operative gynecology, ed. 3, Philadelphia, 1962, J. B. Lippincott Co.)

3. The uterus, tubes, broad ligaments, uterosacral ligaments, rectal wall, sigmoid, and small intestine may be visualized through manipulation of the scope (Fig. 24-37).

4. In the study of sterility, a self-retaining screw-lipped cervical cannula is introduced in the cervical canal, and it is connected by a plastic tube to a syringe containing a dye. If the tube is patent,

the dye solution is seen dripping from the fimbriated end.

5. The culdoscope is withdrawn, the sheath is left in place, and the patient is placed on her side. Pressure is exerted on the abdomen to force the air out of the peritoneal cavity, thereby eliminating postoperative discomfort and potential air embolus. The vaginal wound is not sutured. The patient is returned to bed.

## Excision of Bartholin duct cyst or abscess

DEFINITION. Through the vaginal outlet, the cyst is removed or incised, and/or the gland is drained (Fig. 24-9).

CONSIDERATIONS. A cyst in the vulvovaginal gland usually follows acute infection and is treated by marsupialization when it is quiescent. Such cysts are non-neoplastic and result from retention of glandular secretions due to blockage somewhere in the duct system.

SETUP AND PREPARATION OF THE PATIENT. As for minor vaginal surgery, including dilatation and curettage setup, plus one 10 ml. syringe with a long 15-gauge needle, two culture tubes, two smear slides, and one catheter or soft rubber tube drain.

OPERATIVE PROCEDURE

1. The labia minora are sutured to the perineal skin on each side to expose the vaginal introitus. Silk or plain gut sutures swaged to ⅜-circle, cutting-edge needles on a needle holder, tissue forceps, and suture scissors are needed.

2. An elliptical incision is made in the mucosa, which is distended over the cyst.

3. The cyst wall is dissected, and blunt-pointed scissors complete removal of the gland. A drain may be inserted, and a dressing or perineal pad is applied.

## Colpotomy

DEFINITION. Needle culdocentesis is the insertion of an aspirating needle through the posterior fornix of the vagina. Posterior colpotomy is an incision through the vagina and peritoneum and the removal of pus and blood.

CONSIDERATIONS. Diagnostic needle culdocentesis is done to diagnose ectopic pregnancy or to detect intraperitoneal bleeding or cul-de-sac hematoma. Posterior colpotomy is done to evacuate pus and establish drainage from a cul-de-sac abscess or tubo-ovarian abscess or in a search for blood when a tubal pregnancy is suspected.

SETUP AND PREPARATION OF THE PATIENT. As described for simple vaginal repair, adding the following items:

2 Aspirating needles, 15-gauge, 3½ in.
1 Rochester-Pean hemostat, 10 in.
2 Culture tubes
2 Scissors, angulated blades, right and left
2 Drains, soft rubber tubes

An abdominal setup should also be available.

OPERATIVE PROCEDURE

1. *For needle culdocentesis,* a 15-gauge needle attached to a syringe is inserted through the posterior fornix of the vagina. Suspected intraperitoneal bleeding is confirmed if dark or red blood flows freely into the syringe. Failure to obtain blood does not rule out the possibility of pregnancy completely, but delineates the possibility of intraperitoneal bleeding.

2. *For posterior colpotomy,* a transverse incision, using scissors with angular blades, is made through the vagina and peritoneum behind the cervix at the superior point of the posterior fornix. The cul-de-sac is punctured with a long Rochester-Pean hemostat. The jaws of the hemostat are spread apart to enlarge the opening and permit the flow of liquid from the cul-de-sac. The cavity is explored; drains may be inserted.

3. In either procedure, bleeding of the vaginal wall is controlled by sutures of chromic gut no. 2-0; dressings are applied to the wound surface and held in place with a binder.

## Fothergill-Hunter operation for prolapse of the uterus

DEFINITION. Following dilatation and curettage, a complete repair of the vaginal walls, from above downward toward the vulva, to correct faulty supportive structures of the pelvic floor (a modification of the Manchester operation).

CONSIDERATIONS. The Fothergill-Hunter or similar type of operation may be done in young women with prolapse who desire preservation of the childbearing function.

SETUP AND PREPARATION OF THE PATIENT. As described for dilatation and curettage and vaginal plastic repair.

OPERATIVE PROCEDURE

1. Dilatation and curettage of the uterus is done, as previously described.

2. An inverted V incision is made through the full thickness of the vaginal wall. It extends from the bladder reflection to the urethral meatus, as described previously for anterior vaginal plastic repair.

3. The cervix is circumscribed and bleeding vessels ligated. A knife, Allis-Adair forceps, hemostats, tissue forceps, moist sponges on holders, and chromic gut no. 2-0 ligatures are used.

4. The mucosal flaps are dissected free laterally and posteriorly to expose the cardinal and uterosacral ligaments, which are clamped, cut, and ligated close to the cervical sutures. The cardinal and utero-sacral ligaments containing vesical arteries are secured with chromic gut no. 0 or 2-0 sutures swaged to ½-circle, taper point needles on needle holders.

5. The cervix is amputated at a site to permit shortening of the ligament. The remaining portion of the cervix is grasped with a Jacobs vulsellum forceps. The recto-vaginal septum is exposed by blunt and sharp dissection (Figs. 24-26 and 24-27).

6. The upper portion of a rectocele is repaired, as described for posterior vaginal plastic repair. A wedge-shaped incision is made with a knife in the portion of vaginal wall to be removed (Fig. 24-21). Repair is performed, using an inverting

suture to bring the flaps of the vagina over the sutured fibromuscular tissue of the cervix. Interrupted sutures, chromic gut no. 0 swaged to ½-circle, trocar-point or taper point needles on a needle holder, are placed to approximate the posterior wall.

7. Cardinal ligaments are sutured in the midline with interrupted sutures of chromic gut no. 0 to shorten the parietal connective tissue, thereby permitting them to provide more support of the pelvic floor.

8. An anterior and posterior Sturmdorf-type suture is placed in the upper and lower vaginal wall. Flaps are grasped with Allis forceps, the excised vaginal wall is resected on each side using Metzenbaum scissors, and the anterior vaginal wall is closed and reconstructed, as previously described.

9. A plastic reconstruction of the genital aperture is done, using interrupted chromic gut nos. 0 and 2-0 sutures, as described for vaginal plastic repair. The musculature of the perineum is reconstructed by placement of sutures in such a way that the bulbocavernous and the remaining transverse perineal muscles decrease the genital aperture and add support of the pelvic viscera.

---

Fig. 24-38. Vaginal hysterectomy by ligature method. **A,** Incision of vaginal wall around cervix. Anterior vaginal wall slightly elevated. **B,** Deaver retractor on each side; one Deaver retractor under bladder. Peritoneum opened. **C,** Posterior cul-de-sac opened. Heaney clamp applied to left uterosacral ligament. **D,** Left uterosacral ligament cut and tied. Clamp applied to left cardinal ligament. **E,** Clamp applied to ovarian ligament, round ligament, and fallopian tube. Vaginal hysterectomy by ligature method. Reconstruction of vaginal vault. **F,** Uterosacral ligament, broad ligament, and round ligament shown in their respective normal positions. **G,** Peritoneum closed and cardinal broad ligament and uterosacral ligaments reattached to angle of vagina. Left uterosacral and broad ligaments anchored, **H,** to left angle of vagina, and pubocervical fascia and rectovaginal fascia closed, together with the closure of the vaginal vault. **I,** Closure of vaginal cuff with suture passed through ligaments. **J,** Complete closure of vaginal vault. Repair of pelvic floor (cystocele and rectocele), which is often necessary, done according to technique detailed for vaginal repair. (From Counseller, V. S.: In Lowrie, R. J., editor: Gynecology: surgical techniques, Springfield, Ill., 1955, Charles C Thomas, Publisher.)

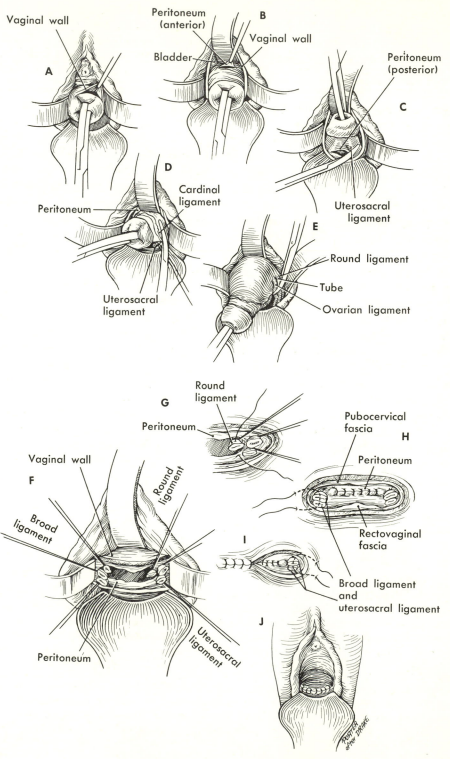

**Fig. 24-38.** For legend see opposite page.

10. A urinary drainage system is established, packing is placed in the vagina, and vaginal dressings are applied.

## Le Fort operation for prolapse of the uterus

Colpocleisis is the closure of the vagina by approximation of the anterior and posterior vaginal walls, with or without an attendant vaginal hysterectomy. The patient must be apprised of the fact that she will no longer possess a functioning vagina. The basic vaginal setup is used.

## Vaginal hysterectomy

**DEFINITION.** Through an incision made in the vaginal wall and the pelvic cavity, the uterus is removed.

**CONSIDERATIONS.** The uterus may be removed through the vaginal outlet except in pelvic malignancy or when a large uterine tumor is present. The vaginal approach is contraindicated in pelvic malignancy because of an inflammatory disease involving the uterine tubes and ovaries. It permits vaginal plastic surgery at the same time.

**SETUP AND PREPARATION OF THE PATIENT.** Instruments include the major vaginal repair setup, adding the dilatation and curettage setup, plus 2 needles, 22-gauge × 3 in., and 2 syringes, 10 ml.

To facilitate dissection and decrease bleeding, the vaginal walls may be infiltrated with saline or local anesthetic (vasoconstrictors optional). A laparotomy setup should also be available.

**OPERATIVE PROCEDURE**

1. The labia are retracted back with sutures of silk or chromic gut no. 2-0 swaged to ⅜-circle, cutting-edge needles held by Crile short needle holders. Tissue forceps and suture scissors are needed. An Auvard or Sims vaginal retractor is inserted to retract the vaginal wall.

2. A dilatation and curettage is performed, as previously described (Fig. 24-29).

3. A Jacobs vulsellum forceps or chromic gut no. 0 suture ligature is placed on both the posterior cervical lips to permit traction on the cervix (Fig. 24-38, *A*).

4. The vaginal wall is incised with a knife. The incision is made anteriorly through the full thickness of the wall. The bladder is pushed off the cervix by the knife handle; the bladder is freed from the anterior surface of the cervix and positioned with Kelly retractors (Fig. 24-38, *B*).

5. The incision is carried around the cervix; the posterior wall flaps are grasped with Allis forceps. The cul-de-sac peritoneum is grasped with two smooth tissue foceps, and the peritoneal cavity is opened with a knife. A suction set and small laparotomy packs may be used. The peritoneal edges are sutured to the posterior wall with silk or chromic traction sutures swaged to ½-circle, taper point needles secured on Crile-Wood needle holders.

6. The uterosacral ligaments containing blood vessels are doubly clamped, ligated, and cut. The ends of the ligatures are left long and tagged with a clamp (Fig. 24-38, *C*).

7. The uterus is drawn downward and the bladder held away with retractors and moist small laparotomy packs. The vesicouterine fold of peritoneum is grasped with tissue forceps and incised with a knife; bleeding vessels are clamped and ligated (Fig. 24-38, *D*).

8. If the bladder is entered, the opening is closed with two layers of interrupted chromic gut no. 4-0 sutures swaged to ½-circle, taper point needles secured to long needle holders. The vesicouterine reflection is sutured to the anterior vaginal wall by means of traction sutures and free ends held in a clamp.

9. The cardinal ligament on each side is doubly clamped, cut, and doubly ligated. The uterine arteries are doubly clamped, cut, and ligated (Figs. 24-4 and 24-5).

10. The fundus is delivered through the posterior route with the aid of a uterine tenaculum.

11. When the ovaries are to be left, a Kocher clamp is placed from below and

two from above to grasp the pedicles, which are then cut and ligated on both sides; the uterus is removed (Fig. 24-38, *E*).

12. The peritoneum between the rectum and vagina is approximated with a continuous suture of chromic gut no. 2-0. The retroperitoneal obliteration of the cul-de-sac is done by sutures that pass from the vaginal wall through the infundibulo-pelvic ligament and round ligament, through the cardinal ligament, and out through the vaginal wall. The suture is tied on the vaginal aspect of the new vault. The uterosacral ligament on each side is sutured in the midline (Fig. 24-38, *F* and *G*). The round, cardinal, and uterosacral ligaments may be individually approximated for additional support.

13. An existing rectocele and the perineum are repaired, as described for vaginal plastic repair (Figs. 24-21 and 24-24). In the presence of prolapse, reconstruction of the pelvic floor is done.

14. An indwelling system of urinary drainage is established; the vagina may be packed; and a perineal pad is applied.

## ABDOMINAL GYNECOLOGICAL SURGERY

### Laparoscopy (peritoneoscopy, celioscopy)

**DEFINITION.** Endoscopic visualization of the peritoneal cavity through the anterior abdominal wall after the establishment of a pneumoperitoneum.

**CONSIDERATIONS.** Laparoscopy provides the gynecologist the same anatomical view of the pelvic organs as is seen at the diagnostic laparotomy. The pathological condition can be seen, and ancillary procedures such as aspiration of cysts, tubal plastics, and tissue biopsies can be performed. Hemostasis can readily be obtained by using the active electrode probe. This procedure may enable the surgeon to avoid unnecessary pelvic surgery.

**SETUP AND PREPARATION OF THE PATIENT.** The patient is placed in the supine position; a general anesthetic is administered; the skin is prepped as for a laparotomy; a

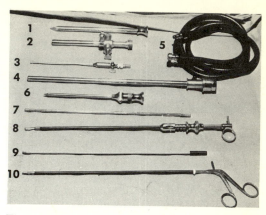

Fig. 24-39. Laparoscope. **1,** Trocar; **2,** valved cannula; **3,** pneumoperitoneal needle; **4,** foroblique vision laparoscope, 135 degrees; **5,** fiberoptic cord; **6,** secondary trocar and cannula; **7,** graduated probe; **8,** Palmer forceps within sheath; **9,** cautery probe; **10,** biopsy forceps. Not shown is the fiberoptic power source, cautery cord, and cautery unit.

Foley catheter is inserted; and the table is placed in extreme Trendelenburg position (apply shoulder braces). Instruments may be placed on a small table. The setup includes the following:

1 Laparoscope set (scope, fiberoptic cord, manipulative probe, biopsy forceps, cautery probe, cautery hook, suction tip) (Fig. 24-39)
1 Syringe, 5 ml.
1 Knife handle no. 3 and blade no. 15
6 Towel clamps
2 Allis forceps, 6 in.
2 Kelly clamps, 5¼ in.
1 Metzenbaum scissors, 5½ in.
1 Needle holder, 6 in.
2 Adson forceps with teeth
2 Skin hooks, single
1 Plain gut suture no. 3-0 swaged to a cutting needle
1 Piece rubber tubing, 3 ft.
  Electrosurgical unit
  Fiberoptic power source
  Gas source for pneumoperitoneum

The lens of the laparoscope may be wiped with sterile pHisoHex to prevent fogging in the warmth of the peritoneal cavity.

**OPERATIVE PROCEDURE**

1. A 1 cm. incision is placed below or to the left of the umbilicus.

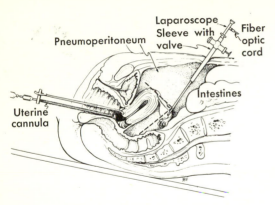

Fig. 24-40. Technique of laparoscopy. (From Cohen, M. R.: J. Obstet. Gynecol. 31:310, 1968.)

2. Elevating the skin with hooks, the trocar and valve sleeve are inserted first subcutaneously, then thrust boldly through the remaining layers of the abdominal wall into the peritoneal cavity. The angle taken by the trocar is approximately 45 degrees toward the concavity of the pelvis (Fig. 24-40).

3. The trocar is removed, the valve sleeve closed, the rubber tubing from the gas source attached, and a pneumoperitoneum produced. Care must be taken to prevent overdistention of the abdomen.

4. After the patient is placed in Trendelenburg position, the laparoscope is introduced and inspection begun. Should the biopsy or cautery forceps be needed, they are introduced by trocar through a separate small incision on the abdomen.

5. The scopes are withdrawn; gas is allowed to escape from the sleeve before it is withdrawn. Subcuticular closure of the skin is followed by the application of a Band-Aid dressing.

### Total abdominal hysterectomy

**DEFINITION.** Through an abdominal incision, the peritoneal cavity is opened, and the entire uterus—including the corpus and the cervix, with or without the adnexa—is removed (Fig. 24-5).

**CONSIDERATIONS.** Total (panhysterectomy or complete) hysterectomy is performed in the presence of fibroids (myomas) of the uterus resulting in uncontrollable bleeding, degeneration, and, in some cases, endometriosis or adenomyosis that is far advanced. Total hysterectomy is also indicated in older women when the bowel and bladder are involved and thereby impair the normal functioning of the urinary and gastrointestinal tracts.

**SETUP AND PREPARATION OF THE PATIENT.** The patient is prepared as described for vaginal and abdominal surgery. Diagnostic dilatation and curettage usually has already been performed. However, a setup should be readily available. Prior to the abdominal skin prep, an internal and external vaginal prep is done. A Foley catheter is inserted to provide constant bladder drainage during the operation. The supine and high Trendelenburg positions are used as described in Chapter 7. Instrumentation includes the abdominal gynecological set; provisions are made to remove from the abdomen and field those instruments used in separating the cervix from the vagina, thereby avoiding vaginal contamination of the pelvis. In performing the abdominal hysterectomy, instrument tables are arranged in relation to the side of the operating table from which the surgeon works.

**OPERATIVE PROCEDURE**

1. As the skin is incised, the head and upper section of the operating table are lowered slowly, approximately 10 degrees at a time. When the peritoneal cavity is opened, as described previously for laparotomy (Chapter 17), the patient is in the desired position for pelvic surgery.

2. In cases of obese patients or for exploration of the upper abdominal cavity, a left rectus or midline incision is made (Chapter 17). For simple hysterectomy, a Pfannenstiel incision may be used. The abdominal layers and the peritoneum are opened as described for laparotomy (Chapter 17).

3. The round ligament is grasped with Allis-Adair forceps, clamped with curved Rochester-Pean hemostats, and ligated with medium silk or chromic gut sutures swaged

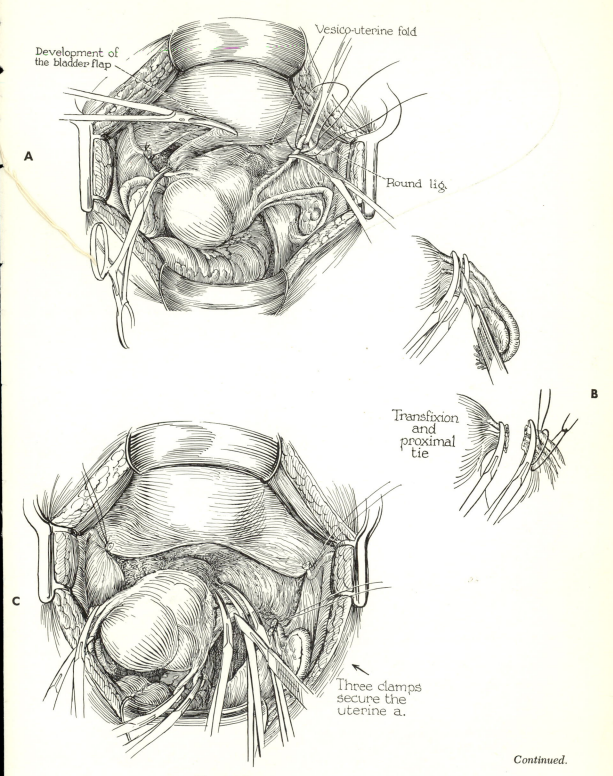

**A**

Development of
the bladder flap

Vesico-uterine fold

Round lig.

**B**

Transfixion
and
proximal
tie

**C**

Three clamps
secure the
uterine a.

*Continued.*

**Fig. 24-41.** For legend see p. 848.

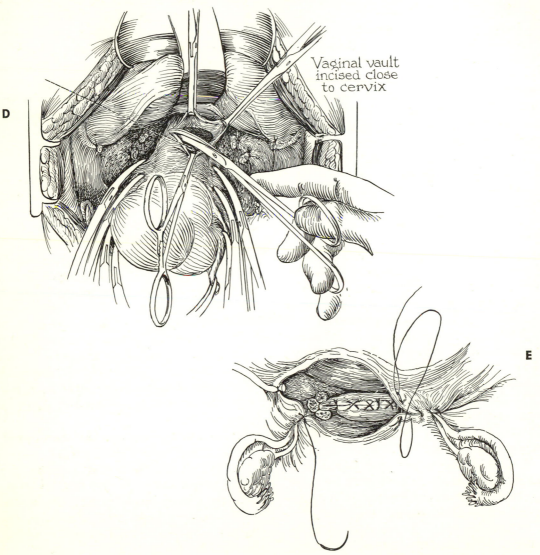

Vaginal vault
incised close
to cervix

D

E

**Fig. 24-41.** Abdominal hysterectomy for simple fibroid uterus. **A,** Peritoneal cavity retracted with self-retaining retractors and organs protected with laparotomy packs saturated in warm normal saline solution. Transverse incision made through uterine peritoneum and carried to each side of uterine attachments of round ligaments. Bleeding vessels clamped and ligated. Round ligament grasped, ligated, and cut. **B,** Tube and ovarian ligaments clamped, cut, and sutured. **C,** Uterus pulled forward, posterior sheath of broad ligaments divided, and uterine artery and veins secured by three heavy curved clamps. Pedicle divided, leaving two hemostats in proximal pedicle. **D,** Bladder separated from cervix and upper vagina. Vaginal vault opened and grasped with Allis forceps. Allis forceps placed on anterior lip of cervix and dissection of cervix carried out, to complete its amputation from vagina. **E,** Three connective tissue thickenings have been anchored to vaginal vault, vaginal mucosa approximated, and vault closed. As shown, peritoneum closed with continuous suture. (From Ball, T. L.: Operative gynecology and urology, ed. 2, St. Louis, 1963, The C. V. Mosby Co.)

to ½-circle, taper point needles on long needle holders. Pedicles are cut with Metzenbaum scissors; sutures are tagged with a hemostat to be used as traction later. The procedure is done on both sides (Fig. 24-41).

4. By use of the surgeon's fingers, the layer of the broad ligament close to the uterus is separated on each side, bleeding vessels are clamped and ligated, and a laparotomy pack is inserted behind the flap. The fallopian tube and the utero-ovarian ligaments are doubly clamped together with Ochsner or Carmalt clamps or Heaney hemostats, cut with a knife, and tied doubly with suture ligatures.

5. The uterus is pulled forward to expose the posterior sheath of the broad ligament, which is incised with knife and Metzenbaum scissors. Ureters are identified. The uterine vessels and uterosacral ligaments are doubly clamped with Ochsner, Heaney, or Carmalt hemostats, divided with a knife at the level of the internal os, and ligated with suture ligatures.

6. The severed uterine vessels are bluntly dissected away from the cervix on each side with the aid of sponges on holders, scissors, and tissue forceps.

7. The bladder is separated from the cervix and upper vagina with a knife or scissors and blunt dissection assisted by sponges on holders.

8. The bladder is retracted with a laparotomy pack and a retractor with an angular blade. The vaginal vault is incised with a knife close to the cervix (Fig. 24-41, *D*).

9. The anterior lip of the cervix is grasped with an Allis or tenaculum forceps. With Metzenbaum scissors, the cervix is dissected and amputated from the vagina. The uterus is removed. Potentially contaminated instruments used on the cervix and vagina are placed in a discard basin and removed from the field (including sponge forceps and suction). Bleeding is controlled with hemostats and sutures.

10. The vaginal vault is reconstructed with chromic interrupted sutures. Angle sutures anchor all three connective tissue ligaments to the vaginal vault. The pedicles, tube, and ovarian ligament are left free of the vault.

11. Vaginal mucosa is approximated with a continuous chromic gut suture swaged to a ⅜-circle needle on a long needle holder. The muscular coat of the vagina is closed with figure-of-eight sutures to make the vault of the vagina firm and provide resistance against prolapse.

12. The peritoneum is closed over the bladder, vaginal vault, and rectum (Fig. 24-41, *E*). The laparotomy packs are removed, and the omentum is drawn over the bowel.

13. The abdominal wound is closed, as described for abdominal closure (Chapter 17).

## Subtotal (supracervical) hysterectomy

**DEFINITION.** Through an abdominal incision, the peritoneal cavity is opened, and the body of the uterus is removed, leaving the cervix in place.

**CONSIDERATIONS.** Subtotal hysterectomy is seldom done in modern gynecology, except in emergencies to terminate a procedure because of shock or cardiac arrest or in abdominal carcinomatosis in conjunction with the removal of the primary tumor in the ovary.

**SETUP AND PREPARATION OF THE PATIENT.** As described for total hysterectomy.

**OPERATIVE PROCEDURE.** As described for total hysterectomy, except that after the uterine arteries are ligated, the corpus of the cervix is amputated and the stump closed with interrupted chromic gut sutures. The pelvis is reperitonealized and the abdominal wound closed, as described in total hysterectomy.

## Abdominal myomectomy

**DEFINITION.** Through an abdominal incision and opening of the peritoneal cavity, the fibromyomas are removed from the uterine wall.

**CONSIDERATIONS.** Myomectomy is usually done in young women with symptoms that indicate the presence of tumors and who

have had no children. The tumors may be removed because of infertility or habitual abortion or because of distortion of the bladder and other organs. Myomectomy may be performed in conjunction with other abdominal pelvic surgery as a prophylactic measure.

SETUP AND PREPARATION OF THE PATIENT. As for vaginal preparation and possible dilatation and curettage, as described previously. The Trendelenburg position and basic abdominal gynecological setup are used, including Bonney's myomectomy clamp.

OPERATIVE PROCEDURE

1. The patient is prepared as described for abdominal hysterectomy. A midline or Pfannenstiel incision is used (Chapter 17); the uterus is exposed.

2. To contract the musculature of the uterine wall, a suitable drug may be injected into the fundus. If the tumor is riding over the bladder or to free it from the tumor, the round ligament is doubly clamped, cut, and ligated, as described for hysterectomy.

3. The fibroid tumor is grasped with a tenaculum. The broad ligament may be opened to determine the course of the ureter or to free the bladder by means of curved hemostats and Metzenbaum scissors.

4. Each tumor is shelled out of its bed, using blunt and sharp instruments. Bleeding vessels are clamped and ligated.

5. The uterus is reconstructed with interrupted chromic gut no. 2-0 sutures swaged to ⅜-circle trocar-point needles held on long needle holders.

6. The round ligament is reapproximated by several interrupted sutures; the anterior sheath of the broad ligament is closed. The perimetrium is closed over the operative site. The abdominal wound is closed, as described for laparotomy closure (Chapter 17).

### Uterine suspension

DEFINITION. Through an abdominal incision and opening of the peritoneum, the ligaments are shortened by being sutured to the muscle structures.

CONSIDERATIONS. Uterine suspension is rarely done today, execept as part of the conservative surgical treatment of some types of pelvic inflammatory disease or endometriosis when the uterus is bound down on the cul-de-sac.

SETUP AND PREPARATION OF THE PATIENT. The vaginal preparation is done as described for vaginal surgery. The laparotomy preparation and a laparotomy abdominal setup, as described for myomectomy, are used.

OPERATIVE PROCEDURE

1. The abdomen is opened, as described for myomectomy.

2. As part of salpingectomy, a modified Coffey suspension may be done to hold the uterus forward and suspend the ovaries so that they cannot prolapse into the cul-de-sac. The round ligaments are sewn toward the bladder. The wound is closed in layers, as described for laparotomy (Chapter 17).

### Oophorectomy and oophorocystectomy

DEFINITION. *Oophorectomy* is the removal of an ovary. *Oophorocystectomy* is the removal of an ovarian cyst (Fig. 24-42).

CONSIDERATIONS. Functional cysts comprise the majority of the ovarian enlargements. Follicle cysts are the most common. Functional cysts develop in the corpus luteum. The corpus luteum cysts are usually larger than are other functional cysts. The true epithelial tumors (serous cystadenomas and pseudomucinous cystadenomas) of the ovary are prone to malignant change.

The choice of operation depends on the patient's age and symptoms, findings on physical examination, and direct examination of the adnexa during exploration. If the ovarian tumor is recognized as benign, only the visibly diseased portions of the adnexa are removed. In the presence of dermoid, follicle, and corpus luteum cysts, the cyst is usually enucleated, and most of the ovarian parenchyma is preserved. In tubal pregnancy the preg-

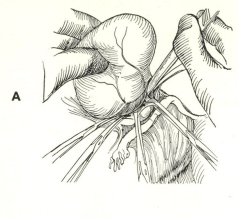

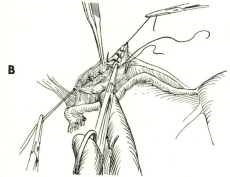

Fig. 24-42. Resection of small cyst from ovary. **A,** Incision made around ovary near junction of cyst wall and normal ovarian tissue. Knife handle is convenient instrument for shelling out cyst. **B,** Wound in ovary closed. (From Ball, T. L.: Operative gynecology and urology, ed. 2, St. Louis, 1963, The C. V. Mosby Co.)

nant tube is removed and, in some cases, the ovary also.

**SETUP AND PREPARATION OF THE PATIENT.** As described for laparotomy, adding the following items:

1 Trocar and cannula with tubing
1 Abdominal suction set
4 Babcock forceps
1 Metzenbaum scissors, 7¼ in.
6 Mayo hemostats, curved
1 Syringe, 10 ml., with 21-gauge needle

**OPERATIVE PROCEDURE**

1. The abdominal peritoneal cavity is opened, as described for laparotomy (Chapter 17).

2A. *For removal of a large ovarian cyst,* a purse-string silk suture is placed in the cyst wall, and a trocar is introduced in its center; the suture is placed around the trocar as the fluid is aspirated. The trocar is removed, and the purse-string suture is tied. All normal ovarian tissue is preserved.

2B. *For removal of dermoid cyst,* the field is protected with laparotomy packs, since the contents of such cysts produce irritation if they are spilled into the peritoneal cavity. An incision is made along the base of the cyst between the wall and normal ovarian tissue. The cystic wall is dissected away. The ovary is closed with interrupted fine chromic gut sutures.

2C. *For decortication of the enlarged ovary and bridge resection,* a large segment of the ovarian cortex opposite the hilum is removed. The cysts are punctured with a needle point and collapsed. A wedge of ovarian stroma, extending deep in the hilum, is resected with a small knife; the cortex of the ovary is closed with interrupted chromic gut no. 3-0 suture.

3. To prevent prolapse of the tube into the cul-de-sac, it may be sutured to the posterior sheath of the broad ligament.

4. The abdominal wound is closed, as described for laparotomy (Chapter 17).

## Salpingo-oophorectomy

**DEFINITION.** Removal of a tube and all or part of the associated ovary.

**CONSIDERATIONS.** Salpingo-oophorectomy may be done in some young women who are anxious to have children after all other methods of treatment have failed to cure chronic salpingo-oophoritis, in patients with ectopic tubal gestation, or in those with tuberculosis of the adnexa or large adnexal cysts. If both tubes and ovaries are diseased, they are removed with total hysterectomy.

**SETUP AND PREPARATION OF THE PATIENT.** As described for myomectomy; in some cases, as described for hysterectomy.

**OPERATIVE PROCEDURE**

1. The abdominal wall and peritoneal cavity are opened, as described for laparotomy.

2. The affected tube is grasped with Allis or Babcock forceps. The infundibulo-pelvic ligament is clamped with Mayo hemostats, cut, and ligated with chromic gut no. 0 or 2-0, swaged to a ½-circle, taper point needle, or no. 2-0 silk on a French-eye needle.

3. The mesosalpinx is grasped with Kelly hemostats and divided with the suspensory ligament of the ovary.

4. The cornual attachment of the tube is excised with a knife or curved scissors. Bleeding vessels are clamped and ligated.

5. The edges of the broad ligament are peritonealized from the uterine horn to the infundibulopelvic ligament, as described for hysterectomy.

6. The wound is closed, as described for laparotomy; dressings are applied and held in place with adhesive or plastic tape.

## Salpingostomy (tubal plasty)

DEFINITION. Removal of the obstructed portion of the tube and suspension of the remaining portion to the side of the pelvic wall or placement of it into the uterine cavity.

CONSIDERATIONS. These procedures are done to restore fertility.

SETUP AND PREPARATION OF THE PATIENT. *For vaginal insertion of cannula,* a Kahn, Calvin, or Rubin set, one Schroeder single-pronged tenaculum, one sponge forceps, two Sims vaginal retractors, and assorted cannulae (as preferred by the surgeon) are needed.

*For abdominal procedure,* a basic abdominal gynecological setup is needed, plus the following:

    2 Iris eye scissors, 1 curved and 1 straight
    2 Razor blades
    2 Adson forceps
    12 Halsted mosquito hemostats, 6 straight and 6 curved
    1 Crile hemostat, curved, rubber-shod
    1 Probe
    2 Crile-Wood needle holders, light with fine tip
    Chromic sutures no. 4-0 or 5-0

Accessory items

    Suction tube and tubing
    Eyedropper with small rubber bulb
    Polyethylene tubing
    Plastic tubing and connectors

OPERATIVE PROCEDURE. One of several techniques is carried out after salpingectomy has been performed. The Estes technique or some modification of it is usually followed. In the Estes technique the convex surface of the ovary is excised, and implantation of the remainder is made into the uterine cornu in an opening made in the myometrium, communicating with the cavity.

## Tubal ligation

DEFINITION. Interruption of fallopian tube continuity, resulting in sterilization of the patient.

CONSIDERATIONS. In general, the indications for sterilization can be divided into three groups: (1) psychiatric, (2) medical, and (3) obstetrical and gynecological. Evaluation and recommendation of sterilization is made by the attending physician. A sterilization permit and a procedure consent form must be signed by both the husband and wife.

The optimum time for sterilization is approximately 24 hours after vaginal delivery, but an objection to this is that the danger of hemorrhage still exists soon after delivery. If a cesarean section is done, the tubes are ligated at this time; with a normal delivery, tubal ligation is done on the first to third postpartum day.

SETUP AND PREPARATION OF THE PATIENT. The patient is placed in a supine position. A catheter is inserted in the bladder. The abdomen is prepared and draped as described for laparotomy (Chapter 17). Instrumentation includes the basic laparotomy setup.

OPERATIVE PROCEDURE

1. The fundus is determined, and a midline incision is made approximately 2 inches below it. The abdomen is opened in the usual manner (Chapter 17).

2. The tube is delivered and grasped with

2 Babcock forceps and clamped with 2 Crile forceps.

3. The section between the Babcock forceps is resected with Metzenbaum scissors and saved for specimen. The tubes are doubly ligated with silk sutures no. 2-0 about 1 inch from the uterine cornu. The sutures on the proximal end of the tube are left long. This tubal stump is then mobilized by dissecting it free from the mesosalpinx.

4. A very small cut is made in the serosa on the posterior surface of the uterus near the cornu, and the musculature is penetrated with a Crile forceps for about ½ inch, spreading the clamp sufficiently to admit the tube.

5. One of the ligatures attached to the tubal stump is threaded on a needle and sutured to the bottom of the pocket and carried out to the uterine surface. The other suture attached to the tubal stump is treated in a similar manner. Traction is placed on the sutures, thus the tubal stump is buried in the uterine musculature.

6. The sutures are tied together, and silk sutures no. 4-0 are used to close the edges of the pocket more tightly about the tube. (The end of the tube may also be buried within the leaves of the broad ligament.)

7. The abdominal incision is closed in layers and the wound dressed.

# OBSTETRICAL SURGERY
## Cesarean section

**DEFINITION.** Delivery of an infant through an incision made in the abdominal and uterine walls.

**CONSIDERATIONS.** Delivery by cesarean section is indicated in instances of previous section, primary and secondary uterine dystocia, cephalopelvic disproportion, placenta previa, abruptio placentae, toxemia, fetal distress (prolapsed cord), diabetes, Rh sensitization, tumors, previous vaginal surgery, abnormal presentation, and many others. In some instances the cesarean section may be scheduled according to the estimated date of confinement,

estimated fetal weight, and definite auscultation of fetal heartbeat at or before 20 weeks from the last menstrual period. At other times, cesarean section may be elected on an emergency basis.

Several methods for abdominal delivery are accepted: classic cesarean section, low or cervical cesarean section, extraperitoneal operation, and cesarean hysterectomy. The low segment section is today considered standard; however, the classic method may be chosen in some circumstances.

**SETUP AND PREPARATION OF THE PATIENT.** The extent of preoperative planning and preparation will depend on the urgency of the delivery and should be paced accordingly. Whole blood should be available. When the patient arrives in surgery, she may or may not be in labor. The circulating nurse should auscultate the fetal heart tone with a fetuscope. The patient is positioned supinely on the table, and restraints are applied; the patient is never left unattended. A Foley retention catheter is inserted and connected to gravity drainage. Choice of anesthetic agent is made by the anesthesiologist after reviewing the condition of the mother and fetus.

Adequate personnel should be available to individually care for the mother and child, since simultaneous urgent needs may arise.

An abdominal prep and drape is done as described in Chapters 4 and 5. A major setup is used with another sterile table prepared for infant resuscitation. Instrumentation includes the abdominal instrument setup and the following (Fig. 24-43):

1 Bandage scissors
8 Pennington clamps, 8 in.
1 Set DeLee vaginal retractors (optional)
1 DeLee delivery forceps (optional)
1 Bulb syringe suction
Oxytocic drugs

**Equipment for care of the infant**
Sterile cotton receiving blankets
Sterile cord clamp or ties
Endotracheal suction catheter
Suction source
Nasogastric tube for lavage

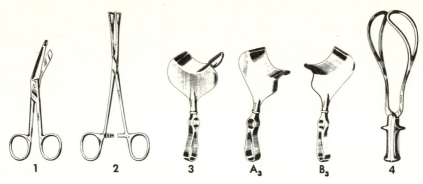

**Fig. 24-43.** Cesarean section instruments. 1, Bandage scissors; 2, Pennington tissue-grasping forceps. DeLee vaginal retractors: 3, universal; A₃, left; B₃, right. 4, DeLee obstetrical forceps. (Courtesy Codman & Shurtleff, Inc., Randolph, Mass.)

Syringes, 10 ml.
Bulb syringe suction
Mucous trap
Infant laryngoscope and endotracheal tubes
Infant resuscitator
Erythromycin (Ilotycin)
Supplies for collecting blood samples
Identification supplies: bracelet and footprint plate
Incubator (warmed)
Supplies for immediate circumcision

**OPERATIVE PROCEDURE**
**(LOW CERVICAL METHOD)**

1. A 12 to 15 cm. long skin incision is made from below the umbilicus to above the symphysis. As the incision is continued through the fascia and rectus muscles to expose the lower portion of the cervix, blood vessels may be clamped with Crile forceps and ligated with plain gut suture no. 3-0.

2. The exposed peritoneum is incised transversely with a scalpel and Metzenbaum scissors between the two round ligaments. By blunt dissection the bladder is freed and retracted with the universal DeLee retractor to expose the lower segment of the uterus.

3. Using a new scalpel blade and bandage scissors, the uterus may be opened either transversely in the manner of Kerr or longitudinally in the manner of Kronig. Using the Kerr technique, a lunar incision is made through the myometrium extend-

ing to within 1 inch of either uterine artery.

4. The membranes are ruptured and suction immediately applied.

5. The fetal head is delivered by inserting a hand between the head and the symphysis, rotating the face posteriorly, and exerting upward traction. (With the Kronig technique, the face is rotated anteriorly.)

6. The fetal body is delivered. The cord is double cross clamped with Rochester-Pean forceps and cut with bandage scissors. The baby is given to the assistant (pediatrician) for resuscitation and care.

7. The placenta and all membranes are manually removed from the uterus.

8. The uterine edges are grasped with Pennington clamps and a layered closure begun. A continuous suture of chromic gut no. 0 or 2-0 is placed through the deep myometrium (and possibly endometrium). A second layer of similar sutures is placed in the superior myometrium and serosa. A sponge count is taken as the uterine cavity is closed.

9. A tubal ligation may be done at this time.

10. The bladder flap of peritoneum is sutured to the visceral layer with a continuous chromic gut suture no. 2-0 swaged to a taper point needle.

11. The fascia and skin are closed as

described for laparotomy in Chapter 17. A pressure dressing is applied to the abdomen and a pad to the perineum.

## REFERENCES

1. Anson, B. J.: An atlas of human anatomy, ed. 2, Philadelphia, 1963, W. B. Saunders Co.
2. Anthony, C. P.: Textbook of anatomy and physiology, ed. 8, St. Louis, 1971, The C. V. Mosby Co.
3. Ball, T. L.: Gynecologic survey and urology, ed. 2, St. Louis, 1963, The C. V. Mosby Co.
4. Brooks, S. M.: Integrated basic science, ed. 3, St. Louis, 1970, The C. V. Mosby Co.
5. Cohen, M. R.: Laparoscopy, culdoscopy, and gynecography, Philadelphia, 1970, W. B. Saunders Co.
6. Costillo, P.: Surgical creation of a vagina, A.O.R.N. Journal 11:41, 1970.
7. Eastman, N., and Hellman, L. N.: William's obstetrics, ed. 13, New York, 1966, Appleton-Century-Crofts.
8. Eaton, C. J.: Technic of uterine aspiration, ed. 2, Berkeley, Calif., 1969, Berkeley Tonometer Co., Bio-Engineering, Inc.
9. Francis, C. C: Introduction to human anatomy, ed. 5, St. Louis, 1968, The C. V. Mosby Co.
10. Goss, C. M., editor: Gray's anatomy of the human body, ed. 28, Philadelphia, 1966, Lea & Febiger.
11. Madden, J. L.: Atlas of techniques in surgery, vol. 1, ed. 2, New York, 1964, Appleton-Century-Crofts.
12. Moyer, C. A., Rhoads, J., Allen, J. G., and Harkins, H. N.: Surgery: principles and practice, ed. 3, Philadelphia, 1965, J. B. Lippincott Co.
13. Novak, E.: Textbook of gynecology, ed. 7, Baltimore, 1965, The Williams & Wilkins Co.
14. Parsons, L. P., and Sommers, S. C.: Gynecology, Philadelphia, 1963, W. B. Saunders Co.
15. Pettit, M. D.: Gynecologic diagnosis and treatment, New York, 1962, The Blakiston Division, McGraw-Hill Book Co., Inc.
16. Sherman, A. I.: Cancer of the female reproductive organs, St. Louis, 1963, The C. V. Mosby Co.
17. Taylor, M. B.: Continuous saline flushing—a modification for vacuum evacuation of the uterus, Am. J. Obstet. Gynecol. **105:** 986, Nov. 15, 1969.
18. TeLinde, R. W.: Operative gynecology, ed. 3, Philadelphia, 1962, J. B. Lippincott Co.
19. Willson, J. R., Beecham, C. T., and Carrington, E. R.: Obstetrics and gynecology, ed. 4, St. Louis, 1971, The C. V. Mosby Co.

# CHAPTER 25

# Pediatric surgery

JUDITH YVONNE JACOBS

The care of ill children has developed in the last 80 years into a specialized area of practice known as pediatrics. Within this area of practice the field of pediatric surgery has more recently evolved as a concomitant discipline in health care for children. Pediatric surgery deals with congenital malformations or defects in the newborn. It also deals with diseases amenable to surgical intervention, some of which are primarily seen in the pediatric age group, whereas others are not age associated. Many specialty areas of surgery (cardiothoracic, genitourinary, plastic, etc.) may be encompassed in the realm of pediatric surgery.

Pediatric surgical success is attributed to recent medical advances that brought about (1) a better understanding of total patient preoperative preparation, (2) a more thorough knowledge of fluid and electrolyte balance, (3) increased knowledge of anesthesia, including new agents and improved techniques, (4) comprehension and implementation of methods effective for postoperative care,* and (5) knowledge about the etiology and physiology of congenital malformations.

## GENERAL CONSIDERATIONS

Contrary to popular belief, a child is not a "miniature adult." His physiological responses are geared toward rapid growth and development. This means that illness and surgery affect and are affected by this physiology. Moreover, the child is undergoing continual developmental changes psychologically and emotionally. These changes may be heightened or lessened by illness and surgery. All events in the life of a child become integral parts in the cycle of his growth and development. Therefore participation in pediatric surgery requires not only the basics of aseptic surgical technique but also an understanding of the child and his pattern of normal growth and development in order to minimize any disruptive effect of surgical intervention on the child's life.

### The child, the hospital, and surgery

The care of the child in the hospital is based on a knowledge of normal patterns of growth and development. Operating room nurses are called on to utilize this knowledge in preoperative patient visits and team planning of surgical nursing care. Preoperative visits include both the parent and the child; the degree of involvement with the child progresses in direct proportion with age. The child will normally harbor fears and anxieties about (1) the substitution of "people" for family, (2) the strange environment, and (3) surgery,

---

*Berry, E. C., and Kohn, M. L.: Introduction to operating room technique, ed. 3, New York, 1966, The Blakiston Division, McGraw-Hill Book Co., p. 147.

which he may percieve as an assault on his physical integrity and body image.

As a result of these fears and anxieties, the first goal of the preoperative visit is to establish rapport with him and his family. Parental participation in preoperative and postoperative care should be explained to the child and encouraged in the parents. Elicit the child's knowledge of the proposed surgery and build on it those facts essential to a good surgical experience. Simplicity and honesty concerning tests, preparations, operation, stitches, and pain allow the child to trust and to be secure in the knowledge that "someone who knows" will be caring for him.

Anxiety concerning the environment may be somewhat alleviated in several ways. Allow the child to see the nurse in scrub attire; provide similar attire for him to inspect and wear. Tours of the operating room and recovery room may be given, depending on the child's age and maturity. Provide medical "toys" that may add to familiarity with the unknown or may allow hostile feelings to be vented. Description of the experience as a "real life adventure" in which he participates may evoke some enthusiasm and more tolerance.

Increasing awareness of his body as a whole may cause the child to view surgery as an assault or mutilation. Explanations and physical demonstrations regarding specific "lumps" to be removed or repaired better define OPERATION. The term *cutting* is avoided, since this connotes damage and pain. An explanation of the dressings and drainage tubes that will be present postoperatively is essential to their remaining in place and to their correct functioning. Assisting the child to bandage a doll or toy may demonstrate this. Introduction to children recovering from similar surgery may bolster his confidence. Do not fail to mention that there will be postoperative discomfort—pain; but do tell him that Mommy and Daddy will be there to help him.

In all these areas, remember to be kind, gentle, and reassuring. Offer the child security in your care. This may be easiest to offer the infant whom you hold and cuddle. With the older child who may be aggressively hostile, patience, tact, acceptance, and firmness may be required.

## Physiological considerations

The basal metabolic rate of children is high to meet the demands of growth and development. Their caloric and fluid needs are correspondingly increased. The stress of surgery adds to these demands. Therefore the child is not given oral nourishment for only a few hours, and feeding is resumed as soon as safely tolerated. During surgical procedures, intravenous fluids are administered to maintain the crucial balance that minimal losses may upset. Oxygen needs are also increased by the elevated basal metabolic rate. Blood gas studies may be used to reveal oxygen levels. Humidity and/or oxygen may be indicated postoperatively and can be provided by use of isolettes, croupettes, face masks, or Plexiglas hoods. A warmed isolette should be ready to receive the neonate.

Maintenance of circulating blood volume is imperative. If more than 10% of the total blood volume (based on 80 to 85 ml./kg.) is lost, replacement is considered. To reduce incidental blood loss, "heel sticks" are often employed to obtain blood samples, meticulous hemostatic technique is used, and sponges and suction contents are weighed or measured. Weighing is accomplished by the use of dry sponges, which are weighed immediately on saturation before the blood dries and evaporation begins. Suction apparatus is calibrated in centimeters for ease in rapidly assessing blood loss. Blood is made available for any procedure in which excessive loss may occur.

During surgery, constant monitoring of the temperature is essential. Wide temperature variations may occur. Considerable heat loss from the body surface can occur. Anesthesia may also cause vasodilatation and heat loss. Undue exposure of the child should be avoided from the time of admis-

sion to the suite until completion of the procedure. If necessary, warmed cotton blankets may be used to prevent body heat loss when the child is admitted to the air-conditioned suite. In conjunction, a warming mattress is placed on the operating table to deter heat loss and maintain body temperature. All fluids that are utilized in pediatric therapy may be warmed before introduction to the body to decrease heat loss. This would include intravenous fluid replacement in large amounts and all blood replacement. Irrigating solutions are used at body temperature. Further conservation of body heat during the procedure may be effected by the use of an adhesive plastic drape that covers all exposed skin surfaces. Thus not only are bacteria from exposed skin denied access to the wound but also the air currents cannot cool the body surface by convection of heat.

Monitoring cardiac and circulatory sufficiency is accomplished by oscilloscope, precardial or esophageal stethoscope, and blood pressure manometer. Choice of the method is dependent on the child's age. Adequate ventilation may also be determined by the stethoscope. Urine production by the kidneys is indicative of circulatory sufficiency.

Anesthetic techniques may vary with the child's age, disease, and the anesthesiologist. Local anesthetics are not frequently employed because the child may not cooperate. Spinal anesthetics are not employed. General anesthesia by intravenous infusion and inhalation is preferred. Frequently an endotracheal tube is inserted to decrease dead space in the anesthesia system and to ensure adequate delivery of oxygen and anesthesia. This tube is an essential guarantee of oxygen supply in the presence of the child's small trachea; even slight hypoxia could have deleterious effects. The anesthetic agent of choice allows rapid induction to surgical levels and equally rapid reversal of effects.

## PATIENT PREPARATION AND SETUP

The surgical environment should be quiet and orderly; distractions should be minimal. The room and surgical team should be ready when the child is admitted to the suite. The child should be positively identified by the surgeon, identification bracelet, chart, and, when possible, verbal response. The operative permit, signed by parent or guardian, should be in order. The child must at all times be accompanied by an adult; if the situation permits, a child may be held. Final preparations should be explained simply and reassuringly. Intravenous fluids may be started before or after induction. Functioning suction equipment should be immediately accessible.

During induction of anesthesia the child is placed in a supine position on the table. The circulating nurse gently holds his arms or hands in a gesture of reassurance. As the level of anesthesia deepens, firmer restraint may be required. (Physical or mechanical restraints frighten the conscious child and may cause him to struggle.) When the child has been anesthetized, he is positioned for surgery, and restraints are applied in a manner that promotes maximum patient safety: freedom of respirations, freedom of circulation, no undue pressure on nerves or bony prominences, support of extremities, and operative accessibility (Chapter 7). An infant or young child may effectively be restrained by wrapping sheet cotton lightly around the extremities and tying these with gauze loops to the table. (The cotton wrapping also conserves body heat.) The thermometer probe is inserted.

Skin preparation seldom includes shaving, with the exception of cranial surgery. A nonirritating chemical disinfectant is applied to the skin over the incisional area. Drapes that expose the operative area and completely cover the operating table are utilized.

Admission to the suite, induction, and operation are enhanced by the immediate availability of equipment and supplies such as the following:

Pediatric table or attachments for regular operating table
Supplies for positioning: pillow, sandbag, sheets
Supplies for restraint: sheet cotton, gauze, circumstraint board

Thermometer probes: rectal and esophageal
Warming blanket
Pediatric-sized intravenous solutions
Microdrip infusion sets
Scalp vein sets or small-gauge needles
Cutdown tray and assorted catheters
Infusion warming coils
Containers graduated in centimeters for accurate measurement: basins, suction bottles
Scale
Warmer for irrigation solutions and unsterile cotton blankets
Pediatric instruments
Pediatric-sized sponges: laparotomy pads and 4 × 4 in. sponge
Assorted fine sutures and needles
Appropriate drugs (vitamin K)
Pediatric recovery bed: isolette, croupette

Instrumentation is similar to that used for adults. However, the instruments themselves are more delicately and finely fashioned for these tender and fragile tissues. Meticulous technique is employed to decrease tissue damage and the possibility of infection. Retraction in particular should be gentle so as not to impair other vital functions. A basic pediatric instrument set would include the following:

### Cutting instruments

2 Knife handles no. 3 with blades no. 10
1 Knife handle no. 7 with blade no. 15
2 Baby dissecting scissors, 5½ in., curved and straight
1 Dura scissors, 4½ in., curved
1 Metzenbaum scissors, 7 in., curved

### Holding instruments

10 Tissue forceps
2 Infant Semkin forceps, 5 in., serrated
2 Infant Semkin forceps, 5 in., with teeth
2 Adson forceps, serrated
2 Adson forceps with teeth
2 Potts-Smith forceps, 7 in.
4 Sponge-holding forceps, 8 in.
12 Backhaus towel clamps, 3 in.
6 Backhaus towel clamps, 5 in.
4 Allis forceps, 6 in.
4 Babcock forceps, 6¼ in.

### Clamping instruments

24 Baby Crile hemostats, 5½ in.
6 Baby Pean forceps, 5½ in.
6 Baby Ochsner forceps, 5½ in.
6 Crile hemostats, 6¼ in.
6 Collier hemostats, 7¾ in.
4 Rochester-Pean forceps, 6¼ in.
4 Ochsner forceps, 6¼ in.
4 Baby Mixter forceps, 7 in.

### Exposing instruments

2 Silver ribbon retractors, ½ and ¾ × 6 in.
2 Baby Deaver retractors, ⅝ and 1 × 8 in.
1 Baby Balfour retractor with center blade
6 Richardson retractors, paired, 1 × ¾, 1¼ × 1, 1½ × 1½ in.
2 U. S. Army retractors
2 Cushing vein retractors
2 Senn retractors, 6¼ in.
1 Weitlaner retractor, 5½ in.

### Suturing items

2 Brown needle holders, 5 in.
2 Crile-Wood needle holders, light, 6 in.
1 Pediatric needle set
Assorted suture materials

### Accessory items

1 Anthony suction tube
1 Yankauer suction tube
1 Frazier suction tube
1 Infant Poole suction tube
Suction tubing
1 Silver probe

SPECIALTY INSTRUMENTS. In general, the names of pediatric-sized specialty instruments are the same as those sized for adults (Payr, Allen, Doyen, Bailey). The instrument shape is also the same. However, the instruments are smaller in size and lighter in weight. Actual instrument size is also determined by the child's age, for example, for use on a 3-month-old or a 9-year-old child. Therefore the child's age and size must be considered together with the type of procedure when selecting instruments.

## PEDIATRIC SURGICAL PROCEDURES

Several surgical procedures that may be designated pediatric have been presented in previous chapters of this book under particular specialty headings. Following are several frequently encountered procedures that have not yet been discussed.

### Venous cutdown

DEFINITION. The exposure and cannulation of a vein in order to administer an infusion.

CONSIDERATIONS. The small size of children's veins and their location in subcutaneous tissue make venipuncture difficult. Direct placement of the catheter ensures

proper infusion and decreases the possibility of infiltration. Venous cutdown may be done preoperatively or in conjunction with surgery after induction. Several veins are accessible for cutdown: cephalic, jugular, and saphenous. The choice of one is dependent on the operative site, the anticipated need for rapid fluid or blood replacement, and the procedure to be performed.

SETUP AND PREPARATION OF THE PATIENT. The child is gently but firmly restrained, and the area of the incision is prepared in the manner previously described. When general anesthesia is not used, a local anesthetic is administered at the incisional site. An eye or circumcision sheet may be used for a drape. The instrument tray includes the following:

1 Knife handle no. 3 with blade no. 15
2 Mosquito forceps, curved
1 Mosquito forceps, straight
2 Adson forceps, 1 plain and 1 with teeth
2 Skin hooks
2 Fine scissors, 3 in., curved and straight
  Plastic catheter

Suturing items

1 Brown needle holder, 5 in.
1 Small cutting needle
1 Package silk suture no. 5-0

OPERATIVE PROCEDURE (specific for saphenous vein)

1. A 1 cm. transverse incision is made, only through the skin, over the internal saphenous vein, which is anterior to the medial malleolus.

2. By blunt dissection with a curved mosquito hemostat, the vein is isolated and a traction silk suture no. 5-0 passed around it.

3. While maintaining traction on the vein via the suture, a V-shaped nick is made into the vein with the scissors. The plastic catheter is threaded into the vein. The distal silk suture ligates the vein to prevent venous bleeding; the proximal suture ties the catheter in the vein.

4. The external end of the catheter is connected to the infusion set.

5. The skin edges are approximated with interrupted silk sutures no. 5-0 on a cutting needle, and a firm pressure dressing is applied.

6. It is wise to label the tape telling the size of the catheter and the date it was inserted. The foot may require some restraint such as taping a small sandbag to the sole of the foot.

### Exchange transfusion in the newborn

DEFINITION AND PURPOSE

1. To remove bilirubin already present, thus preventing its deposition in the tissues, particularly in the brain.

2. To remove sensitized red cells that when destroyed will increase the level of serum bilirubin and replace them with compatible red blood cells.

3. To restore normal cardiac function and to correct anemia without expanding blood volume (packed cells may be used).

4. Less importantly, to remove the maternal antibody from the baby's circulation so that subsequently formed infant's cells will have a chance to survive.

INDICATIONS

1. Rapidly rising serum bilirubin. Most babies with a cord blood bilirubin concentration of 6 mg./100 ml. or over will need an exchange.

2. Cardiac failure or severe anemia that makes the development of cardiac failure likely, cord blood hemoglobin below 11 gm.

3. Any baby whose serum bilirubin has risen above a predetermined "safe" level.

SETUP AND PREPARATION OF THE PATIENT. Prior to exchange transfusion the infant's stomach should be aspirated and his pharynx cleared of mucus. During the procedure the infant must be kept warm and quiet. When immobilizing the infant, care should be taken to prevent undue discomfort from too rigid restraints, and allowance should be made for the administration of external heat, oxygen, suction, auscultation of heart rate, and visual observation of the baby (especially the face). Sugar teats may be helpful in keeping the baby quiet and content. An oxygen source with infant mask, suction set, laryngoscope, and cathe-

ters should be available. The following supplies will be required:

    Circumstraint board
    Disposable exchange transfusion set
    Cutdown tray
    Heat lamp or warming mattress
    Infant nipple and blanket
    Sterile saline
    Supplies for collecting blood samples
    Thermometer
    Apparatus for warming blood

OPERATIVE PROCEDURE. Compatible blood (blood that is free of the antigen that can unite with the maternally produced antibody) is used for the exchange transfusion. Since the destructive antibodies are present in higher titer in the mother's serum than in the baby's, the mother's serum is preferably used to cross match with the donor. In an emergency, group O-negative cells and fresh frozen AB plasma may be used, regardless of the baby's blood group. The safe maximum amount of blood to use in an exchange is 75 ml. per pound of infant weight. Whenever possible, the exchange should be carried out via the umbilical vein with warmed blood (37° C., not higher). After insertion of the catheter, the venous pressure reading is obtained, and, if it is elevated, an appropriate amount of blood is withdrawn. The exchange transfusion is then accomplished by alternate withdrawal and introduction of an equal amount of blood; 10 ml. is usually satisfactory. After each 100 ml. replacement, 1 ml. of 10% calcium gluconate is slowly administered to maintain the blood calcium level, which is lowered by the potassium citrate in the donor blood. Venous pressure readings should be obtained periodically. At completion of the transfusion the infant is placed in an incubator and returned to the nursery for observation.

## Repair of atresia of the esophagus

DEFINITION. Through a right retropleural thoractomy, the tracheoesophageal fistula is closed and the segments of esophagus anastomosed.

CONSIDERATIONS. This congenital anomaly may arise between the third and sixth week of fetal life. Four types are recognized, the most common being an upper segment of esophagus ending in a blind pouch and a lower segment of esophagus communicating by a fistula with the trachea. Ideally, this defect would be recognized in the first hours of life, but more often the diagnosis is made in the first 36 to 48 hours of life. Prompt surgical intervention allows the child to breathe and eat without danger of aspirating mucus, saliva, feedings, or stomach contents. A gastrostomy may first be done to decompress the air-distended stomach, thus facilitating chest movement and ventilation, and to provide nourishment to the infant who is unable to orally ingest food.

SETUP AND PREPARATION OF THE PATIENT. The basic pediatric set is used, adding pediatric rib resection, intestinal, and vascular instruments. Because of the bubbly, gurgling respirations, functioning suction equipment should be at hand. The newborn infant is anesthetized and positioned for a right thoracotomy. Skin preparation and draping are carried out.

OPERATIVE PROCEDURE

1. A right thoracotomy incision is made; a segment of the fourth rib may be removed (Chapter 14), remembering that this is an infant (Fig. 25-1, *A* and *B*). The parietal pleura is carefully separated (Fig. 25-1, *C*). A ribbon retractor holds the lung, covered by the pleura, out of the operative field.

2. The upper and lower esophageal segments are identified. The tracheoesophageal fistula of the lower segment is identified, doubly cross clamped, and cut (Fig. 25-2). The tracheal stump is closed with interrupted silk no. 5-0 sutures, taking care not to cause a tracheal stenosis.

3. The upper segment is freed from adjacent tissues by blunt and sharp dissection; an Allis forceps is applied at the segment's lower tip for downward traction. The lower segment is not extensively freed in order to preserve circulation and viability. The segments are cross clamped with Potts ductus

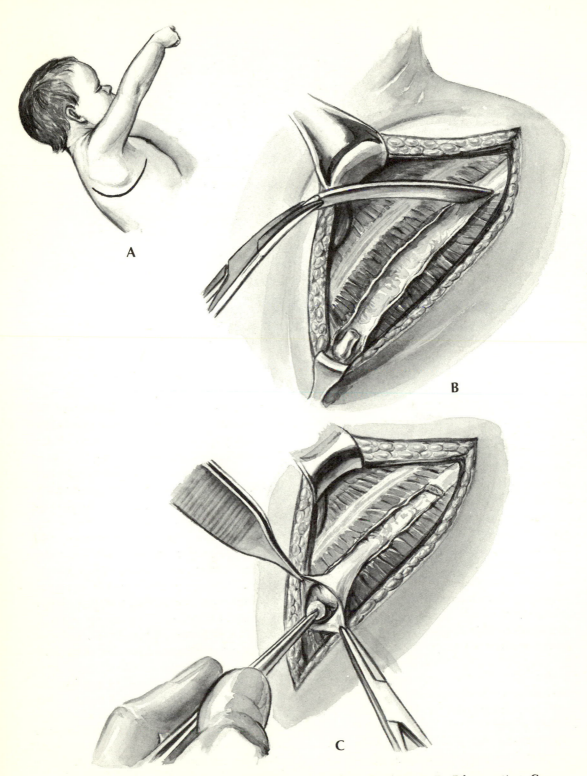

**Fig. 25-1.** Repair of tracheoesophageal fistula. **A,** Right thoracotomy. **B,** Rib resection. **C,** Pleural separation. (From Lewis, J. E.: Atlas of infant surgery, St. Louis, 1967, The C. V. Mosby Co.)

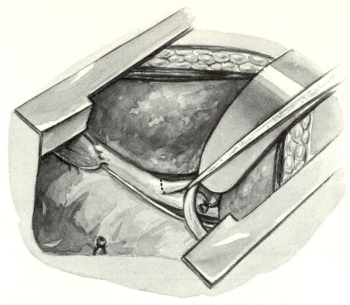

**Fig. 25-2.** Repair of tracheoesophageal fistula. Lower esophageal segment with fistula tract to trachea identified. (From Lewis, J. E.: Atlas of infant surgery, St. Louis, 1967, The C. V. Mosby Co.)

forceps and ends opened; the mucosal and muscular layers are identified.

4. Anastomotic techniques depend on the length of esophagus available. Ideally, the mucosal layer is closed with interrupted silk sutures no. 6-0 swaged on a fine needle, and the muscular layer is closed with interrupted silk sutures no. 5-0 swaged on a fine needle (Fig. 25-3, *A* and *B*). A one-layer closure may be necessary if the segments are extremely short.

5. After establishing a water-tight anastomosis, a chest catheter is placed and the chest closed (Fig. 25-3, *C*). The tube is connected to water-seal drainage and the wound dressed.

## Omphalocele repair

**DEFINITION.** Replacement of the viscera in the abdominal cavity and reconstruction of the abdominal wall.

**CONSIDERATIONS.** Omphalocele is the protrusion of abdominal viscera outside the abdomen into a sac of amniotic membrane and peritoneum at the base of the umbilical cord (Fig. 25-4). There is no skin covering.

Omphalocele occurs when the viscera fail to withdraw from the exocoelomic position and occupy the peritoneal cavity. Treatment at birth consists of applying warm saline or benzalkonium chloride (Zephiran) 1:1000 packs on the sac surface and the insertion of a nasogastric tube to prevent distention. Surgical intervention is necessary to prevent rupture of the sac and/or infection. Should intrauterine rupture of the sac have occurred, the newly delivered child is kept warm, the bowel is inspected for perforation, and torsion and moist warm dressings are applied.

**SETUP AND PREPARATION OF THE PATIENT.** The infant is prepared as discussed previously. The basic setup is used.

**OPERATIVE PROCEDURE.** The sac is protectively covered and the abdominal wall integrity established in one of several ways.

1. In the presence of small defects, the skin edges can be freed, the fascia separated, the sac and contents relocated in the abdomen, and the fascial and skin layers closed.

2. In the presence of larger defects, the

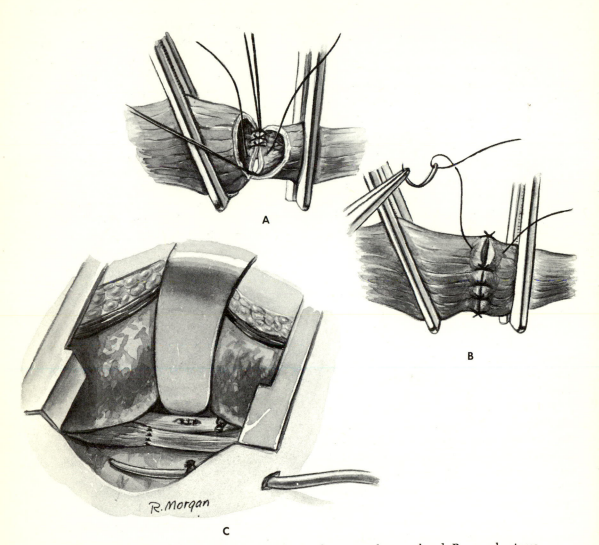

Fig. 25-3. Repair of tracheoesophageal fistula. **A,** Placement of mucosal and, **B,** serosal sutures. **C,** Anastomosis of esophageal segments completed. (From Lewis, J. E.: Atlas of infant surgery, St. Louis, 1967, The C. V. Mosby Co.)

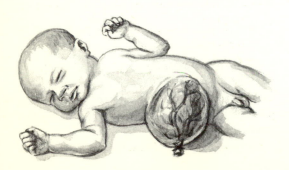

Fig. 25-4. Omphalocele showing sac at the base of umbilical cord. (From Lewis, J. E.: Atlas of infant surgery, St. Louis, 1967, The C. V. Mosby Co.)

skin edges are freed and flaps created. These skin flaps are closed over the sac. Reoperation within a few weeks is done to place the viscera within the abdomen under the rectus muscles and fascia.

3. Omphaloceles encompassing most of the abdomen and possibly containing liver and/or spleen are not easily replaced within the potential abdominal space. Of prime importance is the need for protective covering of the exposed sac and viscera. One technique is the insertion of a sterile Silastic sheeting over the sac and under the skin edges that have been freed. If the defect is too large to allow approximation of the skin edges, the Silastic sheeting may be left exposed. Subsequently it and the surrounding abdomen are dressed with a 0.5% solution of silver nitrate that inhibits bacterial growth. This does not seem to affect the infant's electrolyte balance. During the ensuing weeks, the exposed sheeting is constricted to slowly return the whole viscera to the abdominal cavity. The abdominal wall is repaired in a later-stage operation.

Another technique for treating large omphaloceles is the painting of the sac and surrounding skin with a 2% solution of merbromin (Mercurochrome) until an eschar forms to add strength to the sac and resist infection. Or the sac may be treated with moist 0.5% silver nitrate dressings. The sac membrane gradually contracts, and skin closes the abdominal wall defect. Later surgery then repairs the abdominal musculature.

## Relief of intussusception

**DEFINITION.** Reduction of the invaginated bowel by the hydrostatic pressure of a barium enema or by laparotomy and manual manipulation.

**CONSIDERATIONS.** Intussusception is the telescopic invagination of a portion of intestine into an adjacent part with mechanical and vascular impairment. A frequent site is the ileocecal junction. Intussusception in children is most often idiopathic; other causes may include Meckel's diverticulum, polyps, or hematoma of the bowel. Early diagnosis and reduction are essential to bowel viability.

**SETUP AND PREPARATION OF THE PATIENT.** The child is prepared for surgery as described previously. Reduction by barium enema is first attempted with the full cognizance of the radiologist, surgeon, and pediatrician. Should reduction not be accomplished, a laparotomy must be done. The basic pediatric set is used, with the addition of intestinal instruments.

**OPERATIVE PROCEDURE**

1. A transverse or right paramedian incision is made and the peritoneum entered (Fig. 25-5, *A*).

2. The cecum and ileum are identified; the intussusception is located and elevated in the fingers of the hand (Fig. 25-5, *B* and *C*).

3. If there is no evidence of bowel compromise, manual reduction is performed by gently milking the intussusceptum out of the intussuscipiens in the same direction as the flow of an enema (Fig. 25-5, *D*). No traction or opposing pull is exerted.

4. Should the viability of the bowel be questioned, a resection is done (Chapter 21).

5. The abdomen is closed in layers and the wound dressed.

## Relief of intestinal obstruction

**DEFINITION.** Resection of stenotic or atresic bowel with anastomosis and/or the creation of an ileostomy.

**CONSIDERATIONS.** Intestinal obstruction may occur in the infant for a variety of reasons: atresia, stenosis, congenital aganglionosis, meconium ileus, or malrotation. Surgical intervention is used as indicated.

### Resection and pull-through for Hirschsprung's disease

**DEFINITION.** Removal of the aganglionic portion of the bowel and anastomosis of the colon to the distal rectum after multiple biopsies and frozen section of the muscularis of the bowel.

**CONSIDERATIONS.** Hirschsprung's disease

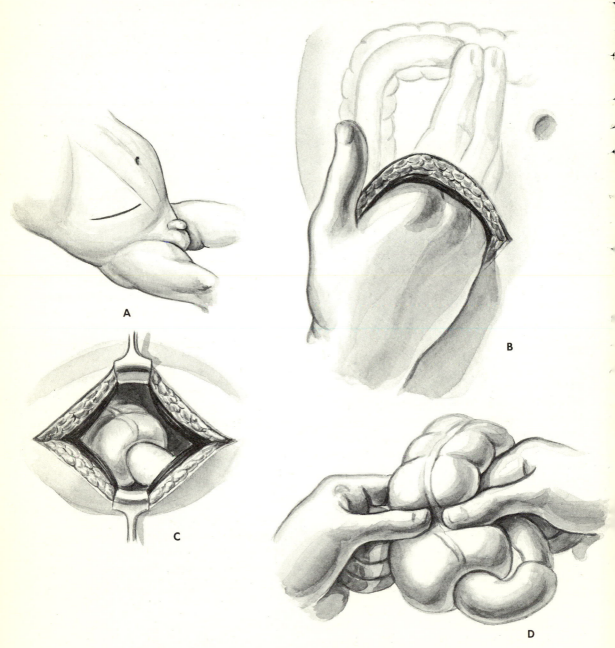

**Fig. 25-5.** Reduction of intussusception. **A,** Transverse abdominal incision. **B,** Location of intussusception. **C,** Mass delivered into incision. **D,** "Milking" reduction. (From Lewis, J. E.: Atlas of infant surgery, St. Louis, 1967, The C. V. Mosby Co.)

is characterized by the presence of a segment of colon that lacks ganglia, resulting in an increase of tone and a lack of peristalsis. Colon contents do not pass through the involved segment but distend the proximal normal colon, causing increasing abdominal distention. The lower colon is most frequently involved, but the disease may encompass the entire colon with a less favorable prognosis. Definitive diagnosis is necessary. Prior to definitive surgery, a colostomy may be made to relieve obstruction and permit the function of the normal bowel. Biopsies of the bowel are taken first to establish diagnosis of aganglionosis and the level at which normal ganglia are present. Definitive therapy is resection of the aganglionic segment and anastomosis.

Several surgical techniques have been devised that remove the aganglionic colon and anastomose the remaining ganglionic colon to a rectal remnant, leaving the anal sphincter intact to maintain continence of stool. The optimum procedure permits ready resection of the diseased bowel with minimal pelvic dissection and potential damage to the pelvic nerves. In addition to the original procedure described by Swenson, modifications by Duhamel, Grob, Martin, Altemeier, Soane, and others have been devised that conserve operating time, minimize blood loss in the infant, preserve the sphincters, and reduce complications.

SETUP AND PREPARATION OF THE PATIENT. The child is prepared as described previously. The basic pediatric set and intestinal instruments are used. Gastrointestinal technique as described in Chapter 21 is followed. The patient is placed in the supine position with legs in a modified "ski" position to facilitate abdominal and perineal approaches. A straight rubber catheter may be inserted to empty the bladder during surgery.

OPERATIVE PROCEDURE (based on Duhamel's retrorectal technique of abdominoperineal pull-through)

1. A left transverse suprapubic incision is made and the abdomen opened in the usual manner.

2. The pelvic peritoneum is opened close to the rectum. The ureters are identified and retracted laterally. The rectum is freed, cross clamped with large right-angled clamps below the level of the pelvic peritoneum, and divided. The clamp remains on the proximal portion to prevent spillage while the distal rectal portion is suctioned clean and sutured closed in layers using chromic gut no. 4-0 sutures on the mucosa and silk no. 4-0 sutures on the serosa.

3. By means of hemostats, Metzenbaum scissors, and ligatures of silk no. 3-0, the portion of aganglionic bowel is dissected free of its mesentery up to the area where biopsies and frozen sections established innervation.

4. Two Ochsner clamps are placed across the bowel at the upper limits of the dissection, the bowel severed by means of a scalpel, and the aganglionic colon removed (Fig. 25-6, *A*).

5. The proximal end of the ganglionated bowel may be closed with chromic gut sutures no. 4-0 and silk sutures no. 4-0 left long. The normal bowel is further freed in order to obtain a sufficient length of colon for the pull-through.

6. Blunt presacral dissection frees the rectum posteriorly from its fascial attachments down to the anal sphincter (Fig. 25-6, *B*).

7. From the perineum, the anal sphincter is divulsed from below and the rectal wall incised posteriorly above the pectinate line (Fig. 25-6, *C*).

8. A uterine dressing forceps passed from the perineum through the rectal opening into the retrorectal space (Fig. 25-6, *D*) grasps and pulls the closed end of the normal colon through the pelvis into the opening of the rectum, taking care not to twist the bowel or its mesentery.

9. The posterior wall of the pull-through segment is anastomosed with silk sutures no. 4-0 to the anal side of the rectal wall; a mucosa-to-mucosa line of chromic gut sutures no. 4-0 is placed (Fig. 25-6, *E*).

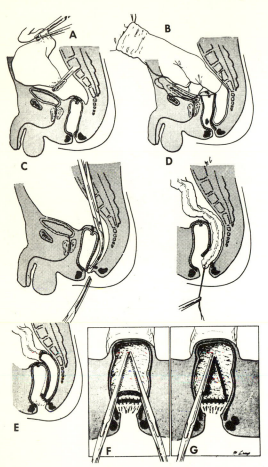

**Fig. 25-6.** Abdominoperineal pull-through resection. **A,** Aganglionic bowel cross clamped and resected. **B,** Blunt dissection of presacral space. **C,** Rectal wall opened through anus. **D,** Colon pulled through pelvis to rectal opening. **E,** Serosal and mucosal suture lines placed in posterior rectum and anterior colon. **F** and **G,** Placement of Ochsner crutching clamps. (From Sieber, W. K., and Kiesewetter, W. B.: Arch. Surg. **87:**112, July, 1963.)

10. Ochsner clamps are applied to the posterior wall of the rectum and the anterior wall of the colon segment up to the apex of the rectal pouch. These will extrude in 5 to 8 days as a result of pressure necrosis; the new rectum will then be created (Fig. 25-6, *F* and *G*).

11. The pelvic floor is peritonized from the abdomen with chromic gut no. 3-0

sutures, leaving the rectal stump beneath the peritoneal closure. A Penrose drain is inserted beneath the peritoneal floor into the presacral space and brought out through the abdomen.

12. The abdominal wound is closed in layers and dressed.

### Repair of rectal atresia

**DEFINITION.** Establishment of colorectoanal continuity through the external sphincter and closure of fistula tracts.

**CONSIDERATIONS.** Congenital atresia of the rectum may present in varied forms. A covered anus may be the only defect, in which case surgical incision and repeated dilatation of the sphincter would be indicated. A blind rectal pouch with or without genitourinary fistulas is the most prevalent type. Herein, the external sphincter is present, and after creation of the anal opening within the sphincter ring, the rectal pouch is brought down within the puborectal portion of the levator sling and sutured to the skin edges around the sphincter; the existing fistulas are closed.

Whatever the distinctive malformation, surgical intervention and repair is indicated within 24 to 48 hours. When the atresia is such that a sacroabdominoperineal pull-through is indicated, a transverse colostomy may be made during these 24 to 48 hours to irrigate the hiatal lumen and to remove meconium plugs while allowing proximal colon function. After the colostomy, further diagnostic studies such as cystograms, vaginograms, and the insertion of dye into the distal colostomy loop may be utilized. Intravenous pyelograms may be helpful. Definitive surgery is performed when the condition and size of the child permits.

**SETUP AND PREPARATION OF THE PATIENT.** The basic pediatric set may be utilized and arranged to facilitate a sacroabdominoperineal approach. Hegar dilators are added to the set. Positional changes will be required, and supplies should be prepared. Positioning and draping are carried out as previously described.

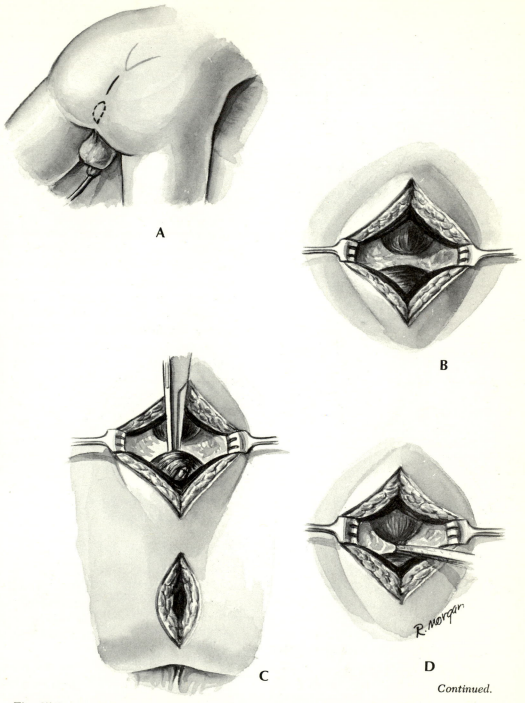

R. Morgan

*Continued.*

**Fig. 25-7.** Sacroabdominoperineal pull-through. **A,** Sacral incision. **B,** Dissection exposing the rectal pouch and levator muscles. **C,** Elevation of puborectal portion of levator preliminary to dilatation of tunnel. **D,** Mobilization of proximal colon after abdominal incision. **E,** Utilizing forceps, the colon is pulled through the rectal pouch and sphincter to the perineum. **F,** Suturing of colon to anal skin edges. (From Lewis, J. E.: Atlas of infant surgery, St. Louis, 1967, The C. V. Mosby Co.)

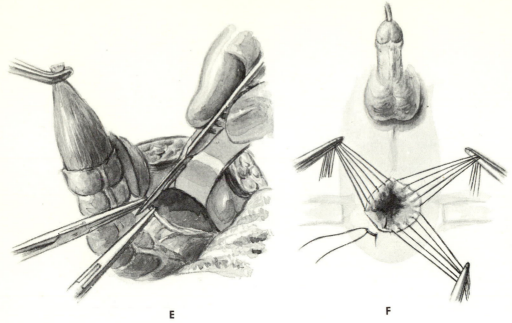

E                                    F

**Fig. 25-7, cont'd.** For legend see p. 869.

OPERATIVE PROCEDURE (endorectal sacro-abdominoperineal pull-through)

1. The patient is placed in a prone position with buttocks taped apart; a metal urethral sound is used to mark the urethra in the male or the vagina in the female; a large rubber catheter is threaded into the distal loop of the transverse colostomy to identify the blind rectal pouch.

2. The skin is incised from the coccyx to the projected anal opening (Fig. 25-7, A). Dissection is carried out in the midline to expose the blind rectal pouch (Fig. 25-7, B) and the puborectal muscle, which is freed from the urethra (or vagina).

3. The perineum is then examined and the external sphincter located. A cruciate incision is made over the sphincter, and it is dissected free from overlying skin and subcutaneous tissue. After making an opening through the center of the muscle, it and the puborectal tunnel are joined and dilated by means of Hegar dilators, taking care not to tear either muscle (Fig. 25-7, C).

4. A Penrose drain is placed through the tunnel up to the rectal pouch. The sacral incision is closed in layers.

5. After repositioning the child to a supine position with legs overhanging the table, the abdomen is incised through a left lower quadrant or transverse incision. The pelvic peritoneum is opened and the rectal pouch identified.

6. After injecting saline into the seromuscular coat of the rectal pouch, the seromuscular layer is circumferentially dissected from the mucosal layer. The mucosa is cross clamped with two Ochsner forceps and divided. The serosal layer is further stripped from the distal blind pouch, and, as fistulas are identified, they are closed.

7. The proximal bowel is mobilized with preservation of the blood supply to allow length for an adequate pull-through (Fig. 25-7, D).

8. A Hegar dilator is inserted through the lumen of the perineal end of the Penrose drain until it reaches the blind rectal pouch. An incision is made through the

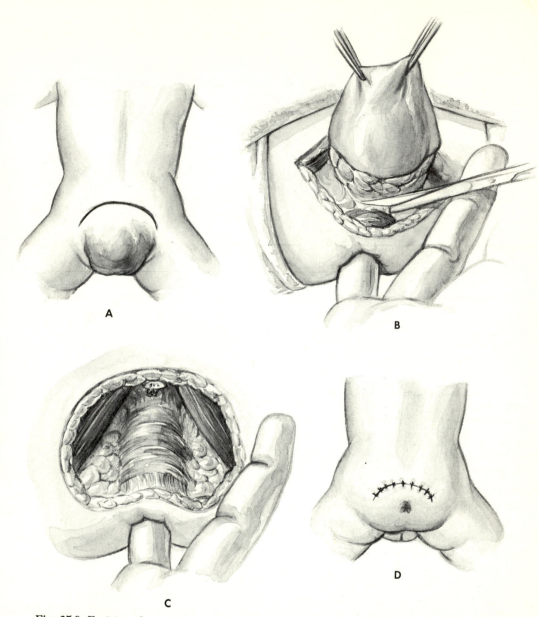

**Fig. 25-8.** Excision of sacrococcygeal teratoma. **A,** ∪-shaped incision. **B,** Dissection of teratoma. **C,** Tumor excised while rectum remains intact. **D.** Closed incisional line. (From Lewis, J. E.: Atlas of infant surgery, St. Louis, 1967, The C. V. Mosby Co.)

pouch over the dilator, and it is removed as the Penrose drain is brought into the pouch.

9. Long Allis forceps are passed along the pathway of the Penrose drain and the edges of the upper segment grasped and pulled out through the pouch and sphinc-ter onto the perineum. The external sphincter may be incised to accommodate the larger colon (Fig. 25-7, *E*).

10. The anal skin edges are then sewn to the mucosal layer of the pull-through segment with silk sutures no. 4-0 (Fig. 25-7, *F*).

11. A drain is placed in the seromuscular layer of the blind pouch and exteriorized through an abdominal stab wound. The serosal layer is loosely attached to the pull-through segment.

12. The pelvis is reperitonized and the abdominal wound closed in the routine manner.

### Resection of tumors

Tumors occur in children as well as adults. As is always the case with tumors, the therapy administered is dependent on the type of tumor. Examination and judicious investigation of all unusual masses is imperative. Thorough diagnostic workup and prompt definitive treatment may result in cure, if the tumor is proved malignant. Malignant tumors in children are distressing to adults, particularly to parents who feel their child has not had a chance to live. Parents will require extra supportive measures from the nursing personnel.

Recent development of chemotherapeutic drugs and radiation therapy are adjuncts to surgical therapy.

*Wilms' tumor* (nephroblastoma) of the kidney is one of the more common childhood neoplasms. The tumor presents as a unilateral, firm, painless mass whose enlargement may laterally distend the abdomen. Radical nephrectomy and the use of chemotherapy and radiation are often combined in the course of treatment.

*Neuroblastomas* are tumors arising from the sympathetic ganglia; the most common site is the adrenal or upper abdominal ganglia. The tumor may present as an irregular enlarging abdominal mass, or a site of distant metastasis may be the first symptom of malignance. A bone marrow biopsy may provide differential diagnosis. Treatment includes excision of the primary tumor mass, chemotherapy, and radiation.

*Sacrococcygeal teratomas* arising in the area of the sacrum and coccyx frequently show external masses but may extend into the pelvis or abdominal cavity. Histologically, these tumors contain a varied array of body tissue. Resection is usually feasible by placing the patient in a Kraske position and excising the tumor mass and coccyx en bloc (Fig. 25-8). Blood should be available. If the pelvic extension is too great, an additional abdominal incision may be necessary.

### REFERENCES

1. Berry, E. C., and Kohn, M. L.: Introduction to operating room technique, ed. 3, New York, 1966, The Blakiston Division, McGraw-Hill Book Co.
2. Bittner, J. S., Freeman, E. L., and Talbert, M. L.: Surgical care of the child: a new challenge for the operating room nurse, A.O.R.N. Journal 9:37, June, 1969.
3. Gellis, S. S., and Kagan, B. M.: Current pediatric therapy, vol. 3, Philadelphia, 1968, W. B. Saunders Co.
4. Haller, J. A., Jr., editor: The hospitalized child and his family, Baltimore, 1967, The Johns Hopkins Press.
5. Harberg, F. J., and Holt, M. B.: Abdominal surgery of the infant and child, A.O.R.N. Journal 1:33, July, 1963.
6. Harberg, F., and Holt, M.: Newborn surgical emergencies, A.O.R.N. Journal 1:64, June, 1963.
7. Harberg, F., and Holt, M.: Surgery for hernia, hydrocele, and undescended testicle, A.O.R.N. Journal 1:47, Sept., 1963.
8. Kiesewetter, W. B.: Imperforate anus: the role and results of sacro-abdomino-perineal operation, Ann. Surg. 164:655, 1966.
9. Lewis, J. E.: Atlas of infant surgery, St. Louis, 1967, The C. V. Mosby Co.
10. Nelson, W. E., editor: Textbook of pediatrics, ed. 8, Philadelphia, 1964, W. B. Saunders Co.
11. Potts, W. J.: Pediatric surgery is growing up, J.A.M.A. 166:462, 1958.
12. Potts, W. J.: The surgeon and the child, Philadelphia, 1959, W. B. Saunders Co.
13. Raffensperger, J. G., and Primrose, R. B.: Pediatric surgery for nurses, Boston, 1968, Little, Brown & Co.
14. Rehbein, F., Moeger, R., Kundert, J. C., and Meier-Tige, W.: Surgical problems in congenital megacolon (Hirschsprung's disease) J. Pediatr. Surg. 6:526, Dec., 1966.
15. Shirkey, H. C., editor: Pediatric therapy, ed. 4, St. Louis, 1972, The C. V. Mosby Co.
16. Sieber, W. K., and Kiesewetter, W. B.: Duhamel's operation for Hirschsprung's disease, Arch. Surg. 87:111, July, 1963.

17. Silverman, W.: Premature infants, ed. 3, New York, 1961, Harper & Row, Publishers.

18. Soane, F.: A new surgical technique for treatment of Hirschsprung's disease, Surgery **56:**1007, Nov., 1964.

19. Soper, R. T., and Miller, F. E.: Modification of Duhamel procedure: elimination of rectal pouch and colorectal septum, J. Pediatr. Surg. **3:**376, June, 1968.

20. Stanley-Brown, E. G.: Pediatric surgery for nurses, Philadelphia, 1961, W. B. Saunders Co.

21. State, D.: Segmental colon resection in the treatment of congenital megacolon, Am. J. Surg. **105:**93, 1963.

22. Stephens, C. R.: Innovations in pediatric anesthesia, A.O.R.N. Journal **9:**41, June, 1969.

23. Ternberg, J.: Personal communications.

# INDEX